NEONATAL CARE

FOR NURSES AND MIDWIVES

NEONATAL CARE

FOR NURSES AND MIDWIVES: PRINCIPLES FOR PRACTICE

2nd Edition

Victoria Kain
RN, MN, NICC, PhD
Senior Lecturer, School of Nursing and Midwifery,
Griffith University, Queensland, Australia

Trudi Mannix
CF, RN, RM, NICC, EdD
Neonatal Nurse, Neonatal Special Care and Intensive Care Units,
Women's and Children's Hospital,
Adelaide, Australia

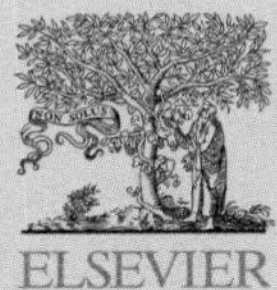

ELSEVIER

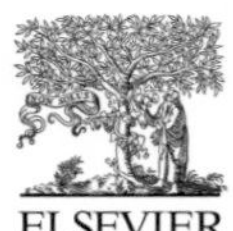

Elsevier Australia. ACN 001 002 357
(a division of Reed International Books Australia Pty Ltd)
Tower 1, 475 Victoria Avenue, Chatswood, NSW 2067

ISBN: 978-0-7295-4389-7

Notice

Practitioners and researchers must always rely on their own experience and knowledge in evaluating and using any information, methods, compounds or experiments described herein. Because of rapid advances in the medical sciences, in particular, independent verification of diagnoses and drug dosages should be made. To the fullest extent of the law, no responsibility is assumed by Elsevier, authors, editors or contributors for any injury and/or damage to persons or property as a matter of product liability, negligence or otherwise, or from any use or operation of any methods, products, instructions or ideas contained in the material herein.

National Library of Australia Cataloguing-in-Publication Data

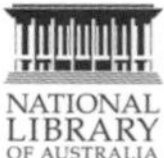

A catalogue record for this book is available from the National Library of Australia

Content Strategist: Libby Houston
Content Project Manager: Fariha Nadeem
Edited by Chris Wyard
Proofread by Annabel Adair
Copyrights Coordinator: Regina Lavanya Remigius
Cover and internal design by Natalie Bowra
Typeset by GW Tech
Printed in India by Multivista Global Pvt. Ltd.

This textbook is dedicated to the memory of my beloved father – Raymond Ward.

Victoria

I dedicate this textbook to my neonatal nursing and midwifery colleagues, my loving partner Tony and my inspirational daughter Sienna.

Trudi

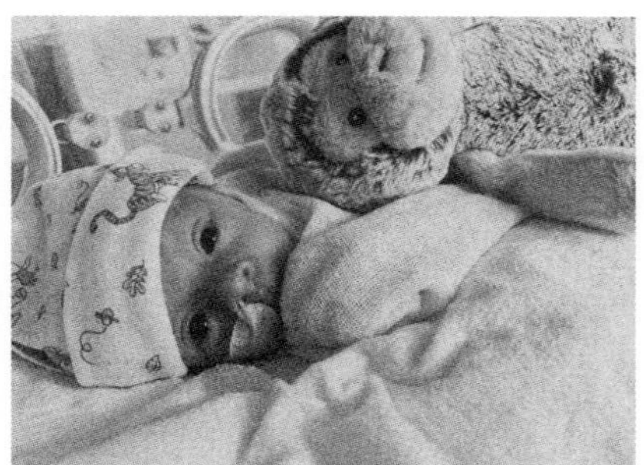

Saynt was born on 20th June 2021 at 33 weeks' gestation and weighed 1.7 kg at birth. As is typical of babies his gestation, he had phototherapy for physiological jaundice twice, but otherwise had an uncomplicated postnatal course. Saynt spent 3 weeks in SCBU, before, at 36 weeks' gestation, and weighing 1.9 kg, he was discharged on the Neonatal Early Discharge program. Today, he is a thriving 9-month-old (7 months corrected), 6.6 kg and still breastfed. Thank you to Saynt and his mother Pixie, for allowing us to use his photo and story for our second edition.

TABLE OF

CONTENTS

PREFACE

We are delighted to be working together again on the second edition of our textbook, bringing together leading neonatal nurses, researchers and midwives to create an exceptional evidence-based guide for the future growth of neonatal and family-centred care. While the central theme to our first edition is enduring – creating a strong scientific foundation for competent family-centred neonatal care – we live in an age where evidence, and therefore practice, is under constant review, and this edition presents that dynamic evidence.

We are eternally grateful to our wonderful neonatal nursing and midwifery colleagues and professional bodies who have helped us along the way by writing, peer reviewing and supporting us. While the second edition represents a labour of love for us, it is also confirmation of the passion and commitment that all contributors feel towards the care of vulnerable newborns and their families. This would not have been accomplished without their assistance. Our appreciation is also extended to the talented and devoted professionals at Elsevier, for guidance in the development of our second edition, and who continue to support us.

Dr Victoria Kain and Dr Trudi Mannix

FOREWORD
BY PROFESSOR KAREN WALKER

It is a privilege to be invited to write a foreword for the second edition of this superb textbook. Dr Trudi Mannix and Dr Victoria Kain have led a team of extraordinary neonatal nurses and midwives who have contributed to updating this key textbook for neonatal nurses and midwives around the world.

So much has changed in the world since the first edition of the textbook was published. Who would have predicted a pandemic in our lifetime? What has made this edition even more impressive is that the writing of this edition has happened during the pandemic, when we are all well aware of the impact this has had on ourselves, our colleagues and the health system. It is a testament to the dedication and resilience of the nurses and midwives who have contributed to these chapters and who leave this legacy for future neonatal nurses/midwives.

The voices of neonatal nurses and midwives are important and I strongly advocate for neonatal nurses/midwives to be integral to every conversation which impacts our professions. One important challenge globally is the provision of specific education for neonatal nurses and midwives regarding the care of the vulnerable newborn. This high-calibre textbook, written by neonatal nurses and midwives for neonatal nurses and midwives, contributes to the body of knowledge that supports this.

This comprehensive revision now has 25 chapters written and updated by many of the previous edition's authors; however, it is gratifying to see new names as authors also. The first chapter is one of the changes in this edition: a new chapter on global perspectives in neonatal nursing/midwifery. Another new chapter describes the care of the normal newborn. The book then proceeds logically through the knowledge required to care for a small or sick newborn, concluding logically with a chapter on discharge planning and follow-up care.

Two chapters I would like to suggest as critical reading just now are Chapter 21 – Family-centred care in the neonatal unit, and Chapter 22 – Developmentally focused neonatal care. I am a chair committee member for the Global Alliance for Newborn Care, an international parent organisation that published the results of a survey detailing the impact of the pandemic on parents, and I recommend that everyone reads this disturbing report. One aspect of the last 2 years which has caused many of us distress has been the exclusion of parents within our neonatal units. As a mother, I cannot imagine not being allowed to see my baby. As a nurse, like many of you, I have had to enforce these rules, understandable though they may be. With these restrictions, having parents in some units has become less common and many new nurses/midwives are not as familiar or comfortable with parents being present and integral partners in care. Some countries are reporting that they have gone back a decade in parental involvement.

I would like to thank Trudi, Victoria and all the authors who have contributed their time and expertise to writing this second edition. As an author I am well aware of the time and effort required, and as an editor I know this workload is amplified exponentially. I would also like to challenge everyone reading this book to believe in yourself and what you can achieve. Any one of you can be a leader in whichever field of neonatal nursing/midwifery you wish to work in. Thank you all.

Professor Karen Walker

ABOUT THE AUTHORS

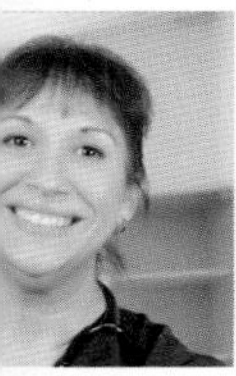

Victoria Kain RN, MN, NICC, PhD
Victoria is a Senior Lecturer in the School of Nursing and Midwifery at Griffith University. Her research interests span several different elements of newborn care, and she has a prominent reputation on an international level in the fields of neonatal and perinatal palliative care. She has a wealth of clinical experience, having worked as a paediatric critical care nurse, a neonatal intensive care nurse and as a nurse educator in neonatal intensive care nursing prior to beginning her academic career. Victoria has written multiple journal papers and book chapters.

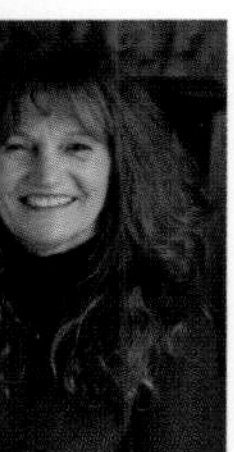

Trudi Mannix CF, RN, RM, NICC, EdD
Trudi currently works as a neonatal nurse in the neonatal special care and intensive care units at the Women's and Children's Hospital in Adelaide. She has taught neonatal intensive and special care nursing for over 30 years both in the hospital setting and in tertiary settings, at Flinders University and the University of South Australia. She is an ex-President of the Australian College of Neonatal Nurses and a Churchill Fellow. Her research interests are in the developmental and parental aspects of neonatal care, and her doctoral research included the development of standards for neonatal intensive care nursing education using the Delphi technique, and a phenomenological study exploring the critical thinking of nurses while at the cot-side in a neonatal unit. Trudi has published in the areas of parental stress and neonatal early discharge. She continues to support and advocate for parents in the neonatal unit.

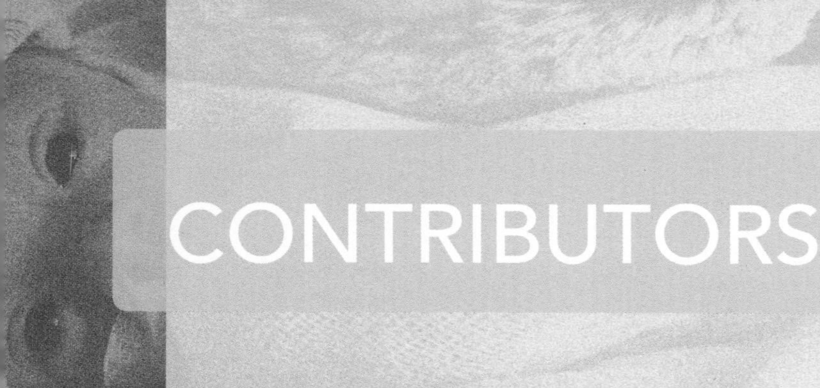

CONTRIBUTORS

Deanne August BSN, GradCertResMeth, PhD
Nurse Researcher
Grantley Stable Neonatal Unit,
University of Queensland,
Brisbane, Queensland
Australia

Laurene Aydon MN
Clinical Nurse Facilitator
Neonatal Directorate;
Nurse Researcher
Department of Nursing Research, CAHS,
Perth Children's Hospital
Nedlands, Western Australia;
Clinical Lecturer, School of Child and Paediatric Health
University of Western Australia
Perth, Western Australia
Australia

Julie Bernardo MN(NP)
Neonatal Nurse Practitioner
Neonatal Intensive Care Unit
Flinders Medical Centre
Adelaide, South Australia
Australia

Patricia Bromley RN, Midwifery, Neonatal Intensive Care, Paediatric, DipTropMed, EdD
Nurse Immuniser
Lecturer, Nursing and Midwifery
School of Health Sciences
University of Tasmania
Hobart, Tasmania
Australia

Carmel Collins RN, RM, NICC, BSocSc(HumServ), GDipPubHlth, PhD, FACNN
Principal Research Fellow
SAHMRI Women and Kids
South Australian Health and Medical Research Centre;
Associate Professor
Discipline of Paediatrics
Adelaide Medical School
The University of Adelaide
Adelaide, South Australia
Australia

Jennifer Dawson RN, MN(Research), PhD
Clinical Trial Co-ordinator
Newborn Research Centre
The Royal Women's Hospital
Melbourne;
Honorary Fellow, Murdoch Children's Research Institute, Parkville;
Honorary Fellow
The University of Melbourne
Melbourne, Victoria
Australia

Glenda Fleming MEd, MAdvN(NP)
Nurse Practitioner (Paediatric Cardiothoracic)
The Children's Hospital at Westmead
Westmead, New South Wales
Australia

Kim Fletcher MAdvNPrac
Neonatal Nurse Practitioner
Monash Newborn
Monash Health
Melbourne, Victoria
Australia

Anndrea Flint RN, RM, AdvNeonatalNursCert, BN, MHlthSci(Health Services Management), GradCertNeonatol, MNursSci(NP)
Neonatal Nurse Practitioner
Maternity/Neonatal Unit Redcliffe Hospital
Redcliffe, Queensland
Australia

Lyn Francis BN, Midwife (non-practising) GradDipTT, LLB, LLM, MHM, PhD
Senior Lecturer
School of Nursing and Midwifery
Western Sydney University
Parramatta, New South Wales
Australia

Kim Gibson RN, BNurs, GCertHealth (NeoIntCare), MNurs
Lecturer in Nursing (Complex Care)
Clinical and Health Sciences
University of South Australia
Adelaide, South Australia
Australia

Janet Green **RN, MN(NEd), MBioethics, MA E-Learning, PhD**
Adjunct Senior Lecturer, Nursing and Midwifery, School of Nursing, College of Health and Medicine, University of Tasmania
Hobart, Tasmania
Australia

Nadine Griffiths **BN, MnClinEd**
Clinical Nurse Consultant Neonatology
Grace Centre for Newborn Intensive Care
Sydney Children's Hospital Network (Westmead)
Westmead, New South Wales
Australia

Deborah Harris **PhD, FCNZ**
Neonatal Nurse Practitioner, Senior Lecturer, Programme Director – Nursing Science, Advanced Practice
School of Nursing, Midwifery and Health Practice
Wellington Regional Hospital
Newtown, Wellington
New Zealand

Denise Harrison **RN, PhD**
Professor
Department of Nursing
School of Health Sciences
Faculty of Medicine, Dentistry and Health Sciences
University of Melbourne
Melbourne, Victoria
Australia;
Honorary Fellow, Murdoch Children's Research Institute and Royal Children's Hospital, Parkville;
Professional Officer, Australian College of Neonatal Nurses

Rebecca May **GradDipPallCare**
Nurse Consultant
Paediatric Palliative Care Service
The Women's and Children's Hospital
Adelaide, South Australia
Australia

Jacqui McGregor **DipApplSci/Nurs, BApplSci/Nurs, GradDipMid, GradDipAdvNurs/NIC, MNurs – Neonates, GradCertHETL**
PG Course Coordinator Masters of Nursing
School of Nursing Midwifery
LaTrobe University
Bundoora, Victoria
Australia

Rhona McInnes **PhD**
Independent Research Consultant
Broadbeach Waters, Queensland
Australia

Judith Needham **RN, RM, BNurs, MNursManagement, EdD**
Senior Lecturer, Director Clinical Placement Office
School of Nursing and Midwifery
Griffith University
Meadowbrook, Queensland
Australia

Karen New **RN, RM, PhD**
Adjunct A/Professor
School of Health and Behavioural Science
University of the Sunshine Coast
Sippy Downs, Queensland
Australia

Fay Presbury **RM, BNurs, NIC Cert, MBus**
Formerly Nursing Director
Newborn Emergency Transport Service Victoria (Paediatric Infant Perineal Emergency Retrieval (PIPER))
The Royal Children's Hospital
Parkville, Victoria
Australia

Kim Psaila **RN, RM, NIDCAP certified, BA, GradDip(CN), GradDip(NE), GradDip(IMH), MA, PhD**
Academic, School of Nursing and Midwifery
Western Sydney University
Parramatta, New South Wales
Australia

Anita Robertson **RIPRN, BNSc, PGCert NSc(Int Care), PGCertNSc(ClinTeach), DipMid, MAdvNPrac, IPN**
Lecturer, Aeromedical Retrieval
School of Public Health, Tropical Medicine and Rehabilitation Sciences
James Cook University;
Flight Nurse
Royal Flying Doctors Service Queensland Section
Townsville, Queensland
Australia

Jackie Smith **RSCN, DipPaed, DipNeo, NNP, MNursSC(NP), DScN**
Neonatal Nurse Practitioner
The Neonatal Unit
The Townsville Hospital
Townsville, Queensland
Australia

Linda Sweet **BN, MNursSci, GradCert Ed, PhD**
Professor
School of Nursing and Midwifery
Deakin University
Burwood, Victoria
Australia

Suza Trajkovski **RN, BN, GradCert(Neonatal), GradCert(Research), GradDipMgt, PhD**
Lecturer
School of Nursing and Midwifery
Western Sydney University
Sydney, New South Wales
Australia

Karen Walker RGN, RSCN, BappSc, MACN, MN, PhD
Neonatal Clinical Nurse Consultant
Royal Prince Alfred Hospital;
President
Council of International Neonatal Nurses;
Honorary Research Fellow
The George Institute for Global Health;
Clinical Professor
Faculty of Medicine and Health
University of Sydney
Sydney, New South Wales
Australia

Lisa-Kim Wright RN, RM, LLB, GCert Health Professional Education, MN (Clinical Nursing, NICU)
Nurse Educator
Nursing/Midwifery Education & Research Unit
Gold Coast University Hospital
Southport, Queensland
Australia

Jeanine Young AM, BSc(Hons, First Class) Nursing Studies, DipAdvNursCare, PhD
Professor of Nursing
School of Nursing, Midwifery and Paramedicine
University of the Sunshine Coast
Petrie, Queensland
Australia

REVIEWERS

Maria Adamopoulos **BAppSci (Nsg, HP), GradCert NICU, GradCert Clinical Teaching**
Neonatal Lecturer, La Trobe University, Melbourne, Victoria, Australia

Jane Bailey **BN(Hons), BAppSc (Health Promotion), GradCert Neonatal Intensive Care Nursing, MCL (Masters in Clinical Leadership)**
Clinical Nurse Consultant (Neonatal)/Acting Director Neonatal Services, The Royal Women's Hospital, Flemington Road, Parkville, Victoria, Australia

Kym Davey **RN, RM, BN**
Lecturer, Monash University, Peninsula Campus, Melbourne, Victoria, Australia

Paula Dellabarca **RN, BN, MCN (Masters in Clinical Nursing), MsC (Dist)**
Neonatal Nurse Practitioner, Neonatal Intensive Care Unit, Wellington Regional Hospital, New Zealand

Dolores Dooley **RN, RM, BN(Hons), MHlthSc (Education)**
Midwifery/Nursing Lecturer, Deakin University, Melbourne, Victoria, Australia

Anna O'Connell **MProfEd&Trng, RN, RM**
Midwifery/Nursing Lecturer, Deakin University, Melbourne, Victoria, Australia

CHAPTER 1

NEONATAL NURSING: GLOBAL PERSPECTIVES

VICTORIA KAIN, TRUDI MANNIX AND KAREN WALKER[a]

Learning objectives

After reading this chapter you will be able to:

- discuss the evolution of neonatal care
- understand the perspectives of neonatal care for First Peoples of Australia and New Zealand
- understand the demographics of neonatal units and the levels of newborn care
- describe the profile of neonatal nurses and midwives globally, and the impact that neonatal nurses and midwives have on neonatal outcomes
- outline newborn epidemiological data
- discuss the emerging role of neonatal simulation and its impact on patient safety
- describe the role of professional organisations for neonatal nurses and midwives
- describe models of governance within the neonatal unit and the organisation
- identify leadership traits and styles to enable change and staff development within the neonatal unit
- discuss components of organisational culture including teamwork and communication
- analyse the impact of evidence for quality improvement within clinical practice.

Key words, terms and abbreviations

Aboriginal Community Controlled Health Service (ACCHS)
Australian and New Zealand Neonatal Network (ANZNN)
Australian College of Neonatal Nurses (ACNN)
Australian Health Practitioner Regulation Agency (AHPRA)
Australian Nursing and Midwifery Accreditation Council (ANMAC)
clinical governance
Congress of Aboriginal and Torres Strait Islander Nurses and Midwives (CATSINaM)
Council of International Neonatal Nurses (COINN)
culture
leadership
National Aboriginal and Torres Strait Islander Health Plan (NATSIHP)
neonatal intensive care unit (NICU)
Neonatal Nurses College of Aotearoa (NNCA)
neonatal nurse practitioner (NNP)
New Zealand Nurses Organisation (NZNO)
nurse practitioner (NP)
safety
special care baby unit (SCBU)
special care nursery (SCN)
organisational culture
teamwork
World Health Organization (WHO)

[a]The authors would like to acknowledge Professor Roianne West, co-author of this chapter in the 1st edition of this book.

INTRODUCTION

Neonatology is considered a relatively new area of medical and nursing specialisation, emerging as a subspecialty of paediatrics in the 1950s. Within a relatively short time frame, neonatology has emerged as one of the fastest growing fields of medical science. Some of the major historical milestones in the field include the impact of exogenous surfactant in the late 1980s, the near eradication of rhesus (Rh) disease and the introduction of antenatally administered corticosteroids, which have all impacted favourably on the morbidity and mortality of neonates globally. While this is largely due to advances in respiratory care and improved nutritional techniques, neonatal nurses/midwives have tirelessly promoted and enforced the fundamental cornerstones of neonatal care, including simple measures for hygiene, warmth and nutrition with the promotion and support of breastfeeding, and have also championed neurodevelopmental and family-centred care.

This chapter considers the context of systems that underpin care of preterm and unwell neonates both within Australia, New Zealand and globally. The evolution of neonatal practice from a historical perspective, the advances in neonatal practice and patient **safety** will be discussed. An introduction to neonatal care is also provided, to give an understanding of neonatal care and the impact that nurses and midwives have had on outcomes. Inclusive to this are the professional organisations that support the development of neonatal care and an overview of the associated framework and theory.

The provision of safe and best practice in the neonatal unit is dependent on the environment and **culture** within the unit and more broadly within the organisation. This chapter will guide neonatal nurses/midwives through the labyrinth of the structure and processes that support their clinical practice. Issues such as **teamwork**, **leadership** and **organisational culture** are discussed with practical information on how they may incorporate the principles into their practice. Processes such as quality improvement, reflection, family-centred care, competency and mandatory skills acquisition are highlighted to enable neonatal nurses/midwives to gain an understanding of their importance when using critical thinking skills and in providing best practice.

TYPES OF NEONATAL UNITS

The **World Health Organization (WHO)** categorises units which provide newborn care into three levels, with level 1 providing basic newborn care, level 2 special care and level 3 intensive care (WHO, 2018). While these three levels of neonatal units are generally accepted, this can vary, from state to state, region to region and country to country. Some jurisdictions have three levels of care while some have up to six levels of care, with levels 1–2 providing care to low-risk neonates, levels 3–5 caring for moderately at-risk neonates and levels 6A and 6B providing tertiary newborn services. In the interests of a consistent approach, however, this text will refer to three levels of care as described here:

- Level 1: neonates admitted to a level 1 unit are considered 'low risk' and do not require complex care.
- Level 2: these neonatal units have facilities to manage mildly or moderately ill neonates. This category of unit is also referred to as a **special care baby unit (SCBU)** or **special care nursery (SCN)**. For the purposes of this chapter, the term 'level 2' will be used.
- Level 3: globally, the level 3 unit (commonly referred to as the **neonatal intensive care unit (NICU)**) may be further classified into levels 4 and above to reflect the level of acuity. Level 3 nurseries and above, or NICUs, are located only in tertiary (or 'teaching') hospitals.

In Australia and New Zealand in 2018, neonates born at less than 32 weeks represented the majority (32.1%) of all neonates admitted to an NICU. Of these neonates, 0.4% weighed less than 500 g at birth, with 26.8% of neonates weighing less than 1500 g (Chow et al., 2020).

EVIDENCE-BASED PRACTICE RESEARCH 1.1

Nurses in Australia come from diverse social and cultural backgrounds, with varying degrees of expertise and experience. It is an appropriate environment to explore the complicated and demanding social dynamics across varied nursing workforces. Social exchanges, organisational culture and power relations shape work-related social relations. This study examined how social relations were established at work for neonatal nurses, guided by the following research questions:

- What are the cultural practices of the neonatal unit?
- How do nurses experience their everyday work life in the neonatal unit?
- How are nurses' social relations of work affected by the neonatal unit?

Data were collected over 18 months in the field by observing 76 nurses and interviewing 65 of them.

To understand the intricacies of social relations between nurses in diverse social situations, intersectionality theory was applied.

How nurses related at work was central to this work. Trust and reciprocity enabled nurses to work together. The assistance of senior nurses and opportunities to learn and improve were deemed essential. A good shift was possible because nurses felt valued, included, encouraged and cared for. However, there was a lack of trust and support among nurses of colour. These nurses were deskilled and faced career difficulties. Nurses of colour seemed to be merely filling in for shortages rather than being valued for their expertise. These activities created a toxic workplace culture for nurses, affecting work–life balance and patient safety. Examining how cultural safety affects social relationships among nurses at work promotes authentic engagement.

Source: Nepali (2020).

THE DESIGN OF THE NEONATAL UNIT

Neonatal units in Australia and New Zealand have a range of designs depending upon the age of the facility and the acuity of the neonates they accommodate. As is the case globally, there are two main designs of neonatal units: the open-bay design, which may also have pods where neonates are grouped together, and single/double family rooms. Fig. 1.1 is an example of an open-bay design. The open-bay environment is a more traditional design that is favoured by some clinicians because it allows for communication and interaction among staff, and also allows for the simultaneous monitoring of multiple neonates.

Since the emergence of the trend incorporating neurodevelopmental care principles into all aspects of neonatal care from the mid 1980s, single rooms (and double rooms for multiple births) and family rooms have been considered superior in terms of providing neurodevelopmentally sound neonatal care and enhancing parental satisfaction (O'Callaghan et al., 2019) (see Fig. 1.2).

This design has been linked to improved outcomes such as increased parental involvement in the care of their baby, reduced rates of sepsis, control of noxious stimuli such as noise, improved sleep patterns for neonates, a decreased length of hospital stay and reduced re-admission to a hospital environment (O'Callaghan et al., 2019). See Chapter 22 for further information.

The single-room design has not been without criticism, however, with a significant increase in the nursing workload and level of isolation reported (Doede et al., 2018). These negative impacts have, on balance, been ameliorated by the increased satisfaction reported by neonatal nurses/midwives upon seeing the benefits to neonates and parents of this design.

EVIDENCE-BASED PRACTICE RESEARCH 1.2

A comparative observational study was conducted to investigate the impact of open-bay and dual-occupancy NICU designs on parent activities and evaluate their opinions of both designs. A parent activity study, parent feedback surveys comparing physical surroundings and parental involvement were all used in the study. To obtain a better understanding of families' experiences in the dual-occupancy NICU, post-transition parent interviews ($n = 10$) were undertaken. Parents spent significantly more minutes per day (24 h) participating in their infant's care in the dual-occupancy NICU than in the open-bay NICU (359.40, 228.70, $p < 0.01$; respectively); similarly, increased participation was recorded in the dual-occupancy special care nursery (SCN) than in the open-bay SCN (295.20, 231.90, $p < 0.01$: respectively). Parents believed that the dual-occupancy design produced a 'home away from home', allowing them to participate in kangaroo care and breastfeeding while attending to their infant's care with minimum interruptions and privacy.

Source: Broom and Kecskes (2020).

AN OVERVIEW OF NEONATAL STATISTICS

There were 315,147 live births in Australia in 2018, and 58,020 live births in New Zealand. In Australia and New Zealand, male births outnumbered female births in 2018,

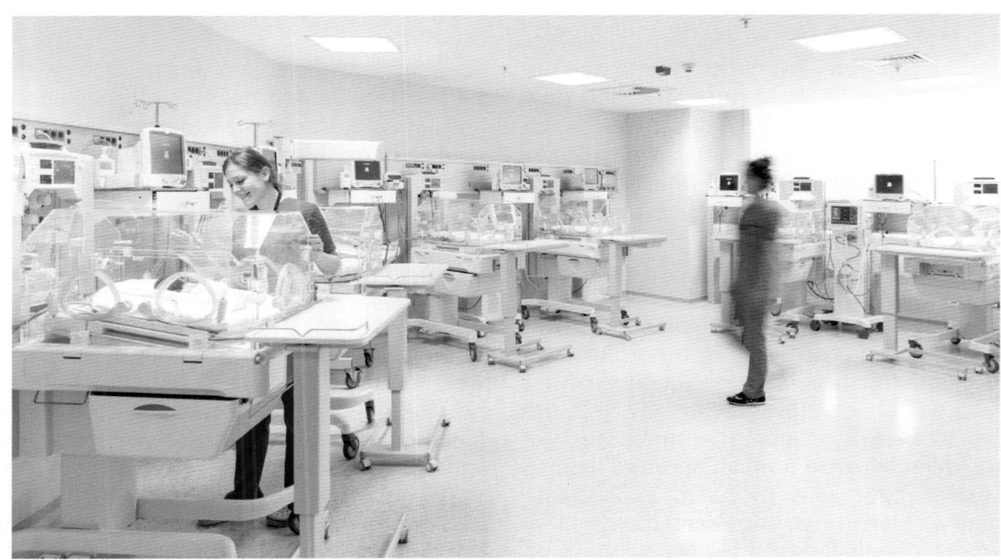

FIGURE 1.1 **A typical neonatal unit in an Australian and New Zealand setting (open-bay design)**
Source: iStockphoto/JazzIRT.

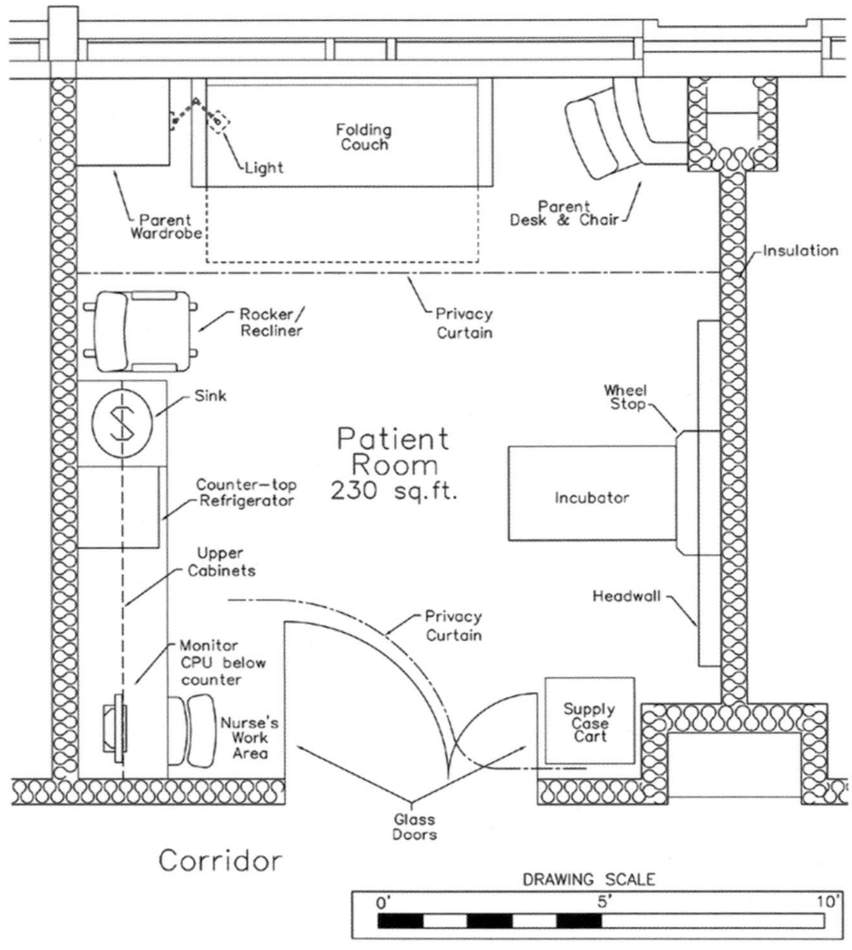

FIGURE 1.2 **Example of a single-room design**

Source: Stevens, D. C., Akram Khan, M., Munson, D. P., Reid, E. J., Helseth, C. C., & Buggy, J. (2007). The impact of architectural design upon the environmental sound and light exposure of neonates who require intensive care: an evaluation of the Boekelheide Neonatal Intensive Care Nursery. Journal of Perinatology, 27(Suppl 2), S20–S28. Reprinted with permission from Springer Nature.

accounting for 51.4% of total live births in both nations. Male births accounted for 58.8% of **Australian and New Zealand Neonatal Network (ANZNN)** registrants, which was higher than the national average. The majority, 55.0% of registrants, born at less than 32 weeks' gestation were male, while 62.4% of births at term were male (Chow et al., 2020).

According to the ANZNN, 10,651 babies were admitted to level 3 NICUs in Australia and New Zealand in 2018 (Chow et al., 2020), representing 2.9% of notified live births. Of these, 80% were delivered in a hospital with tertiary care facilities, with the remainder requiring transfer to a tertiary facility. Of these neonates, 3417 (32.1%) were born at less than 32 weeks' gestation; in Australia, 71.1% of these neonates were delivered from a Caucasian mother, with the second highest ethnicity being Asian (16%). Indigenous neonates were over-represented, with 1 in 13 mothers (7.5%) identifying as of Indigenous descent, which was higher than the proportion of all reported births in Australia in 2018 (4.9%) (Chow et al., 2020).

Although there are many factors that influence perinatal outcomes, one of the most significant is maternal age. In 2018, the ages of mothers of high-risk neonates ranged from 15 to 55 years. Mothers aged 30–34 years had the highest proportion of ANZNN registrants' mothers (33.2%), followed by mothers aged 25–29 years (25.3%). In 2018, they accounted for nearly one-third of all ANZNN registrants' mothers (58.5%) (Chow et al., 2020).

In 2018, 95.9% of ANZNN registrants survived and were discharged home. These records contain babies who were moved to level 2 or level 1 units, as well as those who were transferred to another level 3 unit or to a paediatric hospital. The babies born before 30 weeks' gestation had the highest mortality rate, with a survival rate at discharge rising week by week from 42.1% for babies born before 24 weeks to 95.9% for babies born at 29 weeks.

For 0.8% of registrants, a fatal congenital defect was the cause of death, with the majority of deaths occurring in babies born between 35 and 39 weeks of pregnancy (Chow et al., 2020).

THE GLOBAL NEONATAL AND MIDWIFERY WORKFORCE

Globally, there are challenges for the nursing and midwifery workforce as highlighted in the recent WHO Roadmap on Human Resources for Health Strategies for low- and middle-income countries (WHO, 2020). While this report was not specifically focused on high-income countries, many of the challenges of sustainability of the neonatal workforce are relevant. In many countries, neonatal nursing is not a specialty; however, with increasing survival of small and sick newborns, this is changing and the importance of highly skilled neonatal nurses is becoming more recognised. A sample of the diversity of courses, qualifications and regulatory practices is outlined below.

Australia and New Zealand

In Australia and New Zealand, registered nurses (RNs) and registered midwives (RMs) provide expert care to neonates in the neonatal unit. In both countries, an RN/RM completes a 3-year tertiary degree with a recognised tertiary provider, and, in the case of the latter, the RM may hold a degree in midwifery or both nursing and midwifery. Australian Institute of Health and Welfare (AIHW) and New Zealand Health Workforce (NZHW) data do not capture how many nurses work primarily in neonatal units; however, the majority of clinicians in level 3 units and higher are RNs. In Australia, the **Australian Health Practitioner Regulation Agency (AHPRA)** is the regulating authority for Australia's health practitioners in partnership with the National Boards. For RNs and RMs, this is the Nursing and Midwifery Board of Australia, which is also responsible for developing standards, codes and guidelines for the nursing and midwifery professions, and the **Australian Nursing and Midwifery Accreditation Council (ANMAC)**, which develops and reviews accreditation standards for nursing and midwifery programs of study in Australia.

In order to practise, RNs in New Zealand must be registered with the Nursing Council of New Zealand (which is also the regulatory authority); equally, RMs in New Zealand must be registered with the Midwifery Council of New Zealand. Due to the Trans-Tasman Mutual Recognition Act (TTMRA), those who possess a nursing registration in all states and territories in Australia can apply for registration in New Zealand under the TTMRA, and vice versa with AHPRA.

North America

In North America, nurses may complete a diploma in 2–3 years (a few hospital-based education providers still exist); a 2–3-year Associate Degree in Nursing (ADN) or a 4-year undergraduate Bachelor of Science in Nursing (BSN). After obtaining this nursing education, individuals then sit for the National Council Licensure Exam (NCLEX-RN) and once successful are able to apply for their registered nursing licence. The respective university deans give the student authorisation to test with the Board of Nursing in which they decide to take the exam (each state has its own board). They then take the NCLEX and, if they pass, they receive their RN licensure for that state.

The US Bureau of Labor and Statistics provides data on the employment and wage statistics for nurses and highlights the substantial variance in employment and mean wages for RNs between states (US Department of Labour, 2021). Neonatal nurse certification may be obtained through the American Association of Critical Care Nurses (AACN) or the National Certification Corporation (NCC) for nurses who have worked a minimum specified number of hours/years in the specialty (Registered Nursing.org, 2021). National certification is required for neonatal nurse practitioners to practise, and this is obtained through the NCC.

Midwifery in the US is a postgraduate course, with all programs accredited by the American College of Nurse-Midwives (ACNM) Accreditation Commission for Midwifery Education (ACME) requiring a Bachelor's degree for entry (ACNM, 2021).

While the National Council of State Boards of Nursing (NCSBN) consists of all states' boards of nursing, governance of nurses is administered through individual state nursing boards, with scope of practice defined and regulated by state laws (NCSBN, 2021; Nursing License Map, 2021).

Neonatal nurses in North America are able to join multiple national professional bodies: the National Association of Neonatal Nurses (NANN); the Academy of Neonatal Nursing (ANN); the Association of Women's Health, Obstetric and Neonatal Nurses (AWHONN) as well as the Hawaiian state-based organisation Caring for Hawai'i Neonates, translated in Hawaiian as 'Mālama on Nā Keiki'. In 2017 these organisations held an inaugural meeting in Hawaii and agreed to work together with the Council of International Neonatal Nurses (COINN), and the Alliance of Global Neonatal Nursing (ALIGNN) was formed.

Canada

In Canada, all provinces and territories require nurses to have a Bachelor's degree with the exception of Quebec, where diploma programs are still offered. As of 2015, the 11 provincial/territorial bodies require the successful completion of a standardised Canadian RN entry-to-practice exam. Canada has two advanced practice nursing (APN) roles: the clinical nurse specialist (CNS), and the **nurse practitioner (NP)**, both of which require a minimum of a Master of Nursing degree. A PhD in nursing is the most common requirement for university academic/research positions. A Doctor of Nursing Practice (DNP) is less common, with only one university in Canada, as of 2021, offering this program. There is no national licence in Canada, and each province or territory has regulatory bodies (Canadian Nurses Association (CNA), 2021). Nurses can undertake specialisation in neonatal nursing through programs such as the Canadian Nurses Association Certification Program. The Canadian Association of Neonatal Nurses (CANN) was established in 2006 and is the professional body for neonatal nurses in Canada.

The United Kingdom

In the United Kingdom, the National Health System is responsible for the delivery of healthcare and the training, education and development of health professionals. The professional regulator for nurses and midwives is the Nursing and Midwifery Council (NMC), with which all nurses and midwives must be registered (NMC, 2021a). Nurses and midwives must work within 'The Code', which incorporates the professional standards for practice (NMC, 2021b).

While nurses pay an annual fee for registration, registration must be renewed and revalidated every 3 years. This revalidation process requires evidence of 450 practice hours, 35 hours of continuing professional development, five pieces of practice-related feedback, five written reflections, reflective discussion and declarations of health and character (NMC, 2021c). Neonatal nursing is a recognised specialty and there are postgraduate specialisation courses. The Neonatal Nurses Association (NNA) was established in 1977 (NNA, n.d.).

South Africa

South Africa has a two-tier healthcare system, with the public and private sectors working together. Primary, secondary and tertiary care services are all duplicated. The private healthcare sector caters to those who can afford medical benefits or pay for services privately, while the public healthcare system caters to the majority of the population. Both sectors need neonatal nurse specialists. From 2001 to 2012, specialised neonatal nurses were trained and registered with the South African Nursing Council (SANC). Due to a technicality in the initial approval process, SANC stopped licensing specialist neonatal nurses as an independent specialty in 2012. The cancellation has reportedly had a negative impact on neonatal nurse specialist preparation and availability in South Africa (Maree et al., 2021). The Neonatal Nursing Association of South Africa (NNASA) was established in 2007 by a small group of dedicated neonatal nurses who saw a need to enhance the region's neonatal care by assisting and empowering the nurses who care for these neonates (NNASA, 2018).

The association's goals are to encourage and reward excellence in neonatal care through a national award, to improve skills and knowledge through regional workshops, to foster collaboration and support between nurses in state and private institutions through regional networks, to improve standards of care through the provision of evidence-based best-practice guidelines, and to improve neonatal care through the provision of evidence-based best-practice guidelines.

The neonatal nurse practitioner role

The nurse practitioner (NP) model of an extended scope of practice for the RN has been established internationally since 1966. The **neonatal nurse practitioner (NNP)** position was created in the United States in the 1960s as a result of a physician shortage. This occurred as a result of changes in medical training that decreased time spent in specialist fields and, as a result of the survival of premature babies and advancements in specialised treatment, the demand for neonatal care increased (Forbes-Coe et al., 2020).

In Australia, NPs are RNs with an advanced (Master's) qualification in addition to significant specialist experience in their field of practice. NPs are authorised to practise in an expanded nursing role in clinical settings, including the neonatal setting. In 1990, the first NP committee model was convened in New South Wales and, in 1994, NP pilot projects were established in Australia. The first NPs (and midwifery practitioners) in Australia were authorised to practise in 2000, and neonatal nursing was identified as one of the first areas for an NP model, with South Australia one of the first states to implement the role. Almost two decades later, the neonatal NP model is continuing to establish itself in most level 3 neonatal units in Australia, but uptake has been somewhat slow in some states.

In New Zealand the role was launched by the Ministry of Health and the Nursing Council of New Zealand in May 2001. The development and implementation of the NP role in New Zealand's health and disability sector followed a key recommendation in the report of the Ministerial Taskforce on Nursing (1998). Subsequently, in 1999 a consensus conference of wide-ranging nursing organisations (the College of Nurses Advanced Practice Workshop in Palmerston North) agreed to progress the issue of advanced clinical nursing practice.

The nurse practitioner position is one of the most sought-after senior clinical roles for neonatal nurses because of its many advantages. The provision of autonomy for patients while ensuring stability and continuity of care in the work environment is one of the role's greatest strengths, which prompted its expansion. NNPs initially offered continuity within the workforce, allowing support and education to both medical and nursing personnel during a period of high turnover of medical registrars. The variety of an NNP's clinical experience helps to create a more diverse and stable workforce, which benefits babies and families, and the position offers a previously inaccessible clinical career path at the senior nursing level (Forbes-Coe et al., 2020) (Fig. 1.3).

The position does, however, have some established challenges and limitations. NNPs in Australia do not have a Medicare provider number unless they operate in a private practice, so they must always be countersigned by a medical practitioner when making referrals. The ongoing obligation to work a revolving 24-hour roster, which is usually not needed in other disciplines at this senior level, is one of the key limitations of the current position. Another drawback is that, in many jurisdictions, only a medical practitioner can certify death, which can be difficult for NNPs performing neonatal retrievals (Forbes-Coe et al., 2020).

Neonatal nursing and cultural safety

The **Congress of Aboriginal and Torres Strait Islander Nurses and Midwives (CATSINaM)** considers cultural safety to be the ultimate step in a continuum of nursing

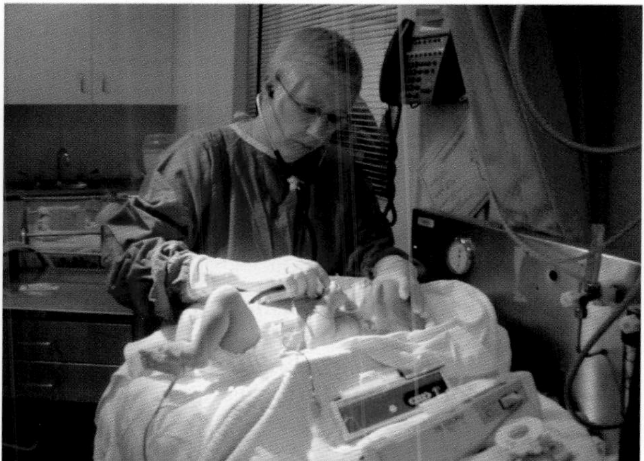

FIGURE 1.3 **A neonatal nurse practitioner in Australia stabilises a neonate pre-retrieval**

Source: Dr Jackie Smith.

and/or midwifery care that encompasses cultural awareness, cultural sensitivity, cultural knowledge, cultural respect and cultural competence. Cultural safety is defined by the recipient and cannot be defined by the care giver. CATSINaM advocates for Aboriginal and Torres Strait Islander peoples by promoting a framework of cultural safety to inform attitudes and behaviours in health professionals' provision of care to Aboriginal and Torres Strait Islander individuals and communities, so that individuals and their families feel culturally secure, safe and respected. Cultural safety must be integrated into all aspects of nursing and midwifery practice in order to achieve this state (CATSINaM, 2014).

In terms of cultural safety training for Australian and New Zealand nurses and midwives, Indigenous health education and cultural safety training is inconsistent across universities. This is the reason for the recently developed Aboriginal and Torres Strait Islander Curriculum Framework (Department of Health, 2021).

Aboriginal and Torres Strait Islander (ATSI) people are significantly under-represented in the health workforce, which potentially contributes to reduced access to health services for the broader Indigenous Australian population (AIHW, 2020). A workforce survey published in 2019 showed that there were 5037 ATSI registered as nurses and midwives, with 4012 currently employed as clinicians (Commonwealth of Australia, 2020). Only 0.8% of Australia's nursing and midwifery workforce identify as Indigenous, and only 1414 are registered nurses (CATSINaM, 2015). Given the over-representation of First Peoples' neonates, a commitment must be made to expand and nurture Indigenous neonatal nurses and/or midwives in order to better reflect the population they serve and to provide culturally safe care in neonatal units. It is currently unknown how many Indigenous nurses and/or midwives work in newborn units. In New Zealand, 7% of registered nurses identify as Māori, and 4% as Pacific ethnicity (NZNO, 2021).

NEONATAL CARE AND INDIGENOUS CONTEXTS

In Australia, the development of Indigenous health as a sector in healthcare occurred at around the same time as neonatal nursing emerged as a specialty field in the 1970s, with the establishment of the first **Aboriginal Community Controlled Health Service (ACCHS)** (National Aboriginal Community Controlled Health Organisation (NACCHO), 2016). The ACCHS's mission is to provide holistic, comprehensive and culturally appropriate healthcare in compliance with the protocols established by the community that governs it. There are presently approximately 150 ACCHSs in Australia's cities, towns and outlying areas (NACCHO, 2016).

There is little research in the field of Māori whānau in New Zealand. However, it is clear that there are many similarities associated with neonatal births among Indigenous women, such as poorer birth outcomes, higher infant mortality and higher rates of low-birthweight and preterm neonates. According to New Zealand statistics from 2016, Asian neonates outnumbered Māori neonates admitted to NICUs and SCBUs. Despite the improvement in the ethnic ratio of admissions to the hospitals, Māori neonates remained over-represented in neonatal and perinatal mortality (National Women's Health, 2020). Clinical care provided to whānau, and whether whānau Māori receive medical and clinical care equivalent to that received by non-Māori families within the neonatal unit, highlights the importance of understanding possible health inequities experienced by Māori in relation to New Zealand's colonial history. In order to improve overall wellbeing, a deeper awareness of health inequities is required, as currently articulated through policies and models such as whānau ora.

PERSPECTIVES OF NEONATAL CARE FOR FIRST PEOPLES

The Indigenous population in Australia accounts for approximately 2.5% of the total population, according to census data. The Council of Australian Governments (COAG) decided in 2009 to be accountable for reaching the six 'Closing the Gap' targets (COAG, 2009). The first goal was to reduce the gap in child mortality. The aims have yielded mixed results; for example, in 2018, the Indigenous infant mortality rate was 141 per 100,000, double the rate for the non-Indigenous population at 67/100,000 (Australian Government, 2020). Since the 'Closing the Gap' target was set in 2008, the Indigenous child mortality rate has improved slightly (by around 7%), but at the same time the mortality rate for non-Indigenous children has improved at a faster rate, so the gap has actually widened (Australian Government, 2020). Continued improvements in important determinants influencing the health of Indigenous neonates, such as access to prenatal care and a decrease in rates of smoking during pregnancy, have the potential to continue to meet this target.

According to census data, Aotearoa/New Zealand's Indigenous population accounts for around 15% of the total population, while the estimated percentage of neonates registered as being of Māori heritage is 30% (Statistics Tatauranga Aotearoa NZ, 2019a). The Indigenous infant mortality rate in New Zealand has fallen since 2008 to 4.9 per 1000 births – close but still not as good as those of European origin (3.8 per 1000 births) (Stats Tatauranga Aotearoa NZ, 2019b). The rates of sudden unexpected death of an infant (SUDI) are significantly higher in the Māori and Pacific Peoples' ethnic groups (Ministry of Health, 2021). To eliminate health disparities for First Peoples' mothers and babies, there has been an increase in demands for more First Peoples' nurses as well as a culturally safe nursing workforce (Taylor et al., 2020).

Given the over-representation of Indigenous neonates in the newborn setting, Indigenous health education and professional development are critical to closing the health outcomes gap between Indigenous and non-Indigenous neonates. The holistic, comprehensive and culturally appropriate care principles used by the Aboriginal Community Controlled Health Services sector should be used in neonatal settings as well. The **Australian College of Neonatal Nurses (ACNN)** and the **Neonatal Nurses College of Aotearoa (NNCA)** articulate the characteristics and qualities expected of neonatal nurses/midwives in Australia and New Zealand in their neonatal nursing standards, which include an expectation that neonatal nurses/midwives provide culturally safe care (NZNO, 2021). This is significant because cultural awareness is essential for providing culturally safe neonatal nursing/midwifery care. More recently, the ability to provide 'culturally appropriate healthcare' has progressed to providing 'culturally safe healthcare' (Department of Health, 2021).

Indigenous health education has advanced significantly in recent years. The Department of Health (2021) authorised a new Aboriginal and Torres Strait Islander Curriculum Framework, which, while aimed at universities, has relevance for service delivery because it intends to equip health professionals to provide culturally safe healthcare. To actively establish stronger cultural safety in health service delivery, the Framework responds to and expands on widespread evidence and recommendations from numerous reports, studies and consultations.

Furthermore, the **National Aboriginal and Torres Strait Islander Health Plan (NATSIHP)** 2013–23 stipulates 'the centrality of culture in the health of Aboriginal and Torres Strait Islander peoples, as well as individuals' rights to a safe, healthy, and empowered existence' (Australian Government, 2013, p. 4). The National Framework for Health Services for Aboriginal and Torres Strait Islander Children and Families is a companion document that articulates a vision and principles for the delivery of child and family health services to Aboriginal and Torres Strait Islander children and families across Australia.

It is critical that neonatal nurses and midwives learn not just 'about', but also 'from' Aboriginal people. Indigenous health education and cultural safety training should be valued in neonatal nursing/midwifery professional development, and they should be recognised as distinct entities.

CLINICAL GOVERNANCE

WHAT IS CLINICAL GOVERNANCE?

Clinical governance is a term widely used to describe systems and processes that support the delivery of safe, high-quality and effective clinical care.

The Australian Commission on Safety and Quality in Health Care (ACSQHC) defines clinical governance as the set of relationships and responsibilities established by a health service organisation between its state or territory department of health, governing body, executive, workforce, patients, consumers and other stakeholders to ensure good clinical outcomes (ACSQHC, 2021).

How does clinical governance work?

Clinical governance originated in the United Kingdom in the late 1990s, with the goal of ensuring that high-quality care is given the same priority as financial control and service performance. There are several examples of inadequate clinical governance leading to negative patient outcomes, including several high-profile failures. There is also a growing body of literature describing specific initiatives to improve patient outcomes, such as antibiotic stewardship and hand hygiene to reduce rates of methicillin-resistant *Staphylococcus aureus*, or the introduction of rapid response teams to reduce hospital-wide mortality and out-of-ICU cardiac arrest (Dwyer, 2019).

Clinical governance is a shared duty that operates at all levels of the organisation and includes a review and improvement program at every level, from the Board to the Executive, the management team, clinicians and non-clinical personnel. A clinical governance framework is subject to the Board's supervision. It must show a commitment to good governance and promote an open and transparent management culture (Dwyer, 2019).

The Chief Executive Officer and the Executive are responsible for leading an organisation in a fair, open and transparent manner while also exhibiting a commitment to strong clinical governance. They must ensure that the essential systems and processes, such as policies and procedures, are in place to enhance clinical quality and patient safety, as well as to report and manage incidents and encourage consumer feedback. They are also in charge of developing a risk management framework that enables the organisation, its patients, employees and visitors to identify, monitor and control hazards. They must ensure that the organisation responds positively and rapidly to change.

Clinical service unit and business unit directors and medical directors are responsible for ensuring that the clinical governance framework is implemented correctly in their domains. This includes maintaining policies and procedures, adhering to organisational standards in work practices, reviewing risks and taking corrective action. They must make certain that employees are properly trained and qualified for their clinical roles. Directors must maintain processes for assessing clinical outcomes and resolving performance concerns.

Within their areas of accountability, unit/department heads and managers are accountable for implementing the governance framework. This entails creating clear lines of responsibility for the quality and safety of the services delivered within each unit or department. Quality business plans should include work plans for continual improvement in systems and content of care, as well as maintaining and embedding organisational policies and procedures in local practice. At this level, managers are responsible for ensuring that incident management systems are properly implemented, and that a systematic response to local issues and performance improvement takes place. Managers should also make certain that adequate training, education and performance evaluation opportunities are available. At the local level, all employees should take ownership of risk management.

Clinical staff members are expected to follow all policies and procedures that pertain to their area of practice, report any occurrences that have or may have an influence on patient safety, and be aware of any legal requirements while doing their duties. They should have a defined scope of practice in their job description, which should be supported by a proper certification process. Employees should have regular performance reviews with their employers, have their scope of practice reviewed on a regular basis, and seek out suitable continued education and training. Clinical staff must participate in the organisation's monitoring systems and processes, as well as initiatives to improve care delivery.

Through the provision of adequate information about the clinical treatment offered, an informed consent procedure and the ability to provide feedback on the care they receive, consumers should be encouraged to be active participants in decisions surrounding their healthcare (Dwyer, 2019). In neonatal units, this responsibility is delegated to parents in the first instance.

Clinical governance in neonatal units

The Australian College of Neonatal Nurses (ACNN, 2019) provides standards of practice to be used as a guide for curricula development and as a tool to measure clinical practice. In New Zealand the National Neonatal Nurses Knowledge and Skills Framework (New Zealand Nurses Organisation, 2014) guides education and provides a structure for the professional development of neonatal nurses, while the Neonatal Nurses College Aotearoa (NNCA) Standards for Neonatal Nursing Practice (2015) represent the standards of practice required to deliver safe and effective neonatal services. The ACNN and NNCA Standards reflect the principles of the ACSQHC (2021) and align neonatal nursing efforts to improving the safety and quality of neonatal nursing care. These standards (currently being revised in 2022) meet the requirement for continuing practice and professional development and the domains are in line with quality improvement standards and the drive for continual improvement in the delivery of clinical care. The specific domains of clinical practice, leadership and teamwork, professional development and research share similar requirements to those described in the Nursing and Midwifery Board of Australia's (NMBA) Registered Nurse Standards for Practice and those of the Nursing Council of New Zealand (NCNZ) respectively. Both frameworks are designed to describe practice domains, work within therapeutic relationships, lifelong professional learning and technical advancement. The accountability for practice extends to all contexts, clinical decision making and provision of care. Both professional colleges and the NMBA and NCNZ link education and skill development as key requirements for nurses and midwives.

Neonatal nursing managers carry the responsibility of leading clinical teams within clinical governance frameworks (Fig. 1.4). Shared governance is a model that extends power, control and authority to front-line teams to promote positive patient outcomes, inclusion and positivity (McKnight & Moore, 2021).

This model supports decision making within clinical units by clinical teams. Similar to other models of governance, the foundational domains of accountability, compliance with legislation, transparent performance reporting and data systems, competence and organisational capacity are necessary for effective implementation. Key organisational goals will include partnerships with families, recognition and management of deteriorating patients, analysis and trending of clinical incidents, recommendations for process improvements, availability of and compliance with clinical practice guidelines (evidence based wherever possible), compliance with legislation, organisational and professional policies and guidelines, continuing professional development support and consumer engagement. These goals are supported by national standards and accreditation systems in Australia and New Zealand and their respective neonatal nursing and midwifery colleges.

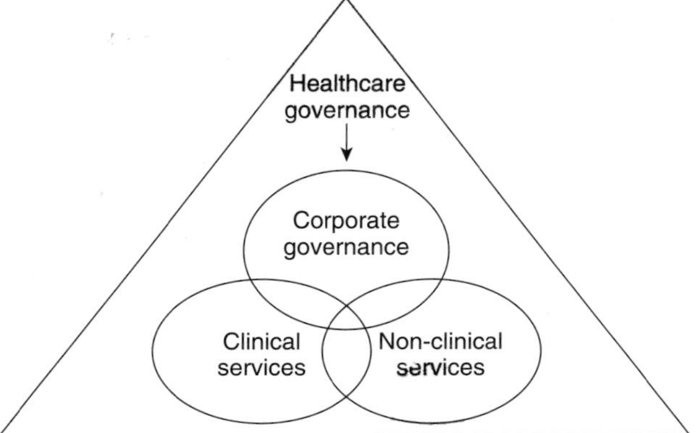

FIGURE 1.4 **Key components of clinical practice**

Source: McSherry and Pearce (2011, Fig. 3.3, p. 55). Reprinted with permission of John Wiley & Sons Inc.

Collaborative working arrangements extend from shared governance and are aimed at supporting organisations to learn from changes that have worked elsewhere. International examples of these neonatal networks include the Vermont Oxford Network (<https://public.vtoxford.org>), whose voluntary membership extends to 1000 neonatal units across the globe and hosts the Neonatal Intensive Care Quality Improvement Collaboratives, aimed at improving care through evidence, and the Cochrane Neonatal Review Group (<http://neonatal.cochrane.org/>), which disseminates systematic reviews to support evidence-based neonatal practice. Application of the learning shows mixed results and may reflect the different levels of reliability in processes in different organisations. The networks focus on key habits of high-reliability organisations and enable the distribution of good practice and the opportunities to learn. The Australian and New Zealand Neonatal Network (ANZNN, 2021) is a collaborative network that includes all level 3 units in both countries and one Singaporean level 3 unit, all New Zealand level 2 units, and an increasing number of level 2 neonatal units in Australia. The collaborative brings together information from a minimum data set to monitor morbidity and mortality and provide an external quality assurance process.

Clinical governance is centred on promoting and achieving continuous improvement within the organisation. Neonatal nurses and midwives need to bring together six key systems and processes to successfully implement clinical governance:

1. risk management
2. performance management
3. quality improvement
4. information
5. accountability
6. communication (McSherry & Pearce, 2011).

Risk management

Risk management frameworks strive to limit, minimise or prevent adverse events occurring. A risk may be described as an event that may potentially occur that prevents an organisation from achieving their objectives (Park & Sharp, 2019). Significant patient risk is described as the high probability of a substantial event that has a demonstrable adverse impact. It is the responsibility of all clinical staff to be able to identify and escalate potential risks so they can be considered by the leadership team. Control, interventions, system changes and treatment actions need to be identified and put in place to treat and mitigate the identified risk. Common risks in the neonatal unit include hospital-acquired infections, medication errors and neonates receiving expressed breast milk from another mother and having an incorrect test due to incorrect identification. Monitoring and preventing the occurrence of adverse events such as these, as well as accessing new knowledge or technology, standardisation of practices based on external guidelines or regulations, and participation in research, has been shown to facilitate innovation and improve and sustain patient care outcomes in NICUs (Cuttini et al., 2020).

CLINICAL PRACTICE 1.1

An important role for neonatal nurses/midwives is to report, monitor and manage incidents. There are several clinical indicators associated with risk that neonatal nurses/midwives are in a position to minimise and prevent. Some of these indicators are:

- unplanned extubation
- central line infections
- nasal integrity
- extravasation injuries
- skin integrity.

Consider your environment and how these potential risks are monitored.

1. When a risk does occur what is the process for review?
2. How can prevention be incorporated into the review and management?
3. How are trends in indicators fed back to the staff in your neonatal unit?

Performance management and quality improvement

This proactive approach strengthens patient safety. Performance management is a responsibility of unit managers and includes the principles of trust, review of consumer feedback and clinical incidents, budget integrity, staff support and development and patient safety. Service performance is shown to be impacted by leadership styles. Leaders who show appreciation, respect and concern for the welfare of others, and who clearly articulate role expectations, set clear team objectives and have a commitment to excellence, enhance performance and patient safety (Kiwanuka et al., 2021).

EVIDENCE-BASED PRACTICE RESEARCH 1.3

In a study of the traditional, collaborative and individualistic managerial models in 51 NICUs in Italy, the authors found that outcomes were better in NICUs that operated under a collaborative model (Fanelli et al., 2020). In the 'traditional' model, the doctor was responsible for the top-down leadership and management of the NICU (and seen as 'above the nurse' in the hierarchy). In the 'individualistic' model, evaluation was left to interested individuals, and there was no focus on organisational effectiveness. In the 'collaborative' model characterised by a participatory leadership model, nurses had autonomy and were involved equally in the decision-making processes. The collaborative model showed the best results in almost all outcomes considered (e.g. quality of care, safety and staff satisfaction), and the traditional model had the worst. The individualistic model was in the middle, although its values were very close to those of the traditional model.

Continuous quality improvement and organisation-wide audit review is the basis of the Australian National Safety and Quality Health Care Standards and those of the

Health Quality and Safety Commission in New Zealand (HQSC, 2021). Accreditation with this or a like organisation is required by Departments of Health in Australia and New Zealand. It is a path to clinical excellence. New Zealand's *Health and Safety at Work Act 2015* (New Zealand Government, 2017), enacted on 4 April 2017, moved from focusing on recording incidents relating to health and safety to a requirement to identify and treat workplace health and safety risks. This pivotal change to include the concept of a 'person undertaking a business or undertaking' pushes the creator of the risk to manage the risk. These concepts are also found in the various Australian Commonwealth and state workplace health and safety acts. The *Safe Work Australia Act 2008* (2009) was adopted to harmonise workplace safety laws across Australian states and territories. Enacting a 'safety culture' involves the willingness of front-line staff to disclose errors, multidisciplinary discussions to highlight potential threats to the safety of the neonatal patient and a safe environment for staff and families to speak up and act in ways that improve safety (Ravi et al., 2021).

Information

High-quality information is required to guide and inform decision making. Clinical teams need to know how they are performing. The Australia and New Zealand Neonatal Network provides an annual report (Chow et al., 2020) that benchmarks neonatal units' performance and describes care given and morbidity and mortality at the unit level against peer care providers. Measures include ventilation rates for gestational age groups, types of assisted ventilation and rates of chronic lung disease and neonatal sepsis, and morbidity data include the prevalence of retinopathy of prematurity and intraventricular haemorrhage. Many neonatal unit teams now participate in service line reporting that measures the acuity, quality, health and safety and human resource indicators. The continued focus on measuring the outcomes that matter most to neonatal patients and contributing factors will move the neonatal unit towards excellence.

Accountability

Accountability is the individual's requirement to be responsible for their professional decisions and actions (Oldland et al., 2020). Accountability at a service level is made possible by clinical pathways. Clinical pathways have been used to improve the quality of healthcare and have four criteria. They include: (1) a structured multidisciplinary plan of care, (2) guidelines and evidence that are translated into local structures, (3) timeframes or a criteria-led progression and (4) standardisation of care for a specific population (Rotter et al., 2019). In Australia, the use of pathways is developing and is mainly focused on term neonates. This ownership of pathways, a zero tolerance for complacency, the will to investigate things that go wrong and managers and clinical staff who are accountable for their performance support a sound basis for continuous quality and cost improvement (Backhouse & Ogunlayi, 2020).

Clinical communication

A key factor in the success of any clinical governance system is communication among carers, parents and families to ensure optimal care for neonates in a neonatal unit. A meta-synthesis regarding the characteristics of adequate communication in NICUs found that communication between parents and healthcare providers should be tailored to each individual (Wreesmann et al., 2021). In their communication framework they emphasised the need to enhance parents' participation in care, regulate parents' emotions and distress, and manage uncertainty about an infant's prognosis. The effective exchange of information about an infant's medical situation facilitates parental empowerment and their independent care of their infant upon discharge. Wreesman et al. (2021, p. 1512) found that 'having regular conversations in a secluded location … increases parents' sense of privacy, their confidence to ask questions' and the feeling of being listened to.

Doctors are trained to communicate concisely, emphasising time-sensitive issues, while nurses tend to be more descriptive in their communication. With the integration of the model of developmentally supportive care in most neonatal units, open and honest communication between healthcare professionals and parents is paramount. Enabling parents to be at the cot-side during rounds, and participate, facilitates this model of open communication.

Healthcare is a high-risk environment. The processes required to support clinical governance are now being refined to support the development of services to become a high-reliability health service provider, as has been achieved by other industries. Such organisations have moved from individual and autonomous roles to multifunctional teams that prioritise clinical excellence and prevention of failure throughout the organisation (Profit et al., 2017). Benchmarking, the review of data and evidence and the quest for excellence and safety will lead organisations towards a culture focused on optimal safety and quality. The challenge to realising this goal is the adoption of standardised processes to achieve a reduction in patient harm.

Throughout the developed world, healthcare costs are growing and healthcare providers are under increasing pressure to reduce costs. The established links between clinical governance and improved clinical outcomes drive greater efficiencies and assist in controlling costs while achieving safer care.

PERSON-CENTRED CARE FRAMEWORK

To be successful, the team needs to believe in the value of clinical governance. Neonatal nursing/midwifery requires a benchmark of good quality and instruments to measure practice, and it needs to make changes to improve practice and then re-measure quality of care. The person-centred care framework developed by McCormack and McCance (2010) is a tool to support improvement to clinical practice.

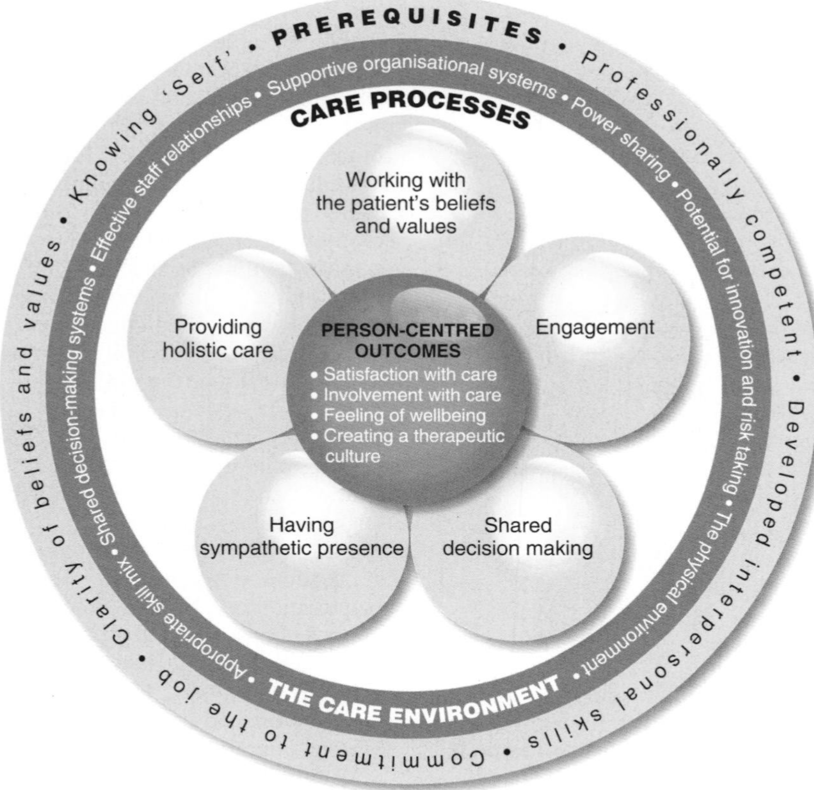

FIGURE 1.5 **Person-centred nursing framework**

Source: McCormack and McCance (2010, Fig 3.2). Republished with permission of John Wiley & Sons Inc.

Person-centred care has been evolving as a concept since the 1980s and is developing in different ways globally (McCormack, 2020). Fig. 1.5 describes the relationships among the four constructs of prerequisites (the attributes of nurses/midwives), the care environment (the context of care delivery), person-centred processes (the activities through which care is delivered) and outcomes (the results when person-centred care is effective). This framework has shaped nursing practice, education, evaluation and policy development across the world and within Australia (McCormack, 2020).

McCormack (2020) argues that person-centredness happens when there is a person-centred culture in place in workplaces, where staff are able to experience person-centredness and are able to work in a person-centred way. When this culture is present, person-centred care will flourish and there will be healthy relationships between care providers and service users. Person-centred care, including the principle of self-determination, is aligned to the principles of family-centred care and partnership models of care that are common to many units. Utilisation of a practice development framework has been shown to improve patient and family engagement, clinical outcomes and staff satisfaction and retention (McCormack, 2020).

EVIDENCE-BASED PRACTICE RESEARCH 1.4

Multidisciplinary safety rounds focus attention on the potential threats to the neonatal patient and address them with input from all members of the team. Practising 'humble enquiry' allows questions to be asked based on genuine curiosity, humility and a willingness to learn. Use of ISBAR (Introduction, Situation, Background Assessment, Recommendation) and adding safety-focused items to a rounding checklist (such as any medications that could be stopped or changed to enteral route, any laboratory work or imaging procedure that could be cancelled, any central line that can be discontinued) offers a structure for the safety rounds.

Source: Ravi et al. (2021, p. 2556).

The successful integration of clinical governance, healthcare standards and quality frameworks will support neonatal clinicians to develop a program of interventions that specifically support their local context. Neonatal nurses/midwives who understand the importance of a broad knowledge of clinical governance and the development of a specific skill set that includes communication, strategic planning and management skills will be equipped to provide high-quality and safe clinical care. The next step is the development of leadership skills to ensure the successful engagement of the team to transform the workplace into a high-resilience care unit.

LEADERSHIP

One of the key principles of neonatal nursing is to provide holistic and family-centred care. To be effective, neonatal nursing managers and those in leadership positions are required to develop and support team members to adapt to change and to inspire colleagues. Managers are often selected on their technical abilities and knowledge. However, in the twenty-first century, managers and staff are required to guide teams through rapidly changing environments, which include electronic medical records, government regulations and changing funding models, the adoption of new technology and evidence that is published at an ever-increasing rate. This is in the context of a clinical environment that requires a high level of sensitivity and emotional intelligence.

Leadership is influential within an organisation and the leadership style will directly influence the culture and job satisfaction (Specchia et al., 2021). Nurse managers and healthcare leaders need to address nursing workload and consider the related variables that can affect a unit's workplace culture (Specchia et al., 2021). In practice, leadership and management are intertwined. The leadership team needs to acknowledge those who value learning. The way nurses/midwives interact with each other while providing care is instrumental in establishing interactions and behaviours that facilitate learning in the clinical context and provide a culture of learning. One example is using a 'buddy' system where a more-experienced nurse/midwife works alongside a less-experienced nurse/midwife while new skills are acquired. Team nursing/midwifery models using innovative strategies such as handover 'huddles' where nurses/midwives spend 2–3 minutes identifying key issues for the shift ahead can contribute to a supportive environment. When there are supportive interactions between the leader and team there are positive contributions to team communication to accomplish the goals of the unit, which in turn enhances job satisfaction (Aldawood et al., 2020).

Contemporary healthcare organisations are focused on ensuring their managers, those that have the day-to-day responsibility for supporting sound clinical governance, budget integrity and meeting activity targets, are developed to become leaders. Nursing and midwifery leaders can become fatigued with the demands of organisational change, and developing skills in leadership, coupled with resilience training, has been shown to enhance critical thinking and decision making, improve the quality of care for patients, contain costs and reduce staff turnover (Spiva et al., 2021).

Styles of leadership including transformational (doing the right thing), considerate (demonstration of concern, respect and welfare for others, display of support and appreciation) and resonant (possessing emotional intelligence) have been associated with significantly higher job satisfaction, which in turn has been associated with lower mortality rates in patients. A systematic review of leadership styles and nurses' job satisfaction found that the transformational style of leadership had the highest positive correlation with nurses' job satisfaction, followed by authentic, resonant and then servant styles (Specchia et al., 2021).

Cope and Murray (2017) encouraged an approach that develops leaders as whole people. Helping people to develop social and emotional intelligence and the capacity for resonant leadership enhances their ability to help others in their intentional change process. Resonant leaders are relationship focused (Specchia et al., 2021), and they coach and inspire those around them, create a positive, trusting work environment and communicate effectively and articulately with teams and colleagues. In a neonatal unit this may include inclusion of teams in decision making, regular meetings and a compassionate approach to understanding others' wants and needs in order to meet individual and team learning agendas.

The influence of leadership on quality-of-care outcomes is widely recognised, using measures such as mortality, family experience and outcomes of infection control such as central-line sepsis. Staff outcomes include morale, productivity and job satisfaction. Kiwanuka et al. (2021) found that a leadership style that promotes information sharing, fosters decision making and acknowledges the contributions of staff in an intensive care unit environment inspires confidence and respect, and enhances quality of care outcomes.

An effective way of leading teams is by supporting a learning organisation. Peter Senge's (2013) seminal management book, *The fifth discipline: the art and practice of the learning organization*, was first published in 1990. It inspired organisations to develop a workplace that nurtures teams to be innovative and successful by working with new ideas, building knowledge, transferring this knowledge and embedding it by developing policies and processes to enable teams to respond to a changing environment. This process requires a supportive learning environment, concrete learning processes and practices and leadership behaviours that provide positive reinforcement (Kwon et al., 2020). Psychological safety is paramount to the success of a learning organisation. This is demonstrated by a blame-free organisation – an environment where seeking feedback, requesting help and reporting mistakes contribute to learning (Kwon et al., 2020). The pillars of the learning environment and learning process and the behaviours of leaders impact the ability of the teams to move to a no-blame culture. Managers need to respond to incident reports in a no-blame manner to enable reporting in the first instance, and then learning about the risk in order to prevent its reoccurrence (Kwon et al., 2020). A multidisciplinary review team should process each incident report and, when the incident is complex, analyse it according to a risk management tool. All employees should be made aware of completed reports using a staff email, and annual statistics should be analysed to observe for trends. In the aftermath of an incident, managers can facilitate reflection, establish a clinical audit or use a systematic debrief to hear alternative points of view and to support the discussion of these ideas in a safe way (Kwon et al., 2020).

Individual leadership capabilities can be learned and improved upon with well-designed leadership training programs (Lacerenza et al., 2018). Neonatal nurses and midwives should be supported in developing leadership and managerial skills and identifying mentors who demonstrate emotional intelligence and resonant leadership. Most major health services have online self-directed learning packages and in-house short courses. Other options include support through professional organisations including the Australian College of Neonatal Nurses and the Neonatal Nurses College Aotearoa (NNCA) and participation in mentoring opportunities through leadership, education and research special interest groups, and ongoing continuing professional development courses and scholarships offered by the respective colleges.

ORGANISATIONAL CULTURE

Organisational culture is influenced by the shared assumptions, values and beliefs that contribute to how people behave within the organisation. Most healthcare organisations have a set of core values that are displayed and available for staff and consumers alike. These values inform the organisational culture, and within health contexts guide the staff to know what to do and what not to do (Mannion & Davies, 2018). This includes how they do their work, how they work together and how they perform their respective roles. A supportive culture can ensure job satisfaction among the employees and ultimately impact on the quality of healthcare.

Organisational culture can be described through the competing values framework (Quinn & Rohrbaugh, 1983), where organisational behaviours are assigned to one of four cultural types (Fig. 1.6).

The model enables leaders to examine their contexts on either an internal or external focus and can identify with stability or flexibility in terms of the effects on the staff, quality care and patients' outcomes. The framework can be applied to the whole organisation or to the specific units within an organisation.

Nursing unit culture

Nursing unit culture is seen as an overriding set of beliefs, assumptions and attitudes, and is reflected in activities, behaviours, practices and interactions. Even if the shared ways of thinking and behaving are dysfunctional, they can be seen as legitimate and acceptable within the workplace or organisation (Braithwaite et al., 2017). The culture has a direct influence on and plays a role in contributing to a happy and healthy work environment when staff members are supportive of each other, and a sense of a cohesive, high-functioning team prevails (Catling et al., 2017). When the culture supports a learning focus and values the contributions of the staff, a healthy and sustained work environment exists, which contributes to good patient outcomes.

When discussing organisational culture, we need to consider how culture can vary across the organisation. Fig. 1.7 shows dominant interlinking cultures within an organisation, where the families in the neonatal unit contribute with their own sets of values and expectations, supported by the nurses and their identified nursing unit culture. This sits within the neonatal unit where the nurses work in a multidisciplinary team that may challenge their

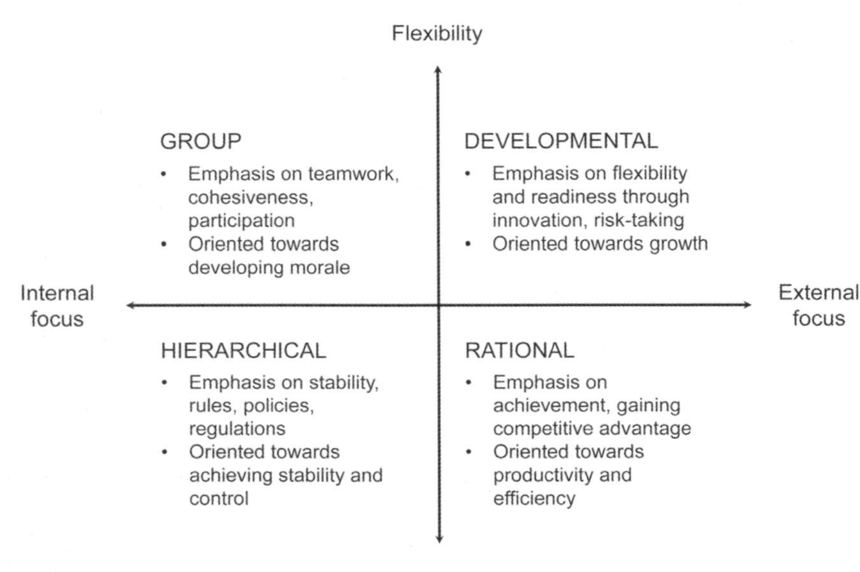

FIGURE 1.6 **Competing values framework of organisational culture**

Source: used with permission: Mahl et al. (2015). Adapted with permission from Quinn & Rohrbaugh (1983).

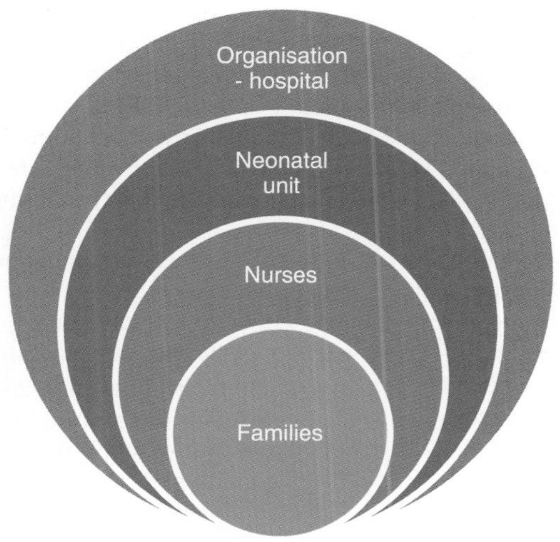

FIGURE 1.7 **Interlinking cultures within an organisation**

assumptions and beliefs. The overarching organisational culture of the hospital can influence the other cultures; however, when there is a mismatch in the beliefs and myths, potential conflict, stress and burnout can occur. This can result in a faster turnover of staff at all levels and disciplines.

In order to capitalise on the intergenerational differences amongst baby boomers, Gen Y and Gen X nurses, leadership practices need to be flexible. Research has shown that Gen Y nurses need more feedback than other generations, and this influences their intention to stay in a neonatal unit (Stevanin et al., 2020). All generations reported a need for flexible rosters and self-scheduling, and all generations agreed that leadership affects their professional development.

Effective teamwork is vital for acute clinical situations such as neonatal resuscitations. Salih and Draucker (2019) found that when each staff member is allocated a task and role according to their proficiency prior to the emergency, including a designated leader, communication improves during a code and outcomes are improved. Nurses/midwives have a key role as they are at the cot-side and coordinating multiple inputs from the patients/parents and multidisciplinary team. This places them in a good position to contribute to the decisions of the day, thereby ensuring they feel part of the team.

REFLECTION

Reflection is a powerful strategy that allows nurses/midwives to review their practice and support their learning. Clinical supervision provides an ideal framework for using reflection. There are different models of clinical supervision, reflecting the differing work contexts and the professional training needs and expectations of staff, and there is no one model of clinical supervision that will suit all occasions.

The NSW Health clinical supervision framework (2015) identifies that consideration should be given to the supervisees' and clinical supervisors' experience and knowledge when determining a particular clinical supervision model/s.

The fundamental components needed to support safe and high-quality patient care through clinical supervision in various clinical/professional settings form four distinct domains. These are:

1. clear concepts and definitions – foundational building blocks that are required in order to provide clarity and understanding about clinical supervision
2. practical tools and resources – practical approaches that would support clinical supervision and enhance clinical practice in various settings
3. positive learning culture and respect – emphasising the importance of two-way feedback, prioritising patient needs and supporting the supervisees in discussing their clinical supervision needs
4. reporting, measuring and monitoring – clear and structured mechanisms for accurately describing and monitoring clinical supervision practices.

For some disciplines, specific requirements such as minimum continuing professional development activities exist to maintain professional registration with the AHPRA.

TEAMWORK

Good teamwork necessitates not only knowledge and use of the team's specific resources and equipment, but also good administration and an acute understanding of the safety culture, or the environment in which the team works. An effective team communicates with the patient and their family in an efficient manner by combining knowledge, skills and decision making to optimise treatment. Interactions between patients, families and clinicians are critical in establishing a therapeutic relationship. This is why, in recent decades, there has been a focus on the quality of communication in the health sector. The neonatal unit environment poses unique challenges because teams are more fluid in composition and experience. In order for neonates to get the best possible care, how the neonatal staff function as a team is vital. Good teamwork requires good communication skills to address the challenges of changing circumstances, such as acute, chronic or complex situations (Sonali & Kaur, 2020). Forbes et al. (2019) found there were significant differences in the perception of communication between doctors and nurses, with nurses having poorer perceptions of the effectiveness of communication between the disciplines. The hierarchical systems that exist in healthcare environments emphasise the power imbalance between doctors and nurses/midwives and emphasise physician authority over decision making (Forbes et al., 2019).

The daily ward round in the neonatal unit is the primary time of interdisciplinary dialogue and communication. The neonatal unit has unique challenges arising from uncertainty about specific neonatal diseases and outcomes. These challenges can be embraced by acknowledging diverse professional perspectives and differing communication styles of the team. A possible option is the use of comprehensive care rounds (CCR) (Boos et al., 2010), which have the potential to significantly lessen the impact of stress caused by complicated/complex cases by fostering good communication and collaboration. The CCR seeks to improve communication by using a systems approach and open communication to identify barriers and identify goals for safe care (Fig. 1.8).

Using such a process enables all members of the team to contribute to patient safety and outcomes. In complex, fast-paced care settings such as the neonatal unit, patients are particularly vulnerable to medical errors. In the neonatal unit, adverse events are common but frequently preventable. Leadership walk-rounds (Sexton et al., 2018) are suggested as a way to improve patient safety through discussions with bedside staff to create a culture of safety. Looking at innovative ways to change requires a group model of organisational culture. However, if care-giver burnout is prevalent, it can be associated with lower perceptions of a patient safety culture (Profit et al., 2017).

WORKPLACE ENVIRONMENT

Evidence-based practice (EBP) is a problem-solving approach for excellence in practice that drives better outcomes for nurses/midwives, members of the healthcare team and their patients. However, to build and sustain EBP, systemic organisational barriers such as staff turnover and movement, insufficient staff and lack of organisational commitment must be overcome (Sharplin et al., 2019). The introduction and integration of changes to practice are driven by the availability of new knowledge or technology, external guidelines, the need to standardise practices, participation in research, adverse events and the desire to improve care (Cuttini et al., 2020). Understanding the culture of the work environment and what the nurses find to be interesting, exciting and frustrating can help in implementing a new model of practice. There are several key components to consider during times of change. These include (Lewis, 2015):

1. organise, plan and improve work efficiencies during the initial phase
2. identify the key elements for improvement in nurse and family satisfaction
3. develop or maintain a healthy work environment
4. establish adequate staffing levels and staff education to successfully care for patient populations following the transition
5. support the staff and patients during the transition.

NEONATAL SIMULATION TRAINING

Simulation in newborn care, especially in newborn resuscitation and stabilisation, has grown at an exponential rate over the last few decades. Simulation is best described as an instructional technique that replaces or enhances real-world experiences with directed experiences that evoke or replicate substantial aspects of the real world in a completely interactive manner. Simulation training has become a critical component of how training is organised to provide better patient care (Garvey & Dempsey, 2020).

The patient safety agenda has a significant impact on the use of simulations-based education. Failures in communication and coordination are often blamed for adverse events and the resulting patient harm. Any of the underlying causes of adverse events can be reduced by practising in virtual learning settings. The term 'fidelity' refers to how closely a simulation resembles life. It also refers to the psychological impact of 'immersion' or 'being there' as well as the degree to which the clinical environment is adequately

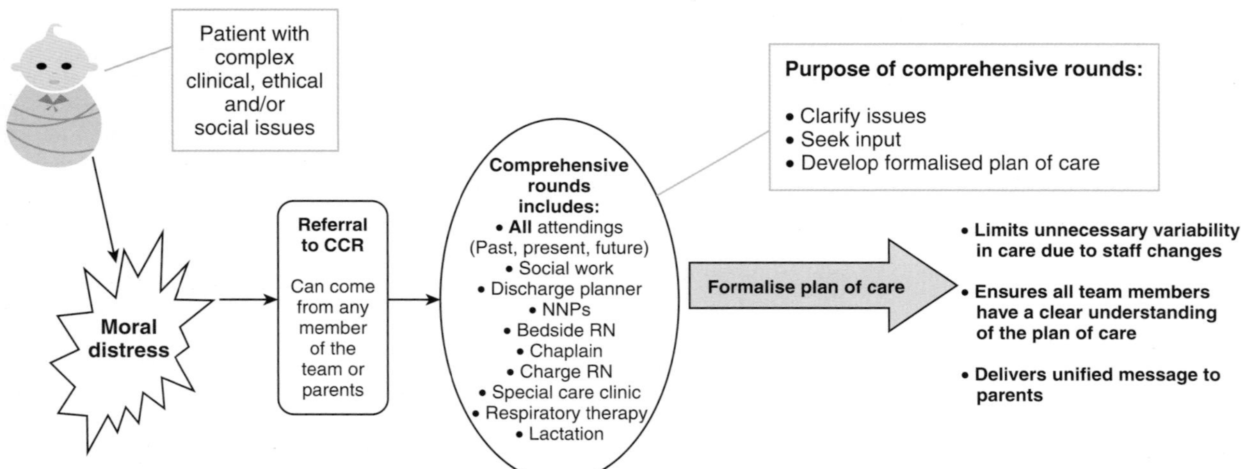

FIGURE 1.8 **Schematic representation of comprehensive care rounds**

Source: Boos et al. (2010).

portrayed. As too much realism and sophistication can distract students, particularly novices, from learning basic skills, the degree of realism of a simulation technique, and hence the choice of simulator device, must be carefully balanced with the educational level.

While simulation has proven to be beneficial, there are a number of obstacles to long-term implementation. Prior to implementation, simulations often necessitate several hours of preparation. Creating concrete learning goals, conducting practice simulations to recognise and solve possible problems such as insufficient materials or realistic equipment and planning sufficient staffing are just a few of the time-consuming challenges. Staff are required to operate the mannequin, act as immersed participants and promote successful pre- and post-briefing, for example. The number of people needed will vary depending on the simulation's fidelity and configuration. A dedicated space is needed to create a suitable environment for the simulation. Finally, getting management and staff on board with simulation may be a challenge. Depending on the cost of materials, staff and equipment, simulation costs can vary from low to high.

While simulation can be expensive, forming an academic–practice relationship can help health systems by distributing resources and exchanging information. The body of knowledge about the advantages of academic–practice collaborations continues to grow. Academic–practice collaborations foster a mutually beneficial collaboration that helps the health system and nursing program enhance patient care and innovate. An academic–practice collaboration could offer an infrastructure to help the health system navigate and incorporate simulation training, as well as several other initiatives to promote long-term quality improvement. Nursing would profit in two ways: practising nurses would improve and advance their expertise, and nursing students would have a seamless transition to practice (Smith et al., 2020).

EVIDENCE-BASED PRACTICE RESEARCH 1.5

The purpose of this study was to see whether simulation-based training influenced self-efficacy, self-perceived leadership qualities and team performance in a neonatal intensive care unit.

A convenience sample of 71 nurses and midwives were studied using a time series approach in a referral neonatal intensive care unit in a general hospital in Flanders, Belgium.

Three simulation-based training sessions were held for participants. A set of validated questionnaires was completed before and after these series to assess the participants' self-efficacy and self-perceived leadership qualities. Each session was recorded, and team performance ($n = 8$) was evaluated.

Participating in repeated high-fidelity in situ simulation-based training resulted in a significant increase in self-efficacy ($p < 0.001$) and self-perceived leadership traits ($p < 0.001$), according to this study. The intervention had no significant effect on team performance ($p < 0.209$).

The study concluded that repeated high-fidelity in situ simulation-based training in the NICU had a positive effect on registered nurses' and midwives' self-efficacy and self-perceived leadership abilities in acute care situations. Participation in simulation-based training on repeated occasions enhanced these results, regardless of the number of years of NICU experience.

Source: Maenhout et al. (2021).

THE ROLE OF NEONATAL NURSING AND MIDWIFERY ORGANISATIONS

Professional organisations and associations in any field of specialty practice are critical for generating energy, flow of ideas and the proactive work needed to maintain a healthy profession that advocates for the needs of its clients and nurses/midwives and the trust of the community.

In terms of professional neonatal organisations, Australia and New Zealand have a vibrant and collegial culture that transects with international neonatal organisations and are affiliate members of the **Council of International Neonatal Nurses (COINN)**. COINN, an affiliate member of the International Council of Nurses (ICN), was officially incorporated in 2005 to act as the global voice for neonatal nursing. It is not an individual membership-driven organisation but rather a group that works on global health policy, advocacy, capacity building and developing regional networks throughout the world, for nurses who specialise in the care of newborn infants and their families. COINN supports countries to form national or local organisations and is a key member of global clinical and advocacy boards including the WHO: <https://www.coinnurses.org/>.

Aboriginal and Torres Strait Islander nurses and midwives are also represented. Neonatal units in Australia and New Zealand should encourage, promote and support all neonatal nurses/midwives to engage in the professional organisations and associations that are available because such organisations contribute to the accountability and voice of the neonatal nursing profession at a societal level.

Organisations in New Zealand

The **Neonatal Nurses College of Aotearoa (NNCA)** is a college within the **New Zealand Nurses Organisation (NZNO)**. The NNCA is committed to Te Tiriti o Waitangi (the Treaty of Waitangi) as the founding document of Aotearoa/New Zealand.

The role of the NNCA is to provide significant benefits to its members, for example:

- promoting the networking of neonatal nurses, nationally and internationally
- providing educational opportunities for neonatal nurses and disseminating information regarding neonatal educational programs

- supporting and encouraging New Zealand neonatal nurses to contribute to the international body of neonatal knowledge
- raising public awareness of issues relating to the care of neonates
- ensuring that the views of neonatal nurses are represented in relevant health policy issues
- disseminating information to neonatal nurses throughout New Zealand via regular newsletters and electronic media
- developing/formalising standards and recommendations for neonatal nursing practice (Neonatal Nurses College of Aotearoa, 2015).

Organisations in Australia

The Australian College of Neonatal Nurses is a national, not-for-profit organisation that serves as the peak professional body for neonatal nurses in Australia. The College is a full member of COINN. The ACNN proudly provides direction and leadership for neonatal nurses, thereby enhancing their professional development within their chosen specialty.

The ACNN is committed to:

- maintaining the highest international standards in clinical practice, teaching and research
- promoting and sustaining a philosophy of family-centred and individualised care for neonates and their families
- advancing the welfare of Australian families, recognising the particular needs of disadvantaged and vulnerable groups
- working with other national and international professional and multidisciplinary bodies to extend and enhance the quality of clinical practice, education and research activities
- maintaining a rewarding environment for the neonatal nursing community through advocating for advancing professional practice within the context of complex and evolving systems of health service provision (ACNN, 2019).

Multinational organisations in Australia and New Zealand

The collaboration of New Zealand and Australia in improving prenatal and postnatal care of the newborn resulted in the foundation of the Perinatal Society of Australia and New Zealand (PSANZ) in 1983. PSANZ is multidisciplinary and includes a wide range of members such as neonatologists, neonatal nurses, obstetricians, midwives, epidemiologists and scientists. The aim of the society is to communicate internationally current research projects and research findings. The society also provides expert advice to governmental bodies on current and future trends in perinatology.

Congress of Aboriginal and Torres Strait Islander Nurses and Midwives

CATSINaM was founded in 1997 to formally represent Aboriginal and Torres Strait Islander nurses and midwives. CATSINaM's primary aim is to increase the numbers of Aboriginal and Torres Strait Islander peoples qualified in nursing and midwifery. CATSINaM is also dedicated to ensuring all nurses/midwives have meaningful cultural safety training to ensure they can provide the best care for Aboriginal and Torres Strait Islander patients, including neonates and their families.

Māori nurses and midwives

Te Rau Matatini is the lead agency for engagement with the Māori health sector providing a strategic focus that is underpinned by Māori workforce development, education, clinical and cultural capability and the capacity for the advancement of Indigenous health and wellbeing for Māori people and their communities.

CONCLUSION

Neonatal nurses and midwives have played a pivotal role in what is arguably the greatest success story in newborn care in the last few decades: dramatically increased preterm neonatal survival. The position of the neonatal nurse/midwife has developed to include the neonatal nurse practitioner (NP) and tertiary level training, recognising the highly specialised nature of this specialty.

Recommended Reading

Forbes-Coe, A., Dawson, J., Flint, A., & Walker, K. (2020). The evolution of the neonatal nurse practitioner role in Australia: a discussion paper. *Journal of Neonatal Nursing, 26*(4), 197–200. doi: 10.1016/j.jnn.2020.01.008.

Online Resources

Academy of Neonatal Nursing: <https:// academyonline.org/>

American Academy of Pediatrics: <https://www.aap.org/en-us/Pages/Default.aspx>

Australian and New Zealand Neonatal Network (ANZNN): <https://npesu.unsw.edu.au/data-collection/australian-new-zealand-neonatal-network-anznn>

Australian College of Neonatal Nurses (ACNN): <https://www.acnn.org.au/>

Australian College of Neonatal Nurses (ACNN). (2019). Australian standards for neonatal nurses (4th ed.).

<https://www.acnn.org.au/resources/resources/ACNN-Standards-for-Practice-4th-Ed.pdf>
Cochrane Neonatal Review Group: <https://.neonatal.cochrane.org/>
Congress of Aboriginal and Torres Strait Islander Nurses and Midwives: <https://catsinam.org.au/>
Council of International Neonatal Nurses: <https://www.coinnurses.org/>
National Association of Neonatal Nurses: <nann.org/>
Neonatal Nurses College of Aotearoa: <https://www.nzno.org.nz/groups/colleges_sections/colleges/neonatal_nurses_college>
Perinatal Society of Australia and New Zealand (PSANZ): <https://www.psanz.com.au/>
Te Rau Matatini: <https://teraumatatini.com/>

References/Acknowledgements

Aldawood, F., Kazzaz, Y., AlShehri, A., Alali, H., & Al-Surimi, K. (2020). Enhancing teamwork communication and patient safety responsiveness in a paediatric intensive care unit using the daily safety huddle tool. *BMJ Open Quality, 9*, e000753. doi: 10.1136/bmjoq-2019-000753.

American College of Nurse-Midwives (ACNM). (2021). About us. <https://www.midwife.org/> (Accessed 2 March 2022).

Australian and New Zealand Neonatal Network (ANZNN). (2021). Improving clinical practice through collaboration. <https://www.anznn.net/> (Accessed 2 March 2022).

Australian College of Neonatal Nurses (ACNN). (2019). *Australian standards for neonatal nurses* (4th ed.). <https://www.acnn.org.au/resources/resources/ACNN-Standards-for-Practice-4th-Ed.pdf> (Accessed 2 March 2022).

Australian Commission on Safety and Quality in Health Care. (2021). Clinical care standards. <https://www.safetyandquality.gov.au/our-work/clinical-care-standards/> (Accessed 2 March 2022).

Australian Government. (2013). *National Aboriginal and Torres Strait Islander Health Plan 2013–2023*. Canberra, ACT: Australian Government.

Australian Government. (2020). *Closing the Gap report 2020; child mortality*. <https://ctgreport.niaa.gov.au/child-mortality> (Accessed 2 March 2022).

Australian Institute of Health and Welfare (AIHW). (2020). Tier 3 – Health system performance. 3.12 Aboriginal and Torres Strait Islander people in the health workforce. <https://www.indigenoushpf.gov.au/measures/3-12-atsi-people-health-workforce> (Accessed 3 March 2022).

Backhouse, A.. & Ogunlayi, F. (2020). Quality improvement into practice. *British Medical Journal, 368*, 865. doi: 10.1136/bmj.m865.

Boos, V. D., Okah, F. A., Swinton, C. H., Wolff, D. M., & Haney, B. (2010). The comprehensive care rounds: facilitating multidisciplinary communication among caregivers of complex patients in the neonatal intensive care unit. *Advances in Neonatal Care, 10*(6), 301–306.

Braithwaite, J., Herkes, J., Ludlow, K., Testa, L., & Lamprell, G. (2017). Association between organisational and workplace cultures, and patient outcomes: systematic review. *BMJ Open, 7*(11), e017708. doi: 10.1136/bmjopen-2017-017708.

Broom, M., & Kecskes, Z. (2020). Exploring the impact of a dual-occupancy NICU design on parental experience. *Journal of Neonatal Nursing, 26*(4), 217–221.

Canadian Nurses Association. (2021). About us. <https://www.cna-aiic.ca/en/home> (Accessed 2 March 2022).

Catling, C. J., Reid, F., & Hunter, B. (2017). Australian midwives' experiences of their workplace culture. *Women and Birth, 30*(2), 137–145. doi: 10.1016/j.wombi.2016.10.001.

Chow, S. S. W., Creighton, P., Chambers, G. M., & Lui, K. (2020). *Report of the Australian and New Zealand Neonatal Network 2018*. Sydney, NSW: ANZNN.

Commonwealth of Australia. (2020). *2019 workforce survey: ATSI nurses and midwives*. <https://hwd.health.gov.au/resources/publications/factsheet-nrmw-atsinrmw-2019.pdf> (Accessed 2 March 2022).

Congress of Aboriginal and Torres Strait Islander Nurses and Midwives (CATSINaM). (2014). *Cultural safety position statement*. Canberra, ACT: CATSINaM. <https://www.aph.gov.au/DocumentStore.ashx?id=0e423afd-5982-4099-ab4b-47559701d5d7&subId=411853> (Accessed 2 March 2022).

Congress of Aboriginal and Torres Strait Islander Nurses and Midwives (CATSINaM). (2015). *Recruitment and retention position statement* (pp. 1–6). Canberra, ACT: CATSINaM.

Cope, V., & Murray, M. (2017). Leadership styles in nursing. *Nursing Standard, 31*(43), 61–70. doi: 10.7748/ns.2017.e10836.

Council of Australian Governments (COAG). (2009). *National Indigenous reform agreement (Closing the Gap)*. Canberra, ACT: Council of Australian Governments.

Cuttini, M., Forcella, E., Rodrigues, C., Draper, E. S., Martins, A. F., Lainé, A., et al. (2020). What drives change in neonatal intensive care units? A qualitative study with physicians and nurses in six European countries. *Pediatric Research, 88*, 257–264. doi: 10.1038/s41390-019-0733-9.

Department of Health (Higher Education Environment). (2021). *Aboriginal and Torres Strait Islander curriculum framework* (updated 2021). <https://www.health.gov.au/sites/default/files/documents/2020/12/aboriginal-and-torres-strait-islander-health-curriculum-framework.pdf> (Accessed 2 March 2022).

Doede, M., Trinkoff, A. M., & Gurses, A. P. (2018). Neonatal Intensive Care Unit layout and nurses' work. *Health Environments Research and Design Journal, 11*(1), 101–118. doi: 10.1177/1937586717713734.

Dwyer, A. (2019). Clinical governance and risk management for medical administrators. In: E. Loh, P. W. Long, & P. Spurgeon (Eds.), *Textbook of medical administration and leadership* (pp. 99–125). Singapore: Springer Singapore.

Fanelli, S., Bellù, R., Zangrandi, A., Gagliardi, L., & Zanini, R. (2020). Managerial features and outcome in neonatal intensive care units: results from a cluster analysis. *BMC Health Service Research, 20*, 957. doi: 10.1186/s12913-020-05796-0.

Forbes, M. P., Iyengar, S., & Kay, M. (2019). Barriers to the psychological well-being of Australian junior doctors: a qualitative analysis. *BMJ Open, 9*(6), e027558. doi: 10.1136/bmjopen-2018-027558.

Forbes-Coe, A., Dawson, J., Flint, A., & Walker, K. (2020). The evolution of the neonatal nurse practitioner role in Australia: a discussion paper. *Journal of Neonatal Nursing, 26*(4), 197–200. doi: 10.1016/j.jnn.2020.01.008.

Garvey, A. A., & Dempsey, E. M. (2020). Simulation in neonatal resuscitation [review]. *Frontiers in Pediatrics, 8*, 59. doi: 10.3389/fped.2020.00059.

Health Quality and Safety Commission New Zealand (HQSC). (2021). Our programmes. <https://www.hqsc.govt.nz/>. (Accessed 2 March 2022).

Kiwanuka, F., Nanyonga, R. C., Sak-Dankosky, N., Muwanguzi, P. A., & Kvist, T. (2021). Nursing leadership styles and their impact on intensive care unit quality measures: an integrative review. *Journal of Nursing Management, 29*(2), 133–142. doi: 10.1111/jonm.13151.

Kwon, C. K., Han, S.-H., & Nicolaides, A. (2020). The impact of psychological safety on transformative learning in the workplace: a quantitative study. *Journal of Workplace Learning, 32*(7), 533–547. doi: 10.1108/JWL-04-2020-0057.

Lacerenza, C. N., Marlow, S. L., Tannenbaum, S. I., & Salas, E. (2018). Team development interventions: evidence-based approaches for improving teamwork. *American Psychologist, 73*(4), 517–531. doi: 10.1037/amp0000295.

Lewis, B. (2015). Leading change evidence-based transition. *Clinical Nurse Specialist, March/April*, E1–E7.

Maenhout, G., Billiet, V., Sijmons, M., & Beeckman, D. (2021). The effect of repeated high-fidelity in situ simulation-based training on self-efficacy, self-perceived leadership qualities and team performance: a quasi-experimental study in a NICU-setting. *Nurse Education Today, 100*, 104849.

Mannion, R., & Davies, H. (2018). Understanding organisational culture for healthcare quality improvement. *British Medical Journal, 363*, k4907. doi: 10.1136/bmj.k4907.

Maree, C., Lubbe, W., Barlow, H., Davidge, R., Prullage, G. S., Scheepers, M., et al. (2021). South African neonatal nurse specialization – is professional licensing justifiable? *Journal of Neonatal Nursing, 27*(2), 69–76. doi: 10.1016/j.jnn.2020.08.004.

McCormack, B. (2020). The person-centred nursing and person-centred practice frameworks: from conceptual development to programmatic impact. *Nursing Standard, 35*(10), 86–89. doi: 10.7748/ns.35.10.86.s40.

McCormack, B., & McCance, T. (2010). *Person-centred nursing: theory and practice*. Oxford: Wiley Blackwell.

McKnight, H., & Moore, S. M. (2021). Nursing shared governance. In: *StatPearls*. Treasure Island, FL: StatPearls Publishing. <https://www.ncbi.nlm.nih.gov/books/NBK549862/> (Accessed 2 March 2022).

McSherry, R., & Pearce, P. (2011). *Clinical governance: a guide to implementation for healthcare professionals* (3rd ed.). Chichester, UK: Blackwell.

Ministerial Taskforce on Nursing. (1998). *Report of the Ministerial Taskforce on Nursing: releasing the potential of nursing*. <https://www.moh.govt.nz/NoteBook/nbbooks.nsf/0/380F282D7CAEDADC4C25669B007C00CA/$file/report-ministerial-taskforce-nursing.pdf> (Accessed 2 March 2022).

Ministry of Health. (2021). Fetal and infant deaths web tool. <https://www.health.govt.nz/publication/fetal-and-infant-deaths-web-tool> (Accessed 2 March 2022).

National Aboriginal Community Controlled Health Organisation (NACCHO). (2016). *Annual report*. <https://f.hubspotusercontent10.net/hubfs/5328468/Resources/Publications%20and%20Resources/Annual%20Reports/J2880-NACCHO-Annual-Report_ACCESSIBLE.pdf> (Accessed 2 March 2022).

National Council of State Boards of Nursing (NCSBN). (2021). About us. <https://www.ncsbn.org/index.htm> (Accessed 2 March 2022).

National Women's Health: Auckland District Health Board. (2020). *National women's health report 2020*. <https://nationalwomenshealth.adhb.govt.nz/assets/Womens-health/Documents/ACR/2020-Annual-Clinical-Report.pdf> (Accessed 2 March 2022).

Neonatal Nurses Association (NNA). (n.d.). About us. <https://nna.org.uk/about-us/> (Accessed 2 March 2022).

Neonatal Nurses College of Aotearea (NNCA). (2015). *Standards for neonatal nursing practice*. <https://www.nzno.org.nz/groups/colleges _sections/colleges/neonatal_nurses_college/ standards> (Accessed 2 March 2022).

Neonatal Nursing Association of South Africa (NNASA). (2018). About us. <https://nnasa.org.za/> (Accessed 2 March 2022).

Nepali, S. (2020). What matters at work: an ethnography of nurses' social relations in a neonatal intensive care unit. Sydney, NSW: University of Sydney, eScholarship database. <https://ses.library.usyd.edu.au/bitstream/handle/2123/24424/Nepali_S_Thesis.pdf?sequence=2> (Accessed 2 March 2022).

New South Wales Health. (2015). *Clinical supervision framework*. Health Education and Training Institute (HETI). NSW, Australia. <http://www.heti.nsw.gov.au/Programs/CSSP/The-NSW-Health-Clinical-Supervision-Framework/> (Accessed 2 March 2022).

New Zealand Government. (2017). *Health and Safety at Work Act 2015*. Wellington: New Zealand Government. <http://www.worksafe.govt.nz/worksafe/hswa> (Accessed 2 March 2022).

New Zealand Nurses Organisation (NZNO). (2021). *NZNO strategy for nursing 2018–2023*. <https://www.nurses.org.nz/nursing_workforce> (Accessed 2 March 2022).

New Zealand Nurses Organisation, Neonatal Nurses College Aotearoa. (2014). *National neonatal nurses knowledge and skills framework*. <http://www.nzno.org.nz/Portals/0/Files/Documents/Groups/Neonatal%20Nurses/2014%20National%20Neonatal%20Nurses%20Knowledge%20and%20Skills%20Framework.pdf> (Accessed 2 March 2022).

Nursing and Midwifery Council (NMC). (2021a). About us. <https://www.nmc.org.uk/about-us/> (Accessed 2 March 2022).

Nursing and Midwifery Council (NMC). (2021b). The code. <https://www.nmc.org.uk/standards/code/> (Accessed 2 March 2022).

Nursing and Midwifery Council (NMC). (2021c). Revalidation. <https://www.nmc.org.uk/revalidation/> (Accessed 2 March 2022).

Nursing License Map. (2021). Nursing licensure by state. <https://nursinglicensemap.com/states/> (Accessed 2 March 2022).

O'Callaghan, N., Dee, A., & Philip, R. K. (2019). Evidence-based design for neonatal units: a systematic review. *Maternal Health, Neonatology and Perinatology, 5*(1), 6. doi: 10.1186/s40748-019-0101-0.

Oldland, E., Botti, M., Hutchinson, A. B., & Redley, B. (2020). A framework of nurses' responsibilities for quality healthcare – exploration of content validity. *Collegian, 27*(2), 150–163. doi: 10.1016/j.colegn.2019.07.007.

Park, S., & Sharp, A. (2019). Improving health and health care efficiency through risk management. *Journal of Hospital Management and Health Policy. 3*, 9. <https://jhmhp.amegroups.com/article/view/5054> (Accessed 2 March 2022).

Profit, J., Sharek, P. J., Kan, P., Rigdon, J., Desai, M., Nisbet, C. C., et al. (2017). Teamwork in the NICU setting and its association with health care-associated infections in very low-birth-weight infants. *American Journal of Perinatology, 34*(10), 1032–1040. doi: 10.1055/s-0037-1601563.

Quinn, R. E., & Rohrbaugh, J. (1983). A spatial model of effectiveness criteria: towards a competing values approach to organizational analysis. *Management Science, 29*, 363–377.

Ravi, D., Tawfik, D. S., Sexton, J. B., & Profit, J. (2021). Changing safety culture. *Journal of Perinatology, 41*, 2552–2560. doi: 10.1038/s41372-020-00839-0.

Registered Nursing.ORG. (2021). Neonatal nurse certification. <https://www.registerednursing.org/certification/neonatal-nurse/> (Accessed 2 March 2022).

Rotter, T., de Jong, R. B., Lacko, S. E., Ronellenfitsch, U., & Kinsman, L. (2019). Clinical pathways as a quality strategy. In: R. Busse, N. Klazinga, D. Panteli, & W. Quentin (Eds.), *Improving healthcare quality in Europe: characteristics, effectiveness and implementation of different strategies* (pp. 309–327). European Observatory on Health Systems and Policies. Health Policy Series, No. 53(12). Copenhagen: WHO Regional Office for Europe. <https://www.ncbi.nlm.nih.gov/books/NBK549262/> (Accessed 2 March 2022).

Salih, Z. N. I., & Draucker, C., B. (2019). Facilitators of and barriers to successful teamwork during resuscitations in a neonatal intensive care unit. *Journal of Perinatology,* 39(7), 974–982. doi: 10.1038/s41372-019-0380-3.

Senge, P. M. (2013). *The fifth discipline: the art and practice of the learning organization.* New York: Crown Business.

Sexton, J. B., Adair, K. C., Leonard, M. W., Frankl, T. C., Proulx, J., Watson, S. M., et al. (2018). Providing feedback following leadership walk rounds is associated with better patient safety culture, higher employee engagement and lower burnout. *BMJ Quality and Safety, 27*, 261–270.

Sharplin, G., Adelson, P., Kennedy, K., Williams, N., Hewlett, R., Wood, J., et al. (2019). Establishing and sustaining a culture of evidence-based practice: an evaluation of barriers and facilitators to implementing the best practice spotlight organization program in the Australian healthcare context. *Healthcare (Basel, Switzerland), 7*(4), 142. doi: 10.3390/healthcare7040142.

Smith, T. S., Dudding, K., Knight, C., Sanders, A., Currie, E., & Shorten, A. (2020). Highlighting simulation practices in the neonatal environment. *Neonatal Network, 5*, 257–262. doi.: 10.1891/0730-0832.39.5.257.

Sonali, S., & Kaur, H. (2020). The human factor: the critical importance of effective teamwork and communication in providing quality and safe care. *Journal of Clinical Engineering, 45*(3), 150–154. doi: 10.1097/JCE.0000000000000404. <https://journals.lww.com/jcejournal/Fulltext/2020/07000/The_Human_Factor__The_Critical_Importance_of.10.aspx> (Accessed 2 March 2022).

Specchia, M. L., Cozzolino, M. R., Carini, E., Di Pilla, A., Galletti, C., Ricciardi, W., et al. (2021). Leadership styles and nurses' job satisfaction. Results of a systematic review. *International Journal of Environmental Research and Public Health, 18*(4), 1552. doi: 10.3390/ijerph18041552.

Spiva, L., Hedenstrom, L., Ballard, N., Buitrango, P., Davis, S., Hogue, V., et al. (2021). Nurse leader training and strength-based coaching: impact on leadership style and resiliency. *Nursing Management, 52*, 42–50. doi: 10.1097/01.NUMA.0000792024.36056.c0.

Stats Tatauranga Aotearoa NZ. (2019a). Demographic tables 2019. Wellington: Statistics New Zealand. <https://www.stats.govt.nz> (Accessed 2 March 2022).

Stats Tatauranga Aotearoa NZ. (2019b). Infant mortality declines. <https://www.stats.govt.nz/news/infant-mortality-rate-declines> (Accessed 2 March 2022).

Stevanin, S., Voutilainen, A., Bressan, V., Vehviläinen-Julkunen, K., Rosolen, V., & Kvist, T. (2020). Nurses' generational differences related to workplace and leadership in two European countries. *Western Journal of Nursing Research, 42*(1), 14–23. doi: 10.1177/0193945919838604.

Taylor, E. V., Lyford, M., Parsons, L., Mason, T., Sabesan, S., & Thompson, S. C. (2020). 'We're very much part of the team here': a culture of respect for Indigenous health workforce transforms Indigenous health care. *PLOS One, 15*(9), e0239207. doi: 10.1371/journal.pone.0239207.

US Department of Labour. (2021). Occupational employment and wage statistics. <https://www.bls.gov/oes/current/oes291141.htm> (Accessed 2 March 2022).

World Health Organization (WHO). (2018). *Survive and thrive: transforming care for every small and sick newborn. Key findings.* Geneva: WHO. WHO/FWC/MCA/18.11. Licence: CC BY-NC-SA 3.0 IGO.

World Health Organization (WHO). (2020). *Human resource strategies to improve newborn care in health facilities in low- and middle-income countries.* Geneva: WHO. Licence: CC BY-NC-SA 3.0 IGO.

Wreesmann, W. W., Lorié, E. S., van Veenendaal, N. R., van Kempen, A. A. M. W., Ket, J. C. F., & Labrie, N. H. M. (2021). The functions of adequate communication in the neonatal care unit: a systematic review and meta-synthesis of qualitative research. *Patient Education and Counselling, 104*(7), 1505–1517. doi: 10.1016/j.pec.2020.11.029.

CHAPTER 2

CARE OF THE NORMAL NEWBORN

VICTORIA KAIN AND RHONA MCINNES

Learning objectives

After reading this chapter you will be able to:

- describe the mother–baby dyad and how it pertains to the normal newborn
- outline the routine care of the normal newborn undergoing a normal transition to the extrauterine environment
- explain the concept of the 'fourth trimester'
- explain methods for determining gestational age and the tools used in assessment of gestational age
- define normal parameters for the normal newborn in terms of sleep–wake cycles, vital signs and measurements
- outline routine care of the normal newborn including hygiene practices
- discuss the early sense capacities of the normal newborn
- identify why newborn screening tests and vitamin K are necessary
- discuss the rationale for administering newborn immunisations
- discuss safe-sleeping practices and how they can be promoted to families
- discuss feeding practices for the healthy newborn, including successful breastfeeding and the composition of breast milk and infant formula.

Key words, terms and abbreviations

Baby Friendly Hospital Initiative (BFHI)
breastfeeding
Dubowitz Score
first bath
fourth trimester
gestational age assessment
mother–baby dyad
nappy dermatitis
New Ballard Score
newborn hearing screening (NHS)
newborn immunisation
newborn screening tests
Prechtl Scale
responsive feeding
safe sleeping
Safe to Sleep
skin to skin
sudden infant death syndrome (SIDS)
sudden unexpected death in infancy (SUDI)
sudden unexpected infant death (SUID)
vitamin K prophylaxis

Kain-Mannix 978-0-729-54389-7/00010

INTRODUCTION

The postpartum period is a critical time for a new mother and her family, and it can be considered a **fourth trimester** (Paladine et al., 2019). The transition to extrauterine life is marked by alterations in circulatory pathways, the initiation of ventilation and oxygenation via the lungs rather than the placenta and other metabolic changes (see Chapter 4 for more information about the transition from intra- to extrauterine life). A newborn must successfully complete the transition to extrauterine life after birth, the act of rapidly transitioning from an aquatic being wholly supported by its mother to an air-breathing human being who exists independently. When placed in an appropriately supportive environment, most newborns born after 36 weeks' gestation will effectively undergo transition within 2–8 hours of birth. The process of rooming in with the mother needs to provide an adequate environment for transition and detecting when the baby is failing to make a proper transition.

INITIAL CARE OF THE NORMAL NEWBORN

For the clinician practising in the neonatal unit, one needs to be reminded that most neonates are born at or near term, require little to no intervention at birth and can be classified as a 'normal newborn'.

The first 60 minutes after birth are crucial for both the mother and the baby (**mother–baby dyad**). This is known as the 'Golden Hour' (Sharma et al., 2017). This is a phase of transition for a newborn from the internal to the external uterine environment. Multiple organ systems, including respiratory, circulatory, metabolic and haemodynamic adaptations, must adapt efficiently within the first hour of life (Sehgal et al., 2021). The Golden Hour guidelines should be followed in the initial care of a normal infant. The three main components of the Golden Hour are maternal–neonatal skin-to-skin contact, delayed cord clamping and **breastfeeding**, all of which promote mother–newborn bonding and neonatal adaptation (Niela-Vilen et al., 2020).

The term 'mother–baby dyad' was coined to promote evidence-based clinical methods of caring for the newborn alongside the mother in the first few hours following birth. The optimal practice at birth is for the newborn to be placed immediately **skin to skin** with the mother. This is important for the transition to extrauterine life as it supports thermoregulation and helps regulate the infant's heart rate, breathing and metabolism. Skin-to-skin care facilitates mother–infant attachment, instinctual pre-feeding behaviours and is the first step to successful breastfeeding (Brimdyr et al., 2020; Cohen et al., 2018; Moore et al., 2016). Ideally skin to skin involves placing the infant on the mother's chest and leaving the infant undisturbed until successful latch at the breast. The infant can be dried in situ and both mother and infant wrapped together in a blanket to keep warm if necessary. During this time, it is important to monitor the mother–baby dyad to ensure that the newborn's face is not inadvertently obstructed and that the newborn is transitioning normally.

Immediately after birth, most babies are at least peripherally cyanotic (acrocyanosis). The baby should be centrally pink during skin-to-skin contact with their mother. If the newborn remains cyanotic, oxygen saturation should be assessed.

If the baby is breathing normally, they can be dried and placed directly onto the mother's chest. While the infant is skin to skin with the mother, observations of breathing and skin colour can be conducted. It is important to continue to support direct skin-to-skin contact while keeping the infant warm. Where mothers do not wish immediate skin to skin, options such as drying the infant first, skin to skin with the birth companion or wrapping the newborn can be discussed. If supported through skin-to-skin care and in the absence of the effects of labour analgesia, most healthy newborns are ready to start feeding at the breast shortly after birth (Safari et al., 2018).

Length, weight and head circumference should be documented as baseline data as soon as possible after birth once the mother–baby dyad have had an opportunity for skin-to-skin contact and a breastfeed.

CLINICAL PRACTICE 2.1

An Australian study investigated the relationship between breastfeeding and new mothers' sleep. The question of whether infants fed breast milk substitutes sleep longer than those solely or partially breastfed is still being debated, and this study wanted to know what this meant for the mother and what were the reasonable expectations for mothers who wanted to breastfeed exclusively.

This study evaluated whether the weekly duration of maternal sleep, sleep disturbance, unpaid housework and free-time activities differed by detailed feeding method, using a unique time use dataset specifically developed to study the time use of new mothers; 156 mothers with infants aged 3, 6 and/or 9 months were recruited through mother's groups, infant health clinics and childcare facilities across Australia. A questionnaire was used to collect sociodemographic and feeding information.

Exclusive breastfeeding was linked to fewer maternal sleep hours (an average of 7.08 h per day).

The study indicated that, in the months following the birth of a newborn, optimal breastfeeding may require realistic maternal sleep expectations and an equitable allocation of paid and unpaid work burdens with other household members.

Source: Smith & Forrester (2021).

GESTATIONAL AGE ASSESSMENT

Gestational age (also referred to as 'menstrual age' or 'postmenstrual age') is defined as the time elapsed since the beginning of the woman's last menstrual period (LMP) and is measured in weeks. Where there has been minimal prenatal care or there appears to be a disparity between birthweight and the expected gestational age at birth, the ability to assess the estimated gestational age of infants at birth is often useful. To differentiate small for gestational age (SGA) from intrauterine growth-restricted (IUGR) infants and preterm infants, examination and assessment are required (see Chapter 3).

Commonly used tools for assessing gestational age

The **Dubowitz Score** for **gestational age assessment** was first developed in 1980 (Dubowitz et al., 1980) and examines physical characteristics and various aspects of neurological function. The physical components of the Dubowitz Score include an assessment of oedema; skin texture, colour and opacity; the presence of lanugo; plantar creases; nipples and breasts; ear form and firmness; and genitals; and the neurological signs include posture, arm recoil, head lag and ankle dorsiflexion. As with all gestational age examinations, it can only reflect the neurological status at the time of the examination, and is affected by seizure activity, anticonvulsants and sedatives (Hawes et al., 2020). The Dubowitz system has been found to have two distinct disadvantages: its overestimation of gestational age in preterm neonates and the large number of criteria that require evaluation, making it difficult to perform on sick or extremely preterm neonates (Lee et al., 2017).

The New Ballard Score

In contemporary practice, the **New Ballard Score** generally replaces the Dubowitz Score and the original Ballard Score; both will be discussed in this chapter. The original Ballard Score was developed in 1979 (Ballard et al., 1979) and subsequently revised to include extremely preterm neonates as the 'New Ballard Score' in 1991 (Ballard et al., 1991). The New Ballard Score is the most used clinical determinant tool for gestational age. The score is based on the neonate's physical and neuromuscular maturity and is considered accurate up to 4 days after birth. In practice, however, the New Ballard Score is usually performed in the first 24 hours of life.

Ballard and colleagues reduced the original Ballard Score to include six neurological and six physical criteria in order to reduce the time required to complete it (Fig. 2.1). Whatever approach is employed, determining gestational age by physical and neurological parameters is only accurate to within 2 weeks, with a tendency to overestimate in extremely premature infants (Lissauer & Hansen, 2020).

The New Ballard Score measures:

- neuromuscular maturation – posture, square window, arm recoil, popliteal angle, scarf sign, heel to ear (see Figs 3.4 and 3.5).
- physical maturity – skin, lanugo, plantar surface, breast, eye/ear, genitals.

NORMAL SLEEP AND WAKE CYCLES

Infants' sleep cycles include active sleep (similar to adults' rapid eye movement (REM) sleep), quiet sleep (analogous to adults' slow-wave sleep (SWS)) and an unclassified type of sleep that is not analogous to any type of adult sleep. Full-term infants spend approximately 50% of their entire sleep duration in active sleep, which decreases with time to approximately 25% by 6 months of age. At birth, infants sleep for around 17 hours per day, dispersed across the day and evening hours; by 1 year of age, infants' sleep is reduced to approximately 14.5 hours, largely occurring at night. By 4 months of age, the circadian rhythm has developed, which is dependent on a day–night cycle as well as external stimuli (Barry, 2021).

Protecting newborn sleep promotes neuronal growth and connectivity, emotional regulation, lowers amygdala activation (which is important for processing fearful and threatening stimuli) and enhances long-term cognitive performance and language development (Jiang, 2019). Premature newborns can sleep for up to 97% of the time, with continuous periods of active sleep thought to consolidate sensorineural plasticity (Georgoulas et al., 2021). Strategies to promote sleep in preterm infants include supportive positioning, nesting, non-nutritive sucking, swaddling and a quiet environment with dimmed lighting (Abdeyazdan et al., 2016).

The level of alertness of a newborn can be classified using the **Prechtl Scale** (Kong et al., 2018) as follows:

- state 1: eyes closed, regular respirations, no movements
- state 2: closed eyes, erratic breathing, no gross movements
- state 3: eyes open, no gross movements
- state 4: open eyes, gross movements, no crying
- state 5: open or closed eyes, crying.

NORMAL VITAL SIGNS

A typical newborn's assessment begins with vital signs, namely heart rate (normal rate, 120–160 beats/min), respiratory rate (normal rate, 30–60 breaths/min), temperature (36.5°C–37.5°C, usually measured as an axillary measurement) and blood pressure (BP) (mean BP is roughly gestational age plus days of life in mmHg – an assessment often reserved for sick infants). A newborn's heart rate should initially be greater than 100 beats per minute (bpm) but less than 180 bpm. Sleeping heart rates in the 85–100 bpm range are appropriate in term newborns, especially postdates neonates (Lissauer & Hansen, 2020). (See Appendix 1 Normal Neonatal Vital Signs.)

MEASUREMENTS

To evaluate if growth is normal, accelerated or delayed for the given gestational age, length, weight and head circumference should be measured and plotted on growth curves (Marcdante & Kliegman, 2019). The website <https://peditools.org/> is a useful online tool for growth

ESTIMATION OF GESTATIONAL AGE BY MATURITY RATING

Neuromuscular Maturity

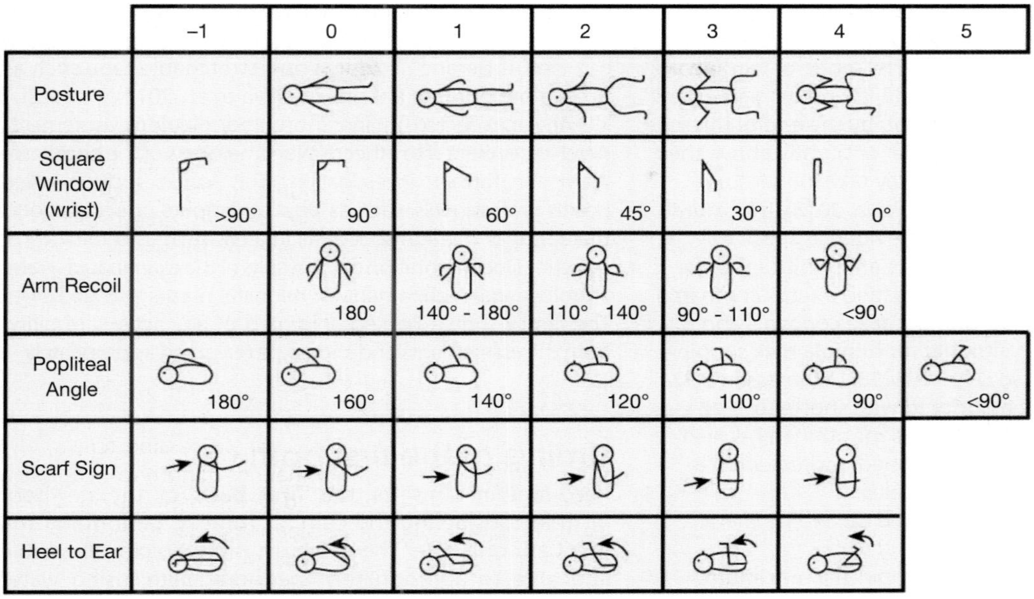

	–1	0	1	2	3	4	5
Posture							
Square Window (wrist)	>90°	90°	60°	45°	30°	0°	
Arm Recoil		180°	140° - 180°	110° 140°	90° - 110°	<90°	
Popliteal Angle	180°	160°	140°	120°	100°	90°	<90°
Scarf Sign							
Heel to Ear							

Physical Maturity

Skin	sticky friable transparent	gelatinous red, translucent	smooth pink, visible veins	superficial peeling &/or rash, few veins	cracking pale areas rare veins	parchment, deep cracking no vessels	leathery cracked wrinkled
Lanugo	none	sparse	abundant	thinning	bald areas	mostly bald	
Plantar Surface	heel–toe 40–50 mm: –1 <40 mm: –2	>50 mm no crease	faint red marks	anterior transverse crease only	creases ant. 2/3	creases over entire sole	
Breast	imperceptible	barely perceptible	flat areola no bud	stippled areola 1–2 mm bud	raised areola 3–4 mm bud	full areola 5–10 mm bud	
Eye/Ear	lids fused loosely: –1 tightly: –2	lids open pinna flat stays folded	sl. curved pinna; soft; slow recoil	well-curved pinna; soft but ready recoil	formed & firm instant recoil	thick cartilage, ear stiff	
Genitals (male)	scrotum flat, smooth	scrotum empty faint rugae	testes in upper canal rare rugae	testes descending few rugae	testes down good rugae	testes pendulous, deep rugae	
Genitals (female)	clitoris prominent labia flat	prominent clitoris, small labia minora	prominent clitoris enlarging minora	majora & minora equally prominent	majora large minora small	majora cover clitoris & minora	

Maturity Rating

score	weeks
–10	20
–5	22
0	24
5	26
10	28
15	30
20	32
25	34
30	36
35	38
40	40
45	42
50	44

FIGURE 2.1 **New Ballard Score**

Source: Ballard, J. L., Khoury, J. C., Wedig, K. et al. (1991). New Ballard Score, expanded to include extremely premature infants, Journal of Pediatrics, 119(3), 418.

chart centiles. The weight, length and head circumference measurement procedures are described here:

1. *Weight measurement:* During the first week of life, a normal neonate may lose up to 10% of their birthweight. However, there are several variables that affect this including birthweight, mode of birth, mode of feeding and maternal and neonatal health (DiTomasso & Paiva, 2018). It is generally believed that, by the end of the second week, the infant should be at or slightly above their birthweight, but some infants may take longer to achieve this goal (DiTomasso & Paiva, 2018). It is important to acknowledge the lack of evidence about expected weight loss because there are significant differences in the pattern among breastfed infants compared with formula-fed infants and because concerns about weight loss are often a trigger for formula milk supplementation (DiTomasso & Paiva, 2018; DiTomasso et al., 2021), which may be associated with shorter overall breastfeeding duration beyond 6 months (Flaherman et al., 2019). The neonate is weighed undressed on a calibrated beam or electronic scales.
   a. The weight should be checked by two neonatal nurses/midwives.
   b. Scales should be easy to zero, with a maximum weight of 20 kg in 1–10-g increments.
2. *Length measurement:*
   a. A calibrated length board with both perpendicular fixed-head and moveable foot pieces should be utilised.
   b. The neonate is placed supine on the board, with the assessor gently aligning the body and placing the head in a neutral position.
   c. One assessor holds the neonate's head in contact with the headboard, while the other extends the left leg with a hand, depressing the left knee and straightening the leg, and moves the footboard to touch the plantar surface of the foot at right angles to the leg (Pereira-da-Silva et al., 2019).
   d. The neonate's length is measured to the nearest millimetre (see Fig. 2.2).
3. *Head circumference measurement:* Head circumference is a proxy for brain volume and, hence, brain growth (Lissauer et al., 2015). These should be compared with standard forms using standardised percentile charts (see Chapter 3).
   a. The measuring tape is positioned just above the eyebrows (glabella), above the ears and around the widest part on the back of the head (the occipital protuberance), using a non-stretchable tape such as a paper tape (Pereira-da-Silva et al., 2019) (Fig. 2.2).

Any unexpected findings in anthropometric measurements need to be referred to other relevant members of the healthcare team for further investigation. This could include allied health professionals, such as physiotherapists or occupational therapists, or medical specialists in areas such as cardiology or genetics. Documentation of the results of the examination is also a professional requirement for neonatal nurses and midwives. The family should be kept informed of any actions resulting from the assessments and should be reassured appropriately.

DAILY CARE

Timing of the first bath

Recommendations for the '**first bath**' of the newborn include considering the cultural context, performing the first bath only after the newborn is physiologically stable and able to appropriately thermoregulate, using water alone or water and an appropriately formulated pH neutral (or acidic) liquid cleanser such as a synthetic detergent or liquid baby cleanser, and wearing gloves if the nurse/midwife is performing the first bath as a demonstration for the parents (Paller & Mancini, 2022).

There is growing evidence to support the delaying of the first bath following birth. Delaying the bath by 12–24 hours has a positive impact on neonatal thermoregulation and glucose metabolism (Chamberlain et al., 2019; Warren et al., 2020). Furthermore, delaying bathing enables the vernix caseosa coating to remain on the newborn's skin, providing a protective barrier against infection, supporting the development of the acid mantle and acting as a moisturiser (Lund, 2016). Delayed bathing can also enable the parents, rather than neonatal nurses or midwives, to perform the first bath, which supports rooming in, bonding and attachment as well as an opportunity for parental learning of care-giving activities (Brogan & Rapkin, 2017) (Fig. 2.3).

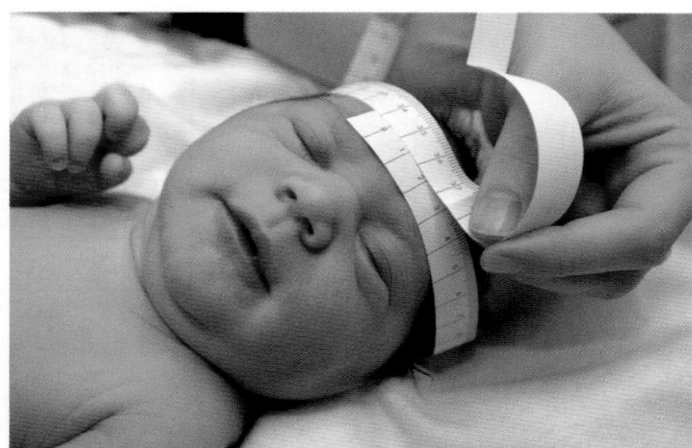

FIGURE 2.2 **Measuring neonatal head circumference**
Source: Shutterstock.com/ChameleonsEye

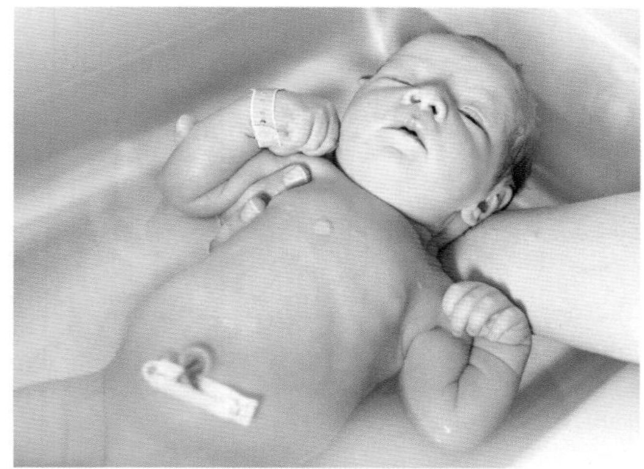

FIGURE 2.3 **Delay the first bath for at least 24 hours**
Source: Shutterstock.com/Kletr.

EVIDENCE-BASED PRACTICE RESEARCH 2.1

The impact of delayed bathing on breastfeeding rates is unclear, with some studies showing no difference in breastfeeding (Long et al., 2020; Turney et al., 2019) while others show increased breastfeeding associated with delayed bathing (Chamberlain et al., 2019; Warren et al., 2020). The difference in these findings could be due to study design and variation in the timings of the first bath before and after the practice change. Nevertheless, the standard of care is shifting towards later, immersion-style baths in the parents' room, performed by the parents, if bathing in the first 24 hours is undertaken at all (Rosen-Carole & Stuebe, 2022).

Skin care

Gentle bathing with a non-toxic, non-abrasive neutral product should be part of skin care. During the 1950s, the use of hexachlorophene-containing products as a prophylactic against *Staphylococcus aureus* infection became commonplace in neonatal skin care. However, due to studies revealing vacuolisation in the central nervous system (CNS) of neonates and laboratory animals after continuous application of these preparations, the use of hexachlorophene preparations as skin cleansers for newborns was prohibited in 1971 (Paller & Mancini, 2022).

There is some evidence that suggests using full-body emollient therapy daily may help to reduce the risk of atopic eczema in high-risk babies with a genetic predisposition to eczema; however, using olive oil or sunflower oil for dry skin in the newborn may negatively affect skin barrier function. According to qualitative research, parents and health professionals alike believe that cleaning baby skin with water alone is the best option (Cooke et al., 2018).

At the very least, neonatal skin care should include the careful removal of blood from the face and head, as well as meconium from the perianal area, through gently rinsing with water. As discussed above, the layer of vernix caseosa should be left intact or perhaps removed only from the face, leaving the remaining vernix to wear off on its own (Paller & Mancini, 2022).

The normal standard of care is to gently wipe and dry the newborn's entire skin surface, which is ideal from a thermoregulatory standpoint (Paller & Mancini, 2022).

In terms of nappy area skin care, research data and technological innovations have increased in recent years, with the use of superabsorbent nappies, baby wipes and wash care products becoming commonplace in many, but not all, countries. **Nappy dermatitis** is a common condition that affects both sexes equally, with a peak incidence around the age of 9–12 months. The incidence of nappy rash and dermatitis is frequently reported to be lower in exclusively breastfed newborns, which may be due to a reduced incidence of infective diarrhoeas and the more acidic composition of the stool compared with formula-fed infants. Applying a high-quality approved barrier product between nappy changes may be beneficial; however, vigorous efforts to remove faeces while cleaning should be avoided as this can harm healing skin (Hugill, 2017) (see Chapter 19).

Cord care

The routine care of the umbilical cord includes the use of an umbilical cord clamp (or, if cord clamps are unavailable, sterile thread may be used) after birth and the washing of the cord with water during the first bath. Monitoring for bleeding, redness, oedema and drainage symptomatic of infection is part of routine care of the umbilical cord site. The area should be kept clean, dry and open to air, if possible. If the area becomes soiled, it should be thoroughly cleaned with simple water and patted dry. Nappies should be folded downward and tucked beneath the umbilical cord stump. The usual time for cord separation is 10–14 days; however, it can take up to 3 weeks (Schmuke, 2018).

Globally, there is no single approach to umbilical cord care that has been shown to reduce bacterial colonisation and disease, and cord care practices vary greatly depending on cultural beliefs and healthcare disparity. Local applications of isopropyl alcohol, triple dye (an aqueous solution of brilliant green, proflavine and gentian violet) and antibacterial drugs such as bacitracin or silver sulfadiazine cream have all been reported. The use of povidone-iodine on a regular basis should be avoided owing to the risk of iodine absorption and transient hypothyroxinaemia or hypothyroidism. A chlorhexidine-containing product is a safer alternative. A recent clinical review suggests considering the use of antimicrobial agents for infants born at home or elsewhere outside of birthing centres or hospitals in resource-limited settings, and reports that their use in high-resource countries or during in-hospital birth has not been shown to provide clear benefit (Paller & Mancini, 2022).

EARLY SENSE CAPACITIES

The normal newborn exhibits a variety of innate and distinct behavioural tendencies. The human face, for example, is preferred by the newborn over objects, colours or patterns. Within a few days, the newborn can visually trace a parent's face. A newborn's hearing, vision and sense of smell are linked to allow them to 'recognise' their mother. It is believed that, after a few weeks, a newborn can visually distinguish between their mother and a stranger (Kyprianou, 2015).

Newborn eyesight

By 26 weeks of gestation, the preterm infant blinks in reaction to light and, by 34 weeks, the newborn may fix and track a bright object for a brief period. By 37 weeks, a newborn has adapted to soft light and is capable of tracking reliably (Feldman & Chaves-Gnecco, 2018). The primary method for assessing visual function in neonates is to observe fixation and following behaviour. At around 30 cm, the human face is the ideal target for fixation. By 9 weeks of age, 90% of infants can fixate on faces (Piña-Garza & James, 2019).

In most newborns, the iris colour is light blue or grey at birth. During the first 6–10 months of life, the iris develops its final colour due to pigmentation. Eye colour is determined by the concentration and location of pigment-containing cells (chromatophores) in the iris's loose vascular connective tissue. The iris appears blue when the melanin pigment is restricted to the pigmented epithelium on the posterior surface of the iris. The eye appears brown if melanin is also distributed throughout the stroma (supporting tissue) of the iris. Changes in the sympathetic innervations of the eye can cause iris heterochromia (mixed colouring) (Moore et al., 2020).

Hearing and newborn hearing screening

Newborns have a reasonable ability to hear, but their hearing is not perfect. A newborn's middle ear is filled with fluid, which affects hearing until the fluid drains. Additionally, the entire auditory system is still developing. Therefore, newborns respond to high-pitched, exaggerated sounds and voices the most.

Hearing loss in newborns is very common. It is estimated that 1–3 out of every 1000 babies suffer from some degree of hearing loss. Certain populations, such as those with a family history of hearing loss, infants with perinatal infection and those requiring a neonatal intensive care unit (NICU) stay, are more vulnerable. Hearing loss is nearly double in NICU patients, at 2–4 per 1000. According to the WHO, 7.5 million children have clinically significant hearing loss (Graham et al., 2021).

Hearing screening prior to the implementation of **newborn hearing screening (NHS)** involved a targeted approach based on the presence of risk factors for permanent hearing loss, such as a family history of hearing loss, a NICU stay of more than 5 days, in utero infections, craniofacial anomalies, syndromes known to include permanent hearing loss, neurodegenerative disorders, postnatal infections associated with hearing loss, head trauma and chemotherapy. Subsequent research has revealed that this method detects only around half of all hearing loss cases (Graham et al., 2021).

The importance of NHS in the early diagnosis of hearing loss cannot be overstated (Fig. 2.4). Prior to the introduction of universal NHS, only approximately 3% of babies in the United States were screened for hearing loss. Without screening, affected children may not be recognised until they exhibit delayed language development; in milder cases of hearing loss, they may go unidentified until they reach school age. According to research, earlier detection of hearing loss leads to earlier intervention, which improves patient outcomes.

The newborn taste system

Taste, also known as gustation, is the sensation that results from chemicals stimulating taste receptors on the dorsum of the tongue and other areas of the oropharynx, such as the larynx, pharynx and epiglottis. The taste system is calibrated to a few perceptual categories of experience, known as 'fundamental tastes', each of which provides critical information about nutrients or harmful substances to the newborn's developing brain. These basic flavours either encourage or prevent eating (sweet, salty and savoury; bitter and sour) (Mennella et al., 2017). Before/at term birth, the taste system is fully matured. Taste buds first form at approximately 7–8 weeks of gestation and begin to resemble adult taste buds morphologically by 13–15 weeks, except for the cornification overlaying the papilla. Before the end of the fourth month of gestation, taste pores are present in fetal fungiform papillae, allowing taste stimuli to interact with taste receptor cells. There is some evidence that the human fetus responds preferentially to different taste stimuli. Clinical observations of differential fetal swallowing after infusions of sweet or bitter chemicals into amniotic fluid imply that the fetus favours sweet and rejects bitter tastes, although these findings are ambiguous owing to methodological difficulties in quantifying fetal reactions (Mennella et al., 2017). This

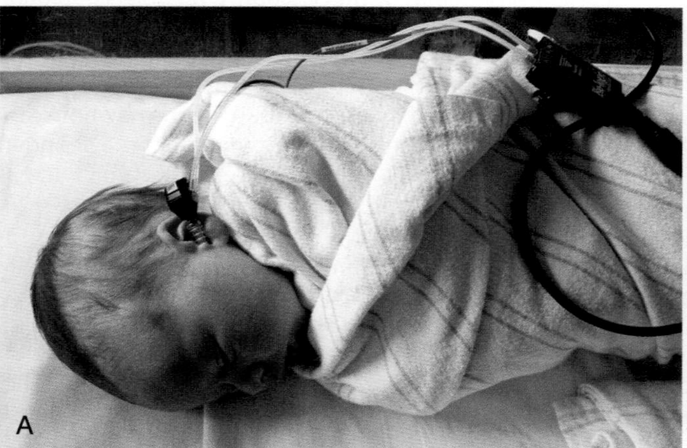

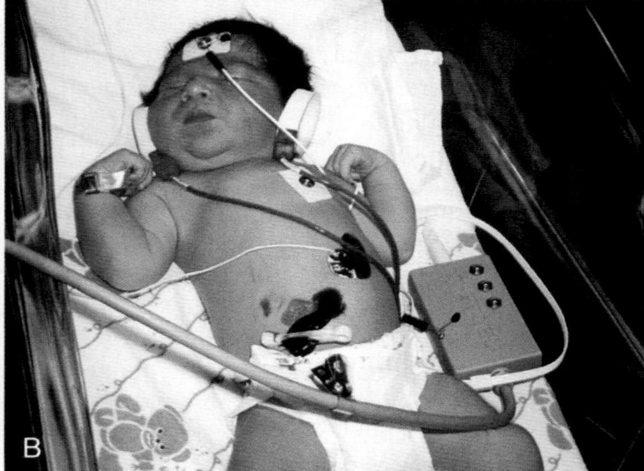

FIGURE 2.4 **Newborn hearing screening**

a *Evoked otoacoustic emissions test.* **b** *Auditory brain response test.*

Source: A, Courtesy Julie and Darren Nelson, Loveland, CO. B, Courtesy Dee Lowdermilk, Chapel Hill, NC.

preference for sweet tastes is utilised in the capacity for the ingestion of oral sucrose (and by extension, breast milk) to increase β-endorphin levels to reduce pain in newborn infants (Tanyeri-Bayraktar et al., 2019).

The newborn olfactory system

Smell, also known as olfaction, occurs when substances trigger olfactory receptors located on a small patch of tissue high in the nasal cavity. The olfactory system's organisation reflects the necessity to recognise a wide variety of aromas and distinguish one from another. The odorant epithelium lines the roof of the nasal cavities, a portion of the nasal septum and the superior (and sometimes middle) turbinate bones. Epithelial plugs restrict the external nares during the first trimester but retreat between 16 and 24 weeks' gestation (Sarnat, 2022).

To reach receptor sites on the cilia of primary olfactory dendrites, volatile chemicals must pass through an aqueous mucous layer covering the olfactory epithelium. The number of bipolar primary olfactory neurons increases dramatically with the creation of the turbinates, which begins about 8 weeks' gestation and allows for a significantly increased surface area of olfactory epithelium in the nasal cavity.

Before 28 weeks' gestation, preterm newborns do not consistently respond to olfactory stimuli. In the neurological evaluation of the term newborn, olfactory reflexes are regarded as well developed. Olfaction can even be semi-quantified in gradients, and sensitivity rises in the first few days after birth. Olfactory development exhibits a broad neuro-ontogenetic concept that does not require complete anatomical maturation for function to begin (Sarnat, 2022). The newborn's heightened olfactory response enables them to locate the mother's areola, hence enabling the first breastfeed (Moore et al., 2016); furthermore, the smell of maternal breast milk can be comforting for the newborn should they be separated from their mother. The olfactory cortices in full-term infants are activated when exposed to maternal breast odour. Neonatal nurses/midwives can encourage mothers to keep cloths against their breasts and then share them with their babies during periods of separation so as to improve bonding (Frie et al., 2020).

NEWBORN SCREENING TESTS

The goal of **newborn screening tests** (also referred to as newborn bloodspot screening) is to identify and treat affected newborns before symptoms appear. The completion of each phase (i.e. specimen collection, transport, testing and result reporting) in a timely manner is crucial for early diagnosis (Sontag et al., 2020). Clinicians need to be aware of the overall screening technique for newborns, as well as screening limitations. A positive result may need a repeat newborn screen or confirmation tests to secure a diagnosis. The time necessary to receive the results varies by country and even across states within the same country. Some metabolic disorders can be severe enough to present clinically before the findings of newborn screening are known. Diagnostic metabolites in milder types of screened disorders, on the other hand, may not exceed a defined threshold to trigger subsequent tests, resulting in a negative newborn screen result and a delayed diagnosis. Negative newborn screening results in a referral to a genetics clinic for additional examination in a patient with symptoms indicative of a metabolic disease (Shchelochkov & Venditti, 2020).

The individual rarity of inborn metabolic errors, the necessity of early detection and the consequent genetic counselling implications together offer a compelling case for universal screening of all newborns. Tandem mass spectrometry of metabolites and digital microfluidics measurement of enzyme activity are now at the heart of neonatal screening. Both procedures include placing a few drops of blood on filter paper and transporting it to a central laboratory for analysis. These approaches can identify a wide range of genetic problems, and the number of disorders that can be screened continues to increase (Shchelochkov & Venditti, 2020).

VITAMIN K PROPHYLAXIS

There is a degree of consensus that all newborn infants have low levels of vitamin K compared with adults. This is thought to be due to inadequate hepatic storage at birth, restricted placental transfer of vitamin K, fluctuating and limited vitamin K content in breast milk, an initially sterile gastrointestinal system or maternal use of drugs that impair vitamin K storage or function (e.g. phenytoin). Comparison of the levels of vitamin K in breast milk compared with formula milk is potentially unhelpful as breast milk is the neonatal biological norm and is specifically designed for newborn metabolic and developmental needs. Conversely, vitamin K is added to infant formula milk as per our perception of need. Vitamin K, which is found in a wide variety of other foods and is synthesised by gut microorganisms (Hamati & Felker, 2022) (see Chapter 11), has an important role in thrombosis.

Vitamin K is offered in order to prevent a rare but serious blood-clotting disorder known as vitamin K deficiency bleeding (VKDB). The incidence of VKBD among babies who don't receive vitamin K is thought to be around 1 per 11,000 live births and most will recover fully with appropriate and timely treatment (Wickham, 2020). The risk of death from VKBD is very low, but is even less likely if the infant receives vitamin K. Infants most at risk are preterm infants and those affected by birth trauma, including difficult instrumental birth.

Bleeding typically begins throughout the first postnatal week. Subarachnoid or intraparenchymal bleeding results in neurological problems (Hamati & Felker, 2022).

Vitamin K prophylaxis can be provided to newborns at birth following discussion with the parents and informed consent. If parents wish, vitamin K can then be administered intramuscularly or orally soon after birth. Administration requires full informed consent from the parents, which includes outlining risks and sequelae in relation to VKBD and the risks associated with vitamin K prophylaxis.

Vitamin K is considered to be safe although there has been limited research into side effects. If administered intramuscularly (IM), it can be painful and may result in bleeding or infection at the injection site (Wickham, 2020).

The American Academy of Paediatrics (AAP) continues to recommend that all neonates receive IM vitamin K (AAP, 2006). This recommendation is based on an examination of surveillance systems in four countries (Australia, Germany, the Netherlands and Switzerland), which found that giving vitamin K orally was less efficacious than administering it IM and may be associated with a higher rate of failure. However, a recent systematic review showed no difference in rates of VKDB following IM compared with oral administration (Jullien, 2021). Furthermore, a 1993 review by the AAP Vitamin K Ad Hoc Task Force effectively addressed concerns that IM vitamin K therapy was linked to juvenile malignancies such as leukaemia (Ng & Loewy, 2018).

A single IM dose of vitamin K (0.5 mg for infants weighing ≤1500 g or 1.0 mg for infants weighing >1500 g) is considered best practice for all newborns within the first 6 hours after birth, following early stabilisation and adequate maternal–newborn interaction. It is also recommended that methods to reduce the procedural pain associated with IM injections be implemented for all neonates (Ng & Loewy, 2018) (Fig. 2.5).

Counselling about the potential risks of VKDB is recommended for parents who do not wish for their baby to receive a vitamin K injection. The option of an oral (PO) dose of 2.0 mg vitamin K at the first feeding, which should be repeated at 2–4 and 6–8 weeks of age, can also be considered (Ng & Loewy, 2018).

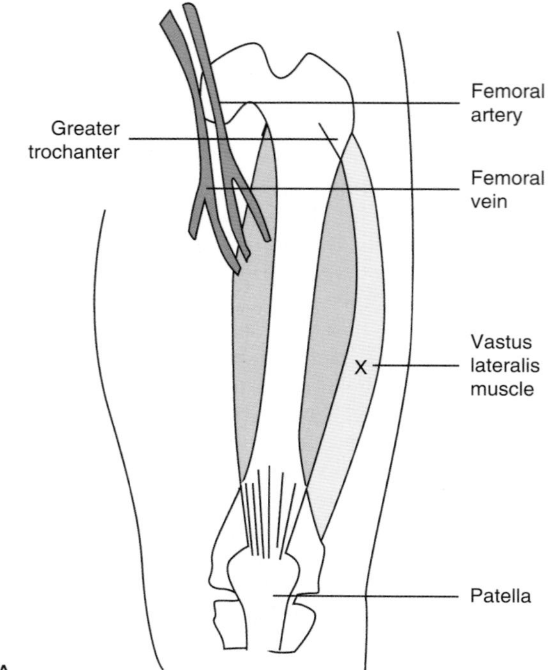

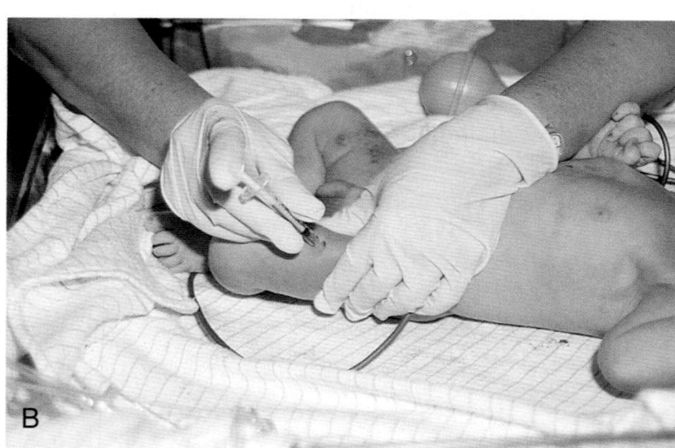

FIGURE 2.5 **Intramuscular Injection**

a *Acceptable intramuscular injection site for newborn infant. X, injection site.* **b** *Infant's leg stabilised for intramuscular injection. Source: A, From Scott PA (2020) Nursing Care of the Newborn and Family. In: Lowdermilk D, Cashion MC, Perry S et al (eds.) Maternity and Women's Health Care, 12th ed, pp. 486–532. St Louis: Elsevier Inc. ; B, Courtesy Marjorie Pyle, Lifecircle, Costa Mesa, CA.*

NEWBORN IMMUNISATIONS

Neonates' underdeveloped immune system makes them more vulnerable to life-threatening infections. However, prior to birth the newborn infant gains immune function from their mother and thereafter breastfeeding transfers maternal immune cells, secretory IgA and an abundance of different types of leukocytes (Laouar, 2020). The development of the neonatal immune response post birth and its association with breastfeeding is not well understood (Laouar, 2020). This emphasises the significance of administering vaccinations in this population, while simultaneously recognising difficulties due to the newborn's own inability to create a protective immune response. Other difficulties include interference from maternal antibodies and an over-reliance on T-helper cell type 2 (Th2) immunity (Chaudhari, 2021).

Newborn immunisation against certain infectious diseases begins during the neonatal period. In some countries (e.g. Australia), the hepatitis B vaccination is routinely administered shortly after birth, and the tuberculosis vaccine bacille Calmette-Guérin (BCG) is administered to high-risk groups such as the indigenous Australian population. In Australia, the first of the routine childhood immunisations (against rotavirus, *Bordetella pertussis*, diphtheria, tetanus, polio, *Haemophilus influenzae*, hepatitis B and pneumococcus) is generally administered at 6–8 weeks of age (Kyprianou, 2015).

SAFE SLEEPING

Sudden infant death syndrome (SIDS) is an unexplained *subset* of **sudden unexpected death in infancy (SUDI)**. When no cause can be found for the infant's death, it is referred to as SIDS, which accounts for around 80% of such deaths.

SIDS is described as the unexpected death of a newborn under the age of 1 year that remains unexplained after a full case investigation, which includes a death scene investigation, autopsy and evaluation of the clinical history. SUDI (also known as **sudden unexpected infant**

death (SUID)) refers to all unexpected infant deaths, which are further classified into explained and unexplained diagnostic groups (Mohan & Maski, 2017).

Around 20% of SUDI have an identifiable cause, such as asphyxia or entanglement, infection, ingestions, metabolic disorders or trauma (accidental or non-accidental). However, distinguishing between SIDS and other causes of SUDI, particularly those that appear to occur during a sleep phase, can be difficult in many cases. Following additional research, some instances initially diagnosed as SIDS have been found to be linked to pathologies such as metabolic abnormalities or heart anomalies (Mohan & Maski, 2017).

The biggest risk factor for SIDS is exposure to cigarette smoke either through maternal smoking or exposure to cigarette smoke during pregnancy or direct neonatal exposure to cigarette smoke after birth. Maternal consumption of alcoholic beverages and illicit drugs are further risk factors that should be avoided during and after pregnancy.

A key campaign to reduce cot deaths has been the 'back to sleep' campaign, now known as '**Safe to Sleep**'. This counters previous advice to place the infant prone to sleep (Sperhake et al., 2018) and recommends that infants should always be laid fully on their backs when sleeping. It is not safe or advisable to place an infant on his or her side. The sleep surface should be specifically designed for infants, firm (e.g. a cot mattress placed in a cot or bassinet) and meet appropriate safety regulations. A soft sleeping surface (e.g. memory foam) can raise the danger of rebreathing or smothering. Other bedding (e.g. pillows, non-fitted sheets), cot bumpers and soft objects (e.g. toys) should be kept away from the sleeping surface (Croke, 2017). Table 2.1 outlines safe-sleeping guidelines for parents and healthcare professionals (infants 0–6 months of age), describing the six key steps to reduce the risk of sudden infant death.

Breastfeeding is protective against SIDS; therefore, practices that support the mother to continue to breastfeed should be encouraged (Thompson et al., 2017). Maternal–infant bed sharing promotes the initiation, duration and exclusivity of breastfeeding and alters the infant regulatory responses, which may affect epigenetic response to stress (Blair et al., 2020). There is no evidence that bed sharing among breastfed infants increases the risk of SIDS where there are no additional risk factors (Blair et al., 2020). During bed sharing the breastfeeding mother has been shown to adopt a protective position in relation to her infant, but this is exhibited less frequently in mothers who have never breastfed (Blair et al., 2020). In recognition of the variation in the risk of bed sharing and the potential impact on breastfeeding, the American Academy of Breastfeeding Medicine have provided updated guidance that focuses on **safe sleeping** rather than proscribing bed sharing entirely

TABLE 2.1 **Safe-sleeping guidelines for parents and healthcare professionals (infants 0–6 months of age): the six key steps to reduce the risk of sudden infant death**

Key steps	Advice and rationale for parents
Always place the baby on their back to sleep	When the baby sleeps on their back, the airway is clear and its defensive reflexes are activated Suffocation, hyperthermia and choking are all reduced when the baby is sleeping on their back
Keep the baby's face and head uncovered	Babies regulate their body temperature through their face and head; therefore, leaving the baby's face and head exposed while sleeping reduces the risk of overheating. It also helps in keeping their airways clear, reducing the risk of suffocation
Keep baby 'smoke free' before and after birth	Smoking during pregnancy and around the baby after birth raises the risk of sudden infant death, as does second-hand smoke If you or your partner smoke, avoid smoking near the baby and never smoke in the same room where the baby sleeps Provide parents with resources to help them stop smoking that are available in your community, e.g. in Australia the Quitline
Safe sleeping environment night and day	The safest location for a baby to sleep is in their own secure environment, which includes a safe mattress and safe bedding. To sleep, the baby should always be laid on their back, with their feet at the bottom of the bassinet or crib • Safe cot: meets Australian standard AS/NZS 2172:2003 or your country's standard • Safe mattress: firm, flat and the correct size for your safe cot, meeting the Australian standard (AS/NZS 8811.1:2013) or the standard in your country • Safe bedding: firmly tucked in and only pulled up to the chest • Secure sleeping bag: well-fitting across the neck and chest, with baby's arms out and no hood
Sleep baby in a safe cot in parents' room for the first 6–12 months	For the first 6–12 months, the safest place for the infant to sleep is in their own safe space, in the same room as their parents or adult care giver
Breastfeed the baby	Breastfeeding has been shown to reduce the risk of sudden infant death

Source: adapted from: Red Nose Safe Sleep Advice Hub. <https://rednose.org.au/section/safe-sleeping> © Red Nose Limited 2020. Updated January 2021.

(Blair et al., 2020). This guidance enables parents to have open, informed discussions with healthcare providers to allow them to plan a safe-sleeping environment and reduce the risk of accidental suffocation when the breastfeeding mother falls asleep with her infant on a couch or sofa. Safe bed sharing with the breastfed infant requires elimination of hazards such as smoking, alcohol, drugs (Croke, 2017) and other hazards in relation to the sleeping surface, bed clothes and bed location. Where bed sharing cannot be done safely, room sharing is advised. Bedside care or cot devices can be considered to support breastfeeding or access to the infant without bed sharing.

There is no robust and consistent evidence that shows pacifier use to be protective against SIDS (Jullien, 2021; Psaila et al., 2017; Smith & Colpitts, 2020). If parents want a pacifier to be provided, if it falls out of the infant's mouth once the infant has fallen asleep it does not need to be replaced. If the pacifier is refused, it should not be forced. The infant's pacifier should not be wrapped around his or her neck or fastened to clothing, soft toys or blankets.

Infants should be dressed appropriately for the sleep environment to avoid overheating. Parents should not cover the infant's face or head with more than one layer of clothing extra to what an adult would wear. It is essential to look for indicators of overheating (e.g. sweating).

Because vaccination may offer some protection against SIDS, newborns should receive the vaccinations recommended by the AAP, the Centers for Disease Control and Prevention (Croke, 2017) and the Australian Children's Education & Care Quality Authority.

Recommendations for minimising the risk of SIDS should be promoted and implemented by healthcare and childcare personnel. During all visits in the first year of an infant's life, healthcare practitioners should screen for and promote safe sleep practices. All healthcare practitioners should be educated on safe infant sleep practices and, as a result, should screen for safe sleep protocols and make recommendations to care givers at each visit. Policies in hospitals should be consistent with current sleeping recommendations, and newborn sleeping surfaces in hospitals should fulfil relevant safety requirements. Persons providing childcare services should be required by their state regulatory agency to complete safe sleep instruction, adhere to safe sleep practices and, if practicable, have written regulations in place (Croke, 2017).

'Safe to Sleep' should be promoted continuously, with professionals actively involved, and should focus on scenarios that raise the risk of SIDS, as well as strategies to reduce the incidence of bed sharing and tobacco smoke exposure, and ways to encourage breastfeeding. Care givers should be targeted for public education (e.g. parents, grandparents, babysitters) (Croke, 2017).

FEEDING THE HEALTHY NEWBORN

The World Health Organization (WHO) recommends exclusive breastfeeding for the first 6 months of life, and this can be continued into the 2nd year and for as long as the mother and infant wish (WHO, 2021). This is supported by the AAP, the Canadian Pediatric Society and the American Academy of Family Physicians who all recommend breastfeeding as the best nutritional source for newborns. Neonatal nurses, midwives and other care givers must always respect the mother's infant-feeding choices and support her to feed her newborn infant. It is important to consider what has informed the mother's feeding choices. For example, has she had any information about infant feeding? How has media advertising influenced her choices? What are the feeding norms in her family? Is she concerned about returning to work, the difficulties of expressing or pumping, or her modesty, or she may perceive breastfeeding to be 'antiquated'? Breastfeeding may go against the mother's cultural and ethnic beliefs. Some Hispanic mothers, for example, are concerned that, by breastfeeding, they might unintentionally pass on unpleasant feelings to their infant. Because Somalian mothers believe that Western medicine and infant formulas have special capabilities, they frequently breastfeed but supplement with formula to guarantee that their infant receives everything that modern medicine has to offer (Seery, 2021).

Breast milk composition and its impact on health

Fresh breast milk is the optimal nutrition for all neonates, including those born preterm where breast milk feeding may reduce the risk of many of the potentially serious long-term effects of prematurity. Growing international evidence supports the significance of human milk in allergy prevention, adult obesity prevention, infection severity and frequency reduction (including infections leading to hospitalisation in affluent countries and death in developing ones), adult metabolic and cardiovascular functioning, and cognitive and intellectual functioning. There are also long-term cost savings to the global economy and to the healthcare system through the use of breast milk, whether the mother's own milk or in combination with, or solely, donor milk for the preterm neonate (Bogen & Whalen, 2019). The global impact of sub-optimal breastfeeding is conservatively estimated at US$341.3 billion per annum (Walters et al., 2019), mainly due to years of life lost. The short- and long-term benefits of both breastfeeding and breast milk feeding have been well documented for mother and neonate (Table 2.2).

Neonatal nurses/midwives working in neonatal units need to have a sound knowledge of the process, science, support and management of expressing and breastfeeding term neonates, to then relate that to the care of sick and/or preterm neonates. This background knowledge can be found in midwifery and lactation texts, and lactation courses. If the neonate is unable to receive breast milk, the mother can store her expressed milk by freezing until her infant is ready for oral nutrition.

There is convincing evidence of the benefits of breast milk, with it both providing passive protection and stimulating the neonate's own immune system (Morrow & Newburg, 2019). The composition of breast milk changes

TABLE 2.2 **Benefits of breastfeeding**

Decreased risk	Protective effect	Improved	Specifically for preterm infants
Otitis media Gastrointestinal illness Urinary tract infections Respiratory tract infections Sudden infant death syndrome Asthma Allergy Some childhood leukaemias Meningitis Dental occlusion Inflammatory bowel disease Coeliac disease Obesity Type 1 diabetes Bacteraemia Meningitis	Cardiovascular health Type 2 diabetes	Cognitive ability	Higher IQ levels Academic achievement Working memory (aged 7 years) Longer-term cardiovascular health Bone health Decreased risk: • Retinopathy of prematurity • Diabetes
For mothers			
Pre- and post-menopausal breast cancer Ovarian cancer Rheumatoid arthritis			

Sources: Belfort et al. (2016); Eidelman et al. (2012); Lucas et al. (2014).

with the needs of the neonate according to the stage of lactation, time of day, gestation and age of the neonate (Ribeiro et al., 2022). While breast milk offers many nutritional benefits, other components of breast milk assist in immune development and provide protection to the gut mucosa. Although the stage of prematurity will influence the development of the gut, breast milk offers protection through lactoferrin, which has prebiotic actions and promotes a healthy microbiome. Also, secretory immunoglobulin A (SIgA) coats the mucosal surface in the gut to suppress pathogens along with non-digestible oligosaccharides, both offering passive protection of the gut and stimulating the neonate's own defence systems (Morrow & Newburg, 2019).

The human milk microbiota is unique in that it contains around 300 bacterial species that have been identified only in human breast and milk microbiome. Historically, mammalian milk was assumed to be sterile unless infected or contaminated during collection or storage. The detection of lactic acid bacteria in breast milk, the surface of the breast and areola and the newborn's mouth and faeces using both culture-dependent and culture-independent methods implies that breast milk may be an important source of lactic acid bacteria for the infant. The human microbiota is made up of roughly 100 trillion microbial symbionts that dwell in the human body as a host symbiont or holobiont. Fundamentally, this indicates that the human body is made up of highly organised biological units, with eukaryotic cells acting as organs and the microbiota living in a variety of microbial habitats on or in the body. The human microbiota plays an important role in the genetic and metabolic variety and functioning of each individual human (Azad, 2019). It directly and indirectly adds to the human host's health and illness. These effects are linked to many microbial habitats in the human body, particularly the microbiota of the human gut. Human milk, with its diverse microbiota and particular nutritional content for human newborns, aids in the establishment of the infant's gut microbiota and has a direct influence on the developing infant's immune system (Ho et al., 2018; Lawrence, 2022a).

The composition of breast milk varies between mothers, across the breastfeeding journey, during a feed and between preterm and term infants. The first milk from the breast after birth is colostrum, which is rich in immunological and developmental factors and is important for priming and protecting the neonatal gut and developing the immune system (Lawrence, 2022b). Colostrum is a viscous fluid and is produced in only very small quantities; because of this, if a mother wishes to express, hand expressing is recommended, though a pump can be offered if a mother does not wish to hand express but needs to stimulate her milk production. Lactogenesis II tends to occur at around days 3–4 after birth; this is where the mother's breast milk is said to 'come in' and is usually experienced as fullness and often copious amounts of milk. Delay in lactogenesis II can be caused by mode of birth, lack of skin-to-skin or breast stimulation, maternal health factors and other adverse events during labour or birth (Huang et al., 2020).

Breast milk is a living fluid perfectly designed for the needs of the individual infant at that time, stage and age. It contains fat, carbohydrates, vitamins, minerals and bioactive factors that affect bodily functions, including growth factors that are important for growth and development and anti-infective and immune-protective factors (Lawrence, 2022b). The dynamic nature of breast milk is visible in the changing amount of fat during a feed. At the start of a feed, breast milk contains only a small amount of fat, which steadily increases so that by the end of a feed the milk has the highest content of fat (Australian Breastfeeding Association (ABA), 2021). This used to be referred to as 'fore' and 'hind' milk, but these terms are *inaccurate* and could potentially be confusing when providing feeding support. The key recommendation is for the infant to finish feeding on one breast to ensure they ingest this fattier milk. Furthermore, emptying the breast at each feed is an important part of local milk production regulation. Ensuring enough milk draining from the breast removes a protein known as the 'feedback inhibitor of lactation' (FiL) from the milk. FiL, as the name implies, inhibits milk supply (Lawrence, 2022c; Peaker & Wilde, 1996).

EVIDENCE-BASED PRACTICE RESEARCH 2.2

Many personal, social and clinical factors interact to influence breastfeeding initiation and duration; however, there is a lack of understanding of in-hospital exclusive breastfeeding (EBF), which is crucial for breastfeeding establishment and duration.

This qualitative study used in-depth, semi-structured interviews to (1) identify facilitators and barriers to in-hospital EBF and (2) investigate breastfeeding assistance available from key stakeholders within the social–ecological model.

The researchers found influences at various levels of the socio-ecological model. At the intrapersonal level, they found maternal perception of insufficient milk supply was a barrier to in-hospital EBF. At the interpersonal level, a personalised and individualised approach to breastfeeding therapy was deemed to be the most helpful in encouraging EBF. Institutional level influences included gaps in prenatal breastfeeding education, a lack of time to deliver comprehensive prenatal teaching to high-risk patients and practical assistance with attaching to the breast and positioning. Community-level services provided added benefits to EBF mothers and were seen as a facilitator, but this was undermined by the provision of vouchers to formula-feeding mothers in hospital. Cultural norms and a diverse patient group have been identified as impediments to providing macrosystem-level support.

Source: Bookhart et al. (2021).

Successful breastfeeding

Breastfeeding is a public health priority, and it is our society's responsibility to provide breastfeeding support services. Breastfeeding is a learned skill and not the 'simple and natural' endeavour that it is often made out to be. Primiparous mothers often have more challenges than multiparous ones, highlighting the importance of providing appropriate support the first time. Breastfeeding assistance begins with prenatal encouragement and instruction. Following birth, in-person lactation care is beneficial in supporting both the initiation and continuation of breastfeeding (Taylor et al., 2018). Successful breastfeeding begins with facilitating skin to skin as discussed earlier. Poor quality or disrupted skin-to-skin contact has a negative impact on the infant's ability to progress through a series of innate pre-feeding behaviours that result in attachment.

An appropriate latch is critical to breastfeeding success because it impacts milk supply, maternal comfort and neonatal feeding behaviours. Achieving a good latch requires:

- the mother and baby to be comfortable, calm and relaxed
- ensuring the infant's head and body are aligned
- nose to nipple, encouraging a wide gape, with tongue down
- bringing the baby to the breast, rather than trying to 'post' the breast to the baby's mouth.

When a baby is correctly latched, their mouth is wide open, with a nearly 180-degree angle between the upper and lower lips (Fig. 2.6). The baby's chin will touch the breast and the nose will be clear. The lips will be everted (flanged) and positioned as far back on the areola as possible and the nipple in the back of the baby's mouth. The quantity of areola visible during a good latch varies owing to the considerable variety in the size of newborns' mouths and mothers' nipples and areolas (Lawrence, 2022a), but more areola should be visible above the baby's top lip than below their lower lip. Signs of a good latch include that it should not be painful, although some mothers may feel some discomfort when first learning to breastfeed; the baby will follow through with a pattern of sucks from short, quick bursts to longer sucks and will

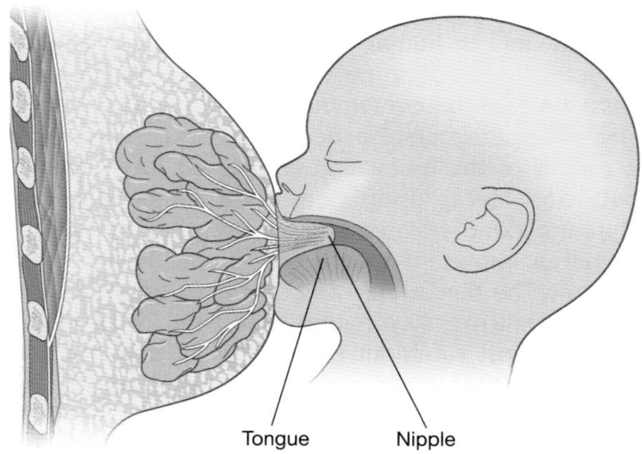

FIGURE 2.6 **Successful latch**

self-release at the end of the feed; the sounds of the infant swallowing might be heard; the mother's breasts will feel softer at the end of the feed.

Signs of a poor latch include nipple pain, and the mother should be supported to detach the baby and reposition. A fussy or unsettled baby might indicate a poor latch and inability to access milk. A nipple that appears flattened when the infant lets go of the breast can indicate that the baby's mouth is not sufficiently opened when feeding. If a woman has prolonged pain when breastfeeding, she should unlatch the infant by placing a finger into the baby's mouth and between the gums and gently pressing down towards the baby's chin. The baby should then be repositioned, and a proper latch should be attempted once more. If the pain persists, the mother–baby dyad should be evaluated during a feeding by a breastfeeding expert, such as a lactation consultant. An insufficient latch can cause breast damage and, over time, reduce milk supply (Balest et al., 2018).

Forcing the infant to the breast, especially by putting pressure on the infant's head or handling the mother's breasts, is an ineffective strategy to support breastfeeding. The first is distressing for the infant and can result in breast rejection. The latter is distressing for the mother, does not enable a good latch and does not empower her to learn how to latch her own infant.

Responsive feeding

The term **responsive feeding** has evolved from demand feeding to baby-led feeding. Responsive feeding means the mother responds to her baby's cues and her own desires to feed or nurture her baby. It also recognises that offering a feed is not solely about nutrition but also about love and comfort. It applies to both breast and bottle feeding (UNICEF UK, 2016).

Indirect breast milk feeding

Where a mother is unable to breastfeed her infant or is separated from her infant for any reason, she should be supported to express her breast milk. This should start as soon after birth as possible and the expressing pattern, where separated, should ideally mimic the expected feeding pattern of the newborn. Hand expressing is particularly recommended in the early days, but a pump can be used if the mother prefers, and pumps are useful later to express larger volumes of breast milk.

Storage of expressed breast milk should be in a sterilised container and can be stored in the fridge for up to 5 days at 4°C or lower (at the back of the fridge rather than in the door), or for 2 weeks in the ice compartment of a fridge or for up to 6 months in a freezer. Frozen milk should be defrosted in the fridge and used straight away once thawed. Milk can be warmed to body temperature before feeding if desired, but never in the microwave as this can cause hot spots, which may cause burns (ABA, 2021). Breast milk can be left at room temperature for 6–8 hours, providing it is in a closed container and the ambient temperature does not exceed 26°C. If refrigeration is available, however, that is preferable (ABA, 2021).

Formula feeding and milk composition

Despite efforts to promote exclusive breastfeeding until the age of 6 months, it is estimated that only half of women continue to breastfeed at 6 months. The decision to use infant formula is often made in pregnancy, but many mothers who start breastfeeding may supplement with infant formula or choose to formula feed entirely in response to their experiences of breastfeeding. In many high-income countries, in-hospital supplementation is common, often as a result of poor breastfeeding support that has led to pain, perceptions of lack of milk and lack of confidence in breastfeeding (Papautsky & Koenig, 2021). Very occasionally, infant formula may be recommended for newborns for whom breast milk consumption is prohibited because of infant variables (e.g. inborn errors of metabolism) or maternal considerations (such as human immunodeficiency virus (HIV), human T-cell lymphotropic virus type 1 (HTLV-1) infection or tuberculosis) where there are no safe alternatives. The use of infant formula as a supplement to increase weight gain in breastfed infants should be a last resort after exploring positioning and attachment and ways to increase milk supply such as skin-to-skin contact, pumping and hand expressing and supporting maternal wellbeing (Lawrence, 2022a).

Infant formula is an inert substance and while nutritionally adequate, does not contain the living cells, anti-infective properties, growth factors or maternal antibodies found in breast milk (Lawrence, 2022b). Infant formula varies by brand, by country and by fluctuations in prices of ingredients. Formula milk sold in high-income countries is generally considered to be safe and nutritionally sound as the sole source of nutrition for healthy infants during their first 6 months of life, although contamination and inappropriate formulation have been reported (Losio et al., 2018). In low–middle-income countries or where there is lack of access to safe water supply, infant formula can be problematic because of cost, storage, risk of contamination, maternal literacy and so forth. In many countries, infant formula comes in ready-to-feed, concentrated liquid and powder formats. Ready-to-feed products typically give 19–20 kcal/30 mL (1 oz) and 64–67 kcal/dL. When concentrated liquid products are diluted according to the manufacturer's directions, they produce a preparation with the same concentration. Powder formulas are available in single or multiple serving sizes, and when mixed according to the instructions they have a similar calorie density (Parks et al., 2020).

When preparing formula and feedings for the newborn, parents should be taught to utilise correct handwashing techniques and provided with up-to-date instructions for making up and storing bottles of formula milk:

- Wash hands and use sterilised equipment and bottles.
- Use fresh boiled and then cooled water – avoid bottled water or water that has been boiled before.
- Only make up one bottle at a time – making several bottles at once and then storing in the fridge is no longer recommended because of contamination risks.

- Follow the manufacturer's instructions and use only manufacturer provided scoops.
- Always check temperature of the formula before feeding.
- Discard any milk left at the end of the feed.
- Discard any bottles that are not used within 2 hours of being made (Department of Health, Western Australia, 2021; Queensland Government, 2017).

Once opened, ready-to-feed and concentrated liquid products should be wrapped in aluminium foil or plastic wrap within their containers and refrigerated for no more than 48 hours. Powder formula should be kept in a cool, dry area; once opened, cans should be covered with the original plastic cap or aluminium foil and the powdered product should be utilised within 4 weeks. Refrigerated prepared formula should be reheated by immersing the container in warm water for around 5 minutes. Despite appearing to be at the correct temperature when tested, formula should not be heated in a microwave as it can heat unevenly and result in burns (Parks et al., 2020).

Formula feedings should be given ad libitum in order to maximise the child's genetic potential for growth and development. In the first 3 months of life, the typical intake to provide for a weight growth of 25–30 g/day is 140–200 mL/kg/day. From 3 to 12 months of age, the rate of weight gain slows (Parks et al., 2020).

CLINICAL PRACTICE 2.2

This quality improvement initiative was carried out at a tertiary care teaching hospital in Delhi, India. The WHO recommends evidence-based strategies that had already benefited over 10,000 mother–baby dyads using the Point of Care Quality Improvement technique. Separation of mothers and newborns after birth was the typical practice in the hospital where this study was conducted. Clinicians would take the normal newborn to the radiant warmer in the resuscitation area for routine care after birth. This was the established care process at their hospital. The staff in the birthing unit embarked on a quality improvement program to identify and document issues that were impeding the delivery of evidence-based practice of providing immediate skin-to-skin care, delayed cord clamping and early breastfeeding within 1 hour of birth. Early newborn mother separation and late transfer of mother from the birthing room to the post-birth observation area were two of the identified hurdles. There was also the issue of a high birth load with differing understanding and provision of skin-to-skin care, as well as drying on the mother's abdomen. This made it difficult to sustain improved care methods.

Using the Plan-Do-Study-Act (PDSA) approach, several effective change ideas were evaluated included pre-birth counselling, avoiding separation of mother and newborn at birth by providing skin-to-skin care immediately after birth, and continuing it in the post-birth observation area, and enlisting the assistance of a family member with the first breastfeed. Multiple iterations, group discussions and feedback were used by the delivery team to adapt to these successful change initiatives. Over a 36-month period, this resulted in improved and sustained compliance with pre-birth counselling, skin-to-skin care, delayed cord clamping and commencing breastfeeding within 1 hour, from minimal compliance to a median compliance of 51%, 56%, 59% and 61% respectively, resulting from this practice change.

Source: Sachan et al. (2021).

The Baby Friendly Hospital Initiative

The **Baby Friendly Hospital Initiative (BFHI)** was created in response to poor breastfeeding outcomes in relation to hospital or facility births, and aimed to reduce hospitals' reliance on artificial infant formulae and to promote, protect and support breastfeeding in these settings. It is now viewed as best practice as a comprehensive program for hospitals to provide a supportive environment with educated and knowledgeable personnel. The program's essentials are described in the Ten Steps. The BFHI program and the evidence for each of the Ten Steps has been re-examined, resulting in the publication of a new guideline: *Protecting, promoting and supporting breastfeeding in facilities providing maternity and newborn services* in 2017 (WHO/UNICEF, 2017) and an updated (2018) implementation guidance for countries implementing the BFHI.

The key clinical practice steps that form part of the 10 steps (steps 3–10) include (note: steps 1 a, b, c and 2 relate to critical management procedures) are as follows:

3. Discuss the importance and management of breastfeeding with pregnant women and their families.
4. Facilitate immediate and uninterrupted skin-to-skin contact and support mothers to initiate breastfeeding as soon as possible after birth.
5. Support mothers to initiate and maintain breastfeeding and manage common difficulties.
6. Do not provide breastfed newborns any food or fluids other than breast milk, unless medically indicated.
7. Enable mothers and their infants to remain together and to practise rooming-in 24 hours a day.
8. Support mothers to recognise and respond to their infants' cues for feeding.
9. Counsel mothers on the use and risks of feeding bottles, teats and pacifiers.
10. Coordinate discharge so that parents and their infants have timely access to ongoing support and care.

<https://www.who.int/teams/nutrition-and-food-safety/food-and-nutrition-actions-in-health-systems/ten-steps-to-successful-breastfeeding>

The achievement of Baby Friendly Hospitals accreditation has been extensive over the world. Progress in the United States and Australia, however, has been slower (Lawrence, 2022d).

Pacifier use

Avoiding pacifiers and artificial teats (sometimes referred to as 'dummies') is one of the guidelines in the Baby Friendly Hospital Initiative's (BFHI) document *The*

Ten Steps to successful breastfeeding (Munn et al., 2016). Systematic review evidence indicates that early use of pacifiers results in sub-optimal breastfeeding outcomes (Buccini et al., 2017). The use of artificial teats and bottles is also associated with poorer outcomes, although this may be due to formula milk feeding or the reason for the supplement in the first place. The potential impact on breastfeeding should be considered and it is recommended that pacifiers are not introduced until breastfeeding is well established (Smith & Colpitts, 2020). There are important baseline characteristics already associated with poorer breastfeeding outcomes which are also associated with women's choices to use pacifiers or supplementary bottle feeds (e.g. lower maternal income, education and being single). In some contexts, however, the use of pacifiers has proved useful. For example, pacifiers as non-nutritive sucking devices can soothe infants and may be useful during painful procedures. For preterm infants in the neonatal unit, pacifiers are part of the developmental care package for soothing and to help to develop the suck reflex during tube feeding, which may hasten the transition to oral feeding (Kaya & Aytekin, 2017; Say et al., 2018). Some research has suggested that pacifiers may be useful in protecting infants against sudden infant death syndrome. According to some reports, pacifiers can interfere with early weaning, increase the likelihood of otitis media and induce dental difficulties. Pacifiers have also been criticised for delaying speech development and interfering with sleeping habits (Caruso et al., 2019).

CASE STUDY

2.1

Sally has given birth to her first child, a female, at 38^2 weeks' gestation. Sally and her partner June named their daughter Ella. Following an uncomplicated vaginal birth, Ella is placed skin to skin on Sally's chest so that Sally and June can bond with their new daughter.

Within a few minutes of birth, Ella is supported by midwife, John, to have her first breastfeed. Supporting the mother–baby dyad, John ensures that Ella is left skin to skin with Sally for the first hour of life as she suckles from the breast and studies her mother's face while he stays unobtrusively nearby to assess Ella's transition and Sally's recovery from the birth.

After an hour or so, Sally asks John if he could weigh Ella. Ella's birthweight is 3650 g; head circumference 35 cm and length 51 cm. Sally and June want to know whether the measurements are 'normal'. John uses the Fenton Growth Chart – available from <https://peditools.org/> – to plot the measurements and respond to this question.

John returns to the room to check on Ella's progress and proceeds to prepare a vitamin K injection for Ella.

Sally and June refuse the vitamin K injection for their daughter because of the risks to their daughter later in life. When John asks them where they heard this information, they respond that they read it on the internet.

1. Outline how John, the midwife, supports the mother–baby dyad in this case study.
2. Using <https://peditools.org/>, plot Ella's measurements and consider how you would respond to Sally and June's question.
3. What are the risks for Ella if she does not receive the vitamin K injection?
4. If you were in John's position, how would you respond to Sally and June's refusal of the vitamin K injection?

CONCLUSION

Maternal care, provided under the guidance of midwives, is best for healthy, term newborns. Standard management should be that the mother and her baby remain together at all times. This supports the normal newborn transition to extrauterine life, maternal–infant bonding and attachment and successful breastfeeding and reduces the risk of cross-infection. It also facilitates the mother's desire to learn how to recognise, respond to and meet every demand of her infant.

Systems of care should be developed to promote the normal newborn as healthy and requiring little intervention beyond breastfeeding support. Interventions for which there is clear evidence that the benefits outweigh the risks should be delivered as discretely as possible so as not to interrupt the mother–baby dyad. Simultaneously, while promoting 'natural' care for these babies, healthcare providers should be on the alert for neonates who are considered 'at risk' of developing health problems.

Recommended Reading

Ekambaram, M., Irigoyen, M. M., Paoletti, A. M., & Siddiqui, I. (2019). Impact of a baby-friendly–aligned pacifier policy on pacifier use at 1 month of age. *Academic Pediatrics, 19*(7), 808–814. doi: doi.org/10.1016/j.acap.2019.02.002.

Malm-Buatsi, E., Anderson, A. G. S., Gubbins, E., Page Phillips, E., Maizels, M., & Washington, K. T. (2020). A qualitative study of parental preferences for post-circumcision care education. *Journal of Pediatric Urology, 16*(1), 46.e41–46.e46. doi: doi.org/10.1016/j.jpurol.2019.10.010.

Online Resources

Academy of Breastfeeding Medicine protocols: <https://www.bfmed.org/protocols>

Australian Breastfeeding Association (ABA): <https://www.breastfeeding.asn.au/>

Australian Children's Education and Care Quality Authority: Safe sleep and rest practices: <https://www.acecqa.gov.au/resources/supporting-materials/infosheet/safe-sleep-and-rest-practices>

Fenton growth charts to report percentiles and Z-scores, with integrated GA calculator and decision support: <https://peditools.org/>

Raising Children: How to breastfeed: <https://raisingchildren.net.au/newborns/breastfeeding-bottle-feeding/how-to-breastfeed/>

UK UNICEF: The baby friendly initiative: <https://www.unicef.org.uk/babyfriendly/>

World Health Organization: Promoting baby-friendly hospitals: <https://www.who.int/activities/promoting-baby-friendly-hospitals>

References/Acknowledgements

Abdeyazdan, Z., Mohammadian-Ghahfarokhi, M., Ghazavi, Z., & Mohammadizadeh, M. (2016). Effects of nesting and swaddling on the sleep duration of premature infants hospitalized in neonatal intensive care units. *Iranian Journal of Nursing and Midwifery Research, 21*(5), 552–556.

American Academy of Pediatrics (AAP). (2006). AAP publications reaffirmed, May 2006. *Pediatrics, 118*(3), 1266–1266. doi: 10.1542/peds.2006-1697.

Australian Breastfeeding Association (ABA). (2021). <https://www.breastfeeding.asn.au/> (Accessed 2 March 2022).

Azad, M. B. (2019). Infant feeding and the developmental origins of chronic disease in the CHILD cohort: role of human milk bioactives and gut microbiota. *Breastfeeding Medicine, 14*(S1), S-22–S-24. doi: 10.1089/bfm.2019.0029.

Balest, A. L., Riley, M. M., & Bogen, D. L. (2018). Neonatology. In: B. J. Zitelli, S. C. McIntire, & A. J. Nowalk (Eds.), *Zitelli and Davis' atlas of pediatric physical diagnosis* (pp. 44–70). Philadelphia, PA: Elsevier.

Ballard, J. L., Novak, K. K., & Driver, M. (1979). A simplified score for assessment of fetal maturation of newly born infants. *Journal of Pediatrics, 95*(5 Pt 1), 769–774.

Ballard, J. L., Khoury, J., Wedig, K., Wang, L., Eilers-Walsman, B., & Lipp, R. (1991). New Ballard score, expanded to include extremely premature infants. *Journal of Pediatrics, 119*(3), 417–423.

Barry, E. S. (2021). What is "normal" infant sleep? Why we still do not know. *Psychological Reports, 124*(2), 651–692. doi: 10.1177/0033294120909447.

Belfort, M. B., Anderson, P. J., Nowak, V. A., Lee, K. J., Molesworth, C., & Thompson, D. K. (2016). Breast milk feeding, brain development, and neurocognitive outcomes: a 7-year longitudinal study in infants born at less than 30 weeks' gestation. *Journal of Pediatrics, 177*, 133–139.e131.

Blair, P. S., Ball, H. L., McKenna, J. J., Feldman-Winter, L., Marinelli, K. A., Bartick, M. C., et al. (2020). Bedsharing and breastfeeding: The Academy of Breastfeeding Medicine Protocol #6, Revision 2019. *Breastfeeding Medicine, 15*(1), 5–16. doi: 10.1089/bfm.2019.29144.psb.

Bogen, D. L., & Whalen, B. L. (2019). Breastmilk feeding for mothers and infants with opioid exposure: What is best? *Seminars in Fetal and Neonatal Medicine, 24*(2), 95–104. doi: 10.1016/j.siny.2019.01.001.

Bookhart, L. H., Joyner, A. B., Lee, K. R., Worrell, N., Jamieson, D. J., & Young, M. F. (2021). Moving beyond breastfeeding initiation: a qualitative study unpacking factors that influence infant feeding at hospital discharge among urban, socioeconomically disadvantaged women. *Journal of the Academy of Nutrition and Dietetics, 121*(9), 1704–1720. doi: 10.1016/j.jand.2021.02.005.

Brimdyr, K., Cadwell, K., Svensson, K., Takahashi, Y., Nissen, E., & Widström, A.-M. (2020). The nine stages of skin-to-skin: practical guidelines and insights from four countries. *Maternal and Child Nutrition, 16*(4), e13042. doi: 10.1111/mcn.13042.

Brogan, J., & Rapkin, G. (2017). Implementing evidence-based neonatal skin care with parent-performed, delayed immersion baths. *Nursing for Women's Health, 21*(6), 442–450. doi: 10.1016/j.nwh.2017.10.009.

Buccini, G. D. S., Perez-Escamilla, R., Paulino, L. M., Araujo, C. L., & Venancio, S. I. (2017). Pacifier use and interruption of exclusive breastfeeding: systematic review and meta-analysis. *Maternal and Child Nutrition, 13*(3). doi: 10.1111/mcn.12384.

Caruso, S., Nota, A., Darvizeh, A., Severino, M., Gatto, R., & Tecco, S. (2019). Poor oral habits and malocclusions after usage of orthodontic pacifiers: an observational study on 3–5 years old children. *BMC Pediatrics, 19*(1), 294. doi: 10.1186/s12887-019-1668-3.

Chamberlain, J., McCarty, S., Sorce, J., Leesman, B., Schmidt, S., Meyrick, E., et al. (2019). Impact on delayed newborn bathing on exclusive breastfeeding rates, glucose and temperature stability, and weight loss. *Journal of Neonatal Nursing, 25*(2), 74–77. doi: 10.1016/j.jnn.2018.11.001.

Chaudhari, T. (2021). Vaccinations in the newborn. *Best Practice and Research: Clinical Obstetrics and Gynaecology, 76*, 66–82. doi: 10.1016/j.bpobgyn.2020.09.004.

Cohen, S. S., Alexander, D. D., Krebs, N. F., Young, B. E., Cabana, M. D., Erdmann, P., et al. (2018). Factors associated with breastfeeding initiation and continuation: a meta-analysis. *Journal of Pediatrics, 203*, 190–196.e121. doi: 10.1016/j.jpeds.2018.08.008.

Cooke, A., Bedwell, C., Campbell, M., McGowan, L., Ersser, S. J., & Lavender, T. (2018). Skin care for healthy babies at term: a systematic review of the evidence. *Midwifery, 56*, 29–43. doi: 10.1016/j.midw.2017.10.001.

Croke, L. M. (2017). SIDS and safe sleeping environments for infants: AAP updates recommendations. *American Family Physician, 95*(12), 806–807.

Department of Health Western Australia. (2021). Safe preparation and use of infant formula. <https://www.healthywa.wa.gov.au/Articles/S_T/Safe-preparation-and-use-of-infant-formula> (Accessed 2 March 2022).

DiTomasso, D., & Paiva, A. L. (2018). Neonatal weight matters: an examination of weight changes in full-term breastfeeding newborns during the first 2 weeks of life. *Journal of Human Lactation, 34*(1), 86–92. doi: 10.1177/0890334417722508.

DiTomasso, D., Wambach, K. A., Roberts, M. B., Erickson-Owens, D. A., Quigley, A., & Newbury, J. M. (2021). Maternal worry about infant weight and its influence on artificial milk supplementation and breastfeeding cessation. *Journal of Human Lactation, 38*(1), 177–189. doi: 10.1177/08903344211000284.

Dubowitz, L. M., Dubowitz, V., Palmer, P., & Verghote, M. (1980). A new approach to the neurological assessment of the preterm and full-term newborn infant. *Brain Development, 2*(1), 3–14. doi: 10.1016/s0387-7604(80)80003-9.

Eidelman, A., Schanler, R., & Johnston, M. (2012). Breastfeeding and the use of human milk. *Pediatrics, 129*(3), e827–e841.

Feldman, H. M., & Chaves-Gnecco, D. (2018). Developmental/behavioral pediatrics. In: B. J. Zitelli, S. C. McIntire, & A. J. Nowalk (Eds.), *Zitelli and Davis' atlas of pediatric physical diagnosis* (pp. 71–100). Philadelphia, PA: Elsevier.

Flaherman, V. J., Cabana, M. D., McCulloch, C. E., & Paul, I. M. (2019). Effect of early limited formula on breastfeeding duration in the first year of life: a randomized clinical trial. *Journal of the American Medical Association: Pediatrics, 173*(8), 729–735. doi: 10.1001/jamapediatrics.2019.1424.

Frie, J., Bartocci, M., & Kuhn, P. (2020). Neonatal cortical perceptions of maternal breast odours: a fNIRS study. *Acta Paediatrica (Oslo, Norway: 1992), 109*(7), 1330–1337. doi: 10.1111/apa.15114.

Georgoulas, A., Jones, L., Laudiano-Dray, M. P., Meek, J., Fabrizi, L., & Whitehead, K. (2021). Sleep–wake regulation in preterm and term infants. *Sleep, 44*(1), zsaa148. doi: 10.1093/sleep/zsaa148.

Graham, M. E., Dedhia, K., & Park, A. H. (2021). Early detection and diagnosis of infant hearing impairment. In: P. W. Flint, H. W. Francis, B. H. Haughey, M. M. Lesperance, V. J. Lund, K. T. Robbins, et al. (Eds.), *Cummings otolaryngology: head and neck surgery* (pp. 2887–2897.e2883). Philadelphia, PA: Elsevier.

Hamati, A. I., & Felker, M. V. (2022). Neurological complications of systemic disease: children. In: J. Jankovic, J. C. Mazziotta, S. L. Pomeroy, & N. J. Newman (Eds.), *Bradley and Daroff's neurology in clinical practice* (pp. 882–896.e884). Philadelphia, PA: Elsevier.

Hawes, J., Bernardo, S., & Wilson, D. (2020). The neonatal neurological examination: improving understanding and performance. *Neonatal Network, 39*(3), 116–128.

Ho, N. T., Li, F., Lee-Sarwar, K. A., Tun, H. M., Brown, B. P., Pannaraj, P. S., et al. (2018). Meta-analysis of effects of exclusive breastfeeding on infant gut microbiota across populations. *Nature Communications, 9*(1), 4169. doi: 10.1038/s41467-018-06473-x.

Huang, L., Xu, S., Chen, X., Li, Q., Lin, L., Zhang, Y., et al. (2020). Delayed lactogenesis is associated with suboptimal breastfeeding practices: a prospective cohort study. *Journal of Nutrition, 150*(4), 894–900. doi: 10.1093/jn/nxz311.

Hugill, K. (2017). Revisiting infant nappy dermatitis: causes and preventive care. *British Journal of Midwifery, 25*(3), 150–154. doi: 10.12968/bjom.2017.25.3.150.

Jiang, F. (2019). Sleep and early brain development. *Annals of Nutrition and Metabolism, 75*(suppl 1)(1), 44–54. doi: 10.1159/000508055.

Jullien, S. (2021). Vitamin K prophylaxis in newborns. *BMC Pediatrics, 21*(1), 350. doi: 10.1186/s12887-021-02701-4.

Kaya, V., & Aytekin, A. (2017). Effects of pacifier use on transition to full breastfeeding and sucking skills in preterm infants: a randomised controlled trial. *Journal of Clinical Nursing, 26*(13–14), 2055–2063. doi: 10.1111/jocn.13617.

Kong, A. H. T., Lai, M. M., Finnigan, S., Ware, R. S., Boyd, R. N., & Colditz, P. B. (2018). Background EEG features and prediction of cognitive outcomes in very preterm infants: a systematic review. *Early Human Development, 127*, 74–84. doi: 10.1016/j.earlhumdev.2018.09.015.

Kyprianou, K. (2015). Routine neonatal care. In: M. Permezel, S. Walker, & K. Kyprianou (Eds.), *Beischer & MacKay's obstetrics, gynaecology and the newborn* (pp. 592–596). Chatswood, NSW: Elsevier Australia.

Laouar, A. (2020). Maternal leukocytes and infant immune programming during breastfeeding. *Trends in Immunology, 41*(3), 225–239.

Lawrence, R. A. (2022a). Maternal nutrition and supplements for mother and infant. In: R. A. Lawrence & R. M. Lawrence (Eds.), *Breastfeeding: a guide for the medical profession* (9th ed., pp. 247–277). Philadelphia, PA: Elsevier.

Lawrence, R. A. (2022c). Biochemistry of human milk. In: R. A. Lawrence & R. M. Lawrence (Eds.), *Breastfeeding: a guide for the medical profession* (9th ed., pp. 93–144). Philadelphia, PA: Elsevier.

Lawrence, R. A. (2022d). Breastfeeding support groups and community resources. In: R. A. Lawrence & R. M. Lawrence (Eds.), *Breastfeeding: a guide for the medical profession* (9th ed., pp. 710–718). Philadelphia, PA: Elsevier.

Lawrence, R. M. (2022b). Host-resistance factors and immunologic significance of human milk. In: R. A. Lawrence & R. M. Lawrence (Eds.), *Breastfeeding: a guide for the medical profession* (9th ed., pp. 145–192). Philadelphia, PA: Elsevier.

Lee, A. C. C., Panchal, P., Folger, L. Whelan, H., Whelan, R., Rosner, B., et al. (2017). Diagnostic accuracy of neonatal assessment for gestational age determination: a systematic review. *Pediatrics, 140*(6), e20171423. doi: 10.1542/peds.2017-1423.

Lissauer, T., & Hansen, A. (2020). Physical examination of the newborn. In: R. J. Martin, A. A. Fanaroff, & M. C. Walsh (Eds.), *Fanaroff and Martin's neonatal-perinatal medicine* (9th ed., pp. 440–457). Philadelphia, PA: Elsevier.

Lissauer, T., Fanaroff, A. A., Miall, L., & Fanaroff, J. (2015). *Neonatology at a glance*. Oxford, UK: Wiley-Blackwell.

Long, K., Rondinelli, J., Yim, A., Cariou, C., & Valdez, R. (2020). Delaying the first newborn bath and exclusive breastfeeding. *MCN: American Journal of Maternal/Child Nursing, 45*(2), 110–115.

Losio, M. N., Pavoni, E., Finazzi, G., Agostoni, C., Daminelli, P., Dalzini, E., et al. (2018). Preparation of powdered infant formula: could product's safety be improved? *Journal of Pediatric Gastroenterology and Nutrition, 67*(4), 543.

Lucas, R., Paquette, R., Briere, C., & McGrath, J. (2014). Furthering our understanding of the needs of mothers who are pumping breast milk for infants in the NICU: an integrative review. *Advances in Neonatal Care, 14*(4), 241–252.

Lund, C. (2016). Bathing and beyond: current bathing controversies for newborn infants. *Advances in Neonatal Care, 16*, 513–520. doi: 10.1097/ANC.0000000000000336.

Marcdante, K. J., & Kliegman, R. M. (2019). Assessment of the mother, fetus, and newborn. In: K. J. Marcdante & R. M. Kliegman (Eds.), *Nelson essentials of pediatrics* (8th ed., pp. 217–235). Philadelphia, PA: Elsevier.

Mennella, J. A., Bobowski, N., & Liem, D. G. (2017). Taste and smell. In: K. F. Swaiman, S. Ashwal, D. M. Ferriero, N. F. Schor, R. S. Finkel, A. L. Gropman, et al. (Eds.), *Swaiman's pediatric neurology* (6th ed., pp. e134–e149). Philadelphia, PA: Elsevier.

Mohan, M. A., & Maski, K. P. (2017). Apparent life-threatening event and sudden infant death syndrome. In: K. F. Swaiman, S. Ashwal, D. M. Ferriero, N. F. Schor, R. S. Finkel, A. L. Gropman, et al. (Eds.), *Swaiman's pediatric neurology* (pp. e1555–e1563). Philadelphia, PA: Elsevier.

Moore, E. R., Bergman, N., Anderson, G. C., & Medley, N. (2016). Early skin-to-skin contact for mothers and their healthy newborn infants. *Cochrane Database of Systematic Reviews, 11*. <https://www.cochrane.org/CD003519/PREG_early-skin-skin-contact-mothers-and-their-healthy-newborn-infants> (Accessed 2 March 2022).

Moore, K. L., Persaud, T., & Torchia, M. G. (2020). Development of eyes and ears. In: K. L. Moore, T. Persaud, & M. G. Torchia (Eds.), *The developing human* (pp. 395–413). Philadelphia, PA: Elsevier.

Morrow, A. L., & Newburg, D. S. (2019). Human milk oligosaccharide. In: J. Neu, & B. Poindexter (Eds.), *Gastroenterology and nutrition: neonatology questions and controversies* (3rd ed., pp. 43–57). Philadelphia, PA: Elsevier.

Munn, A. C., Newman, S. D., Mueller, M., Phillips, S. M., & Taylor, S. N. (2016). The impact in the United States of the Baby-Friendly Hospital Initiative on early infant health and breastfeeding outcomes. *Breastfeeding Medicine*, *11*(5), 222–230. doi: 10.1089/bfm.2015.0135.

Ng, E., & Loewy, A. D. (2018). Guidelines for vitamin K prophylaxis in newborns. *Paediatrics and Child Health*, *23*(6), 394–397. doi: 10.1093/pch/pxy082.

Niela-Vilen, H., Axelin, A., & Flacking, R. (2020). The golden hour in Finnish birthing units – an ethnographic study. *Midwifery, 89*, 102793.

Paladine, H. L., Blenning, C. E., & Strangas, Y. (2019). Postpartum care: an approach to the fourth trimester. *American Family Physician*, *100*(8), 485–491.

Paller, A. S., & Mancini, A. J. (2022). Cutaneous disorders of the newborn. In: A. S. Paller & A. J. Mancini (Eds.), *Paller and Mancini – Hurwitz clinical pediatric dermatology* (6th ed., pp. 11–41.e15). St Louis, MO: Elsevier. doi: 10.1016/B978-0-323-54988-2.00011-3.

Papautsky, E. L., & Koenig, M. D. (2021). A mixed-methods examination of inpatient breastfeeding education using a human factors perspective. *Breastfeeding Medicine, 16*(12), 947–955. doi: 10.1089/bfm.2021.0087.

Parks, E. P., Shaikhkhalil, A., Sainath, N. N., Mitchell, J. A., Brownell, J. N., & Stallings, V. A. (2020). Feeding healthy infants, children, and adolescents. In: R. M. Kliegman, J. W. St Geme, N. J. Blum, S. S. Shah, R. C. Tasker, & K. M. Wilson (Eds.), *Nelson textbook of pediatrics* (21st ed., pp. 321–331.e321). Philadelphia, PA: Elsevier.

Peaker, M., & Wilde, C. J. (1996). Feedback control of milk secretion from milk. *Journal of Mammary Gland Biology and Neoplasia, 1*(3), 307–315.

Pereira-da-Silva, L., Virella, D., & Fusch, C. (2019). Nutritional assessment in preterm infants: a practical approach in the NICU. *Nutrients*, *11*(9), 1999. doi: 10.3390/nu11091999.

Piña-Garza, J. E., & James, K. C. (2019). Disorders of the visual system. In: J. E. Piña-Garza & K. C. James (Eds.), *Fenichel's clinical pediatric neurology* (8th ed., pp. 313–325). Philadelphia, PA: Elsevier.

Psaila, K., Foster, J. P., Pulbrook, N., & Jeffery, H. E. (2017). Infant pacifiers for reduction in risk of sudden infant death syndrome. *Cochrane Database of Systematic Reviews,* 4(4), CD011147. doi: 10.1002/14651858.CD011147.pub2.

Queensland Government. (2017). Infant formula feeding. <http://conditions.health.qld.gov.au/HealthCondition/condition/8/31/325/infant-formula-feeding> (Accessed 2 March 2022).

Ribeiro, K., Fernandes Assunção, D., Maia Amorim, N. C., & de Oliveira, P. G. (2022). Vitamin E nutrition in pregnancy and the newborn infant. In: R. A. Polin, S. H. Abman, D. H. Rowitch, W. E. Benitz, & W. W. Fox (Eds.), *Fetal and neonatal physiology* (6th ed., pp. 295–302.e293). Philadelphia, PA: Elsevier.

Rosen-Carole, C., & Stuebe, A. M. (2022). Practical management of the nursing "dyad". In: R. A. Lawrence & R. M. Lawrence (Eds.), *Breastfeeding: a guide for the medical profession* (9th ed., pp. 206–246). Philadelphia, PA: Elsevier.

Sachan, R., Srivastava, H., Srivastava, S., Behera, S., Agrawal, P., & Gomber, S. (2021). Use of point of care quality improvement methodology to improve newborn care, immediately after birth, at a tertiary care teaching hospital, in a resource constraint setting. *BMJ Open Quality*, *10*(suppl 1), e001445. doi: 10.1136/bmjoq-2021-001445.

Safari, K., Saeed, A. A., Hasan, S. S., & Moghaddam-Banaem, L. (2018). The effect of mother and newborn early skin-to-skin contact on initiation of breastfeeding, newborn temperature and duration of third stage of labor. *International Breastfeeding Journal, 13*, 32. doi: 10.1186/s13006-018-0174-9.

Sarnat, H. B. (2022). Development of olfaction and taste in the human fetus and neonate. In: R. A. Polin, S. H. Abman, D. H. Rowitch, W. E. Benitz, & W. W. Fox (Eds.), *Fetal and neonatal physiology* (9th ed., pp. 1455–1464.e1453). Philadelphia, PA: Elsevier.

Say, B., Simsek, G. K., Canpolat, F. E., & Oguz, S. S. (2018). Effects of pacifier use on transition time from gavage to breastfeeding in preterm infants: a randomized controlled trial. *Breastfeeding Medicine, 13*(6), 433–437. doi: 10.1089/bfm.2018.0031.

Schmuke, A. D. (2018). Current practices and cultural variations in umbilical cord care. *International Journal of Childbirth Education*, *33*(2), 18–20.

Seery, A. (2021). Normal infant feeding. In: R. D. Kellerman & D. P. Rakel (Eds.), *Conn's current therapy 2021* (pp. 1276–1283). Philadelphia, PA: Elsevier.

Sehgal, A., Allison, B. J., Miller, S. L., Polglase, G. R., McNamara, P. J., & Hooper, S. B. (2021). Impact of acute and chronic hypoxia–ischemia on the transitional circulation. *Pediatrics, 147*(3), e2020016972. doi: 10.1542/peds.2020-016972.

Sharma, D., Sharma, P., & Shastri, S. (2017). Golden 60 minutes of newborn's life. Part 2: term neonate. *Journal of Maternal, Fetal and Neonatal Medicine, 30*(22), 2728–2733. doi: 10.1080/14767058.2016.1261399.

Shchelochkov, O. A., & Venditti, C. P. (2020). An approach to inborn errors of metabolism. In: R. M. Kliegman, J. W. St Geme, N. J. Blum, S. S. Shah, R. C. Tasker, & K. M. Wilson (Eds.), *Nelson textbook of pediatrics* (21st ed., pp. 688–695. e681). Philadelphia, PA: Elsevier.

Smith, J. P., & Forrester, R. (2021). Association between breastfeeding and new mothers' sleep: a unique Australian time use study. *International Breastfeeding Journal, 16*(1), 7. doi: 10.1186/s13006-020-00347-z.

Smith, R. W., & Colpitts, M. (2020). Pacifiers and the reduced risk of sudden infant death syndrome. *Paediatrics and Child Health, 25*(4), 205–206. doi: 10.1093/pch/pxz054.

Sontag, M. K., Miller, J. I., McKasson, S., Sheller, R., Edelman, S., Yusuf, C., et al. (2020). Newborn screening timeliness quality improvement initiative: impact of national recommendations and data repository. *PloS One*, *15*(4), e0231050.

Sperhake, J., Jorch, G., & Bajanowski, T. (2018). The prone sleeping position and SIDS. Historical aspects and possible pathomechanisms. *International Journal of Legal Medicine, 132*(1), 181–185. doi: 10.1007/s00414-017-1749-5.

Tanyeri-Bayraktar, B., Bayraktar, S., Hepokur, M. & Güzel Kıran, G. (2019). Comparison of two different doses of sucrose in pain relief. *Pediatrics International, 61*: 797–801. doi: 10.1111/ped.13914.

Taylor, J. A., Wright, J. A., & Woodrum, D. (2018). Newborn nursery care. In: C. A. Gleason, & S. E. Juul (Eds.), *Avery's diseases of the newborn* (10th ed., pp. 312–331.e316). Philadelphia, PA: Elsevier.

Thompson, J. M. D., Tanabe, K., Moon, R. Y., Mitchell, E. A., McGarvey, C., Tappin, D., et al. (2017). Duration of breastfeeding and risk of SIDS: an individual participant data meta-analysis. *Pediatrics, 140*(5). doi: 10.1542/peds.2017-1324.

Turney, J., Lowther, A., Pyka, J., & Fields, W. (2019). Delayed newborn first bath and exclusive breastfeeding rates. *Nursing for Women's Health, 23*(1), 31–37.

UNICEF UK. (2016). UNICEF UK Baby Friendly Initiative info sheet: *Responsive feeding–supporting close and loving relationships.* <https://www.unicef.org.uk/babyfriendly/wp-content/uploads/sites/2/2017/12/Responsive-Feeding-Infosheet-Unicef-UK-Baby-Friendly-Initiative.pdf> (Accessed 2 March 2022).

Walters, D. D., Phan, L. T. H., & Mathisen, R. (2019). The cost of not breastfeeding: global results from a new tool. *Health Policy and Planning, 34*(6), 407–417. doi: 10.1093/heapol/czz050.

Warren, S., Midodzi, W. K., Allwood Newhook, L.-A., Murphy, P., & Twells, L. (2020). Effects of delayed newborn bathing on breastfeeding, hypothermia, and hypoglycemia. *Journal of Obstetric, Gynecologic and Neonatal Nursing, 49*(2), 181–189. doi: 10.1016/j.jogn.2019.12.004.

Wickham, S. (2020). Seven things every parent needs to know about vitamin K. <https://www.sarawickham.com/articles-2/information-about-vitamin-k/> (Accessed 2 March 2022).

World Health Organization (WHO). (2021). Breastfeeding. <https://www.who.int/health-topics/breastfeeding#tab=tab_2> (Accessed 2 March 2022).

World Health Organization (WHO)/UNICEF (2017) and updated in 2018: Promoting baby-friendly hospitals. <https://www.who.int/activities/promoting-baby-friendly-hospitals> (Accessed 2 March 2022).

CHAPTER 3

NEONATAL ASSESSMENT

TRUDI MANNIX AND VICTORIA KAIN

Learning objectives

After reading this chapter you will be able to:

- demonstrate an understanding of how perinatal history is linked to findings from the neonatal physical examination
- perform physical and neurological examinations, using a systematic cephalocaudal approach, interpreting both normal and abnormal characteristics
- coordinate neonatal management with the multidisciplinary team based on examination findings, while sharing information with the parents and involving them in all aspects of their baby's care
- identify the different neonatal classifications, based on maturity and growth, with a knowledge of implications for practice in each group.

Key words, terms and abbreviations

extremely low birthweight (ELBW)
gestational diabetes mellitus (GDM)
intrauterine growth restriction (IUGR)
low birthweight (LBW)
selective serotonin reuptake inhibitor (SSRI)
small for gestational age (SGA)
teratogens
very low birthweight (VLBW)

INTRODUCTION

Physical examination of the newborn is a vital component of neonatal care, as subsequent findings help to guide management and ongoing care. The neonatal nurse/ midwife is in the unique position of being able to perform the examination and interpret data using a systematic head-to-toe (cephalic–caudal) approach, considering information obtained from the perinatal history, along with assessment of growth and maturity. This chapter offers an insight into the various perinatal issues that may impact on the neonate's health, development and wellbeing, in addition to providing a general introduction to the physical and neurological examination (detailed information about normal and aberrant findings can be located in the comprehensive tables). The physical examination of the neonate is important for the family as it offers the opportunity for the neonate's capacity for interaction, however limited, to be assessed (Fig. 3.1). If further investigation is required, parents are fully involved in the decision-making process and the appropriate multidisciplinary specialists are integrated into the ongoing care. Further discussion occurs around the various classifications of the neonate, their implication for practice, with a focus on **intrauterine growth restriction (IUGR)** and the methods used to determine gestational age, which is especially useful if the mother's dates are uncertain.

THE IMPACT OF PERINATAL HISTORY ON THE GROWING FETUS

Complex interactions between the fetal and maternal systems during pregnancy are designed to promote normal growth and development, with efficient gas exchange and optimal nutrient transfer by the placenta as required (Parrettini et al., 2020). The proper formation of the organs (organogenesis) early in pregnancy is necessary for a healthy neonatal outcome. During this critical period of development, the fetus is vulnerable to noxious exposures, such as maternal diseases, trauma, infections, chemicals, drugs and other environmental **teratogens**. Depending on the nature of the exposure, the fetus may be affected in the short term but often there can be lasting consequences (Woo et al., 2020).

It is essential that the neonatal clinician is able to anticipate the newborn's needs with a sound knowledge of the perinatal history, so that physical findings are validated. Informed decisions for ongoing care, considering the wishes and needs of the family, can therefore be undertaken (Australian College of Neonatal Nursing (ACNN), 2019; Neonatal Nurses College Aotearoa (NNCA), 2015). The following sections provide an overview of the maternal influences and environmental factors that may impact on the development of the fetus.

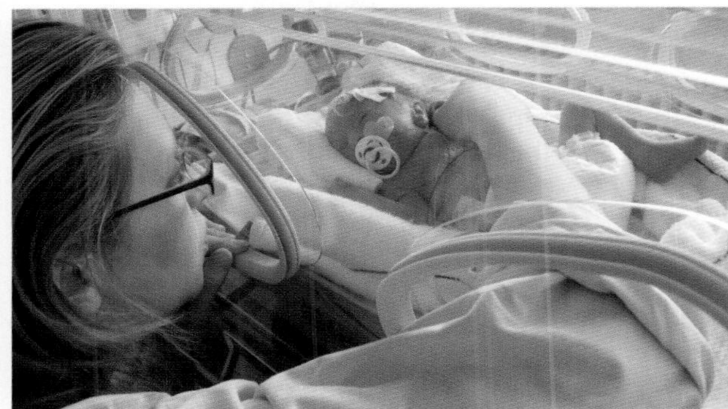

FIGURE 3.1 **A mother with her preterm infant**
Source: iStockphoto/metinkiyak.

MATERNAL DISEASE

Diabetes

The incidence of diabetes, including **gestational diabetes mellitus (GDM)**, is increasing globally because of its link to obesity (Woo et al., 2020). GDM increases the risk for poor maternal and neonatal outcomes, with the mother predisposed to preeclampsia, kidney and vascular disease and a high rate of caesarean section. Potential consequences seen in the neonate include **low birthweight (LBW)**, macrosomia, birth trauma and metabolic, cardiovascular and neurological disorders (Woo et al., 2020). Its prevalence is higher in Australian and New Zealander Indigenous populations, with studies demonstrating that maternal and neonatal outcomes are worse for those who are disadvantaged, of lower socioeconomic status and in a minority group (Power et al., 2021).

Hypertension

Four categories of hypertension in pregnancy have been described: chronic, gestational, preeclampsia (a hypertensive disease specific to pregnancy) and preeclampsia superimposed on chronic hypertension (Kenner & Lott, 2019). Hypertension causes vasoconstriction of the uteroplacental circulation, which reduces placental perfusion. Growth restriction, being born **small for gestational age (SGA)** and a potential risk of stillbirth should be anticipated (Kenner & Lott, 2019). Severe pregnancy-induced hypertension can lead to HELLP syndrome, whereby the mother presents with **h**aemolysis, **e**levated **l**iver enzymes, **l**ow **p**latelets and impaired renal function, with emergent birth necessary regardless of gestational age (Woo et al., 2020).

Infection

Viral infections in the mother are well-known teratogens, which can have devastating effects on the fetus (Cornish et al., 2020). Manifestations include chorioretinitis, sensorineural hearing loss, seizures, cerebral calcification, hepatosplenomegaly, thrombocytopenia, jaundice and rash, with a high chance of severe anaemia-induced fetal demise from maternal parvoviral infection.

Group B streptococcus (GBS) is the most prevalent bacterial infection, resulting in respiratory distress and overwhelming sepsis (Woo et al., 2020). Up to 15% of pregnant women carry GBS in the vagina, with prolonged rupture of membranes (PROM) and maternal pyrexia being associated with a higher risk of infection (Dai et al., 2019).

Sexually transmitted infections can cause poor reproductive health outcomes for the mother, with inflammatory pelvic disease and infertility common, while untreated syphilis leads to cardiovascular and neurological complications in the neonate (Griffiths et al., 2020). Notification rates for both chlamydia and gonorrhoea have increased in Australia over the past decade, with most cases being seen in young Aboriginal and Torres Strait Islander females (Griffiths et al., 2020).

Maternal medications and SSRIs

The Food and Drug Administration (FDA) warned in 2005 that using paroxetine, a **selective serotonin reuptake inhibitor (SSRI)**, during the first trimester of pregnancy could raise the risk of cardiac abnormalities. The link between maternal SSRI usage during pregnancy and congenital abnormalities in neonates has been the topic of much debate since then. Gao et al. (2018) conducted a comprehensive analysis of the links between the use of SSRIs during early pregnancy and the risk of congenital abnormalities, with a focus on potential confounding by indication.

The evidence points to a low incidence of congenital abnormalities and refutes the idea that SSRIs have a significant teratogenic effect. Making decisions on whether to continue or stop taking SSRIs during pregnancy should be done with caution (Gao et al., 2018).

REFLECTION

Consider how much you know about the management of mental illness in pregnancy. How well equipped are you to anticipate reactions in the newborn to maternal medications used to treat these problems? Do you need to improve your knowledge in this area?

Obesity

The prevalence of obesity is increasing in Australia and New Zealand, with approximately 50% of pregnant women in 2013 being either overweight (BMI >25) or obese (BMI >30), and these percentages are rising (Royal Australian and New Zealand College of Obstetricians and Gynaecologists (RANZCOG), 2017). The problems experienced include thromboembolism, gestational diabetes, preeclampsia, shoulder dystocia, postpartum haemorrhage, instrumental birth and caesarean section, with a higher incidence of congenital anomalies, prematurity, macrosomia, stillbirth and childhood obesity being observed (Australian Institute of Health and Welfare (AIHW), 2021).

SOCIAL BEHAVIOURS

Substance abuse

Australia and New Zealand have a pervading problem of alcohol, tobacco and illicit drug use, with recent data showing increasing trends for those in their childbearing years (RANZCOG, 2018). Alcohol crosses the placenta easily and is responsible for the features of fetal alcohol syndrome, skeletal anomalies and both behavioural and developmental problems, while vasoconstriction to the placenta caused by smoking usually culminates in a low birthweight pregnancy (Woo et al., 2020). The illicit drugs used in Australia and New Zealand include heroin, cannabis, cocaine, amphetamines and, more recently, ice/crystal methamphetamine, the use of which is on the rise (RANZCOG, 2018). Cannabis can impair fetal growth and negatively impact on neurobehaviour, as can stimulants (Roncero et al., 2020). 'Tell-tale' signs of substance abuse may include 'meth mouth', with severe tooth decay and gingivitis, which can trigger preterm delivery, preeclampsia and GDM (Hartnett et al., 2016). Methadone has been an acceptable pharmaceutical therapy for opiate dependency in pregnancy over the past four decades and is considered to be relatively safe for the fetus, although it is also associated with neonatal abstinence syndrome (Smith et al, 2020). (Refer to Chapter 20 for further information.)

Domestic violence

In Australia and New Zealand, domestic violence is a significant public health and social issue, with women being more at risk during pregnancy and in early parenthood (AIHW, 2020). Studies have shown that susceptibility to abuse includes violence prior to pregnancy, low educational status, unplanned pregnancy and low socioeconomic ranking (Gardner & Voos, 2020). Domestic violence is any behaviour that causes physical, psychological or sexual abuse within an intimate partnership. It is acknowledged as a serious risk factor for poor pregnancy outcomes, with physical injury resulting in neonatal death, preterm labour, low birthweight neonates, intrauterine growth restriction and other neonatal problems. Substance abuse is common in this group (Records, 2015). The prevalence of domestic violence is greater in rural Australia and among Indigenous communities, with rates much higher than in non-Indigenous populations (Douglas & Fitzgerald, 2018). The time around pregnancy may afford obstetric health professionals opportunities for counselling if abuse is suspected, bearing in mind that the sensitive nature of this topic and the different cultural beliefs and customs is paramount.

EVIDENCE-BASED PRACTICE RESEARCH 3.1

Pregnancy, delivery and the postpartum period are all affected by violence against women (VAW). Domestic violence (DV) or intimate partner violence (IPV) may rise during pregnancy and have an impact on the birthing process.

Consideration of violence throughout pregnancy and the postpartum period is critical to providing women with the best possible treatment. Therefore, midwives need to be able to recognise women who are suffering from VAW (Siller et al., 2022).

The inclusion of VAW screening in midwifery has been linked to midwives acting as active advocates of the women under their care. To the woman, this means being intuitive, helpful and empowering as a midwife (Siller et al., 2022).

The professional role of midwives in actively protecting women is crucial. Neglecting DV detection during pregnancy, childbirth and puerperium can result in DV being silenced.

Maternal age

The age of pregnant women at either end of the spectrum (<19 and >35 years) has been linked with neonatal and maternal morbidities (Von Kohler, 2015). In the adolescent, hypertensive disorders with preterm and low birthweight are more likely, whereas the older mother may be more likely to have infertility, a Down syndrome baby, GDM, hypertension or placenta praevia (Von Kohler, 2015). Further information on all these considerations in the perinatal history is discussed in more detail in other chapters.

Having a healthy term baby is reliant on good placental function and a well mother. With the public health issues of today and more complicated maternal disease processes, the clinician is met with many challenges. Fortunately, antenatal screening technologies continue to be 'fine tuned' for accurate determination of fetal wellbeing and diagnoses. However, it is equally important for clinicians to be familiar with the maternal perinatal history.

Congenital abnormalities

Malformations and genetic conditions can be caused by chromosomal abnormalities, multifactorial disorders and abnormalities from teratogenic exposures (Matthews & Robin, 2020). Antenatal morphology scans are essential for early identification of problems. This allows time for parents to prepare themselves psychologically and for the clinician to be able to plan appropriate care (Gardner & Carter, 2020).

FAMILY-CENTRED CARE 3.1

When a baby with a congenital abnormality is born, good communication with parents as partners in the decision-making process is essential, as is being culturally aware and sensitive to the needs of our increasingly multicultural society (Gardner & Voos, 2020; NNCA, 2015 (Standard 1.5)).

PHYSICAL ASSESSMENT OF THE NEWBORN

The first assessment of the newborn is immediately after birth, with two aims: to quickly determine the adequacy of the neonate's adaptation to extrauterine life and, all being well, to follow with an unobtrusive assessment of normal physical findings and obvious defects prior to placing the newborn safely on the mother's chest for skin-to-skin contact and a breastfeed. The first complete physical assessment of the newborn is a critical event that should be performed in all newborns within the first 24 hours of life. The neonatal assessment should include a review of the duration of labour and of ruptured membranes, the mode of delivery, the neonate's gestational age and condition at birth and the need for resuscitation (McKee-Garrett, 2021). While there are specific occasions when the newborn examination is performed, periodic physical assessments are also conducted for a variety of reasons, such as when there is a deterioration in the neonate's condition, prior to discharge or transfer, and at home by the neonatal outreach team if the neonate has been sent home on a neonatal early-discharge program.

Whenever possible the neonate's parents, or at the least the mother, should be present for the assessment to meet the family-centred care principles described in both the ACNN Standards 1 and 5 (ACNN, 2019) and NNCA Standard 3 (NNCA, 2015). The neonatal nurse/midwife should communicate with the parents throughout the steps of the examination, allow them to participate and ask questions, and provide teaching as needed. If any concerns arise, the parents should be provided with reassurance and a clear plan of action. Having both parents present also provides the neonatal nurse/midwife with an opportunity to observe the level of interest they show in their baby, indicating their degree of attachment. Aside from these bonding behaviours between the parents and the baby, the clinician can observe interactions between each parent, to add to a risk assessment for child protection if concerns have been raised.

FAMILY-CENTRED CARE 3.2

When conducting the head-to-toe examination of the neonate, consider strategies to involve the parents in a meaningful way. The neonatal nurse/midwife can begin with 'Tell me about your baby' and, later in the examination, ask 'What have you observed?' to encourage interactive dialogue during the exam.

A warm environment is essential to prevent the neonate becoming cold. The room should be warm, or an overhead heat source should be used (e.g. a heating lamp or a radiant warmer). Draughts of cold air should be prevented by closing doors and windows. The neonate should be examined on a warm surface and ideally be completely undressed. A good light is important so that the examiner can see the neonate well. To begin the examination, the neonatal nurse/midwife needs to attend to hand hygiene.

The physical assessment of a neonate should proceed in an orderly fashion, beginning with observation without disturbing the neonate, then progressing from the least intrusive to the more 'hands-on' components. The neonatal nurse/midwife should aim to conduct the examination

TABLE 3.1 **Newborn examination findings prior to handling: normal and abnormal**

Observation	Normal findings	Abnormal findings
Colour	Pink with acrocyanosis (blue discoloration of the hands and feet, which is normal in the first 24 h)	Central cyanosis Plethora Jaundice Bruising Ecchymosis Pallor
Position/tone	Appropriate limb flexion according to gestational age If breech, then limbs may be extended	Hypotonia (extended and flaccid) Hypertonia (flexed and rigid) Hyper-reflexive fingers and toes when resting Opisthotonos (arching of the back) Asymmetry of the limbs
Cry	Vigorous and sustained Lessens with settling	Weak High-pitched Hoarseness or aphonia Continuous
Skin	Mild peripheral peeling Soft Vernix (see Fig. 3.2)	Widespread peeling Petechiae (rashes) Blisters
Pigmentation and skin lesions	Lanugo Naevus flammeus Mongolian blue spot Milia Erythema toxicum Harlequin line	Haemangioma Pigmented patches Meconium staining
Level of consciousness	Asleep Awake	Nonresponsive Unable to sleep

Source: adapted from Women's and Children's Health Network (2014).

quickly but thoroughly in a warm environment, while gently handling the neonate. Documentation of the assessment is essential, as is referral to a paediatrician in the case of any unusual findings in order to plan the appropriate care for the neonate and provide support for the parents.

The examination is best conducted while the neonate is in the quiet and alert state of consciousness when hunger or tiredness will not impact on the findings. The observations of the neonate's colour, position (reflecting tone), skin and level of consciousness described in Table 3.1 should be conducted prior to handling the neonate. Auscultation of heart and lung sounds is best performed next while the neonate is the most settled.

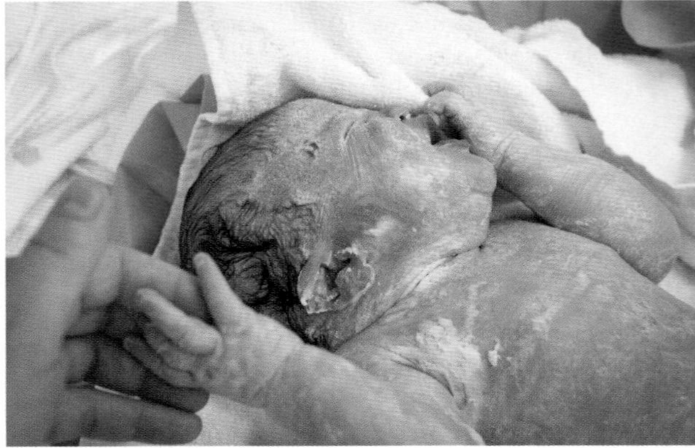

FIGURE 3.2 **Vernix**
Source: Shutterstock.com/Dave Clark Digital Photo.

The head-to-toe examination then proceeds as detailed in Table 3.2, in this order:

1. head (including size, shape, fontanelles, sutures and hair)
2. face (including eyes, ears, nose and mouth)
3. neck (including mobility, masses and clavicles)
4. chest (including shape, breast tissue, breath sounds and work of breathing)
5. heart (including heart sounds, pulses and perfusion)
6. abdomen (including shape and bowel sounds)
7. groins and umbilicus
8. genitalia
9. extremities (including feet, limbs, hands and hips).

And then turn the neonate over to examine the:

10. spine and anus.

Once the head-to-toe assessment is complete, the neurological examination should follow, including observation of the neonate's alertness, motor activity, tone, muscle strength and primitive reflexes. Table 3.3 outlines the expected findings from this examination, and deviations from normal.

As well as the head-to-toe examination, anthropometric measurements should be checked within hours of birth. Thereafter, the frequency of weight checks is determined by the gestation, postnatal age and condition of the neonate while head circumference and length are generally checked weekly. Head circumference measurement, often referred to as OFC (occipital frontal circumference), is a valuable technique for tracking and monitoring brain growth and development. The typical growth in head circumference during the first year of life is 0.9–1.0 cm/week (Pereira-da-Silva et al., 2019).

The infant's length should also increase by 1 cm a week if growth is normal. Once measurements are confirmed, they are plotted on the relevant percentile chart. Evidence and management of growth failure may be found early if these increments are measured and charted correctly. Weight, length and head circumference measurement procedures are described in Chapter 2. Assessment of gestational age tools is also described in Chapter 2.

Text continued on p. 52

TABLE 3.2 **Newborn head-to-toe examination findings: normal and abnormal**

Body part	Examination procedures	Normal findings	Abnormal findings
HEAD			
Size	Palpate Observe	Size depends on many factors – ethnic group, gestational age and growth in utero Cranial moulding or oedema of the scalp may affect the size or shape of the head, but should revert to normal within a few days of birth Normal term range head circumference is 31–38 cm	Hydrocephalus (bulging fontanelles; 'split' sutures; swollen scalp veins) Microcephaly
Shape	Palpate	Moulding Caput succedaneum	Cephalhaematoma Plagiocephaly/asynclitism Scaphocephaly Subgaleal haemorrhage
Fontanelles	Palpate	Vary in size Anterior – diamond-shaped, soft, flat and admits the tip of the small finger Posterior – triangular in shape and may be closed at birth	Bulging (raised ICP) Depressed (dehydration) Too small or too large Subgaleal haemorrhage – soft fluctuant feel, crosses suture lines and may displace ears
Sutures	Palpate	Ballotable (mobile)	Rigid and fixed, i.e. craniosynostosis Widely separated Craniotabes (usually harmless in newborns unless associated with other problems such as rickets or osteogenesis imperfecta)
Hair	Observe and palpate	Soft One colour	Low hair line Coarse hair Coloured tufts Cutis aplasia (areas of skin loss, usually only the epidermis, usually on the scalp) Overly abundant
FACE	Observe and palpate	Symmetrical	Facial palsies (after forceps application) Dysmorphic features
EYES	Observe	Position – space between eye/nose/eye = one-third each	Hypotelorism (fetal alcohol syndrome) Hypertelorism
Sclera	Observe	White and clear	Inflamed Excessive lacrimation Discoloration (jaundice) Scleral haemorrhages due to birth (should fade within days)
Pupils	Penlight test Observe	Red eye reflex – a penlight is used to shine a bright light on the lens of the eye. A clear red colour should be reflected back from the retina Pupils should react equally and constrict briskly to light Size and shape look normal Pupils are parallel	Opaque with absent red-light reflex Cataract Unequal or slow to react to light Non-parallel Brushfield spots ('speckles' on the iris, frequently seen in trisomy 21)
Eyelids	Observe	Lid oedema Eyelids may be fused in the extremely preterm neonate	Unusual slant or size Epicanthal folds Excessive oedema
Vision	Penlight test	Reacts to light with squints and blinks	Does not react to visual stimulation
EARS	Observe	Position – the pinna should be located above a line extended from the inner to outer canthus of the eye	Low-set ears Ears posteriorly rotated more than 10 degrees from the vertical axis of the head Skin tags
Shape	Observe Palpate	Curved pinna considering familial variation Patent meatus Equal	Skin tag or sinus Large, small or malformed ears Unequal

Continued

TABLE 3.2 **Newborn head-to-toe examination findings: normal and abnormal—cont'd**

Body part	Examination procedures	Normal findings	Abnormal findings
Hearing	Test (clap or formal test)	Reacts to auditory stimulus	No reaction to auditory stimulus
NOSE	Observe	Shape – may be squashed or off to one side due to birth process. This should return to normal within a few days of birth Both nares patent No discharge	Unusually thin or broad Depressed nasal bridge Choanal atresia (uni- or bilateral) Discharge
MOUTH	Observe Palpate	Movement – symmetrical	Asymmetrical
Jaw	Observe	Mandible and maxillae should fit together and open at equal angles bilaterally Asynclitism	Micrognathia
Palate	Observe Palpate	Epstein's pearls Hard and soft palate intact Gentle arch Moves with gag reflex	Cleft or high-arched palate Bifid uvula Decreased mobility
Tongue	Observe	Contained in the mouth Can protrude Loose frenulum	Large or protruding (hyperglossia) Tight frenulum
Teeth	Observe Palpate	None	Natal teeth
Mucous membranes	Observe	Epithelial pearls Pink Moist	Thrush Cysts Dry
Saliva	Observe	Manageable amount	Excessive amount causing airway obstruction
NECK	Observe Palpate	The normal neck is short	Long neck Torticollis (wry neck) Webbing Nuchal fold (excessive skin on the back of the neck)
Mobility/ movement	Palpate	Ear to shoulder and chin to shoulder	Restricted movement
Masses	Palpate	Cervical lymph nodes may be palpable	Cystic hygroma Lymphangioma
Clavicles	Palpate Observe	Symmetrical	Asymmetrical Tender to touch Crepitus
CHEST	Observe	Shape – cylindrical Symmetrical	Asymmetrical Hyper-expanded Prominent sternum Short sternum
Breast tissue	Observe Palpate	2 nipples – symmetrical and in the mid-clavicular line Space between nipples Nipple areola visible Dry or small secretions ('witch's milk')	Asymmetrical Widely spaced nipples >2 cm breast tissue Supernumerary nipples
LUNGS	Auscultate	Clear bilateral and equal breath sounds although some rales may be heard for a few hours after birth Respiratory rate <60 breaths per minute Periodic (irregular) breathing	Cough Snore Grunt Stridor Tachypnoea Apnoea Cyanosis

TABLE 3.2 **Newborn head-to-toe examination findings: normal and abnormal—cont'd**

Body part	Examination procedures	Normal findings	Abnormal findings
Effort	Observe	Effortless	Nasal flaring Retractions – intercostal, substernal, suprasternal Tracheal tug
HEART	Auscultate	Heart sounds best heard along the left sternal border Physiological murmurs may be heard in the first few days of life Heart rate 100–160 bpm Rate regular	Pathological murmurs, i.e. PDA Tachycardia (>160 bpm) Bradycardia (<100 bpm) Irregular rhythm Apex shifted to the right or left
Pulses	Palpate	Palpation of femoral pulses should be routine, whereas a more extensive cardiac examination should include palpation of axillary, palmar, brachial, radial, popliteal and posterior tibial pulses Pulses should be present bilaterally, with a regular rhythm	Irregular rhythm Weak or absent Bounding Pulse deficit (difference between heart rate counted by pulse and that counted by auscultation)
Perfusion	Palpate	Capillary refill <2 seconds Pulses palpable Warm to touch	Capillary refill >2 seconds Cool or cold peripheries Non-palpable or bounding pulses
ABDOMEN	Observe Palpate Auscultate	Shape is gently rounded Symmetrical Liver palpable (<1 finger below ribs) Bowel sounds absent at birth but, after crying and sucking, they are present within 15 minutes	Distended Scaphoid Asymmetrical Palpable mass Separation of abdominal muscles (prune belly syndrome) Gastroschisis (herniation of bowel contents through the abdominal wall – exposed bowel)
GROIN	Palpate	No masses Strong bilateral and equal femoral pulses	Mass (inguinal hernia) Diminished femoral pulses (coarctation of the aorta)
UMBILICUS	Observe	Two umbilical arteries and 1 vein Translucent in colour Wharton's jelly	Single umbilical artery Herniation of bowel contents through the cord (exomphalos) Yellow or green meconium staining Bilirubin staining
GENITALIA – MALE	Observe		Ambiguous genitalia – bifid scrotum, micropenis, cryptorchidism in a phenotypic male
Testes	Observe Palpate	2 testes in scrotal sac Equal size	Undescended testes – cryptorchidism (ectopic or arrested in the line of normal descent)
Penis and urethra	Observe Palpate	Urethral opening is at the tip and centre of the glans Foreskin complete and non-retractile Shaft straight	Hypospadias – the urethral opening is on the underside (ventral surface) of the penis Epispadias – the urethral opening is on the upper surface (dorsal surface) of the penis Chordee (penis bent downwards or upwards)
Scrotum	Observe Palpate	2 testicles in the scrotal sac	Hydrocele (fluid-filled sac surrounding a testicle causing swelling in the scrotum) Trauma (swelling and/or bruising) after breech presentation Torsion of testes (sudden onset of swelling and discoloration)

Continued

TABLE 3.2 **Newborn head-to-toe examination findings: normal and abnormal—cont'd**

Body part	Examination procedures	Normal findings	Abnormal findings
GENITALIA – FEMALE	Observe Palpate		Ambiguous genitalia – palpable gonads in a phenotypic female
Hymen	Observe	Patent hymen Hymenal tag	Imperforate hymen Labial adhesions
Labia	Observe	Labia majora cover the labia minora in term neonates In preterm neonates, the clitoris and labia minora are prominent	Fused labia
Vagina and vulva	Observe	White mucoid or scant blood discharge due to exposure to maternal oestrogen Skin tags	
EXTREMITIES			
Feet	Observe Palpate	Full range of movement Equal size Full, rounded heel 10 toes and toenails	Talipes equinovarus (foot is internally rotated at the ankle) Talipes calcaneovalgus (foot is externally rotated at the ankle) Unequal size Metatarsus adductus (the front half of the foot turns inwards) Saddle toe (Down syndrome) Rocker bottom feet Hypoplastic toenails Polydactyly (supernumerary toes) Syndactyly (webbing or fusion of toes) Amputations Amniotic bands
Limbs	Observe Palpate	Equal, symmetrical and spontaneous movement Full range of movement Equal size and length	Asymmetrical reflex movement Unequal size or length Joint contractures (arthrogryposis) Amelia/phocomelia
Palms of hands, fingers and fingernails	Observe	Multiple creases 10 fingers and 10 fingernails	Single palmar crease (simian) Hypoplastic fingernails Polydactyly (supernumerary fingers) Syndactyly (webbing or fusion of fingers) Amputations Amniotic bands
Hips	Palpate	Ortolani's and Barlow's manoeuvre (may be accredited skills) Symmetrical Full range of movement	Congenital subluxation or dislocation of the hip Decreased range of movement
SPINE	Observe Palpate	Symmetrical Smooth contours	Curvatures Masses (cystic) Sacral cleft or dimple Pigmented patches Tufts of hair Myelo/meningocele
ANUS	Observe	Patent Active tone	Imperforate anus Inactive and patulous

ICP, intracranial pressure; PDA, patent ductus arteriosus.

Source: adapted from Women's and Children's Health Network (2014).

TABLE 3.3 **Newborn neurological examination findings: normal and abnormal**

Criterion	Normal findings	Abnormal findings
Alertness	Depends on time after birth and whether the neonate is hungry or sleepy	Persistent irritability Lethargy
Motor activity	Movements should be smooth, symmetrical and spontaneous	Jitteriness Tremors Convulsions
Tone	Moderate flexion in all limbs at rest Minimal head lag in the pull-to-sit manoeuvre	Hypotonia Hypertonia Extension of limbs Pronounced head lag in the pull-to-sit manoeuvre
Muscle strength	Should be able to weight bear on lower extremities when held in a vertical position with feet on a flat surface	Unable to weight bear while attempting to stand
Primitive reflexes		
Moro (startle)	One hand is placed under the neonate's shoulders and the other hand under the head. The head is suddenly dropped several centimetres – the normal response is symmetrical extension and abduction of the arms and opening of the hands, followed by flexion of the upper extremities in an embracing movement. An audible cry may follow	Asymmetry may suggest a brachial palsy or bone injury Adduction is variable in neonates at 34 weeks Extension is seen at 30 weeks No response at 26 weeks
Palmar/plantar grasp	Pressure is applied to the palm of the hand or sole of the foot and fingers/toes then flex The finger closing and clinging provides a firm and equal grasp If traction is applied, the neonate should be able to lift their head	The reflex appears at 28 weeks' gestation and is well established at 32 weeks' gestation – an absent, diminished or exaggerated response is abnormal
Tonic neck reflex	The head is turned to one side and the arm and leg on that side extend	Reflex should appear at 35 weeks' gestation – an absent, diminished or exaggerated response is abnormal
Stepping reflex	The neonate is held upright and leaning forwards slightly, with feet gently touching a flat surface. The neonate's feet will move in an alternating stepping motion	Reflex should appear at 35–36 weeks' gestation – an absent, diminished or exaggerated response is abnormal
Rooting reflex	Tactile stimulation is provided to the cheek at the corner of the mouth. The neonate should turn their head towards the stimulation and open the mouth (Fig. 3.3)	Reflex should appear at 28 weeks' gestation and is well established at 32–34 weeks' gestation – an absent, diminished or exaggerated response is abnormal
Doll's eye	The head is rotated from side to side. As the head is moved to the right or left, the eyes should move in the opposite direction	The reflex is well established at 24–25 weeks. If abnormal, the eyes will move in the same direction as the head
Babinski reflex	This reflex occurs when the sole of the neonate's foot is firmly stroked. The big toe should move upwards or towards the top surface of the foot. The other toes should fan out This is a normal reflex in children up to 2 years old, but may disappear as early as 12 months	An absent Babinski reflex may indicate central nervous system disease or spinal cord damage

Source: adapted from Women's and Children's Health Network (2014).

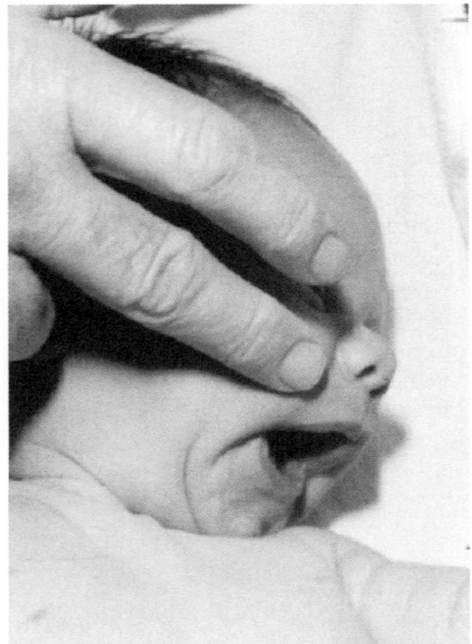

FIGURE 3.3 **Rooting reflex**
Source: Howlett and Jangaard (2011).

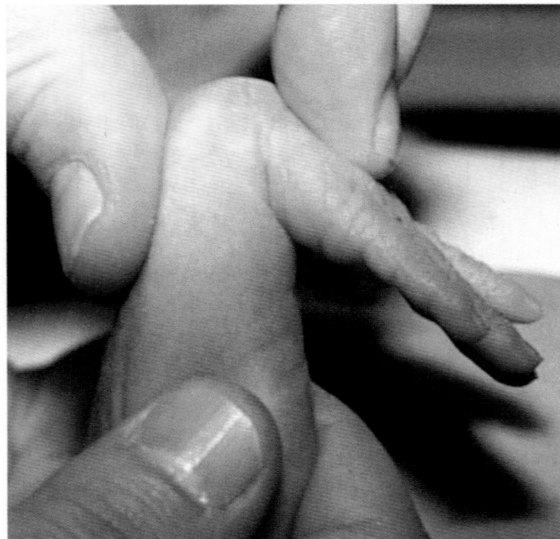

FIGURE 3.4 **Neonatal square window**
Source: Zitelli et al. (2018).

EVIDENCE-BASED PRACTICE RESEARCH 3.2

The PEA POD is an air displacement plethysmography (ADP) system that uses whole-body densitometry to determine the body composition (fat and fat-free mass) in neonates weighing between 1 and 8 kg. A systematic review was undertaken by Wiechers et al. in 2019 on neonatal body composition determined by air displacement plethysmography in healthy infants. The findings revealed different body composition results for infants from different ethnic or socioeconomic backgrounds. Gender seemed to affect not only bodyweight, but also body composition. Increasing postnatal age during the first 96 postnatal hours did not seem to affect body fat percentage, but was associated with decreased bodyweight at assessment and fat-free mass.

Neuromuscular maturation

Posture

As maturation progresses, the fetus gradually assumes increasing passive flexor tone that proceeds in a centripetal direction, with lower extremities slightly ahead of upper extremities. To test posture, the neonate is placed supine and the examiner waits until the neonate settles into a relaxed posture. Hip flexion without adduction results in the frog-leg position as depicted in posture 3 in Fig. 3.6a. Hip adduction accompanying flexion is depicted by the acute angle at the hips in posture 4. The figure that most closely depicts the neonate's preferred posture is selected.

Square window

Wrist flexibility and/or resistance to extensor stretching are responsible for the resulting angle of flexion at the wrist. The examiner straightens the neonate's fingers and applies gentle pressure to the back of the hand, close to the fingers. From extremely preterm to post term, the resulting angle between the palm of the neonate's hand and forearm is estimated as: >90 degrees, 90 degrees, 60 degrees, 45 degrees, 30 degrees or 0 degrees. As wrist flexibility and resistance to extensor stretching are responsible for the resulting angle of flexion at the wrist, preterm neonates will demonstrate less flexion at the wrist than term infants (Fig. 3.4).

Arm recoil

This test focuses on passive flexor tone of the biceps muscle by measuring the angle of recoil following very brief extension of the upper extremity.

With the neonate lying supine, the examiner places one hand beneath the neonate's elbow for support. Taking the neonate's hand, the examiner briefly sets the elbow in flexion, then momentarily extends the arm before releasing the hand. The angle of recoil to which the forearm springs back into flexion is noted, and the appropriate square is selected on the score sheet. The extremely preterm neonate will not exhibit any arm recoil.

Popliteal angle

With the neonate's thigh pressed against the abdomen, the popliteal angle can be measured by moving the foot gently towards the head until you meet resistance. At this point, measure the angle behind the knee in the popliteal area. Term neonates are less flexible, with about a 90-degree angle. With very preterm neonates, the leg straightens to a 180-degree angle.

Scarf sign

The scarf sign is assessed by grasping the neonate's hand and attempting to cross the arm over the body at the neck. The arms of term neonates meet resistance before crossing

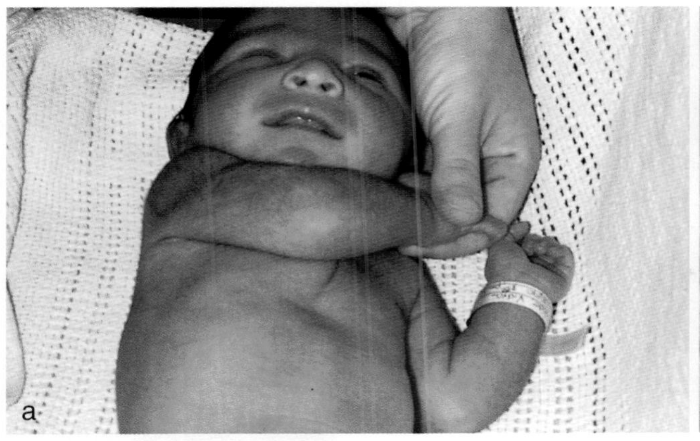

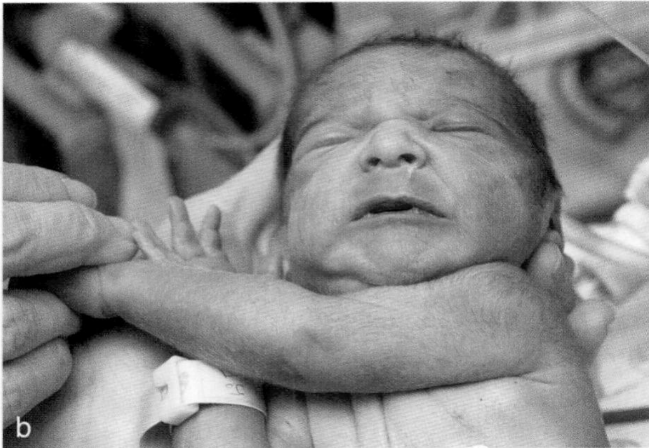

FIGURE 3.5 **Neonatal scarf sign**
Source: Zitelli et al. (2018).

the midline, while preterm neonates cross the elbow past the midline (Fig. 3.5).

Heel to ear

Assess heel to ear by raising the neonate's heel towards the head in an attempt to bring the foot to the ear. It is important not to raise the buttocks off the surface. Stop when you meet resistance and measure the degree of extension of the leg. With preterm neonates, you will come close to touching the heel to the ear, while you will meet resistance almost immediately with term neonates.

Refer to Fig. 3.6 for a summary of neuromuscular maturity scores.

Physical maturation

Skin

The skin ranges from translucent and friable in preterm neonates to leathery, cracked and wrinkled in post-term neonates. Assess the skin for transparency, cracks, veins, peeling and wrinkles.

Lanugo

Extremely preterm neonates will not have lanugo. During the middle of the third trimester, most fetuses have plentiful lanugo. Closer to term, this body hair begins to thin. Term neonates have very little, and it is nearly absent in post-term neonates (Fig. 3.7).

Plantar surface

Inspect the plantar surface of the foot for creases. Term neonates have creases over the entire plantar surface, whereas the creases of a preterm neonate range from absent to faint red markings.

Breasts

Inspect the breasts to assess the size of the breast bud in millimetres and the development of the areola. Preterm neonates will lack developed breast tissue. Term neonates have a raised to a full areola with breast buds that are 3–10 mm in diameter.

Eye/ear

The eye/ear assessment is an analysis of the ear cartilage and shape of the pinna. The pinna is less curved in preterm neonates, whereas term neonates have a well-curved pinna with firm cartilage. Determine ear recoil by folding the pinna down and assessing how quickly it returns to its previous position. Very preterm neonates may have fused eyelids. Score the degree of fusion for these neonates.

Genitals

Observe the genitals for physical maturity. With males, the testes usually descend near term and rugae (ridges or folds) are visible on the scrotum. Palpate the testes to determine whether they have descended and note the rugae. With extreme prematurity, the scrotum is flat and smooth.

With female neonates at term, the labia majora are larger than the clitoris and the labia minora. Preterm female neonates have a prominent clitoris and small labia minora. Base your scores on the degree of development of the labia.

Refer to Fig. 3.8 for a summary of physical maturity scores.

CLASSIFICATION ACCORDING TO GROWTH AND MATURITY

Fetal growth should increase six-fold between 22 and 40 weeks' gestation, with the mother, the placenta and the fetus all playing their part (Fenton & Kim, 2013). Maternal disease, placental dysfunction and problems occurring in the fetus can all interfere with growth and/or interrupt the length of normal gestation. The newborn's birthweight and gestational age are the determinants used in categorising the newborn into a specific group, which helps to guide management and allows for prognostic predictions in the long term (Gomella, 2020).

a. Posture

SIGN	NEURO-MUSCULAR MATURITY SCORE							SIGN SCORE
	–1	0	1	2	3	4	5	
Posture								

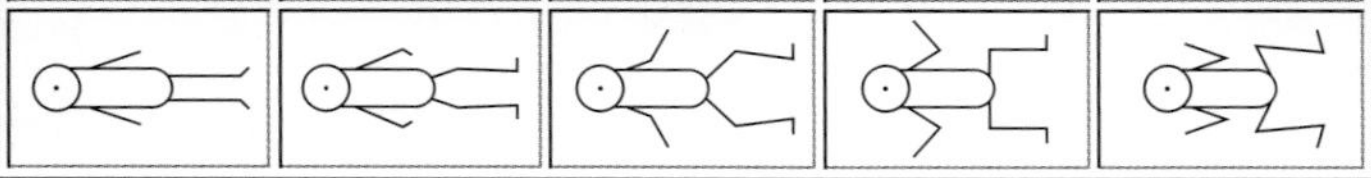

b. Square window

SIGN	NEURO-MUSCULAR MATURITY SCORE							SIGN SCORE
	–1	0	1	2	3	4	5	
Square Window	>90°	90°	60°	45°	30°	0°		

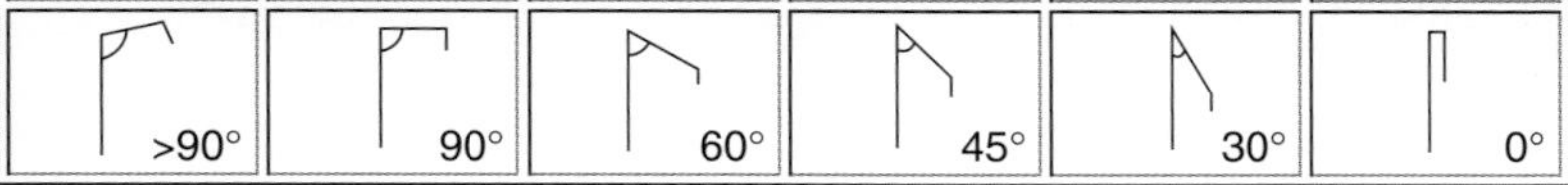

c. Arm recoil

SIGN	NEURO-MUSCULAR MATURITY SCORE							SIGN SCORE
	–1	0	1	2	3	4	5	
Arm Recoil		180°	140°–180°	110°–140°	90°–110°	<90°		

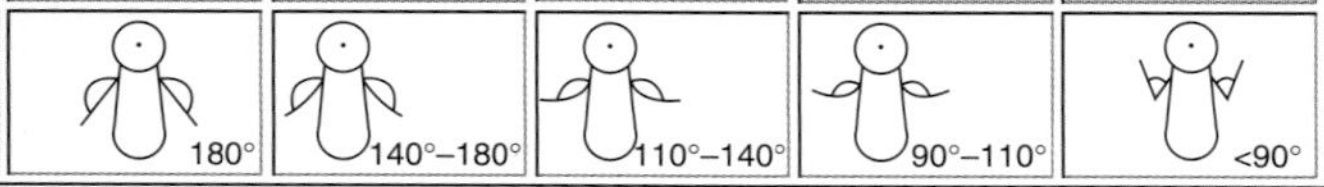

d. Popliteal angle

SIGN	NEURO-MUSCULAR MATURITY SCORE							SIGN SCORE
	–1	0	1	2	3	4	5	
Popliteal Angle	180°	160°	140°	120°	100°	90°	<90°	

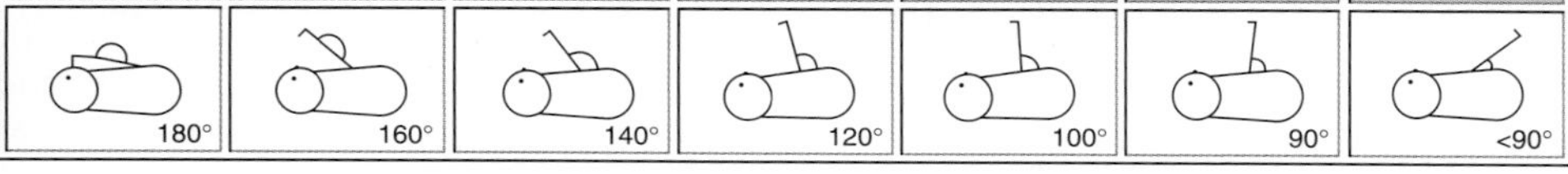

e. Scarf sign

SIGN	NEURO-MUSCULAR MATURITY SCORE							SIGN SCORE
	–1	0	1	2	3	4	5	
Scarf Sign								

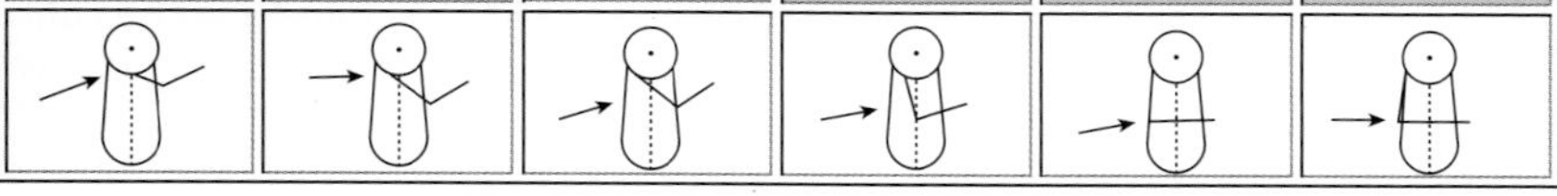

f. Heel to ear

SIGN	NEURO-MUSCULAR MATURITY SCORE							SIGN SCORE
	–1	0	1	2	3	4	5	
Heel To Ear								

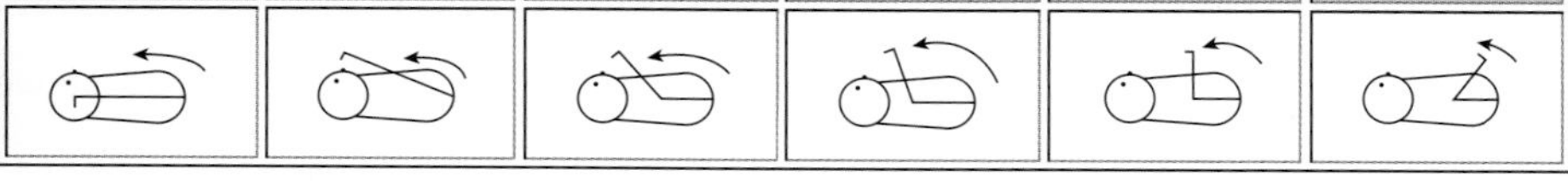

FIGURE 3.6 **Neuromuscular maturity scores**

Source: Ballard et al. (1991).

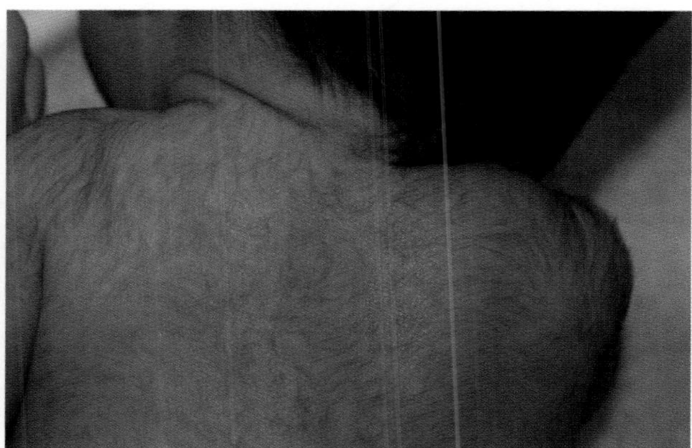

FIGURE 3.7 **Lanugo**
Source: Lam and Wong (2015).

medical centre were included in a population-based cohort analysis. Post-term and term deliveries (37 0/7 to 41 6/7 weeks' gestation) were compared in terms of pregnancy and perinatal outcomes. Preterm births, gestational age unknown, congenital abnormalities and multiple pregnancies were all ruled out.

The analysis covered 226,918 deliveries during the course of the study period. Ninety-five percent (n = 217,544) were term, while 4.1% (n = 9374) were post term. Oligohydramnios, macrosomia, meconium-stained amniotic fluid, shoulder dystocia, low Apgar scores and hysterectomy were all more common in post-term pregnancies. Post-term delivery was found to involve higher rates of adverse perinatal outcomes and was independently associated with significant perinatal mortality.

Source: Or Maoz et al. (2019).

Neonatal classifications

Neonatal classification is based on gestational age, birthweight and both gestational age and birthweight together, with further subdivision to encompass all categories for the neonate (see Table 3.4) (Lissauer & Steer, 2013).

GESTATIONAL AGE AND BIRTHWEIGHT

An SGA neonate's birthweight is below the tenth percentile for gestational age, meaning that 10 out of 100 newborns (10%) have a lower weight-for-age in the reference population. Unfortunately, the definition of SGA does not distinguish between a constitutionally small newborn (i.e. when the newborn is small because of genetics or ethnicity; symmetrically growth restricted) and an infant who is growth restricted and small. Fetal growth restriction and intrauterine growth restriction (IUGR) are interchangeable descriptors for a fetus that has not reached its full growth potential, owing to genetic or environmental factors. Similarly, LGA neonates, defined as having a birthweight greater than the 90th percentile for age, have a 10% higher weight-for-age than their counterparts (Divon, 2017). These definitions are useful as they pinpoint the neonates 'at risk' for poor outcomes, without having to base decisions on birthweight alone (Mari, 2021). The IUGR fetus and neonate can encounter several adverse effects, largely as a result of the impact of placental insufficiency, but are also highly susceptible to fetal and/or perinatal demise (Mari, 2021). LGA babies may have obstetric complications and long-term metabolic effects that increase the propensity for obesity and insulin resistance (Mandy, 2017).

EVIDENCE-BASED PRACTICE RESEARCH 3.3

In 2019, a study investigated whether post-term pregnancy (≥42 0/7 weeks' gestation) increased the risk for adverse perinatal outcome. All singleton deliveries in a tertiary

Brain sparing in intrauterine growth restriction

As discussed, IUGR is most commonly caused by placental insufficiency. In a phenomenon known as 'brain sparing', the fetus can adapt its circulation to preserve oxygen and nutrient supply to the brain. Although brain sparing may not completely avoid the negative effects of IUGR on brain development, it is linked to better neurological outcomes than when no brain sparing occurs. Furthermore, even after controlling for various confounding factors, mortality is higher in IUGR with symmetric growth. The Doppler pulsatility index (PI) in the middle cerebral artery (MCA) can be used to detect brain sparing prenatally; PI is reduced by decreased cerebral resistance, which permits a greater fraction of the cardiac output to perfuse the brain. However, this compensatory blood distribution process might become 'decompensatory' if the increased brain blood flow and blood volume become harmful in and of themselves. Understanding when and how relative cerebral blood flow changes from a compensatory to a decompensatory response is critical for developing the most effective interventions and therapies (Fleiss et al., 2019).

EVIDENCE-BASED PRACTICE RESEARCH 3.4

Symmetrical and asymmetrical growth restriction

A prospective study was undertaken to identify the various risk factors for IUGR and its neonatal outcome (Manandhar et al., 2018). Depending on the onset or aetiology of a given prenatal injury, IUGR has been classified as symmetrical or asymmetrical: symmetrical, in which the newborn is symmetrically small and has normal head to abdomen and femur to abdomen ratio, and asymmetrical, in which head and long bones are spared compared with the abdomen and viscera. In the case of symmetrical growth restriction, an early insult could cause a reduction in cell quantity and size, as well as a corresponding reduction in

a. Skin

SIGN	PHYSICAL MATURITY SCORE							SIGN SCORE
	−1	0	1	2	3	4	5	
Skin	sticky, friable, transparent	gelatinous, red, translucent	smooth pink, visible veins	superficial peeling &/or rash, few veins	cracking, pale areas, rare veins	parchment, deep cracking, no vessels	leathery, cracked, wrinkled	

b. Lanugo

SIGN	PHYSICAL MATURITY SCORE							SIGN SCORE
	−1	0	1	2	3	4	5	
Lanugo	none	sparse	abundant	thinning	bald areas	mostly bald		

c. Plantar surface

SIGN	PHYSICAL MATURITY SCORE							SIGN SCORE
	−1	0	1	2	3	4	5	
Plantar surface	heel-toe 40–50mm: −1 <40mm: −2	>50mm no crease	faint red marks	anterior transverse crease only	creases ant. 2/3	creases over entire sole		

d. Breast

SIGN	PHYSICAL MATURITY SCORE							SIGN SCORE
	−1	0	1	2	3	4	5	
Breast	imperceptible	barely perceptible	flat areola no bud	stippled areola 1–2mm bud	raised areola 3–4mm bud	full areola 5–10mm bud		

e. Eye and Ear

SIGN	PHYSICAL MATURITY SCORE							SIGN SCORE
	−1	0	1	2	3	4	5	
Eye / Ear	lids fused loosely: −1 tightly: −2	lids open pinna flat stays folded	sl. curved pinna; soft; slow recoil	well-curved pinna; soft but ready recoil	formed & firm instant recoil	thick cartilage ear stiff		

f. Genitals – male

SIGN	PHYSICAL MATURITY SCORE							SIGN SCORE
	−1	0	1	2	3	4	5	
Genitals (male)	scrotum flat, smooth	scrotum empty, faint rugae	testes in upper canal, rare rugae	testes descending, few rugae	testes down, good rugae	testes pendulous, deep rugae		

g. Genitals – female

SIGN	PHYSICAL MATURITY SCORE							SIGN SCORE
	−1	0	1	2	3	4	5	
Genitals (female)	clitoris prominent & labia flat	prominent clitoris & small labia minora	prominent clitoris & enlarging minora	majora & minora equally prominent	majora large, minora small	majora cover clitoris & minora		

FIGURE 3.8 **Physical maturity scores**

Source: Ballard et al. (1991).

TABLE 3.4 **Neonatal classifications**

Classification	Gestational age
Preterm	Born before the 37th completed week of gestation
Term	Born from the 38th to the 42nd week of gestation
Late preterm	Born between 34 and 36 + 6 weeks of gestation
Post term	Born >42 weeks
	Birthweight
Extremely low birthweight (ELBW)	Birthweight <1000 g
Very low birthweight (VLBW)	Birthweight <1500 g
LBW	Birthweight <2500 g
	Gestational age and birthweight
SGA	Small for gestational age
AGA	Appropriate for gestational age
LGA	Large for gestational age

Source: Lissauer and Steer (2013).

head and body size. A late-pregnancy injury may result in asymmetrical growth restriction due to preferential shunting of oxygen and nutrients to the brain, allowing normal brain and head growth, also known as brain sparing. The fetal brain is usually quite large, while the liver is quite small. Asymmetrical fetuses are considered to be preferentially protected from the full effects of growth restriction owing to brain-sparing effects.

This study found that symmetrical neonates were proportionately small, but asymmetrical neonates showed disproportionately lagging abdominal growth. An early injury in the case of symmetrical growth restriction could result in a reduction in cell number and size. Symmetrically grown IUGR neonates had low risks for perinatal asphyxia and neonatal hypoglycaemia, as well as lowered growth measurements from early in pregnancy, a normal ponderal index, brain growth proportional to body size and a normal ponderal index.

Asymmetrical growth restriction was associated with late-onset growth failure, a low ponderal index, brain sparing and an increased risk of prenatal hypoxia and neonatal hypoglycaemia. Asymmetrical prenatal growth restriction indicated highly disordered growth, but symmetrical growth restriction indicated normal, genetically determined reduced height more likely.

In this study, 7 (11.66%) of the participants had no signs of IUGR after delivery, while the remaining 53 (88.33%) had IUGR, of which 9 (16.98%) were symmetrical IUGR and 44 (83.01%) were asymmetrical IUGR.

Source: Manandhar et al. (2018).

Figs 3.9 to 3.11 depict various percentile charts that demonstrate growth. Fig. 3.9 shows normal growth percentiles for a male neonate who was born with measurements on the 50th percentile, which were appropriate for his gestational age of 33 weeks.

Brain sparing is demonstrated in the percentiles of a female neonate at 37 weeks' gestation in Fig. 3.10, where a defect in the hypertrophic stage of growth has led to compensatory head growth and, subsequently, a head circumference that is normal while other measurements are below the 50th percentile. This late-onset insult results in *less cytoplasm in each cell*, rather than a reduction in the number of cells in the organism and leads to *asymmetrical* growth failure.

The final graph (Fig. 3.11) shows the growth parameters of a male neonate born at 39 weeks' gestation whose insult to growth occurred in early pregnancy, resulting in a reduction in the size in all measurements. Brain sparing is not demonstrated in this late-onset insult to hyperplasia, which results in a reduction in the *number* of cells in the organism and leads to *symmetrical* growth failure.

Despite improved survival rates for **extremely low birthweight (ELBW)** and **very low birthweight (VLBW)** neonates with advancements in both obstetric and neonatal care, this group is still at a higher risk of psychomotor disabilities, behavioural issues and neurodevelopmental problems, the last being attributed to nutritional deficits and suboptimal growth (Mandy, 2021). The generally accepted goal in preterm neonates is for growth to continue at intrauterine rates (Fenton & Kim, 2013). However, delayed feeding, resulting in inadequate protein and calorie intake, in addition to being born into an early extrauterine life which physiologically they are not equipped for, contributes to faltering weight (Andrews et al., 2019). Hence, the cornerstone of neonatal care nowadays is focused on improving their postnatal growth, by individualising nutritional support, optimising health and monitoring growth closely (Rochow et al., 2016).

GROWTH CHARTS

All neonates should be assessed for maturity and patterns of growth at birth. Anthropometric measurements are plotted on a population-based neonatal growth chart (Andrews et al., 2019). Currently, the charts available in clinical practice are fetal growth curves and postnatal growth charts for term neonates (Ohuma & Altman, 2019). Lubchenco et al. developed the first one in 1963. Since then, numerous intrauterine charts have been published, the most commonly used being the following: Usher and McLean (1969); Niklasson et al. (1991); Beeby et al. (1996), who suggested periodic review to account for different multicultural groups and changing socioeconomic circumstances; Fenton (2003), who updated data from Babson and Benda's 'fetal–infant growth graph' to include preterm neonates at 22 weeks' gestation; and the gender specific growth curves of

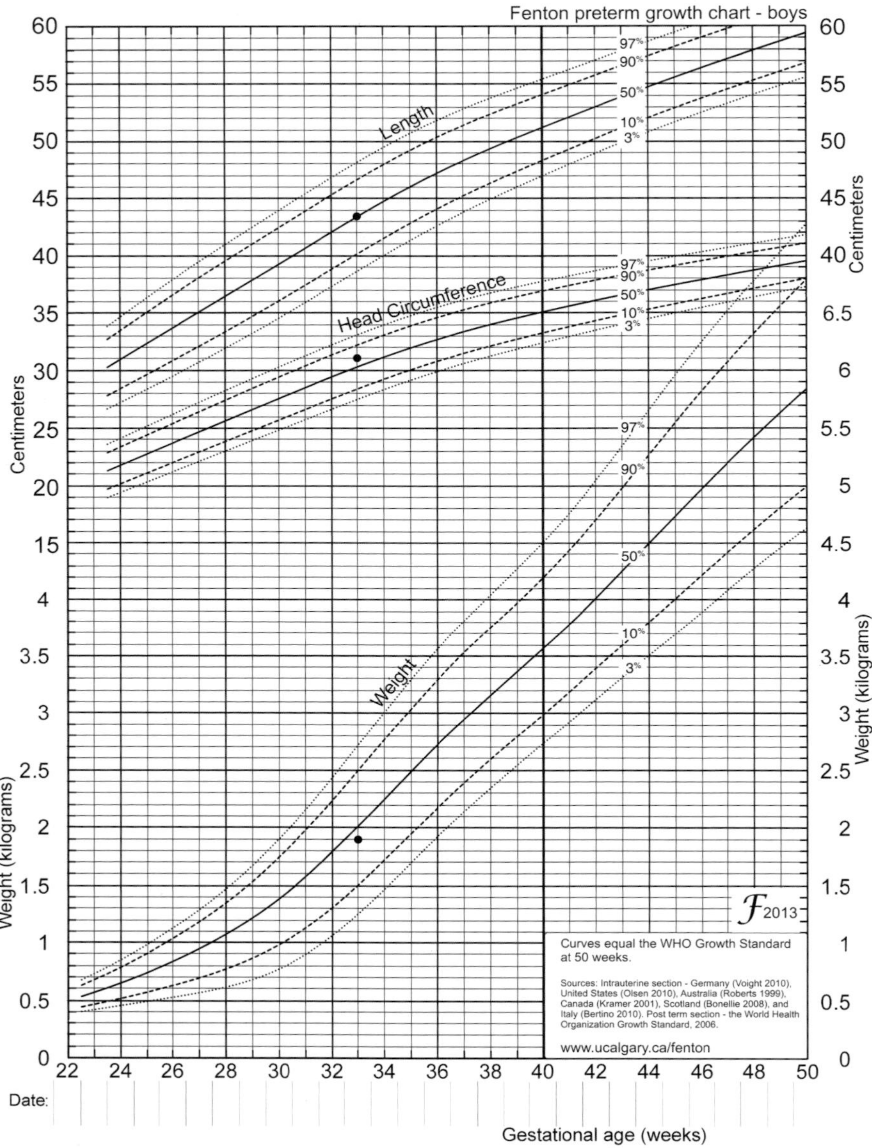

FIGURE 3.9 **Average gestational age percentiles for a male infant at 33 weeks' gestation**

Source: adapted from Fenton and Kim (2013).

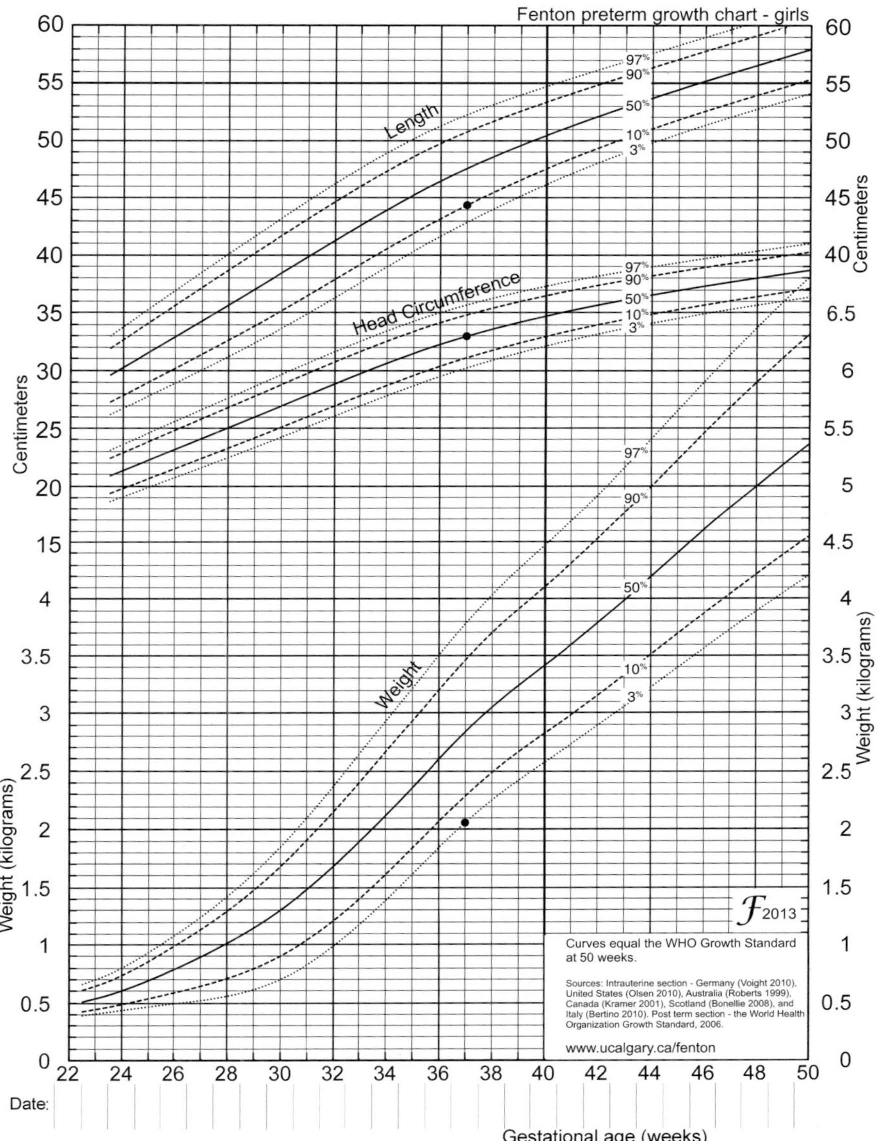

FIGURE 3.10 **Percentiles for an IUGR female infant born at 37 weeks' gestation with brain sparing and asymmetrical growth failure**

Source: adapted from Fenton and Kim (2013).

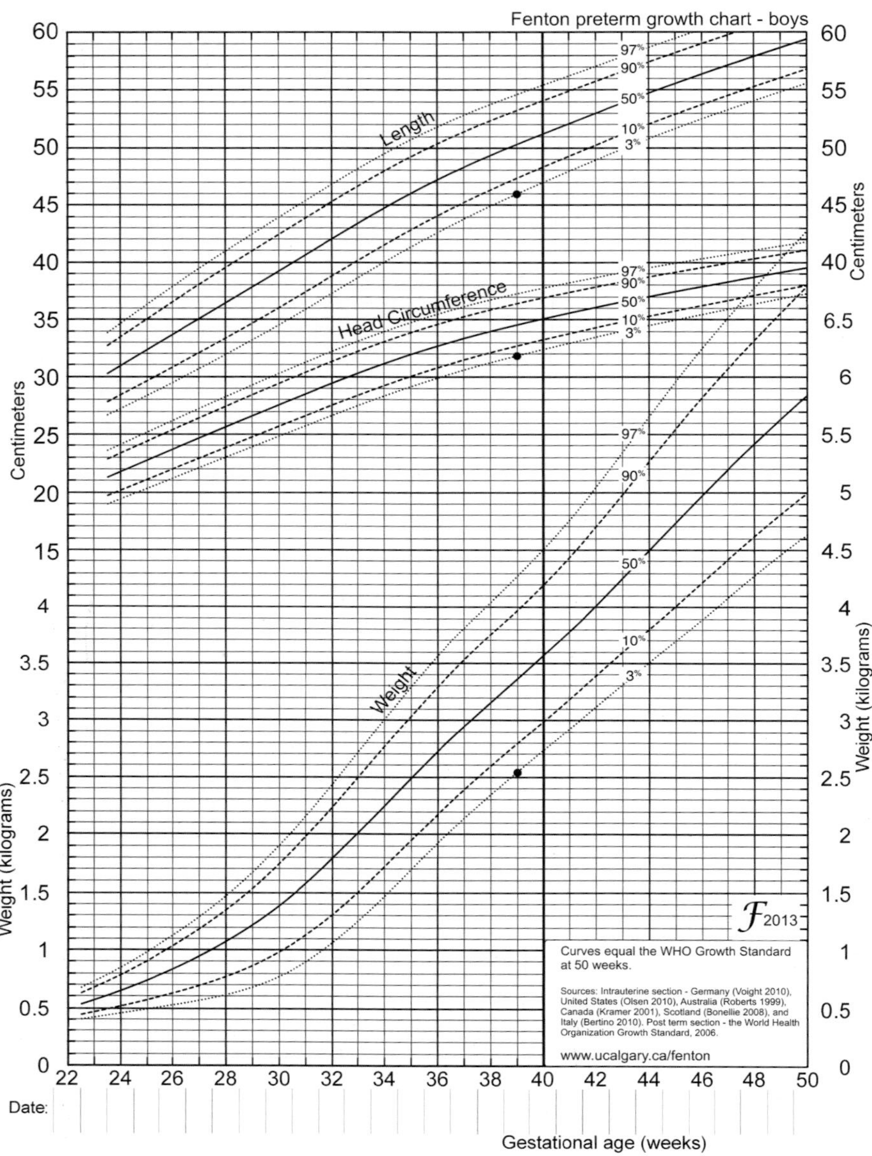

FIGURE 3.11 **IUGR without brain sparing in a 39 weeks' gestation newborn male**

Source: adapted from Fenton and Kim (2013).

Olsen et al. (2010). Ultrasound imaging of the fetus, with accurate maternal dating and history, has formed the foundation for these (Andrews et al., 2019). See Figs 3.12 and 3.13 for female and male intrauterine growth charts, respectively.

Two types of growth chart are available: the 'growth reference' chart, which describes actual growth from birth, and the 'growth standard' chart, reflecting growth in a population, selected from a group of healthy individuals (Bertino et al., 2012). In 2006, the World Health Organization (WHO) published the first international growth standard, replacing the growth references, developed by the Centers for Disease Control and Prevention (CDC), and these were adopted as the 'gold standard' (Rabner et al., 2014). In 2013, Fenton and Kim, however, integrated their charts with those recommended by WHO, with measurements being plotted for exact age rather than completed week, a trend used in previous growth curves, hence affecting their interpretation (Fenton & Kim, 2013).

Customised growth charts were developed to account for maternal influences on fetal growth, such as height, weight, ethnicity and parity, with the supposition that there would be differences between constitutional and pathological smallness (Tudehope et al., 2012). Studies showed that SGA newborns seem to be at risk of long-term adverse cardio-metabolic health outcomes, irrespective of the use of customised or population birthweight charts, and therefore the implementation of customised charts to select neonates at risk of long-term adverse outcomes cannot be recommended (Erkamp et al., 2019).

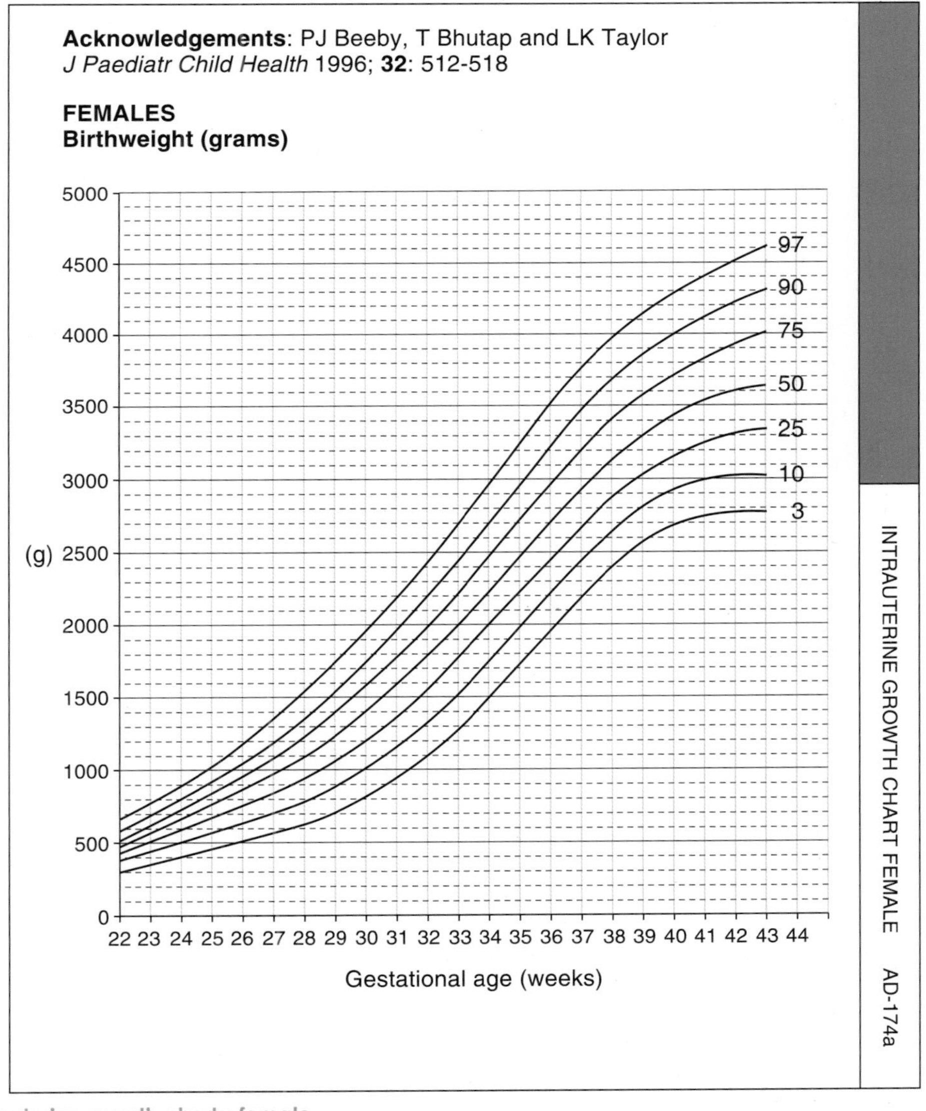

FIGURE 3.12 **Intrauterine growth charts: female**

Source: Beeby et al. (1996).

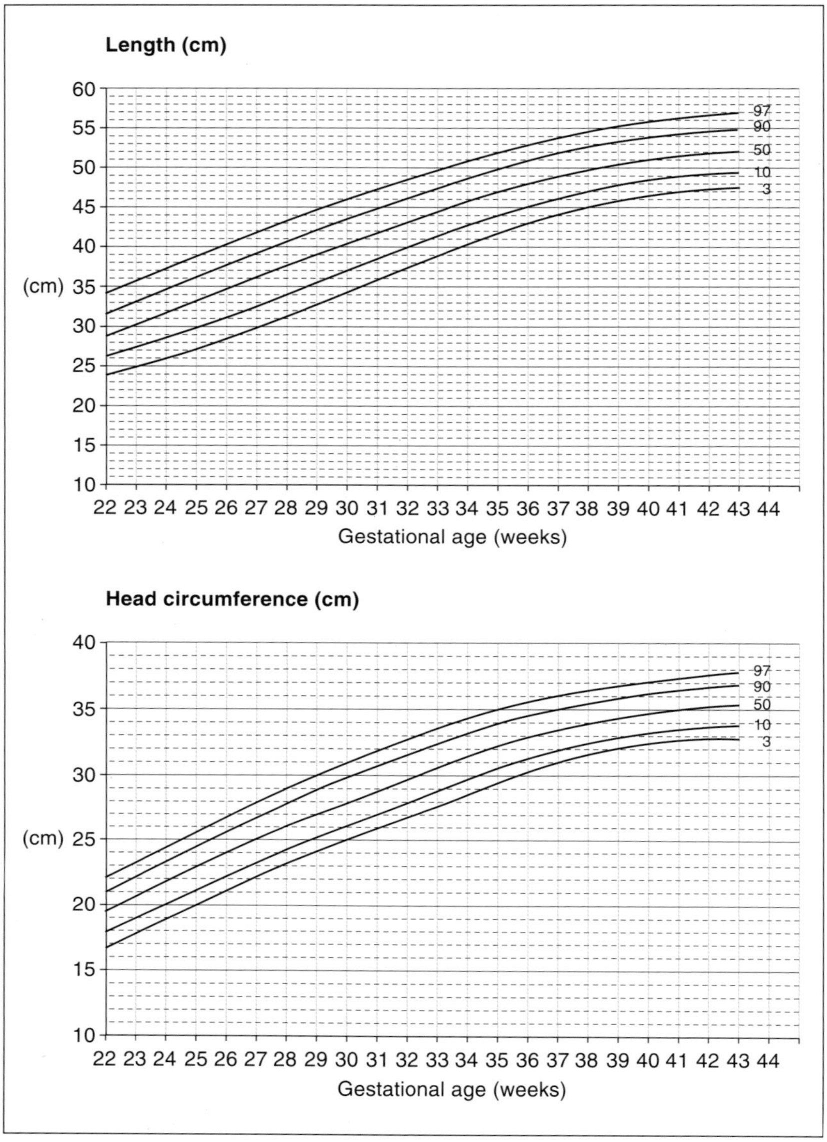

Length (cm)

Gestational age (weeks)

Head circumference (cm)

Gestational age (weeks)

FIGURE 3.12 cont'd

CASE STUDY

3.1

Luke was born at 33 weeks' gestation, weighing 1.02 kg. On examination after birth, the neonatal nurse/midwife found that he had a single umbilical artery. Luke's head circumference and length were 26 cm and 36 cm, respectively. This symmetrical growth failure was assumed to be the result of deficient placental blood flow due to the single artery, as described in the systematic review conducted by Kim et al. (2017).

Luke's Apgar scores were 7^1 and 9^5 and he was admitted to the neonatal special care unit for observation. His initial axillary temperature was 36°C and he was placed in a prewarmed incubator. An early blood glucose level revealed hypoglycaemia, and a 10% glucose infusion was commenced. Luke had low oxygen saturations on admission to the neonatal unit, which normalised after a few hours in 23% oxygen.

The neonatal nurse/midwife admitting Luke to the neonatal unit uses their knowledge of the potential problems of growth-restricted neonates such as Luke to plan his care and anticipate his needs.

1. Explain the significance of a single umbilical artery.
2. Explain why neonates with IUGR are susceptible to hypoglycaemia.

CLINICAL PRACTICE 3.1

INTERGROWTH-21st project is an internationally multicentric, multiethnic population-based project formed to develop new gender-specific 'prescriptive' standards for optimal fetal, preterm and neonatal growth (Villar et al., 2019). The INTERGROWTH-21st project has many interconnected studies with the primary goal of evaluating growth, health, nutrition and neurodevelopment in children aged less than 14 weeks to 2 years, using the same conceptual framework as the WHO Multicentre Growth Reference Study. Prescriptive international criteria for fetal growth, neonatal size and body composition and postnatal growth of preterm newborns have been developed by the Project. The standards are an excellent addition to the existing WHO Child Growth Standards, demonstrating that participants in the INTERGROWTH-21st Project were carefully chosen to meet WHO prescriptive requirements for optimal human growth and neurodevelopment.

Based on WHO-recommended techniques, investigations have found strong evidence of skeletal growth similarities from early pregnancy to 2 years of age. However, beyond skeletal growth, the scientific concept of commonalities across non-isolated groups needs to be expanded to include indices of neurodevelopment. This is warranted because cognition, attentional issues, language, motor and visual capacity are core human capabilities, and their development reflects the brain's rapid growth and maturation, which happens in tandem with fetuses and newborns' rapid skeletal growth.

Source: Villar et al. (2019).

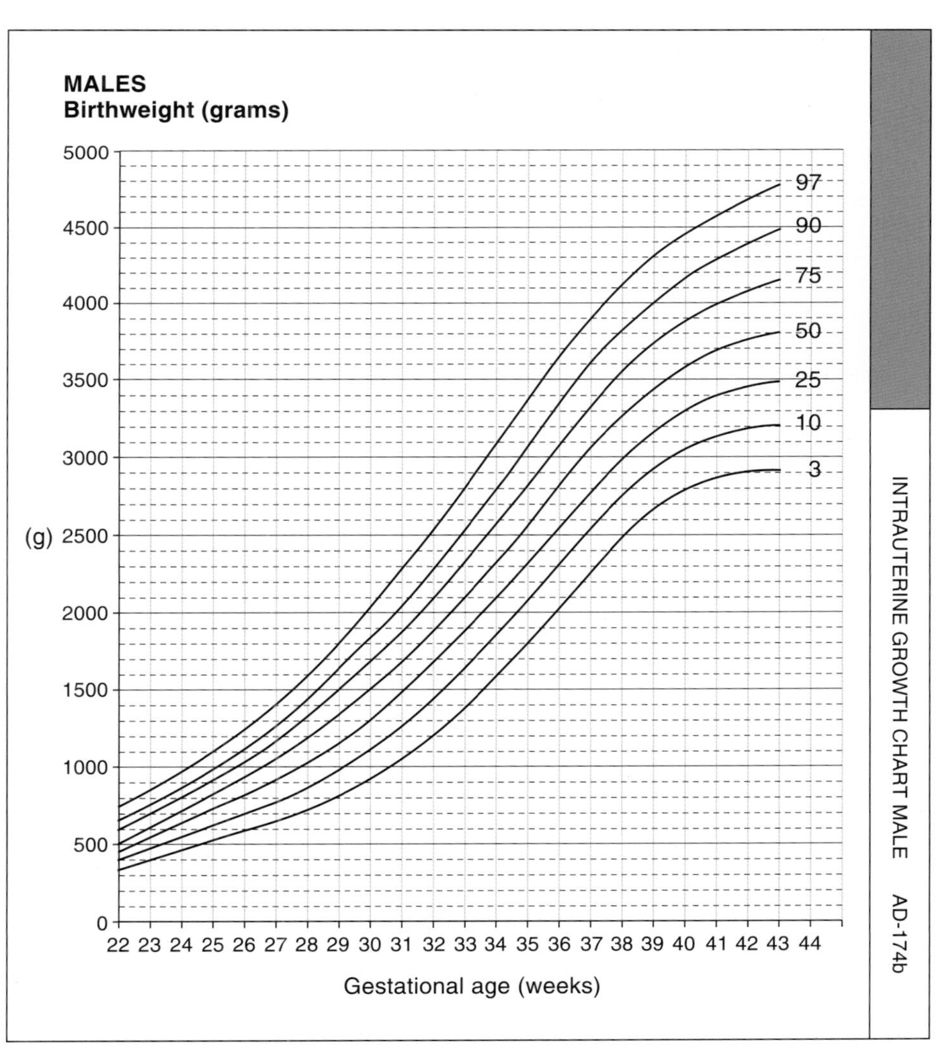

FIGURE 3.13 **Intrauterine growth charts: male**

Source: Beeby et al. (1996).

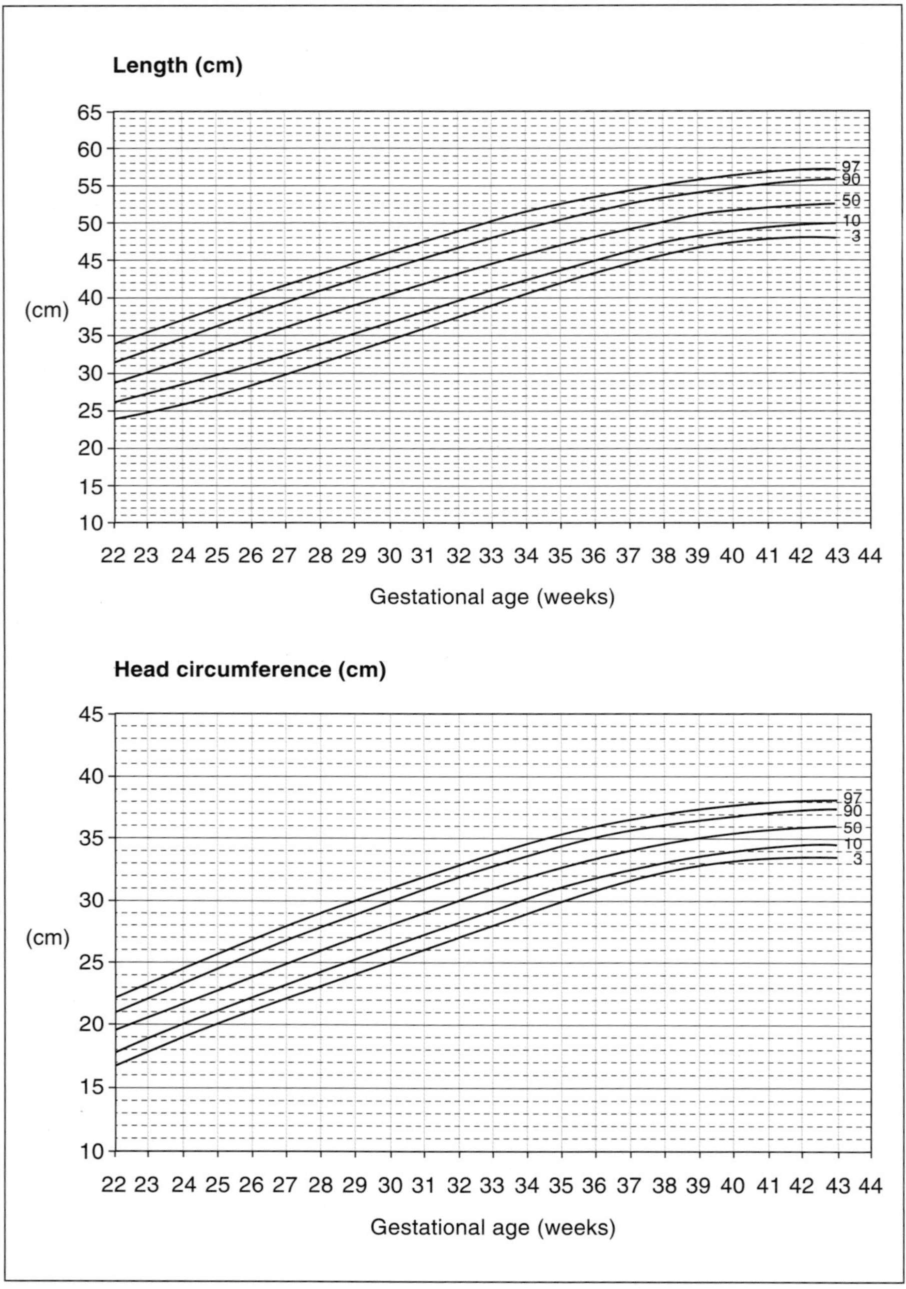

FIGURE 3.13 cont'd

CONCLUSION

This chapter has described the potential impacts that elements of family and maternal medical and obstetric history can have on the neonate. Gestational age assessment can provide important clues about the neonate's capacity for self-regulation, communicating with care givers and feeding. The neonatal nurse/midwife is perfectly placed to conduct the comprehensive newborn examination, having gained substantial evidence-based information, and should then communicate the findings to both the parents and the multidisciplinary team. With the ongoing acquisition of knowledge and repeated practice, these skills should become more familiar and well honed.

Recommended Reading

Gardner, S., & Niermeyer, S. (2020). Immediate newborn care after birth. In: S. L. Gardner, B. S. Carter, M. E. Enzman-Hines, & S. Niermeyer (Eds.), *Merenstein and Gardner's handbook of neonatal intensive care* (9th ed., Ch 5, pp. 93–136). St Louis, MO: Elsevier.

References/Acknowledgements

Andrews, E. T., Ashton, J. J., Pearson, F., Beattie, R. M., & Johnson, M. J. (2019). Early postnatal growth failure in preterm infants is not inevitable. *Archives of Disease in Childhood. Fetal and Neonatal Edition, 104*(3), F235–F241.

Australian College of Neonatal Nursing (ACNN). (2019). *Australian standards for neonatal nurses* (4th ed.). Camperdown, NSW: ACNN. <https://www.acnn.org.au/resources/resources/ACNN-Standards-for-Practice-4th-Ed.pdf> (Accessed 13 March 2022).

Australian Institute of Health and Welfare (AIHW). (2020). Health impacts of family, domestic and sexual violence. <https://www.aihw.gov.au/reports/australias-health/health-impacts-family-domestic-and-sexual-violence> (Accessed 3 March 2022).

Australian Institute of Health and Welfare (AIHW). (2021). *Australia's mothers and babies*. <https://www.aihw.gov.au/getmedia/bba093ef-a623-4cfd-818b-1bb5af9f0d20/Australia-s-mothers-and-babies.pdf.aspx?inline=true> (Accessed 3 March 2022).

Ballard, J., Khoury, J., Wedig, K., Wang, L., Eilers-Walsman, B., & Lipp, R. (1991). New Ballard Score expanded to include extremely premature infants. *Journal of Pediatrics, 119*(3), 417–423. doi: 10.1016/s0022-3476(05)82056-6.

Beeby, P. J., Bhutap, T., & Taylor, L. K. (1996). New South Wales population-based birthweight percentile charts. *Journal of Paediatrics and Child Health, 32*, 512–518.

Bertino, E., Coscia, A., Arslanoglu, S., Cresi, F., Sabatino, G., Guiliani, F., et al. (2012). Critical appraisal of different anthropometric charts to evaluate postnatal growth of preterm infants. *Journal of Biological Regulators and Homeostatic Agents, 26*(3 suppl), 5–7.

Cornish, E. F., Filipovic, I., Åsenius, F., Williams, D. J., & McDonnell, T. (2020). Innate immune responses to acute viral infection during pregnancy. *Frontiers in Immunology, 11*, 572567. doi: 10.3389/fimmu.2020.572567.

Dai, W., Zhang, Y., Xu, Y., Zhu, M., Rong, X., & Zhong, Q. (2019). The effect of group B streptococcus on maternal and infants' prognosis in Guizhou, China. *Bioscience Reports, 39*(12), BSR20191575. doi: 10.1042/BSR20191575.

Divon, M. Y. (2017). Fetal growth restriction: screening and diagnosis. In: D. Levine & V. A. Barss (Eds.), *UpToDate*. Waltham, MA: UpToDate. <http://www.uptodate.com/contents/fetal-growth-restriction-diagnosis> (Accessed 3 March 2022).

Douglas, H., & Fitzgerald, R. (2018). The domestic violence protection order system as entry to the criminal justice system for Aboriginal and Torres Strait Islander people. *International Journal for Crime, Justice and Social Democracy, 7*(3), 41.

Erkamp, J. S., Jaddoe, V. W. V., Mulders, A. G. M. G. J., et al. (2019). Customized versus population birth weight charts for identification of newborns at risk of long-term adverse cardio-metabolic and respiratory outcomes: a population-based prospective cohort study. *BMC Medicine, 17*, 186. doi: 10.1186/s12916-019-1424-4.

Fenton, T. R. (2003). A new growth chart for preterm babies: Babson and Benda's chart updated with recent data and a new format. *BMC Pediatrics, 3*, 1–10. doi: 10.1186/1471-2431-3-13.

Fenton, T. R., & Kim, J. H. (2013). A systematic review and meta-analysis to revise the Fenton growth chart for preterm infants. *BMC Pediatrics, 13*, 59.

Fleiss, B., Wong, F., Brownfoot, F., Shearer, I. K., Baud, O., Walker, D. W., et al. (2019). Knowledge gaps and emerging research areas in intrauterine growth restriction-associated brain injury. *Frontiers in Endocrinology, 10*, 188. doi: 10.3389/fendo.2019.00188. [Review.]

Gao, S. Y., Wu, Q. J., Sun, C., Zhang, T. N., Shen, Z. Q., Liu, C. X., et al. (2018). Selective serotonin reuptake inhibitor use during early pregnancy and congenital malformations: a systematic review and meta-analysis of cohort studies of more than 9 million births. *BMC Medicine, 16*(1), 205. doi: 10.1186/s12916-018-1193-5.

Gardner, S. L., & Carter, B. S. (2020). Grief and perinatal loss. In: S. L. Gardner, B. S. Carter, M. E. Enzman-Hines, & S. Niermeyer (Eds.), *Merenstein and Gardner's handbook of neonatal intensive care* (9th ed., Ch 30, pp. 1096–1140). St Louis, MO: Elsevier.

Gardner, S. L., & Voos, K. (2020). Families in crisis: theoretical and practical considerations. In: S. L. Gardner, B. S. Carter, M. E. Enzman-Hines, & S. Niermeyer (Eds.), *Merenstein and Gardner's handbook of neonatal intensive care* (9th ed., Ch 29, pp. 1039–1095). St Louis, MO: Elsevier.

Gardner, S. L., Carter, B. S., Enzman-Hines, M. E., & Niermeyer, S. (Eds.), *Merenstein and Gardner's handbook of neonatal intensive care* (9th ed.). St Louis, MO: Elsevier.

Gomella, T. L. (2020). Gestational age and birth weight classification. In: T. L. Gomella (Ed.), *Neonatology: management, procedures, on-call problems, diseases, and drugs* (8th ed., Ch 6). New York: McGraw-Hill Education.

Griffiths, E., Marley, J. V., & Atkinson, D. (2020). Preconception care in a remote Aboriginal community context: what, when and by whom? *International Journal of Environmental Research and Public Health, 17*(10), 3702. doi: 10.3390/ijerph17103702.

Hartnett, D., Carr, A., Hamilton, E., & O'Reilly, G. (2016). The effectiveness of functional family therapy for adolescent behavioural and substance misuse problems: a meta-analysis. *Family Process, 56*(3), 607–619. doi: 10.1111/famp.12256.

Howlett, A. A., & Jangaard, K. A. (2011). Evaluating the newborn: diagnostic approach. In: R. Goldbloom (Ed.), *Pediatric clinical skills* (4th ed., Ch 4, pp. 28–55). London: Saunders.

Kenner, C., & Lott, J. W. (Eds.) (2019). *Comprehensive neonatal nursing care* (6th ed.). New York: Springer.

Kim, H. J., Kim, J. H., Chay, D. B., Park, J. H., & Kim, M. A. (2017). Association of isolated single umbilical artery with perinatal outcomes: systemic review and meta-analysis. *Obstetric and Gynecologic Science, 60*(3), 266–273. doi: 10.5468/ogs.2017.60.3.266.

Lam, J. M., & Wong, L.-C. (2015). Hair disorders. In: L. F. Eichenfield, I. J. Frieden, A. Zaenglein, & E. Mathes (Eds.), *Neonatal and infant dermatology* (3rd ed., pp. 510–526). London: Elsevier Health Sciences.

Lissauer, T., & Steer, P. (2013). Size and physical examination of the newborn infant. In: J. M. Fanaroff (Ed.), *Klaus and Fanaroff's care of the high-risk neonate* (6th ed., pp. 105–131). Philadelphia, PA: Elsevier.

Manandhar, T. Prashad, B., & Nath Pal, M. (2018). Risk factors for intrauterine growth restriction and its neonatal outcome. *Gynecology and Obstetrics, 8*(2), 464.

Mandy, G. T. (2017). Large for gestational age newborn. In: L. E. Weisman & L. Wilkie (Eds.), *UpToDate*. Waltham. MA: UpToDate. <http://www.uptodate.com/contents/large-for-gestational-age-newborn> (Accessed 3 March 2022).

Mandy, G. T. (2021). Infants with fetal (intrauterine) growth restriction. In: L. E. Weisman & L. Wilkie (Eds.), *UpToDate*. Waltham. MA: UpToDate. <https://www.uptodate.com/contents/infants-with-fetal-intrauterine-growth-restriction#!> (Accessed 16 March 2022).

Mari, G. (2021). Fetal growth restriction: evaluation and management. In: C. J. Lockwood, D. Levine, & V. A. Barss (Eds.), *UpToDate*. Waltham, MA. <https://www.uptodate.com/contents/fetal-growth-restriction-evaluation-and-management?search> (Accessed 3 March 2022).

Matthews, A. L., & Robin, N. H. (2020). Genetic disorders, malformations and inborn errors of metabolism. In: S. L. Gardner, B. S. Carter, M. E. Enzman-Hines, & S. Niermeyer (Eds.), *Merenstein and Gardner's handbook of neonatal intensive care* (9th ed., Ch 27, pp. 969–995). St Louis: Elsevier.

McKee-Garrett, T. M. (2021). Assessment of the newborn infant. In: R. Martin & T. K. Duryea (Eds.), *UpToDate*. Waltham, MA. <https://www.uptodate.com/contents/assessment-of-the-newborn-infant?search=McKee%20Assessment%20of%20the%20newborn%20infant&source=search> (Accessed 3 March 2022).

Neonatal Nurses College Aotearoa (NNCA). (2015). *NNCA standards for neonatal nursing practice*. Wellington, NZ: New Zealand Nurses Organisation.

Niklasson, A., Ericson, A., Fryer, J. G., Karlberg, J., Lawrence, C., & Karlberg, P. (1991). An update of the Swedish reference standards for weight, length and head circumference at birth for given gestational age (1977–1981). *Acta Paediatrica Scandinavica, 80*, 756–762.

Ohuma, E. O. & Altman, D. G. (2019). Design and other methodological considerations for the construction of human fetal and neonatal size and growth charts. *Statistics in Medicine, 38*(19), 3527–3539.

Olsen, I. E., Groveman, S. A., Lawson, M. L., Clark, R. H., & Zemel, B. S. (2010). New intrauterine growth curves based on United States data. *Pediatrics, 125*, e214–e224.

Maoz, O., Wainstock, T., Sheiner, E., & Walfisch, A. (2019). Immediate perinatal outcomes of post term deliveries. *Journal of Maternal–Fetal & Neonatal Medicine, 32*, 11, 1847–1852. doi: 10.1080/14767058.2017.1420773.

Parrettini, S., Caroli, A., & Torlone, E. (2020). Nutrition and metabolic adaptations in physiological and complicated pregnancy: focus on obesity and gestational diabetes. *Frontiers in Endocrinology, 11*, 611929. doi: 10.3389/fendo.2020.611929.

Pereira-da-Silva, L., Virella, D., & Fusch, C. (2019). Nutritional assessment in preterm infants: a practical approach in the NICU. *Nutrients, 11*(9), 1999. doi: 10.3390/nu11091999.

Power, T., Wilson, D., East, L., Cashman, B., Wannell, J., & Jackson, D. (2021). Indigenous women's experiences of diabetes in pregnancy: a thematic synthesis. *Collegian, 28*(5), 541–550. doi: 10.1016/j.colegn.2021.01.004.

Rabner, M., Meurling, J., Ahlberg, C., & Lorch, S. A. (2014). The impact of growth curve changes in assessing premature infant growth. *Journal of Perinatology, 34*, 49–53.

Records, K. (2015). Intimate partner violence. In: S. Mattson & J. E. Smith (Eds.), *Core curriculum for maternal-newborn nursing* (5th ed., pp. 417–434). Philadelphia, PA: Elsevier.

Rochow, N., Raja, P., Liu, K., Fenton, T., Landau-Crangle, E., Gottler, S., et al. (2016). Physiological adjustment to postnatal growth trajectories in healthy preterm infants. *Pediatric Research, 79*(6), 870–879.

Roncero, C., Valriberas-Herrero, I., Mezzatesta-Gava, M., Villegas, J. L., Aguilar, L., & Grau-López, L. (2020). Cannabis use during pregnancy and its relationship with fetal developmental outcomes and psychiatric disorders. A systematic review. *Reproductive Health, 17*(1), 25. doi: 10.1186/s12978-020-0880-9.

Royal Australian and New Zealand College of Obstetricians and Gynaecologists (RANZCOG). (2017). *Management of obesity in pregnancy*. C-Obs 49, <https://ranzcog.edu.au/RANZCOG_SITE/media/RANZCOG-MEDIA/Women%27s%20Health/Statement%20and%20guidelines/Clinical-Obstetrics/Management-of-obesity-(C-Obs-49)-Review-March-2017.pdf?ext=.pdf> (Accessed 3 March 2022).

Royal Australian and New Zealand College of Obstetricians and Gynaecologists (RANZCOG). (2018). *Substance use in pregnancy*. C-Obs 55, <https://ranzcog.edu.au/RANZCOG_SITE/media/RANZCOG-MEDIA/Women%27s%20Health/Statement%20and%20guidelines/Clinical-Obstetrics/Substance-use-in-pregnancy-(C-Obs-55)-March-2018.pdf?ext=.pdf> (Accessed 3 March 2022).

Siller, H., König-Bachmann, M., Perkhofer, S., & Hochleitner, M. (2022). Midwives perceiving and dealing with violence against women: is it mostly about midwives actively protecting women? A modified grounded theory study. *Journal of Interpersonal Violence, 37*(3–4), 1902–1932. doi: 10.1177/0886260520927497.

Smith, J., Lafferty, M., Boelig, R. C., Carola, D., Adeniyi-Jones, S., Kraft, W. K., et al. (2020). Is maternal methadone dose associated with the severity of neonatal abstinence syndrome? *American Journal of Perinatology*. doi: 10.1055/s-0040-1721693. [Online ahead of print.]

Tudehope, D., Gibbons, K., Cormack, B., & Bloomfield, F. (2012). Growth monitoring of low-birth-weight infants: what references to use? *Journal of Paediatrics and Child Health, 48*, 759–767.

Usher, R., & McLean, F. (1969). Intrauterine growth of live-born Caucasian infants at sea level: standards obtained from measurements in 7 dimensions of infants born between 25 and 44 weeks of gestation. *Journal of Pediatrics, 74*, 901–910.

Villar, J., Fernandes, M., Purwar, M., Staines-Urias, E., Di Nicola, P., Cheikh Ismail, L., et al. (2019). Neurodevelopmental milestones and associated behaviours are similar among healthy children across diverse geographical locations. *Nature Communications, 10*(1), 511. doi: 10.1038/s41467-018-07983-4.

Von Kohler, C. (2015). Age-related concerns. In: S. Mattson & J. E. Smith (Eds.), *Core curriculum for maternal-newborn nursing* (5th ed., pp. 123–134). St Louis, MO: Elsevier.

Wiechers, C., Kirchhof, S., Maas, C., Poets, C. F., & Franz, A. R. (2019). Neonatal body composition by air displacement plethysmography in healthy term singletons: a systematic review. *BMC Pediatrics, 19*(1), 489. doi: 10.1186/s12887-019-1867-y.

Women's and Children's Health Network. (2014). *WHCN multidisciplinary clinical guideline: newborn examination*. Adelaide, SA: WHCN, SA Health. (Accessed via the Clinical Governance Intranet.)

Woo, J., Carrington, S. M., & Ambia, A. (2020). Prenatal environment: effect on neonatal outcome. In: S. L. Gardner, B. S. Carter, M. E. Enzman-Hines, & S. Niermeyer (Eds.), *Merenstein and Gardner's handbook of neonatal intensive care* (9th ed., Ch. 2, pp. 17–44). St Louis, MO: Elsevier.

Zitelli, B. J., McIntire, S. C., & Nowalk, A. J. (2018). *Zitelli and Davis' atlas of pediatric physical diagnosis* (7th ed.). Philadelphia, PA: Elsevier, Inc.

CHAPTER 4

STABILISATION AND RESUSCITATION OF THE NEONATE

JULIE BERNARDO AND JENNIFER DAWSON

Learning objectives

After reading this chapter, you will be able to:

- understand the physiology of the transition from intrauterine to extrauterine life
- anticipate the neonate who may need resuscitation at birth and in the neonatal period
- identify neonates requiring assistance to breathe in the birthing suite
- identify the equipment needed for neonatal resuscitation
- use the neonatal resuscitation algorithm to manage the newly born neonate who requires assistance to breathe
- describe the management of the neonate requiring resuscitation in the neonatal period
- describe the after care of a neonate who has received resuscitation
- explain how to support parents whose infant requires resuscitation
- explain the complications of neonatal resuscitation
- describe the education and training needed to ensure that neonatal nurses/midwives are competent at performing neonatal resuscitation
- discuss the major ethical issues around initiating and discontinuing resuscitation.

Key words, terms and abbreviations

arterial oxygen saturation (PaO_2)
birthing suite
endotracheal tubes (ETTs)
functional residual capacity (FRC)
heart rate (HR)
intermittent positive pressure ventilation (IPPV)
intraosseous (IO)
laryngeal mask airway (LMA)
oxygenation
peak inspiratory pressure (PIP)
peripheral oxygen saturation (SpO_2)
positive end expiratory pressure (PEEP)
positive pressure ventilation (PPV)
pulse oximeter (PO)
resuscitation

INTRODUCTION

> 'Resuscitation is undertaken to establish independent respirations and heartbeats, to treat depressed respiratory effort or to correct metabolic disturbances.'
>
> Australian Institute of Health and Welfare (AIHW, 2021, p. 44)

Resuscitation interventions range from airway suction to ventilation and external cardiac massage. In Australia in 2019, 91% of neonates were born at term (37–41 weeks) (AIHW, 2021). Between 75% and 85% of live-born neonates born in Australia in 2019 did not require active resuscitation immediately after birth (AIHW, 2021). Of those neonates who required an intervention in the **birthing suite**, approximately one-third (38%) received **intermittent positive pressure ventilation (IPPV)** with less than 1% of newborn infants receiving external cardiac massage and ventilation to initiate breathing and maintain oxygenation (AIHW, 2020). Of the babies included in the 2019 report from the Australian and New Zealand Neonatal Network (ANZNN), 13.9% of babies required intubation in the birthing suite (Chow et al., 2021). Effective resuscitation is important in reducing mortality and severe morbidity in infants who do not sustain breathing at birth (World Health Organization (WHO), 2012).

The International Liaison Committee on Resuscitation (ILCOR) reviews the scientific evidence and makes recommendations for basic life support and advanced resuscitation every 5 years. Where there is no new evidence, the guidelines may reflect evidence evaluation from previous reviews. National bodies use the ILCOR recommendations (Wyckoff et al., 2020) to formulate guidelines in their country (ANZCOR, 2021; Aziz et al., 2020; Madar et al., 2021).

RESUSCITATION AT BIRTH

The transition from fetal life is the most complex physiological adaptation across the life span. The transition depends upon successful lung aeration, which acts as a trigger for the critical change from fetal to neonatal circulation that is essential for postnatal life.

A small number of neonates who do not breathe at birth can develop hypoxic damage to their heart, lungs, liver, gut or kidneys, but damage to the brain is the most serious cause of morbidity and mortality.

The Apgar score, named after obstetric anaesthetist Dr Virginia Apgar, who developed the scoring method in 1952, is a clinical indication of the neonate's condition shortly after birth and should be calculated contemporaneously. The measure is based on the assessment of five characteristics of the neonate including skin colour, pulse, breathing, muscle tone and reflex irritability. Each characteristic is given between 0 and 2 points, with a total possible score between 0 and 10 points. An Apgar score of 7 or more at 5 minutes after birth indicates that the neonate adapted well to the extrauterine environment; a score between 4 and 6 indicates moderate respiratory depression. Neonates with a score of 0 to 3 are considered to have had severe respiratory depression and required immediate resuscitation (Pinheiro, 2009). In 2019 in Australia, 2% of babies had an Apgar score of less than 7 at 5 minutes, an increase from 0.9% in 2004 (AIHW, 2021).

REFLECTION

Have you been at the birth of a neonate who had a low Apgar score? Can you remember what the neonate looked like and what was required to help them to breathe?

Fetal circulation

Fetal circulation (Fig. 4.1) is significantly different to adult circulation. In utero, the placenta functions as the organ of gas exchange for the fetus. Following cord clamping and separation from the placenta, the neonate is dependent on achieving an oxygenated circulation by establishing and maintaining normal lung aeration and postnatal cardiovascular adaptation.

The fetal circulation is comprised of the placenta, two umbilical arteries and an umbilical vein. This ensures supply of oxygenated blood to the fetus and removal of carbon dioxide (CO_2) and other waste gases. The fetus has an **arterial oxygen saturation (*PaO_2*)** of 25–30 mmHg, compared with an adult PaO_2 of 80–100 mmHg. Despite a low PaO_2, the fetus remains oxygenated because of several factors. Firstly, the presence of fetal haemoglobin helps maintain oxygen delivery in the fetus despite low oxygen partial pressures. Fetal haemoglobin has a higher affinity for binding oxygen; this means that the partial pressure of oxygen that corresponds to 50% saturation in the fetus is 19 mmHg, compared with an adult, who needs a partial pressure of approximately 27 mmHg to achieve the same level of oxygen binding. Fetal haemoglobin can be 80% saturated and this meets the metabolic needs of the fetus. Fetal haemoglobin is present for approximately 6 months after birth. The presence of fetal haemoglobin coupled with high ventricular output helps maintain oxygen delivery in the fetus despite the low partial pressure of oxygen (Fernandes, 2017). Secondly, blood with the highest oxygen level flows preferentially to vital organs including the brain, heart and liver. Lastly, the fetus has decreased metabolic and oxygen consumption compared with a neonate. The fetus does not require energy to maintain thermoregulation: this is maintained by the mother. The physiological functions of the respiratory, gastrointestinal and renal systems are decreased in the fetus; therefore, tissue oxygen consumption is reduced (Fernandes, 2017).

In the fetus the low vascular resistance of the placenta, high pulmonary vascular pressure and the fluid-filled lungs create an environment of high vascular resistance. These factors are responsible for the differences in the way blood circulates through the fetus compared with the adult.

Oxygenated blood from the placenta enters the fetus via the umbilical vein (UV). The UV bifurcates at the level of the liver, with some blood perfusing the hepatic

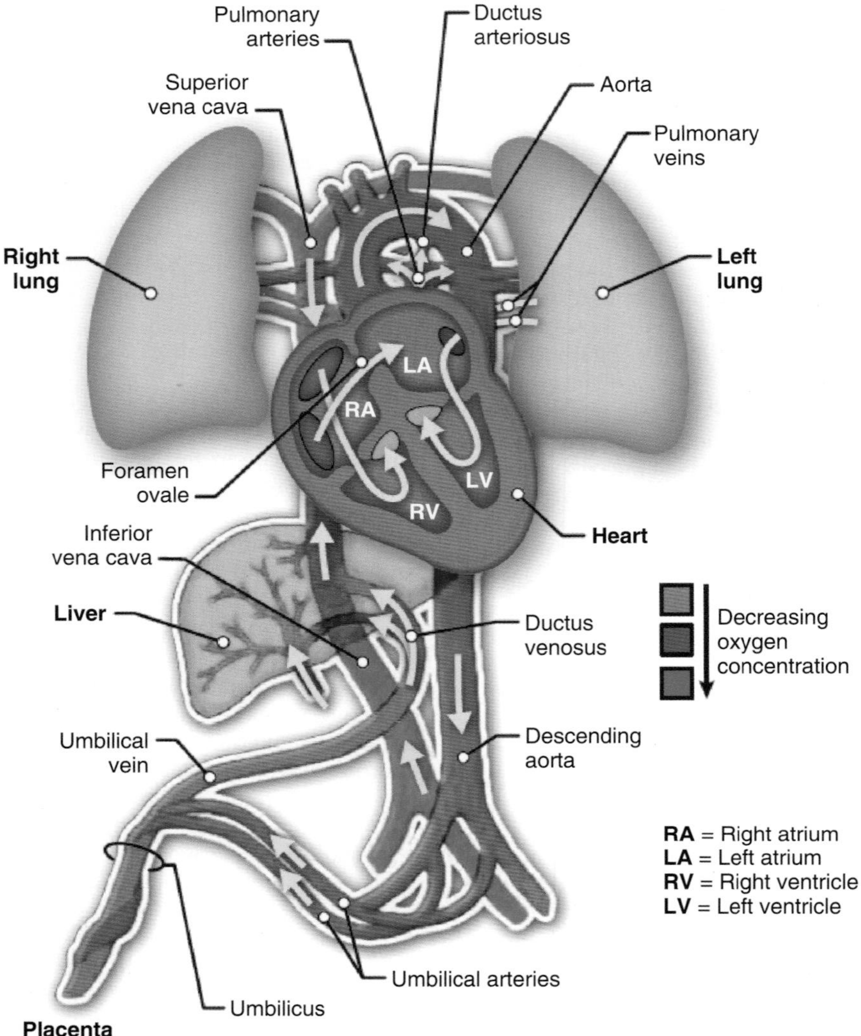

FIGURE 4.1 **Fetal circulation**

Adapted from: Rychik and Tian (2012).

circulation and the remainder entering the *ductus venosus* and combining with deoxygenated blood in the inferior vena cava. Most of the blood from the inferior vena cava is directed across the foramen ovale to the left atrium (LA) because pressure in the right atrium is higher than the pressure in the left atrium. Oxygenated blood from the inferior vena cava mixes with deoxygenated blood from the superior vena cava entering the right atrium. Some blood will travel from the right atrium to the right ventricle and into the pulmonary artery. A small amount of blood (about 10%) will flow into the pulmonary circulation. However, due to the high pulmonary pressure, 90% of the blood will bypass the lungs and move directly to the descending aorta via the *ductus arteriosus*. This results in higher oxygen concentration in the preductal arteries. These arteries originate from the aorta prior to the junction with the *ductus arteriosus*, compared with the postductal arteries (Fernandes, 2017).

TRANSITION FROM FETAL TO EXTRAUTERINE LIFE

After birth, the neonate must undergo a series of physiological events to enable successful transition from reliance on the placenta for gas exchange to aerating the amniotic fluid-filled lungs. The lungs must expand, alveolar fluid must be cleared and changes to the circulation must occur to close intracardiac (*foramen ovale*) and extracardiac shunts (*ductus venosus, ductus arteriosus*).

Breathing and aeration of the lungs trigger an increase in pulmonary blood flow, and increased alveolar oxygen pressure causes vasodilation in the pulmonary blood vessels. The umbilical cord is clamped, inducing constriction of the umbilical vein and umbilical arteries. In postnatal life these become the *ligamentum teres* and medial umbilical ligaments respectively. Within a few minutes to hours after birth the *ductus arteriosus* constricts and will become the *ligamentum arteriosum*. Increased pressure in the left atrium due to increased pressure in the systemic circulation and decreased pressure in the right atrium due to reduced pressure in the pulmonary circulation cause the foramen ovale to close and become the *fossa ovalis*. The *ductus venosus* contracts and will become the *ligamentum venosum*. It may take several months for the *ductus arteriosus* to become anatomically closed. In the preterm neonate, or in neonates who suffer severe hypoxia around the time of birth, the *ductus arteriosus* may remain functionally open for minutes to days after birth (Van Woudenberg et al., 2012).

Cells lining the epithelium of the lungs produce fluid to distend the airways to a volume approximating **functional residual capacity (FRC)** (30 mL/kg) during fetal life, to facilitate normal lung development. This liquid fills the airways before birth, and must be cleared to enable the lungs to inflate. Several mechanisms are involved in clearing lung fluid. Once labour is initiated, an increase in catecholamines (mainly adrenaline (epinephrine) and vasopressin) results in a rapid reversal of the production of lung fluid and a switch to absorption of this fluid from the lumen of the lungs into the fetal lymphatic circulation. Catecholamines secreted during labour have an additional role in activating amiloride-sensitive sodium (Na^+) channels. Activation of this mechanism results in Na^+ moving from the lung lumen into the interstitial compartment. The movement of Na^+ changes the osmotic gradient, resulting in reabsorption of lung liquid (Hooper et al., 2010).

The primary mechanism for airway liquid clearance at birth is the increased transpulmonary pressure generated by inspiration. Inspiration or lung inflation provides a hydrostatic pressure gradient that drives liquid movement from the airways and into the surrounding tissue (Hooper et al., 2015). Lung fluid pushed into lung tissue is reabsorbed into the lymphatic and pulmonary circulation over the next few hours. The thoracic squeeze that occurs during a vaginal birth will aid in removing approximately one-third of fetal lung fluid. This does not occur during a caesarean section birth, and may explain why this group of neonates may need assistance to transition to establish breathing (Hillman et al., 2012). However, thoracic squeeze is thought to play a minor role in fetal lung fluid clearance (Jha et al., 2022). If transition is impeded by any number of factors, the neonate will require assistance to ensure adequate onset of respiration and transition occur.

With the onset of breathing, negative pressure is exerted on the lungs, the alveoli expand and surfactant is released. Alveolar surface tension decreases, compliance improves and FRC is established.

Identifying the at-risk neonate

It is imperative that all clinicians attending a birth are able to identify neonates at risk for problems with transition, to enable them to prepare for potential resuscitation. The most common indications for an at-risk neonate are outlined in Box 4.1. Risk factors are identified by taking a clinical history from the mother or by seeking this information from the obstetric team.

BOX 4.1 **Maternal and neonatal risk factors for neonates at risk for requiring resuscitation**

Maternal risk factors

- Substance abuse (drugs and alcohol), heavy smoker
- No antenatal care
- Previous fetal or neonatal death
- Chronic illness (congenital or acquired heart disease, renal disease, hypertension, type 1 diabetes)
- Drug therapies (methadone, buprenorphine, adrenergic blocking agents, lithium, magnesium, sedation)
- Maternal infection, chorioamnionitis, maternal pyrexia
- Pregnancy-induced hypertension
- Antepartum haemorrhage (abruption, placenta praevia, vasa praevia, placenta accreta/increta)
- Prolonged rupture of membranes (>18 hours)

Neonatal risk factors

- Multiple gestation (twins, triplets etc)
- Preterm birth (increased need for resuscitation if <35 weeks)
- Prolonged pregnancy (>41 weeks)
- Fetal growth anomalies (intrauterine growth restriction, large for gestational age)
- Congenital abnormalities that may affect successful transition post birth
- Polyhydramnios, oligohydramnios
- Intrauterine infection
- Alloimmune haemolytic (that may lead to fetal anaemia or hydrops fetalis)
- Reduced fetal movement prior to labour

Intrapartum risk factors

- Abnormal fetal presentation (breech, transverse lie etc)
- Cord prolapse
- Precipitous or prolonged labour
- Non-reassuring fetal heart rate pattern on cardiotocography (CTG)
- Intrapartum haemorrhage
- Meconium-stained liquor
- Instrumental birth (ventouse, forceps)
- Maternal pain relief in labour (narcotics <4 hours pre-birth)
- Lower-segment caesarean section (LSCS) via general anaesthetic
- Shoulder dystocia

Source: adapted from Australian and New Zealand Council on Resuscitation (ANZCOR) (2021).

If an at-risk neonate is identified, there should be clear communication among obstetric, midwifery and neonatal teams. A coordinated approach to the management of the pregnant woman and her baby should be formulated. The parents need clear, consistent and appropriate communication regarding risk factors and potential management of their baby. Parents should be included in the decision-making process (ANZCOR, 2021).

Preparation of the room and equipment

Being prepared is the first and most important step in effective neonatal resuscitation. The resuscitation cot, equipment and medications for resuscitation should be checked every day and again before each birth, including the correct functioning of each piece of equipment. A list of the equipment that should be available is outlined in Box 4.2. Preparation includes turning on the overhead heater and lights on the resuscitator and assembling the equipment that might be required. This includes ensuring that the face mask, **endotracheal tubes (ETTs)**, laryngoscope handle and blade and suction catheters are the right size for the neonate. Preterm neonates will require a smaller-sized mask appropriate for their gestational age (O'Shea et al., 2015). The globe in the laryngoscope should be checked for brightness, and fit if it is a screw-in version as opposed to a fibreoptic light source.

Preparation of the neonatal team

Every member of the team responsible for the neonate should be able to perform basic life support. Basic life support in the birthing suite includes positioning the neonate correctly to open the airway, clearing the airway of secretions if they are blocking the airway, providing positive pressure inflations via a mask and, if required, chest compressions.

For births where a neonate has been determined to be at high risk for requiring higher-level skills (e.g. endotracheal intubation, umbilical cannulation and the administration of drugs or fluids), additional personnel with these skills should be in attendance (ANZCOR, 2021; Aziz et al., 2020; Madar et al., 2021). However, some neonates may deteriorate rapidly, so a system to call for help quickly should be in place.

An important step in preparing for the birth of an at-risk neonate is to nominate a team leader and to discuss anticipated interventions and delegate responsibilities for procedures such as **positive pressure ventilation (PPV)**, auscultating the **heart rate (HR)** and breath sounds and placing the **pulse oximeter (PO)** sensor. When a prolonged or complex resuscitation is anticipated, a member of the team is allocated to record interventions and the neonate's response (HR and **peripheral oxygen saturation (SpO_2)**) (ANZCOR, 2021; Aziz et al., 2020; Madar et al., 2021).

BOX 4.2 **Equipment for resuscitation of the neonate**

Thermoregulation

- Warm, absorbent wraps
- Plastic bag (for neonates <1250 g)
- Overhead heater/Resuscitaire®

Equipment for management of airway and breathing

- T-piece resuscitator with circuit
- Self-inflating bag with reservoir bag and appropriate gas tubing
- Wall source or cylinders of air and oxygen
- Twin-o-vac suction unit with pressure gauge
- Oxygen/air blender, standard flow meter and tubing
- Clean suction tubing with Y catheter size FG10 attached
- Suction catheters, sizes 5FG/6FG/8FG/10FG (2 each) OR a neonatal Yankauer sucker
- Face masks, sizes 00/01/2 (1 each)
- Infant laryngoscope handle
- Straight laryngoscope blades, sizes 1/0/00 (1 each)
- Battery AA × 2
- End-tidal CO_2 detector
- Uncuffed endotracheal tubes (ETTs), sizes 2.5 mm/3.0 mm/3.5 mm/4.0 mm (2 each)
- Laryngeal mask airway size 1
- Meconium aspirator
- Stylet (sterile) × 1
- Clean suction tubing
- Duoderm and tapes to fix an ETT
- Pulse oximeter and sensors
- Posey wrap
- Paediatric stethoscope

Equipment for management of circulation and fluid administration

- Syringes, 20 mL/10 mL/5 mL/3 mL/2.5 mL/1 mL
- Needles, 25G 16 mm/23G 25 mm/18G 38 mm drawing up (2 each)
- Tape
- Drugs
- Adrenaline (epinephrine), 1:10,000
- Naloxone
- Sodium chloride 0.9% vials, 10 mL or 100 mL mini bag
- Water for injection, 10 mL
- Umbilical vein catheter (UVC) single lumen, 3.5FG/5FG/8FG
- IV cannula 24G 14 mm/24G 19 mm/22G 25 mm/16G 30 mm
- Butterfly needle, 23G 19 mm
- Negative uncrossed-matched blood and blood giving equipment suitable for emergency neonatal transfusion needs to be readily available for a profoundly anaemic neonate

Source: adapted from Australian and New Zealand Council on Resuscitation (ANZCOR) (2021).

FAMILY-CENTRED CARE 4.1

Preparation for resuscitation includes preparing the parent/s. If a neonate has been identified as at risk, ensure that the parents and family members present at the birth know what to expect in terms of the number of people in the room and what is likely to happen when their baby is born. If admission to the neonatal unit is anticipated (e.g. preterm birth or a neonate with a congenital anomaly), the parents should be given the opportunity to tour the neonatal unit prior to the birth of their baby.

Thermoregulation

Neonates exposed to cold stress at birth have a greater likelihood of morbidity and death (ANZCOR, 2021). Preterm neonates are especially predisposed to heat loss due to their immature skin, increased surface area-to-weight ratio and reduced stores of subcutaneous fat. The suggested optimal temperature for the birthing suite is 23–25°C (Madar et al., 2021). In preparation for the birth, doors and windows should be closed to reduce the possibility of convective heat loss. To prevent conductive heat loss, a radiant warmer should be set to pre-warm. Additional equipment to keep the neonate warm should be assembled, including a woollen hat and pre-warmed blankets. A prewarmed transport cot should be available if the infant needs transport to the neonatal unit. Management of thermoregulation in the newly born neonate is described in Chapter 8.

SUPPORTING TRANSITION AND NEONATAL RESUSCITATION

Newly born neonates rarely require resuscitation but sometimes require assistance during the process of postnatal transition. The term 'support of transition' has been introduced to better distinguish between interventions that are needed to restore vital organ functions (resuscitation) and those required to support transition to extrauterine life (Wyllie et al., 2015).

One such example of interventions that support transition is the timing of cord clamping. The question of when to clamp the umbilical cord after birth has received renewed attention in recent years. Compelling evidence has been published supporting the practice of waiting for placental perfusion, which aids the neonate's physiological transition to extrauterine life (McDonald et al., 2014). ANZCOR recommends a delay of a minimum of 1 minute, or until the cord stops pulsating, prior to clamping the umbilical cord in term or late preterm infants born at >34 weeks' gestation (ANZCOR, 2021). For infants born at less than 34 weeks' gestational age who do not require immediate resuscitation after birth, ANZCOR suggests deferring clamping the cord for at least 30 seconds (ANZCOR, 2021). If the neonate appears to have acute, profound hypoxia (as demonstrated by an HR of less than 60 beats per minute (bpm) and poor muscle tone), or if meconium is present and the neonate is apnoeic, the umbilical cord should be clamped and severed and the neonate immediately transferred to the resuscitation cot.

Research surrounding the benefit of delayed versus immediate cord clamping is ongoing, with most studies defining 'delayed' as greater than or equal to 60 seconds. The latest systematic review and meta-analysis (Fogarty et al., 2018) examined delayed cord clamping only (without cord milking) in preterm infants. They concluded that delayed clamping reduces mortality in preterm infants without increasing maternal morbidity. They confirmed findings from earlier studies that demonstrated delayed clamping reduced the number of blood transfusions required in preterm infants.

A potential rationale for improved outcomes with delayed cord clamping includes increasing red cell volume and increasing oxygen-carrying capacity, which leads to higher oxygen saturation. Lower oxygen saturations increase mortality in the very preterm infant. Cord milking (also referred to as 'cord stripping'), an alternative to delayed clamping of the cord, is not recommended in infants <28 weeks' gestation where there is a higher risk of intraventricular haemorrhage (IVH) when the cord is milked (Aziz et al., 2020).

Most preterm infants, if gently stimulated, will begin spontaneous breathing within 60 seconds. Delaying cord clamping may allow the breathing infant to transition from a fetal to a neonatal circulation, allowing them to maintain cardiac output, **oxygenation** and optimum arterial blood pressure. This may reduce the requirement for endotracheal intubation and invasive ventilation (Kluckow & Hooper, 2015).

CLINICAL PRACTICE 4.1

In any neonate receiving extensive resuscitation, the umbilical cord clamp should be applied at least 3 cm away from the skin. This allows easier access if the umbilical vessels need to be accessed for the administration of fluids/ medications.

Initial management of the newly born neonate

As soon as the neonate is born, they should be assessed for breathing, muscle tone and HR. The neonate's degree of cardiorespiratory depression is used to dictate the need for respiratory support and procedures, as outlined in the ANZCOR (2021) neonatal resuscitation flow chart (Fig. 4.2).

The following apply when assessing for breathing, muscle tone and HR:

- If the neonate is at/near term gestation and breathing or crying, with good muscle tone (moving limbs with a flexed position), they can be dried and placed on the mother's chest for skin-to-skin contact. Ensure that the neonate's face is visible so as to observe colour and is not obstructed by the mother's neck or breasts.

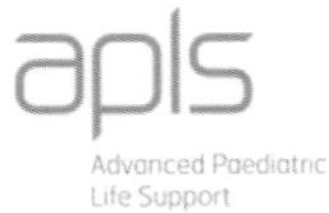

Newborn life support

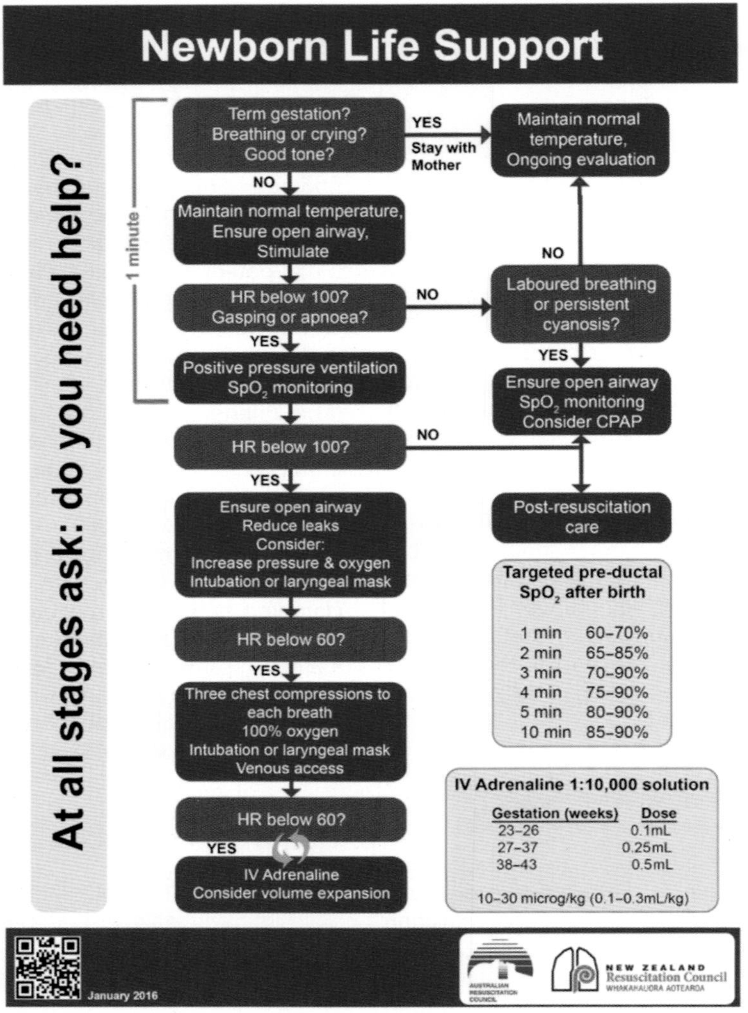

FIGURE 4.2 **Newborn Life Support Algorithm**

Source: Australian and New Zealand Council on Resuscitation (ANZCOR) (2021).

- If the neonate has laboured breathing, gasping respirations or poor muscle tone, they must be stimulated to breathe. This can be done by gently drying and rubbing the neonate with a warm dry towel, including the trunk and face. Gaertner and colleagues have shown that truncal stimulation is the most effective method of eliciting a positive response; flicking the infant's foot is the least effective method for stimulating an infant to breathe (Gaertner et al., 2018).
- To ensure that the airway is not obstructed, the neonate's head and neck are maintained in a 'sniffing' position (Fig. 4.3) (ANZCOR, 2021). Suction is applied to the mouth and nose only if there is a concern that secretions are occluding the airway.

EVIDENCE-BASED PRACTICE RESEARCH 4.1

Research has shown that routine suctioning of the oropharynx and nasopharynx of the neonate at birth can have harmful effects, including vagal stimulation resulting in bradycardia and apnoea, and trauma to the mucous membranes (Foster et al., 2017; Wyckoff et al., 2020). There is no benefit of routine suctioning of neonates at birth, including those born by caesarean section.

If suctioning is required to clear the airway, a size 10–12FG catheter is used for a term neonate. Negative pressure of no more than 100 mmHg (133 cm H_2O, 13 kPa, 1.9 psi)

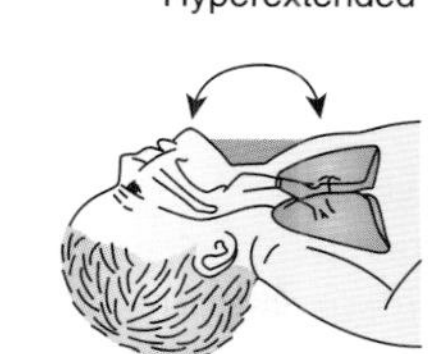

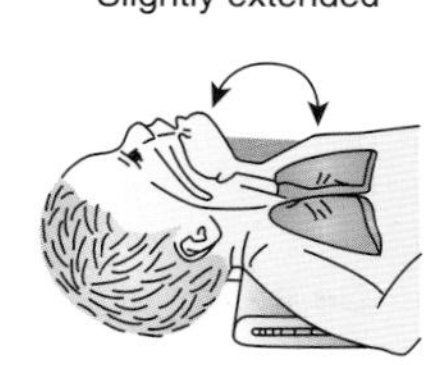

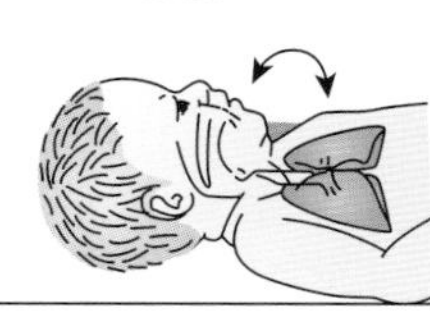

FIGURE 4.3 **Recommended sniffing position used to open the neonate's airway**

The slightly extended or sniffing position illustrated in the middle panel results in optimal airway patency for resuscitation.

is applied for a term neonate (Australian Resuscitation Council (ARC), 2010). The length of the suction catheter to be passed into the oropharynx is equal to the distance from the corner of the mouth to the tragus of the ear. The oropharynx is aspirated prior to the nasopharynx (suctioning the nose first may cause the neonate to gasp and aspirate any vomit/mucus present into the pharynx). Suction is applied for about 5 seconds while withdrawing the catheter.

CLINICAL PRACTICE 4.2

If a neonate is not breathing effectively at birth, and does not respond to stimulation, they are in secondary apnoea and require positive pressure ventilation immediately.

The neonate's breathing and HR continue to be assessed. The HR should be checked every 30 seconds. The HR is estimated by auscultating the HR with a stethoscope, counting the number of beats over 6 seconds and multiplying by 10. If the neonate is breathing (no evidence of gasping or laboured respirations) and has an HR above 100 bpm, they need to be observed and assessed at least every 30 seconds. Uncompromised neonates may take up to 10 minutes to become centrally pink (Dawson et al., 2010).

If the neonate remains centrally cyanosed, has good muscle tone and is breathing well in the first few minutes after birth, the administration of supplemental oxygen should be determined by pulse oximetry measurements of oxygen saturation. If SpO_2 measurements are low, free-flow oxygen can be given with a T-piece resuscitator, flow-inflating bag or oxygen tubing held close to the neonate's face with a cupped hand. Only some types of self-inflating bags can be used to give free-flowing oxygen (Dawson et al., 2007). In some models of self-inflating bags, valves within the bag can restrict the flow of gas, allowing oxygen to be administered only when the bag is squeezed. Clinicians need to be aware of limitations in the devices available in their clinical setting.

If the neonate is breathing spontaneously, HR remains above 100 bpm, with good muscle tone, they are likely to be stable and no further medical intervention will be required. The neonate's breathing and HR continue to be assessed for at least the first 10 minutes after birth.

Positive pressure ventilation in the birthing suite

If the neonate has bradycardia, defined as an HR less than 100 bpm, and has laboured breathing, positive pressure ventilation is recommended. Aerating the lungs is the most important and effective step in cardiopulmonary resuscitation of the compromised neonate. PPV can be provided with a self-inflating bag, flow-inflating bag or a T-piece resuscitator (Fig. 4.4) (ANZCOR, 2021). Each of these devices has advantages and limitations (Table 4.1); therefore, it is important for the clinician to be competent with whichever device is available in the clinical setting. If PPV is required, it is suggested that the neonatal nurse/midwife call for help early by whatever system is in place in their setting.

Mask ventilation

Successful mask ventilation requires an airtight seal between the rim of the mask and the neonate's face (Fig. 4.5) (ANZCOR, 2021). Achieving this can be difficult; hence, an ineffective seal is the most common reason for failure of mask ventilation. The face mask should be applied using a rolling motion from chin to nose bridge

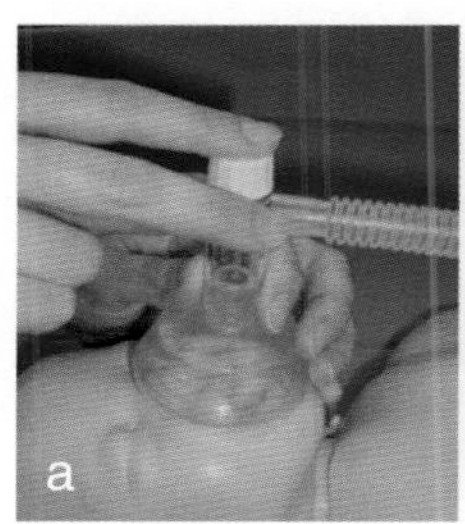

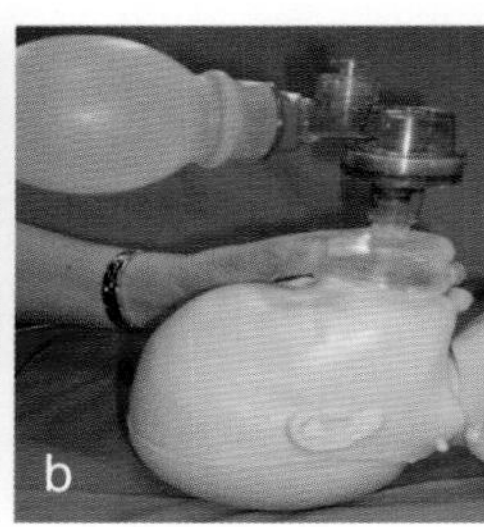

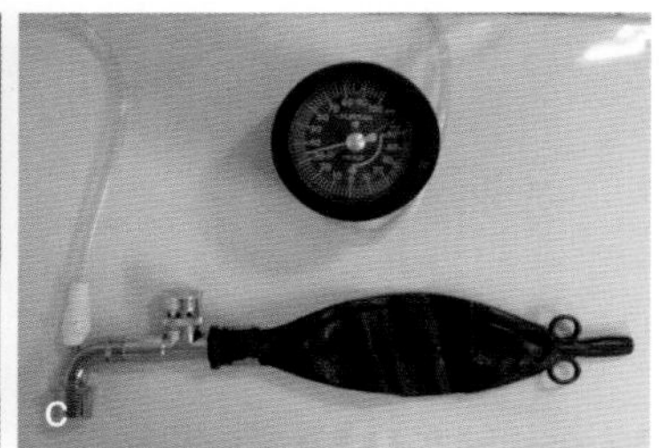

FIGURE 4.4 **Devices suitable for positive pressure ventilation**

a T-piece resuscitator; **b** self-inflating bag; **c** flow-inflating bag.

TABLE 4.1 **Devices and their limitations for providing respiratory support**

Type of device that can be used to give respiratory support	Ability to free-flow O_2	Ability to administer CPAP/PEEP	Easy to use
T-piece	Yes	Yes	Yes
Self-inflating bag[a]	Yes	No	Yes
Flow-inflating bag	Yes	Yes	No

CPAP, continuous positive airway pressure; PEEP, positive end expiratory pressure.
[a] Not all self-inflating bags can be used to deliver free-flow oxygen.

and held in place using a suitable grip that minimises leaks. Effectiveness of mask ventilation is judged by observing the chest rise and an increase in HR. A correctly sized mask should cover the nose and mouth, without extending beyond the tip of the chin or covering the eyes (WHO, 2016). Inflations should be given at a rate of 40–60 per minute.

CLINICAL PRACTICE 4.3

To achieve the correct number of inflations, count aloud: 'breathe-two-three, breathe-two-three', inflating the lungs each time you say 'breathe' and allowing the neonate to exhale on the count of 'two-three'.

The amount of pressure to give with inflations is determined by the neonate's gestation and underlying respiratory physiology. American Heart Association (AHA, 2020) guidelines for neonatal life support recommend, when using a T-piece resuscitator to ventilate a neonate who is born at term gestation, using an initial **peak inspiratory pressure (PIP)** of 30 cm H_2O and a **positive end expiratory pressure (PEEP)** of 5 cm H_2O. In preterm neonates, lower pressures are usually required – for example, a PIP of 20–25 cm H_2O and a PEEP of 5 cm H_2O (Aziz et al., 2020). Higher pressures may be required if the infant does not respond. If a self-inflating bag is used, the bag is squeezed with only enough pressure to make the chest rise.

Laryngeal mask airway

A laryngeal mask or supraglottic airway (Fig. 4.6) is an alternative airway to mask ventilation when face-mask ventilation is unsuccessful and tracheal intubation is unsuccessful or not feasible (Luba & Cutter, 2010). The smallest **laryngeal mask airway (LMA)** available, size 1, is suitable only for neonates over 34 weeks' gestation, or who are over 2 kg and up to 5 kg. It can be useful in securing an airway in term or near-term neonates if face-mask ventilation is unsuccessful and tracheal intubation is unsuccessful or not feasible (ANZCOR, 2021). There is a variety of brands of LMA available (see Fig. 4.6). Clinicians should be familiar with the type of LMA available at their site.

EVIDENCE-BASED PRACTICE RESEARCH 4.2

Current recommendations are to give inflations at 40–60 per minute if PPV is required. However, these inflations are very short and may not be long enough to open the lungs in very preterm neonates with stiff lungs. There is some evidence that a longer or sustained inflation is preferred to facilitate lung fluid clearance and to aerate the lungs. The AHA recommends an inflation time of ≤ 1 second (AHA, 2020). A sustained inflation greater than 10 seconds in the preterm infant is not recommended and is potentially harmful (Aziz et al., 2020; Wyckoff et al., 2020).

When to cease positive pressure ventilation

PPV can be ceased when the neonate is breathing and the HR remains over 100 bpm. The HR and breathing should continue to be observed at least every 30 seconds. If the neonate is breathing effectively and the HR remains over 100 bpm, they are likely to be stable and not require further assistance, and can be placed on the mother's chest for skin-to-skin contact.

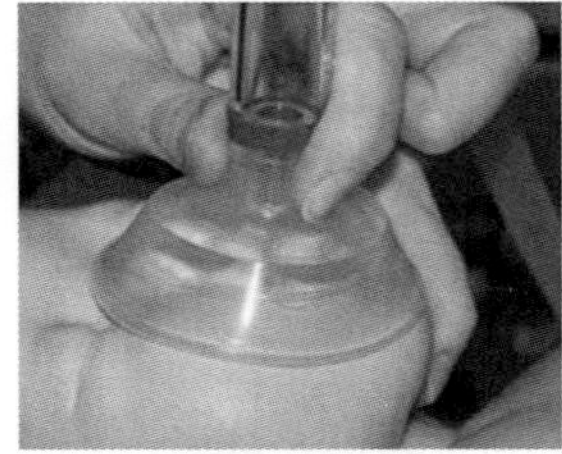
The stem hold

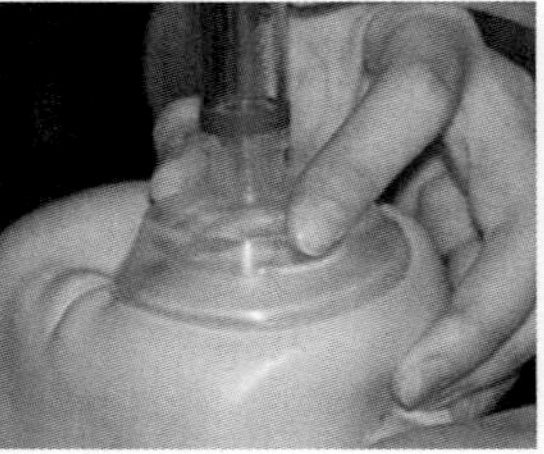
The two-point top hold

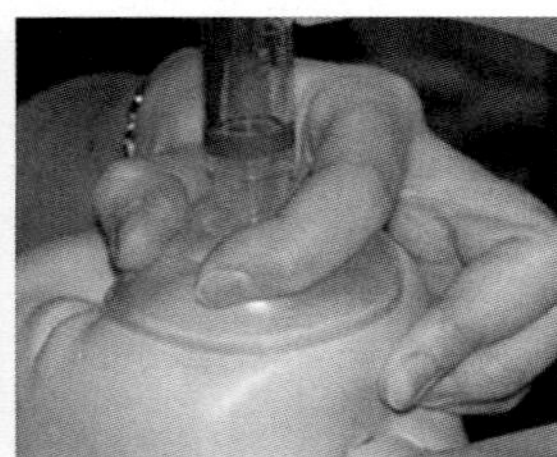
The OK rim hold

FIGURE 4.5 **Techniques to apply a mask to a neonate's face during positive pressure ventilation**
The recommended technique for a commonly used mask is the two-point top hold.
Source: Wood et al. (2008). With permission from BMJ Publishing Group Ltd.

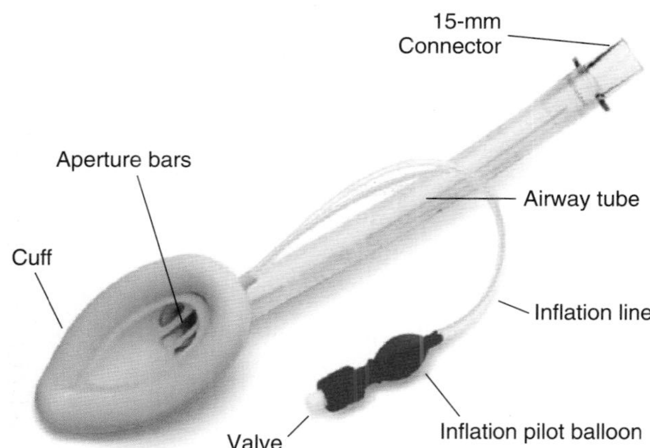

FIGURE 4.6 **Laryngeal mask airway**
Source: Tracy et al. (2018).

The use of oxygen with positive pressure ventilation in the birthing suite

During the first minutes of life, SpO_2 increases from intrapartum levels of 30–40% (East et al., 2014) to 95–100% by 5–10 minutes after birth (Dawson et al., 2010). Clinical assessment of the neonate is important before starting oxygen therapy. However, clinical assessments of colour and HR are subjective and unreliable (ANZCOR, 2021). Many healthy neonates do not appear centrally pink until several minutes after birth; this is normal and does not mean that they need oxygen. A pulse oximeter with the sensor placed in a preductal position on the neonate's right hand/wrist provides continuous measurement of oxygen saturation and HR. When the sensor is applied correctly, it provides measurements within 90 seconds of birth (ANZCOR, 2021). Suggested target oxygen saturation measurements at intervals after birth have been recommended (ANZCOR, 2021) (see Box 4.2). The goal is to avoid hypoxia and hyperoxia, particularly in extremely preterm neonates.

In term neonates receiving respiratory support at birth with PPV, it is recommended to begin with air (21%) rather than 100% oxygen (Welsford et al., 2019a; Wyckoff et al., 2020). If, despite effective ventilation, there is no increase in HR or oxygenation (guided by oximetry wherever possible) remains inadequate, a higher concentration of oxygen is used to achieve preductal oxygen saturation targets (Madar et al., 2021). If increased oxygen concentrations are used, they should be weaned as soon as possible to prevent hyperoxia. For preterm neonates less than 32 weeks' gestation at birth, oxygen concentration is initiated between 21% (air) and 30% (Aziz et al., 2020; Madar et al., 2021; Welsford et al., 2019b; Wyckoff et al., 2020).

CLINICAL PRACTICE 4.4

The first priority in resuscitation of the newly born neonate is to ensure adequate ventilation of the lungs, before increasing the concentration of inspired oxygen.

Cardiac compressions in the birthing suite

Very few neonates will require chest compressions because the circulation is almost always maintained until all respiratory activity ceases. Cardiac compressions are recommended if the HR is less than 60 bpm despite at least 30 seconds of adequate PPV. The oxygen is increased to 100% if cardiac compressions are required (ANZCOR, 2021; Aziz et al., 2020; Madar et al., 2021). The neonatal nurse/midwife must anticipate and prepare for intubation and securing vascular access. If there is no one skilled at intubation, the neonatal nurse/midwife must continue PPV.

CLINICAL PRACTICE 4.5

If chest compressions are required, access to the neonate can be facilitated by moving the neonate so that their body lies across the cot instead of the traditional 'head at the end of the cot' position.

There are two methods to administer cardiac compressions: the two-thumb and the two-finger technique. The two-thumb technique is the preferred method as greater pressure can be applied, generating higher systolic and coronary perfusion pressure (Solevåg & Schmölzer, 2017). Additionally, it is less tiring for the clinician administering compressions (see Fig. 4.7). This method requires the clinician to use both hands to encircle the neonate's chest with the thumbs on the sternum (thumbs are superimposed or side by side) and the fingers under the neonate's back. In the two-finger technique, the resuscitator places the tips of their first two fingers (or the middle and ring fingers) in a perpendicular position over the sternum and direct pressure is applied downwards (see Fig. 4.8). This technique is useful when there is only

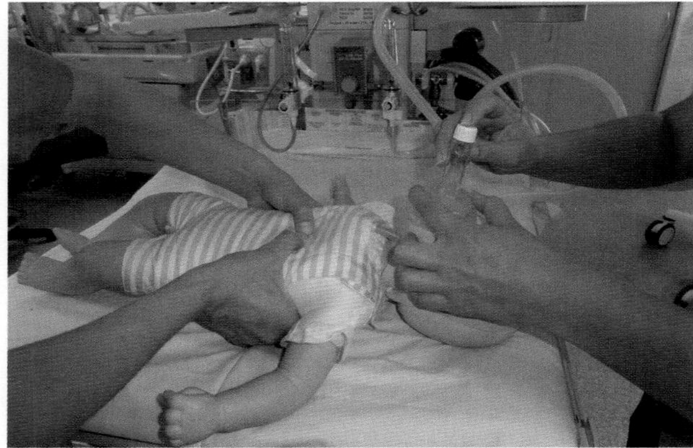

FIGURE 4.7 **The two-thumb technique of cardiac compressions**

Note how the neonate has been repositioned sideways on the resuscitation surface for easier access.

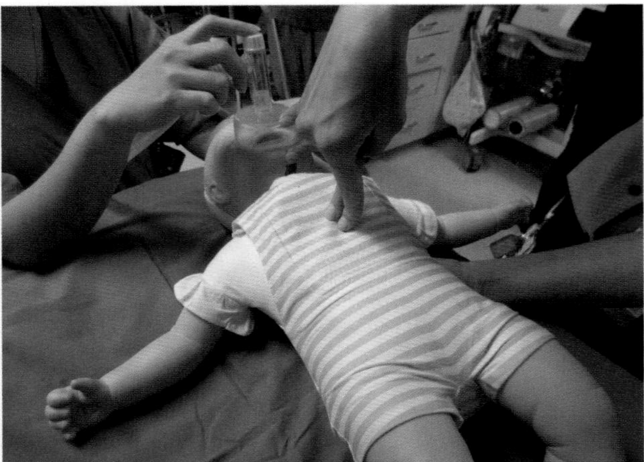

FIGURE 4.8 **The two-finger technique of cardiac compressions**

one person available for resuscitation, as the mask can be held in place with one hand while the other hand applies compressions. It also provides clearer access to the neonate's umbilical vein if administration of fluids and/or adrenaline is required (ANZCOR, 2021; Aziz et al., 2020; Madar et al., 2021).

CLINICAL PRACTICE 4.6

The correct ratio of compressions to ventilations is 3:1. The aim is to deliver 90 compressions and 30 inflations per minute.

Whichever technique is used, the fingers/thumbs of the clinician should not lift from the neonate's chest between compressions, so that no pressure is applied to the chest between or after compressions to allow the heart chambers to fill. Pressure is applied to the lower one-third of the sternum, just below an imaginary line drawn between the nipples, with fingers surrounding the lateral and posterior chest and approximately two finger-widths above the xiphoid process. With each compression, the chest should be depressed to one-third of the anterior–posterior diameter of the chest, then released to allow time for the heart to refill. The aim is to deliver 90 compressions and 30 breaths per minute at a ratio of 3:1 (compressions:inflations) in a coordinated approach. A slight pause after every third compression allows for lung inflation. To enable a coordinated approach and to maintain the correct rhythm, the person performing the compressions should count aloud: 'one-and-two-and-three-and-breathe'. Compressions are given at each count and ventilations given at 'breathe' to give the person managing the airway time to give the inflation.

The neonate's HR and respiratory rate are reassessed at least every 30 seconds. If the HR is greater than 60 bpm, compressions can be ceased. However, PPV is continued until the neonate has adequate spontaneous breathing and the HR remains greater than 100 bpm. It is important to continue reassessing the HR every 30 seconds to be sure that the HR remains above 60 bpm. Cardiac compressions are recommenced if the HR falls below 60 bpm (ANZCOR, 2021; Aziz et al., 2020; Madar et al., 2021).

CLINICAL PRACTICE 4.7

Minimise interruption to compressions. Stop compressions only for ongoing assessment of HR and respiratory effort, or if other treatments are required.

Intubation in the birthing suite

Endotracheal intubation allows for direct PPV to the lungs. A person skilled at intubation should be present for the birth of any neonate identified as high risk during transition. Additionally, endotracheal intubation should be considered if it is anticipated that PPV will be ongoing – for example, in the case of an extremely preterm neonate or for a neonate with a congenital diaphragmatic hernia. Other situations where intubation is recommended include when PPV via mask or laryngeal mask ventilation is inadequate, when chest compressions are required or for administration of medication via an ETT (ANZCOR, 2021).

In older children and adults, the ETT is cuffed and inserted using a curved blade. In contrast, in the neonatal population ETTs are uncuffed and inserted using a laryngoscope with a straight blade. The tube is positioned with the tip of the ETT at the third to fourth thoracic vertebrae (T3–T4) confirmed by chest X-ray. In the birthing suite it might not be possible to obtain an X-ray quickly. The alternative is to use an estimate of the neonate's weight and/or gestation with the '7-8-9 rule' to guide oral placement of the ETT. Using the data in Table 4.2, a 30–32 weeks' gestation neonate weighing approximately 1 kg will need the ETT inserted to approximately 7 cm at the lips (ANZCOR, 2021).

CLINICAL PRACTICE 4.8

The neonatal nurse/midwife has an important role when a neonate requires intubation. The nurse's/midwife's role includes assembling, checking, preparing and passing the equipment, monitoring the neonate's HR and oxygen saturation during the procedure, and assisting with stabilising and taping the endotracheal tube once it is in place. Neonatal nurse practitioners with advanced training can undertake neonatal intubation.

VERIFICATION OF ENDOTRACHEAL TUBE PLACEMENT

During resuscitation it is not practical to confirm that the ETT is in the correct position with a chest X-ray. Other observations can be made to verify the tube is in the trachea, such as the chest rising with each inflation, the

TABLE 4.2 **Endotracheal tube placement**

Corrected gestation (weeks)	Actual weight (kg)	ETT size	ETT at the lip (cm)	ETT at the nares	Laryngoscope blade size
23–24	0.5–0.6	2.0–2.5	5.5	6.0	00
25–26	0.7–0.8		6.0	6.5	
27–29	0.9–1.0		6.5	7.0	
30–32	1.1–1.4	3.0	7.0	7.5	0
33–34	1.5–1.8		7.5	8.0	
35–37	1.9–2.4	3.5	8.0	8.5	1
38–40	2.5–3.1		8.5	9.0	
41–43	3.2–4.2	3.5–4.0	9.0	9.5	

Adapted from: Australian and New Zealand Council on Resuscitation (ANZCOR) (2021).

HR increasing above 100 bpm and improving oxygen saturations. Other positive signs include condensation in the ETT, symmetrical air entry on auscultation of the lungs and change in colour of the end-tidal CO_2 detector. The CO_2 detector attaches to the end of the ETT and, in the presence of CO_2, it will change from purple to yellow over approximately 4–6 breaths. However, if cardiac output and pulmonary blood flow are low, the detector may not change colour despite the correct placement of the tube (ANZCOR, 2021).

Medications and fluids used in resuscitation

It is rare to need medications during resuscitation in the neonate, as adequate ventilation usually improves the HR and oxygenation. However, if the HR remains less than 60 bpm despite adequate ventilation and cardiac compressions, adrenaline may be needed.

ROUTES OF ADMINISTRATION FOR MEDICATIONS IN THE BIRTHING SUITE

Medications can be given via the intravascular route (via the umbilical vein) or via the ETT. The intravascular route is the most effective for delivery of adrenaline; however, it can take several minutes to gain vascular access. While there is little evidence to support the effectiveness of adrenaline delivered via the ETT, it can be administered via this route while venous access is acquired.

Umbilical venous access is recommended as the optimal method of vascular access in the birthing suite. If umbilical access is not possible, the **intraosseous (IO)** route could be used as an alternative (Wyckoff et al., 2020).

A peripheral intravenous cannula can be difficult to secure as these types of neonates are often hypovolaemic. An umbilical venous catheter (UVC) is the quickest method to achieve intravenous access. The umbilical vein is easily visualised and cannulated; it is large and patulous. The catheter is primed with 0.9% sodium chloride solution and inserted 4–5 cm. Once good backflow of blood is achieved, the catheter can be curled slightly on the abdomen and secured with sterile transparent dressing to prevent accidental dislodgement. Medications can then be administered via the catheter (ANZCOR, 2021).

MEDICATIONS

If the HR remains below 60 bpm despite effective ventilation with cardiac compressions, adrenaline 1:10,000 (100 μg/mL) undiluted is recommended. The dose via the ETT is 1 mL/kg administered as a rapid push.

The dose via the UVC route is 0.1–0.3 mL/kg (10–30 μg/kg) (Wyckoff et al., 2020). It is administered as a rapid push, followed by a 0.5 mL 0.9% sodium chloride flush. If the HR remains below 60 bpm despite effective ventilation and cardiac compressions, repeat doses can be given every few minutes. Subsequent doses are administered via the umbilical vein at 0.1–0.3 mL/kg (10–30 μg/kg) (Wyckoff et al., 2020).

VOLUME EXPANSION

If the neonate is in shock (as indicated by poor perfusion, pallor and weak pulses), has not responded to adequate resuscitation or blood loss is suspected, intravascular volume expansion should be considered. An isotonic crystalloid solution (0.9% sodium chloride or Hartmann's solution) is administered over several minutes via the UVC at 10 mL/kg (ANZCOR, 2021). If critical blood loss from the neonate is suspected (this is rare as blood loss is usually from the mother), red cells (O negative) can be given at 10 mL/kg (Wyllie et al., 2015). It is rare that preterm neonates require volume as part of resuscitation and fluids should be administered with caution. Rapidly infused volume may be associated with intraventricular and pulmonary haemorrhages (Wyllie et al., 2015).

EVIDENCE-BASED PRACTICE RESEARCH 4.3

Historically, sodium bicarbonate was used in resuscitation when PPV and cardiac massage were required. It was thought to reverse metabolic acidosis and improve myocardial function. However, there is insufficient evidence for this practice and, if ventilation is inadequate, the administration of sodium bicarbonate may exacerbate intracellular hypercarbia and impair myocardial and cerebral function. As a result, sodium bicarbonate is not recommended as a neonatal resuscitation medication unless resuscitation is prolonged (Wyckoff et al., 2020). If resuscitation is prolonged and the neonate is unresponsive to other therapies, a dose of sodium bicarbonate 1–2 mmol/kg, diluted 1:1 with water for injection, may be given slowly via the venous route only. It is imperative that adequate ventilation is sustained (Madar et al., 2021).

CLINICAL PRACTICE 4.9

Naloxone is a specific opiate antagonist used to reverse respiratory depression in a neonate whose mother received opiate medication within 4 hours of birth. However, Kattwinkel, in the 2010 ILCOR update, stated, 'there is no evidence of benefit and substantial evidence of risk, naloxone cannot be recommended during delivery room resuscitation' (Kattwinkel et al., 2010).

Establishing adequate respiratory support, using the principles outlined in the ANZCOR (2021) Newborn Life Support algorithm (see Fig. 4.2), is the most important component of resuscitation and supporting transition in this population.

If administered to a neonate whose mother is narcotic dependent, this may initiate abrupt withdrawal and seizures. However, if naloxone has been administered, the neonate should be admitted to the neonatal unit for cardiorespiratory monitoring for at least 4 hours to observe for signs of rebound respiratory depression. Dosing is 100 μg/kg/dose IM.

Continuing care after resuscitation

The type of care required after resuscitation will depend on the neonate's gestation, any comorbidities and the types of interventions the neonate has received. The mnemonic S.T.A.B.L.E.® helps clinicians remember components of care after resuscitation. It stands for:

S = sugar; consider testing for hypoglycaemia
T = thermoregulation; prevent hypo/hyperthermia
A = airway; is the neonate breathing normally? Is respiratory support required to maintain oxygenation and ventilation?
B = blood pressure (BP); monitor skin perfusion, heart rate, and blood pressure to evaluate for shock
L = laboratory work; is the neonate at risk for sepsis? Is a septic screen or antibiotics required?
E = emotional support for the family; communicate with the family. They will be anxious and need to be kept involved and informed about their baby's progress and need for continuing care (Karlsen 2013).

FAMILY-CENTRED CARE 4.2

Neonates who have required no or minimal resuscitation (drying and stimulation or short period of PPV) and have recovered quickly can stay with their mothers for skin-to-skin contact but should continue to have their breathing, HR and temperature monitored.

Discontinuing resuscitation

The time to discontinue resuscitation is controversial, as the effectiveness of resuscitation interventions throughout 10 consecutive minutes may not have been optimal, and evidence from hypothermia trials shows increasing numbers of intact survivors after those neonates experienced 10 minutes of an Apgar score of 0 (Natarajan et al., 2013). However, in large epidemiological studies, at birth an Apgar score of 0 at 10 minutes has been shown to be a strong predictor of mortality or morbidity in late-preterm and term neonates (Cnattingius et al., 2017).

At birth and in the neonatal unit, if there are no signs of life after prolonged continuous and adequate resuscitative efforts (10–20 minutes), it may be justifiable to discontinue resuscitation (Wyllie et al., 2015). This decision should be individualised and made by the most senior medical officer present in discussion with the consultant responsible for the neonate's care (Wyckoff et al., 2020) and the family.

BIRTHING SUITE MANAGEMENT OF NEONATES WITH ADDITIONAL REQUIREMENTS

Preterm neonates

Preterm neonates have both structural and functional lung immaturity compared with term neonates, making them more likely to require respiratory support in the birthing suite. Interventions in the birthing suite may affect short-term and long-term outcomes for preterm neonates. The approach to the management of preterm neonates is changing from being interventional and invasive to being observational and gentle. Nevertheless, preterm neonates are still likely to need oxygen supplementation because of their lung immaturity. However, their antioxidant defences to high levels of oxygen are reduced until the third trimester. There is a precarious balance between the need for oxygen and oxygen toxicity that can result in damage to the neonate's eyes and lungs from oxidative stress. For preterm neonates, ILCOR recommends commencing resuscitation either using room air or blended air and oxygen up to an oxygen concentration of 30% (Wyckoff et al., 2020). The percentage of oxygen is adjusted according to oxygen saturation measured by pulse oximetry. The ANZCOR (2021) Newborn Life Support algorithm (see Box 4.2) outlines the SpO_2 target range for each minute after birth. If the oxygen saturation measurement is outside the target range, the percentage of oxygen is adjusted until the target range is reached (Wyckoff et al., 2020). Individual hospitals may differ in how these adjustments are made.

CASE STUDY

4.1

Ms Smith is a primigravida who is now 27 weeks pregnant with twins. Her labour is induced because of evolving preeclampsia. You are called to the birthing suite to assist with managing these neonates.

1. What will you need to prepare to manage these very preterm neonates in the birthing suite? How will you prepare the:
   a. equipment
   b. personnel
   c. parent/s?

Twin 1 is male. He looks to weigh about 900 g. He is moving all his limbs, is crying and has an HR of 100 bpm. At 1 minute after birth his Apgar score is 7.

2. What is the immediate management for this male neonate?

Twin 2 is female, who looks to weigh about 800 g and is not breathing well. Her HR is 70 bpm. At 1 minute after birth her Apgar score is 5.

3. What is the immediate management for this female neonate? What is your rationale?

Neonate born through meconium-stained liquor

If meconium-stained liquor is present, it is recommended that a clinician with skill in endotracheal intubation is present at the birth; however, the neonatal nurse/midwife must be able to resuscitate the neonate until skilled help arrives. Regardless of the consistency of the meconium, the management of the newly born neonate is the same. If the neonate is vigorous – that is, breathing or crying with good tone – routine care is provided. Suction or endotracheal intubation is not required to clear the airway (Wyllie et al., 2015). If the neonate is not vigorous, has poor tone, minimal respiratory effort or HR less than 100 bpm, and there is meconium in the airway, then suction is required. Care should be taken to avoid stimulating the neonate by drying or excessive handling. Oropharyngeal suction could be considered: first the mouth, then the nose and providing PPV. Excessive or deep suction can induce a vasovagal response and should be avoided; the emphasis is on establishing respirations (Aziz et al., 2020). The current recommendation suggests against routine immediate direct laryngoscopy with or without tracheal suctioning (Wyckoff et al., 2020).

CLINICAL PRACTICE 4.10

If the nose is suctioned before the mouth, the neonate may gasp when the catheter is inserted into the nares and aspirate any secretions sitting in the oropharynx. A tip to help you to remember the order for suctioning the mouth and nose of the neonate is to remember that 'M' comes before 'N' in the alphabet. Suction the **m**outh before you suction the **n**ose.

If a skilled person is available to intubate the neonate, suction can be applied to the trachea after intubation. Suction can be performed through a meconium aspirator connected to the ETT, using a negative pressure less than 100 mmHg (133 cmH_2O, 13 kPa, 1.9 psi). The potential benefit of removing meconium from the trachea needs to be weighed against what is likely to be an urgent need for other resuscitation manoeuvres (Wyckoff et al., 2020).

EVIDENCE-BASED PRACTICE RESEARCH 4.4

In a large randomised clinical trial of over 1000 neonates, Vain and colleagues showed that routine intrapartum oropharyngeal and nasopharyngeal suctioning of term neonates born through meconium-stained amniotic fluid did not prevent meconium aspiration syndrome (Vain et al., 2004).

In a meta-analysis of four randomised clinical trials, vigorous term neonates born through meconium-stained liquor showed no benefit from tracheal suctioning (Halliday & Sweet, 2001).

Pneumothorax

A spontaneous pneumothorax in neonates is a rare complication. A pneumothorax is a collection of air or gas in the pleural space of the lung, causing the lung to collapse. It can occur most commonly in preterm neonates who have received PPV. However, neonates born at term can also develop a pneumothorax in response to the large negative pressure generated with their first few breaths after birth. Signs of a pneumothorax include decreased breathing sounds on the affected side and respiratory distress (nasal flaring, expiratory grunting, cyanosis, intercostal recession). If the neonate does not respond to resuscitation, consider the possibility of a pneumothorax. In the birthing suite, treatment of a pneumothorax can include needle aspiration or insertion of an intercostal drain (Kitsommart et al., 2012).

Choanal atresia

Congenital choanal atresia (CCA) is a very rare abnormality of the nares that occurs when there is no communication between the nasal cavity and the nasopharynx. The blockage can be either unilateral or bilateral but, when it is bilateral, it becomes a life-threatening medical emergency in the obligatory nasal-breathing neonate. Signs of CCA include respiratory distress following birth, which may result in cyanosis, unless the neonate is crying. In affected neonates, there will be an inability to pass a catheter through the nares. The neonate will have difficulty with sucking feeds and breathing at the same time. In the birthing suite, if the blockage is unilateral the neonate may not require additional support; however, if the defect is bilateral the neonate will require oral intubation (Andaloro and Mantia, 2021).

Congenital diaphragmatic hernia

Congenital diaphragmatic hernia (CDH) occurs when there is a defect in the diaphragm. Organs in the abdomen (i.e. stomach, bowels, liver, etc.) may fill the chest, thereby compressing the lungs and preventing normal development. Severe respiratory distress can occur as a result of lung hypoplasia. The level of assistance the neonate requires to breathe after birth is determined, in part, by the size of the lungs. If the lungs are hypoplastic, respiratory support and oxygen will be required in the birthing suite (Snoek et al., 2016).

A consortium of neonatal specialists, the Congenital Diaphragmatic Hernia (CDH) EURO Consortium, has published a standardised neonatal treatment protocol. Their recommendations for management of neonates with CDH in the birthing suite include targeting a preductal oxygen saturation of between 80% and 95% and postductal oxygen saturations >70% to prevent hypo/hyperoxia. Intubation is recommended as the optimal initial ventilation strategy, to reduce the amount of gas that enters the stomach and bowel. However, to avoid damage to the affected lung, low peak pressures, preferably <25 cmH_2O, are recommended. An orogastric or nasogastric tube with continuous or intermittent suctioning is inserted to avoid bowel distension and any additional ipsilateral lung compression (Snoek et al., 2016).

Abdominal wall defects

The two most common abdominal defects are omphalocoele and gastroschisis (Fig. 4.9). These are explained in more detail in Chapter 12. Immediate birthing suite management of either an omphalocoele or gastroschisis is to protect the exposed viscera and prevent hypothermia by wrapping the defect with clear plastic wrap or placing the lower half of the neonate's body into a plastic bag. An orogastric tube should be inserted to allow for gastric decompression to avoid distension of the gastrointestinal tract (Ferguson, 2017).

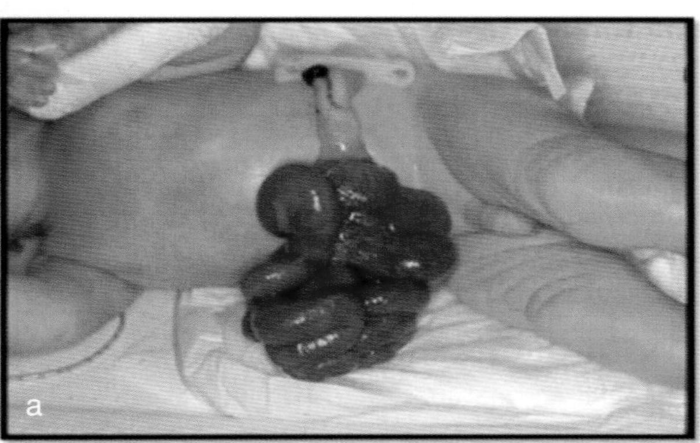

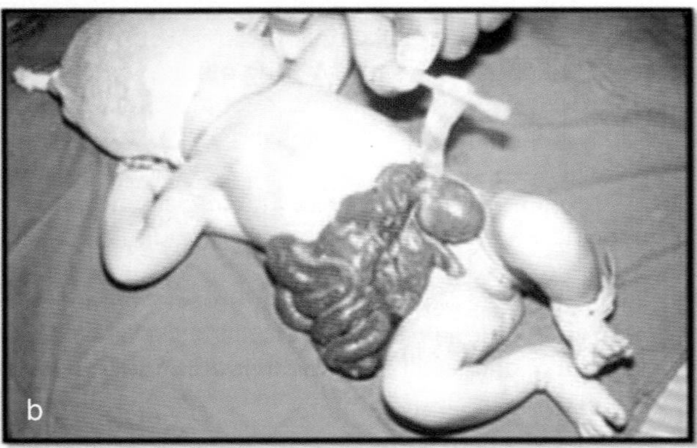

FIGURE 4.9 **Gastroschisis**
Source: Lakshminarayanan and Lakhoo (2014). Copyright © 2014 Elsevier Ltd.

RESUSCITATION IN THE NEONATAL SPECIAL CARE UNIT AND POSTNATAL WARDS

Other areas where an infant during the neonatal period might require intervention are the neonatal special care unit and the postnatal ward. The initial steps for assessment and management of the neonate should follow the Newborn Life Support algorithm provided as Fig. 4.2.

CLINICAL PRACTICE 4.11

In the neonatal intensive care unit, the nurse/midwife caring for an intubated infant needs to be able to determine quickly if the ETT becomes dislodged. Signs of a dislodged tube include increased oxygen requirement, decreased oxygen saturation, decreased HR, hearing the neonate cry and/or reduced breath sounds.
If an end-tidal CO_2 detector is available, this can be used to determine placement of the ETT. If the ETT has been dislodged it will NOT change colour during expiration.
If an ETT does become dislodged the neonate should be managed according to the Newborn Life Support algorithm (see Fig. 4.2).

Documentation

At the beginning of the resuscitation, one person should be allocated the task of documenting the time, interventions and the neonate's response to interventions. Documentation should be comprehensive and contemporaneous (ANZCOR, 2021). A standardised neonatal resuscitation record can be helpful to document birthing suite management; it should include an explanation of interventions performed and their timing (Kattwinkel et al., 1999).

Debriefing

Team debriefing immediately after a neonatal resuscitation is recommended (Wyckoff et al., 2020). The aim is to discuss what worked well and what could have been done better. It provides members of the resuscitation team with an opportunity to identify questions about the resuscitation. It may also be appropriate to plan for a later debriefing with relevant teams if needed. For staff distressed after participating in resuscitation, the hospital/health service should provide access to counselling services.

REFLECTION

Being present at the birth of a neonate who requires resuscitation can be a distressing experience for nurses/ midwives caring for the neonate and their family. How might you support yourself and colleagues after a stressful event?

Ethical issues and resuscitation

Neonatal nurses/midwives may be confronted with ethical issues around resuscitation. These issues may include initiating, withholding or discontinuing resuscitation. Examples of situations where active resuscitation might not be recommended are neonates diagnosed in the antenatal period with anencephaly or other life-limiting malformations. For some extremely preterm neonates for whom there is little possibility of intact survival, there should be a discussion with the parent/s regarding the possibility that initiation of active resuscitation might not be in the best interests of the neonate and the family (Byrne et al., 2008; Safer Care Victoria, 2020).

The decision about when to discontinue resuscitation may be influenced by the gestation of the neonate, presence of complications and the parents' expressed views regarding an acceptable risk of morbidity. When withdrawing or withholding resuscitation, care should be focused on the neonate's and family's comfort, privacy and dignity. The ethical issues around discontinuing care are discussed in greater detail in Chapter 23.

Parents and resuscitation

Parents may find witnessing the resuscitation of their baby distressing regardless of outcome. In contrast, many parents find it reassuring to see what was done to help their baby (Sawyer et al., 2015). Neonatal nurses/midwives need to, whenever possible, prepare parents for resuscitation if it is anticipated. They will be responsible for explaining to parents who and how many doctors/nurses/midwives are likely to be called to manage the resuscitation of their baby. The neonatal nurse/midwife can help by explaining the types of interventions that the neonate is likely to receive. If it is anticipated that the neonate will be transferred to the neonatal unit, this should be explained to the parents.

Parents must be kept informed during the resuscitation. A neonatal nurse/midwife can take on the role of liaising between the clinical team and the parents. She/he can talk with the parents about what the team is doing, answering questions and being present with the parents. The nurse/ midwife can also be with the parents when they first see their baby. Additionally, if the parents wish to have photos of their newly born baby, the neonatal nurse/midwife can facilitate this for them.

After resuscitation, an experienced clinician involved in the resuscitation should discuss with the parents what was involved in the resuscitation, expected future management and outcomes.

EDUCATION AND TRAINING IN NEONATAL RESUSCITATION

One of the key requirements for any healthcare professional who attends births is to have knowledge, clinical skills training and competency assessment in neonatal resuscitation undertaken annually (Council of International Neonatal Nurses (COINN), 2019). Nursing and midwifery registration authorities in many countries have identified the importance of registered nurses/midwives maintaining skills within their area of practice. Nurses and midwives are responsible for their continuing professional development (CPD). This includes updating knowledge related to administration of interventions, treatments, medications and best-practice guidelines within their area of practice. Additionally, the significance of CPD is recognised in the standards for neonatal nursing practice in international (COINN, 2019) and relevant national bodies – for example, Australia (ACNN, 2019) and New Zealand (NNCA, 2015). There are similar international (ICM, 2011) and national (NMBA, 2018) standards for midwives working with newly born infants.

Neonatal resuscitation requires the application of a combination of cognitive, technical and behavioural skills (Halamek, 2013). Organised programs to develop and maintain standards, skills and teamwork are required for neonatal resuscitation and are essential for healthcare providers and institutions caring for mothers and neonates at the time of birth (ANZCOR, 2021).

The traditional way of training for neonatal resuscitation has involved classroom-type settings with lectures, small group discussions and performing technical skills with mannequins. Assessment has been measured with oral and written examinations. Competency has been measured by nurses/midwives performing technical tasks at skill stations. An alternative to this low-fidelity style of learning is high-fidelity simulation. High-fidelity training for neonatal resuscitation, involving testing clinical skills and team simulation, is a powerful tool for evaluating individual and team performance (Halamek, 2013).

CONCLUSION

In this chapter the transition at birth from fetal to neonatal circulation was reviewed. Most neonates transit from intrauterine to extrauterine life without any assistance. However, some neonates require assistance to breathe. This chapter outlined the skills required to assist neonates to breathe, highlighting the provision of adequate and appropriate ventilation as the priority when the neonate is not breathing. All staff members involved in the care of

neonates must be familiar with equipment that might be required and should have regular training and assessments of competency in basic resuscitation techniques. Resuscitation guidelines are updated at least every 5 years. (Nurses/midwives must keep up to date with current evidence for practices used in neonatal resuscitation.) The neonatal nurse/midwife has a responsibility to communicate with and support parents when their baby requires resuscitation.

References/Acknowledgements

American Heart Association (AHA). (2020). Highlights of the 2020 American Heart Association Guidelines for CPR and ECC. Dallas, TX: AHA. <https://cpr.heart.org/-/media/CPR-Files/CPR-Guidelines-Files/Highlights/Hghlghts_2020_ECC_Guidelines_English.pdf> (Accessed 13 March 2020).

Andaloro, C., & La Mantia, I. (2021). Choanal atresia. In: StatPearls [Internet]. Treasure Island, FL: StatPearls Publishing. <https://www.ncbi.nlm.nih.gov/books/NBK507724/>.

Australian and New Zealand Council on Resuscitation (ANZCOR). (2021). Guidelines 13.1–13.10. <https://resus.org.au/guidelines/index/> (Accessed 18 February 2022).

Australian College of Neonatal Nurses (ACNN). (2019). *Standards for practice* (4th ed.). Camperdown, NSW: ACNN. <https://www.acnn.org.au/resources/resources/ACNN-Standards-for-Practice-4th-Ed.pdf> (Accessed 18 February 2022).

Australian Institute of Health and Welfare (AIHW). (2020). *Australia's mothers and babies 2018 – in brief*. Perinatal statistics series no. 36. Cat no. PER 108. Canberra, ACT: AIHW.

Australian Institute of Health and Welfare (AIHW). (2021). *Australia's mothers and babies*. Cat. no. PER 101. Canberra, ACT: AIHW. <https://www.aihw.gov.au/reports/mothers-babies/australias-mothers-babies> (Accessed 18 February 2022).

Australian Resuscitation Council (ARC). (2010). *Guideline 13.4: Airway management and mask ventilation of the newborn infant*. <http://www.nzrc.org.nz/assets/Uploads/New-Guidelines/guideline-13-4dec10.pdf> (Accessed 18 February 2022).

Aziz, K., Lee, H. C., Escobedo, M. B., Hoover, A. V., Kamath-Rayne, B. D., Kapadia, V. S., et al. (2020). Part 5: neonatal resuscitation: 2020 American heart association guidelines for cardiopulmonary resuscitation and emergency cardiovascular care. *Circulation, 142*(16_Suppl_2), S524–S550.

Byrne, S., Szyld, E., & Kattwinkel, J. (2008). The ethics of delivery-room resuscitation. *Seminars in Fetal and Neonatal Medicine, 13*, 440–447.

Chow, S. S. W., Creighton, P., Chambers, G. M., & Lui, K. (2021). *Report of the Australian and New Zealand Neonatal Network 2019*. Sydney, NSW: UNSW.

Cnattingius, S., Norman, M., Granath, F., Petersson, G., Stephansson, O., & Frisell, T. (2017). Apgar score components at 5 minutes: risks and prediction of neonatal mortality. *Paediatric and Perinatal Epidemiology, 31*(4), 328–337.

Council of International Neonatal Nurses (COINN). (2019). International Neonatal Nursing Competency Framework. *Journal of Neonatal Nursing, 25*, 58–264.

Dawson, J. A., Davis, P. G., O'Donnell, C. P., Kamlin, C. O., & Morley, C. J. (2007). Free-flow oxygen delivery to newly born infants. *Archives of Disease in Childhood. Fetal and Neonatal Edition, 92*(2), F132–F134.

Dawson, J. A., Kamlin, C. O., Vento, M., Wong, C., Cole, T. J., Donath, S. M., et al. (2010). Defining the reference range for oxygen saturation for infants after birth. *Pediatrics, 125*, e1340–e1347.

East, C. E., Begg, L., Colditz, P. B., & Lau, R. (2014). Fetal pulse oximetry for fetal assessment in labour. *Cochrane Database of Systematic Reviews, 10*, CD004075. doi: 10.1002/14651858.CD004075.pub4.

Ferguson, M. (2017). Nursing management of gastroschisis in the newborn. *Journal of Neonatal Nursing, 23*(1), 40–45.

Fernandes, C. J. (2017). Physiologic transition from intrauterine to extrauterine life. *UpToDate*. Walters Kluwer. <http://www.uptodate.com/contents/physiologic-transition-from-intrauterine-to-extrauterine-life?source=search> (Accessed 18 February 2022).

Fogarty, M., Osborn, D. A., Askie, L., Seidler, A. L., Hunter, K., Lui, K., et al. (2018). Delayed vs early umbilical cord clamping for preterm infants: a systematic review & meta-analysis. *American Journal of Obstetrics and Gynecology, 218*(1), 1–18.

Foster, J. P., Dawson, J. A., Davis, P. G., & Dahlen, H. G. (2017). Routine oro/nasopharyngeal suction versus no suction at birth. *Cochrane Database of Systematic Reviews, 4*, CD010332.

Gaertner, V. D., Flemmer, S. A., Lorenz, L., Davis, P. G., & Kamlin, C. O. (2018). Physical stimulation of newborn infants in the delivery room. *Archives of Disease in Childhood. Fetal and Neonatal Edition, 103*(2), F132–F136.

Halamek, L. P. (2013). Simulation as a methodology for assessing the performance of healthcare professionals working in the delivery room. *Seminars in Fetal and Neonatal Medicine, 18*, 369–372.

Halliday, H. L., & Sweet, D. G. (2001). Endotracheal intubation at birth for preventing morbidity and mortality in vigorous, meconium-stained infants born at term. *Cochrane Database of Systematic Reviews, 1*, CD000500. doi: 10.1002/14651858.CD000500.

Hillman, N., Kallapur, S. G., & Jobe, A. (2012). Physiology of transition from intrauterine to extrauterine life. *Clinics in Perinatology, 39*(4), 769–783. doi: 10.1016/j.clp.2012.09.009.

Hooper, S. B., Te Pas, A. B., Lewis, R. A., & Morley, C. J. (2010). Establishing functional residual capacity at birth. *Neo Reviews, 11*(9), c474–c482.

Hooper, S. B., Te Pas, A. B., Lang, J., van Vonderen, J. J., Roehr, C. C., Kluckow, M., et al. (2015). Cardiovascular transition at birth: a physiological sequence. *Pediatric Research, 77*(5), 608–614.

International Confederation of Midwives (ICM). (2011). *Global standards for midwifery regulation*. The Hague, Netherlands: ICM. <https://www.internationalmidwives.org/assets/files/general-files/2018/04/global-standards-for-midwifery-regulation-eng.pdf> (Accessed 18 February 2022).

Jha, K., Nassar, G. N., & Makker, K. (2021). Transient tachypnea of the newborn. In: StatPearls [Internet]. Treasure Island, FL: StatPearls Publishing. <https://www.ncbi.nlm.nih.gov/books/NBK537354/>.

Karlsen, Kristine A. (2013). The S.T.A.B.L.E. Program – post-resuscitation/pre-transport stabilization care of sick infants. 6ed. Stableprogram.org. Salt Lake City, UT; S.T.A.B.L.E., Inc.

Kattwinkel, J., Niermeyer, S., Nadkarni, V., Tibballs, J., Phillips, B., Zideman, D., et al. (1999). Resuscitation of the newly born infant: an advisory statement from the pediatric working group of the International Liaison Committee on resuscitation. *Resuscitation, 40*, 71–88.

Kattwinkel, J., Perlman, J. M., Aziz, K., Colby, C., Fairchild, K., Gallagher, J., et al. (2010). Part 15: Neonatal resuscitation. *Circulation, 122*(18 suppl 3), S909–S919.

Kitsommart, R., Martins, B., Bottino, M. N., & Sant'Anna, G. M. (2012). Expectant management of pneumothorax in preterm infants receiving assisted ventilation: report of 4 cases and review of the literature. *Respiratory Care, 57*(5), 789–793.

Kluckow, M., & Hooper, S. B. (2015). Using physiology to guide time to cord clamping. *Seminars in Fetal and Neonatal Medicine, 20*(4), 225–231.

Lakshminarayanan, B., & Lakhoo, K. (2014). Abdominal wall defects. *Early Human Development, 90*(12), 917–920.

Luba, K., & Cutter, T. (2010). Supraglottic airway devices in the ambulatory setting. *Anesthesiology Clinics, 28*(2), 295–314. doi: 10.1016/j.anclin.2010.02.004.

Madar, J., Roehr, C. C., Ainsworth, S., Ersdal, H., Morley, C., Rüdiger, M., et al. (2021). European Resuscitation Council Guidelines 2021: Newborn resuscitation and support of transition of infants at birth. *Resuscitation, 161*, 291–326. doi: 10.1016/j.resuscitation.2021.02.014.

McDonald, S. J., Middleton, P., Dowswell, T., & Morris, P. S. (2014). Effect of timing of umbilical cord clamping of term infants on maternal and neonatal outcomes. *Evidence-Based Child Health: A Cochrane Review Journal, 9*(2), 303–397.

Natarajan, G., Shankaran, S., Laptook, A. R., Pappas, A., Bann, C. M., McDonald, S. A., et al. (2013): Apgar scores at 10 min and outcomes at 6–7 years following hypoxic-ischaemic encephalopathy. *Archives of Disease in Childhood. Fetal and Neonatal Edition, 98*(6), F473–F479.

Neonatal Nurses College Aotearoa (NNCA). (2015). *Standards for neonatal nursing practice*. <https://www.nzno.org.nz/groups/colleges_sections/colleges/neonatal_nurses_college> (Accessed 18 February 2022).

Nursing and Midwifery Board of Australia (NMBA). (2018). Midwife standards for practice. Canberra, ACT: NMBA, Australian Health Practitioner Regulation Agency. <https://www.nursingmidwiferyboard.gov.au/Codes-Guidelines-Statements/Professional-standards/Midwife-standards-for-practice.aspx> (Accessed 18 February 2022).

O'Shea, J. E., Thio, M., Owen, L. S., Wong, C., Dawson, J. A., & Davis, P. G. (2015). Measurements from preterm infants to guide face mask size. *Archives of Disease in Childhood. Fetal and Neonatal Edition, 101*(4), F294–F298. doi: 10.1136/archdischild-2014-307350.

Pinheiro, J. M. (2009). The Apgar cycle: a new view of a familiar scoring system. *Archives of Disease in Childhood. Fetal and Neonatal Edition, 94*(1), F70–F72.

Rychik, J., & Tian, Z. (2012). *Fetal cardiovascular imaging: a disease-based approach*. Philadelphia, PA: Saunders. Fig. 1.1.

Safer Care Victoria. (2020). *Extreme prematurity guideline – clinical guidance*. Melbourne, Vic: Victoria State Government.

Sawyer, A., Ayers, S., Bertullies, S., Thomas, M., Weeks, A. D., Yoxall, C. W., et al. (2015). Providing immediate neonatal care and resuscitation at birth beside the mother: parents' views, a qualitative study. *BMJ Open, 5*(9), e008495.

Snoek, K. G., Reiss, I. K., Greenough, A., Capolupo, I., Urlesberger, B., Wessel, L., et al. (2016). Standardized postnatal management of infants with congenital diaphragmatic hernia in Europe: the CDH EURO consortium consensus, 2015 update. *Neonatology, 110*(1), 66–74.

Solevåg, A. L., & Schmölzer, G. M. (2017). Optimal chest compression rate and compression to ventilation ratio in delivery room resuscitation: evidence from newborn piglets and neonatal manikins. *Frontiers in Pediatrics, 5*, 3.

Tracy, M. B., Priyadarshi, A., Goel, D., Lowe, K., Huvanandana, J., & Hinder, M. (2018). How do different brands of size 1 laryngeal mask airway compare with face mask ventilation in a dedicated laryngeal mask airway teaching manikin? *Archives of Disease in Childhood. Fetal and Neonatal Edition, 103*, F271–F276.

Vain, N. E., Szyld, E. G., Prudent, L. M., Wiswell, T. E., Aguilar, A. M., & Vivas, N. (2004). Oropharyngeal and nasopharyngeal suctioning of meconium-stained neonates before delivery of their shoulders: multicentre, randomised controlled trial. *Lancet, 364*, 597–602.

Van Woudenberg, C., Wills, C., & Baas Rubarth, L. (2012). Newborn transition to extrauterine life. *Neonatal Network, 31*(5), 317–322.

Welsford, M., Nishiyama, C., Shortt, C., Isayama, T., Dawson, J. A., Weiner, G., et al. (2019a). Room air for initiating term newborn resuscitation: a systematic review with meta-analysis. *Pediatrics,143*(1), e20181825. doi: https://doi.org/10.1542/peds.2018-1825.

Welsford, M., Nishiyama, C., Shortt, C., Weiner, G., Roehr, C. C., Isayama, T., et al. (2019b). Initial oxygen use for preterm newborn resuscitation: a systematic review with meta-analysis. *Pediatrics, 143*(1), e20181828. doi: 10.1542/peds.2018-1828.

Widström, A.-M., Brimdyr, K., Svensson, K., Cadwell, K., & Nissen, E. (2019). Skin-to-skin contact the first hour after birth, underlying implications and clinical practice. *Acta Paediatrica, 108*, 1192–1204. doi: 10.1111/apa.14754.

Wood, F. E., Morley, C. J., Dawson, J. A., Kamlin, C. O., Owen, L. S., Donath, S., et al. (2008). Improved techniques reduce face mask leak during simulated neonatal resuscitation: study 2. *Archives of Disease in Childhood. Fetal and Neonatal Edition, 93*, F230–F234.

World Health Organization (WHO). (2012). *Guidelines on basic newborn resuscitation*. Geneva: WHO.

World Health Organization (WHO). (2016). *WHO technical specification of neonatal resuscitation devices*. Geneva: WHO. <https://www.who.int/publications/i/item/9789241510264> (Accessed 18 February 2022).

Wyckoff, M. H., Wyllie, J., Aziz, K., de Almeida, M. F., Fabres, J., Fawke, J., et al. on behalf of the Neonatal Life Support Collaborators (2020). Neonatal life support 2020. International consensus on cardiopulmonary resuscitation and emergency cardiovascular care science with treatment recommendations. *Circulation, 142* (suppl 1), S185–S221.

Wyllie, J., Bruinenberg, J., Roehr, C. C., Rüdiger, M., Trevisanuto, D., & Urlesberger, B. (2015). European Resuscitation Council guidelines for resuscitation, 2015. *Resuscitation, 95*, 249–263.

CHAPTER 5

NUTRITION AND FLUID MANAGEMENT IN THE NEONATAL UNIT

TRUDI MANNIX, KIM GIBSON AND CARMEL COLLINS

Learning objectives

After reading this chapter you will be able to:

- describe the anatomical development of the gastrointestinal tract
- calculate the fluid, energy, electrolyte, macronutrient and micronutrient requirements of the preterm neonate
- describe the advantages and risks of the administration of total parenteral nutrition
- discuss the use of human milk fortifier and donor milk for preterm neonates
- describe the initiation and advancement of enteral feeds, and the assessment of feeding tolerance and growth.

Key words, terms and abbreviations

breast milk
donor breast milk
expressed breast milk (EBM)
feeding tolerance
growth
intravenous (IV) catheters
minimal enteral feeds (MEF)
necrotising enterocolitis (NEC)
parenteral nutrition (PN)
parenteral nutrition-associated liver disease (PNALD)
small for gestational age (SGA)
total parenteral nutrition (TPN)
umbilical venous catheters (UVCs)
very low birthweight (VLBW)

INTRODUCTION

The nutritional management of preterm neonates presents an ongoing challenge to clinicians. Postnatal **growth** failure remains a common consequence of preterm birth and is associated with adverse neurodevelopmental outcomes. The last trimester of pregnancy is a time of rapid fetal growth and active transplacental nutrient transfer. With preterm birth and the interruption of placental nutrient transfer and limited nutrient stores of the neonate, a significant nutrient deficit can rapidly develop, affecting postnatal growth and cognitive function. Due to the immaturity of the preterm neonate, establishing enteral feeds takes time and parenteral (intravenous) nutrition forms an integral part of care. Although the ideal postnatal rate of weight gain and body composition for preterm neonates is not known, in the absence of a 'gold standard', current nutritional management is directed towards achieving a postnatal growth rate similar to intrauterine growth (Izquierdo Renau et al., 2019). Achieving this goal, however, is difficult, with many controversies and limited high-quality evidence.

DEVELOPMENT OF THE GASTROINTESTINAL TRACT

The anatomical development of the gastrointestinal tract commences around the fourth week of gestation with partitioning of the yolk sac and the formation of the primitive gut, and is complete by 20 weeks' gestation (Ditzenberger 2018). During the second trimester the fetus begins to swallow amniotic fluid, which is important for gastrointestinal tract development – see Chapter 12. By 25 weeks' gestation the fetal intestine can digest and absorb milk but to a more limited degree than the more mature infant (Brown et al., 2021). The preterm neonate's ability to feed enterally is limited by the immature mechanical function of the gastrointestinal tract, including the suck–swallow reflex, gastric emptying and gastric motility. A mature suck–swallow–breathe pattern starts to develop at around 32 weeks' gestation (Hair, 2021), and is fully mature between 34 and 37 weeks of gestation (Bakker et al., 2021); from 25 to 30 weeks' gestation, gastric motility is 'disorganised', developing to a mature pattern by 36 weeks (Henderickx et al., 2021); gastric emptying is slower in preterm than term infants and gastric enzymes are present but in low concentrations (Brown et al., 2021). There is increasing evidence that the intestinal microbiome plays important roles in nutrition and the developing immune system, influencing disease development and health outcomes. The gut microbiome is composed of trillions of microorganisms, with between 500 and 3000 species and 5 million unique genes. Mode of birth (caesarean or vaginal), antibiotic use and type of enteral feeding (**breast milk** or formula) all contribute to the balance of the gut microbiome (Pérez-Cano, 2020).

STANDARDISED FEEDING PROTOCOLS AND AUDITS

The introduction of evidence-based, standardised feeding protocols in neonatal units has the potential to reduce variation in practice, resulting in increased use of breast milk, earlier introduction of feeds, reduced time to achieve full enteral feeds, improved growth and a reduction in serious outcomes including **necrotising enterocolitis (NEC)** (McLeod et al., 2021). Inconsistencies among neonatal units in the feeding management of preterm neonates persist, with evidence-based interventions often not applied uniformly to daily practice (Bakker et al., 2021). Audits of nutritional management form an essential part of ongoing care, with findings consistently highlighting the difference between what clinicians think is happening and what is actually administered.

CLINICAL PRACTICE 5.1

Consider forming a core nutrition support team (NST) in your unit. Include interested representatives from each discipline, including neonatologists, neonatal nurses, midwives, dietitians, pharmacists and parents. This team can take responsibility for continuing education, updating and auditing standardised feeding protocols and advising on nutritional issues.

Vlug et al. (2020) have described NSTs as the development of multidisciplinary teams focused on the management of patients receiving PN.

On a day-to-day basis, include parents in the planning and management of their infant's nutrition.

Fluid and electrolytes

Fluid supplementation is based on meeting maintenance needs, replacing ongoing losses (insensible and sensible water losses), and environmental conditions. In the first 24–48 hours postnatally, oliguria is present, followed by natriuresis (excretion of sodium in the urine), then diuresis and weight loss in days 2–3 as contraction of extracellular fluid occurs, followed by a post-diuretic phase on days 4–5 characterised by varied urine output (Ringer, 2020). The early postnatal weight loss (10–15% of birthweight) reflects a combination of physiological weight loss and weight loss associated with catabolism (Ringer, 2020).

Fluid volumes commence at approximately 60 mL/kg/day, as indicated in Table 5.1, and are gradually increased by 20–30 mL/kg/day to an average maximum of 150 mL/kg/day (Bolisetty et al., 2020), although regimens should vary to meet the requirements of individual neonates, as well as between neonatal units. During the period of extracellular fluid contraction (in the first 24–48 hours of life), sodium intake should be restricted (1.0 mmol/kg/day), then increased to a maximum of 4.6 mmol/kg/day in the preterm and 3.4 mmol/kg/day in near-term and term infants; potassium supplementation is

TABLE 5.1 **Fluid intake days 1–6 in mL/kg/day**

Day of life	Birthweight	
	<1500 grams	≥1500 grams
1	80–90	60–80
2	100–110	80–100
3	120–130	100–120
4	130–150	120–150
5	140–160	140–160
6	160–180	140–160

Source: adapted from Koletzko et al. (2005).

2.7–3.0 mmol/kg/day depending on gestational age, commenced once plasma potassium levels are within normal ranges (Bolisetty et al., 2020). It is important to monitor and control sodium intake in preterm neonates as they are at risk of early hypernatraemia and later hyponatraemia because of their immature renal system. (See Chapter 14 for more information about renal function in preterm neonates.) Sodium deficiency is associated with poor growth, and measurements of sodium in urine and serum may be necessary to guide sodium supplementation, and then reduce sodium intake once levels are corrected (Givens-Bell, 2021).

Fluids are calculated using birthweight until birthweight has been regained. Fluid requirements should be re-calculated at the commencement of each shift to ensure that the volume being administered is the same as that ordered. An accurate, cumulative hourly record of intake and output needs to be maintained. Regular monitoring of electrolytes, glucose and urea is also required.

EVIDENCE-BASED PRACTICE RESEARCH 5.1

The incidence of patent ductus arteriosus (PDA) and NEC is reduced if fluid intake is restricted judiciously during the first 24–48 hours of life (so that physiological needs are met without dehydration) (Rutledge et al., 2021). The rationale for fluid restriction to prevent PDA is to reduce the left atrial overload associated with left-to-right ductal shunting. In neonates with a PDA and a large left-to-right shunt, blood flow to the intestines is reduced (the 'steal' phenomenon), which increases the risk of NEC (Diez et al., 2020).

TOTAL PARENTERAL NUTRITION

Intravenous total parenteral nutrition (TPN) is necessary for nutritional support of preterm and high-risk neonates when enteral intake is not possible or fails to provide sufficient energy and protein to meet requirements. TPN provides amino acids, glucose and electrolytes, lipids and vitamins. As Table 5.2 demonstrates, volumes to be administered commence at 60 mL/kg/day. If neonates receiving standardised TPN formulations require higher fluid volumes, this can be achieved by adding extra fluid using a 'piggyback' line.

TPN solution can be prescribed on an individualised basis or using standardised formulations. In Australia and New Zealand, consensus has been gained on the standardisation of TPN solutions. This includes a 'starter' formulation for use in the first 1–2 days and a 'standard' formulation for stable preterm neonates <32 weeks and/or <1500 g within the first 12 hours of life (Bolisetty et al., 2020). Standardised TPN has been shown to reduce practice variation and labour costs, and may minimise errors in TPN prescribing. Compared with individualised TPN solutions, it is readily available, minimising the delay in commencing nutritional support, and it provides adequate nutrition to the majority of neonates (Bolisetty et al., 2020). See Table 5.3 for 'starter' and 'standard' TPN formulations.

CLINICAL PRACTICE 5.2

Total parenteral nutrition is generally required in neonates born at <30 weeks' gestation or those born at >30 weeks' gestation and unlikely to achieve full enteral feeds (150 mL/kg/day enteral) by day 5 of life. Umbilical venous lines provide convenient short-term access for nutrition, but central lines are safer for long-term intravenous infusions.

Administration of total parenteral nutrition

Intravenous (IV) catheter

The use of **intravenous (IV) catheters** for the delivery of **parenteral nutrition (PN)** is usually temporary until central venous access can be established. PN is generally restricted to infants with central venous catheter (CVC)

TABLE 5.2 **Total parenteral nutrition intake**

	Volume of fluid (mL/kg/d)	Standardised TPN formulation	Protein (g/kg/d)	Lipid emulsion (g/kg/d)
Day 1	60	Starter	2	1
Days 2–3	80–90	Starter – standard	3	2
Days 4–6	120	Standard	4	3–4
Day 7	150	Standard	4	3–4

Source: adapted from Bolisetty et al. (2014).

TABLE 5.3 **Australasian consensus on standardised parenteral nutrition formulations**

	Starter PN birth to 24–48 h	Standard preterm PN After 24–48 h	High sodium preterm PN	7.5% Dextrose preterm PN	34 weeks to term PN after 24–48 h
Concentration/litre					
AA (g)	37.5	30	30	30	23
Glucose (g)	100	100	100	75	120
Na (mmol)	20	34	60	34	25
K (mmol)	0	22	22	22	20
Cl (mmol)	10.1	12.7	30.7	12.7	28.2
Ca (mmol)	17	17	17	17	7
Mg (mmol)	1.5	1.5	1.5	1.5	1.5
P (mmol)	10	13	13	13	4
Acetate (mmol)	0	26	34	26	16.2
Zinc (μg)	3270	3270	3270	3270	1900
Selenium (μg)	20	20	20	20	20
Iodine (μg)	8.16	8.16	8.16	8.16	8.16
Heparin (units)	500	500	500	500	500
Osmolarity (mosm/L)	933	944	996	805	957
At 135 mL/kg/d					
Energy (kcal/kg/d)[a]		70	70	57	77
AA (g/kg/d)		4.1	4.1	4.1	3.1
Glucose (g/kg/d)		13.5	13.5	10.1	16.2
Na (mmol/kg/d)		4.6	8.1	4.6	3.4
K (mmol/kg/d)		3	3	3	2.7
Cl (mmol/kg/d)		1.7	4.1	1.7	3.8
Acetate (mmol/kg/d)		3.5	4.6	3.5	2.2
Ca (mmol/kg/d)		2.3	2.3	2.3	0.9
P (mmol/kg/d)		1.8	1.8	1.8	0.5
Mg (mmol/kg/d)		0.2	0.2	0.2	0.2

[a]Energy rates are based on estimated 4kcal per each gram of glucose and protein.
AA, amino acids; PN, parenteral nutrition.
Source: Bolisetty et al. (2020).

access owing to the osmolarity of the infusate that when infused peripherally can cause phlebitis and extravasation. This may further result in tissue necrosis and permanent damage (Murphy et al., 2019). Close monitoring of the IV site is *essential* during the short-term delivery of TPN and any hyperosmolar dextrose fluid to prevent extravasation injury.

Umbilical venous catheter

Umbilical venous catheters (UVCs) are utilised for unwell or preterm infants and are generally the first choice in venous access shortly after birth. Radiological confirmation of catheter tip placement is required *prior* to the commencement of TPN. The UVC tip should be located at the junction of the inferior vena cava (IVC) and right atrium (RA), above the diaphragm, which coincides with T8 to T9 using X-ray (Hoellering et al., 2018). UVCs should be managed aseptically to prevent catheter-associated bloodstream infection (BSI). Cohort studies have demonstrated an association between catheter dwell-times from 4 to 10 days and UVC-associated BSI (Levit et al., 2020). UVCs should be removed as soon as possible when no longer needed and replaced with a peripherally inserted central catheter (PICC) to prevent UVC-associated BSI. Other adverse events associated with UVCs are tip malposition and migration which may cause damage to surrounding tissue and organs, compounded by infusing hyperosmolar fluids causing extravasation (Selvam et al., 2018). Routine serial radiological surveillance is essential to ensure that the correct location of the catheter tip is maintained to avoid such sequelae (Gibson et al., 2021).

Peripherally inserted central catheter

PICCs often replace UVCs to provide ongoing central venous access to deliver PN. They are inserted percutaneously in the cephalic or basilic vein. For PICCs inserted into the upper extremities, the tip of the catheter should be positioned at the junction of the superior vena cava (SVC) and right atrium, and, for PICCs inserted into the lower limbs, beyond the origin of the IVC proximal to the ascending lumbar arteries (Sharma et al., 2019). Common adverse events associated with PICCs are BSI and catheter tip migration into the cardiac silhouette, causing effusions and extravasation injury (Sertic et al., 2018). Unlike UVCs, extended PICC dwell-time is not associated with increased risk of central-line-associated BSI (Sanderson et al., 2017). The use of chlorhexidine for skin antisepsis and maximum sterile barriers when inserting and accessing PICCs are preventive strategies commonly adopted into standard PICC care to prevent BSI (Schmid et al., 2018). Adequate securement of the PICC, in addition to routine radiological surveillance, is essential to ensure the correct location of the catheter tip is maintained (Acun et al., 2021).

CLINICAL PRACTICE 5.3

Due to the potential risks of photodegradation and oxidation of the TPN solution, the infusion set (tubing) and bag should be protected from light. Adding filters can remove particulate matter, fungi, bacteria and endotoxins (depending on the size of the filter), and minimising opportunities to break the line will also reduce the risk of sepsis (National Institute for Health and Care Excellence (NICE), 2020).

Complications associated with total parenteral nutrition administration

Sepsis (bacterial or fungal), occlusion, thrombosis, pulmonary embolism, accidental removal or damage, electrolyte disturbances, renal anomalies, metabolic bone disease, micronutrient deficiencies and liver disease are all known risks of PN (Mantagazza et al., 2018). For neonates on prolonged TPN with no or minimal enteral intake, the risk of **parenteral nutrition-associated liver disease (PNALD)**, with its associated features of cholestasis and cholestatic jaundice and metabolic bone disease, is increased (Gura & Elisofon, 2021). Although the exact mechanism of PNALD is unknown, multifactorial causative factors closely correlated to the disease include the actual components of PN (specifically a soy-based lipid emulsion that is more associated with liver injury than a fish-oil based emulsion), bacterial endotoxins and the lack of enteral feeding. General measures to reduce the risk of PNALD include maximising enteral feeding, limiting soy-based lipids if a prolonged course of PN (>21 days) is anticipated and preventing catheter-related sepsis (Gura & Elisofon, 2021).

Energy (calorie) intake

Energy intake must replace energy expenditure (resting metabolic rate, activity, thermoregulation) and provide what is needed for growth. To meet the preterm neonate's minimal energy requirements, 50–60 kcal/kg/day are needed. To achieve growth (i.e. maximal protein accretion) a higher calorie intake is needed; in the neonate fed parenterally, 90–100 kcal/kg/day are required (Bolisetty et al., 2020). Both protein and energy are needed for growth; however, there needs to be sufficient energy so that protein is used for *growth*, and not to provide energy.

Amino acids

Adequate amounts of both protein and energy and the optimal blend of essential and non-essential amino acids are required for growth. There is no available evidence to guide the timing of the introduction of amino acid solutions (early (within 24 hours of birth) versus late (more than 24 hours after birth)) in terms of its effects on mortality, growth and neurodevelopment; however, early initiation of amino acids is associated with improved short-term growth outcomes (Griffin, 2021). Australasian consensus guidelines recommend commencing amino acids within the first 24 hours at 2 g/kg/day, with an incremental increase in amino acid infusions over 3–5 days up to a maximum of 4 g/kg/day (see Table 5.2) (Bolisetty et al., 2020). The amino acid dose associated with important clinical outcomes, including neurodevelopment, is yet to be resolved and will require large randomised controlled trials.

Carbohydrates

Glucose is the primary source of energy in the body and the primary substrate for the brain. Preterm neonates are at risk for both hypo- and hyperglycaemic episodes, and, as such, glucose regulation can be challenging (see Chapter 15). Glucose infusion should not exceed glucose oxidation, as glucose infusion rates >10–11 mg/kg/min generally result in hyperglycaemia (Armentrout, 2021). Blood sugar levels are checked several times a day in infants receiving intravenous glucose to detect hypo- or hyperglycaemia (Olsen et al., 2021). Glucose administration should commence at 5–8 mg/kg/min (Griffin, 2021). Australasian 'standard' TPN (10% dextrose) provides 13.5 g/kg/day (9.4 mg/kg/min) of glucose when infused at 135 mL/kg/day, and 12% dextrose provides 17 g/kg/day (11.8 mg/kg/min) at 135 mL/kg/day (Bolisetty et al., 2020).

Fat

Intravenous lipid emulsions provide essential fatty acids (linoleic and alpha-linolenic acids) and are an important source of high-density calories (9 calories/g). Fatty acids and their metabolites are also important in platelet function, immune response, inflammation (Radzikowska et al., 2019) and neural and visual development (Ditzenberger, 2018). Commencing lipids on day one of TPN administration appears to be safe and well tolerated (Bolisetty et al., 2020); however, regular triglyceride monitoring is required to avoid hyperlipidaemia.

Intravenous lipids used in neonatal care include those based on 100% soybean oil (e.g. Intralipid 20%), mixed olive oil (80%), soybean oil (20%) (e.g. Clinoleic 20%) and emulsions containing fish oil (e.g. SMOFlipid, 20% (**S**oybean oil (6%), **M**edium-chain triglyceride oil (6%), **O**live oil (5%), **F**ish oil (3%)) and Omegaven, 100% fish oil based). These lipids all appear to be well tolerated (Edward et al., 2018). Fish oil-containing lipids have theoretical advantages as they do not contain phytosterols (associated with impaired biliary secretion), have a high concentration of vitamin E, may reduce oxidative stress, maintain omega-3 fatty acid levels and reduce parenteral nutrition-associated liver disease (Gura & Elisofon, 2021). See Table 5.4 for the characteristics of commercially available intravenous lipid emulsions. Vitamins, water and fat soluble, are added to the lipid emulsion (Bolisetty et al., 2020).

CLINICAL PRACTICE 5.4

The vascular anatomy and physiology of preterm infants, particularly those weighing less than 1 kg, pose unique challenges for vascular access. Hugell and van Rens (2020, p. S16) have some tips for advancing a central catheter when resistance is met:

- Advance and hold the PICC 'under slight pressure' for a few seconds.
- Massage the PICC by stretching the skin in the direction of flow.
- Reposition the limb.
- Gently flush the catheter while advancing.
- Support the infant to reposition into their preferred position.

Trace elements and minerals

Trace minerals include zinc, copper, selenium, manganese, chromium and carnitine, and are necessary for normal physiological processes, optimal growth, development and health (Zemrani et al., 2018). They are not important if the TPN is going to be required for only a short period, but the longer that TPN continues, the more important they become (Griffin, 2021). Zinc, selenium and iodine are added to TPN solutions, but not starter TPN because of

TABLE 5.4 **Characteristics of commercially available intravenous lipid emulsions**

	Emulsion (year of introduction)				
	Intralipid 20% SO (1960s)	ClinOleic 20% OO/SO (1990s)	Lipofundin 20% MCT/SO (1980s)	SMOFlipid 20% multicomponent FO-containing (2000s)	Omegaven 10% FO (1990s)
	Oil source, %				
Soya bean	100	20	50	30	0
MCT	0	0	50	30	0
Olive	0	80	0	25	0
Fish	0	0	0	15	100
	Fatty acids, % of total fatty acids				
Linoleic acid	53	18.7	29.1	37.2	4.4
Arachidonic acid	0.1	0.5	0.2	1.0	2.1
α-Linolenic acid	8	2.3	4.5	4.7	1.8
Eicosapentaenoic acid	0	0	0	4.7	19.2
Docosahexaenoic acid	0	0	0	4.4	12.1
ω-6: ω-3 ratio	7:1	9:1	7:1	2.5:1	1:8
Phytosterols (mg/L) based on Angsten et al. (39)[a]	348 ± 33	237 ± 8	NA	47.6	0
Phytosterols (mg/L) based on Xu et al. (27)[b]	439.07 ± 5.72	274.38 ± 2.60	278.14 ± 5.09	207	No phytosterols, squalene 26.7 mg/L
α-Tocopherol (mg/L)	38	32	85 ± 20	200	150–296

FO, fish oil; MCT, medium-chain triglycerides; OO, olive oil; SO, soya bean oil.
[a]Data in the table are the mean value when an interval is given from the manufacturer (39).
[b]Independently evaluated concentration of 9 different phytosterols and squalene (27).
Source: Hojsak et al. (2016).

incompatibility concerns. Infants requiring exclusive TPN for more than 2–4 weeks with minimal enteral intake can have copper, manganese and molybdenum added to their TPN formulation (Bolisetty et al., 2020).

In a recent survey of neonatal units in Australasia, supplements of iron, folic acid, calcium and phosphate were routine, despite the fact that there is no recommended range for their doses and a lack of evidence to support supplementations (Oliver et al., 2019).

Vitamins

Vitamins are essential for normal metabolism, but the precise biological roles of vitamins have not been established in preterm infants. Vitamin C is important for enhancing iron absorption from the gastrointestinal (GI) tract, vitamin K for preventing haemorrhagic disease in the newborn (see Chapter 11), vitamin D for absorbing calcium and preventing rickets, and vitamins A and E for their antioxidant properties (Brown et al., 2021). Preterm infants are especially at risk of micronutrient deficiencies, and most require vitamin supplementation soon after birth (Oliver et al., 2019). Fat- and water-soluble vitamins are therefore added to SMOF lipid emulsion.

ENTERAL NUTRITION

Due to the risks associated with intravenous cannulation and the prolonged administration of TPN, a significant goal in the nutritional management of preterm neonates is to reduce intravenous therapies and achieve full enteral feeds as quickly and safely as possible. Initially, enteral feeds are delivered via a naso- or orogastric feeding tube, and then suck feeds are gradually introduced via the breast or bottle according to each neonate's individual tolerance and capacity. The transition from intravenous to enteral tube feeds, and then to full suck feeds, is a significant developmental task for preterm neonates.

Feeding tube placement

Enteral feeding tubes can be placed nasally or orally, with practice varying among neonatal units. Orally placed tubes may be more difficult to secure and may cause vagal stimulation, whereas nasal placement partially obstructs the nares and may compromise respiration. An early study by Watson and McGuire (2013) found that the route of tube placement (oral or nasal) did not appear to affect the time taken to reach full enteral feeds, or compromise respiration. More recently, a pilot randomised clinical trial found that preterm infants who received bolus nasogastric feeds achieved full oral feeds earlier and had less aspiration events than did infants who received bolus orogastric feeds (Badran et al., 2020). For more detail, see Evidence-based Practice 5.2. Yet, in the absence of high-quality trials, the route of placement is still based on local preference. Enteral feeding tubes can be placed either into the stomach (gastric tube feeding) or lower, into the upper small bowel (transpyloric tube feeding). Generally, a size 5 or 6FG feeding tube has a sufficient bore to facilitate tube feeds for a preterm neonate, while still being relatively comfortable.

EVIDENCE-BASED PRACTICE RESEARCH 5.2

Badran et al. (2020) conducted a pilot unblended, randomised clinical trial on 98 stable preterm infants (aged between 31 and 35 weeks' gestation) comparing orogastric bolus feeds with nasogastric bolus feeds, to ascertain which infants reached full enteral feeding quicker and which route was safer.

They found that preterm infants who were fed by bolus nasogastric tubes achieved full enteral feeding sooner than the infants fed by bolus orogastric tubes. The incidence rates of aspiration and feeding tube displacement were significantly higher in the bolus orogastric tube group than in the bolus nasogastric tube group.

There was no difference in the incidence rates of apnoea, NEC, bradycardia, oxygen desaturation and gastric residual between the two groups.

Source: Badran et al. (2020).

There are two methods to achieve an accurate insertion distance for a nasogastric tube. The first uses the distance from the tip of the nose to the ear lobe, to the midway point between the xiphoid and the umbilicus, as seen in Fig. 5.1. This is based on the acronym 'NEMU' – **n**ose/**e**ar/**m**id/**u**mbilicus (Parker et al., 2018). The other is the 'ARHB' method – **a**ge-**r**elated, **h**eight-**b**ased length, as shown in Table 5.5 (Dias et al., 2020). This calculation is based on the equation:

$$\text{insertion length} = 1.950\text{ cm} + 0.372 \times \text{length (cm)}$$

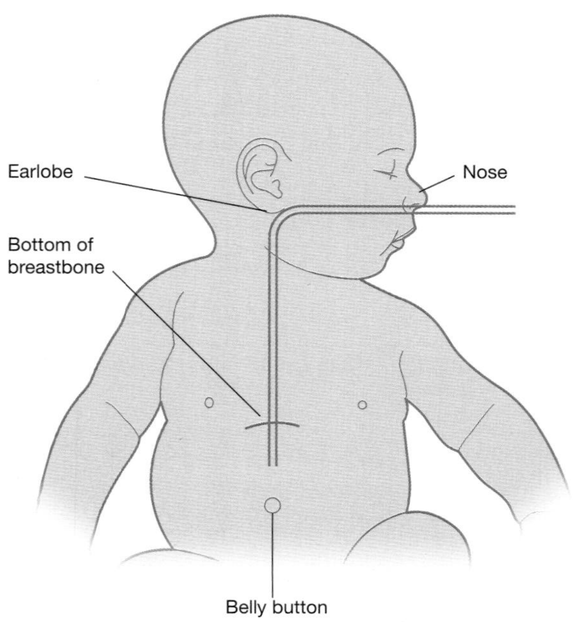

FIGURE 5.1 **Measuring the distance of the nasogastric tube using NEMU (nose/ear/mid/umbilicus)**

TABLE 5.5 **Nasogastric tube insertion length based on neonatal length**

Neonate's length (cm)	*Nasogastric tube insertion length (cm)*
35.0–35.5	15.0
36.0–37.0	15.5
37.5–38.0	16.0
38.5–39.5	16.5
40.0–41.0	17.0
41.5–42.0	17.5
42.5–43.5	18.0
44.0–45.0	18.5
45.5–46.5	19.0
47.0–47.5	19.5
48.0–49.0	20.0
49.5–50.5	20.5
51.0–51.5	21.0
52.0–53.0	21.5
53.5–54.5	22.0
55.0–55.5	22.5
56.0–56.5	23.0

Source: Ellett et al. (2011).

Dias et al. (2020) found that using the weight-based equation was the most reliable method for correct placement in the gastric body (NEMU 67.5% versus 91.5% when using the ARHB equation).

EVIDENCE-BASED PRACTICE RESEARCH 5.3

In a retrospective cohort study of 368 extremely low birthweight (ELBW) infants, Wallenstein et al. (2019) found that early transpyloric tube (TPT) feeding (initiated soon after birth) was associated with a *reduced* risk of death or bronchopulmonary dysplasia (chronic lung disease). They cited a study by Farhath et al. (2006), who found pepsin, a marker of gastric content, in 92% of tracheal aspirate samples in ventilator-dependent infants of less than 32 weeks' gestation. Shimokaze et al. (2021) evaluated the effect of TPT feeding in 33 ventilated infants with a mean gestation of 25.4 weeks, and found that TPT feeding prevented deterioration in oxygenation and was without major complications. However, insertion of TPTs, and maintenance of TPT feeds, requires considerable expertise and is therefore recommended only in high-level neonatal settings (Banait et al., 2020).

Commencing and increasing feeds

The aim is to achieve full enteral feeds (an enteral intake of ≈ 150–200 mL/kg/day) in infants born weighing 1000–1500 g by approximately 1 week of age, and by 2 weeks of age in neonates born weighing <1000 g. As enteral intake is increased, parenteral intake is decreased.

CLINICAL PRACTICE 5.5

Urashima et al. (2019) conducted a randomised trial investigating cow's milk atopy induced by cow's milk formula in term infants, and followed 302 infants at risk of atopy (due to parental history of atopic diseases such as asthma) for 2 years. They concluded that cow's milk formula should be avoided for at least the first 3 days of life to prevent the development of allergies in later childhood. As a consequence, neonates born after 35 weeks' gestation to mothers who wish to exclusively breastfeed and require supplementary feeds at the Women's and Children's Hospital in South Australia now receive 5% glucose water rather than non-hydrolysed infant formula in the first 72 hours of life (Andersen et al., 2021).

Human breast milk (from the mother of the baby) is the feed of choice, followed by donor human milk and then preterm formula (Banait et al., 2020). Enteral feeds should be commenced within 6 hours of life in the medically stable preterm infant to help stimulate the development of the gastrointestinal tract (Hair, 2021). Enteral feeds are commenced 2–6 hourly at 10–15 mL/kg/day (and are known as **minimal enteral feeds (MEF)** or 'trophic feeds'). MEF stimulates GI motility and hormone secretion without burdening the GI tract with additional volume (Parker et al., 2021). There has been no association found between feeds commenced before 4 days of age and NEC (Hair, 2021). There is insufficient evidence to recommend how long to maintain minimal enteral feeds; therefore, feeds should be increased as tolerated. In neonates weighing <1000 g, feeding volumes are increased by 15–20 mL/kg/day, and 30 mL/kg/day for neonates born weighing ≥1000 g. The results of the SIFT (**S**peed of **I**ncreasing milk **F**eeds: a randomised controlled **T**rial), increasing feeds by 30 mL/kg/day versus 18 mL/kg/day, were that there was no difference in survival, late-onset sepsis or NEC; also, less time was taken to reach full feeds, with less time requiring TPN, when feeds were increased at the faster rate of 30 mL/kg/day in preterm or VLBW infants (Dorling et al., 2019). A recently published systematic review suggested that increasing enteral feed volumes slowly (up to 24 mL/kg/day), compared with faster rates, probably does not reduce the risk of NEC, death or feeding intolerance in very preterm infants or VLBW infants (Oddie et al., 2021).

Frequency and mode of feeds

While older studies suggest that neonates born weighing >1250 g can be fed 3-hourly, and those born weighing <1250 g show greater feed tolerance and reduced time to full enteral feeds if fed 2-hourly (Dutta et al., 2015), a recent Cochrane review suggests that there may be no clinically important differences between 2- and 3-hourly feeding intervals in preterm infants (Ibrahim et al., 2021). Intermittent tube feeds can be push or gravity fed.

EVIDENCE-BASED PRACTICE RESEARCH 5.4

Different approaches to delivering tube feedings are practised, with some units advocating push feeds (using a syringe to gently push milk through the tube) and others gravity gavage feeds (using the open barrel of the syringe and allowing milk to flow by gravity). There is still insufficient evidence on which to base recommendations about the mode of delivery – push or gravity – for gavage feeds (Dawson et al., 2021).

Neonates who receive their milk by continuous perfusor feeding delivered using a syringe on a driver pump may reach full enteral feeds earlier than neonates who are fed intermittently (Sadrudin Premji et al., 2021). However, as continuous feeds require a syringe pump and continuous supervision, they may not be feasible in all neonatal units (Banait et al., 2020).

EVIDENCE-BASED PRACTICE RESEARCH 5.5

In a systematic review of continuous perfusor feeds versus intermittent feeds in infants with birthweights between 1000 and 1500 grams, the researchers found little to no difference in rate of weight, length or head circumference gain, feeding interruptions or risk of NEC (Sadrudin Premji et al., 2021). Infants receiving continuous perfusor feeds took 1 day longer to reach full enteral feeds, but the evidence was of low certainty.

FAMILY-CENTRED CARE 5.1

Parents holding their baby skin to skin during tube feeds is a regulating experience for preterm infants, and promotes bonding and emotional stability in the mother. One study combined tube feeding with skin-to-skin contact (SSC) after the woman **expressed breast milk (EBM)**. While being tube-fed, the mother manually dripped her breast milk onto the baby's lips, and the baby tasted and became familiar with breast milk. Non-nutritive breast sucking was discovered to be beneficial to the transition from tube feeding to breastfeeding, which in turn was beneficial to breastfeeding. As the infant matured, they naturally approached the breast during SSC, triggering instinctive breastfeeding behaviour, promoting the coordination of sucking and swallowing, initiating their first nutritive sucking earlier, and increasing the duration of sucking, which fulfilled the infant's instinctive desire to suck.

Source: based on Li, L., Wang, L., Niu, C., Liu, C., Lv, T., Ji, F., ... & Hu, X. (2021). Early skin contact combined with mother's breastfeeding to shorten the process of premature infants ≤ 30 weeks of gestation to achieve full oral feeding: the study protocol of a randomized controlled trial. Trials, *22(1), 1-10.*

Non-nutritive sucking during tube feeds reduces the time that neonates need to transit from tube to full oral feeding, and the time from the start of oral feeding to full oral feeding. It also reduces the length of hospital stay. Non-nutritive sucking on an emptied breast has been shown to improve sucking skills, increase milk supply, promote mother–infant bonding and increase exclusive breastfeeding rates at discharge (Fucile et al., 2021). Time at the breast and contact with the breast is important, even if the neonate is not yet ready for fully functional suck feeds. The gradual introduction of sucking feeds is described later in this chapter.

Feeding small for gestational age infants

Small for gestational age (SGA) infants with abnormal antenatal umbilical artery ultrasound (absent or reversed end diastolic flow (AREDF)) are at an increased risk of developing NEC. With AREDF the blood flow to the brain is preserved at the expense of other organs. A retrospective cohort study of preterm infants with REDF by Aradhya et al. (2020) found that feeds could be commenced early (at 24 hours) without increasing the risk of NEC if abdominal examination was normal.

Mother's own milk is the first choice of feeds for SGA infants as it is protective against NEC, followed by pasteurised donor human milk, both with nutrient supplementation (Banait et al., 2020).

EVIDENCE-BASED PRACTICE RESEARCH 5.6

In the absence of other signs of feed intolerance in preterm LBW neonates, neither routine pre-feed abdominal circumference nor pre-feed gastric residue estimation is recommended for assessment of tolerance to enteral feeds.

Source: Banait et al. (2020, p. 29).

Donor human milk

If mother's own milk is unavailable, pasteurised donor human milk is the next best choice and is associated with better outcomes than using preterm formula. Use of mother's own breast milk, or combined with donor human milk, has been shown to significantly reduce the incidence of NEC in **very low birthweight (VLBW)** neonates compared with neonates receiving formula (Quigley et al., 2019).

The European Milk Bank Association (EMBA) recommend donor human milk should be used only from a source that has safety guidelines for screening donors, and collecting and processing, handling, testing and storing the milk (Weaver et al., 2019).

A census conducted as part of a systematic review found 572 milk banks around the world, but inequities exist in access to donated breast milk between high- and low-income countries because of the high set-up and maintenance costs of human milk banks (Altobelli et al., 2020). In Australia, human milk sharing in maternity hospitals was common prior to the 1980s (Lording, 2006) and informal human milk sharing between individual women has been documented since the 1940s and is still occurring through groups such as Human Milk 4 Human Babies. Formal human milk banks are now operating at maternity hospitals in Western Australia, Victoria and Queensland, and the Australian Red Cross Blood Service has established human milk banks (Lifeblood Milk Banks) in New South Wales, Queensland and South Australia, and is implementing a pilot project for a national human milk bank; in New Zealand there is one formal milk bank in Christchurch.

The role of donor milk banks involves collecting breast milk from donors, then providing it to individual neonates following specific protocols and, generally, only to preterm or sick neonates in neonatal units. Donor milk, screened and collected through milk banks, will be pasteurised (at 62.5°C for 30 minutes), destroying bacteria and viruses, but also affecting some properties of breast milk. Pasteurisation has been found to reduce the concentration of immunoactive compounds, particularly cytokines and growth factors (Moro et al., 2019).

EVIDENCE-BASED PRACTICE RESEARCH 5.7

Pasteurisation reduces fat and energy content; freezing prior to and following pasteurisation, and then thawing, of the milk also reduces fat, protein and energy content (Păduraru et al., 2019).

Perceptions of the use of donor milk

While donor milk has many benefits over formula, and is shown to reduce the risk of NEC and other infections, there may also be apprehension and aversion from women to giving **donor breast milk** to their babies. Klein et al. (2021) found, when donor milk was an option for supplementing mothers' own EBM, women were not concerned about the quality and safety risks of *giving* donor breast milk, but were concerned when 'someone else's breast milk' was being used for their infant. Comprehensively discussing the benefits and giving parents time to reflect on their feelings before asking for consent helped parents in their decision making about the use of donor breast milk. A positive outcome of the implementation of a donor milk program in one setting in the USA was that women provided more milk for their infants and there was an increased awareness of the benefits of breastfeeding and breast milk for their baby (Parker, 2019). Education on the benefits of breast milk and the use of donor milk when required influenced this outcome (Parker, 2019).

Human milk fortifier

Human milk is the feed of choice but may not meet the preterm neonate's nutrient requirements, and then nutrient supplements (fortification) are required.

EVIDENCE-BASED PRACTICE RESEARCH 5.8

Moltu et al. (2021) published a position paper on behalf of the European Society of Paediatric Gastroenterology, Hepatology and Nutrition (ESPGHAN) Committee on Nutrition which detailed the nutritional management of the critically ill neonate. The Committee recommended that during critical illness, nutritional care should be adapted according to the different phases of the metabolic stress response, and that it was important to recognise the hepatic transition to anabolic protein metabolism when growth reoccurs. This would help avoid inappropriate nutrition, especially overfeeding during the early (catabolic) phase of illness and underfeeding during recovery. They believed it would be prudent to consider nutritional support in three different phases: the early acute phase, the late acute phase and the recovery phase.

Fortifiers provide additional protein, typically 1.0–1.5 g/100 mL EBM (McLeod et al., 2021). Fortifiers raise the energy density of breast milk from 67 to 80 kcal/100 mL EBM, and provide additional electrolytes, microminerals and vitamins, with some providing additional fatty acids. The amounts of nutrients vary considerably between different fortifiers. Available fortifiers include bovine-derived fortifier and human milk-derived fortifier (HMF). There appears to be no difference in feeding tolerance, postnatal growth and morbidity, including NEC, between bovine-derived fortifier and human milk-derived fortifier (Premkumar et al., 2019). While showing promise in reducing NEC, larger trials are required before practice change can be recommended (Arslanoglu et al., 2019). Individualised targeted fortification of breast milk is also an increasing practice, and has been shown to enhance the quality of nutrition and growth, and be feasible in neonatal clinical routines (Rochow et al., 2021).

Artificial feed thickener

Thickening feeds is an effective treatment for gastroesophageal reflux, to enhance weight gain and prevent aspiration in preterm infants (Koo et al., 2019). Most neonatal units in Australia and New Zealand use artificial feed thickener (AFT) (usually carob bean gum), although caution is recommended for the use of thickening agents for preterm neonates <37 weeks' gestation because of the risk of NEC (Oliver et al., 2019). Practical issues arise for neonatal nurses and midwives administering thickened feeds because of their viscosity, which causes them to clog feeding tubes and slow down gavage feeds, as well as creating difficulties for bottle-fed infants struggling to extract thickened feeds from a teat. Prewarming thickened feeds can help to ameliorate these issues.

Probiotics

Probiotics are live microorganisms that have been administered to preterm neonates at risk of developing NEC to promote the growth of normal flora in the gut and, hence, control the growth of pathogenic flora that may contribute to the development of NEC. Most neonatal units use probiotics, but brands, bacterial strains and dosing regimens differ across sites (McLeod et al., 2021). (See Chapter 12 for more information about probiotics in the prevention of NEC.)

Vitamin and mineral supplementation

Breast milk does not contain adequate vitamins for the growth of the preterm neonate. Preterm formula and human milk fortifiers are supplemented with vitamins and minerals; however, the amount varies between products. Products (see Table 5.4) should therefore be checked against recommended intakes. Multivitamin supplementation is generally not required for neonates receiving fortified breast milk or preterm formula, but, due to variation in products, further supplements may be required. When fortifier or preterm formula is no longer used, infants should receive a multivitamin supplement. Vitamin D should be supplemented to 400–1000 IU/day (*not per kg*) (Oliver et al., 2019), according to their vitamin D status. Most needs are met by fortified breast milk or preterm formula once the feeding volume is greater than 150 mL/kg/day, but the majority of neonatal units in the Australian/New Zealand survey supplement infants with vitamin D, and one-third supplement vitamin E (Oliver et al., 2019).

There is no consensus about when prophylactic enteral iron supplementation should be commenced, but iron supplements commencing at a dose of 2 mg/day from 6 weeks to 6 months of age (earlier in ELBW infants) was shown to reduce the risk of iron deficiency anaemia effectively (Moreno-Fernandez et al., 2019). Some fortifiers and preterm formulas may provide sufficient iron. High enteral iron intakes have been associated with possible adverse effects; therefore, intakes >5 mg/kg/d should be avoided (Moreno-Fernandez et al., 2019). A summary of the recommended intakes of micro- and macronutrients is provided in Table 5.6.

TABLE 5.6 **Recommended intakes of micro- and macronutrients**

	Per kg per day	Per 100 kcal
Fluid (mL)	135–200	
Energy (kcal)	110–135	
Protein (g for <1 kg bodyweight)	4.0–4.5	3.6–4.1
Protein (g for 1–1.8 kg bodyweight)	3.5–4.0	3.2–3.6
Lipids (g, of which MCT <40%)	4.8–6.6	4.4–6.0
Linolenic acid (mg)[a]	385–1540	350–1400
α-Linolenic acid (mg)	>55 (0.9% of fatty acids)	>50
DHA (mg)	12–30	11–27
AA (mg)[b]	18–42	16–39
Carbohydrate (g)	11.6–13.2	10.5–12
Sodium (mg)	69–115	63–105
Potassium (mg)	66–132	60–120
Chloride (mg)	105–177	95–161
Calcium salt (mg)	120–140	110–130
Phosphate (mg)	60–90	55–80
Magnesium (mg)	8–15	7.5–13.6
Iron (mg)	2–3	1.8–2.7
Zinc (mg)[c]	1.1–2.0	1.0–1.8
Copper (μg)	100–132	90–120
Selenium (μg)	5–10	4.5–9

	Per kg per day	Per 100 kcal
Manganese (μg)	<27.5	6.3–25
Fluoride (μg)	1.5–60	1.4–55
Iodine (μg)	11–55	10–50
Chromium (ng)	30–1230	27–1120
Molybdenum (μg)	0.3–5	0.27–4.5
Thiamin (μg)	140–300	125–275
Riboflavin (μg)	200–400	180–365
Niacin (μg)	380–5500	345–5000
Pantothenic acid (mg)	0.33–2.1	0.3–1.9
Pyridoxine (μg)	45–300	41–273
Cobalamin (μg)	0.1–0.77	0.08–0.7
Folic acid (μg)	35–100	32–90
L-ascorbic acid (mg)	11–46	10–42
Biotin (μg)	1.7–16.5	1.5–15
Vitamin A (μg RE, 1 μg ~ 3.33 IU)	400–1000	360–740
Vitamin D (IU/d)	800–1000	
Vitamin E (mg (α-tocopherol equivalents))	2.2–11	2–10
Vitamin K1 (μg)	4.4–28	4–25
Nucleotides (mg)		≤5
Choline (mg)	8–55	7–50
Inositol (mg)	4.4–53	4–48

AA, arachidonic acid; DHA, docosahexaenoic acid; IU, international unit; MCT, medium-chain triacylglycerols.
Note: Calculation of the range of nutrients expressed per 100 kcal is based on a minimum energy intake of 110 kcal/kg.
[a] The linoleic acid-to-α-linolenic acid ratio is in the range of 5 to 15:1 (wt/wt).
[b] The ratio of AA to DHA should be in the range of 1.0–2.0 to 1 (wt/wt), and eicosapentaenoic acid (20:5ω-3) supply should not exceed 30% of DHA supply.
[c] The zinc-to-copper molar ratio in infant formulas should not exceed 20.
Source: Agostoni et al. (2010).

Long-chain fatty acid supplementation

Long-chain polyunsaturated fatty acids are significant in brain development, and infants born preterm miss out on the in utero accretion of the omega-3 long-chain polyunsaturated fatty acid docosahexaenoic acid (DHA). While earlier randomised controlled trials providing DHA at the in utero accretion rate of ~60 mg/kg/day showed improved neurodevelopment at 18 months' corrected age, the effect was no longer apparent at 7 years' corrected age, and supplemental DHA did not reduce, and may increase, the risk of bronchopulmonary dysplasia (chronic lung disease) in extremely preterm neonates (Gould et al., 2021). Therefore, additional DHA beyond that present in the breast milk of women consuming a Western diet or present in preterm infant formula (providing ~20–30 mg/kg/day) is not required.

Assessing feeding tolerance

Feeding tolerance is strongly related to the degree of prematurity but not to the type of human milk fortification (Eibensteiner et al., 2019). Feeding intolerance (discussed in more detail in Chapter 12) is extremely common in the preterm neonate; however, the decision to withhold feeds needs to be carefully considered as stopping feeds contributes to poor neonatal growth. Feeding tolerance requires regular assessment and a complete clinical examination should be undertaken before the decision is made to stop feeds (Hair, 2021).

Feeds should be stopped when NEC is suspected – that is, where there is clear abdominal pathology (abdominal distension, ileus with visible loops of bowel, blood in the stool, heavily bile-stained or large gastric residuals or vomiting) – or when gastrointestinal symptoms are associated with apnoea, bradycardia or poor perfusion (Kim, 2021) (see also Chapter 12).

Gastric residuals are usually a result of the preterm neonate's immature gut and low motility, and on their own should not lead to cessation of feeds. The effect of increasing gastric residual volumes on clinical outcomes such as mortality, pneumonia, vomiting and length of hospital stay could not be determined in a recent systematic review (Yasuda et al., 2021). Banait et al. (2020) recommend that gastric residuals and abdominal girth should not be checked routinely in the absence of other signs of feeding intolerance. However, the aspiration of gastric residuals to evaluate gastrointestinal tolerance remains common practice, with frequency varying according to local practice, despite little evidence for this practice in diagnosing feeding intolerance or NEC (Dorling et al., 2020). There is not enough quality evidence to support or refute the practice of re-feeding gastric residuals in preterm infants, and more trials are needed to ascertain whether the practice is beneficial or harmful (Abiramalatha et al., 2019).

Assessing growth

Nutritional adequacy is monitored by assessing changes in weight, length and head circumference. Weight is generally measured daily to assess changes in fluid status as well as growth. However, serial weekly measurements of length and head circumference are important, as weight may fluctuate owing to changes in fluid rather than lean or adipose tissue accretion. Birthweight should be regained by about 14 days of life and expected weight gain is 15–20 g/day from 23 to 36 weeks' gestation, and then, once the infant reaches 2 kg, the goal is 20–30 g/day (Hair, 2021). Accurate length measurement requires two people and use of a length board. Expected length and head circumference gain is 1.0 cm/week. Weight, length and head circumference should be plotted on preterm infant growth charts for regular review by the neonatal team. While various growth charts are in use across the world, Fenton growth charts and accompanying z-scores (which allow for correction of early weight loss due to the contraction of extracellular water) are recommended to monitor preterm infants' growth up to 50 weeks post-menstrual age (McLeod et al., 2021).

BREAST MILK EXPRESSION

For mothers of preterm neonates, expressing breast milk is necessary until the baby is able to attach and suckle at the breast. Expressing can be challenging for the mother with a sick or preterm neonate; she will be anxious and worried about her baby as well as separated from her baby in intensive or special care. Emotional support and encouragement to participate in her baby's care, skin-to-skin contact and a welcoming environment in the neonatal unit are all strategies that can engage the mother and help her feel connected to her baby. Early initiation and frequent and effective breast milk expression can increase the success of longer-term lactation, ensuring the benefits of her baby receiving breast milk and later breastfeeding. Maternal–infant bonding, including skin-to-skin contact between mother and baby, will enhance oxytocin release, the important hormone for stimulating the release of breast milk, while also offering an easier transition to breastfeeding (Uvnäs Moberg et al., 2020). A systematic review of kangaroo mother care (skin-to-skin) and neonatal outcomes confirmed the many benefits of early skin-to-skin contact, including the promotion of exclusive breastfeeding (Gupta et al., 2021).

Social support may influence the amount of breast milk a mother is able to express for her preterm baby; however, the availability of appropriate policies and practices of staff may have a greater effect. The access to hospital grade breast pumps, bedside expressing, information and education on expressing, consistent professional support, rooming-in, skin to skin, on-demand breastfeeding, availability of lactation consultants and, importantly, the mother's intent to breastfeed all have an impact (Theurich et al., 2021). Support from staff, comfortable surroundings and education all impact on how positive the mother will feel about her experience of expressing. While standardised protocols and procedures around breastfeeding and expressing, peer counsellors and training of healthcare providers in breastfeeding and expression for preterm neonates are all essential to increasing positive outcomes, breastfeeding support must also be woman centred and individualised (Ericson & Palmér, 2018). Education on early expressing and the benefits of breast milk and breastfeeding are, where possible, given to parents prior to the neonate's birth, along with other information about the care of the preterm baby and the importance of the mother–infant relationship.

Expressing methods and techniques

The initiation of expressing as soon as possible, certainly within the first hours following the birth, will both provide the neonate with colostrum and improve the mother's ability to maintain her supply and consequently longer-term breastfeeding (Maastrup et al., 2021).

Early and frequent hand expression within the first 6 hours after birth, and 6–10 times over 24 hours, including overnight, will increase the volume of milk produced in the following weeks. Higher volumes of milk were associated with frequent and early expression when mothers expressed at least five times each day in the first 3 days, with a maximum interval of 7 hours between expressions (Lai et al., 2020). Recent studies have shown that using electric breast pumps within 6 hours of delivery facilitates more milk production than hand expression (Ru et al., 2020). Once lactogenesis II occurs at around day 3, double pumping using a hospital grade electric breast pump will increase prolactin levels and reduce the time required for expressing. Massaging the breast during expression also has a positive effect on the amount of milk produced and reduces pain associated with breast problems such as mastitis (Anderson, 2019). When hand expression is combined with electric pumping, both milk production and fat content of the expressed milk are increased (Boss et al., 2018). Expressing and storing of breast milk is well described in the Australian Breastfeeding Association (ABA) booklet *Breastfeeding: expressing and storing breastmilk* (ABA, 2020).

Opportunities for the mother to have skin-to-skin contact with her baby, who has contact with the nipple while expressing, will stimulate both oxytocin and prolactin release, enabling the mother to increase the amount of milk she expresses (Fewtrell et al., 2016).

Many mothers experience times when the amount they express is less than the requirements of their babies. The reasons can include recovery from her labour and birthing, separation from her baby and concern and worry for the medical condition of her baby, all of which affect the amount of milk she is able to express and her ability to express effectively. A low milk supply is also common during 36–40 weeks' postmenstrual age, when neonates are often discharged, and during the period where the mother and partner have sole responsibility for their baby (Wilson et al., 2015). Strategies to increase her supply can include post-discharge support (Wilson et al., 2015), advice about pumping regularly seven to eight times a day, having pictures or a DVD of baby to watch while expressing, bedside pumping, rest, reducing visitors and housework, spending time with baby and skin-to-skin contact. Pharmacological methods can also be used in conjunction with these methods to increase milk supply. Domperidone, a dopamine antagonist, is commonly used to enhance prolactin levels and does not cross the blood–brain barrier; therefore, it has fewer side effects (Wada et al., 2019).

EVIDENCE-BASED PRACTICE RESEARCH 5.9

The Baby-Friendly Hospital Initiative (BFHI) was launched in neonatal units worldwide in 1991, with modifications made to the Ten Steps for Successful Breastfeeding in 2018 to include preterm and sick infants. 'Infant stability' is now recognised as the only criterion for early initiation of breastfeeding, which is an important shift in practice away from criteria related to postmenstrual age or weight (Maastrup et al., 2019).

Transition to the breast

Deciding when a preterm neonate is ready for breastfeeding depends on a number of factors. These include the neonate's oral motor development, tolerance of milk feeds by gavage, the neonate's overall condition, their ability to maintain body temperature and whether they exhibit feeding cues such as the rooting reflex, hand-to-mouth activity and mouth opening. The implementation of skin-to-skin contact as early as practicable will enable an easier transition to breastfeed. The closeness to the breast will improve suckling ability and promote earlier breastfeeding. There are now several instruments for determining feeding readiness (Çamur & Çetinkaya, 2021). Sucking feeds are generally introduced at around 32–34 weeks' postmenstrual age.

Once sucking feeds begin, they are increased gradually, usually beginning with once a day and increasing as the neonate demands or is assessed as ready to progress. As the number of sucking feeds increases, the number of tube feeds decreases until sucking feeds alone provide sufficient intake for growth and development. It is not always possible for a mother to be available to breastfeed during this transition period. At times after a breastfeed, the amount of milk that the neonate has received is assessed, and a 'top up' with EBM or formula may be required.

When bringing their milk to the hospital from home, mothers need advice about hygienic methods of expression, storage and transport conditions. The pump kit needs to be washed after every use, dried with a paper towel and disinfected daily. Milk can be kept in the fridge (at the back, at up to 4°C) for 48 hours before freezing. Once frozen it can be kept in a freezer in the fridge for 2 weeks, or in a freezer with a separate door for 3 months. Milk should be transported to the neonatal unit in an insulated food container with gel or cold packs (rather than ice) (Rodrigo et al., 2021).

EVIDENCE-BASED PRACTICE RESEARCH 5.10

During transition from gavage to breast feeds, five studies used cup feeding, one used tube feeding and one used a novel teat when supplemental feeds were required. The primary outcome of self-reported exclusive breastfeeding rates was assessed at hospital discharge and at 3 and 6 months after discharge. Use of non-bottle feeding devices instead of a bottle correlated with a higher percentage of exclusive breastfeeding at hospital discharge. Compared with cup feeding, bottle feeding was associated with a 39% decreased likelihood of exclusive breastfeeding at hospital discharge. Similarly, cup feeding was associated with a 17% lower risk of breastfeeding cessation at 3 months after discharge (Milano & Menzel, 2021).

Important considerations to promote successful breastfeeding include realistic expectations, the mother's position, skin-to-skin contact, the neonate's position, expressing to begin the oxytocin release, recognising correct attachment, stimulating the neonate's rooting reflex, allowing the neonate to stay at the breast and not limiting feeds. Other helpful strategies include the Dancer hold if the neonate is having difficulty staying at the breast because of uncoordinated suckling, recognising milk transfer and treating any nipple damage (Fig. 5.2). The Dancer hand position supports the breast, as well as the neonate's jaw, decreasing the workload of maintaining a proper latch while helping prevent the neonate from slipping off the breast. The mother can use the hand that is supporting her breasts, using three fingers and her palm to support the breast, and the index finger and thumb on her baby's cheeks forming a U-shape upon which to rest their chin.

The use of ultra-thin nipple shields can help the preterm neonate with attachment and aid milk transfer when breasts are engorged, but nipple shields have also been associated with less breastfeeding at discharge (Heller et al., 2021). Findings related to the use of a dummy, or pacifier, are contradictory. Some studies have found that use of a dummy is associated with an earlier transition to excusive breastfeeding, while others have found that exclusive breastfeeding is more successful when the use of dummies is minimised (Maastrup et al., 2021). Using a cup instead of a bottle increases the extent and duration of breastfeeding in preterm neonates, but is associated with prolonged hospital stays (World Health Organization (WHO), 2019).

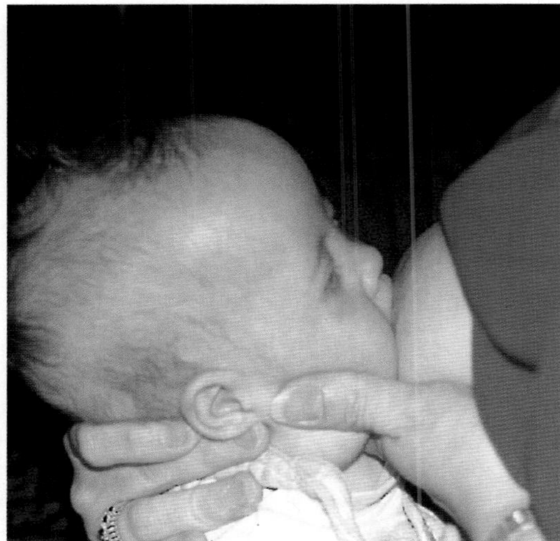

FIGURE 5.2 **The Dancer hold**

Source: © 2017 Wilson-Clay and Hoover, from The breastfeeding atlas. *6th ed.*

The preterm neonate's feeding limitations

Table 5.7 summarises the limitations experienced by the preterm neonate transitioning to full enteral feeds, and the neonatal nursing/midwifery strategies to support them during this period.

CASE STUDY 5.1

Baby Lily

Baby Lily was born at 23 weeks' gestation to Zoe, after preterm labour of unknown aetiology was unable to be halted. She weighed 628 g at birth and, with Apgar scores of 6^1 and 8^5, she was actively resuscitated. Her postnatal course was complicated by hyaline membrane disease, hypoglycaemia and a grade 2 intraventricular haemorrhage.

1. What deleterious effects does early and optimal nutritional management aim to prevent in Lily's first week of life?
2. What nutritional deficits does Lily have that may impede her growth?

At birth, Lily was administered prophylactic surfactant in the birthing suite and, when hyaline membrane disease developed, she received high-frequency oscillatory ventilation, then high-frequency jet ventilation, and she finally was weaned to synchronised intermittent mechanical ventilation and nasal CPAP over a period of the next month. Apnoea of prematurity was treated with intravenous and then oral caffeine. Blood transfusions were required for anaemia of prematurity. Despite the grade 2 intraventricular haemorrhage, Lily's neurobehaviour seemed appropriate for her gestational age.

3. What nutritional management would be utilised in Lily's first weeks of life?
4. What medications would Lily most likely receive in the neonatal unit that have implications for her gastrointestinal function?

By day 86, Lily was at 35 weeks' corrected age. Her measurements were all average for gestational age: weight of 2330 g, length of 44 cm, head circumference of 32 cm. Sadly, Zoe was unable to maintain the breast milk supply for Lily and her enteral feeds consisted of preterm formula.

5. What nutritional management is now needed to ensure Lily is receiving 100% of her calorie requirements?

TABLE 5.7 **Issues and strategies for feeding preterm neonates**

Issue	Strategy
Easily overwhelmed by environmental stimuli	• Feed in a low-stimuli environment, i.e. a quiet room with minimal interruptions • Neonate may not be able to manage multiple modes of input at once, so it may be best to feed the neonate without making direct eye contact or talking to them at the same time • Initiate skin to skin to calm the neonate before the feed
Tires easily	• Feed when awake and alert • If sleepy, massage the neonate's body, back and front, drop some milk onto the neonate's lips, and encourage non-nutritive sucking to wake them up • Restrict length of time taken for suck feeds until energy levels increase • Include rest periods during feeding sessions • Assess the neonate's readiness for feeding by observing cues such as rooting, mouthing, hand-to-mouth activity, and respond to them • Provide pre-feed oral stimulation • A nipple shield may be useful for neonates who have difficulty attaching to the nipple or who tire easily • Encourage the mother to gently hand massage the breast to encourage milk flow while her baby sucks
Potential for neck flexion and airway compromise during feeding	• Ensure the neonate is held in a supportive position, upright with airway neutral during skin to skin, and during feeding episodes
Potential for hypothermia while feeding	• Position the neonate skin to skin, or ensure they are wrapped or swaddled gently and loosely (muslin cloth is useful) • Ensure the neonate's temperature is normal prior to feed
Small mouth and comparatively large nipple size/flat nipples	• Ensure the neonate is attached correctly • Stimulate the rooting reflex. Ensure the mouth is wide open. Bring the neonate to the breast quickly • Soften full breasts by expressing them and then make a 'sandwich' shape with the breast to enable the neonate to draw the nipple to the back of the mouth • If a nipple shield has been used, once the mother's nipple protrudes, remove the shield and latch the neonate directly to the breast
Weak suck reflex, inability to create a strong vacuum and poorly coordinated suck/swallow/breathe	• Promote early and frequent breast contact, even before sucking coordination is functional • Encourage the rooting reflex • Feed on demand (a limit will need to be set initially)
Breast milk supply low	• Encourage mothers to express 8–12 times every 24 hours in the first 2 weeks postpartum, including overnight • Teach mother how to hand express and then how to use the breast pump • Do not offer a bottle to a neonate whose mother wishes to breastfeed

Source: Mannix (unpublished).

CONCLUSION

The importance of the nutritional management of preterm neonates cannot be underestimated. Postnatal growth failure is common and is associated with poorer longer-term developmental outcomes. Increased calories and protein received in the first week after birth and during hospitalisation are associated with enhanced body composition and neurodevelopmental outcomes for preterm infants (Ramel et al., 2020). Careful attention to the nutritional needs of preterm neonates is required in order to optimise outcomes. The implementation of standardised feeding guidelines reduces variation in clinical practice and improves postnatal growth.

Breastfeeding and breast milk have been clearly demonstrated to be the most appropriate and beneficial nutrition for neonates, and specifically for preterm neonates. With the many challenges that preterm neonates encounter, having access to their mother's fresh breast milk and subsequent breastfeeding assists in the development of their immune system as well as decreasing risk for many illnesses. Preterm formula may be the only option if the mother is unable to breastfeed or provide breast milk, or when donor milk is not available.

Supporting mothers with expressing, breastfeeding and skin-to-skin contact with their baby is paramount for them to feel confident and involved in their baby's care. Early initiation and frequent, effective expression have longer-term benefits of lactation success. Advocacy of neonatal nurses and midwives in encouraging breastfeeding, expressing and skin-to-skin contact will have longer-term benefits for the mother–child relationship and breastfeeding. The implementation of skin-to-skin contact as early as practicable enables an easier transition to breastfeed, improves suckling ability and promotes earlier breastfeeding.

Recommended Reading

Neu, J., & Patton, L. (2021). The microbiome as a therapeutic target in preterm nutrition. *World Review of Nutrition and Diet, 122*, 180–190. doi: 10.1159/000514737.

Poindexter, B. B., & Martin, C. R. (2020). Nutrient requirements/nutritional support in premature neonate. In: R. J. Martin, A. A. Fanaroff, & M. C. Walsh (Eds.), *Fanaroff and Martin's neonatal–perinatal medicine* (pp. 670–689). Philadelphia, PA: Elsevier.

Online Resources

Australian Breastfeeding Association. (2016). Breastfeeding your premature baby: <https://www.breastfeeding.asn.au/bf-info/premature>

Kam, R. (2016). Breastfeeding a premature baby – 7 great tips: <https://www.bellybelly.com.au/breastfeeding/breastfeeding-premature-baby/>

References/Acknowledgements

Abiramalatha, T., Thanigainathan, S., & Balakrishnan, U. (2019). Re-feeding versus discarding gastric residuals to improve growth in preterm infants. *Cochrane Database of Systematic Reviews, 7*, CD012940. doi: 10.1002/14651858.CD012940.pub2.

Acun, C., Baker, A., Brown, L. S., Iglesia, K. A., & Sisman, J. (2021). Peripherally inserted central catheter migration in neonates: incidence, timing and risk factors. *Journal of Neonatal and Perinatal Medicine, 14*(3), 411–417. doi: 10.3233/NPM-200684.

Agostoni, C., Buonocore, G., Carnielli, V. P., De Curtis, M., Darmaun, D., Decsi, T., et al. (2010). Enteral nutrient supply for preterm infants: commentary from the European Society of Paediatric Gastroenterology, Hepatology and Nutrition Committee on Nutrition. *Journal of Pediatric Gastroenterology and Nutrition, 50*(1), 85–91.

Altobelli, E., Angeletti, P. M., Verrotti, A., & Petrocelli, R. (2020). The impact of human milk on necrotizing enterocolitis: a systematic review and meta-analysis. *Nutrients, 12*(5), 1322. doi: 10.3390/nu12051322.

Andersen, C., French, J., Stock, L., & Crompron, A. (2021). *Change of practice: WAB's WCH – Neonatal Feeding Pathway: 5% glucose for infants equal to or greater than 35 weeks gestational age requiring supplementary feeds*. Adelaide, SA: WCH.

Anderson, L. (2019). Breast massage: can it keep mothers breastfeeding longer? *JBI Database of Systematic Reviews and Implementation Reports, 17*(8), 1550–1551. doi: 10.11124/JBISRIR-D-19-00233.

Aradhya, A. S., Mukhopadhyay, K., Saini, S. S., Sundaram, V., Dutta, S., & Kumar, P. (2020). Feed intolerance in preterm neonates with antenatal reverse end diastolic flow (REDF) in umbilical artery: a retrospective cohort study. *Journal of Maternal–Fetal and Neonatal Medicine, 33*(11), 1846–1852. doi: 10.1080/14767058.2018.1531123.

Armentrout, D. (2021). Glucose management. In: M. T. Verklan, M. Walden, & S. Forest (Eds.), *Core curriculum for neonatal intensive care nursing* (6th ed., pp. 144–151). St Louis, MO: Elsevier.

Arslanoglu, S., Boquien, C. Y., King, C., Lamireau, D., Tonetto, P., Barnett, D., et al. (2019). Fortification of human milk for preterm infants: update and recommendations of the European Milk Bank Association (EMBA) working group on human milk fortification. *Frontiers in Pediatrics, 7*, 76. doi: 10.3389/fped.2019.00076.

Australian Breastfeeding Association (ABA). (2020). Expressing and storing breastmilk. South Melbourne, Vic: ABA. <https://www.breastfeeding.asn.au/bf-info/breastfeeding-and-work/expressing-and-storing-breastmilk> (Accessed 3 March 2022).

Badran, A. T., Hashish, M., Ali, A., Shokeir, M. A., & Shaaban, A. (2020). Nasogastric versus orogastric bolus tube feeding in preterm infants: pilot randomized clinical trial. *American Journal of Perinatology, 38*(14), 1526–1532. doi: 10.1055/s-0040-1713865.

Bakker, L., Jackson, B., & Miles, A. (2021). Oral-feeding guidelines for preterm neonates in the NICU: a scoping review. *Journal of Perinatology, 41*, 140–149. doi: 10.1038/s41372-020-00887-6.

Banait, N., Basu, S., Desai, P., Dutta, S., Kumar, A., Kumar, J., et al. (2020). Feeding of low birth weight neonates. *Journal of Neonatology, 34*(1–2), 28–51. doi: 10.1177/0973217920938522.

Bolisetty, S., Osborn, D., Sinn, J., & Lui, K.; the Australasian Neonatal Parenteral Nutrition Consensus Group. (2014). Standardised neonatal parenteral nutrition formulations: an Australasian group consensus 2012. *BMC Pediatrics, 14*, 48.

Bolisetty, S., Osborn, D., Schindler, T., Sinn, J., Deshpanda, G., Wong, C. S., et al. (2020). Standardised neonatal parenteral nutrition formulations – Australasian neonatal parenteral nutrition consensus update 2017. *BMC Pediatrics, 20*(1), 59. doi: 10.1186/s12887-020-1958-9.

Boss, M., Gardner, H., & Hartmann, P. (2018). Normal human lactation: closing the gap. *F1000 Research*, 7, F1000 Faculty Rev-801. doi: 10.12688/f1000research.14452.1.

Brown, L. D., Hendrickson, K., Evans, R., David, J., & Hay, W. W. (2021). Enteral nutrition. In: S. L. Gardner, B. S. Carter, M. Enzman-Hines, & S. Niermeyer (Eds.), *Merenstein & Gardner's handbook of neonatal intensive care* (pp. 480–533). St Louis, MO: Elsevier.

Çamur, Z., & Çetinkaya, B. (2021). The validity and reliability study of the Turkish version of the Preterm Oral Feeding Readiness Assessment Scale (T-POFRAS). *Journal of Pediatric Research, 8*(3). doi: 10.4274/jpr.galenos.2020.35682.

Dawson, J. A., Summan, R., Badawi, N., & Foster, J. P. (2021). Push versus gravity for intermittent bolus gavage tube feeding of preterm mature and low birth weight infants. *Cochrane Database of Systematic Reviews, 8*(8), CD005249.

Dias, F., Jales, R. M., Alvares, B. R., Caldas, J. P., & Carmona, E. V. (2020). Randomized clinical trial comparing two methods of measuring insertion length of nasogastric tubes in newborns. *Journal of Parenteral and Enteral Nutrition, 44*(5), 912–919.

Diez, S., Tielesch, L., Weiss, C., Halbfass, J., Müller, H., & Besendörfer, M. (2020). Clinical characteristics of necrotizing enterocolitis in preterm patients with and without persistent ductus arteriosus and in patients with congenital heart disease. *Frontiers in Pediatrics, 8*, 257.

Ditzenberger, G. R. (2018). Gastrointestinal and hepatic systems and perinatal nutrition. In: S. Blackburn (Ed.), *Maternal, fetal and neonatal physiology: a clinical perspective* (5th ed., pp. 387–420). St Louis, MO: Elsevier.

Dorling, J., Abbott, J., Berrington, J., Bosiak, B., Bowler, U., Boyle, E., et al. (2019). Controlled trial of two incremental milk-feeding rates in preterm infants. *New England Journal of Medicine, 381*(15), 1434–1443.

Dorling, J., Tume, L., Arch, B., Woolfall, K., Latten, L., Roper, L., et al. (2020). Gastric residual volume measurement in British neonatal intensive care units: a survey of practice. *BMJ Paediatrics Open, 4*, e000601. doi: 10.1136/bmjpo-2019-000601.

Dutta, S., Singh, B., Chessell, L., Wilson, J., Janes, M., McDonald, K., et al. (2015). Guidelines for feeding very low birth weight infants. *Nutrients, 7*(1), 423–442.

Edward, R. R., Innes, J. K., Marino, L. V., & Calder, P. C. (2018). Influence of different intravenous lipid emulsions on growth, development and laboratory and clinical outcomes in hospitalised paediatric patients: a systematic review. *Clinical Nutrition, 37*, 765–783.

Eibensteiner, F., Auer-Hackenberg, L., Jilma, B., Thanhaeuser, M., Wald, M., & Haiden, N. (2019). Growth, feeding tolerance and metabolism in extreme preterm infants under an exclusive human milk diet. *Nutrients, 11*(7), 1443.

Ellett, M. L., Cohen, M. D., Perkins, S. M., Smith, C. E., Lane, K. A., & Austin, J. K. (2011). Predicting the insertion length for gastric tube placement in neonates. *Journal of Obstetric, Gynecologic, and Neonatal Nursing, 40*, 412–421. doi: 10.1111/j.1552-6909.2011.01255.x.

Ericson, J., & Palmér, L. (2018). Mothers of preterm infants' experiences of breastfeeding support in the first 12 months after birth: a qualitative study. *Birth, 46*(1), 129–136.

Farhath, S., Aghai, Z. H., Nakhla, T., Saslow, J., He, Z., Sounder, S., et al. (2006). Pepsin, a reliable marker of gastric aspiration, is frequently detected in tracheal aspirates from premature ventilated neonates: relationship with feeding and methylxanthine therapy. *Journal of Pediatric Gastroenterology and Nutrition, 43*(3), 336–341. doi: 10.1097/01.mpg.0000232015.56155.03.

Fewtrell, M. S., Kennedy, K., Ahluwalia, J. S., Nicholl, R., Lucas, A., & Burton, P. (2016). Predictors of expressed breast milk volume in mothers expressing milk for their preterm infant. *Archives of Disease in Childhood. Fetal and Neonatal Edition, 101*(6), F502–F506. doi: 10.1136/archdischild-2015-308321.

Fucile, S., Wener, E., & Dow, K. (2021). Enhancing breastfeeding establishment in preterm infants: a randomized clinical trial of two non-nutritive sucking approaches. *Early Human Development, 156*, 105347. doi: 10.1016/j.earlhumdev.2021.105347.

Gibson, K., Sharp, R., Ullman, A., Morris, S., Kleidon, T., & Esterman, A. (2021). Risk factors for umbilical vascular catheter–related adverse events: a scoping review. *Australian Critical Care, 35*(1), 89–101. doi: 10.1016/j.aucc.2021.02.010.

Givens-Bell, S. (2021). Fluid and electrolyte management. In: M. T. Verklan, M. Walden, & S. Forest (Eds.), *Core curriculum for neonatal intensive care nursing* (6th ed., pp. 131–143). St Louis, MO: Elsevier.

Gould, J. F., Roberts, R. M., & Makrides, M. (2021). The influence of omega-3 long-chain polyunsaturated fatty acid, docosahexaenoic acid, on child behavioural functioning: a review of randomized controlled trials of DHA supplementation in pregnancy, the neonatal period and infancy. *Nutrients, 13*(2), 415. doi: 10.3390/nu13020415.

Griffin, I. J. (2021). Parenteral nutrition in premature infants. In: S. A. Abrams (Ed.), *UpToDate*. Walters Kluwer. <https://www.uptodate.com/contents/parenteral-nutrition-in-premature-infants?search> (Accessed 3 March 2022).

Gupta, N., Deierl, A., Hills, E., & Banerjee, J. (2021). Systematic review confirmed the benefits of early skin-to-skin contact but highlighted lack of studies on very and extremely preterm infants. *Acta Paediatrica, 110*, 2310–2315. doi: 10.1111/apa.15913.

Gura, K. M., & Elisofon, S. A. (2021). Intestinal failure-associated liver disease in infants. In: S. A. Abrams & E. B. Rand (Eds.), *UpToDate*. Walters Kluwer. <https://www.uptodate.com/contents/intestinal-failure-associated-liver-disease-in-infants?search> (Accessed 3 March 2022).

Hair, A. B. (2021). Approach to enteral nutrition in the premature infant. In: S. A. Abrams (Ed.), *UpToDate*. Walters Kluwer. <https://www.uptodate.com/contents/approach-to-enteral-nutrition-in-the-premature-infant?search> (Accessed 3 March 2022).

Heller, N., Rüdiger, M., Hoffmeister, V., & Mense, L. (2021). Mother's own milk feeding in preterm newborns admitted to the neonatal intensive care unit or special-care nursery: obstacles, interventions, risk calculation. *International Journal of Environmental Research and Public Health, 18*(8), 4140. doi: 10.3390/ijerph18084140.

Henderickx, J. G. E., Zwittink, R. D., Renes, I. B., van Lingen, R. A., van Zoeren-Grobben, D. L. J. G., et al. (2021). Maturation of the preterm gastrointestinal tract can be defined by host and microbial markers for digestion and barrier defence. *Science Reports, 11*, 12808. doi: 10.1038/s41598-021-92222-y.

Hoellering, A., Tshamala, D., & Davies, M. W. (2018). Study of movement of umbilical venous catheters over time.

Journal of Paediatric and Child Health, 54(12), 1329–1335.

Hojsak, I., Colomb, V., Braegger, C., Bronsky, J., Campoy, C., Domellöf, M., et al. (2016). ESPGHAN Committee on Nutrition Position Paper. Intravenous lipid emulsions and risk of hepatotoxicity in infants and children: a systematic review and meta-analysis. *Journal of Pediatric Gastroenterology and Nutrition, 62*(5), 776–792.

Hugill, K., & van Rens, M. (2020). Inserting central lines via the peripheral circulation in neonates. *Journal of Nursing, 29*(19), S12–S18. doi: 10.12968/bjon.2020.29.19.S12.

Ibrahim, N. R., Van Rostenberghe, H., Ho, J. J., & Nasir, A. (2021). Short versus long feeding interval for bolus feedings in very preterm infants. *Cochrane Database Systemic Review, 8*(8), CD012322. doi: 10.1002/14651858.CD012322.pub2.

Izquierdo Renau, M., Aldecoa-Bilbao, V., Balcells Esponera, C., Del Rey Hurtado de Mendoza, B., Iriondo Sanz, M., & Iglesias-Platas, I. (2019). Applying methods for postnatal growth assessment in the clinical setting: evaluation in a longitudinal cohort of very preterm infants. *Nutrients, 11*(11), 2772. doi: 10.3390/nu11112772.

Kim, J. H. (2021). Neonatal necrotizing enterocolitis: pathology and pathogenesis. In: S. A. Abrams (Ed.), *UpToDate*. Walters Kluwer. <https://www.uptodate.com/contents/neonatal-necrotizing-enterocolitis-pathology-and-pathogenesis?search> (Accessed 3 March 2022).

Klein, L. D., Keir, A. K., Cruz, M., & Rumbold, A. (2021). 'I wish I'd had the option': views about donor human milk among parents with babies born moderate–late preterm. *Journal of Paediatrics and Child Health, 57*(8), 1334–1335.

Koletzko, B., Goulet, O., Hunt, J., Krohn, K., & Shamir, R., for the Parenteral Nutrition Guidelines Working Group. (2005). Guidelines on paediatric parenteral nutrition of the European Society of Paediatric Gastroenterology, Hepatology and Nutrition (ESPGHAN) and the European Society for Clinical Nutrition and Metabolism (ESPEN), Supported by the European Society of Paediatric Research (ESPR). 6. Fluid and electrolytes (Na, Cl and K). *Journal of Pediatric Gastroenterology and Nutrition, 41*, S33–S38.

Koo, J. K., Narvasa, A., Bode, L. & Kim, J. H. (2019). Through thick and thin: the in vitro effects of thickeners on infant feed viscosity. *Journal of Pediatric Gastroenterology and Nutrition, 69*(5), e122–e128. doi: 10.1097/MPG.0000000000002470.

Lai, C. T., Rea, A., Mitoulas, L., Kent, J. C., Simmer, K., Hartmann, P. E., et al. (2020). Short-term rate of milk synthesis and expression interval of preterm mothers. *Archives of Disease in Childhood. Fetal and Neonatal Edition, 105*(3), 266–269.

Levit, O. L., Shabanova, V., & Bizzarro, M. J. (2020). Umbilical catheter-associated complications in a level IV neonatal intensive care unit. *Journal of Perinatology, 40*(4), 573–580.

Li, L., Wang, L., Niu, C., Liu, C., Lv, T., Ji, F., et al. (2021). Early skin contact combined with mother's breastfeeding to shorten the process of premature infants ≤30 weeks of gestation to achieve full oral feeding: the study protocol of a randomized controlled trial. *Trials, 22*(1), 1–10.

Lording, R. J. (2006). A review of human milk banking and public health policy in Australia. *Breastfeeding Review, 14*(3), 21–30.

Maastrup, R., & Haiek, L. N.; The Neo-BFHI Survey Group. (2019). Compliance with the "baby-friendly hospital initiative for neonatal wards" in 36 countries. *Maternal and Child Nutrition, 15*, e12690. doi: 10.1111/mcn.12690.

Maastrup, R., Rom, A. L., Walloee, S., Sandfeld, H. B., & Kronborg, H. (2021). Improved exclusive breastfeeding rates in preterm infants after a neonatal nurse training program focusing on six breastfeeding-supportive clinical practices. *Plos One, 16*(2), e0245273. doi: 10.1371/journal.pone.0245273.

Mantegazza, C., Landy, N., Zuccotti, G. V., & Köglmeier, J. (2018). Indications and complications of inpatient parenteral nutrition prescribed to children in a large tertiary referral hospital. *Italian Journal of Pediatrics, 44*(1), 66. doi: 10.1186/s13052-018-0505-x.

McLeod, G., Farrent, S., Gilroy, M., Page, D., Oliver, C. J., Richmond, F., et al. (2021). Variation in neonatal nutrition practice and implications: a survey of Australia and New Zealand neonatal units. *Frontiers in Nutrition, 8*, 445. doi: 10.3389/fnut.2021.642474.

Milano, K., & Menzel, E. (2021). Does bottle feeding in the newborn period in addition to breastfeeding decrease breastfeeding success? *Evidence-Based Practice, 24*(2), 29–30.

Moltu, S. J., Bronsky, J., Embleton, N., Gerasimidis, K., Indrio, F., & Köglmeier, J.; ESPGHAN Committee on Nutrition. (2021). Nutritional management of the critically ill neonate: a position paper of the ESPGHAN Committee on Nutrition. *Journal of Pediatric Gastroenterology and Nutrition, 73*(2), 274–289. doi: 10.1097/MPG.0000000000003076.

Moreno-Fernandez, J., Ochoa, J. J., Latunde-Dada, G. O., & Diaz-Castro, J. (2019). Iron deficiency and iron homeostasis in low birth weight preterm infants: a systematic review. *Nutrients, 11*(5), 1090. doi: 10.3390/nu11051090.

Moro, G. E., Billeaud, C., Buffin, R., Calvo, J. Cavallarin, L., Christen, L., et al. (2019). Processing of donor human milk: update and recommendations from the European Milk Bank Association (EMBA). *Frontiers in Pediatrics, 7*, 49. doi: 10.3389/fped.2019.00049.

Murphy, A. D., Gilmour, R. F., & Coombs, C. J. (2019). Extravasation injury in a paediatric population. *Australia and New Zealand Journal of Surgery, 89*, E122–E126. doi: 10.1111/ans.14104.

National Institute for Health and Care Excellence (NICE). (2020). *Neonatal parenteral nutrition*. NICE guideline 154. <https://www.nice.org.uk/guidance/ng154/resources/neonatal-parenteral-nutrition-pdf-66141840283333> (Accessed 3 March 2022).

Oddie, S. J., Young, L., & McGuire, W. (2021). Slow advancement of enteral feed volumes to prevent necrotising enterocolitis in very low birth weight infants. *Cochrane Database Systemic Review, 8*(8), CD001241. doi: 10.1002/14651858.CD001241.pub8.

Oliver, C., Watson, C., Crowley, E., Gilroy, M., Page, D., Weber, K., et al. (2019). Vitamin and mineral supplementation practices in preterm infants: a survey of Australian and New Zealand neonatal intensive and special care units. *Nutrients, 12*(1), 51. doi: 10.3390/nu12010051.

Olsen, S. L., Oschman, A., & Tracy, K. (2021). Total parenteral nutrition. In: S. L. Gardner, B. S. Carter, M. Enzman-Hines, &

S. Niermeyer (Eds.), *Merenstein & Gardner's handbook of neonatal intensive care* (pp. 459–479). St Louis, MO: Elsevier.

Păduraru, L., Zonda, G. I., Avasiloaiei, A. L., Moscalu, M., Dimitriu, D. C., & Stamatin, M. (2019). Influence of refrigeration or freezing on human milk macronutrients and energy content in early lactation: results from a tertiary centre survey. *Paediatric Child Health, 24*(4), 250–257. doi: 10.1093/pch/pxy164.

Parker, L. A. (2019). Donor human milk. *Journal of Perinatal and Neonatal Nursing, 33*(3), 216–218. doi: 10.1097/JPN.0000000000000425.

Parker, L. A., Withers, J. H., & Talaga, E. (2018). Comparison of neonatal nursing practices for determining feeding tube insertion length and verifying gastric placement with current best evidence. *Advances in Neonatal Care, 18*(4), 307–317.

Parker, L. A., Desorcy-Scherer, K., & Magalhaes, M. (2021). Feeding strategies in preterm very low birth-weight infants. *Advances in Neonatal Care, 21*(6), 493–502. doi: 10.1097/ANC.0000000000000849.

Pérez-Cano, F. J. (2020). What does influence the neonatal microbiome? *Nutrients, 12*(8), 2472. doi: 10.3390/nu12082472.

Premkumar, M. H., Pammi, M., & Suresh, G. (2019). Human milk-derived fortifier versus bovine milk-derived fortifier for prevention of mortality and morbidity in preterm neonates. *Cochrane Database of Systematic Reviews, 11*, CD013145. doi: 10.1002/14651858.CD013145.pub2.

Quigley, M., Embleton, N. D., & McGuire, W. (2019). Formula versus donor breast milk for feeding preterm or low birth weight infants. *Cochrane Database of Systematic Reviews, 7*, CD002971. doi: 10.1002/14651858.CD002971.pub5.

Radzikowska, U., Rinaldi, A. O., Çelebi Sözener, Z., Karaguzel, D., Wojcik, M., Cypryk, K., et al. (2019). The influence of dietary fatty acids on immune responses. *Nutrients, 11*(12), 2990. doi: 10.3390/nu11122990.

Ramel, S. E., Haapala, J., Super, J., Boys, C., & Demerath, E. W. (2020). Nutrition, illness and body composition in very low birth weight preterm infants: implications for nutritional management and neurocognitive outcomes. *Nutrients, 12*(1), 145. doi: 10.3390/nu12010145.

Ringer, S. (2020). Fluid and electrolyte therapy in newborns. In S. A. Abrams & T. K. Mattoo (Eds.), *UpToDate*. Waltham, MA: UpToDate. <https://www.uptodate.com/contents/fluid-and-electrolyte-therapy-in-newborns?search=> (Accessed 16 March 2022).

Rochow, N., Fusch, G., Ali, A., Bhatia, A., So, H., Iskander, R., et al. (2021). Individualized target fortification of breast milk with protein, carbohydrates, and fat for preterm infants: a double-blind randomized controlled trial. *Clinical Nutrition, 40*(1), 54–63. doi: 10.1016/j.clnu.2020.04.031.

Rodrigo, R., Amir, L. H., Forster, D. A., McEgan, K., & Opie, G. (2021). Human milk expression, storage, and transport by women whose infants are inpatients at a tertiary neonatal unit in Melbourne, Australia. *Advances in Neonatal Care, 21*(6), E199–E208. doi: 10.1097/ANC.0000000000000825.

Ru, X., Huang, X., & Fang, Q. (2020). Successful full lactation achieved by mothers of preterm infants using exclusive pumping. *Frontiers in Pediatrics, 8*, 191. doi: 10.3389/fped.2020.00191.

Rutledge, A., Murphy, H. J., Harer, M. W., & Jetton, J. G. (2021). Fluid balance in the critically ill child section: "How bad is fluid in neonates?" *Frontiers in Pediatrics, 9*, 651458. doi: 10.3389/fped.2021.651458.

Sadrudin Premji, S., Chessell, L., & Stewart, F. (2021). Continuous nasogastric milk feeding versus intermittent bolus milk feeding for preterm infants less than 1500 grams. *Cochrane Database of Systematic Reviews, 6*, CD001819. doi: 10.1002/14651858.CD001819.pub3.

Sanderson, E., Yeo, K. T., Wang, A. Y., Callander, I., Bajuk, B., Bolisetty, S., et al.; NICUS Network. (2017). Dwell time and risk of central-line-associated bloodstream infection in neonates. *Journal of Hospital Infection, 97*(3), 267–274. doi: 10.1016/j.jhin.2017.06.023.

Schmid, S., Geffers, C., Wagenpfeil, G., & Simon, A. (2018). Preventive bundles to reduce catheter-associated bloodstream infections in neonatal intensive care. *GMS Hygiene and Infection Control, 13*, Doc10. doi: 10.3205/dgkh000316.

Selvam, S., Humphrey, T., Woodley, H., English, S., & Kraft, J. K. (2018). Sonographic features of umbilical catheter-related complications. *Pediatric Radiology, 48*(13), 1964–1970.

Sertic, A. J., Connolly, B. L., Temple, M. J., Parra, D. A., Amaral, J. G., & Lee, K. S. (2018). Perforations associated with peripherally inserted central catheters in a neonatal population. *Pediatric Radiology, 48*, 109–119. doi: 10.1007/s00247-017-3983-x.

Sharma, D., Farahbakhsh, N., & Tabatabaii, S. A. (2019). Role of ultrasound for central catheter tip localization in neonates: a review of the current evidence. *Journal of Maternal–Fetal and Neonatal Medicine, 32*(14), 2429–2437. doi: 10.1080/14767058.2018.1437135.

Shimokaze, T., Yamamoto, K., Miyamoto, Y., Toyoshima, K., Katsumata, K., & Saito, T. (2021). Acute respiratory effect of transpyloric feeding for respiratory exacerbation in preterm infants. *Journal of Perinatal Medicine, 49*(3), 383–387. doi: 10.1515/jpm-2020-0243.

Theurich, M. A., McCool-Myers, M., & Koletzko, B. (2021). Supporting breastfeeding of small, sick and preterm neonates. *Seminars in Perinatology, 45*(2), 151387.

Urashima, M., Mezawa, H., Okuyama, M., Urashima, T., Hirano, D., Gocho, N., et al. (2019). Primary prevention of cow's milk sensitization and food allergy by avoiding supplementation with cow's milk formula at birth: a randomized clinical trial. *JAMA Pediatrics, 173*(12), 1137–1145. doi: 10.1001/jamapediatrics.2019.3544.

Uvn äs Moberg, K., Ekström-Bergström, A., Buckley, S., Massarotti, C., Pajalic, Z., Luegmair, K., et al. (2020). Maternal plasma levels of oxytocin during breastfeeding – a systematic review. *PLoS One, 15*(8), e0235806. doi: 10.1371/journal.pone.0235806.

Vlug, L. E., Nagelkerke, S., Jonkers-Schuitema, C. F., Rings, E., & Tabbers, M. M. (2020). The role of a nutrition support team in the management of intestinal failure patients. *Nutrients, 12*(1), 172. doi: 10.3390/nu12010172.

Wada, Y., Suyama, F., Sasaki, A., Saito, J., Shimizu, Y., Amari, S., et al. (2019). Effects of domperidone in increasing milk production in mothers with insufficient lactation for infants in the neonatal intensive care unit. *Breastfeeding Medicine, 14*(10), 744–747.

Wallenstein, M. B., Brooks, C., Kline, T. A., Beck, R. Q., Yang, W., Shaw, G. M., et al. (2019). Early transpyloric vs gastric feeding in preterm infants: a retrospective cohort study. *Journal of Perinatology, 39*, 837–841. doi: 10.1038/s41372-019-0372-3.

Watson, J., & McGuire, W. (2013). Nasal versus oral route for placing feeding tubes in preterm or low birth weight infants. *Cochrane Database of Systematic Reviews, 2*, CD003952.

Weaver, G., Bertino, E., Gebauer, C., Grovslien, A., Mileusnic-Milenovic, R., Arslanoglu, S., et al. (2019). Recommendations for the establishment and operation of human milk banks in Europe: a consensus statement from the European Milk Bank Association (EMBA). *Frontiers in Pediatrics, 7*, 53.

Wilson, E., Christensson, K., Brandt, L., Altman, M., & Bonamy, A. K. (2015). Early provision of mother's own milk and other predictors of successful breast milk feeding after very preterm birth: a regional observational group. *Journal of Human Lactation, 3*(3), 393–400.

Wilson-Clay, B., & Hoover, K. (2017). *The breastfeeding atlas* (6th ed.). Manchaca, TX: Lactnews Press.

World Health Organization. (2019). Cup-feeding for low-birth-weight infants unable to fully breastfeed. <https://www.who.int/elena/titles/cupfeeding_infants/en/> (Accessed 3 March 2022).

Yasuda, H., Kondo, N., Yamamoto, R., Asami, S., Abe, T., Tsujimoto, H., et al. (2021). Monitoring of gastric residual volume during enteral nutrition. *Cochrane Database of Systematic Reviews, 9*, CD013335. doi: 10.1002/14651858.CD013335.pub2.

Zemrani, B., McCallum, Z., & Bines, J. E. (2018). Trace element provision in parenteral nutrition in children: one size does not fit all. *Nutrients, 10*(11), 1819. doi: 10.3390/nu10111819.

CHAPTER 6

CARE OF THE EXTREMELY LOW BIRTHWEIGHT NEONATE

JEANINE YOUNG AND VICTORIA KAIN

Learning objectives

After reading this chapter you will be able to:

- prioritise care requirements, including associated equipment, in preparation for the admission of an extremely low birthweight (ELBW) neonate
- identify the needs, best-practice principles and evidence-based protocols that support the neonatal nursing/midwifery care of ELBW neonates
- recognise common complications that are likely to be experienced by an ELBW neonate, and the strategies to reduce adverse sequelae
- discuss key principles in effective communication with parents of an ELBW neonate
- demonstrate strategies that foster an interdisciplinary and collaborative approach between health professionals and the family in the care of an ELBW neonate.

Key words, terms and abbreviations

continuous positive airway pressure (CPAP)
extremely low birthweight (ELBW)
gestational age (GA)
golden hour protocol (GHP)
intrauterine growth restriction (IUGR)
intraventricular haemorrhage (IVH)
necrotising enterocolitis (NEC)
small for gestational age (SGA)
very low birthweight (VLBW)

INTRODUCTION

Birthweight is important because it is one of the strongest predictors of neonatal morbidity and mortality (Anil et al., 2020; Park et al., 2021). At the population level, the proportion of neonates with a low birthweight (LBW) is an indicator of a multifaceted public health problem that includes long-term maternal malnutrition, poor health outcomes, low socioeconomic background and a lack of antenatal care during pregnancy (Bellizzi & Padrini, 2020; Marete et al., 2020; Patton et al., 2017). At the individual level, LBW is an important predictor of neonatal health and survival and is strongly associated with a higher risk of infant mortality and, to a lesser degree, childhood developmental problems and the risk of developing certain adulthood diseases (Anil et al., 2020; Brumbaugh et al., 2019; Schneider, 2017). Small neonates who are admitted to neonatal units are usually born preterm or may be **small for gestational age (SGA)** due to growth restriction in utero and comprise a considerable proportion of neonates cared for in the neonatal unit. Of neonates admitted in 2018 to neonatal units that participated in the Australian and New Zealand Neonatal Network Registry, approximately 60% were low birthweight (<2500 grams), approximately 11% were **extremely low birthweight (ELBW)** (<1000 grams) while approximately 36% of neonates were born at <32 weeks' gestation (Chow et al., 2020). The rates of preterm and LBW births have stabilised, with preterm birth rates ranging from 8.2% to 8.6% between 2009 and 2019, and rates of LBW ranging from 6.2% to 6.6% between 2009 and 2019 (Australian Institute of Health and Welfare (AIHW), 2021).

This chapter will focus on the ELBW neonate and will discuss key health issues more commonly experienced by LBW neonates, using definitions and epidemiology relevant to the Australian and New Zealand context. Care needs of the LBW and ELBW neonate will focus on thermoregulation, fluid and electrolyte management, nutrition, developmental care and support of the family. Finally, a brief overview of the ethical and legal issues and economic impact will be discussed relating to care of ELBW neonates.

This chapter will complement several other chapters that explore specific issues and aspects of neonatal nursing/midwifery management in greater detail for all neonates admitted to the neonatal unit.

'Low birthweight': definitions and classifications

Accurate classification and understanding of the factors that contribute to a low birthweight are important in predicting outcomes and in anticipating the issues that these vulnerable neonates may experience. With this understanding, optimal evidence-based management that aims to improve survival while reducing adverse sequelae can be instituted that meets the specific needs of the individual neonate.

The international definition for low birthweights, accepted in both developing and developed countries (World Health Organization (WHO), 2021), is a neonate born weighing <2500 grams (up to and including 2499 grams). A 2-kg neonate at birth would be considered SGA or LBW. Tables 6.1 to 6.3 provide commonly used definitions for grouping neonates according to birthweight, maturity at birth or size for **gestational age (GA)**.

A newborn or neonate is defined by the World Health Organization as being under 28 days of age (WHO, 2018a). A neonate may be born LBW, including VLBW or ELBW, due to being born preterm or may be SGA, primarily due to **intrauterine growth restriction (IUGR)**. However, fetal growth restriction is not synonymous with being SGA. While growth restricted neonates may be SGA, 50–70% of SGA neonates are 'constitutionally small', meaning that their

TABLE 6.1 **Definitions according to birthweight**

Definition	Birthweight (grams)	Weight range (grams)
LBW: low birthweight	<2500	≤2499
VLBW: very low birthweight	<1500	U≤1499
ELBW: extremely low birthweight	<1000	≤999

Source: Stark & Eichenwald (2021).

TABLE 6.2 **Neonatal descriptive classifications based on maturity at birth**

Definition of maturity at birth	Completed weeks of gestation
Extremely preterm	<28
Very preterm	28 to <32
Moderate-to-late preterm	32 to <37
Term	37 to 41
Post-term	≥42 weeks

Source: World Health Organization (2018b).

TABLE 6.3 **Neonatal classification of size for gestational age**

Classification of size for gestational age	Position on the centile chart
Large for gestational age (LGA)	>90th centile
Small for gestational age (SGA)	<10th centile
Severe IUGR	<3rd centile

Source: Royal College of Obstetricians and Gynaecologists (RCOG) (2019).

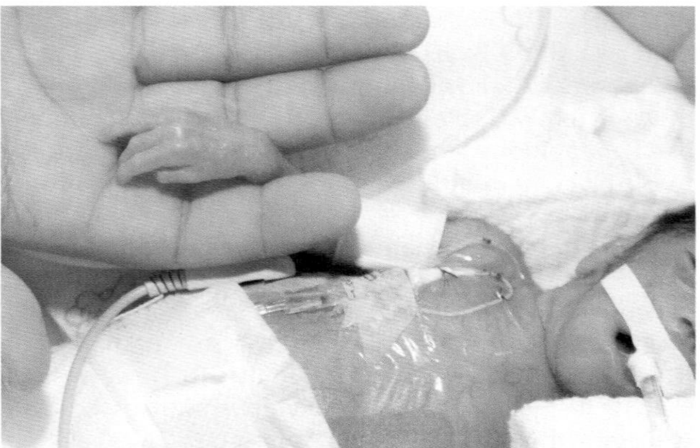

FIGURE 6.1 **An extremely low birthweight neonate (25 weeks 6 days, <400 grams)**

Source: iStockphoto/herjua.

fetal growth is appropriate for maternal size and ethnicity (Royal College of Obstetricians and Gynaecologists (RCOG), 2019). Fig. 6.1 depicts an ELBW neonate.

For accurate classification, the birthweight and GA of all neonates should be plotted according to an appropriate standard (Dobbin et al., 2012). Maternal weight, height, ethnicity, parity and gender have each been found to be significantly associated with normal variation in birthweight in Gardosi's seminal work (Gardosi, 2006). For example, the average birthweight for neonates born at term in Australia is 3355 g (AIHW, 2021) while the average 40 weeks' gestation neonate in India is 2790 g (Marete et al., 2020).

These variables can be adjusted to calculate true growth potential, which can be represented as individually customised fetal growth curves and birthweight percentiles (see <https://www.perinatal.org.uk> hosted by the Perinatal Institute). This method for calculating growth potential was validated in seminal work by Gardosi (2006) and has been shown to be more effective in identifying small neonates at higher risk of morbidity and mortality than those identified by population centiles (Gardosi et al., 2018).

With epidemiological changes within populations, particularly with regard to maternal characteristics, periodic review of national growth charts has been advised (Gardosi et al., 2018). In Australia, the World Health Organization Childhood Growth Standards (WHO, 2006) remain the preferred standard used within most states and territories, and are recommended for use in New Zealand (Ministry of Health, 2020). Local and state guidelines frequently refer to the Fenton Growth Chart for Preterm Infants, WHO Growth Standards (Fenton & Kim, 2013) and Australian national birthweight percentiles by GA (Dobbin et al., 2012). Some Australian states suggest use of gestation calculators that are continually being updated for different populations and countries, depending on availability of databases from which coefficients can be derived (Gardosi et al., 2018).

EVIDENCE-BASED PRACTICE RESEARCH 6.1

Multi-ethnic growth standards

The International Fetal and Newborn Growth Consortium for the 21st Century (INTERGROWTH-21st) has published international anthropometric standards (weight, length and head circumference by GA and sex based on healthy fetal growth) to assess newborn size, designed for use in routine clinical practice (Villar et al., 2016). These standards are intended to complement the WHO child growth standards (WHO, 2006) and allow comparisons across multi-ethnic populations (Villar et al., 2014). These standards and comprehensive training tools were validated in further research using population samples from ten low- and middle-income countries (Kozuki et al., 2015) and have been used as reference guides in recent New Zealand reports for maternity clinical indicators (Ministry of Health, 2020). The availability of such standards that draw on comparisons across multi-ethnic populations has increasing relevance in contemporary Australian and New Zealand multicultural societies.

Survival rates

While the number of neonates born at <27 weeks' gestation admitted to neonatal units has not increased in recent years, survival rates to discharge continue to improve (Chow et al., 2020). Australian and New Zealand data report survival rates of approximately 70–89% for neonates born at 24–26 weeks of gestation, and greater than 94% for neonates over 27 weeks. Survival rates generally increase proportionally to completed weeks of gestation (Chow et al., 2020). Management and long-term developmental sequelae of these small neonates are resource intensive and present a challenge for neonatal care. Long-term follow-up of neonates following their discharge from the neonatal unit is addressed in Chapter 25.

The threshold of viability

Neonates born at the threshold of viability pose care challenges in terms of the neonate's physical and developmental care needs, family support and ethico-legal considerations. Where the threshold of viability lies is the subject of much debate, nationally and internationally (Smith, 2019), with variation among countries, and sometimes states or regions within the same country. Available data on survival rates and outcomes of extremely low GA neonates (22–25 weeks' gestation), who are additionally likely to be ELBW, also display wide variation by country (Smith, 2019). A systematic review by Guillén et al. (2015) looked at choices in management in the birth suite care of extremely low GA neonates. Of 47 highly developed countries (rated by the United Nations Development Programme's Human Development Index), 34 guidelines from 23 countries and four international groups were identified. Of those guidelines, 31 had specific management recommendations, 21 (68%) supported comfort care at 22 weeks' and 20 (65%) supported active care at 25 weeks' gestation. Between 23 and 24 weeks' gestation, greater variation was seen (Guillén et al., 2015). In Australia, there is no statutory or common law definition of viability or of when resuscitation should or should not be provided (Queensland Health, 2020). While GA is the most important determinant of viability, all decisions regarding the neonate's birth, active resuscitation and the decision to withdraw or withhold care require consideration of individual circumstances, likely prognosis and parental preferences (Lee & Lee, 2019; Queensland Health, 2020). Models of care and local facility data from various regional areas of Australia and New Zealand, including local hospital guidelines that may also consider the neonate's weight and respiratory effort at birth, will also contribute to these decisions. If an ELBW neonate is anticipated, a tour of the neonatal unit where parents will have the opportunity to speak with senior members of staff is optimal. These discussions should ideally include information about the gestation and presenting condition, unit-specific information, parental presence and family support options in the neonatal unit, feeding preferences and contact details of relevant staff. Ethical and legal issues that arise in neonatal units in the care of vulnerable neonates, and particularly those born ELBW and on the threshold of viability, will be explored in Chapter 23.

CLINICAL PRACTICE 6.1

Identify the standard used in your neonatal unit to identify neonates of extremely low birthweight who may also be SGA. Does your unit utilise criteria that are similar to these?

- preterm: <37 completed weeks' gestation
- late preterm: born between 34 weeks and $<36^{+6}$ weeks
- low birthweight: <2500 g at birth
- extremely low birthweight <1000 g at birth
- SGA: <10th percentile of birthweight for appropriate gestation at birth

REFLECTION

The following articles provide a historical perspective of the perceptions relating to neonatal birthweight that continue to influence contemporary practice:

Wilcox, A. J. (2001). On the importance – and the unimportance – of birthweight. *International Journal of Epidemiology, 30*(6), 1233–1241.

McCowan, L., Stewart, A. W., Francis, A., & Gardosi, J. (2004). A customised birthweight centile calculator developed for a New Zealand population. *Australian and New Zealand Journal of Obstetrics and Gynaecology, 44*, 428–431.

FACTORS CONTRIBUTING TO NEONATES BEING BORN AT LOW BIRTHWEIGHT

In addition to preterm birth and IUGR, key factors contributing to low birthweight, including ELBW neonates, include complications with the pregnancy (RCOG, 2019) and congenital anomalies. Poor maternal nutrition, insufficient weight gain throughout the pregnancy, incomplete or absent antenatal care, preeclampsia, essential hypertension, diabetes, renal disease, thrombophilia, autoimmune and connective tissue diseases and maternal substance use may also contribute to this population of vulnerable neonates (RCOG, 2019).

In Australia, approximately 1 in 16 neonates was born at a low birthweight (approximately 6%), with this proportion relatively unchanged in the period 2013–18 (AIHW, 2021). ELBW neonates (<1000 grams) contribute approximately 11% to the 60% of neonates born LBW who are admitted to Level III neonatal units in Australia and New Zealand each year (Chow et al., 2020). The proportion of LBW and ELBW is higher among neonates born female, twins or higher multiples, those with mothers who smoked during pregnancy, neonates of Aboriginal and Torres Strait Islander mothers, Māori and Pacific Islander mothers and neonates born in public hospitals (AIHW, 2021; Ministry of Health, 2020).

Placental disease (including that associated with preeclampsia) and smoking are common causes of poor fetal growth leading to SGA neonates. Appropriate management of women at increased risk of SGA (those with a past history of SGA, hypertension or obesity, and those who smoke) may reduce the risk (RCOG, 2019). Timely detection of poor fetal growth in those women with or without risk factors for SGA may also reduce the risk of stillbirth by presenting the opportunity for enhanced surveillance and early birth (RCOG, 2019).

Neonates who are born SGA are at an increased risk of morbidity and mortality, reduced growth during childhood, lower childhood neurodevelopmental scores, reduced educational attainment and increased lifetime risk of impaired glucose tolerance, including diabetes and cardiovascular disease (Ludvigsson et al., 2018). Risk of neonatal mortality is highest when a neonate is born both preterm and SGA (Sania et al., 2018); essentially, the lower the birthweight of the neonate, the greater is the risk of complications and mortality.

Critical factors in differentiating preterm LBW from more mature growth-restricted LBW neonates are accurate obstetrical history, neonatal physical assessment and examination of maturational age (Osuchukwu & Reed, 2021). Morbidity for **very low birthweight (VLBW)** neonates is associated with aetiology and severity of intrauterine growth restriction, while survival for ELBW is closely correlated with GA at birth (Brumbaugh et al., 2019). See Chapter 3 for more information about growth failure.

EVIDENCE-BASED PRACTICE RESEARCH 6.2

Recent research has highlighted the importance of the prenatal period as a gateway for maternal and neonatal health and has called for renewed focus on and action during this period. Increased access for women to high-quality prenatal care is required in order to provide greater opportunities for children to be born well (Bellizzi & Padrini, 2020). For low-birthweight neonates, and especially ELBW neonates, when early birth is inevitable, the key to optimising health outcomes and promoting neuroprotection is preparation for the birth through close interdisciplinary teamwork that takes into consideration the individual presenting needs of the neonate and family (e.g. administration of antenatal corticosteroids to reduce respiratory distress syndrome and intraventricular haemorrhage (IVH), administration of magnesium sulfate for neuroprotection, antibiotic treatment of maternal infection and consideration of caesarean section based on fetal indicators) (Kim et al., 2019; Queensland Health, 2020).

FAMILY-CENTRED CARE 6.1

Parents, who are frequently stressed and anxious following the often-unanticipated early birth and admission of their baby to a neonatal unit, require considerable support as they manage further uncertainty about short- and long-term outcomes for their ELBW preterm baby. Provision of parent information regarding both preterm birth and care of their baby after admission to the neonatal unit will assist in reducing high levels of anxiety and facilitate parental knowledge and understanding. Providing multiple opportunities to repeat key information, ask questions and check parental understanding is also very important, as parents are likely to be overwhelmed and less able to retain information during this stressful life event. Neonatal nurses/midwives have a key role in assessing and coordinating the need for referral to, and involvement of, multidisciplinary healthcare team members in the care of the family.

NEONATAL TRANSPORT DECISIONS

Very preterm and LBW neonates born outside of tertiary centres are at a higher risk of adverse outcomes than neonates born in tertiary facilities (Helenius et al., 2019). Regionalisation of perinatal care has been introduced in many parts of the world to improve outcomes as current evidence clearly demonstrates that skilled care and developmentally supportive environments provided in the first days and weeks of life have a significant impact on survival and long-term health outcomes for these vulnerable and often physiologically fragile neonates (Helenius et al., 2019).

Mothers make the best transport incubators. It is recommended that high-risk preterm neonates be transferred in utero where possible to a tertiary facility. However, often this is not feasible, and consideration should be given to transport of neonates <1750 g birthweight. Transport of VLBW and ELBW preterm neonates is associated with an increased incidence and severity of **intraventricular haemorrhage (IVH)** (Shipley et al., 2019). The decision to transport will be influenced by the expertise of the regional neonatal intensive care unit and the safety and availability of transportation. A detailed overview of neonatal nursing/midwifery considerations in the retrieval and transport of a neonate requiring the specialist services of a tertiary centre can be found in Chapter 7.

'SMALL BABY' PROTOCOLS

Survival without impairment remains the common goal of neonatal care. Survival rates for VLBW and ELBW neonates have improved, but many are discharged from hospital with significant challenges (Brumbaugh et al., 2019; Kaempf & Gautham, 2022). Extreme prematurity is not recognised as a cause of death or morbidity, but rather a cluster of conditions such as cardiorespiratory failure, brain injury, renal failure with non-oliguric hyperkalaemia and multi-organ failure (Morris et al., 2015). Over the past decade, significant advancements have been made in improving survival rates and neurodevelopmental outcomes for neonates through the establishment of 'small baby' protocols (Fathi et al., 2021; Kaempf & Gautham, 2022; Nationwide Children's Hospital, 2020).

A small baby protocol or small baby program is a standardised protocol comprised of evidence-based clinical guidelines and/or a series of practical algorithms for areas of clinical practice in the early care of extremely preterm neonates that are likely to be responsible for early mortality and increased morbidity in the ELBW preterm neonate – for example, ventilation and thermoregulation (Kaempf & Gautham, 2022; Nationwide Children's Hospital, 2020). Small baby protocols may vary across units; however, they usually include multiple aspects that address care provided in the: (1) birth suite (e.g. initial steps, thermoregulation; transport to the neonatal intensive care unit (NICU)), (2) admission and first days of life (e.g. cardiorespiratory stabilisation, thermoregulation, fluid and electrolyte balance, protection from brain injury) and (3) weeks after the neonate's birth (e.g. maintenance of skin integrity, developmental care).

A small baby protocol is usually developed through a process of consensus among all members of the professional healthcare team who care for ELBW neonates and families, in order to provide a uniform, interdisciplinary approach to family-centred care of these neonates. Evidence-based protocols are often accompanied by the level of evidence supporting the interventions that underpin the guidelines. It has been recognised that many practices utilised in the care of small preterm neonates have not been adequately studied and large variations are common across neonatal unit environments (Kaempf & Gautham, 2022).

Small baby protocols are designed to improve neonatal outcomes by standardising the approach to treatment, which ensures that key treatments are not overlooked and are implemented in a timely fashion and excludes practices with the potential for harm (Puchalski, 2011). Reducing variation in treatment minimises the risk of errors, reduces potentially noxious stimili and is reported to reduce costs by streamlining services and reducing length of hospital stay (Fathi et al., 2021). Concerns have been raised that protocols reduce nursing/midwifery and medicine to a 'cookbook' approach and minimise individualised care, with the risk of lowering the standard of care for an individual and increasing opportunities for litigation if a protocol is not followed (Puchalski, 2011). Historically, evidence-based protocols have moved more care to the obligation of skilled neonatal nurses/midwives, especially regarding infection control and safe oxygen use, with careful observation of oxygen saturation levels and follow-up care (Sola et al., 2008).

Clearly, the most effective protocols build in opportunities for customising care to address patient circumstances and identified special needs. The protocol's framework for interventions should be grounded in evidence, emphasise safe practice factors and communication and systematically build in measures for impact on mortality and morbidity. Application of these principles to the care of the VLBW or ELBW neonate acknowledges the unique vulnerabilities in this cohort and improves practices that specifically address and reduce the risks of morbidity and mortality (Fathi et al., 2021; Kaempf & Gautham, 2022).

Seven key areas that most impact the ELBW neonate during the first 14 days of life are outlined here and in Table 6.4. Further evidence-based information on these conditions can be found in related chapters to inform the care of this vulnerable population of neonates. These considerations and conditions are recommended for inclusion in a small baby protocol:

1. thermoregulation needs and skin care (Chapters 8 and 19)
2. neuroprotection and neurodevelopment (Chapters 13 and 22)
3. cardiorespiratory and haematological (Chapters 9, 10 and 11)
4. fluid and nutritional requirements (Chapter 5)
5. infection prevention (Chapter 16)
6. family integration and support (Chapter 21)
7. birth suite stabilisation and transport (Chapters 3 and 7).

TABLE 6.4 **A summary of conditions recommended for inclusion in a small baby protocol**

Condition/ consideration	Key principles
Skin care/thermoregulation	
Immature thermoregulatory mechanisms	Achieving and maintaining a neutral thermal environment is one of the key physiological challenges critical to the care and survival of neonates, more so for those born preterm
Lack of brown fat and adipose tissue	Brown adipose tissue (BAT), also known as brown fat, is required in the neonate as the metabolism of BAT generates heat. BAT, however, is not present before 25 weeks' gestation. It does not significantly increase until during the third trimester (Knobel, 2014). The lower the gestation at birth, the less brown adipose tissue, so neonates born at <32 weeks' gestation have inadequate stores of BAT to produce enough heat by non-shivering thermogenesis, increasing their risk of hypothermia (Symonds, 2013). Neonates born ELBW and <28 weeks are particularly at risk of hypothermia. Care provided to reduce risks of hypothermia during the first hour of birth has important long-term implications for an ELBW neonate
Skin immaturity	The junction between the epidermis and dermis is weaker in preterm and term skin causing layers of skin to separate from each other easily (Amer et al., 2021)
	Vernix protects the integrity of the developing skin from exposure in utero to amniotic fluid, and in the perinatal period plays an important role in skin hydration (Visscher & Narendran, 2014). While this substance is produced from 20 weeks' gestation, and is most visible from 33 to 34 weeks, it is not seen on the skin of preterm neonates
Dehydration from insensible water loss	Incubator humidification remains 'best practice' for improved growth and thermal stability and also decreases fluid and electrolyte imbalances (including transepidermal water loss (TEWL)) for neonates of <34 weeks' gestation
Neuroprotection/neurodevelopment	
Intraventricular haemorrhage (IVH)	IVH is caused by a haemorrhagic disorder affecting the germinal matrix of the brain (Bruschettini et al., 2016). This can lead to brain injury, cognitive delay, disability, hydrocephalus and death. The germinal matrix is present only in the preterm brain and is no longer present from 33 weeks' gestation. The incidence of IVH is inversely proportional to gestation, with most neonates born in Australia and New Zealand who experience severe IVH (grade 4) being born at <26 weeks' gestation and of ELBW (Chow et al., 2020)

TABLE 6.4 **A summary of conditions recommended for inclusion in a small baby protocol—cont'd**

Condition/ consideration	Key principles
Periventricular leucomalacia (PVL)	The most prevalent ischaemic brain injury in preterm neonates, it occurs in the border zone at the end of arterial vascular distributions. The ischaemia of periventricular leucomalacia occurs in the white matter adjacent to the lateral ventricles. The condition commonly leads to cerebral palsy
Neurodevelopmental considerations	Neonates born preterm face many potential risk factors that may contribute to abnormal brain development. For example, neonates admitted to a neonatal intensive care unit (NICU) and special care nursery (SCN) are more likely to have been resuscitated at birth and have a higher prevalence of seizures, severe respiratory disease requiring ventilator support, intraventricular haemorrhage, congenital anomalies and/or the need for surgical intervention (Jarjour, 2015)
	Physical closeness and emotional closeness are crucial to the physical, emotional and social wellbeing of both the parent and the neonate (Flacking et al., 2012). The ability to form bonds through cues is controlled by a complex physiological mechanism, developed during evolution, in order to maximise the species' chances of survival (Kommers et al., 2016). Preterm birth alters these cues and, therefore, bonding (Kommers et al., 2016). Preterm neonates' cues are often unrecognisable as, due to their physical immaturity, they are not capable of expressing their internal states in the way that term neonates can (Feldman et al., 2014)
Cardiorespiratory and haematological	
Depleted surfactant	Neonates born preterm during the late canalicular period of fetal development have immaturely structured airways and surfactant deficiency, as the type II alveolar cells are just beginning to develop (Rubarth & Quinn, 2015). This leads to a surfactant deficiency
Anaemia	Whereas physiological anaemia is considered a normal process in term neonates, anaemia of prematurity is a pathological anaemia occurring in preterm neonates (von Lindern & Lopriore, 2014). Preterm neonates (born at <1000 g) are likely to develop anaemia of prematurity because placental iron transport and fetal erythropoiesis are incomplete
Hyperbilirubinaemia	Hyperbilirubinaemia is more commonly present in preterm neonates, who have more-immature livers and often have higher amounts of haemoglobin. The most common jaundice is unconjugated jaundice as the immature liver has difficulty conjugating the volume of bilirubin; the risk of unconjugated jaundice is kernicterus
Apnoea of prematurity	Premature neonates are at risk of apnoea
Patent ductus arteriosus (PDA)	The ductus arteriosus is a structure in the fetal circulation that diverts the blood flow from the pulmonary artery to the aorta (a right-to-left shunt), bypassing the lungs. In the preterm neonate after birth the ductal flow is generally left to right from the aorta to the pulmonary arteries, leading to increased blood flow to the lungs and decreased blood flow in the systemic circulation; the majority of ELBW will have a PDA at some point in their clinical course (Philip et al., 2019)
Fluid/nutritional	
Maintaining optimal growth	The essential fatty acids (FAs) arachidonic acid (ARA) and docosahexaenoic acid (DHA) are deficient in extremely preterm newborns in current dietary treatment (DHA). ARA and DHA supplementation may help to promote brain development and prevent inflammation-related disorders. If ARA and DHA supplementation reduces the frequency of serious newborn morbidities, it will have a significant influence on future premature infants (Wendel et al., 2021)
Meeting caloric needs	To meet the preterm neonates' minimal energy requirements 50–60 kcal/kg/d are needed. To achieve growth (i.e. maximal protein accretion) a higher calorie intake is needed; in the neonate fed parenterally 90–100 kcal/kg/d are required (Bolisetty et al., 2014)
Milk fortifiers	Human milk (HM) is the best source of nutrition for both term and preterm newborns, providing short- and long-term health benefits. When fed at the recommended feeding quantities, unfortified HM does not offer enough nourishment to VLBW infants. To meet the high requirements of this group of preterm newborns, human milk should be supplemented (fortified) with nutrients in short supply, particularly protein, calcium and phosphate (Arslanoglu et al., 2019)
Infection prevention	
Infection	Infection is a major contributor to mortality and morbidity in the ELBW neonate. Neonatal sepsis is more commonly experienced in neonates born of lower gestational age. Of neonates admitted to New Zealand and Australian level III neonatal units diagnosed with sepsis, 46.3% were born at <28 weeks, while 69.9% were born at <32 weeks' gestation (Chow et al., 2020). The most common causes of infection are group B streptococcus (GBS), *Escherichia coli* (*E. coli*), *Staphylococcus aureus* (*S. aureus*) and *Candida albicans*, with GBS and *E. coli* being causes of early-onset infection. Late-onset infections are most commonly (but not always) caused by nosocomial infections such as coagulase-negative *Staphylococcus*, *S. aureus* and *C. albicans*

Continued

TABLE 6.4 **A summary of conditions recommended for inclusion in a small baby protocol—cont'd**

Condition/ consideration	Key principles
Necrotising enterocolitis (NEC)	NEC is an inflammation caused by bacteria, viruses and normal gut flora of the gastrointestinal tract (Alsaied et al., 2020). Up to 90% of those diagnosed with NEC are born preterm (Shah & Sinn, 2012). In 2018, of ANZNN registrants, 1.6% of neonates were confirmed with NEC, with 54.9% of these neonates being born at <28 weeks' gestation and of VLBW or ELBW (Chow et al., 2020). This disease continues to be the foremost cause of preterm neonatal morbidity and mortality (Alsaied et al., 2020). There is a strong association between neonates who receive only human milk and reduction in NEC: 90% of neonates who develop NEC have been fed, and more neonates fed formula develop NEC than neonates who are fed breast milk (de la Cruz & Bazacliu, 2018)
Family integration and support	
Promotion of parent/ neonate attachment	Preterm neonates often spend weeks, even months, in hospital, which makes them particularly vulnerable to the effects of separation from their parents. Research suggests families with neonates in the neonatal unit are at greater risk for disturbances in the development of maternal newborn attachment (Flacking et al., 2012)
	Parents often struggle with the highly technical, busy, overcrowded and noisy neonatal unit environment (Venkataraman et al., 2018)
	In the NICU, maternal distress manifests as a mix of depression, anxiety, trauma and posttraumatic stress symptoms. The symptoms appear on a range and manifest themselves differently in each woman. A NICU stay and a perceived disruption in the transition to parenthood are both antecedents to maternal distress. Issues with forming a good mother–infant relationship, unfavourable newborn development and decreased maternal quality of life are all consequences of maternal distress in the NICU (Staver et al., 2019)
Birth suite/golden hour and transport	
Transport	Wherever possible, in utero transfer of the ELBW neonate should be facilitated for birthing in tertiary units. This early intervention improves survival rates in comparison with those who are born outside of tertiary centres (Boland et al., 2016)
Resuscitation	For preterm neonates, the Australian and New Zealand Committee on Resuscitation (ANZCOR) recommends commencing resuscitation using either room air or blended air and oxygen up to an oxygen concentration of 30% (ANZCOR, 2021)
	Preterm neonates – in particular ELBW neonates – are far more likely to require resuscitation at birth (ANZCOR, 2021)
Golden hour protocol (GHP)	ELBW and VLBW neonates are vulnerable to their environment during the first hour after birth. The use of a GHP provides an organised approach to admission procedures and care. By using a checklist and recording intervention times, care givers become more aware of time management for each intervention and potentially decrease time to initiation of interventions such as intravenous fluids and antibiotics (see Clinical Practice 6.3 for more information)

CLINICAL PRACTICE 6.2

Identify and discuss the rationale/s supporting nursing and midwifery strategies to minimise the risk of IVH in an ELBW neonate.

Which behaviours might you identify while caring for a neonate in the neonatal unit who has recently been diagnosed with grade IV IVH and how would you respond to these behaviours?

FAMILY-CENTRED CARE 6.2

Integration of the family into the care of their baby from admission is integral to supporting optimal short- and long-term outcomes for the ELBW neonate and their family. Increasing parent involvement and understanding of their baby's needs through family-centred small baby protocols and pathways facilitates parents' understanding of their baby's progress and physiological maturation. Family-centred care models support and empower parents to develop confidence and self-efficacy in caring for their baby and do not assume parents wish to take on quasi-professional roles, particularly when caring for ELBW neonates who require high levels of technical support. This is achieved through open communication and negotiation with individual families. Evaluations of family-centred neonatal discharge planning, which commences from admission to the neonatal unit, have demonstrated notable positive outcomes including parent satisfaction and a significant reduction in emergency department visits and healthcare usage post discharge (Balasundaram et al., 2021; Gupta et al., 2019).

Effective implementation of a small baby protocol requires multidisciplinary consensus while developing the protocol, education of all members of the healthcare team involved in the care of small neonates and monitoring of compliance and effectiveness of the protocol with respect to key neonatal health outcomes.

EVIDENCE-BASED PRACTICE RESEARCH 6.3

Results from evaluations of small baby protocols comprising integrated evidence-based guidelines, before and after implementation, have been promising (Fathi et al., 2021). A unique program called the small baby unit has been established to care for EBLW neonates born at <28 weeks and weighing <1000 grams. Neonatal health outcomes and resource utilisation were compared before and after the implementation of the standardised approach of evidence-based guidelines and a checklist was provided by a core multidisciplinary team that participated in ongoing educational and process improvement collaboration. Results demonstrated reduced proportions of neonates with chronic lung disease, and significantly reduced hospital-acquired infection rates, neonatal growth restriction at discharge and resource utilisation (Morris et al., 2015). More-recent studies have demonstrated improved survival, reduced incidence of short-term morbidities and improved neurodevelopmental outcomes for extremely premature babies (Fathi et al., 2021).

CASE STUDY 6.1

You are caring for an 11-week-old female neonate, Taylor, in the neonatal unit. Taylor was born at 25 weeks and 2 days' gestation with a birthweight of 760 grams. Taylor's discharge from hospital is planned to take place in approximately 1 week.

1. What is Taylor's corrected age today? Taylor's parents are looking forward to discharge and have asked if there is anything they can do to monitor or prevent apnoea episodes from occurring at home.
2. As the neonatal nurse/midwife caring for Taylor, which elements of the 'family-centred care' philosophy would you utilise to respond to these parental concerns?
3. What safe-sleeping parent education should Taylor's parents have received during her admission to the neonatal unit? How has Taylor's sleep position changed as she has developed and become independent of respiratory support?

CASE STUDY 6.2

You are caring for Emily, a female neonate who was born at 23 weeks' gestation. Emily is now a corrected age of 28 weeks' gestation and is receiving **continuous positive airways pressure (CPAP)** with 25% oxygen. Emily's parents have asked if they can be more involved in her care and, as they have observed nurses and midwives undertaking CPAP care, they would like to be taught how to change the CPAP prongs and be involved in the airway suctioning of their baby.

1. How would you respond to their request?

PREPARATION FOR ADMISSION OF THE ELBW NEONATE

Ideally, neonates are admitted to the neonatal unit from the birth suite, but many neonates require transfer by a retrieval team. Preparation for a neonate admitted by retrieval is the same as for a neonate who is admitted from the birth suite. However, a retrieved neonate has been inundated with a series of stressors that may lead to the neonate being unstable on admission and remaining so over the next several days.

The personnel involved in the admission should have the 'core' skills (Gurung et al., 2019) and experience to facilitate a smooth transition for the neonate to postnatal life. Some Australian and New Zealand neonatal units have developed guidelines that define requirements for skill sets and/or experience levels in staff members who are required to attend the resuscitations of and support preterm and LBW neonates to assist this critical transition to promote optimal outcomes and reduce long-term sequelae. Please refer to your local hospital guidelines if this applies to your clinical setting. Quality improvement initiatives, such as the development of a small baby unit (Fathi et al., 2021) or 'drills' and simulation activities for maintaining neonatal resuscitation skills (Gurung et al., 2019), are examples of the interventions that can lead to improved neurodevelopmental outcomes for the ELBW neonate.

Most neonatal units will have a protocol or guidelines for the care of these neonates that will set out the expectations of the team. The equipment needs to be prepared for a rapid and easy admission: incubators with humidification for neonates of <29 weeks' gestation, monitoring equipment and respiratory support. Respiratory support is likely to be unit specific as some units will provide CPAP from birth and others ventilation. It is good practice to prepare for the insertion of the umbilical or central lines and set up the initial infusion fluids.

Admission procedures should aim to be completed swiftly and competently: resuscitation, thermoregulation, antibiotic administration (especially to those neonates whose mothers have features of chorioamnionitis or a history of GBS), timely parenteral nutrition administration and ensuring euglycaemia. Fig. 6.2 demonstrates stabilisation prior to admission of the ELBW neonate.

CLINICAL PRACTICE 6.3

The golden hour protocol for the ELBW neonate

Extremely preterm newborns are at risk of developing hypothermia and hypoglycaemia quickly after their birth. A multidisciplinary team established a program standardising evidence-based care practices during the first hour after birth to lower local rates of these morbidities.

The **golden hour protocol (GHP)** was established for all inborn newborns of 27 weeks' gestation using quality

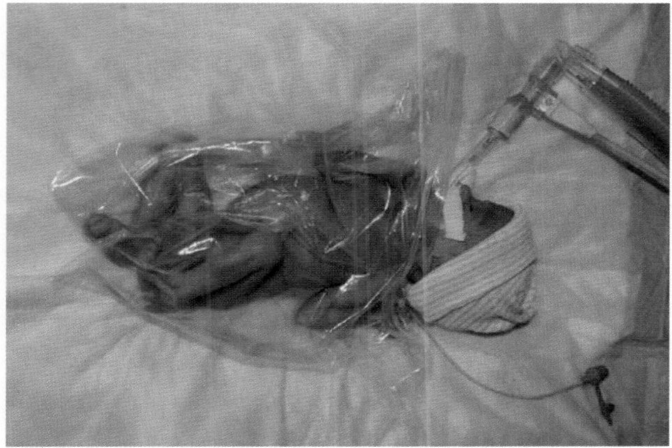

FIGURE 6.2 **Stabilisation of the ELBW neonate**
Source: Cheryl Briggs.

improvement techniques. Data were collected during three phases from 2012 to 2017: pre-protocol (n = 80), phase I (n = 42) and phase II (n = 92).

There were no notable changes in the characteristics of the infants. There were improvements in hypothermia (59% vs 26% vs 38%; p = 0.001), hypoglycaemia (18% vs 7% vs 4%; p = 0.012) and minutes to complete stabilisation (median (Q1, Q3) 110 (89,138) vs 111 (94,135) vs 92 (74,129; p = 0.0035).

The GHP, which is evidence based, is a successful intervention for lowering hypothermia and hypoglycaemia in severely preterm newborns (Croop et al., 2020).

The 'golden hour' is a term derived from adult trauma, emphasising the notion that the first hour of care is critical to optimal outcomes. In newborn care, what happens in the first hour of life for all neonates as they transition from their in-utero environment can lead to short- and long-term consequences, affecting neurodevelopmental outcomes and mortality. Narendran and Hoath (1999) first applied the term to neonates in 1999. A standardised interdisciplinary approach or 'principles' for the care of compromised neonates in the first hour of life can lead to more-efficient care delivery and contribute to improved outcomes (Qu et al., 2020). These improved outcomes include (Arora et al., 2020):

- a significant increase in admission temperature
- a decrease in the incidence of retinopathy of prematurity and chronic lung disease
- significant improvement in time to surfactant administration and time to administration of dextrose and amino acids to prevent hypoglycaemia
- significant decrease in time to start intravenous fluids and antibiotics with intravenous/intra-arterial lines being placed faster
- a decrease in the incidence of IVH
- significant reduction in culture proven sepsis
- significant reduction in mechanical ventilation days without affecting mortality or other comorbidities.

Despite the relatively small number of neonatal intensive care units (NICUs) within Australia and New Zealand, little is known about the consistency of practice in the first hour of life for a compromised neonate, or whether neonatal units within Australia and New Zealand have a protocol for the first hour of life to guide practice and contribute to the best possible outcomes.

Does your unit have a policy or guideline based on a GHP?

FAMILY-CENTRED CARE 6.3

Family partnership and support

The birth of an ELBW neonate is associated with profound stress to the family dynamic. Parents and families will often experience a range of emotions as their neonate progresses through the various levels of the neonatal unit. Parents and the family unit may also experience all five stages of grief, from denial through to acceptance.

The birth of an ELBW neonate can place strain on parental relationships and great care must be taken by care givers to be considerate of the myriad of emotions experienced by parents while care is provided to their baby. As care givers, neonatal nurses/midwives should be prepared to provide additional support to the family, which may include:

- providing realistic information/preparation for seeing their ELBW neonate
- consideration of cultural needs of the parents and family members
- conveying information in a manner that supports understanding
- care of siblings/extended family within the newborn care unit environment
- inclusion of parents in all aspects of decision making
- providing education about neonatal behavioural cues (see Chapter 21 for more information)
- inclusion of parents in care provision where possible. Negotiation of care is also important and scheduling care – such as bathing and nappy changes – around parental visits
- providing skin-to-skin time for the parents and their neonate (Fig. 6.3)
- discussion of quality-of-life issues where appropriate.

Refer to Chapter 21 for more information about facilitating family-centred care in the neonatal unit.

EVIDENCE-BASED PRACTICE RESEARCH 6.4

A Cochrane review comprising a meta-analysis of 24 eligible randomised and quasi-randomised controlled trials (AlFaleh & Anabrees, 2014) concluded that enteral probiotic supplementation prevents severe **necrotising enterocolitis (NEC)** and all-cause mortality in VLBW preterm neonates, whereas data relating to potential benefits and adverse effects for the ELBW population were insufficient to make recommendations. A further meta-analysis of 37 eligible

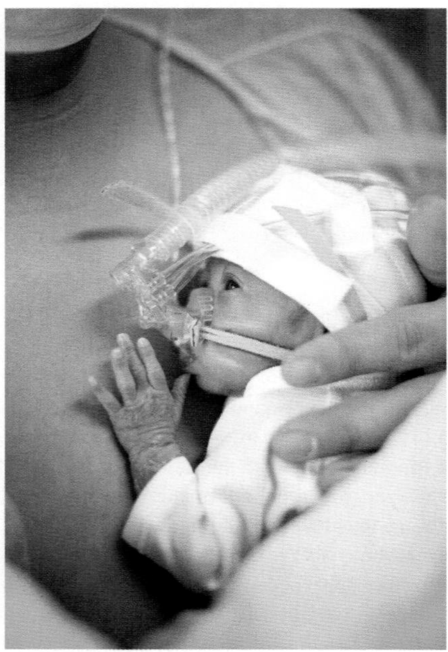

FIGURE 6.3 **Skin-to-skin contact of an ELBW neonate with their mother**

Source: Alamy/Phanie/Alamy Stock Photo.

randomised controlled trials by Rao and colleagues published in 2016, which excluded studies with a high risk of bias, confirmed the benefits of probiotic use in significantly reducing late-onset sepsis (LOS) in preterm neonates 1500 grams. Subgroup analysis of extremely preterm neonates (born at <28 weeks' gestation or <1000 g) revealed no significant benefits of probiotic supplementation in reducing LOS, but the sample size was small (Rao et al., 2016). In 2021 the American Academy of Pediatrics Committee on Fetus and Newborn, which provides clinical care guidance to physicians, advised that, although recent studies support probiotic use to reduce risk of NEC and late-onset infection, these studies have used multiple different probiotic formulations and diverse preterm populations (Poindexter et al., 2021). Most of these trials have not demonstrated a reduction in NEC in infants at highest risk for this disease: those <1000 grams. The authors concluded that current evidence does not support routine, universal administration of probiotics to preterm infants particularly those <1000 grams. Recommendations relating to monitoring outcomes, adverse events and safety were made for centres choosing to administer probiotics (Poindexter et al., 2021). Further studies are required to develop specific recommendations for this vulnerable population.

CONCLUSION

While many neonates will survive neonatal unit admission, some of them will have impairments, which may be physical, behavioural and/or intellectual, that may have a lifelong impact. As discussed in this chapter, this cohort is at increased risk for cerebral palsy, developmental delay, visual problems (including blindness), hearing impairment, chronic lung disease and sudden unexpected death in infancy (see Chapter 2).

The cost of being born at ELBW is both economic and personal. Care of families is particularly important as the clinical trajectory of these neonates can be prolonged and extend far beyond the neonatal unit with the need for continuing healthcare, education, social services and other societal resources.

The long-term follow-up of this cohort of neonates is imperative, and further information about this aspect can be found in Chapter 25.

Online Resources

Australian College of Neonatal Nurses (ACNN). (2019). *Australian standards for neonatal nurses* (4th ed.). <https://www.acnn.org.au/resources/resources/ACNN-Standards-for-Practice-4th-Ed.pdf>.

National Institute for Health and Care Excellence (NICE). (2019). Preterm labour and birth. <https://www.nice.org.uk/guidance/ng25>.

Queensland Health. (2016). Guideline supplement: Term small for gestational age (SGA) infant. <www.health.qld.gov.au/__data/assets/pdf_file/0015/140163/s-sga.pdf>.

Royal Prince Alfred Hospital, New South Wales, Australia. Small baby guideline: management of infants <27 weeks gestation. <www.slhd.nsw.gov.au/rpa/neonatal/html/newprot/small_baby.html>.

World Health Organization. (2015). WHO recommendations on interventions to improve preterm birth outcomes. <http://apps.who.int/iris/bitstream/handle/10665/183037/9789241508988_eng.pdf;jsessionid=06DADA3191DE2A70A598EA4360D6B5F1?sequence=1>.

References/Acknowledgements

AlFaleh, K., & Anabrees, J. (2014). Probiotics for prevention of necrotizing enterocolitis in preterm infants. *Cochrane Database of Systematic Reviews, 4*, CD005496. doi: 10.1002/14651858.CD005496.pub4doi: 10.1002/14651858.CD005496.pub4.

Alsaied, A., Islam, N., & Thalib, L. (2020). Global incidence of necrotizing enterocolitis: a systematic review and meta-analysis. *BMC Pediatrics, 20*(1), 1–15.

Amer, Y., Bridges, C., & Marathe, K. (2021). Epidemiology, pathophysiology, and management strategies of neonatal wound care. *Neoreviews, 22*(7), e452. doi: 10.1542/neo.22-7-e45.

Anil, K. C., Lal Basel, P., Singh, S. (2020). Low birth weight and its associated risk factors: health facility-based case–control study. *PLoS One, 15*(6), e0234907. doi: 10.1371/journal.pone.0234907.

Arora, S., Yada, P., Bajaj, H., Thakur, A. S., Mittal, M., Gupta, M. R., et al. (2020). Improving clinical outcomes of very low birth weight infants: implementation of standardized management guidelines in tertiary care hospital in Haryana. *International Journal of Pediatric Adolescent Medicine, 7*(4), 174–180. doi: 10.1016/j.ijpam.2019.08.002.

Arslanoglu, S., Boquien, C., King, C., Lamireau, D., Tonetto, P., Barnett, D., et al. (2019). Fortification of human milk for preterm infants: update and recommendations of the European Milk Bank Association (EMBA) working group on human milk fortification. *Frontiers in Pediatrics, 7*, 76. doi: 10.3389/fped.2019.00076.

Australian and New Zealand Committee on Resuscitation (ANZCOR). (2021). *Guideline 13. Neonatal resuscitation*. <https://www.nzrc.org.nz/guidelines/#Section-13-Guidelines>, <https://resus.org.au/guidelines/anzcor-guidelines/> (Accessed 18 February 2022).

Australian Institute of Health and Welfare (AIHW). (2021). *Australia's mothers and babies*. <https://www.aihw.gov.au/reports/mothers-babies/australias-mothers-babies/contents/summary> (Accessed 18 February 2022).

Balasundaram, M., Porter, M., Miller, S., Sivakumar, D., Fleming, A., & McCallie, K. (2021). Increasing parent satisfaction with discharge planning: an improvement project using technology in a Level 3 NICU. *Advances in Neonatal Care*, Feb 4. doi: 10.1097/ANC.0000000000000841. [Online ahead of print]

Bellizzi, S., & Padrini, S. (2020). Quality utilization of antenatal care and low birth weight: evidence from 18 demographic health surveys. *East Mediterranean Health Journal, 26*(11), 1381–1387. doi: 10.26719/emhj.20.055.

Boland, R. A., Davis, P. G., Dawson, J. A., & Doyle, L. W. (2016). Outcomes of infants born at 22–27 weeks' gestation in Victoria according to outborn/inborn status. *Archives of Disease in Childhood. Fetal and Neonatal Edition, 102*, F153–F160. doi: 10.1136/archdischild-2015-310313.

Bolisetty, S., Osborn, D., Sinn, J., & Lui, K.; Australasian Neonatal Parenteral Nutrition Consensus Group. (2014). Standardised neonatal parenteral nutrition formulations: an Australasian group consensus 2012. *BMC Pediatrics, 14*, 48.

Brumbaugh, J. E., Hansen, N. L., Bell, E. F., Sridhar, A., Carol, W. A., Hintz, S. R., et al. (2019). Outcomes of extremely preterm infants with birth weight less than 400 grams. *JAMA Pediatrics, 173*(5), 434–445. doi: 10.1001/jamapediatrics.2019.0180.

Bruschettini, M., Romantsik, O., Zappettini, S., Banzi, R., Ramenghi, L. A., & Calevo, M. G. (2016). Heparin for the prevention of intraventricular haemorrhage in preterm infants. *Cochrane Database of Systematic Reviews, 5*, CD011718. doi: 10.1002/14651858.CD011718.pub2.

Chow, S. S. W., Creighton, P., Chambers, G. M., & Lui, K. (2020). *Report of the Australian and New Zealand Neonatal Network 2018*. Sydney: ANZNN.

Croop, S., Thoyre, S. M., Aliaga, S., McCaffrey, M. J., & Peter-Wohl, S. (2020). The Golden Hour: a quality improvement initiative for extremely premature infants in the neonatal intensive care unit. *Journal of Perinatology, 40*(3), 530–539. doi: 10.1038/s41372-019-0545-0.

de la Cruz, D., & Bazacliu, C. (2018). Enteral feeding composition and necrotizing enterocolitis. *Seminars in Fetal and Neonatal Medicine, 23*(6), 406–410. doi: 10.1016/j.siny.2018.08.003.

Dobbin, T. A., Sullivan, E. A., Roberts, C. L., & Simpson, J. M. (2012). Australian national birthweight percentiles by sex and gestational age, 1998–2008. *Medical Journal of Australia, 197*(5), 291–294. doi: 10.5694/mja11.11331.

Fathi, O., Nelin, L. D., Shepherd, E. G., & Reber, K. M. (2021). Development of a small baby unit to improve outcomes for the extremely premature infant. *Journal of Perinatology, 42*(2), 157–164. doi: 10.1038/s41372-021-00984-0.

Feldman, R., Rosenthal, Z., & Eidelman, A. I. (2014). Maternal–preterm skin-to-skin contact enhances child physiologic organization and cognitive control across the first 10 years of life. *Biology of Psychiatry, 75*(1), 56–64.

Fenton, T. R., & Kim, J. H. (2013). A systematic review and meta-analysis to revise the Fenton growth chart for preterm infants. *BMC Pediatrics, 13*, 1–13. doi: 10.1186/1471-2431-13-59.

Flacking, R., Lehtonen, L., Thomson, G., Axelin, A., Ahlqvist, S., Moran, V. H., et al. (2012). Closeness and separation in neonatal intensive care. *Acta Paediatrica, 101*(10), 1032–1037. doi: 10.1111/j.1651-2227.2012.02787.x.02787.

Gardosi, J. (2006). New definition of small for gestational age based on fetal growth potential. *Hormone Research, 65*(suppl 3), 15–18. doi: 10.1159/000091501.

Gardosi, J., Francis, A., Turner, S., & Williams, M. (2018). Customized growth charts: rationale, validation, and clinical benefits. *American Journal of Obstetrics and Gynaecology, 218*(2S), S609–S618. doi: 10.1016/j.ajog.2017.12.011.

Guillén, U., Weiss, E. M., Munson, D., Maton, P., Jefferies, A., Norman, M., et al. (2015). Guidelines for the management of extremely premature deliveries: a systematic review. *Pediatrics, 136*(2), 343–350. doi: 10.1542/peds.2015-0542.

Gupta, M., DeWayne, M. P., & Smith, V. C. (2019). Preparing for discharge from the neonatal intensive care unit. *Pediatrics, 143*(6), e20182915. doi: 10.1542/peds.2018-2915.

Gurung, R., Gurung, A., Sunny, A. K., Basnet, O., Shreshtha, S. K., Gomo, O. H., et al. (2019). Effect of skill drills on neonatal ventilation performance in a simulated setting-observation study in Nepal. *BMC Pediatrics, 19*, 387. doi: 10.1186/s12887-019-1723-0.

Helenius, K., Longford, N., Lehtonen, L., Modi, N., & Gale, C. (2019). Association of early postnatal transfer and birth outside a tertiary hospital with mortality and severe brain injury in extremely preterm infants: observational cohort study with propensity score matching. *British Medical Journal, 367*, l5678. doi: 10.1136/bmj.l5678.

Jarjour, I. T. (2015). Neurodevelopmental outcome after extreme prematurity: a review of the literature. *Pediatric*

Neurology, 52, 143–152. doi: 10.1016/j.pediatrneurol.2014.10.027.

Kaempf, J. W., & Gautham, K. (2022). Do small baby units improve extremely premature infant outcomes? *Journal of Perinatology, 42*(2), 281–285. doi: 10.1038/s41372-021-01076-9.

Kim, J. K., Chang, Y. S., Sung, S., & Park, W. S. (2019). Mortality rate-dependent variations in the survival without major morbidities rate of extremely preterm infants. *Scientific Reports, 9*(1), 7371. doi: 10.1038/s41598-019-43879-z.

Knobel, R. B. (2014). Fetal and neonatal thermal physiology. *Newborn and Infant Nursing Reviews, 14*(2), 45–49.

Kommers, D., Oei, G., Chen, W., Feijs, L., & Bambang Oetomo, S. (2016). Suboptimal bonding impairs hormonal, epigenetic, and neuronal development in preterm infants, but these impairments can be reversed. *Acta Paediatrica, 105*, 738–751.

Kozuki, N., Katz, J., Christian, P., Lee, A. C., Liu, L., Silveira, M. F., et al.; Child Health Epidemiology Reference Group Preterm Birth–SGA Working Group. (2015). Comparison of US birth weight references and the International Fetal and Newborn Growth Consortium for the 21st Century standard. *JAMA Pediatrics, 169*(7), e151438. doi: 10.1001/jamapediatrics.2015.1438.

Lee, J., & Lee, J. H. (2019). A clinical scoring system to predict the need for extensive resuscitation at birth in very low birth weight infants. *BMC Pediatrics, 19*, 197. doi: 10.1186/s12887-019-1573-9.

Ludvigsson, J. F., Lu, D., Hammarström, L., Cnattingius, S., & Fang, F. (2018). Small for gestational age and risk of childhood mortality: a Swedish population study. *PLoS Medicine, 15*(12), e1002717. doi: 10.1371/journal.pmed.1002717.

Marete, I., Ekhaguere, O., Bann, C. M., Bucher, S. L., Nyongesa, P., Patel, A. B., et al. (2020). Regional trends in birth weight in low- and middle-income countries 2013–2018. *Reproductive Health, 17*(suppl 3), 176. doi: 10.1186/s12978-020-01026-2.

Ministry of Health. (2020). *New Zealand maternity clinical indicators 2018*. Wellington, NZ: Ministry of Health. <https://www.health.govt.nz/publication/new-zealand-maternity-clinical-indicators-2018> (Accessed 18 February 2022).

Morris, M., Cleary, J. P., & Soliman, A. (2015). Small baby unit improves quality and outcomes in extremely low birth weight infants. *Pediatrics, 136*, e1007. doi: 10.1542/peds.2014-3918.

Narendran, V., & Hoath, S. B. (1999). Thermal management of the low birth weight infant: a cornerstone of neonatology. *Journal of Pediatrics, 134*(5), 529–531. doi: 10.1016/S0022-3476(99)70232-5.

Nationwide Children's Hospital. (2020). Small Baby Program – Nationwide Children's Hospital, Columbus, Ohio. <http://www.nationwidechildrens.org/small-baby-guidelines> (Accessed 18 February 2022).

Osuchukwu, O. O., & Reed D. J. (2021). Small for gestational age. In: *StatPearls*. Treasure Island, FL: StatPearls Publishing. <https://www.ncbi.nlm.nih.gov/books/NBK563247/> (Accessed 18 February 2022).

Park, H. W., Park, S. Y., & Kim, E. A. (2021). Prediction in in-hospital mortality after 24 hours in very low birth weight infants. *Pediatrics, 147*(1), 1–9. doi: 10.1542/peds.2020-004812.

Patton, D., Costich, J. F., & Lidströmer, N. (2017). Paid parental leave policies and infant mortality rates in OECD countries: policy implications for the United States. *World Medical and Health Policy, 9*(1), 6–23. doi: 10.1002/wmh3.214.

Philip, R., Towbin, J. A., Sathanandam, S., Goldberg, J., Yohannan, T., Swaminathan, N., et al. (2019). Effect of patent ductus arteriosus on the heart in preterm infants. *Congenital Heart Disease, 14*(1), 33–36.

Poindexter, B., & Committee on Fetus and Newborn. (2021). Use of probiotics in preterm infants. *Pediatrics, 147*(6), e2021051485. doi: 10.1542/peds.2021-051485.

Puchalski, M. L. (2011). Protocol vs individual care: what's best for VLBW infants? *Medscape*. <https://www.medscape.com/viewarticle/755574> (Accessed 18 February 2022).

Qu, W., Yue, Q., Wang, Y., Yang, J. L., Jin, X., Huang, X., et al. (2020). Assessing the changes in childbirth care practices and neonatal outcomes in Western China: pre-comparison and post-comparison study on early essential newborn care interventions. *BMJ Open, 10*, e041829. doi: 10.1136/bmjopen-2020-041829.

Queensland Health. (2020). *Queensland clinical guidelines. Perinatal care of the extremely preterm baby*. Guideline No. MN20.32-V2-R25. <http://www.health.qld.gov.au/qcg> (Accessed 18 February 2022).

Rao, S. C., Athalye-Jape, G. K., Deshpande, G. C., Simmer, K. N., & Patole, S. K. (2016). Probiotic supplementation and late-onset sepsis in preterm infants: a meta-analysis. *Pediatrics, 137*(3), e20153684.

Royal College of Obstetricians and Gynaecologists (RCOG). (2013, updated 2019). *The investigation and management of the small-for-gestational-age fetus* (2nd ed.). London: RCOG. <https://www.rcog.org.uk/globalassets/documents/guidelines/gtg_31.pdf> (Accessed 18 February 2022).

Rubarth, L. B., & Quinn, J. (2015). Respiratory development and respiratory distress syndrome. *Neonatal Network, 34*(4), 231.

Sania, A., Smith, E. R., Manji, K., Duggan, C., Masanja, H., Kisenge, R., et al. (2018). Neonatal and infant mortality risk associated with preterm and small for gestational age births in Tanzania: individual level pooled analysis using the intergrowth standard. *Journal of Pediatrics, 192*, 66–72.e4. doi: 10.1016/j.jpeds.2017.09.007.

Schneider, E. B. (2017). Fetal health stagnation: have health conditions in utero improved in the United States and Western and Northern Europe over the past 150 years? *Social Science and Medicine, 179*, 18–26. doi: 10.1016/j.socscimeddoi: 10.1016/j.socscimed.2017.02.018.

Shah, D., & Sinn, J. K. H. (2012). Antibiotic regimens for the empirical treatment of newborn infants with necrotising enterocolitis. *Cochrane Database of Systematic Reviews, 8*, CD007448. doi: 10.1002/14651858.CD007448.pub2doi: 10.1002/14651858.CD007448.pub2.

Shipley, L., Gyorkos, T., Dorling, J., Tata, L. J., Szatkowski, L., & Sharkey, D. (2019). Risk of severe intraventricular haemorrhage in the first week of life in preterm infants transported before 72 hours of age. *Pediatric Critical Care Medicine, 20*(7), 638–644. doi: 10.1097/PCC.0000000000001937.

Smith, L. (2019). Comparing international survival rates of extremely preterm infants: the impact of variation in reporting signs of life. *Infant, 15*(2), 62–64.

Sola, A., Saldeño, Y., & Favareto, V. (2008). Clinical practices in neonatal oxygenation: where have we failed? What can we do? *Journal of Perinatology, 28*(suppl 1), S28–S34.

Stark, A. R., & Eichenwald, E. C. (2021). Bronchopulmonary dysplasia: prevention. In: R. Martin, G. Redding, & M. S. Kim (Eds.). *UpToDate*. Walters Kluwer. <https://www.uptodate.com/contents/bronchopulmonary-dysplasia-prevention#!> (Accessed 18 February 2022).

Staver, M. A., Moore, T. A., & Hanna, K. M. (2019). Maternal distress in the neonatal intensive care unit: a concept analysis. *Advances in Neonatal Care, 19*(5), 394–401.

Symonds, M. E. (2013). Brown adipose tissue growth and development. *Scientifica, 13*, 1–14.

Venkataraman, R., Kamaluddeen, M., Amin, H., & Lodha, A. (2018). Is less noise, light and parental/caregiver stress in the neonatal intensive care unit better for neonates? *Indian Pediatrics, 55*(1), 17–21.

Villar, J., Ismail, L. C., Victora, C. G., Ohuma, E. O., Bertino, E., Altman, D. G., et al. (2014). International standards for newborn weight, length, and head circumference by gestational age and sex: the Newborn Cross-Sectional Study of the INTERGROWTH-21st Project. *Lancet, 384*(9946), 857–868. doi: 10.1016/S0140-6736(14)60932-6.

Villar, J., Giuliani, F., Fenton, T., Ohuma, E., Cheikh Ismail, L., & Kennedy, S. (2016). INTERGROWTH-21st very preterm size at birth reference charts. *Lancet, 387*(10021), 844–845. doi: 10.1016/S0140-6736(16)00384-6.

Visscher, M., & Narendran, V. (2014). Vernix caseosa: formation and functions. *Newborn and Infant Nursing Reviews, 14*(4), 142–146.

von Lindern, J., & Lopriore, E. (2014). Management and prevention of neonatal anaemia: current evidence and guidelines. *Expert Review of Hematology, 7*(2), 195–202.

Wendel, K., Pfeiffer, H., Fugelseth, D., Nestaas, E., Domellöf, M., Skålhegg, B. S., et al. (2021). Effects of nutrition therapy on growth, inflammation and metabolism in immature infants: a study protocol of a double-blind randomized controlled trial (ImNuT). *BMC Pediatrics, 21*(1), 19. doi: 10.1186/s12887-020-02425-x.

World Health Organization (WHO) Multicentre Growth Reference Study Group. (2006). Assessment of differences in linear growth among populations in the WHO Multicentre Growth Reference Study. *Acta Paediatrica, 450*, 56–65.

World Health Organization. (2018a). Newborn health. <http://www.who.int/topics/infant_newborn/en/> (Accessed 18 February 2022).

World Health Organization. (2018b). Preterm birth. <https://www.who.int/news-room/fact-sheets/detail/preterm-birth> (Accessed 18 February 2022).

World Health Organization (WHO). (2021). Global Health Observatory (GHO) data repository. Low birth weight, prevalence (%) (child malnutrition). <http://apps.who.int/gho/data/view.main.LBWCOUNTRYv>. Preterm birth fact sheet. <http://www.who.int/mediacentre/factsheets/fs363/en/> (Accessed 18 February 2022).

CHAPTER 7

NEONATAL RETRIEVALS AND TRANSPORT

FAY PRESBURY AND ANITA ROBERTSON

Learning objectives

After reading this chapter you will be able to:

- describe how the geographical landscape impacts on the provision of neonatal retrieval and transport services
- identify the neonate who requires retrieval or transport
- outline the process for coordinating and undertaking a neonatal retrieval
- identify the various modes of transport used for a neonatal retrieval
- outline specific equipment required for a neonatal retrieval
- outline the principles of neonatal stabilisation for transport
- outline the physiological and logistic considerations of a neonate requiring aeromedical or road retrieval
- discuss parental and family support prior, during and following neonatal retrieval and transport
- identify the purpose and process of back transfers.

Key words, terms and abbreviations

back transfer
neonatal retrieval
neonatal transports
sea level (also known as ground level)
transport mode

This chapter is dedicated to Jo Kent Biggs, who made a lifelong contribution to developing and advancing neonatal nursing in Australia. Jo was passionate about everything she did in nursing, and in particular about advanced nursing practice for neonatal retrieval nurses.

INTRODUCTION

Neonatal retrieval services vary in their functionality and resourcing internationally. Some neonatal retrieval services are located and resourced within hospital neonatal units, others are part of combined neonatal/paediatric retrieval services that are more autonomous, with dedicated standalone buildings, staff, equipment and vehicle resources, and others are part of a general retrieval structure that combines adult, perinatal, paediatric and neonatal retrievals into one service.

Neonatal retrieval nurses and midwives require specific qualities compared with a hospital-based neonatal nurse/midwife practising in a clinical environment. The neonatal retrieval nurse/midwife must have the ability to be practical and adaptable in unfamiliar environments, have excellent communication skills, practise collaboratively with retrieval medical staff and referral teams, troubleshoot transport equipment, plan for and manage the unknown and be able to travel in confined spaces in the different modes of transport and under varying environmental conditions. The nurse/midwife should have extensive experience and/or qualifications in neonatal intensive care, with a broad range of understanding of neonatal conditions and a sound knowledge of the effects of transport on the neonate. The key elements for a good outcome for neonates requiring transport are comprehensive clinical handover/referral, timely advice, planning, resourcing, equipment and stabilisation. In addition to the specialised care of the neonate, careful communication strategies are required for the parents and family to ensure an holistic approach before, during and after transport (Kronforst, 2016).

DATA INFORMING CLINICAL CARE FOR NEONATAL RETRIEVALS

Neonatal retrieval medicine is a clinical and logistical process based on quality and research. All neonatal retrieval services collect varying sources of data to enable these services to provide best practice in clinical care and appropriate human and clinical resources.

Table 7.1 outlines key data that are collected.

More-comprehensive clinical and logistical evidence collected in neonatal retrievals will provide improved practices and outcomes.

TABLE 7.1 **Key data collection**

Logistical	Clinical	Other
Mobilisation time Response time Stabilisation time Mission time Transport platforms Referring hospital, level of care Interstate referrals Retrieval activity Concurrent referrals Clinical classification Overflow transports, tertiary to tertiary centres	Diagnosis Maternal history Mode of delivery Adverse events Clinical interventions Patient gestation, weight, age Observations Ventilation modes Outcomes	Parent feedback Education and training in referring hospitals

GEOGRAPHICAL CONSIDERATIONS AND LEVELS OF CARE

Aeromedical retrievals have become a cornerstone of healthcare expectations owing to population clustering near major cities, vast distances, geographical considerations and centralisation of services. While healthcare services are provided at regional centres, the levels of maternity and newborn care vary. Chapter 1 outlines the varying levels of care.

The distances and geographies provide a challenge to the availability of appropriate medical and hospital resources for emergency maternity and newborn care outside of large cities. The utilisation of road ambulance transportation, rotary wing (helicopter) and fixed wing (aeroplane) transport plays an important role in providing equal access to healthcare resources.

Neonatal emergency transport services have evolved since the 1970s to be a highly specialised branch of the aeromedical and retrieval systems. Global centralisation of perinatal and neonatal services into tertiary centres has led to major improvements in maternal and neonatal outcomes but has also driven an increase in demand for the retrievals of sick neonates into these centres (Trevisanuto et al., 2020). There is risk with any aeromedical retrieval and even higher risk with preterm infants, who are at a higher risk of morbidity and mortality, especially with decreasing gestational age (Sharpe & Davies, 2018). In response to this, there has been a proactive move through regionalised perinatal care and referral systems to facilitate in utero transfer for birthing in the tertiary units. This early intervention improves survival rates in comparison with those who are born outside of tertiary centres (Watson et al., 2020). Despite best intentions, there will be the fetus for whom the opportunity to transfer in utero is not appropriate and a neonatal retrieval is required (Thompson et al., 2016).

The retrieval and transport of the neonate is a complex process with many factors to consider. The process begins with the recognition of the need for transfer by the referring centre and ends with admission into a higher level of care.

TASKING AND CLINICAL COORDINATION

When a neonate has been born outside of the level of service required, transportation is required.

A centralised coordination centre is pivotal to this process to ensure optimisation of resources. While there are varying types of coordination services internationally, the fundamental principles are the same. The centralised coordination centre acts as the single point of contact between the referring centre, the retrieval team and the receiving centre to provide safe, consistent patient care that is equitable, cohesive and efficient for all involved. For neonatal retrievals, experienced clinicians conference call with specialised neonatologists who provide initial advice and determine the priority of tasking, retrieval team and transport frame to be used. Box 7.1 outlines a guide to clinical information required to begin the retrieval process.

The centralised or tertiary hospital retrieval services have information on the referring hospitals that comprises helipad availability, level of neonatal care, neonatal clinical equipment, diagnostic equipment, pathology and blood transfusion resources and medical and nursing capabilities. This information allows the retrieval service personnel to understand the referring hospital staff's capacity for care during the stabilisation period prior to transport.

The role of telehealth or telemedicine

Telehealth or telemedicine plays an important role in retrieval medicine and is rapidly expanding with the benefit for the neonate, family and healthcare services, significantly outweighing any perceived challenges (Azzuqa et al., 2021). For some neonates, large distances mean that retrieval is time consuming and rapid transport is not feasible. The use of telemedicine/teleconferencing supports the roles of healthcare providers within the current model of neonatal care to include:

- supporting clinical decision making by allowing direct remote visual and diagnostic assessment via video of neonates prior to retrieval
- providing remote advice to support the early intervention and management of the neonate while the retrieval team are en route
- supporting staff at referring hospitals by providing otherwise unavailable educational and upskilling opportunities at a distance
- reducing the potentially avoidable or unnecessary transfer of infants who are not ill or who have transient self-limited conditions (Curfman et al., 2020; Haynes et al., 2020).

Criteria and priority for tasking

For each case presentation, following a telephone handover and assessment to determine the clinical condition of the neonate, a *priority* or *triage classification* is applied. Globally, various organisations have developed retrieval criteria and tasking priorities that are best suited to their service, geographical location and demographics. Table 7.2 shows an example of a priority classification system.

Most retrieval services only very occasionally task a neonatal retrieval team to attend births of high-risk and/or preterm neonates in rural hospitals. It would always be preferable to transfer the pregnant mother rather than for a preterm neonate to be out-born. Currently, it is not standard practice to depart on a retrieval if the neonate is not yet born. However, some neonatal emergency retrieval services, such as the Paediatric Infant Perinatal Emergency Retrieval (PIPER) in Victoria Australia, aim to be present at all births of neonates under 29 weeks in non-tertiary hospitals so as to resuscitate and stabilise the neonate (Boland et al., 2017).

The criteria for a neonatal retrieval are vast and based on the premise that reduced mortality and improved

BOX 7.1 **Clinical details for retrieval referrals**

Contact details of the referring hospital
Contact details of the receiving hospital and name of the accepting medical officer
Maternal details:

- Name, date of birth and location
- Weight (if transfer is by air)
- Antenatal and intrapartum history and current management

Perinatal history
Neonatal details:

- Neonate's name, date of birth, weight, gender, gestation and current location
- Summary of resuscitation
- Current condition – vital signs and management
- Results of any diagnostic tests (if applicable)

Interventions that may be required during transfer

TABLE 7.2 **Paediatric Infant Perinatal Emergency Retrieval neonatal retrieval classification**

Urgency	Timing
Time critical	Departs within 15 minutes
Urgent	Departs within 25 minutes
Non-urgent	Departs within 60 minutes if required
Elective and return	Booked time

Source: Royal Children's Hospital, Melbourne. (2021). Standard and defined transfer processes for newborn. <https://www.rch.org.au/uploadedFiles/Main/Content/piper/PIPER%20Retrieval%20Team%20Response%20Time%20v2ms.pdf>.

outcome for the neonate will outweigh the risk of transfer (Haynes et al., 2020). The following is a list of neonatal conditions, though not exhaustive, that would require retrieval to a tertiary level of care:

- extreme prematurity
- bodyweight <1500 grams
- ongoing active resuscitation
- respiratory disorders – respiratory distress from any cause where the care exceeds local capabilities
- central nervous system disorder:
  - neonatal encephalopathy
  - neonatal seizures
- infection or suspected infection
- metabolic disorders – e.g. hyperbilirubinaemia or persistent hypoglycaemia
- malformations – e.g. malrotation
- cardiac/cyanosis – suspected or confirmed congenital heart disease
- congenital abnormalities – severe or multiple congenital abnormalities
- conditions requiring surgical interventions – e.g. bowel obstruction, tetralogy of Fallot, diaphragmatic hernia, gastroschisis.

CLINICAL PRACTICE 7.1

While Covid-19 is diagnosed less frequently in neonates, infected individuals are a risk to healthcare workers, especially owing to the close proximity of the retrieval environment. Infection control and monitoring during inter-hospital transport and retrieval of critically ill neonates are crucial owing to the highly infectious nature of the novel coronavirus. Recently published European consensus guidelines recommend strategies to prevent transmission and maintain safety for the neonate and team of a neonate with suspected or proven Covid-19 (Terheggen et al., 2021). They include determining the Covid-19 status of the patient at referral, the retrieval team wearing full personal protective equipment (PPE) after training in donning and doffing PPE procedures, using high-efficiency particulate air (HEPA) filters on the expiratory limb on the ventilatory circuit, and assuring that staff have a secure and dedicated pathway for entering the receiving unit (Terheggen et al., 2021, p. 1096).

Transport platforms

The choice of transport platforms used for neonatal retrievals generally is road, rotary wing (helicopter) or fixed wing (fixed-wing aircraft). The type of platform selected for a tasking is dependent on a variety of factors. These include the neonate's clinical diagnosis, anticipated or potential complications, time to anticipated definitive care and transport criticality. This information needs to be linked with knowledge of the distance between the referring and receiving facilities, local weather, traffic and geographical considerations. Table 7.3 compares the advantages and disadvantages of the different types of transport platforms.

Crew configuration

The retrieval of the neonatal patient, irrespective of transport platform, with two specialised skilled practitioners is associated with improved neonatal outcomes (Jordán Lucas et al., 2021). Neonatal retrieval teams vary depending on the Retrieval Service Clinical Governance structure. The teams may consist of specialist neonatologists, neonatal fellows, senior registrars, neonatal nurse practitioners, neonatal nurses/midwives and registered nurses, all of who have specialised in neonatal and paediatric nursing. This is further supported by the finding of Patel et al. (2020) that the use of specialised nurses improved outcomes. Historically, Orr et al. (2009) have provided strong evidence that using specialised transport teams results in fewer adverse events and increased survival (23% versus 9% for specialised versus non-specialised teams) during inter-hospital transfers.

Neonatal teams offer the advantage of taking intensive care level skills to the neonate with a philosophy of implementing clinical interventions at the referral hospital in a controlled manner ('stay and play' mantra), as opposed to rushing back to the neonatal intensive care unit (NICU) ('scoop and swoop'). Orr et al. (2009) demonstrated that the neonatal retrieval teams that adhered to the 'stay and play' mantra spent nearly twice as long at the scene but had better outcomes.

EVIDENCE-BASED PRACTICE RESEARCH 7.1

Dedicated transport teams

Throughout the literature, there is much discussion comparing specialist transport teams with non-specialist transport teams for aeromedical retrievals for the paediatric population; however, evidence of outcomes specifically for neonatal retrievals is limited.

A Cochrane database systematic review in 2015 by Chang et al. was neonatal specific and aimed to find the impact a specialist versus a non-specialist team had on neonatal morbidity or mortality during transport to an NICU. The study, unfortunately, identified no eligible trials to be included in the review. The authors concluded that additional research from cluster trials or non-randomised study designs is required to answer the question.

Although the review by Chang et al. (2015) provided no evidence to support the use of specialist teams for neonatal retrievals, De Vries et al. (2011) identified that the use of a dedicated neonatal service with specialised transport teams was beneficial as opposed to use of on-call hospital-based NICU staff. The overall availability and mobilisation time with the dedicated neonatal retrieval service and teams improved, with response times within 30 minutes increasing from 11.7% to 46.6%.

In 2016, a study published by Foronda et al. focused on handover and transport of paediatric patients and included **neonatal transports**. Foronda et al. (2016) suggested that handover and transport of critically ill children is a process

TABLE 7.3 **Characteristics and requirements of transport platforms**

	Road	Rotary wing	Fixed wing
Transport platform	FIGURE 7.1 **Road ambulance** *Source: iStock photo/Bossiema.*	FIGURE 7.2 **Augusta Bell 412** *Source: iStock photo/PomlnOz.*	FIGURE 7.3 **King Air B200** *Source: iStock photo/PomlnOz.*
Response times	2–10 min	2–10 min	15–30 min
Range/distance	100 km	100–350 km	>350 km
Speed	60–120 km/h	200–300 km/h	350–800 km/h
Secondary transfer	Door to door	Door to door[a]	Secondary road transfer
Landing capabilities	Not applicable	Can land at the scene	Airstrip required
Space	FIGURE 7.4 **Road platform with transport cot** *@ ZOOM Photography & Video Productions.*	FIGURE 7.5 **Helicopter with transport cot** *@ ZOOM Photography & Video Productions.*	FIGURE 7.6 **Internal RFDSQ aircraft** *Source: Royal Flying Doctor Service of Australia.*
Weather	Minimal impact	Limited by weather	Limited by weather
Altitude		0–10,000 ft (3048 m)	0–35,000 ft (3048 m)
	Not applicable	Non-pressurised	Pressurised
Patient access	No limitation	Limited	Limited
Cost	Low cost	Very high cost	High cost

[a]**Note:** sometimes secondary transfer is required.

that is associated with a high risk of complications. One of the key findings from this review was the fact that the use of specialised teams and standardised communication was associated with improved outcomes. This has since been validated by a study conducted by VanGraafeiland et al. (2019), who state that handovers from team to team improve understanding of roles, communication and safety.

Health and safety

Within the retrieval environment there are increased health and safety risks. Retrieval teams are often exposed to challenges to safe manual handling principles while working in unfamiliar or small, cramped environments. Systems such as patient-loading systems and mandatory training within individual retrieval services should be in place to mitigate these risks.

Fatigue in the retrieval environment is due to a combination of flight stressors, shift work and human factors (tiredness, hunger, stress, etc.), and is one of the causes of errors in clinical decision making and skill performance (Nosker et al., 2020). To minimise risk and address fatigue, retrieval organisations must adopt a robust fatigue risk management system (FMS) that includes self-reporting of fatigue in combination with a flight risk assessment (FRA) tool that is applicable to all clinical and operational staff (Nosker et al., 2020).

Education and training

Every retrieval organisation provides a formal induction or orientation program at the commencement of employment with the overall aim to equip the retrieval team with the necessary expertise and knowledge to conduct a safe retrieval in its area of specialty. The training should include the educational requirements outlined in Box 7.2.

In addition to an induction or orientation process into an aeromedical retrieval environment, registered nurses/registered midwives/flight nurses must have a commitment to continuous professional development, training and education; tertiary level postgraduate and master's level courses in neonatal care and generic aeromedical retrieval are available in hospitals and universities globally. A neonatal nurse practitioner model has been developed and implemented into many neonatal retrieval services throughout the world (Forbes-Coe et al., 2020).

BOX 7.2 **Educational requirements**

Organisational
- Organisational structure
- Clinical governance
- Documentation

Logistics
- Initiation and response
- Coordination
- Communication
- Transport platforms
- Responsibilities

Equipment
- Respiratory support
- Circulatory support
- Transport cot
- Interface to transport platform
- Pharmacology

Clinical issues
- Effects of transport
- Flight physiology and stressors of flight
- Stabilisation and optimisation for transfer
- Patient preparation and scenarios
- Neonatal and paediatric advanced life support
- Crew resource management and safety management
- Aircraft safety and emergency procedures
- Aircraft abandonment
- Sea and land survival
- Helicopter underwater escape training (HUET)
- Aircraft cabin environment
- Fire and evacuation
- Manual handling
- Personal protection equipment

Source: Aeromedical Society of Australasia (ASA) (2020).

Professional industry bodies are strong supporters and advocates for flight/retrieval nursing services that provide opportunities for ongoing professional development, and include:

- Aeromedical Society of Australasia, <https://www.aeromedsocaustralasia.org/>
- Air & Surface Transport Nurses Association, <https://www.astna.org/>
- College of Air and Surface Transport Nursing, <https://www.nzno.org.nz/groups/colleges_sections/colleges/college_of_air_surface_transport_nurses/about_us>
- Flight Nurses Australia, <https://www.flightnursesaustralia.com.au/>

EQUIPMENT

The challenge for neonatal retrievals is to replicate equivalent care to that provided in the neonatal unit.

Equipment, both personnel and patient related, is the foundation for any retrieval service. The equipment and supplies available must reflect the needs of the neonatal population. They need to be highly flexible to cater for the majority of clinical situations as well as provide some redundancy if the primary equipment fails while out on a retrieval. The essential neonatal transport equipment includes portable transport incubators that are fitted with transport ventilators, humidified gases, oxygen, air, high-flow nitric oxide, suction, vital signs monitors, phototherapy units and syringe pumps. Other additional equipment includes basic and advanced resuscitation and procedural equipment and drugs.

Considerations for the retrieval environment include the excessive weight of the equipment, the interface with the transport platform and stretchers, an adequate power supply as well as air and oxygen gas consumption requirements.

Transport incubator

The neonatal intensive care transport incubator is a vital component for the transportation of sick neonates. Transport incubator technology has evolved to enable improved safety features and adaptability, to care for a broad range of neonatal medical requirements. The incubators are designed to be interchangeable so they can interface with different modes of transport and environments. The transport incubator provides a neutral thermal environment and protection from extreme environmental conditions of heat and cold, achieved with the use of double walls and thermal blankets. The transport incubators should have independent lighting, adequate oxygen, low-pressure suction and a power supply with long battery life. To secure the neonate, inbuilt safety harnesses are essential.

Transport vital signs monitors

Assessing and monitoring the neonate during retrieval pose several challenges due to the environment and stresses during transport. Vital signs monitoring is essential and should include:

- temperature (non-invasive or invasive)
- heart rate

- respiratory rate
- blood pressure (non-invasive or invasive)
- oxygen saturation
- transcutaneous CO_2
- end-tidal CO_2.

Respiratory support/transport ventilators

Oxygen can be delivered via the incubator, at low flow via nasal prongs or via a neonatal transport ventilator. Modes of respiratory support can include:

- high-flow gases
- nasal continuous positive airway pressure (NCPAP)
- intermittent positive airway pressure (IPPV)
- high-frequency oscillation ventilation (HFOV).

Nitric oxide

Nitric oxide can be administered via a ventilator for neonates with a diagnosis of persistent pulmonary hypertension of the newborn (PPHN). This gas is utilised under strict safety procedures on the various modes of transport. Delivery of nitric oxide is environmentally monitored (refer to Chapter 9).

Phototherapy

Phototherapy can be performed during aeromedical and road transports with the use of portable phototherapy units that are attached to the transport cot and illuminated to the exposed neonate directly.

Syringe pumps

Syringe pumps are a standard component of the equipment for neonatal retrievals; at times, multiple pumps are required for high-acuity neonates and/or twin retrievals.

Retrieval packs

As there are different levels of care for neonates globally, referring hospitals have diverse equipment availability. The retrieval teams must have all the equipment that is required to stabilise and care for the sick neonate during all phases of the retrieval. Examples of clinical equipment carried by retrieval teams include that needed for vascular access, air-trapping drainage, blood gas sampling, emergency hand ventilation and thermoregulation. Retrieval packs are designed to be interchangeable so that the appropriate equipment is provided depending on the mode of transport, twin transports, equipment for cooling a neonate with hypoxic ischaemic encephalopathy (HIE) (see Chapter 13) and other equipment depending on the diagnosis of the neonate and location.

Medications

Medication packs and retrieval bags are pre-packed to ensure a rapid response to a referral. The medications stocked for retrievals are designed to cover a broad range of critical clinical conditions. Some medications require refrigeration, such as surfactant and prostaglandins, and these drugs will require special refrigerated packs for the transport.

Diagnostic specimens, blood products and expressed breast milk

During road and aeromedical transfers, the transport of any diagnostic specimens (e.g. blood, urine, cerebrospinal fluid, placenta), blood products and expressed breast milk must be stored in the appropriate packaging according to the International Air Transport Association (IATA) Dangerous Goods Regulations (2021). The packaging must consist of three components: a leak-proof primary receptacle, secondary leak-proof packaging and outer packing to prevent the loss of the contents. Immediately inform the pilot and maintenance personnel if there is any spillage of these products owing to their corrosive properties and therefore the potential risk to the aircraft structure (IATA, 2021).

NEONATAL STABILISATION FOR RETRIEVALS

As many countries need to incorporate the challenges of long distances and/or logistical transport difficulties, the referring hospital has the challenge of resuscitating and stabilising the neonate. Through the coordination centre, advice regarding stabilisation and ongoing clinical support can be provided via telephone until the retrieval team arrives.

Principles of stabilisation

The principles of stabilisation should include identification of the neonate's immediate needs, initiation of therapeutic interventions and diagnostic investigations, prevention of/recognition of deterioration and establishment and maintenance of ongoing communication with the parent(s) (Queensland Health, 2018).

Prior to the retrieval team's arrival, and stabilisation of the neonate has occurred, a number of interventions can be commenced by the referring hospital. Refer to Clinical Practice 7.2.

CLINICAL PRACTICE 7.2

Nursing care of the neonate prior to the retrieval team arriving

While waiting for the retrieval team, the neonatal nurse/midwife can limit the therapeutic vacuum by preparing the neonate for transfer. Essential preparation includes the following:

- communicating with the parents and significant others about the pending retrieval and obtaining consent for treatment
- preparing the neonate
- attaching two secure identification bands with the name, date and time of birth, gender and patient record number
- continuous monitoring of vital signs and oxygenation saturation

- inserting a size 6–8 orogastric or nasogastric tube and connecting to free drainage
- keeping the neonate nil by mouth
- ensuring all intravenous (IV) lines are labelled, patent and secured
- ensuring IV maintenance fluids of 10% glucose are in progress
- administering antibiotics as ordered
- initiating neurodevelopmental care
- commencing adequate pain medication and/or sucrose
- completing relevant documentation
- referral letter
- neonatal medical records, observations, medication chart, fluid administration chart, pathology (if able)
- perinatal data collection form
- maternal notes to include antenatal and intrapartum information
- parental contact details – phone numbers and address
- consent for transport and clinical interventions
- consent for pacifier
- additional information
- Infant Personal Health Record
- any neonatal pathological specimens collected to be labelled and packaged appropriately for transfer
- placenta collected, labelled and packaged appropriately for transfer (see Appendix)
- photos for the parents
- directions and contact details of receiving hospital
- social worker contact or assistance with accommodation.

When the retrieval team arrives at the referring hospital, a comprehensive handover using the standard clinical handover tool of ISBAR (**i**dentify, **s**ituation, **b**ackground, **a**greed plan and **r**ead back) is required to understand the full perinatal and neonatal clinical history (Wilson et al., 2017). A consent form for treatment is provided for the retrieval team, which covers medical interventions, drugs, expressed breast milk (EBM) and pacifiers.

The use of checklists is becoming increasingly routine through all phases of the retrieval. Examples of checklist use include equipment checking, intubation and handover. A uniform approach in the dynamic environment reduces the cognitive load and ensures that items, critical sequences or tasks are not forgotten.

Written or electronic clinical documentation, from both the referring hospital and the retrieval team, that is contemporaneous and comprehensive is essential.

Procedures for stabilisation include:

- airway support
- appropriate oxygenation and cardiovascular support
- thermoregulation strategies
- maintenance of fluid and electrolyte balance
- administration of medications
- infection control measures
- diagnostic interventions (X-ray/blood gases)
- vital signs observations
- specific management for surgical/congenital conditions
- ensuring airway and intravenous and arterial lines are labelled and secured, as the effect of vibration can be a risk during transport
- minimal handling
- parental support.

The retrieval team aims to have the neonate as stable as possible prior to departing the referring hospital, as clinical interventions are challenging in the unstable transport environment.

PHYSIOLOGICAL CONSIDERATIONS FOR THE NEONATE DURING TRANSPORT

In any mode of transport, the common challenges are acceleration and deceleration, continuous motion in the vehicle, inadequate lighting, cramped conditions and variations in temperature control in the cabin of the **transport mode**. All of these components create challenges for observing the neonate and providing care and create potential risks for equipment, power and gas dislodgement. The neonatal nurse/midwife has the ability to multitask and is continuously reviewing the neonate and the work environment.

Aeromedical aviation physiology

The use of rotary and fixed-wing transport platforms is a common mode of transport for the sick neonate owing to various factors as previously discussed. Note that this is not without risk: a very real but often unrealised complication is the stress of altitude that can affect both the already-compromised neonate and the flight crew. Table 7.4 outlines the main concerns.

Through a robust understanding of the environment, the neonatal retrieval nurse/midwife will anticipate the effects of the stresses associated with altitude and ensure that strategies are in place to alleviate the impacts to ensure a safe and uneventful transport.

TABLE 7.4 **Effects on the cabin environment of aviation gas laws and stresses associated with aeromedical retrievals**

	Gas laws	Stresses of flight
Hypoxia	✓	✓
Gas expansion	✓	
Temperature	✓	
Noise		✓
Vibration		✓
Decreased humidity		✓
Acceleration and deceleration		✓

Effects of gas laws

Boyle's law

Boyle's law states that, at a constant temperature, the volume of a gas is inversely proportional to the pressure (Fig. 7.7). In practical terms, as the aircraft's altitude increases the atmospheric pressure decreases; therefore, any volume within a space will increase (Table 7.5).

Dalton's law

Dalton's law states that the total pressure of a mixture of gases is equal to the sum of the partial pressures of each gas in the mixture (Fig. 7.8). The implications for the neonate and crew as well as strategies for oxygenation are shown in Table 7.6.

> **CLINICAL PRACTICE 7.3**
>
> **Hypoxia at altitude**
>
> Oxygen makes up 21% of the total atmospheric pressure regardless of altitude. During flight, as the altitude increases and the atmospheric pressure drops, the oxygen molecules move further apart, which results in a reduction in the availability of oxygen. The overall effect is hypoxia (Perry, 2021).
>
> In clinical practice, a neonate who does not require supplemental oxygen (on the ground) prior to aeromedical transfer may require additional oxygen during flight to maintain the same oxygen saturations.

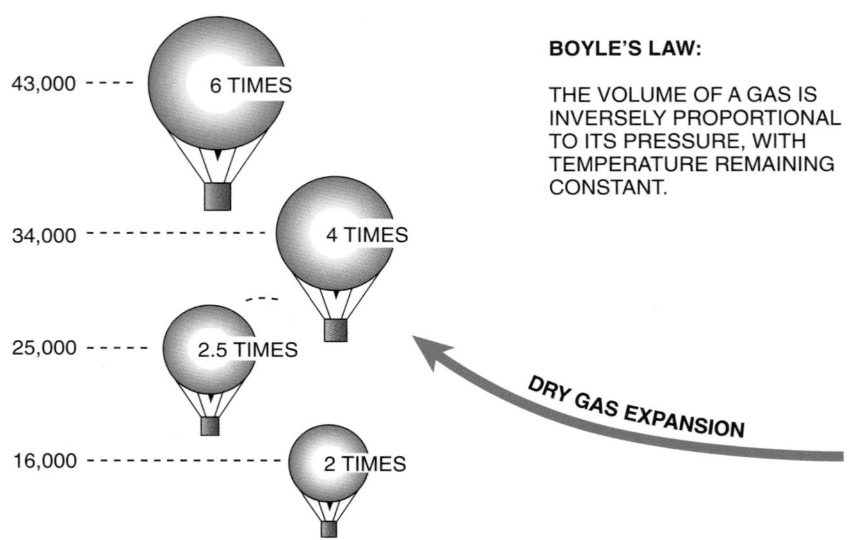

FIGURE 7.7 **Boyle's law**

Adapted from: Pilot Friend, <http://www.pilotfriend.com>

TABLE 7.5 **Implications, complications and strategies for transfers at altitude**

Clinical implications for the neonate	Complications of altitude	Strategies
Lung injury – pneumothorax	Small pneumothorax at sea level may increase or even tension	1 Needle decompression 2 Intercostal drain with Heimlich valve 3 Sea level cabin
Gastrointestinal space/bowel – bowel obstruction	Obstruction of intestinal air may increase and cause ischaemia, necrosis or perforation Could cause tension on the diaphragm and affect ventilation	1 Nasogastric or orogastric tube on free drainage 2 Sea level cabin
Implications for the crew		Strategies
1 Sinus 2 Middle ear 3 Teeth 4 Flatulence	Barosinusitis Barotitis media Barodentalgia	1 Avoid flying with colds or sinus complaints 2 Avoid flying with ear infections 3 Avoid flying for 48–72 h after dental treatment involving deep restoration 4 Avoid foods and drinks that are gas producing

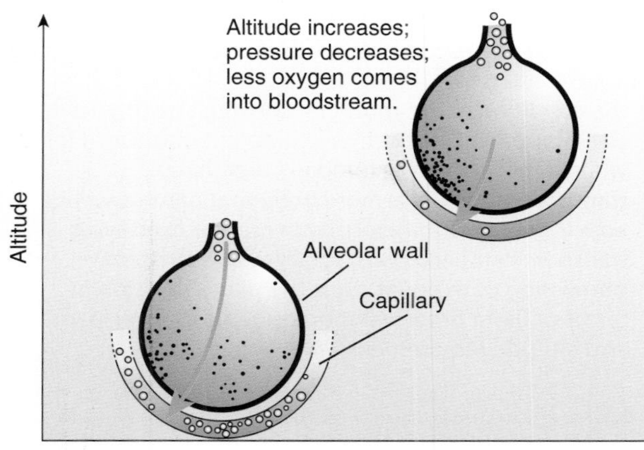

FIGURE 7.8 **Dalton's law.**
Effects on oxygen transfer.

TABLE 7.6 **Implications and strategies for oxygenation**	
Clinical implications for the neonate	Strategies
Oxygenation requirements increase – hypoxia	1 Supplemental oxygen 2 Cabin altitude restriction
Implications for the crew	Strategies
Fatigue	1 Fatigue management protocols 2 Appropriate rostering 3 Adequate nutrition and hydration

Temperature or thermal changes

An increase in altitude results in a decrease in the ambient temperature, that is, the temperature in the surrounding environment. For every 1000 ft (≈305 m) in altitude, the temperature will decrease by 2°C.

In practical terms, if at **sea level** (also known as ground level) the temperature is 35°C, then at 10,000 ft the temperature will be 15°C. In pressurised aircraft (fixed wing), maintaining ambient temperature is achievable (Table 7.7).

TABLE 7.7 **Implications and strategies for temperature or thermal changes**	
Clinical implications	Strategies
For the neonate: inability to maintain temperature control	1 Use a transport cot to provide a neutral thermal environment 2 Minimise the amount of exposure to low environmental temperatures 3 Use transport cot covers 4 Warm ambient temperatures of the aircraft 5 Frequent temperature monitoring of the neonate
For the crew: hypothermia/hyperthermia	1 Appropriate clothing rated to the aviation environment

Stresses of flight

Noise

Helicopters produce more noise than fixed-wing aircraft. Noise levels can reach up to 125 dB during the cruise in aeromedical retrievals. Excess noise may cause stress and discomfort to the infant. Strategies to ensure noise reduction in the neonate include the use of the transport cot and earmuffs during the aeromedical retrieval (Fig. 7.9). Noise levels for the retrieval crew can be fatiguing and, if long term, exposure may contribute to hearing loss.

Strategies for hearing protection and health: these include the use of protective noise-attenuating headsets and fatigue management guidelines.

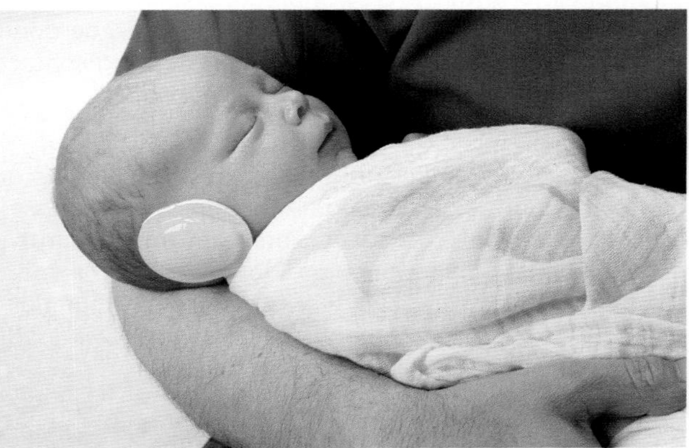

FIGURE 7.9 **Earmuffs (Newmatic Medical™)**
Source: Newmatic Medical™, <https://www.newmaticmedical.com/product/Neonatal-Noise-Guards-NNG>.

Offer the options of earplugs, headsets or helmets to the parents who escort the neonate during the aeromedical transfer.

Clinical equipment implications: auscultation using a stethoscope is almost impossible secondary to the noise. The use of pulse oximetry and astute clinical observations is necessary.

Humidity

Temperature is inversely proportional to altitude; therefore, an increase in altitude produces a decrease in temperature and therefore humidity (Araiza et al., 2021). In practice, as altitude is increased the humidity decreases, causing the environment to be dry.

Dehydration is a concern at altitude for both the neonate and the crew.

Clinical implications for the neonate: nursing care in a transport cot with humidified oxygen will assist to mitigate the effects of low humidity.

Implications for the crew: dehydration is minimised by continuing to drink fluids throughout the retrieval.

Vibration

Vibration is the motion of objects relative to a reference point. Vibration may come from the transport platform and the environment. In ground transport, vibration levels in transit may exceed adult limits of vibration tolerance (Perry, 2021).

In practice, fixed-wing vibration originates from the turbulence through which the aircraft flies. Rotary-wing vibration increases with airspeed and transitioning to the hover position (Araiza et al., 2021).

Clinical implications for the neonate: vibrations are not usually detrimental to the infant owing to transportation in insulated cots. However, Bailey et al. (cited in Perry, 2021) found that using a gel-filled mattress, with or without a foam pad, resulted in a decrease in vibrations experienced by an infant during transport.

Implications for the crew: vibrations can cause fatigue and decreased ability to concentrate. Little can be done about vibrations apart from avoiding or reducing contact with the aircraft frame, and adequate seat padding.

Acceleration and deceleration

Acceleration and deceleration (G-forces) usually occur during take-off and landing. Although these stresses of flight usually do not cause significant impact on the neonatal patient, the optimal positioning of the transport cot is limited to the retrieval service vehicle configuration. Securing all of the equipment and passengers will assist with acceleration and deceleration forces.

PARENTAL FAMILY SUPPORT

For any parents the birth of a new baby should be a joyous, exciting time in their lives. However, with the prospect of a sick baby that needs to be transferred to another hospital away from their home and social support network, it could be the most frightening, confusing and difficult experience.

Family-centred care is essential, with communication starting as soon as practically possible. All communication should be clear, consistent, honest and open with the reasons for the transfer shared and explained. Treat parental wishes and expectations with the utmost respect, along with their cultural and religious views.

The retrieval team should introduce themselves and establish early on an ongoing communication with the family. Parents need information regarding the neonate's condition, with the anticipated management plan and possible prognosis. They should be encouraged to be present throughout the stabilisation (Lefevre et al., 2021). The family should be provided with the opportunity to see, touch and take photographs of the baby prior to departing, and information on the destination, location and phone numbers if travelling with the neonate is not possible for them.

In recent times, there has been a cultural shift in attitude towards allowing a parent to travel with the neonate. While this is possible and even encouraged with some transport platforms, consider the following factors for any parental escort (Whyte & Jefferies, 2015), including but not limited to:

- the condition of the mother – she must be physically stable; retrieval services have different guidelines for when a mother can accompany their baby
- transport mode – it is more likely that parents will be able to travel with their baby in road or fixed-wing transport compared with rotary-wing transport
- permission of the pilot – it is the pilot's decision in terms of flight time, weight requirements, fuel loads and altitude requirements.

FAMILY-CENTRED CARE 7.1

Family-centred care concepts are common in NICUs, but there is less emphasis for acute neonatal transports. Providing family-centred care during neonatal transports presents unique challenges to the transport team, particularly due to the time constraints.

Parents and other family members find neonatal transport traumatic and psychologically distressful. Here are some recommendations to reduce anxiety in the parents and extended family:

- Bring the baby to the mother and family to touch and see them.
- Give clear and concise information about the baby's condition and timeframes for the transport and ensure that the referring hospital supports the same approach.
- Transport a parent where possible with the baby.
- Contact the mother, father and other family members once you arrive at the receiving hospital.
- Provide a receiving hospital information booklet and photographs to the parents.
- Understand how the mother wishes to feed the baby once their condition allows and communicate this to the receiving hospital.
- Where possible, allow parents to be part of the care.

Transferring neonates closer to home ('back transfers')

Once neonates do not require intensive care, consider transporting them to a health service with the appropriate facilities closer to the family home. This is known as **back transfer**, or step-down and/or return transfer, and is an important part of the neonate's journey to discharge home. Communicating about and preparing parents for the transport of the neonate to another hospital will reduce stress and improve confidence in the care the neonate will receive. These transfers have become a specialty within the large, centralised retrieval services, with a high demand to move neonates closer to home for continuation of care, and they enable the family to be closer to home while their baby is prepared for discharge. With discharge from the tertiary level of care, they also provide effective and efficient use of bed availability in the intensive care units.

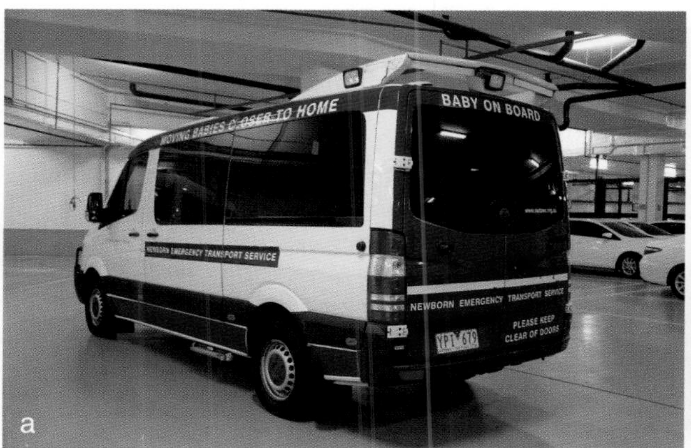

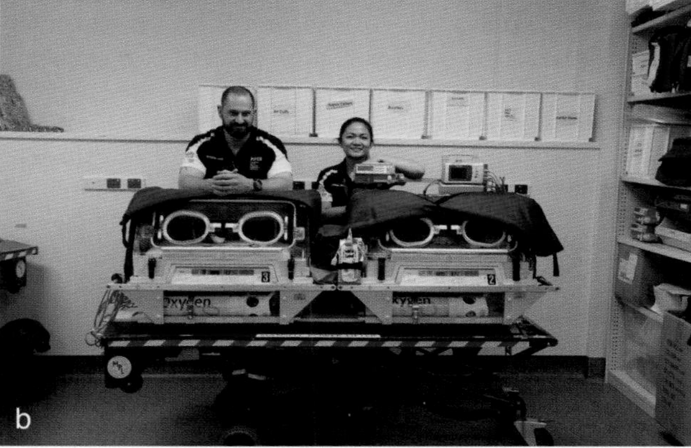

FIGURE 7.10 **a Specially designed return transport vehicle. b Return transport incubators**
Source: © PIPER (Paediatric Infant Perinatal Emergency Retrieval), Royal Children's Hospital, Melbourne. Photo by Chris Fry.

Back transfers can occur via road ambulance or air (Fig. 7.10) and are dependent on the location of the referring hospital relative to the receiving facility. The evolution of back transfers in some states of Australia has seen the introduction of specifically designed road ambulances and specialised nursing staff dedicated to these transfers. Replicate the nursing care and monitoring for the neonate to be transported so that the same level of care is provided during the road or air transportation.

CASE STUDY

7.1 THE NEONATE REQUIRING AEROMEDICAL TRANSFER

It is a quiet afternoon in the central coordination centre. A phone call is received from a junior medical officer requesting assistance for a neonatal retrieval. The handover given is a 38-weeks' gestation female birthed vaginally 24 hours ago. The Apgar scores were 9 and 10, and the neonate's weight is 3 kg. The neonate was breastfed within the first 20 minutes of life. In the past hour, the neonate has been vomiting and her abdomen is becoming increasingly distended. The medical officer has ordered an abdominal X-ray and there are dilated loops of bowel. The provisional diagnosis is a bowel obstruction. Her vital signs are temperature per axilla – 36.2°C, heart rate – 155 bpm, respiratory rate – 50 breaths/minute, and oxygen saturation – 96% in room air.

1. What information given to the clinical coordination centre would assist in determining the priority and timing of tasking and the type of transport platform?
2. Who would be part of the retrieval team and why?
3. What type of training and skills would you expect a neonatal retrieval nurse/midwife to have to be part of this team?
4. What type of equipment would you expect the retrieval team to require for this case?
5. What are the priorities for stabilisation of this neonate?
6. What would be the aeromedical considerations for this neonate's transport?

CONCLUSION

The retrieval of a neonate is a process that commences with the identification of the sick neonate at a referring hospital and involves many clinical and logistical considerations. Potentially, it is a time during which the family unit might be separated and all the impacts of this must be continually considered and addressed. The use of centralised retrieval coordination centres has streamlined the retrieval process with clear and concise communication between all parties involved, and with the dedicated neonatal retrieval teams focusing on implementing appropriate clinical stabilisation procedures and transportation of the neonate. Throughout the retrieval process, the effects of the environment can be a key factor influencing the retrieval. A neonatal retrieval nurse/midwife requires specific skills and has a unique role within neonatal care.

Recommended Reading

Aeromedical Society of Australasia (ASA). (2020). *Standards for aeromedical services*. Final version 1.0.

Online Resources

Health Victoria procedures: <https://www2.health.vic.gov.au/hospitals-and-health-services/patient-care/perinatal-reproductive/neonatal-ehandbook/procedures>

References/Acknowledgements

Aeromedical Society of Australasia (ASA). (2020). Standards for Aeromedical Services Final Version 1.0. <https://www.aeromedsocaustralasia.org/img.ashx?f=f&p=standards_2020%2fASA_Aeromedical_Standards+Final12020.pdf>.

Araiza, A., Duran, M., Surani, S., & Varon, J. (2021). Aeromedical transport of critically ill patients: a literature review, *Cureus, 13*(5), e14899. doi: 10.7759/cereus.14899.

Azzuqa, A., Makkar, A., & Machut, K. (2021). Use of telemedicine for subspecialty support in the NICU setting, *Seminars in Perinatology, 45*(5), 151425. doi: 10.1016/j.semperi.2021.151425.

Boland, R. A., Davis, P. G., Dawson, J. A., & Doyle, L. W. (2017). Outcomes of infants born at 22–27 weeks' gestation in Victoria according to outborn/inborn status. *Archives of Disease in Childhood. Fetal and Neonatal Edition, 102*(2), F153–F161. doi: 10.1136/archdischild-2015-310313.

Chang, A. S., Berry, A., Jones, L. J., & Sivasangari, S. (2015). Specialist teams for neonatal transport to neonatal intensive care units for prevention of morbidity and mortality. *Cochrane Database Systematic Review, 10*, CD007485. doi: 10.1002/14651858.CD00745.pibs.

Curfman, A., Groenendyk, J., Markham, C., Quayle, K., Turmelle, M., Tieken, B., et al. (2020). Implementation of telemedicine in pediatric and neonatal transport. *Air Medical Journal, 39*, 271–275. doi: 10.1016/j.amj.2020.04.008.

De Vries, S., Wallis, L. A., & Maritz, D. (2011). A retrospective evaluation of the impact of a dedicated obstetric and neonatal transport service on transport times within an urban setting. *International Journal of Emergency Medicine, 4*, 28. doi: 10.1186/1865-1380-4-28.

Forbes-Coe, A., Dawson, J., Flint, A., & Walker, K. (2020). The evolution of the neonatal nurse practitioner role in Australia: a discussion paper, *Journal of Neonatal Nursing, 26*, 197–200. doi: 10.1016/j.jnn.2020.01.008.

Foronda, C., VanGraafeiland, B., Quon, R., & Davidson, P. (2016). Handover and transport of critically ill children: an integrative review. *International Journal of Nursing Studies, 62*, 207–225. doi: 10.1016/j.ijnurstu.2016.07.020.

Haynes, S., Dharmar, M., Hill, B. C., Hoffman, K. R., Donohue. L. T., Kuhn-Riordon, K. M., et al. (2020). The impact of telemedicine on transfer rates of newborns at rural community hospitals, *Academic Pediatrics, 20*, 636–641. doi: 10.1016/j.acap.2020.02.013.

International Air Transport Association (IATA). (2021). *Dangerous Goods Regulations*. <https://www.iata.org/publications/dgr/Pages/index.aspx>.

Jordán Lucas, R., Boix H., Sánchez García, L., Cernada, M., de las Cuevas, I., & Couce, M. L. (2021). Recommendations on the skills profile and standards of the neonatal transport system in Spain. *Anales de Pediatría (English Edition), 94*, 6, 420–431.

Kronforst, K. D. (2016). Interhospital transport of the neonatal patient. *Clinical Pediatric Emergency Medicine, 17*(2), 140–146. doi: 10.1016/j.cpem.2016.03.003.

Lefevre, N. C., Jarrier, L., Normand, A., De Luca, D., & Jourdain, G. (2021). Parental presence during pediatric retrieval: the caregiver's perspective. *European Journal of Pediatrics, 180* (5), 1637–1640. doi: 10.1007/s00431-020-03893-0.

Nosker, J. L., Cornelius, A., Lassen, M., Bragg, T., & Killeen. J. (2020). Fatigue in aeromedicine: a validity study of the Flight Risk Assessment Tool. *International Journal of Aerospace Physiology, 30*, 1-2, 69–75. doi: 10.1080/24721840.2020.1735939.

Orr, R. A., Felmet, K. A., Han, Y., McCloskey, K. A., Dragotta, M. A., Bills, D. M., et al. (2009). Pediatric critical care specialized transport teams compared with non-specialized teams are associated with fewer unplanned events and improved survival rates. *Paediatrics, 124*(1), 40–48.

Patel, M., Hebber., K., Dugan., M., & Petrillo, T. (2020). A survey assessing pediatric transport team composition and training. *Pediatric Emergency Care*, 36(5), 263–267. doi: 10.1097/PEC.0000000000001655.

Perry, S. E. (2021). Fifty years of progress in neonatal and maternal transport for specialty care. *Journal of Obstetric, Gynecologic and Neonatal Nursing, 50*(6), 774–788. doi: 10.1016/j.jogn.2021.04.013.

Queensland Health. (2018). Maternity and Neonatal Clinical Guidelines. *Neonatal stabilization for retrieval*, <https://www.health.qld.gov.au/__data/assets/pdf_file/0017/144026/g-stabil.pdf>.

Royal Children's Hospital, Melbourne. (2021). Standard and defined transfer processes for newborn. <https://www.rch.org.au/uploadedFiles/Main/Content/piper/PIPER%20Neonatal%20-%20Defined%20Transfer%20Process%20v4.pdf>.

Sharpe, J. B., & Davies, M. W. (2018). Does earlier arrival of the retrieval team improve short-term outcomes in outborn extremely premature infants? *Journal of Paediatric Child Health. 54*(11),1234–1241. doi: 10.1111/jpc.14064.

Terheggen, U., Heiring, C., Kjellberg, M., Hegardt, F., Kneyber, M., Gente, M., et al. (2021). European consensus recommendations for neonatal and paediatric retrievals of positive or suspected COVID-19 patients. *Pediatric Research, 89*(5), 1094–1100. doi: 10.1038/s41390-020-1050-z.

Thompson, K., Gardiner, J., & Resnick, S. (2016). Outcome of outborn infants at the borderline of viability in Western Australia: a retrospective cohort study. *Journal of Paediatrics and Child Health, 52*, 728–733. doi: 10.1111/jpc.13187.

Trevisanuto, D., Cavallin, F., Loddo, C., Brombin, L., Lolli, E., Doglioni, N., et al. (2020). Trends in neonatal emergency transport in the last two years. *European Journal of Paediatrics, 180*, 635–641. doi: 10.1007/s00431-020-03908-w.

VanGraafeiland, B., Foronda, C., Vanderwagem, S., Allan, L., Bernier, M., Fishe, J., et al. (2019). Improving the handover and transport of critically ill pediatric patients. *Journal of Clinical Nursing, 28*, 56–65. doi: 10.1111/jocn.14627.

Watson, H., McLaren, J., Carlisle, N., Ratnavel, N., Watts, T., Zaima, A., et al. (2020). All the right moves: why *in utero* transfer is both important for the baby and difficult to achieve and new strategies for change. *F1000Research*, 9, F1000 Faculty Rev-979. doi: 10.12688/f1000research.25923.1.

Whyte, H. E. A., & Jefferies, A. L. (2015). The interfacility transport of critically ill newborns. *Paediatric Child Health, 20*(5), 265–269.

Wilson, D., Kochar, A., Whyte-Lewis, A., Whyte, H., & Lee, K. (2017). Evaluation of situation, background, assessment, recommendation tool during neonatal and pediatric interfacility transport. *Air Medical Journal, 36*, 182–187. doi: 10.1016/j.amj.2017.02.013.

APPENDIX

The Consultative Council on Obstetric and Paediatric Mortality (CCOPMM) state that the placenta should be sent for pathological examination in any of the following circumstances:

- neonatal hypoxic ischaemic encephalopathy
- small for gestational age
- preterm delivery under 34 weeks
- antepartum haemorrhage
- suspected chorioamnionitis
- diabetes
- preeclampsia
- macroscopic placental abnormalities
- early neonatal death
- fetal death.

Source: Department of Health and Human Services (2017) Consultative Council on Obstetric and Paediatric Mortality and Morbidity. <https://www2.health.vic.gov.au/hospitals-and-health-services/quality-safety-service/consultative-councils/council-obstetric-paediatric-mortality>.

CHAPTER 8

NEONATAL THERMOREGULATION

KAREN NEW AND JACKIE SMITH

Learning objectives

After reading this chapter you will be able to:

- describe the physiology of thermoregulation
- identify physiological and physical mechanisms of thermoregulation in the neonate
- describe the mechanisms of heat transfer
- describe neonatal temperature ranges and the different methods and devices for obtaining a neonatal temperature, including the associated advantages and disadvantages of each method
- discuss the risk factors for hypo- and hyperthermia and actions for rewarming and cooling neonates
- describe strategies to support thermoregulation in neonatal care
- review the evidence base for thermoregulation practices
- understand the importance of and describe strategies to involve the family in the care of their infant, ensuring best thermoregulation practice.

Key words, terms, abbreviations

air control
brown adipose tissue (BAT)
cold stress
conduction
convection
core temperature
evaporation
free fatty acids (FFAs)
hyperthermia
hypothermia
metabolic rate (MR)
neutral thermal environment (NTE)
non-shivering thermogenesis (NST)
radiation
servo-control
thermogenesis
thermoregulation
transepidermal water loss (TEWL)

INTRODUCTION

While temperature regulation in all humans is important for survival, for neonates it is a critical physiological function in which they are unable to protect themselves owing to their physical immaturity, environmental factors and, at times, illness (Brand & Shippey, 2021). As early as the 1830s, the first double-walled incubator was developed to provide a warm environment for preterm infants, and in the 1880s a link between cold exposure and increased mortality was made, resulting in the discovery that neonates kept warm in incubators resulted in a reduction in mortality rates (Gardner & Cammack, 2021). Nevertheless, **hypothermia** remains a common problem for low birthweight (LBW) infants, and continues to be a major contributor worldwide to neonatal mortality (McCall et al., 2018; Pinheiro, 2018). The 2018 report of the Australian and New Zealand Neonatal Network (ANZNN) states that the median admission temperature to neonatal intensive care units for all admissions (n = 10,556) was 36.6°C. However, the range was between 36.0°C and 37.1°C in gestational age groups between 24 and 36 weeks, with little variation between groups (Chow et al., 2020). This highlights that even the smallest of neonates can be kept warm when there is focused attention on **thermoregulation**, and that even heavier and more mature newborns can become cold when there is not. Being cold on admission and day 1 are increased risks for mortality, where for each decrease in admission temperature of 1°C below 36°C the mortality increases by 28% (Cavallin et al., 2020).

A **neutral thermal environment (NTE)** is one where body temperature is maintained at a point that minimises oxygen consumption required for heat maintenance, thereby conserving energy for other basic functions and growth (Gardner & Cammack, 2021). Achieving and maintaining an NTE is one of the key physiological challenges critical to the care and survival of neonates, more so for those born preterm. The World Health Organization (WHO) defines neonatal temperature ranges taken per axilla as normal between 36.5°C and 37.5°C, hypothermia as less than 36.5°C and **hyperthermia** as greater than 37.5°C. The WHO degrees of hypothermia are mild (36.0–36.4°C), moderate (32.0–35.9°C) and severe (less than 32°C) (Nyandiko et al., 2021). These reference ranges are used for this chapter.

The risk of hypothermia is greatest at the time of birth when heat exchange through the placenta ceases and the neonate is exposed to environmental temperatures. Heat is lost through four primary mechanisms: **conduction**, **convection**, **evaporation** and **radiation**. Understanding these mechanisms and the interventions to minimise heat loss is key to reducing mortality (Brand & Shippey, 2021). These mechanisms and the physiology of thermoregulation, risk factors for hypo- and hyperthermia, prevention of thermal instability and the importance of family involvement in the maintenance of normothermia are discussed in this chapter.

All aspects of care of the neonate and their family should be underpinned and guided by standards for neonatal nursing practice and/or competencies for neonatal nursing and for midwifery practice. The Council of International Neonatal Nurses (COINN) has produced an international neonatal nursing competency framework (2019) to guide both novice and competent neonatal nurses. Similarly, the International Confederation of Midwives (ICM) *Essential competencies for midwifery practice 2018 update* (2019) should be used to guide midwives in the care of the normal newborn. Many countries have standards produced by their own professional bodies such as the Australian College of Neonatal Nurses (ACNN) (2019) and the Neonatal Nurses College of Aotearoa (NNCA) (2015), New Zealand's peak neonatal nursing professional body. Reference is made to these standards throughout this chapter.

PHYSIOLOGY OF THERMOREGULATION

Humans are homeothermic. This means they can regulate their **core temperature** within a narrow range, by physiologically and behaviourally balancing heat loss with heat gain to maintain a normal body temperature (Douglas, 2020). Thermoregulation is achieved by a complex system managed by the hypothalamus. Central and peripheral thermoreceptors sense a change in body temperature, which is a response by the homeostatic system with effectors and detectors that are aimed at preserving body temperature. Effectors are heat production by **thermogenesis**, evaporation, vasomotor response and behavioural response. Detection is made by the core and skin thermoreceptors, which is then fed back to the hypothalamus.

The body uses three responses to process this thermoregulatory information: afferent thermal sensing (afferent means to receive), central regulation (hypothalamus) and efferent responses (efferent means to act) (Osilla et al., 2021).

MECHANISMS OF THERMOREGULATION

The uterus provides a stable thermal environment for the fetus, whose temperature is maintained approximately 0.3–0.5°C higher than maternal temperature under optimal conditions; a gradient that allows the fetus to offload heat to the mother (Blackburn, 2017). While maternal factors and placental blood flow control fetal temperature, thermoregulatory processes in the fetus are suppressed. Consequently, changes in maternal factors or placental blood flow can impact on the fetus. For example, if the mother has an elevated temperature (i.e. from exercise or illness), the maternal–fetal temperature gradient is reduced, leading to an increase in the temperature of the fetus (Blackburn, 2017). Maternal fever in labour (>38°C) in non-infected women has been linked to lower Apgar scores, tachycardia, hypotonia, hypoxia and an increased need for resuscitation and oxygen at birth (Brand & Shippey, 2021).

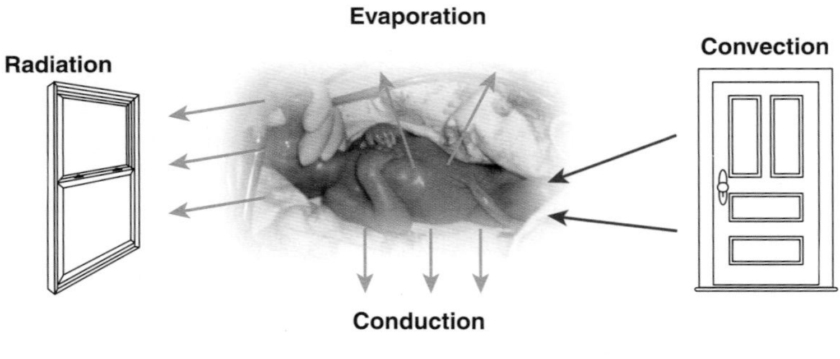

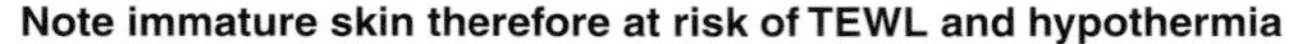

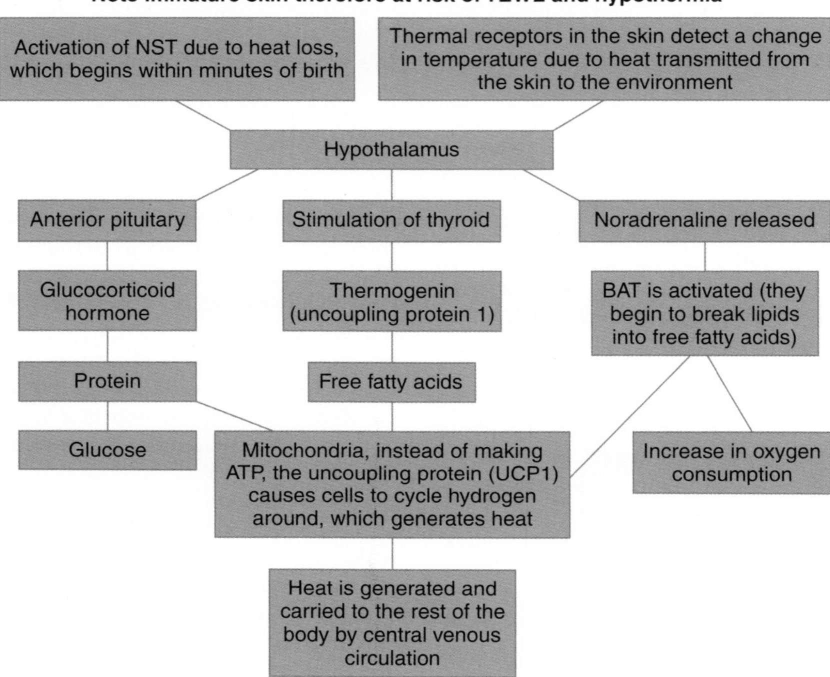

FIGURE 8.1 **Heat loss and non-shivering thermogenesis**

At birth, exposure to the cooler environment and separation from the placenta trigger thermogenesis and activate heat production. This thermogenic response commences as soon as the neonate is born and can continue for many hours. It encompasses two processes: **non-shivering thermogenesis (NST)** (Fig. 8.1), known as the endocrine control of the onset of thermogenesis, and an increased **metabolic rate (MR)**. For heat to be generated by NST, **brown adipose tissue (BAT)**, also known as brown fat, is required. It is the metabolism of BAT that generates heat. BAT is located around the interscapular region, kidneys and mediastinum (Fig. 8.2) and can be identified as early as 25 weeks' gestation. It significantly increases during the third trimester, comprising about 1–2% of bodyweight at birth, and contains thermogenin, a key enzyme that regulates NST (Brand & Shippey, 2021). Consequently, the lower the gestation at birth, the less BAT there is, so neonates born at less than 32 weeks' gestation have inadequate stores of BAT to produce enough heat by NST, increasing their risk of hypothermia (Brand & Shippey, 2021).

With a drop in body temperature below 35–36°C, a sequence of responses is activated as the hypothalamus receives messages via the central thermoreceptors, stimulating sympathetic nerve activity and leading to the release of noradrenaline (norepinephrine). Noradrenaline attaches to adrenergic receptors on the brown fat cell membrane, stimulating the release of **free fatty acids (FFAs)**. FFAs are derived from triglycerides that are hydrolysed into glycerol (adrenaline (epinephrine) stimulates the formation of glucose from glycogen), using the energy from adenosine triphosphate (ATP), which is made in the mitochondria (powerhouse of the cell), by use of glycogen stores. Once FFAs have been released, combustion occurs in the mitochondria of brown fat cells that oxidises the FFAs, which results in the generation of

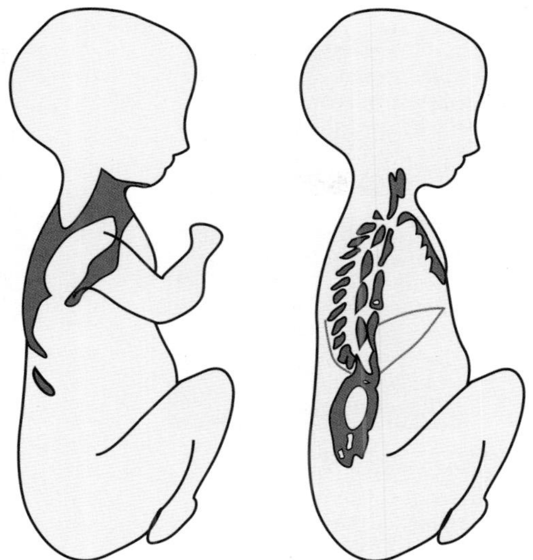

FIGURE 8.2 **Location of brown fat**

Source: Aherne and Hull (1964).

heat. This heat is then circulated around the body via the systemic blood flow. For combustion to occur, uncoupling of protein 1 is required, which is an enzyme that is key to NST heat production (Jastroch et al., 2021). Thyroxine (T4), when changed to triiodothyronine (T3), is also capable of initiating a thermogenic response (see Fig. 8.1 and Fig. 8.3).

The second mechanism by which the neonate produces heat is as a by-product of the metabolism of fat, glucose and/or protein. The basal metabolic rate (BMR) is the rate at which the body uses energy while at rest to maintain vital functions such as breathing and keeping warm. 'Term neonates can increase their BMR by 200–300% ... whereas VLBW infants may only be able to increase it by 25%, and ELBW infants may not be able to respond at all' (Brand & Shippey, 2021, p. 91).

All neonates are at risk of **cold stress**, defined as whenever heat loss requires an increase in metabolic heat production. Cold stress is more likely to occur at temperatures less than 36.4°C, but can occur at higher temperatures when there is a difference of more than 2°C between core and peripheral skin temperatures (Brand & Shippey, 2021) (see section on temperature measurement). An early response to cold stress is for vasoconstriction of the peripheries to reduce blood flow so as to minimise heat loss. At greater risk are those born preterm and/or requiring resuscitation, owing to the diminished capacity for metabolic heat production, high surface-area-to-weight ratio and high evaporative heat losses within a cool environment (Lubkowska et al., 2019). When cold stressed, the body undergoes several physiological changes: a rise in MR, vasoconstriction, increased oxygen consumption, metabolic acidosis due to persistent vasoconstriction (decrease in tissue perfusion and oxygenation) and pulmonary vasoconstriction (reducing pulmonary perfusion). A rise in MR in an attempt to produce heat requires glucose, which can lead to hypoglycaemia. Preterm neonates and those with respiratory distress, who are hypothermic and attempting to produce heat, will markedly increase oxygen consumption. This may result in worsening respiratory distress as glycogen stores become depleted and oxygen utilisation increases,

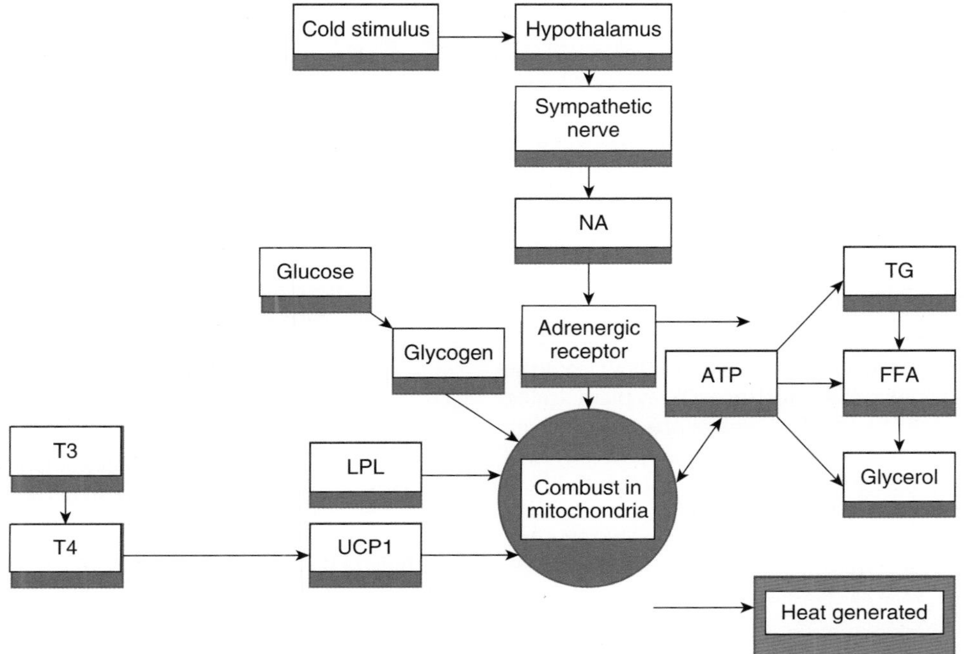

FIGURE 8.3 **Function of brown fat and heat generation**

ATP, adenosine triphosphate; FFA, free fatty acids; LPL, lipoprotein; NA, noradrenaline; T3, triiodothyronine; T4, thyroxine; TG, triglycerides; UCP1, uncoupling protein 1.

Behavioural changes
Hypotonia
Apnoea
Lethargy
Weak cry
Poor tolerance of feeds

Birth, Resuscitation & Transport
Delay transition from fetal to neonatal circulation

Oxygenation
Oxygen uptake is affected
Increase in pulmonary resistance, causing a decrease in surfactant production

Glucose
Increased uptake of glucose leads to hypoglycaemia
Decreased energy for growth

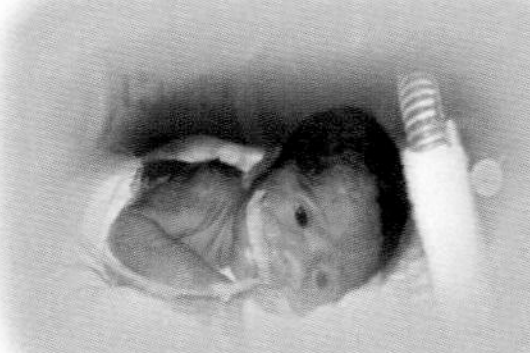

Surfactant production
Surfactant production is decreased
Decreased ability to act as a surface tension lowering agent (temp <35°) causing atelectasis
Worsening hypoxia

Perfusion
Perfusion can become prolonged causing anaerobic metabolism
Can lead to worsening acidosis

Acidosis
Increase in pulmonary artery pressure causing a decrease in blood flow, thereby affecting blood flow to the lungs

FIGURE 8.4 **Effects of cold stress on the neonate**

resulting in anaerobic metabolism to produce heat. This results in metabolic acidosis (due to the accumulation of lactic and pyruvic acids), pulmonary vasoconstriction, decreased surfactant production and hypoxia (Brand & Shippey, 2021). This sequence of events can impact on the transition from fetal to neonatal circulation. Physiological and behavioural changes are outlined in Fig. 8.4.

MECHANISMS OF HEAT TRANSFER

Heat transfer occurs between the neonate and the environment via four mechanisms: conduction, convection, evaporation and radiation (Trevisanuto et al., 2018) (see Fig. 8.1). The amount of heat transfer is determined largely by the difference in temperature between the neonate and the environment.

Conduction

Conduction is the transfer of heat between two solid surfaces that are in direct contact. Heat will flow from the warm body to a cooler surface such as an X-ray plate, scales, stethoscope or cold hands. The greater the temperature difference between the surfaces, and the larger the area of contact between the two surfaces, the greater is the heat flow. Conduction can also be utilised to effectively transfer heat to the neonate – for example, with the use of warming mattresses and warm wraps.

Convection

Convection is the transfer of heat between the neonate and either air or liquid. Heat is lost when cooler air moves across the skin surface, or to water – for example, if the bath water is cooler than the neonate's body temperature.

Evaporation

The skin, as the largest organ of the body, plays a major role in thermoregulation, in particular in **transepidermal water loss (TEWL)** by evaporative heat losses. Neonates of less than 30 weeks' gestation are at increased risk of high water loss through the skin, leading to temperature instability, dehydration and electrolyte imbalance, as well as heat and calorie loss. Evaporative heat loss is the most significant heat loss at birth, as amniotic fluid and water from the skin and mucous membranes evaporates. The more premature the neonate, the thinner is the stratum corneum of the skin, thus increasing the potential for evaporative heat and transepidermal water losses.

Radiation

Radiation involves the transfer of radiant energy from the warm neonate to cooler surrounding surfaces, such as an incubator inside wall or a window, that are not in direct contact with the neonate. Radiant heat loss can be up to 60% depending on the coldness of the surrounding surfaces.

It is the neonate's susceptibility to temperature instability that needs to be recognised and understood in order to appropriately manage and limit the effects of heat loss (Table 8.1) (Brand & Shippey, 2021). Equally, temperature measurement is a critical component of neonatal care.

REFLECTION

Take a moment to reflect on how your body responds to cold and heat. Now consider the limitations of the neonate in relation to these responses and what measures you could take to prevent cold stress from occurring in the neonatal setting.

TABLE 8.1 **Potential heat loss methods and solutions for thermal management of neonates**

Problem	Solution(s)
Heat loss via conduction	Use of warm sheets and blankets Prewarmed incubator surface or warm mattress Warm objects like X-ray plates and scales Skin-to-skin contact with mother/father
Heat loss via evaporation	Plastic wrap or bag for VLBW infants Dry neonate with warmed towels, especially the head Limit the use of radiant warmer Place in a preheated and humidified incubator Bath water temperature must be 38–40°C Prewarm any solutions, lotions or soaks
Heat loss via radiation	Ensure neonates are not placed near doors, windows, air vents or cold exterior walls Radiant warmer for resuscitation or procedures Prewarmed double-walled incubators Dress the neonate when possible
Heat loss via convection	Protect the neonate from draughts Plastic wrap or bag for VLBW infants Prewarm the incubator Wrap in warm linen Place a hat Use warmed humidified oxygen Prewarm the birth suite Ensure bath water is 38–40°C Prewarm breast milk
Environmental temperature is low	Increase room temperature prior to birth
Transepidermal water loss (TEWL)	Plastic wrap/bag Limit use of radiant warmer Place in humidified incubator as soon as possible Neonates with open lesions are at high risk of TEWL. Open lesions must be wrapped in plastic (according to your unit protocol) as soon as the neonate is born
External heat source prior to birth	Ensure the radiant warmer is turned on prior to birth
Parental bonding	It is very important for the parents to see and touch their infant (if stable) prior to transfer to the neonatal unit Breastfeed as soon as possible. If not possible, provide caloric intake to support heat generation

TEMPERATURE MEASUREMENT

Temperature is one of the vital signs that require close observation as it is often one of the first signs of a change in a neonate's clinical condition (see Clinical Practice 8.1). Internal body temperature, also referred to as core temperature, is usually steadier and stable over time. Core temperature is measured directly from a body cavity (rectum, oesophagus, tympanic membrane, pulmonary artery or bladder). Indirect temperature measurements are a measure of the skin's surface temperature, and are taken from locations such as the axilla and abdomen, or from peripheral locations such as the foot or hand. Per axilla temperatures have shown good correlation with core temperatures (Nadkarni et al., 2021). In this chapter, the term 'core temperature' will be used when referring to internal body temperature.

CLINICAL PRACTICE 8.1

Assessment of the neonate and obtaining a thorough history of the immediate post-birth period will alert the neonatal nurse/midwife to the risk factors for thermal instability and the need to develop management strategies to prevent hypo- and hyperthermia (Brand & Shippey, 2021). Obtaining accurate temperature measurements is an integral part of caring for neonates (ACNN, 2019; COINN, 2019; ICM, 2019; NNCA, 2015).

The most accurate and appropriate method of measuring core and skin temperatures remains debated, and there is conflicting data on whether rectal or axillary temperatures are ideal methods for measuring temperature in this population (McCarthy & O'Donnell, 2021). The different routes for measuring neonatal temperature are outlined in Table 8.2. The National Institute for Health and Care Excellence (NICE) recommends axillary measurement using a digital axillary thermometer and discourages the measurement of temperature via the oral and rectal routes in neonates owing to safety concerns (NICE, 2019).

Rectal temperature is not recommended because of the potential for trauma to the rectum and the potential for infection secondary to perforation. However, for newborns undergoing therapeutic cooling for hypoxic ischaemic encephalopathy, continuous rectal temperature measurements using a device such as a thermistor probe are recommended (Brand & Shippey, 2021). Therapeutic cooling, by either whole-body or selective head cooling, to 32–34°C has been shown to reduce neurological sequelae without adverse effects. This procedure decreases the temperature of the vulnerable deep brain structures, therefore reducing the amount of damage to the brain cells by decreasing cerebral metabolism, inflammation, oxidative damage and cellular apoptosis (Wassink et al., 2019). Refer to Chapter 13 for further information.

The most common and preferred method to measure a neonate's skin temperature intermittently is the axillary method using a digital thermometer (NICE, 2019). To measure an axillary temperature, turn the thermometer on, place the tip end of the thermometer under the armpit, making sure it touches skin and not clothing. The thermometer will signal when the neonate's temperature is reached, usually after 3–5 minutes. This method is non-invasive, accurate and easy to use, although it can cause distress from the additional handling (Gardner & Cammock, 2021). Studies using the tympanic method, in which a digital tympanic thermometer is placed snugly into the ear

TABLE 8.2 **Comparison of methods for measuring neonatal temperature**

Rectal	Axillary
Oldest method but now used infrequently High chance of cross-contamination if thermometer not cleaned effectively Danger of rectal perforation Can cause distress Contraindicated in patients with thrombocytopenia Resistant to changes in ambient temperature Inaccurate temperature due to the presence of faeces, depth of insertion, timing, NEC, infection and blood flow There can be a lag in core temperature at times Shown to closely approximate core temperature Parents and staff may view this method as invasive	Non-invasive – minimal cross-infection Easily accessible Easy to use Can cause distress to the neonate due to additional handling Can be affected by ambient temperature, humidity and radiant warmer Poor tracking of core temperature in neonates with hypothermia due to vasoconstriction (not continuous, does not track the trend) Has been shown to elevate temperature owing to the presence of brown fat Needs accurate placement Placement time needs to be consistent Recommended as standard practice (AAP)
Tympanic	Forehead
Convenient access Non-invasive Close proximity to the hypothalamus Inter-user variability Temperature can vary depending on ambient temperature Ear open to the environment may be subject to temperature variation Some studies suggest the size of the ear probe affects accuracy Can cause distress due to the ear 'tug' Ear canal must be free of obstruction Continuous research is required for this method	Non-contact No cross-contamination Quick and easy to use No distress Only use on clean, dry, hairless skin Forehead is supplied by the superficial temporal artery, receives high blood flow from the carotid artery Poor agreement with other methods Can underestimate temperature, especially hyperthermia Affected by ambient temperature More research needed in both preterm and term neonates
Skin (by sensor probe)	Oesophageal
Non-invasive method Easy to use Continuous trend Does not cause any distress Neonate usually responds to cold stress by vasoconstriction; therefore, it will monitor a fall in temperature Can cause skin irritation due to the tape securing the probe Probe placement needs to be secure to obtain an accurate temperature More research is required in both term and preterm neonates	Invasive Only used in intubated, surgical and anaesthetised patients Not yet used in the neonatal population but currently research trials are active in the use of this temperature method Neonates have minimal thermal insulation between the oesophagus and the trachea–bronchial tree Central temperature measurement More research needed on the use of the oesophageal method

NEC, necrotising enterocolitis.

canal, have shown mixed results for use in neonates, with this method being less reliable owing to the curvature of the ear canal, hyperaemia and ear wax, which may affect the accuracy of the readings. The small size of the ear of preterm infants precludes tympanic measurement (Hodson, 2018).

The type of thermometer used and preferred measurement site are workplace specific. Given the importance of temperature measurements in the neonatal population, it is imperative that nurses and midwives are skilled in using the devices in their workplace.

REFLECTION

Take a moment to reflect on the temperature measuring devices used in your workplace. What key points would you convey to a novice colleague and a parent in demonstrating how to take a temperature with the devices in your workplace?

Intermittent temperature measurements do not reveal how much energy the neonate may be utilising to maintain normothermia or indicate if cold stress is occurring. In cold stress the peripheral body parts (hands, feet) will cool before the more central parts such as the abdomen. Standard care in most NICUs involves continuous recording with a digital readout of skin temperatures via a skin probe on the abdomen or back, with 3–4-hourly checks of the infant's axillary temperatures to detect cold stress.

A skin temperature sensor (probe or thermistor) needs to be repositioned regularly to prevent skin irritation and pressure areas. Sensors should be placed to avoid BAT areas (see Fig. 8.5) as this may cause detection of higher temperatures. Sensors are usually placed on the abdomen or flank and are not sited over bony prominences. Observations of the sensor site are undertaken to ensure that the sensor does not become detached, resulting in a lower skin reading, which causes the incubator or radiant

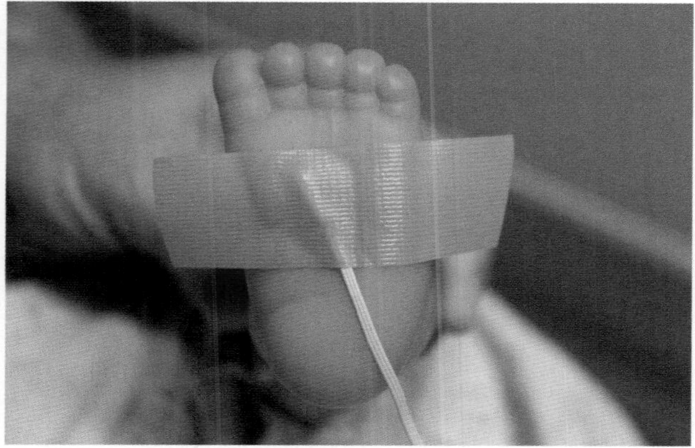

FIGURE 8.5 **Peripheral temperature sensor**

warmer to increase the cot temperature and overheat the neonate when used in the **servo-control** mode. The ability of the incubator or radiant warmer to adjust its heating output in response to the skin temperature is called servo-control. Servo-controlled systems use an electronic feedback loop to adjust the air temperature or radiant warmer output automatically to maintain the skin temperature at a set point. Therefore, it is essential that the skin sensor is placed and secured correctly to avoid hyperthermia. Other risks of the servo-controlled system are the failure to detect the early signs of sepsis, as alterations in body temperature are masked (Blackburn, 2017). Some neonatal unit policies describe how they wean infants off servo-control onto manual air temperature control once certain criteria are met (Gardner & Cammack, 2021, p. 148). Placement, securement and repositioning timeframes for skin temperature sensors are usually workplace specific and outlined in current standard practice guidelines.

An alternative to servo-controlled systems is air or manual cot temperature control. This occurs when the incubator or radiant warmer air temperature is manually set and the incubator or radiant warmer maintains this set air temperature irrespective of the skin temperature. There is less variability in air temperature when this mode is used (Brand & Shippey, 2021).

REFLECTION

Reflect on your workplace standard practice guideline for the use of servo- or air control modes. What are the advantages and disadvantages of each mode?

Hypothermia

Prevention of hypothermia is an essential role for the neonatal nurse/midwife caring for the at-risk newborn. Table 8.1 outlines the strategies to meet this goal. Conventional practice to prevent hypothermia after birth in the normal newborn is to provide a warm environment for birth, dry the neonate, especially the head, with prewarmed linen, place a covering on the head (e.g. a woollen hat), position them skin to skin with the mother (preferably) or father/support person and cover the neonate with dry, warm linen. Full-term healthy neonates should then be able to maintain their core temperature; however, if left wet and uncovered, heat loss will exceed heat production, and the risk of hypothermia is high. Body temperature can drop between 0.1°C and 0.3°C every 5 minutes in the absence of immediate thermo-protective action (McCall et al., 2018).

The following characteristics (as pictured in Fig. 8.6) place newborns at a greater risk of heat loss:

- being born wet and into an environment cooler than the uterus
- additional factors for premature and very low birth-weight infants include:
  - limited substrate (glycogen) for heat production
  - an inability to flex to reduce exposed surface area
  - less brown fat
  - less subcutaneous tissue
  - at increased risk of other complications (e.g. respiratory distress) and needing interventions which compromise thermal stability
- large surface area-to-body ratio, with the head accounting for one-fifth of the total body surface area
- decreased insulating subcutaneous fat
- immature skin with increased permeability to water
- greater body water content
- immature metabolic mechanisms, which impact on the ability to generate heat via NST
- resuscitation
- increased handling
- neonates undergoing surgery as analgesics and anaesthesia decrease the MR, compromising the ability to generate heat
- birth asphyxia, which decreases the effect of noradrenaline in NST, causing a delayed metabolic response to cold stress and delayed vasoconstriction
- inability to shiver.

While signs of hypothermia are often either absent or non-specific in the neonate, clinical findings may include lethargy, hypotonia, apnoea, restlessness, tachypnoea, poor feeding or decreased weight gain (Blackburn, 2017). The hypothermic neonate appears pale and/or mottled with cool extremities as the body responds by vasoconstriction. If left uncorrected, this leads to a chain of responses: metabolic acidosis and anaerobic metabolism (the production of energy in the cells in the absence of oxygen), pulmonary vasoconstriction (pulmonary arterioles constrict in the presence of hypoxia) and respiratory acidosis, hypoglycaemia, hypoxia and death (Demtse et al., 2020).

There is limited information available about the safest and most effective method of rewarming hypothermic neonates (Brand & Shippey, 2021). Rewarming should not occur too quickly in the moderate to severe hypothermic neonate as this could potentially cause apnoea, hypotension secondary to vasodilation, a decrease in blood pressure and increased oxygen consumption

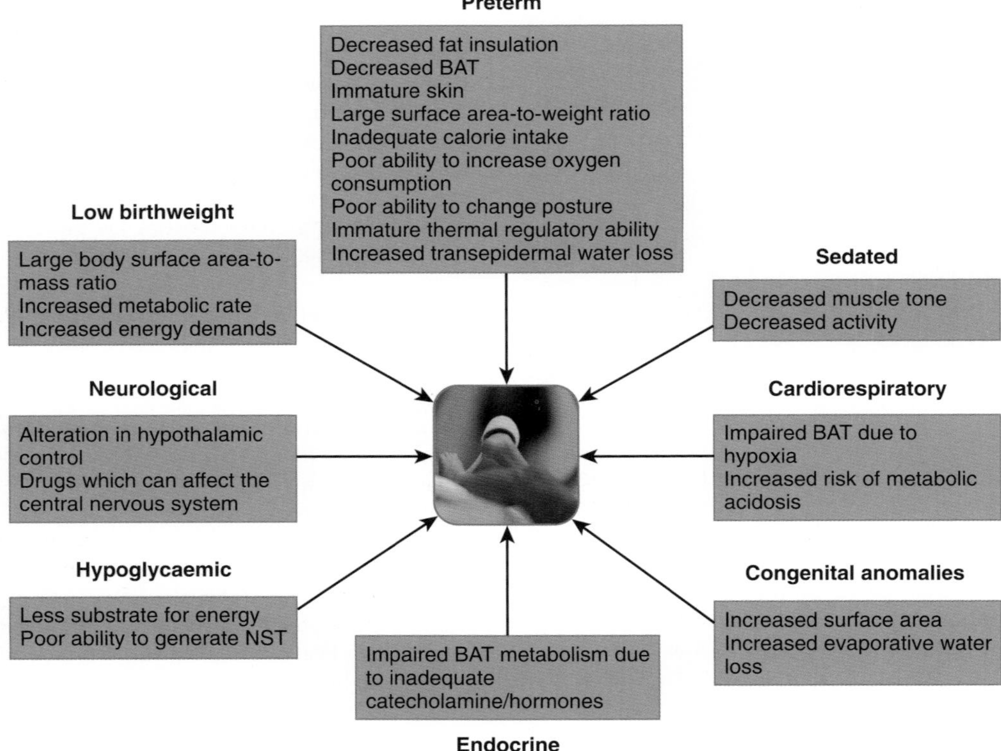

FIGURE 8.6 **Neonates at increased risk of hypothermia**

(Brand & Shippey, 2021). Procedures to rewarm a cold neonate should be commenced immediately. The following guidelines (Morassutti et al., 2015) should be used in conjunction with your workplace specific protocols.

Rewarming the mildly hypothermic neonate (36°C to 36.4°C):

- feed (if appropriate)
- place skin to skin, the head covered with a warm hat and a warm wrap/blanket covering them and the parent
- recheck axillary temperature every 30 minutes and document as required.

Rewarming the moderately hypothermic neonate (32°C to 35.9°C):

- use the appropriate warming device available in your workplace – incubator, radiant warmer, warming mattresses (see equipment section)
- as recommended, set the temperature of the warming device 1°C above the neonate's skin temperature
- use a skin sensor and peripheral temperature sensor (if possible) to continuously measure the temperature
- monitor and document temperature every 30 minutes
- note that a set temperature of 36°C should provide a heat-gaining environment for neonates with a skin temperature of 35°C
- do not increase the incubator temperature faster than 0.5°C every 15–30 minutes (if the temperature remains suboptimal)
- commence humidity if temperature less than 35°C
- measure oxygen saturations (hypothermic neonates are sometimes hypoxic)
- check blood glucose levels (metabolic stress may induce hypoglycaemia) (Blackburn, 2017).

Hyperthermia

Hyperthermia (an axillary temperature of greater than 37.5°C) is usually caused by being born to a pyrexial mother or, more frequently, due to iatrogenic reasons such as overwrapping, positioning a neonate in an incubator in direct sunlight, placing a neonate in an incubator where the air temperature is too high, phototherapy, or when the skin temperature sensor has become detached and the servo-control system has increased temperature output. Drug withdrawal, sepsis, CNS injury and medication side effects (e.g. prostaglandin) can also cause hyperthermia in the neonate (Brand & Shippey, 2021). Similar to hypothermia, hyperthermia also increases the risk for neonatal mortality and morbidity in newborns of all gestational ages (Trevisanuto et al., 2018). McCarthy and O'Donnell (2021) found that axillary temperature measurements were less sensitive at detecting hyperthermia than hypothermia; however, frequent per axilla temperature monitoring remains the key to early detection of any thermal instability.

When overheated, hypothalamic receptors sense the increase in body temperature above the 'set point' and send out signals to activate heat dissipation (Blackburn, 2017). Vasodilation occurs in an attempt to increase heat transfer to the environment, by increasing the blood flow to the extensive capillary and venous network. Sweating can occur in term and late preterm neonates of greater than 35 weeks' gestation, thereby increasing heat loss via evaporation. Neonates of less than 35 weeks' gestation have a reduced or no ability to sweat, and a limited ability to vasoconstrict, so it is highly probable that they have a limited ability to vasodilate when too warm (Gardner & Cammack, 2021).

Overheating manifests in the neonate as tachycardia, tachypnoea, restlessness or lethargy, warm skin, flushing and apnoea (Brand & Shippey, 2021). The consequences of hyperthermia are presented in Fig. 8.7, and include hypotension secondary to vasodilation and fluid and electrolyte imbalance secondary to dehydration. Seizures, apnoea, shock, diarrhoea, disseminated intravascular coagulation and renal and hepatic failure will also occur in overheated neonates if their temperature is not regulated to within normal limits (Brand & Shippey, 2021).

The procedure to cool a hyperthermic neonate should be commenced immediately and includes:

- cool slowly by reducing the environmental temperature by 0.5°C every 30 minutes, and measuring and documenting axillary temperatures every 30 minutes
- remove excessive clothes (woollen hat), wraps, blankets and bundling
- consider non-environmental causes such as infection
- if the cot is on air control, check and reduce the set air temperature by no more than 1°C each hour
- check that the servo-controlled system is functioning correctly and that the skin temperature sensor has not become dislodged
- monitor oxygen saturation levels (increase in MR so you may see an increase in oxygen consumption)
- monitor blood pressure (can become hypotensive).

STRATEGIES TO SUPPORT THERMOREGULATION IN NEONATAL CARE

Irrespective of climate or whether born in high-resource or low-resource settings, every neonate requires interventions to support thermoregulation. Neonates in both birth settings (e.g. birthing suites, operating suites, resuscitation areas, in the home) and postnatal care settings (e.g. neonatal and maternity units) are at risk of hypothermia. Hence, providing warmth is a basic need to ensure the wellbeing of all neonates, and it is essential that nurses and midwives react responsively, initiating care within an individualised, developmentally supportive, family-centred care framework.

The following actions for supporting thermal stability need to be applied according to the nurses' and midwives' assessment and interpretation of the clinical status of the neonate:

- Eliminate draughts from fans, air conditioners, open windows and doors (prevents the loss of heat to air currents moving past the body surface, which are dependent on air velocity and temperature – *convection*).
- Increase the temperature of, or warm, birthing rooms and operating theatres for all neonates of less than 35 weeks' gestation to 21–23°C to improve outcomes (Trevisanuto et al., 2018).
- Place the neonate on the mother's abdomen or chest (this transfers heat from the mother's warm skin to the cooler skin surface of the neonate – *conduction*).
- Use a warm towel or cloth to dry the neonate, gently rubbing the head, body, arms and legs (this prevents loss of heat through evaporation of water from the skin – *evaporation*).
- Remove all damp or wet cloths from the neonate.
- Continue skin-to-skin contact between the mother and the neonate, or another family member if the mother is not able to be involved at this time, covering both with warm dry towels or blankets.
- Ensure that the neonate's head is covered with a woollen hat.

Those neonates requiring resuscitation and stabilisation are particularly at risk of hypothermia. Minimising heat loss should include the above, with additional consideration given to:

- warming resuscitation areas and eliminating draughts from this area if possible
- prewarming resuscitation contact surfaces (prevents loss of heat to a cooler object in direct contact with the neonate – *conduction*)
- using a polyethylene (plastic) wrap or bag for preterm neonates of less than 28 weeks' gestation (see Fig. 8.8).

Plastic wraps have been shown to be effective in reducing evaporative heat loss and hypothermia (Travers et al., 2021). These coverings are used to create a microenvironment in an attempt to reduce evaporative heat loss, TEWL and interstitial water loss. The concept is that the neonate's body is not dried (the head is dried), and the trunk and limbs are placed in the wrap, still moist. If access is required to the umbilicus, the goal should be to keep as much of the wrap in place as possible, making a small hole in the wrap near the umbilical area (see Fig. 8.8). Care needs to be taken when instigating a number of interventions as to the potential cumulative effects. Reports of hyperthermia with the use of plastic wraps have been published, although it was not an issue in the randomised controlled trial conducted by Travers et al. (2021).

Positioning and skin-to-skin care

As discussed previously, neonates have a large surface area-to-bodyweight ratio and, therefore, the more extended the neonate, the more surface area is exposed to potential heat losses by conduction, convection, evaporation and radiation. Nesting and positioning the neonate in a flexed

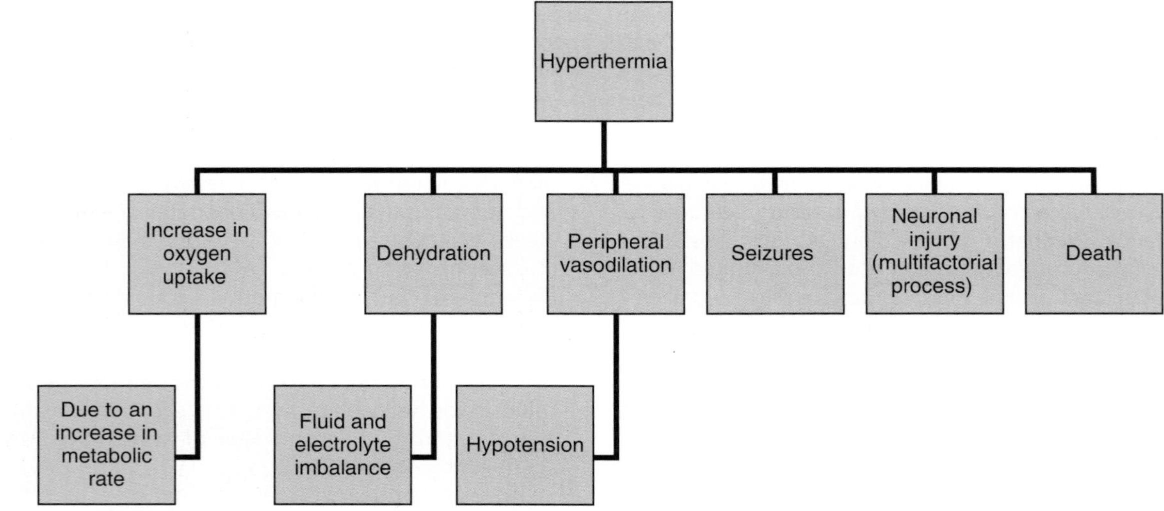

FIGURE 8.7 **Consequences of hyperthermia in the neonate**

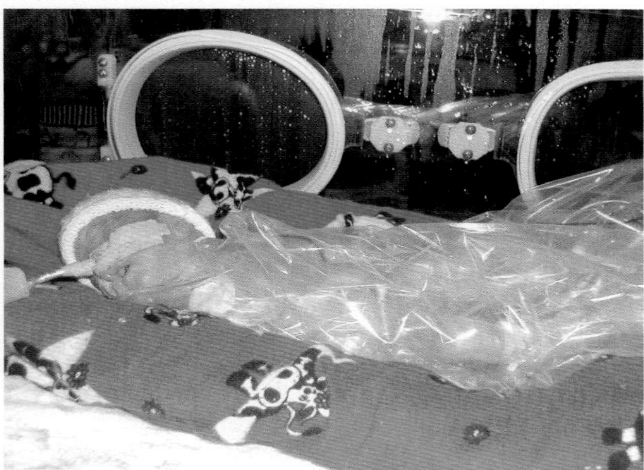

FIGURE 8.8 **Neonate in a plastic wrap**

position reduces surface area exposure and thereby assists thermoregulation (McCall et al., 2018).

Skin-to-skin or kangaroo care has been shown to be effective and life saving in both high- and low-resource countries (see Evidence-based Practice Research 8.1) and should commence preferably at birth and continue for at least 1 hour. If the neonate has to be separated from the mother for stabilisation, skin-to-skin care should be commenced after stabilisation, and preferably within the first 24 hours of life (Ramani et al., 2018).

EVIDENCE-BASED PRACTICE RESEARCH 8.1

'Kangaroo care' was a concept first implemented in Bogota, Colombia, in 1978 in response to a shortage of incubators, where neonates were placed on their mother's chest to be kept warm. The World Health Organization now includes the provision of kangaroo mother care (KMC) in its 10-step 'warm chain' guidelines (Nyandiko et al., 2021). Despite the success of KMC in reducing the risks of hypothermia and hence mortality in low birthweight stable neonates, especially in low-resource settings, it requires intensive staffing support, resources and parent participation. NICU infants should be continuously monitored during KMC, and infants who need a high-humidity environment may need to have KMC delayed until they are more stable (Hodson, 2018).

Equipment

Incubators and radiant warmers

Incubators are set to servo-control or **air control**, adjusting heat and maintaining humidity parameters, to create a microclimate for neonates requiring intensive or high-dependency care. These 'convective' incubators draw room air in via a filter system, and warm and circulate the air around the incubator. Newer incubators are 'double walled', with an inner wall of plastic that sits securely on both long sides of the incubator. This allows for air to circulate between the outer and inner walls, thereby reducing heat losses. In addition, many newer incubators have an 'air curtain' so that, when the incubator sides are opened, a 'curtain' of warm air is circulated from the bottom towards the top of the incubator, preventing significant heat loss from within the incubator. With advancements in technology and design of incubators, the humidity delivery systems are computer controlled by the selection of a humidity percentage on the control panel of the incubator. Water is placed in the purpose-built water reservoir in the incubator and the circulating air is actively humidified via vaporisation.

Likewise, radiant warmers allow the provision of a thermoneutral environment. A perceived benefit of these open-care systems is that they provide easier access to the neonate, not only for provision of care, but also for enhancing family engagement without the barrier created by the closed incubator environment. Radiant warmers increase insensible water losses by 40–50% compared with incubators; however, the use of polyurethane bags or wraps during resuscitation of the preterm infant below 30 weeks' gestation can ameliorate these effects, and still allow access for resuscitative interventions (Gardner & Cammack, 2021). A number of studies have demonstrated potential limitations, including a lack of consistency in the amount of heat generated between commercially available radiant warmers and a lack of consensus on the temperature of exposure and the level of radiant warmer power needed (Trevisanuto et al., 2018). The performance of the heater can also be affected by the environmental temperature, humidity and air movement surrounding its location (Trevisanuto et al., 2018).

Warming mattresses

A number of different transwarmer devices such as heated thermal pads or heated water-filled mattresses are available as an alternative to incubators or to assist neonates with the transition to open cots, or when caring for the infant in surgery (see Evidence-based Practice Research 8.2). Exothermic chemical gel mattresses are also an available source of heat for use in transporting preterm infants between the birth suite and the neonatal nursery and during retrievals. However, caution is advised around the use of such mattresses, as a number of studies have demonstrated an increased risk of hyperthermia (Trevisanuto et al., 2018).

EVIDENCE-BASED PRACTICE RESEARCH 8.2

A Cochrane review (McCall et al., 2018) presents the evidence from three studies involving 157 infants comparing skin-to-skin care or thermal mattress with routine care; and from four studies involving 196 infants comparing a thermal mattress with a plastic wrap or bag; and plastic bags and thermal mattresses versus plastic bags only. The authors reported that skin-to-skin care 'was shown to be effective in reducing risk of hypothermia when compared with conventional incubator care for infants with birthweight ≥1200 and ≤2199 grams' (McCall et al., 2018, p. 2). Transwarmer mattresses 'significantly kept infants ≤1500 grams warmer and reduced the incidence of hypothermia' (p. 67), as did plastic wraps or bags on admission to the NICU. Caution is required and infants need to be monitored closely for hyperthermia, particularly if a combination of interventions is used such as a plastic wrap and warming mattress.

EVIDENCE BASE FOR THERMOREGULATION PRACTICES

Plastic coverings and wraps

A plastic bag/wrap applied immediately after birth reduces evaporative and conductive heat losses in infants <28 weeks' gestation and is now recommended by the World Health Organization and the International Liaison Committee on Resuscitation (ILCOR) (Travers et al., 2021). However, they are not without risks, and further research is needed to support their use. Despite the inclusion of 18 studies investigating the use of plastic wraps or bags in the updated Cochrane review (McCall et al., 2018), the evidence that plastic wraps or bags significantly reduced important outcomes such as in-hospital deaths or other major morbidities remains insufficient. While plastic wraps or bags reduced hypothermia, their use was also associated with increased episodes of hyperthermia.

Humidity

As early as 1933 the literature reported that high ambient humidity improved preterm neonates' survival rates (Glass & Valdez, 2020). Evaporative heat losses are the largest source of heat loss for preterm and low birthweight neonates, where 'for each millilitre of water that evaporates from the skin, 560 calories of heat is lost' (McCall et al., 2018, p. 8). By increasing the water content in the air of the incubator, evaporative heat and water losses are reduced and temperature stability achieved (Gardner & Cammack, 2021). Blackburn (2017, p. 492) stated that 'an ambient humidity of 85% eliminates almost all evaporative losses'. Brand and Shippey (2021) recommend starting at 70% or greater for the first 7 days of life and then gradually decreasing the humidity to 50% until the infant is either 28 days old or 30–32 weeks' gestation.

Glass and Valdez (2020) published a recent systematic review in which 12 studies were included; however, they found no studies conducted since 2014, hence the conclusions remain unchanged from that of Knobel, who in 2014 suggested that large randomised controlled trials are still needed.

Transition from incubator to open cot

For many years the determination for well, stable preterm neonates to transfer from an incubator or radiant warmer to an open cot was based upon reaching the arbitrary weight of 1800 g.

Berger et al. (2014, cited in Hobson 2018) stated that preterm neonates can be safely transferred to open cots at 1500 g, without adverse effects to thermal stability and weight gain. Hodson (2018) further recommends that infants of 1500 g can be transferred to open cots if the room temperature is 26–28°C.

INVOLVING THE FAMILY IN BEST THERMOREGULATION PRACTICE

It is imperative that families are partners in the care of their infant, and that they receive information about why neonates cannot maintain their temperature and prevention strategies for avoiding hypothermia and overheating. Families should be engaged in best thermoregulation practices while in hospital and in preparation for the home environment (see Family-centred Care 8.1). Parental education should include the following factors:

- Skin-to-skin contact is the most beneficial in keeping the neonate warm.
- A neonate's head is large compared with the rest of the body and is a source of a large amount of heat loss.
- The head can be kept covered with a woollen or cotton hat to stop heat loss when it is safe to do so (e.g. neonate awake, outside, while in hospital). At home, safe-sleeping practices should be practised (e.g. sleep baby with head and face uncovered).
- Prolonged periods of having the neonate undressed or exposed should be avoided.
- Different climates and times of day affect the way the neonate should be dressed and wrapped. The neonate requires one additional layer of clothing than parents need to remain comfortable.
- Prolonged bath times should be avoided.
- The water temperature for bathing should be 38°C to 40°C and the room temperature between 26°C and 27°C (Association of Women's Health, Obstetric and Neonatal Nurses, 2018). The bath temperature should be tested with the elbow or wrist and should not feel hot to the skin.
- The neonate should be kept away from draughts from air conditioners, fans, windows and doors.
- An overhead heater may be required if the maternity or neonatal environment is cool.

FAMILY-CENTRED CARE 8.1

Bathing is a significant risk factor for hypothermia, particularly in the early neonatal period. But bathing is an important time as it provides an opportunity for families to bond with and interact with their baby. Teaching parents to bath their baby, while proactively controlling environmental factors to minimise heat loss during bathing, teaches parents how to minimise the risk of hypothermia and significantly benefits the parents and their infant (ACNN, 2019; COINN, 2019; ICM, 2019; NNCA, 2015).

CASE STUDY 8.1

A full-term neonate, Adam, was born to Rachel by spontaneous vaginal delivery. He was in a good condition at birth, with Apgar scores of 9^1 and 10^5, and required no resuscitation. Rachel was gravida 4, para 3 and her serology was unremarkable. Adam was breastfed and then transferred to the postnatal ward with Rachel and her partner Joel. At 12 hours of age, Adam was bathed by his parents. A few hours later, Rachel noticed that Adam was quiet, he didn't want to feed, he was jittery and he felt cold to the touch. The midwife measured his per axilla temperature with a digital thermometer, which had a reading of 35.3°C.

1. Why might Adam be hypothermic?
2. Why is he quiet and not feeding well?
3. Why might Adam be 'jittery'?

Adam was subsequently admitted to the neonatal unit. On admission his oxygen saturations were 95%, he had a respiratory rate of 65 breaths per minute and his per axilla temperature was 35°C.

4. What are your nursing care priorities?
5. What actions will you take to help Adam increase his body temperature?
6. What education should be conveyed to the parents on thermoregulation of the neonate?

CONCLUSION

All neonates, but more so those of lower gestational age or weight, are challenged by the demands of heat production and, consequently, balancing heat loss. Given the potentially detrimental consequences of hypo- and hyperthermia, close monitoring of the thermoregulatory needs of the neonate is essential. Maintaining an NTE should be the aim at all times. This chapter highlights the importance of understanding the mechanisms of heat transfer and how these can be managed. The importance of avoiding neonatal cold stress to prevent health problems and increased morbidity and mortality is stressed. Temperature is one of the vital signs that needs ongoing assessment, prompt recognition and subsequent action to correct emerging thermoregulatory problems to prevent harmful consequences. Neonatal nurses/midwives have primary responsibility for the maintenance of the thermal stability of neonates in their care.

Recommended Reading

Glass, L., & Valdez, A. (2020). Preterm infant incubator humidity levels: a systematic review. *Advances in Neonatal Care, 21*(4), 297–307. doi: 1097/ANC.0000000000000791.

McCall, E., Alderdice, F., Halliday, H., Vohra S., & Johnston L. (2018). Interventions to prevent hypothermia at birth in preterm and/or low birthweight infants. *Cochrane Database of Systematic Reviews, 2*, CD004210. doi: 10.1002/14651858.CD004210.pub5.

Pinheiro, J. M. (2018). Preventing hypothermia in preterm newborns – simple principles for a complicated task. *Journal of Pediatrics (Rio Journal), 94*, 337–339.

References/Acknowledgements

Aherne, W., & Hull, D. (1964). The site of heat production in the newborn infant. *Proceedings of the Royal Society of Medicine, 57*, 1172.

Association of Women's Health, Obstetric and Neonatal Nurses. (2018). *Neonatal skin care evidence based clinical practice guideline* (4th ed.). Washington, DC: Association of Women's Health, Obstetric and Neonatal Nurses.

Australian College of Neonatal Nursing (ACNN). (2019). *Standards for practice* (4th ed.). Camperdown, NSW: ACNN. <https://www.acnn.org.au/resources/resources/ACNN-Standards-for-Practice-4th-Ed.pdf> (Accessed 2 March 2022).

Blackburn, S. T. (2017). *Maternal, foetal, and neonatal physiology: a clinical perspective* (5th ed.). Melbourne, Vic: Elsevier Australia.

Brand, M. C., & Shippey, H. A. (2021). Thermoregulation. In: AWHONN, M. T. Verklan, M. Walden, & S. Forest (Eds.). *Core curriculum for neonatal intensive care nursing* (6th ed., pp. 86–98). St Louis, MO: Elsevier.

Cavallin, F., Calgaro, S., Brugnolaro, V., Seni, A., Hussein A., Muhelo, et al. (2020). Impact of temperature change from admission to day one on neonatal mortality in a low-resource setting. *BMC Pregnancy and Childbirth, 20*(1), 1–646. doi: 10.1186/s12884-020-03343-7.

Chow, S., Creighton, P., Chambers, G., & Lui, K. (2020). *2018 Report of the Australian and New Zealand Neonatal Network*. Sydney, NSW: ANZNN. <https://www.anznn.net/Portals/0/AnnualReports/Report%20of%20the%20Australian%20and%20New%20Zealand%20Neonatal%20Network%202018.pdf> (Accessed 2 March 2022).

Council of International Neonatal Nurses (COINN). (2019). International neonatal nursing competency framework. *Journal of Neonatal Nursing, 25*, 258–264.

Demtse, A. G., Pfister, R. E., Nigussie, A. K., McClure, E. M., Ferede, Y. G., Tazu Bonger, Z., et al. (2020). Hypothermia in preterm newborns: impact on survival. *Global Pediatric Health, 7*, 1–8. doi: 10.1177/2333794X20957655.

Douglas, C. (2020). Vital signs: using a primary survey approach for patient assessment. In: J. Crisp, D. Clint, G. Rebeiro, & D. Waters (Eds.), *Potter & Perry's fundamentals of nursing – ANZ edition* (6th ed., pp. 326–371). Melbourne, Vic: Elsevier.

Gardner, S. L., & Cammack, B. H. (2021). Heat balance. In: S. L. Gardner, B. S. Carter, M. I. Enzman-Hines, & S. Niermeyer (Eds.), *Merenstein & Gardner's handbook of neonatal intensive care: an interprofessional approach* (9th ed., pp. 105–125). St Louis, MO: Elsevier.

Glass, L., & Valdez, A. (2020). Preterm infant incubator humidity levels: a systematic review. *Advances in Neonatal Care, 21*(4), 297–307. doi: 10.1097/ANC.0000000000000791.

Hodson, W. (2018). Temperature regulation. In: C. A. Gleason & S. E. Juul (Eds.), *Avery's diseases of the newborn* (10th ed., pp. 361–367). Philadelphia, PA: Elsevier.

International Confederation of Midwives (ICM). (2019). *Essential competencies for midwifery practice: 2019 update*. The Hague, Netherlands: ICM. <https://www.internationalmidwives.org/our-work/policy-and-practice/essential-competencies-for-midwifery-practice.html> (Accessed 2 March 2022).

Jastroch, M., Polymeropoulos, E. T. & Gaudry, M. J. (2021). Pros and cons for the evidence of adaptive non-shivering thermogenesis in marsupials. *Journal of Comparative Physiology B, 191*(6), 1085–1095. doi: 10.1007/s00360-021-01362-0.

Lubkowska, A., Szymański, S., & Chudecka, M. (2019). Surface body temperature of full-term healthy newborns immediately after birth – pilot study. *International Journal of Environmental Research and Public Health, 16*(8), 1312. doi: 10.3390/ijerph16081312.

McCall, E., Alderdice, F., Halliday, H., Vohra S., & Johnston L. (2018). Interventions to prevent hypothermia at birth in preterm and/or low birthweight infants. *Cochrane Database of Systematic Reviews, 2*, CD004210. doi: 10.1002/14651858.CD004210.pub5.

McCarthy, L. K., & O'Donnell, C. P. F. (2021). Comparison of rectal and axillary temperature measurements in preterm newborns. *Archives of Disease in Childhood. Fetal and Neonatal Edition, 106*(5), 509–513. doi: 10.1136/archdischild-2020-320627.

Morassutti, R. F., Cavaliin, F., Zaramella, P., Bortolus, R., Parotto, M., & Trevisanuto, D. (2015). Association of rewarming rate on neonatal outcomes in ELBW infants with hypothermia. *Journal of Pediatrics, 167*, 557–561. doi: 10.1015/j.jpeds.2015.06.008.

Nadkarni, K. P., Mayo, Z., Laux, J. P., McRea, A., Angelillo, D., Meitzen, R., et al. (2021). Axillary thermometry demonstrates greater reliability compared with rectal thermometry in healthy neonates. *Clinical Pediatrics, 60*(6–7), 298–303. doi: 10.1177/00099228211005293.

National Institute for Health and Care Excellence (NICE). (2019). *Fever in under 5's: assessment and initial management. NICE guideline [NG 143]*. <http://www.nice.org.uk/guidance/ng143> (Accessed 2 March 2022).

Neonatal Nurses College Aotearoa (NNCA). (2015). *NNCA standards for neonatal nursing practice*. Wellington, NZ: New Zealand Nurses Organisation.

Nyandiko, W. M., Kiptoon, P. & Lubuya, F. A. (2021). Neonatal hypothermia and adherence to World Health Organization thermal care guidelines among newborns at Moi Teaching and Referral Hospital, Kenya. *PLoS One, 16*(3), e0248838. doi: 10.1371/journal.pone.0248838.

Osilla, E. V., Marsidi, J. L., & Sharma, S. (2021). Physiology, temperature regulation. In: *StatPearls*. Treasure Island, FL: StatPearls Publishing. <https://www.ncbi.nlm.nih.gov/books/NBK507838/> (Accessed 2 March 2022).

Pinheiro, J. M. (2018). Preventing hypothermia in preterm newborns – simple principles for a complicated task. *Journal of Pediatrics (Rio Journal), 94*, 337–339.

Ramani, M., Choe, E. A., Major, M., Newton, R., Mwenechanya, M., Travers, C. P., et al. (2018). Kangaroo mother care for the prevention of neonatal hypothermia: a randomised controlled trial in term neonates. *Archives of Disease in Childhood, 103*(5), 492–497. doi: 10.1136/archdischild-2017-313744.

Travers, C. P., Ramani, M., Gentle, S. J., Schuyler, A., Brown, C., Dills, M. M., et al. (2021). Early skin-to-skin care with a polyethylene bag for neonatal hypothermia: a randomized clinical trial. *Journal of Pediatrics, 231*, 55–60.e1. doi: 10.1016/j.jpeds.2020.12.064.

Trevisanuto, D., Testoni, D. & de Almeida, M. F. (2018). Maintaining normothermia: why and how? *Seminars in Fetal and Neonatal Medicine, 23*(5), 333–339.

Wassink, G., Davidson, J. O., Dhillon, S. K., Zhou, K., Bennet, L., Thoresen, M., et al. (2019). Therapeutic hypothermia in neonatal hypoxic-ischemic encephalopathy. *Current Neurology and Neuroscience Reports, 19*(2), 2. doi: 10.1007/s11910-019-0916-0.

CHAPTER 9

CARE OF THE NEONATE WITH A RESPIRATORY DISORDER

VICTORIA KAIN AND TRUDI MANNIX[a]

Learning objectives

After reading this chapter you will be able to:

- understand respiratory embryology and the stages of fetal lung development
- understand the aetiology, pathophysiology, diagnosis and clinical presentation and the medical, pharmacological and neonatal nursing and midwifery management of the common respiratory disorders of the neonate
- undertake a systematic approach to a neonatal respiratory assessment
- analyse and interpret respiratory-related laboratory, imaging and non-invasive respiratory monitoring
- describe the ventilator technologies that are utilised to support a neonate with a respiratory illness.

Key words, terms, abbreviations

Australian and New Zealand Neonatal Network (ANZNN)
blood oxygen saturation levels (SpO_2)
carbon dioxide (CO_2)
chronic lung disease (CLD)
continuous positive airway pressure (CPAP)
endotracheal tube (ETT)
extracorporeal membrane oxygenation (ECMO)
functional residual capacity (FRC)
high-flow nasal cannula (HFNC)
high-frequency jet ventilation (HFJV)
high-frequency oscillatory ventilation (HFOV)
inhaled nitric oxide (iNO)
intermittent positive pressure ventilation (IPPV)
meconium-stained amniotic fluid (MSAF) aspiration
minimally invasive surfactant therapy (MIST)
oxygen (O_2)
oxygenation
partial arterial pressure of carbon dioxide ($PaCO_2$)
partial arterial pressure of oxygen (PaO_2)
partial pressure of carbon dioxide (PCO_2)
partial pressure of oxygen (PO_2)
peak inspiratory pressure (PIP)
positive end expiratory pressure (PEEP)
pulmonary interstitial emphysema (PIE)
respiratory distress syndrome (RDS)
tidal volume (TV)
transcutaneous monitoring (TCM)
transient tachypnoea of the newborn (TTNB)
ventilation

[a]The authors would like to acknowledge Melissah Burnett and Sara Willmore, co-authors of this chapter in the 1st edition of this book.

INTRODUCTION

In 2018, 97.5% of all neonates registered on the **Australian and New Zealand Neonatal Network (ANZNN)** (which incorporates all level 3 and higher neonatal intensive care units and a number of level 2 units) received some form of respiratory support. **Respiratory distress syndrome (RDS)** remained the most common indication for respiratory support at 41.5%. Non-specific respiratory distress accounted for 34.4% of babies, surgery for 3.8%, while **meconium-stained amniotic fluid (MSAF) aspiration** and congenital anomaly each accounted for 3.3%. For neonates at 37 weeks' gestation or less, RDS remained the most common indication for respiratory support, at 59.7%. Non-specific respiratory distress accounted for 46.6% of neonates, and MSAF aspiration accounted for 9.0% (Chow et al., 2020).

These statistics indicate that respiratory compromise is responsible for the majority of admissions to the neonatal unit. As such, neonatal nurses/midwives need to be familiar with respiratory disease processes to provide effective and appropriate care to sick neonates.

This chapter will discuss lung embryology, pathophysiology, diagnosis and management of common respiratory conditions, as well as modes of respiratory support.

EMBRYOLOGICAL DEVELOPMENT OF THE RESPIRATORY SYSTEM

The embryonic lung does not play a role in gas exchange in utero but is responsible for the production of some amniotic fluid. The lungs develop from 28 days' gestation through to childhood in five distinct stages: embryonic, pseudoglandular, canalicular, saccular (terminal sac) and alveolar (Table 9.1).

The lung epithelium is derived from the gut and as such is endodermal in origin, as the bud develops into the surrounding mesoderm, which gives rise to the cartilage and smooth muscle of the respiratory conduction pathways. At approximately 5 weeks' gestation, the tracheal bud bifurcates into lateral outgrowths (the bronchial buds), which give rise to the left and right main bronchi. From 6 weeks' gestation, respiratory development enters the pseudoglandular stage, so called because, histologically, the lungs resemble a gland during this stage (Leslie & Wick, 2018).

It is during this stage that lung-specific type II alveolar cells (pneumocytes) begin to appear, the cells that will produce surfactant. By 16 weeks, the entire respiratory tree has formed and the canalicular stage begins, which leads to the development of the terminal bronchioles, the alveolar ducts and the terminal sacs. From the last trimester, whole clusters of sacs form on the terminal bronchioles, which represent the last subdivision of the passages that supply air. In the saccular phase, the last generation of air spaces in the respiratory part of the bronchial tree are formed. At the end of each respiratory tract passage, smooth-walled sacculi form, coated with type I and type II pneumocytes. The alveoli are primitive at this time and, consequently, extrauterine life is not possible before 22 weeks. It is during the saccular stage (also known as the terminal sac period), from 25 weeks to birth, that many neonates cared for in the neonatal unit are delivered (Fig. 9.1). Neonates born prematurely during the late canalicular period have immaturely structured airways and surfactant deficiency, as the type II cells are only just beginning to develop (Jackson, 2018).

TABLE 9.1 **Stages of fetal lung development**

Stage	Fetal time period	Development event
Embryonic	3–7 weeks	• Respiratory bud forms • Initial branching of bronchial tree • Trachea and larynx form
Pseudoglandular	6–16 weeks	• Branching of the bronchial tree continues • Development of the terminal bronchioles – ongoing • Closure of the pleuroperitoneal folds
Canalicular	16–24 weeks	• Development of respiratory bronchioles – formation of some alveolar ducts and terminal ducts • Lung tissue vascularisation • Gas exchange occurs at ≈24 weeks
Saccular (terminal sac)	24–28 weeks	• Terminal sacs become abundant • Lung epithelium thins • Development of type I and II pneumocytes
Alveolar	36 weeks–≈3 years	• 'True' alveoli develop and increase in number • Secondary septation

Source: adapted from Rubarth and Quinn (2015).

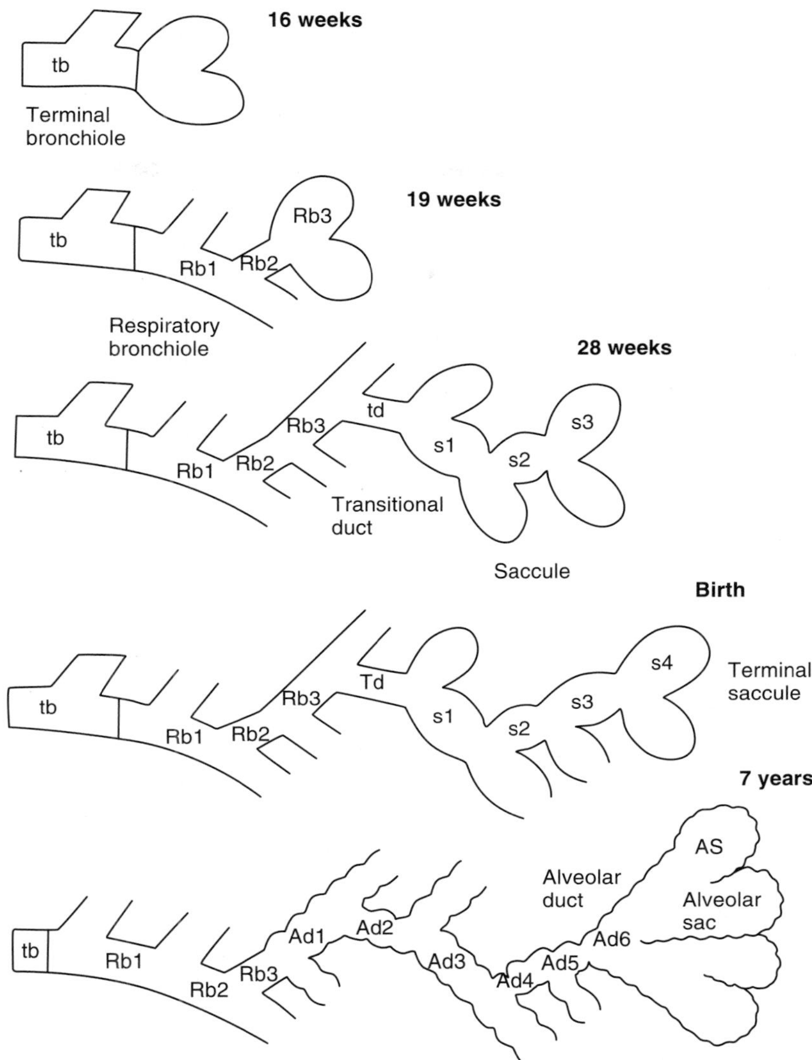

FIGURE 9.1 **Embryological development of the fetal lung into childhood**

Source: modified from Dilly (1984). © Mark Hill. <https://embryology.med.unsw.edu.au/embryology/images/4/43/Lung_alveoli_development_cartoon.jpg>.

SIGNS AND SYMPTOMS OF RESPIRATORY DISEASE

Regardless of underlying respiratory aetiology, there are four aspects that should be considered when evaluating the neonate for signs and symptoms of respiratory distress: clinical signs of respiratory distress, blood chemistry, chest radiography and basic pulmonary physiology (Gleason & Juul, 2018).

In terms of the clinical signs of respiratory distress, a comprehensive overview of respiratory assessment is provided in Chapter 3. Respiratory rate, retraction of the chest wall, skin colour and presence of grunting and air entry into the lungs should all be assessed by the neonatal nurse/midwife during the evaluation. Tachypnoea is a classic sign of respiratory distress and results from a compensatory reaction to hypoxia; chest wall retraction, grunting and poor airway entry, however, are indicative of abnormal lung mechanics. Grunting is a sound produced on expiration through partially closed vocal cords, in an attempt to maintain **functional residual capacity (FRC)** and prevent alveolar atelectasis (Martin, 2021a). The presence of cyanosis might be either central or peripheral. Central cyanosis is most often due to right-to-left cardiopulmonary shunting, while peripheral cyanosis beyond 24 hours of life is an indicator of poor tissue **oxygenation** and might be seen in neonates with acidosis, heart failure, shock or hypothermia (Gleason & Juul, 2018).

CLINICAL PRACTICE 9.1

The Silverman–Anderson Index is an assessment scoring system that evaluates five criteria of the work of breathing and assigns a numerical score for each parameter (Silverman & Andersen, 1956).

Each category is scored as '0' for normal, '1' for moderate impairment or '2' for severe impairment.

Parameters assessed include retractions of the upper chest, lower chest and xiphoid, nasal flaring and expiratory grunt.

Neonates who are breathing normally should have a cumulative score of 0, whereas critically ill and severely depressed neonates with a respiratory illness will have scores closer to 10 (Fig. 9.2).

REFLECTION

Consider the neonates you have previously cared for with respiratory distress. Reflect upon the clinical signs and symptoms that you observed.

OXYGENATION IN THE NEONATE

Oxygen consumption is typically higher in a neonate than an adult, as reflected by an increased respiratory rate and higher metabolic rate resulting from the additional work required due to the neonate's less compliant lungs.

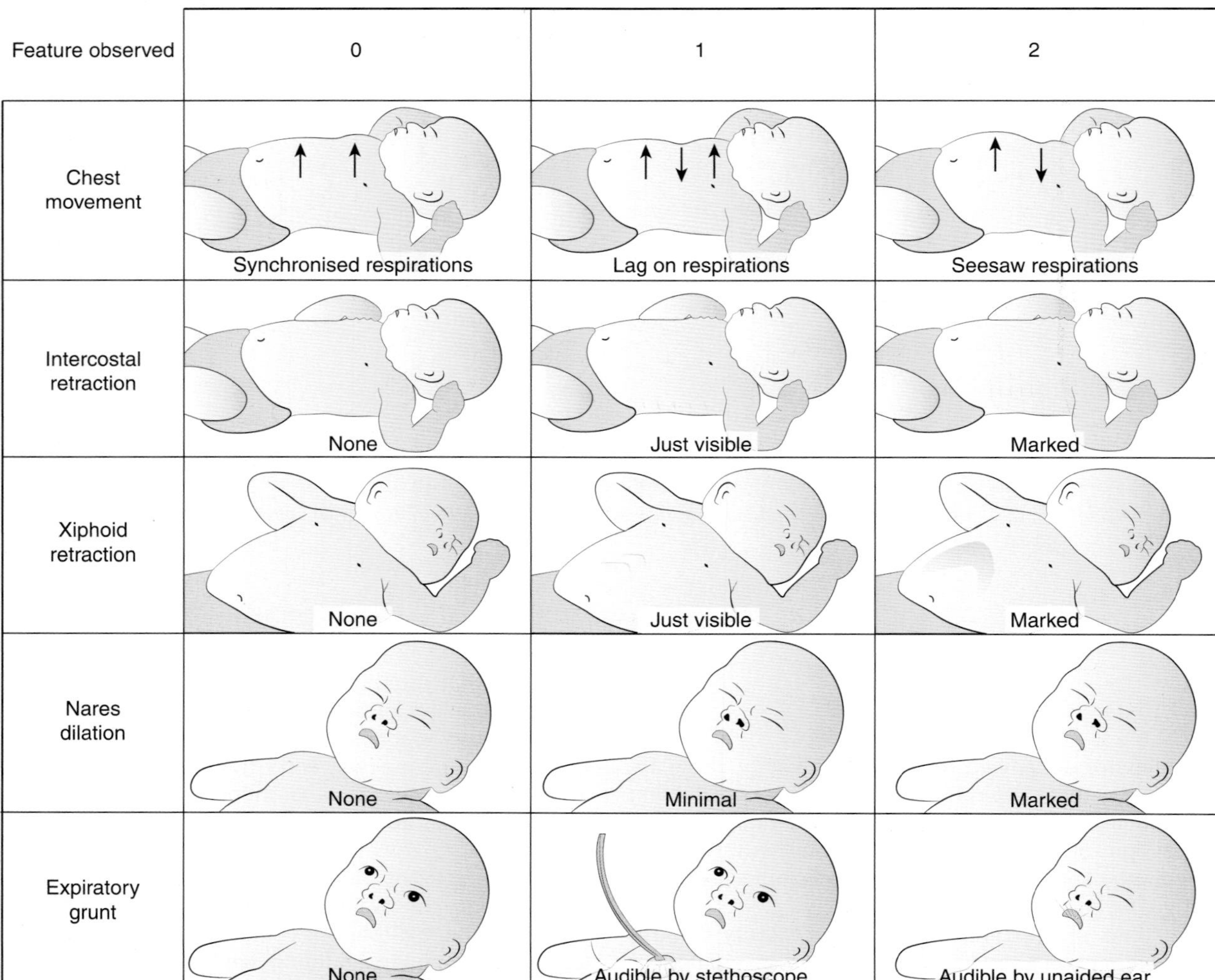

FIGURE 9.2 **Grading of neonatal respiratory distress using the Silverman–Anderson Index**
Source: adapted from Silverman and Andersen (1956).

Tissues require **oxygen (O_2)** for survival and, at a cellular level, individual cells take up O_2 from their environment continuously to support aerobic metabolism. Oxygen is essential for the production of adenosine triphosphate (ATP), a molecule that stores and releases energy. Without ATP, anaerobic metabolism occurs, which produces lactic acid leading to metabolic acidosis (Sunil et al., 2017).

Delivery of O_2 to the tissues and cells is dependent on adequate pulmonary and alveolar **ventilation**, gas exchange and circulatory distribution (cardiac output). Tissue hypoxia is defined as arterial hypoxaemia and/or the failure of the O_2 haemoglobin transport system. Low content of O_2 in inspired air, alveolar hypotension, ventilation perfusion (*V/Q*) mismatch (explained later in this chapter) and right-to-left shunting can cause arterial hypoxaemia. Inadequate tissue perfusion with low blood volume or hyperviscosity, low haemoglobin concentration, abnormal oxyhaemoglobin dissociation (also explained later in this chapter), acid–base imbalance and temperature are all contributing factors.

The oxygen cascade

The oxygen cascade is the process by which oxygen is transported from the atmosphere to the mitochondria in cells (Fig. 9.3). The distribution of oxygen to systemic tissues is based on the passive movement of gas along decreasing partial pressure gradients, with the **partial pressure of oxygen (PO_2)** falling at each stage in the cascade. The key point to note is that oxygen is required for normal cellular function, and the rate and degree of gas transfer are determined by partial pressure (Tomkins, 2020).

Generally, gases move from an area of high concentration (pressure) to areas of low concentration, as defined by Dalton's law of partial pressures. Oxygen diffuses across an interface until the PO_2 in each area is equal. Oxygen moves along a gradient from a relatively high level in air to the interface levels in the respiratory tract and alveoli, the arterial blood, capillaries and finally the cell. The partial pressure of oxygen (PO_2) reaches the lowest level in the mitochondria (the structures in cells responsible for energy production). This decrease in PO_2 from air to the mitochondrion is known as the oxygen cascade, and any change in oxygenation under pathological circumstances may result in hypoxia. **Carbon dioxide (CO_2)** is transported from cells to tissues and moves similarly along a partial pressure gradient across the same interfaces. CO_2 is excreted as a waste product and carried to the lungs (van Kaam et al., 2021).

The normal process that will allow uptake of O_2 and elimination of CO_2 is dependent upon: adequate uptake in the lung, movement of gas along conducting airways, gas exchange between alveoli and pulmonary capillaries, global delivery from lung to tissue with adequate cardiac output and carrying capacity of O_2 on the haemoglobin molecule, diffusion from capillaries to cells and the cellular use of O_2 (van Kaam et al., 2021).

Ventilation/perfusion (*V/Q*) mismatch

In normal lungs all alveoli would receive an equal distribution of alveolar ventilation, and the pulmonary capillaries that surround different alveoli would receive an equal distribution of cardiac output – that is, ventilation (*V*) and perfusion (*Q*) would be perfectly matched.

The neonatal lung, however, is unique as there may be a marked mismatch between ventilation and perfusion owing to prematurity and/or lung disease as a result of a number of factors including: limited number of alveoli; collapsed, over-distended or damaged alveoli; shunting of blood due to persistent pulmonary hypertension; or shunting through open ducts in the circulation. Adequate pulmonary ventilation does not guarantee adequate cellular oxygenation – for example, in persistent pulmonary hypertension and circulatory collapse states such as shock (Dassios et al., 2017).

Oxygen transport and haemoglobin

Oxygen is transported in the blood bound to haem on the haemoglobin molecule and there is a very small amount dissolved in the plasma (Fig. 9.4).

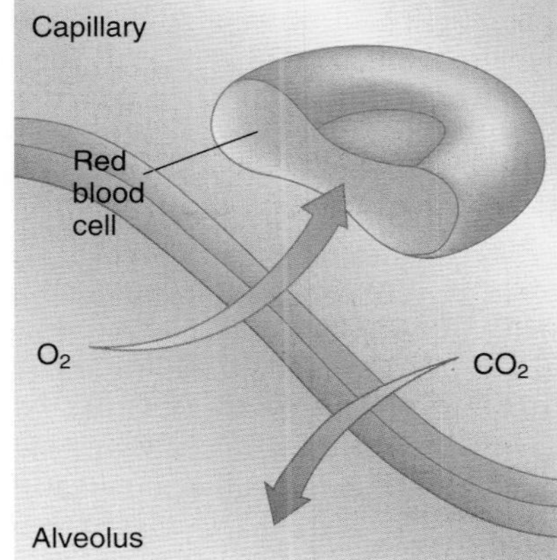

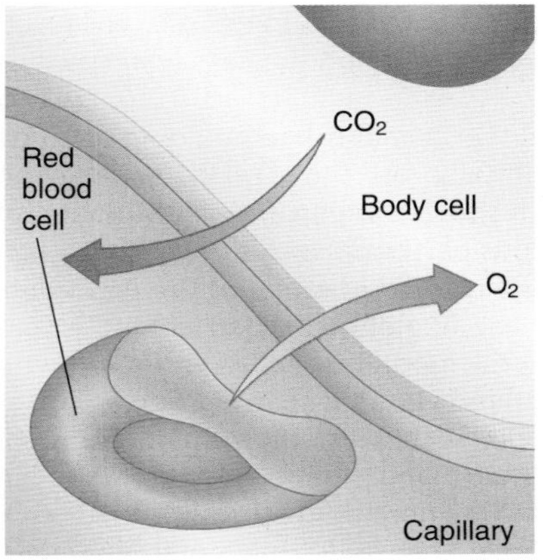

FIGURE 9.3 **The oxygen cascade**

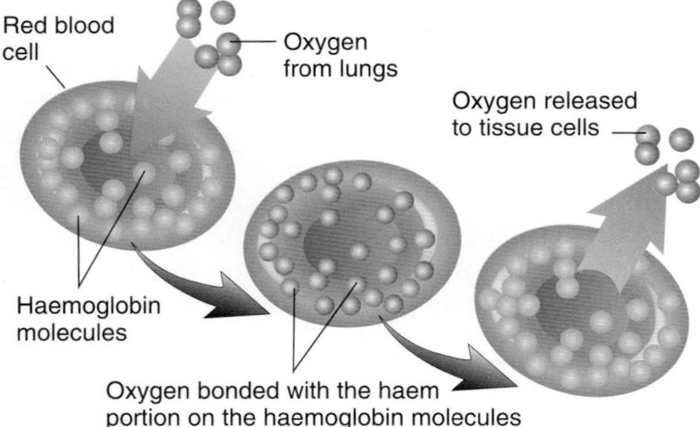

FIGURE 9.4 **Oxygen transport**

Source: Craft, J. (2018). Understanding pathophysiology ANZ. *[ClinicalKey Student]. Figure 24.21.*

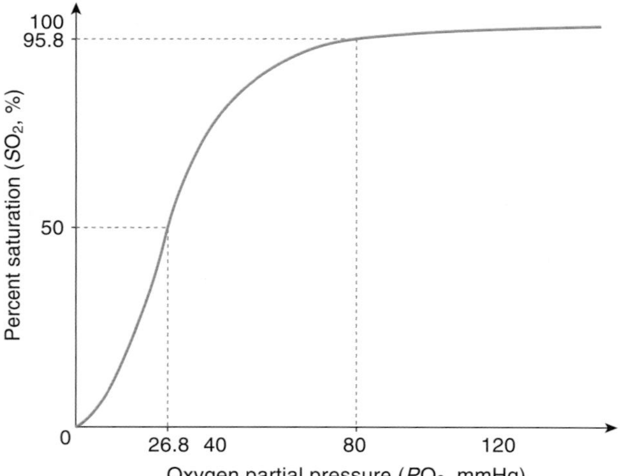

FIGURE 9.5 **Oxygen dissociation curve**

Source: Wikipedia/Diberri. CC BY SA 3.0.

The amount of O_2 carried in blood is not only dependent on the haemoglobin concentration but also on the percentage saturation of the haemoglobin (Verklan & Walden, 2020). Problems of anaemia where there is inadequate haemoglobin to carry O_2 to the cells will result in inadequate levels of O_2 reaching the cells (van Kaam et al., 2021).

The affinity that O_2 has for haemoglobin can be demonstrated graphically as the O_2/Hb dissociation curve (Fig. 9.5), which shows the percentage saturation of haemoglobin at various partial pressures of O_2. This graph is most commonly interpreted in terms of the *P*50 value, an abbreviation for haemoglobin–oxygen affinity – that is, the PO_2 when the haemoglobin is 50% saturated with oxygen (normally 26.8 mmHg, as seen in Fig. 9.5).

Fetal haemoglobin (HbF) is the major form of haemoglobin in utero. The fetus has a high Hb concentration (up to 40% more than an adult), and the O_2 affinity of HbF is higher than adult haemoglobin (HbA), allowing efficient transfer of O_2 across the placenta. The

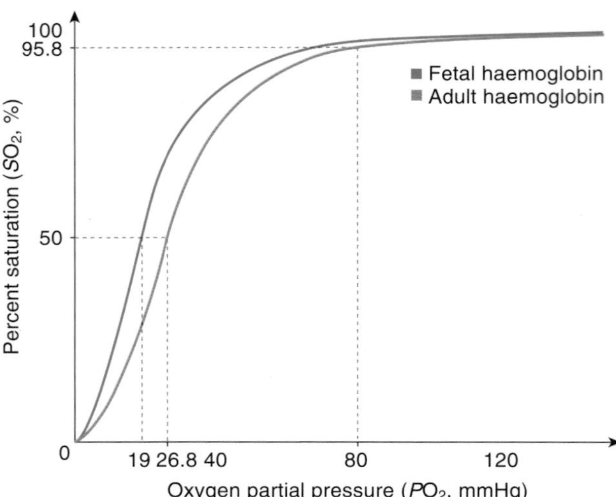

FIGURE 9.6 **Oxygen saturation and partial pressure**

Source: Wikipedia/Diberri. CC BY SA 3.0.

O_2–Hb dissociation curve for HbF is different from that of HbA in that it is shifted to the left (Sunil et al., 2017). The fetus is in a relatively hypoxic environment compensated for by this left shift, where the O_2 haemoglobin saturation is greater at lower partial O_2 pressures and there is a higher percentage of haemoglobin bound to O_2 at a lower O_2 tension (van Kaam et al., 2021).

In Fig. 9.6, the *y*-axis plots percentage of O_2 saturation and the *x*-axis plots the oxygen partial pressure, and it is clear that HbF has a lower *P*50 (18–20 mmHg) than HbA (26.6 mmHg) (van Kaam et al., 2021).

Fetal haemoglobin is not able to deliver O_2 to the tissues as efficiently as HbA because the oxygen–haemoglobin dissociation curve is shifted to the left causing O_2 to be bound more tightly to haemoglobin. Neonates, however, have a higher haemoglobin concentration (40% more than adults), and blood volume per kg, together with an increased cardiac output per kg, compensates for the decreased release of O_2 from haemoglobin to the tissues.

Between 32 and 36 weeks' gestation the production of HbA increases, with a sharp decline in HbF production so that from 32–34/40 weeks there is a mean of 90% HbF, and by term a mean of 70–80% HbF. The *P*50 rapidly increases with a right shift at the same time that the HbF is replaced by HbA, and this ensures efficient oxygenation to the tissues. The gradual decrease in O_2-carrying capacity in the first few months of life as Hb levels fall is thus well tolerated by normal, healthy infants (van Kaam et al., 2021).

In the neonatal period there are multiple factors that affect the affinity for O_2, moving the curve to the right or to the left, including temperature, pH and haemoglobin structure. Hyperthermia, acidosis, hypercarbia and adult haemoglobin may result in a right shift, meaning *more* O_2 is needed to achieve the same saturation. Hypothermia, alkalosis, hypocarbia and fetal haemoglobin may result in a left shift, meaning *less* O_2 is needed to achieve the same saturation (Gardner et al., 2020).

COMMON DISORDERS OF THE RESPIRATORY SYSTEM

Respiratory problems are responsible for the majority of morbidity and mortality in the neonatal period. Globally, 45% of inborn and 80% of neonates transferred to a neonatal unit will experience some degree of respiratory problems at birth. Positive neonatal outcomes correlate with a good understanding of the basic physiology, pathology and biochemistry of common neonatal respiratory disorders.

Respiratory distress syndrome

Aetiology

Respiratory distress syndrome (RDS) is the most common indication for respiratory support in Australia and New Zealand (41.5%) (Chow et al., 2020). RDS, also referred to as hyaline membrane disease, is a disease of prematurity due to the lack of pulmonary surfactant with accompanying functional and structural immaturity of the cardiopulmonary system. The manifestation of the disease process is dependent upon the size and gestation of the neonate and the presence of the clinical signs of respiratory distress. Tachypnoea, shallow breathing, nasal flaring (thought to be a compensatory symptom that increases upper airway diameter and reduces resistance and work of breathing) (Monica et al., 2017), grunting, apnoea and cyanosis may be present shortly after birth, potentially increasing in severity in the first few days of life and typically resolving within a week. Sepsis is the most common differential diagnosis and should always be excluded first but, in general, the symptoms of respiratory distress and chest radiography identifying a 'ground-glass' appearance and small lung volumes either at or shortly after birth will confirm the diagnosis (Jackson, 2018).

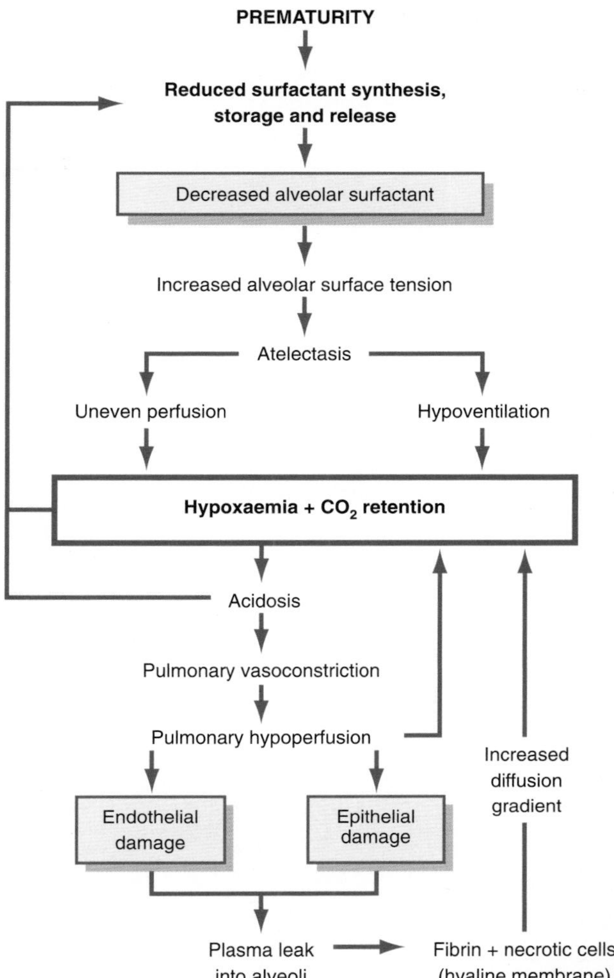

FIGURE 9.7 **Flow chart of RDS pathophysiology**

Source: Mitchell et al. (2017).

Pathophysiology

As stated, RDS is primarily caused by a deficiency of the lipoprotein surfactant (Fig. 9.7).

Surfactant reduces the surface tension within the alveoli, which increases alveolar expansion and optimises gas exchange. Surfactant greatly assists in the maintenance of functional residual capacity (FRC). FRC refers to the volume of air remaining in the lung at the end of expiration to prevent alveolar collapse and provides a balance between the decreasing surface area of the lung on expiration and the re-inflation upon inspiration. The FRC is calculated by adding the residual volume (RV) and expiratory reserve volume (ERV) of the lungs. Pulmonary compliance refers to the elasticity of the lungs and the capability to expand with ventilation. During expiration, compliance is decreased owing to the reduction in alveolar pressure and increased intrapleural pressure. Therefore, a decreased FRC results in reduced lung compliance; hence, surfactant will subsequently improve lung compliance by maintaining the FRC.

Surfactant is composed of phospholipids, neutral lipids (cholesterol) and surfactant proteins – giving it a soapy, slippery texture. During the canalicular phase of respiratory development, type II pneumocytes in the epithelial lining of the alveoli produce and store surfactant from approximately 22 weeks' gestation (Ruaro et al., 2021). In the neonate with RDS, surfactant deficiency greatly reduces lung compliance and increases alveolar collapse (atelectasis). The reduced amount of surfactant can lead to intrapulmonary shunting, which leads to hypoxaemia, hypercarbia and acidosis (Jackson, 2018). Surfactant deficiency also causes lung inflammation and damage to the respiratory epithelium, leading to pulmonary oedema and increased airway resistance (Martin, 2021a). Post-mortem inspection of the lungs of affected neonates reveals them to be airless and ruddy red, rather like liver. On radiographic inspection, progressive alveolar collapse, barotrauma or 'volutrauma' (arising from ventilation) and oxygen toxicity damage to the cells lining the distal airways result in exudation of a fibrinous matrix derived from blood, known as

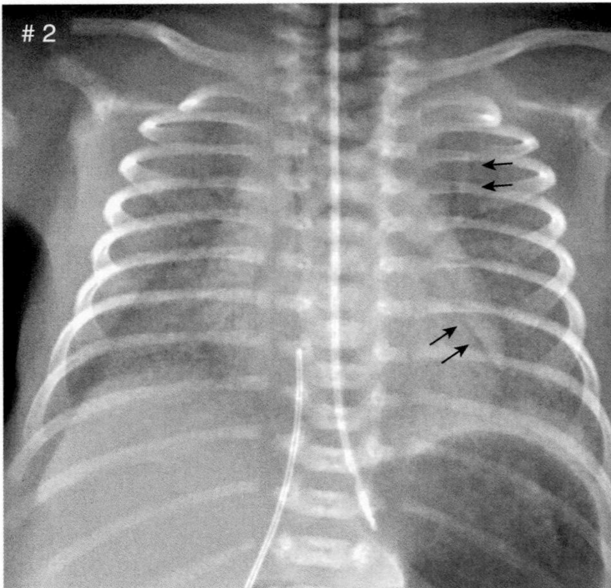

FIGURE 9.8 **Air bronchograms on the radiograph**
Source: Goldsmith et al. (2017).

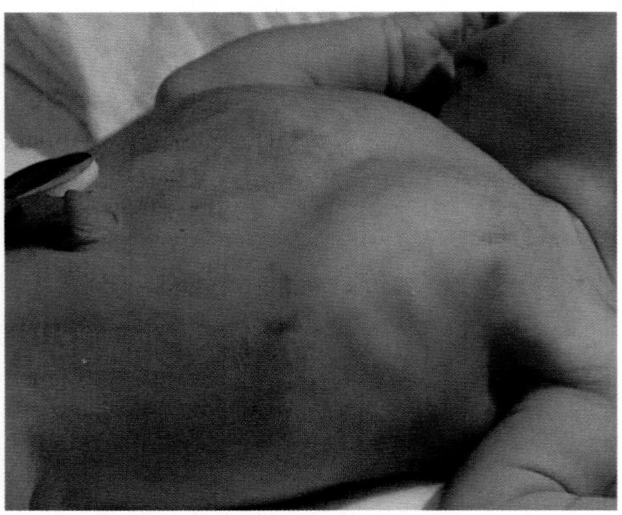

FIGURE 9.9 **Intercostal retractions in a neonate with RDS**
Source: © Janelle Aby, MD.

hyaline membranes – hence the common term 'hyaline membrane disease'. This characteristic radiographic finding may appear in as little as half an hour after birth. Air bronchograms (Fig. 9.8) are another common finding on the chest radiograph of a neonate affected by RDS and refer to the phenomenon of air-filled bronchi (appearing dark) being made visible by the opacification of surrounding alveoli (appearing grey/white). Intercostal retractions are a common sign of the increased work of breathing experienced by neonates with this condition (Fig. 9.9).

Prevention

Antenatal corticosteroids administered to women who are likely to deliver before 34 weeks' gestation is the first-line strategy to mature the fetal lung. In Australia and New Zealand, 89.5% of women who delivered before 34 weeks received one or more doses of antenatal corticosteroids (Chow et al., 2020). A typical clinical course is at least one dose of antenatal corticosteroids, with the first dose given more than 24 hours and less than 8 days before the neonate's birth to women at risk of preterm delivery, including threatened premature labour, antepartum haemorrhage and premature rupture of membranes or any other condition requiring elective preterm delivery. Antenatal steroids are associated with significant reductions in the rates of RDS, neonatal death, intraventricular haemorrhage and necrotising enterocolitis.

EVIDENCE-BASED PRACTICE RESEARCH 9.1

Women who give birth before 34 weeks should be given prenatal corticosteroids, according to current consensus. Rescue courses are recommended, but not repeated, serial, repetitive or weekly courses. Antenatal corticosteroids are used to treat a variety of clinical conditions, including preterm premature rupture of membranes, multiple pregnancies, extreme preeclampsia/HELLP syndrome and fetal growth restriction (Briceño-Pérez et al., 2019).

Management

The overall aim of management of RDS is twofold: to maintain respiratory function while minimising potential adverse effects. Exogenous surfactant administered to neonates with moderate to severe RDS has been shown to reduce the severity of the disease, ventilation requirements and the risk of air leaks. Exogenous surfactant can be administered for both preventative and curative reasons. In 2018, almost 27% of the Australian and New Zealand Neonatal Network (ANZNN) registrants received exogenous surfactant (Chow et al., 2020).

EXOGENOUS SURFACTANT

In Australia and New Zealand, the natural surfactants poractant alfa (Curosurf®, an extract of natural porcine lung surfactant) and beractant (Survanta®, a modified bovine pulmonary surfactant) are the most commonly utilised surfactants for neonatal use. Poractant alfa has become more commonly used in neonatal units in Australia and New Zealand because it delivers more surfactant with less volume. **Minimally invasive surfactant therapy (MIST)** has become a mainstay since 2013 because, in this method, surfactant delivery can occur via a narrow-bore tracheal catheter and be administered via **continuous positive airway pressure (CPAP)**, thereby negating the need for endotracheal intubation (Dargaville et al., 2014).

The dosage varies and is dependent upon type and brand of surfactant, hospital policy and whether it is required for treatment or prophylaxis.

CLINICAL PRACTICE 9.2

Dosage and administration of surfactant

Poractant alfa (Curosurf)

Respiratory distress syndrome

- Loading dose: 200 mg/kg
- Repeat dose of 100 mg/kg when required every 6–12 hours
- Maximum of 3 doses

Meconium-stained amniotic fluid (MSAF) aspiration

- Single dose: 200 mg/kg
- Further doses can be given as below if required:
  - 2nd dose: 200 mg/kg
  - 3rd dose: 100 mg/kg
  - 4th dose: 100 mg/kg
- These doses can be administered at 6-hourly intervals

Beractant (Survanta®)

- 100 mg/kg birthweight (4 mL/kg)

For all surfactant types, follow the manufacturer's guidelines for administration, but in general terms:

- *Intratracheal technique*: beractant and poractant alfa solutions can be administered intratracheally by instillation through a size 5 French end-hole catheter by passing the catheter through a neonatal suction valve attached to the **endotracheal tube (ET)** (so that ventilation is not interrupted) (Barkhuff & Soll, 2019).
- *The 'Hobart method' of MIST*: the Hobart method is an alternative and novel MIST technique using a narrow-bore vascular catheter made from fluorinated ethylene propylene polymer. This catheter is stiff enough to allow guidance towards and beyond the vocal cords, while also having sufficient elasticity and softness to avoid damage to the vocal cords and vital structures. Magill's forceps are not necessary. Surfactant can then be administered in one or several boluses, and respiratory support continued with nasal CPAP (Dargaville et al., 2014). A video of the technique can be accessed at the OPTIMIST-A trial website: <https://youtu.be/ULHyMFpK5GA>.

The administration of prophylactic surfactant remains an area of ambiguity in clinical practice. The complications of surfactant administration include blockage of the endotracheal tube (ETT), bradycardia and hypoxic events, pneumothorax and, rarely, pulmonary haemorrhage. Observations should be regularly performed post administration.

The mainstay of treatment for RDS continues to be CPAP via mask or nasal prongs to maintain functional residual capacity (Gleason & Juul, 2018). Heated humidified high-flow nasal cannula (HHHFNC) is increasingly used as a non-invasive form of respiratory support (Miller et al., 2020). These strategies have superseded positive pressure ventilation, but if mechanical ventilation is necessary, excessive **tidal volume (TV)** should be avoided because of the risk of barotrauma and volutrauma. Intubation is usually indicated only for neonates who are unresponsive to positive pressure ventilation by mask or nasal prongs, or those requiring administration of surfactant: in these situations, intubation is limited to the administration of surfactant.

FAMILY-CENTRED CARE 9.1

RDS is a very common condition in the neonatal unit. For parents, however, the condition is unique and anxiety provoking. Watching their baby struggle for breath can cause intense emotional distress for parents and families. The neonatal nurse/midwife should explain RDS to parents who may experience the following emotions:

- emotional distress, including feelings of guilt, anger and depression
- anxiety about their baby's future
- a feeling of a lack of control over the situation
- distress learning about problems relating to their baby while they are in the neonatal unit
- fatigue
- frustration that they cannot breastfeed right away and that they will need support to pump and store breast milk for later use.

Transient tachypnoea of the newborn

Aetiology

One of the most common respiratory disorders seen in the neonate, **transient tachypnoea of the newborn (TTNB)** arises from pulmonary oedema secondary to inadequate or delayed clearance of fetal alveolar fluid and is sometimes referred to as 'wet lung'. The condition itself is self-limiting and usually resolves by 48–72 hours. It mimics other common respiratory disorders and, as such, it is important to differentiate it from other illnesses, particularly pneumonia (Levin et al., 2020).

Epidemiology

As stated, the disorder is relatively common at 5.7 per 1000 births in term neonates. There is a higher incidence in neonates delivered via elective caesarean delivery without labour, with the incidence tripling in this cohort (Tefera et al., 2020). Other risk factors include neonates who are large for gestational age, whose mother has maternal diabetes or asthma, twin pregnancy and male neonates.

Pathophysiology

During pregnancy, the fetal lung epithelium actively secretes chloride (Cl^-) ions into the alveolar space, which due to their charge, are then passively followed by sodium (Na^+) ions and water to create a fluid unique to the fetal lungs. The production of this fetal lung fluid is vital for normal lung growth and function, facilitating the development of a FRC ready for gaseous exchange after birth. The secretion of fetal alveolar fluid declines in the days leading up to delivery, when the fetal lungs switch from actively secreting Cl^- ions to actively resorbing Na^+ ions, which reverses the osmotic gradient in order to withdraw fluid from the lungs and reduce the amount of fluid present at birth (Alhassen et al., 2020). The changes in electrolyte secretion and resorption are precipitated by the hormonal changes that occur with spontaneous labour, especially the surge of catecholamines and endogenous steroids (Magnani & Donn, 2020). It was once thought that the compression of the neonatal thorax in the birth canal played a role in lung fluid resorption, but this is actually a minor factor. Fetal adrenaline (epinephrine) is also triggered by the stress of labour and birth, which activates the epithelial Na^+ channels (ENaC) and reverses the process of lung fluid secretion to fluid absorption (Alhassen et al., 2020). In elective caesarean sections when spontaneous labour does not occur, there is a higher incidence of TTNB (Bruschettini et al., 2020).

Presentation

TTNB is a diagnosis of exclusion which is made when all other causes of respiratory distress have been eliminated. Neonates with TTNB typically present with symptoms associated with reduced lung compliance and pulmonary oedema. On physical assessment, tachypnoea and signs of respiratory distress due to increased work of breathing, including expiratory grunting, nasal flaring and retractions, are seen. Clinical signs of hypoxaemia and respiratory acidosis will be demonstrated with an O_2 requirement (usually $<40\%$), together with hypercapnoea and respiratory failure. TTNB is often a self-limiting condition; however, CPAP, HFNC, fluid restrictions and the use of diuretics may be implemented. The majority of neonates respond well to these treatment modalities and the condition generally resolves within 24–48 hours of life although, in some neonates, symptoms persist beyond 72 hours of life (Jackson, 2018).

Diagnosis

While ultrasound may be useful in the diagnosis of TTNB, chest radiography is most commonly used. The chest radiograph will reveal perihilar streaking (a 'sunburst' pattern) due to the engorgement of the periarterial lymphatics and fluid-filled interlobar fissures. The lung fields take on a characteristic 'wet' appearance, hence the original term of 'wet lung'. Fluid-filled alveoli appear as fluffy bilateral infiltrates. Atelectasis and pleural effusion can also be seen (Jackson, 2018).

Management

Given the transient nature of TTNB, management is supportive, with CPAP or HFNC $\pm$ O_2 occasionally indicated. Differentiation of other disorders, however, is important and, as such, most neonates will receive antibiotics until blood cultures are found to be negative. Diuretics such as frusemide have been found to play no role in the treatment of TTNB (Alhassen et al., 2020). Nursing and midwifery care for TTNB primarily focuses on monitoring, particularly **blood oxygen saturation levels (SpO_2)**, measured by pulse oximetry), respiratory rate and signs of respiratory distress.

Pneumonia

Aetiology

Neonatal pneumonia is classified depending upon the timing of the presentation of clinical signs (Gallacher et al., 2016):

- Early: the neonate presents as symptomatic within the first 3 days of life. There are two subcategories of early pneumonia:
  - congenital: acquired in utero and presents immediately following delivery
  - perinatal: acquired through aspiration of infected amniotic fluid; an ascending infection through intact or ruptured membranes.
- Late: the neonate becomes symptomatic after 3 days of life and is usually due to a nosocomial infection.

Epidemiology

Contributing to significant morbidity and mortality, neonatal pneumonia is especially prevalent in developing countries (Nair et al., 2018). In developed countries, however, the incidence is considerably less at between 1% in term neonates and 10% in low birthweight neonates.

Pathophysiology

Bacterial, viral and fungal agents can all cause pneumonia; however, the aetiological cause is generally related to the timing of the pneumonia (Gallacher et al., 2016):

- Early (within 48 hours of birth, as defined by the Australian New Zealand Neonatal Network (Chow et al., 2020)) – group B streptococcus (GBS), plus:
  - Congenital:
    - Viral agents: adenovirus, enterovirus, mumps and rubella
    - Bacterial: syphilis
    - Parasitic: toxoplasmosis
    - Fungal: *Candida*, especially in preterm infants
  - Perinatal:
    - Viral: herpes simplex acquired during labour is the most common.
- Late – usually caused by nosocomial agents:
  - Bacterial: staphylococcus species, including coagulase-negative staphylococci and *Staphylococcus aureus*, *Streptococcus pyogenes*, *Streptococcus pneumoniae*, *E. coli*, *Klebsiella*, *Serratia*, *Enterobacter cloacae*, *Pseudomonas*, *Bacillus cereus* and *Citrobacter*
  - Fungal: *Chlamydia trachomatis* is acquired during labour, but does not manifest until 2 to 4 weeks of life
  - Viral: respiratory syncytial virus (RSV) (most common), adenovirus, enteroviruses, parainfluenza, rhinoviruses and influenza viruses.

Diagnosis

A common adage in neonatal care is to consider sepsis before coming to what may appear to be an 'obvious' diagnosis and this is particularly true of neonatal pneumonia. Early-onset neonatal pneumonia presents similarly to TTNB, RDS and MSAF aspiration, as well as cardiac lesions. Radiographic findings, which include non-specific findings such as unilateral or bilateral streaky densities, diffuse granulation and air bronchograms, cannot differentiate pneumonia from these disorders.

Symptomatically, late-onset pneumonia presents with non-specific changes in the overall condition of the neonate. These can include bouts of apnoea, a change in feeding (including intolerance), temperature instability, respiratory distress and cardiovascular instability. A sepsis work-up, therefore, is paramount to arrive at a timely diagnosis (Gleason & Juul, 2018).

Management

When pneumonia is suspected, management with antibiotic therapy is usually started before isolation of the organism (Abdelhamid, 2017). Once identification of the causative organism has been established, antibiotic therapy can be tailored if necessary. If the pneumonia is uncomplicated, 10–14 days of therapy are usually sufficient.

Supportive care is also necessary, and this may involve circulatory support with fluids and inotropes in the acute phase. Mechanical ventilation and O_2 may also be required to correct hypoxaemia. Electrolyte imbalance, acidosis and hypoglycaemia may also be evident and require specific management. If feeding intolerance is an issue, total parenteral nutrition and lipids may be indicated to provide adequate nutrition and prevent protein catabolism (refer to Chapter 12 for further information).

EVIDENCE-BASED PRACTICE RESEARCH 9.2

Severe acute respiratory syndrome coronavirus 2 (SARS-CoV-2) appears to affect children less severely than adults. However, there has been a scarcity of information about the virus's impact on babies in the first 28 days following birth. In terms of virus exposure, neonates are expected to differ from older groups: while they can contract SARS-CoV-2 through close personal contact in the same manner that other groups can, they may also contract the virus vertically before or at birth. Because the newborn immune system differs from that of older children and adults, neonates may be more susceptible to infection or disease.

Infection with SARS-CoV-2 in newborns has been found to be uncommon in hospitals. Infection with SARS-CoV-2 during neonatal admission after delivery to a woman with perinatal SARS-CoV-2 infection is considered unlikely, and vertical transmission also unlikely, confirming international guidance to keep mother and baby together (Gale et al., 2021).

Persistent pulmonary hypertension of the newborn

Aetiology

Once referred to as 'persistent fetal circulation', the term 'persistent pulmonary hypertension of the newborn' (PPHN) is more descriptive of the failure of normal transition of the circulatory system that occurs at birth. The condition is characterised by pulmonary hypertension resulting in marked hypoxaemia due to the right-to-left shunting of circulating blood, and occurs primarily in term or late preterm infants ≥34 weeks' gestation (Stark & Eichenwald, 2021). The acute pulmonary vasoconstriction that occurs is due to an acute perinatal event: acute pulmonary vasoconstriction, pulmonary hypoplasia or idiopathic pulmonary hypertension (Mathew & Lakshminrusimha, 2017), as described here:

- Acute pulmonary vasoconstriction, where the pulmonary structures and branching are normal, but the smooth muscle in the pulmonary circulation is constricted (Mandell et al., 2021):
  - MSAF aspiration (see later in this chapter)
  - hypoventilation from asphyxia
  - hypothermia
  - hypoglycaemia.
- Pulmonary hypoplasia, where disease processes lead to significant alterations in vasculogenesis or angiogenesis, resulting in hypoplasia of the pulmonary vascular bed (Mandell et al., 2021):
  - diaphragmatic hernia (see Chapter 17)
  - oligohydramnios leading to hypoplastic lungs.
- Idiopathic pulmonary hypertension (pulmonary vascular remodelling), where underlying pathology maintains pulmonary vasoconstriction with an increase in pulmonary artery pressure for a prolonged period (Mandell et al., 2021):
  - closure of the ductus arteriosus in utero
  - exposure to nonsteroidal anti-inflammatory drugs (NSAIDs) in utero (third trimester).

Epidemiology

PPHN affects term or late preterm neonates and occurs in 2:1000 live births (Martinho et al., 2020). Male neonates are more predisposed than females, race does not appear to play a role, and there is a higher incidence in neonates with Down syndrome with otherwise normal hearts (Bush et al., 2018). Morbidity and mortality have decreased significantly since the advent of **inhaled nitric oxide (iNO)** therapy to reduce pulmonary vasoconstriction and **extracorporeal membrane oxygenation (ECMO)** to allow the lungs (particularly in pulmonary hypoplasia) to recover. Despite these advances, mortality associated with the condition remains at 10% (Mandell et al., 2021).

Pathophysiology

To review the haemodynamic alterations that occur at birth, refer to Chapter 4. When pulmonary vascular resistance fails to decrease for any reason and remains elevated, a right-to-left shunt across the ductus arteriosus and/or the foramen ovale may occur resulting in pulmonary hypertension.

Mechanisms that contribute to the high pulmonary vascular resistance that causes PPHN are low O_2 concentrations, either in utero or ex utero, the decreased production of endogenous vasodilators (endogenous nitric oxide and prostaglandins) and the increased production of endothelins (peptides that constrict blood vessels to raise the blood pressure) (Mandell et al., 2021).

EVIDENCE-BASED PRACTICE RESEARCH 9.3

In a study from six Asian countries to identify mortality risk factors in neonates with PPHN, a total of 369 infants with PPHN were identified. The incidence of PPHN ranged from 1.2 to 4.6 per 1000 live births. The mortality rate was 20.6% (76 of 369). Meconium aspiration syndrome was the primary cause of PPHN (24.1%). This study found that the incidence of PPHN was higher than in Western settings.

Prematurity, neonatal infection and lower socioeconomic conditions are all risk factors that are more common in low–middle income countries. In developed countries, lower rates of complications from diseases like PPHN were directly attributed to advanced treatment modalities like iNO and ECMO, which are not available in many low-income setting centres (Nakwan et al., 2020).

Diagnosis

The neonate with PPHN will present with cyanosis, tachypnoea and respiratory distress due to hypoxaemia. Hypotension and signs of shock are often evident. Upon auscultation a loud, single second heart sound (S2) or a harsh systolic murmur secondary to tricuspid regurgitation may be heard. Cardiac echocardiography is used to diagnose the presence of a shunt at the ductus arteriosus and foramen ovale level and can provide an estimation of pulmonary vascular resistance. A **partial arterial pressure of oxygen (PaO_2)** difference of 20 mmHg or more between the right radial artery (pre-ductal) and preferably the umbilical artery confirms a right-to-left shunt at the ductus arteriosus level (Mandell et al., 2021).

Management

Oxygen is a powerful vasodilator, so most infants with PPHN require intubation and assisted ventilation to maintain oxygen saturation levels. Hypercarbia and acidosis increase pulmonary vascular resistance, so ventilation parameters must strike a balance between maintaining normal PaO_2, PCO_2 and pH, while minimising lung injury associated with high tidal volumes (Stark & Eichenwald, 2021). Inhaled nitric oxide (a potent, targeted pulmonary vasodilator) therapy is often indicated, which reduces the need for extra-corporeal membrane oxygenation (ECMO) in most cases. High frequency ventilation (HFV) ± nitric oxide is frequently indicated, particularly where there is underlying parenchymal lung disease (Dassios et al., 2020). These ventilation treatment modalities are explained elsewhere in this chapter.

Management is tailored towards increasing and maintaining the systemic blood pressure, which often requires inotropic support, while decreasing pulmonary vascular resistance, optimising oxygenation and reducing the iatrogenic effects of high inspired O_2 and the necessary ventilator support. Inotropic support with dopamine, dobutamine and/or milrinone is often necessary to maintain adequate cardiac output and blood pressure while avoiding excessive volume administration. There is an emphasis on minimal handling and support of parents and family.

Pulmonary air leaks

Aetiology

Pulmonary air leaks occur more commonly in the neonatal period than at any other period of life. Air leak syndromes commonly include:

- pneumothorax (Fig. 9.10)
- pneumomediastinum
- pulmonary interstitial emphysema
- pneumopericardium.

Less commonly seen in the neonate are:

- pneumoperitoneum
- subcutaneous emphysema.

Air leaks can occur spontaneously (Deepthi & GiriDhar, 2020) but are most likely to occur in neonates with underlying lung pathology (such as MSAF aspiration, pneumonia, RDS, diaphragmatic hernia and pulmonary hypoplasia). Positive pressure ventilation often plays a role and, with the introduction of surfactant treatment of RDS, the incidence of air leaks has decreased.

Epidemiology

The incidence of air leaks increases with decreasing gestational age, and they are most common in neonates delivered at $>$24 weeks' gestation (12.6%) (Chow et al., 2020). Prior to the judicious use of ventilatory support, air leaks were a common iatrogenic effect of positive pressure ventilation. Ventilation strategies play a significant role in the development of pneumothorax: high peak inspiratory pressures (PIP), especially in the 24 hours preceding

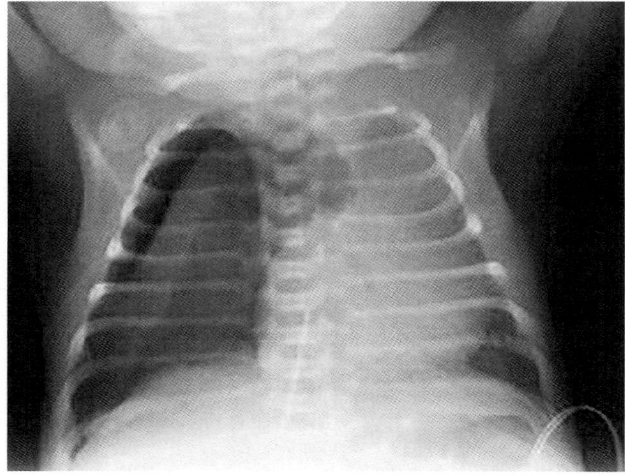

FIGURE 9.10 **Right tension pneumothorax with mediastinal shift to the left and flattening of the right hemidiaphragm**

Source: © Phillip Silberberg.

pneumothorax, long inspiratory time (>0.5 seconds) and frequent suctioning all contribute to neonatal deterioration due to pneumothoraces. A spontaneous pneumothorax is rare and seen in 1–2% of term/near-term neonates who have never been ventilated, owing to high opening pressures (James & Rajan, 2020). These neonates typically have had a history of fetal distress requiring resuscitation.

Pathophysiology

Preterm neonates are particularly vulnerable to air leaks due to a less dissectible interstitium. In conditions such as MSAF aspiration, due to plugging of the small airways, an unequal distribution of gases coupled with high transpulmonary pressures also increases the risk of air leaks.

When the alveoli become over-distended, they are prone to rupture into the perivascular bundle. Air can then track towards the hilum or pleura, resulting in a pneumomediastinum (where air leaks into the hilum) or a pneumothorax (where air leaks into the potential space between the parietal and visceral pleura). Air from the ruptured alveoli can remain in the perivascular sheets, resulting in **pulmonary interstitial emphysema (PIE)**, which can affect one or both lungs and on radiograph demonstrates a characteristic cystic appearance over the affected field.

Pneumopericardium is seen almost exclusively in ventilated neonates, resulting from air dissecting into the pericardial sac. The condition is asymptomatic until the air accumulates to the extent where the heart tamponades, resulting in cardiovascular collapse.

Less-common neonatal air leaks include pneumoperitoneum and subcutaneous emphysema. Pneumoperitoneum results from air dissecting into the peritoneum. The condition is not considered clinically significant unless the cause is from a ruptured abdominal viscus, which becomes a surgical emergency.

Subcutaneous emphysema is seen most commonly over chest wall drain sites owing to air tracking into the subcutaneous space. While the condition itself is generally asymptomatic, the underlying cause requires attention because of the possibility of visceral injury or re-emergence of a pneumothorax (Masand & Hauptfleisch, 2018).

Presentation

The presentation of the neonate with an air leak depends upon the type and severity. Infants with a small pneumothorax may be asymptomatic (Fernandes, 2021). In an acute pneumothorax, the neonate presents with a sudden deterioration accompanied by respiratory distress including tachypnoea, grunting, nasal flaring and significant retractions. Hypoxaemia and hypercapnia are also evident. On examination, the neonate will have diminished air entry on the affected side, and hyperinflation of the chest wall. This is due to the downward displacement of the diaphragm. The cardiac apex is often displaced away from the affected side (dextroposition) and the trachea may also be deviated away from the affected side. Bradycardia and hypotension can arise even in a moderate pneumothorax.

If not associated with a pneumothorax, a pneumomediastinum is often asymptomatic. If the air dissects through the anterior mediastinum, subcutaneous emphysema may be palpable in the neonate's face, neck or the area of the supraclavicular notch.

Pneumopericardium arises from air trapped in the limited pericardial space, which can rapidly deteriorate to cardiac tamponade, which decreases venous return and cardiac output. The neonate will often demonstrate a markedly narrow pulse pressure and a clinical picture indistinguishable from other air leaks: signs of respiratory distress, hypotension, bradycardia, pallor and/or cyanosis. On auscultation, heart sounds will be muffled, and a pericardial rub may be heard.

Pneumoperitoneum is often asymptomatic and may be seen serendipitously on radiographic evaluation. The most common cause of pneumoperitoneum is necrotising enterocolitis (Villamil et al., 2018). A ruptured viscus needs to be ruled out, however, but these neonates are usually symptomatic with signs and symptoms of peritonitis (Ravikumar et al., 2019).

Diagnosis

Transillumination of the chest assists as a handy bedside diagnostic tool; however, it requires radiographic confirmation. Transillumination involves a fibreoptic light source that is placed against the neonate's chest wall in a darkened area of the neonatal unit, or in an area where the lights can be dimmed. In the presence of an air leak such as an acute pneumothorax, the chest wall on the affected side will be illuminated, while the unaffected side will have diminished transillumination. This technique is effective only for pneumothoraces, and radiographic investigation is required to detect other air leaks (Arya & Verma, 2017).

On radiographic evaluation, if a large or tension pneumothorax has occurred, air will clearly be seen accumulating between the parietal and visceral pleura, with flattening of the diaphragm on the affected side and a mediastinal shift away from the pneumothorax (Fernandes, 2021).

As with other air leaks, pneumomediastinum can be diagnosed only on chest radiograph; elevation of the edge of the thymus from the pericardium will be seen. A large pneumomediastinum can be differentiated from a pneumothorax by a lateral decubitus radiograph, which causes the air to rise so that a definitive diagnosis can be made.

Pneumopericardium can be diagnosed on a chest radiograph and appears as free air surrounding the heart. It can be difficult to differentiate from a large pneumomediastinum, and, as such, it is the presence of air between the heart and the diaphragm that is diagnostic of pneumopericardium.

Pulmonary interstitial emphysema (PIE) is evident on a chest radiograph as a coarse, cystic image. Hyperinflation on the affected side also persists even after positive pressure ventilator support is weaned (Gronbach et al., 2018).

CLINICAL PRACTICE 9.3

If you have the opportunity in the clinical environment, practise using the transilluminator in your neonatal unit on a stable neonate. A normal chest will have a small glowing halo around the light source, which extends less than 1 cm from the light source and is symmetrical. This is considered normal. Compare both sides of the chest (Puri, 2020).

Knowing what is normal when you perform transillumination will assist you in recognising an air leak should it occur in a neonate in your care.

Management

Treatment of a pneumothorax will be dependent on the clinical presentation of the neonate. If the neonate is asymptomatic and there is no underlying pulmonary disease, no treatment is generally required, and the pneumothorax will typically resolve in 1 or 2 days (Fernandes, 2021). In the event of a spontaneous pneumothorax in term neonates, up to 100% O_2 has been administered for a prescribed period to promote 'nitrogen washout', although the effectiveness of this approach is highly questionable (Gregory et al., 2019).

Thoracentesis (needle aspiration of air with a syringe attached to a 23- or 25-gauge scalp vein needle, or 18–20-gauge angiocatheter) with or without a chest drain is indicated for emergency evacuation of a pneumothorax in unstable, symptomatic neonates. Initial management often includes prompt weaning of the PIP and **positive end expiratory pressure (PEEP)** to reduce further air leak while chest tube placement is prepared. The chest tube (trocar) needs to be inserted under aseptic technique by a suitably skilled practitioner. Pigtail catheters, however, have been found to be a safe and effective alternative to traditional chest tubes as their insertion is quick and relatively easy, and they are particularly useful for preterm neonates who require immediate air drainage (Panza et al., 2020). The position of the tube – whether a trocar or a pigtail catheter – should then be confirmed by anteroposterior and lateral chest radiographs. Management of PIE involves a treatment strategy that aims to decrease mean airway pressures while tolerating higher CO_2 levels and determining an O_2 requirement that allows for collapse of the dilated cystic lesions and expansion of normal alveoli. High-frequency oscillatory ventilation is a common strategy for PIE as it does not rely on the inflating volumes that tend to worsen the condition. Treatment of PIE is challenging, and different strategies have been attempted, including single-lung ventilation in unilateral cases. If the PIE ruptures and becomes a pneumothorax, the air can be evacuated using thoracentesis (Gregory et al., 2019).

Meconium-stained amniotic fluid aspiration

Aetiology

Meconium-stained amniotic fluid (MSAF) aspiration primarily affects term and post-term neonates who pass meconium during the process of labour. During early fetal life, the intestinal contents pass into the amniotic fluid until innervation of the anal sphincter is complete, at about 20 weeks' gestation (Rohrer et al., 2020). Meconium is comprised of desquamated fetal intestinal cells, bile acids, minerals and enzymes, as well as swallowed amniotic fluid, lanugo, skin cells and vernix. The texture is thick and sticky; aspiration of meconium during labour and delivery poses significant risk to the neonate.

Epidemiology

MSAF aspiration is relatively common, occurring in approximately 13% of normal pregnancies. Of these neonates, 7% will go on to develop respiratory distress (Monica et al., 2017). There are several risk factors for MSAF aspiration including post maturity (after 41 weeks' gestation), neonates who are small for gestational age (SGA) and in utero conditions including placental insufficiency and cord compression. An ageing placenta, especially >40 weeks' gestation, decreases the amount of O_2 to the fetus and reduces the volume of amniotic fluid concentrating the meconium. Therefore, MSAF aspiration is rarely seen in preterm neonates and more commonly occurs in neonates born after their due date.

Pathophysiology

Increased parasympathetic activity arising from fetal distress appears to play a role in MSAF aspiration, causing increased peristalsis and relaxation of the anal sphincter secondary to enhanced vagal output during cord compression (Martin et al., 2019). The exact mechanism that causes MSAF aspiration, however, is not clearly understood.

As the fetus breathes in utero, fluid in the lungs moves outwards from the airways and into the oropharynx. If the fetus experiences asphyxia in utero, gasping can occur leading to the aspiration of amniotic fluid and particulate matter into the large airways. At delivery, any meconium aspirated by the fetus may be visible in the trachea. Once the neonate commences air breathing, especially gasping respirations, the meconium will rapidly be inhaled into the lungs. Neonates at risk of meconium aspiration during delivery will have clear signs of thick MSAF, a non-reassuring fetal heart tracing and a low Apgar score (Martin et al., 2019).

The aspiration of meconium damages the lung tissues because of the complete or partial obstruction of airways when, on inspiration, the airways dilate and air moves around the particulate meconium, and then, on expiration, the airways narrow and air is trapped distally in a process known as the ball-valve effect. This leads to over-distension and alveolar rupture, resulting in air leaks (Garcia-Pratts, 2021). Sepsis, inflammation, complement activation and cytokine production, inhibition of surfactant synthesis and function, apoptosis of epithelial cells and increased pulmonary vascular resistance can also occur as inflammatory pneumonitis and infection arise as a reaction to the components of meconium (Martin et al., 2019).

Presentation

Neonates with MSAF aspiration are typically post mature: the skin may be cracked and peeling, the fingernails long and there may be heavy staining of the nails, skin and umbilical cord with a yellowish pigment. The neonate will demonstrate respiratory depression secondary to the hypoxic insult that precipitated the passage of meconium, with perinatal asphyxia occurring in 20–33% of infants born through MSAF (Garcia-Pratts, 2021). Respiratory distress will be accompanied by cyanosis, grunting, nasal flaring and marked chest retractions, and tachypnoea is often seen.

On radiograph, the chest will have an overinflated, barrel-like appearance, chest sounds will be coarse on auscultation and rales are often heard. X-ray will also show high lung volumes (secondary to small airway obstruction) and asymmetric, patchy pulmonary opacities. Air leaks including pneumothorax and pneumomediastinum are common.

Right-to-left shunting at the ductus arteriosus and foramen ovale level is common in neonates who have aspirated meconium, characterised by hypoxaemia and hypercapnia. The development of PPHN, which frequently accompanies MSAF aspiration, contributes substantially to morbidity.

Management

When MSAF is observed, a collaborative effort by the obstetric and neonatology teams represents best practice. Women who are considered at risk, in particular those with a gestational age of 41 weeks or greater with thick meconium-stained liquor with or without a non-reassuring fetal heart tracing, require careful monitoring. Amnioinfusion of the amniotic fluid with warm, sterile saline to dilute the meconium has not been found to be effective (Daskalakis, 2018). Intrapartum suctioning following delivery of the fetal head, once a mainstay of treatment, is no longer recommended (Nangia et al., 2017). In the absence of MSAF, fetal scalp oximetry improves the accuracy of detecting neonates at risk (Martin et al., 2019). The administration of oxygen and surfactant may be utilised as a management strategy, although surfactant has not been found to impact upon mortality. In severe cases of MSAF aspiration, the neonate may require intubation and ventilation, and subsequent administration of inhaled nitric oxide, sedation and paralysis. The increased pulmonary pressures and right-to-left shunting may result in a haemodynamic impact with changes to the blood pressure, and subsequently inotropic support may be initiated to achieve stability. In rare situations, ECMO may be required to achieve haemodynamic stability, adequate oxygenation and gas exchange.

CLINICAL PRACTICE 9.4

When aspiration of meconium occurs, intubation and immediate suctioning of the airway before stimulation to breathe are recommended to remove as much of the aspirated meconium as possible. Minimal handling is essential for these neonates, as they are easily agitated. If the neonate becomes agitated, an increase in pulmonary hypertension and right-to-left shunting, leading to additional hypoxia and acidosis, can occur. As such, sedation is often indicated.

Surfactant therapy may reduce the severity of disease and is sometimes used to replace displaced or inactivated surfactant and as a detergent to remove meconium; however, the evidence on this is sparse and inconsistent (Abdelaal et al., 2020).

Pulmonary haemorrhage

Aetiology

Prematurity is most commonly associated with pulmonary haemorrhage, a serious complication associated with high mortality and morbidity in neonates with RDS. In serious cases, a sudden spurt of blood via the ETT in intubated neonates presents with a sudden and often-profound deterioration, which requires increased ventilatory support (specifically an increase in PEEP) and blood product transfusion (Omansky, 2019).

Epidemiology

The incidence of pulmonary haemorrhage is 3–5% of preterm infants needing respiratory support, usually at 1–3 days of age (Jackson, 2018). There are several risk factors including extreme prematurity, surfactant administration due to a sudden improvement in pulmonary vascular resistance, patent ductus arteriosus (particularly in the resolution phase when pulmonary vascular resistance may suddenly improve) with left-to-right (acyanotic) shunting, multiple birth and male gender. Other risk factors include coagulopathy and asphyxia. More than 80% of cases of serious pulmonary haemorrhage occur within the first 72 hours of life.

Pathophysiology

A pulmonary haemorrhage is more likely to be haemorrhagic pulmonary oedema than a 'true' haemorrhage, given that the haematocrit is lower in the pulmonary fluid than in the circulating blood and the concentration of proteins is higher than in the plasma (Jackson, 2018). Pulmonary haemorrhage is most likely secondary to a sudden decrease in pulmonary vascular resistance (as often happens after the administration of surfactant), causing increased left-to-right shunting and pulmonary vascular engorgement, pulmonary oedema and, ultimately, the rupture of pulmonary capillaries. Pulmonary haemorrhage can also occur in neonates who have not received surfactant or have had a patent ductus arteriosus. Endotracheal suctioning may also play a role (McKinley et al., 2018).

Presentation

The neonate with a pulmonary haemorrhage will often present with blood-stained ETT aspirate, cyanosis, bradycardia, apnoea, gasping and hypotension as a result of shock, increased work of breathing, hypoxia and hypercapnia, requiring increased ventilatory support. Chest radiographs will reveal bilateral fluffy infiltrates, escalating to complete whiteout in severe cases (Jackson, 2018).

Management

Increased ventilation support, especially PEEP, is indicated and serves two purposes: to maintain adequate ventilation and oxygenation and also to effectively tamponade and stop the bleeding. Although maintenance of the airway is paramount, suctioning of the ETT should be limited during the acute haemorrhagic phase. Transfusion of blood products and correction of underlying or secondary coagulopathy is an essential component of treatment. Pulmonary haemorrhage can deactivate surfactant stores and exogenous surfactant administration has been used successfully (Martin et al., 2019).

EVIDENCE-BASED PRACTICE RESEARCH 9.4

Mechanically ventilated infants in the neonatal intensive care unit (NICU) may develop a superimposed bacterial infection of the small airways and lung parenchyma, known as ventilator-associated pneumonia (VAP). VAP is a form of infection linked to healthcare settings (nosocomial infection). Healthcare-associated infections are increasingly being scrutinised as potentially preventable contributors to poor hospitalisation results and rising inpatient care costs.

VAP is difficult to diagnose in a neonate, so a high index of suspicion is necessary. The definition of VAP first appeared in adult ICU literature, where intrusive airway sampling by bronchial brushings or lavage can help with a particular aetiological diagnosis – techniques that are seldom used in the NICU. The fact that infected infants also have persistent pulmonary inflammation and dysfunction due to prematurity and respiratory support, which can complicate the diagnostic impression and make infection difficult to detect, adds to the difficulty of detecting VAP in the neonate. Finally, as with neonatal infection in general, babies with VAP have fewer localising signs and symptoms than do older children and adults, and often present with general deterioration that may not be directly due to VAP (Hooven & Polin, 2019).

Nevertheless, as the role of VAP in poor NICU outcomes has become more commonly known, recommendations for diagnosis, management and prevention have been developed and refined.

Pleural effusions

Aetiology

Pleural effusions are rare in the neonatal period and are usually associated with other clinical conditions (Perez et al., 2020). The condition arises as a result of an abnormal fluid collection within the pleural space. Treatment decisions depend on the effect of the effusion on the respiratory status of the neonate and the cause and chronicity of the condition. Iatrogenic causes, such as perforation from thoracentesis, can also be a cause of pleural effusion (Liu et al., 2020).

Pathophysiology

As previously described, the pleural space is bound by the visceral and parietal pleura membranes that line the chest wall (parietal) and the lung surface (visceral). The small volume of fluid that is always present in the pleural space results from a balance of fluid production, thought to be produced by the visceral pleura and absorption by the lymphatics of the parietal pleura. When the production of pleural fluid is in excess of absorption, pleural effusion occurs as fluid collects in the pleural space (Liu et al., 2020). This can result from overproduction of fluid and/or reduced absorption, depending on the underlying cause. The arrows in Fig. 9.11 indicate the presence of bilateral pleural effusions on a chest radiograph (or X-ray). Causes of antenatal pleural effusion include congenital heart disease, infection and chylothorax, while postnatally they occur in response to injury to the thoracic duct (e.g. during central venous catheter placement), pneumonia or haemothorax (Philips, 2021).

Presentation and management

Neonates with small pleural effusions may be asymptomatic, and the incidental diagnosis is confirmed on X-ray (Philips, 2021). The neonate with a pleural effusion will present with increased work of breathing, cyanosis, tachypnoea and feeding difficulties. The underlying cause of the pleural effusion will determine treatment. Treatment strategies are aimed at the underlying cause of the effusion. In cases where the neonate is symptomatic, thoracentesis is commonly required.

Where chylothorax is the underlying cause, cessation of enteral feedings and use of total parenteral nutrition, or a formula that contains medium-chain triglycerides to reduce the chyle flow, can lead to closure of the thoracic duct and resolution of pleural effusion (Dehghan, 2019).

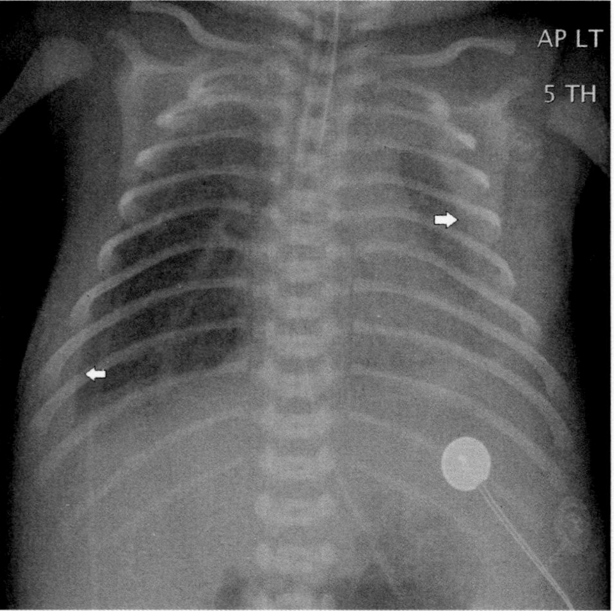

FIGURE 9.11 **Neonate with bilateral chylothoraces**

Radiograph demonstrates bilateral pleural effusions (see arrows).

Source: Adam et al. (2015, Figure 76.17).

Apnoea

Aetiology

One of the most common problems diagnosed in the newborn care unit is apnoea of prematurity (AoP), which is characterised as a cessation of breathing for 10–20 seconds and is often followed by bradycardia and/or hypoxia (Cramer et al., 2021). Apnoea is sub-classified into central (where inspiratory efforts are absent: 10–25% of cases), obstructive (where inspiratory efforts persist, but are ineffective due to upper airway obstruction: 10–25% of cases) or mixed (where upper airway obstruction precedes or follows central apnoea: 50–75% of cases) (Martin, 2021b; Montealegre-Pomar et al., 2020). These distinctions are becoming less clear, however, with evidence that central apnoea can occur with airway obstruction.

Pathophysiology

AoP (central apnoea) is a developmental disorder due to immature respiratory control in preterm infants. The incidence of AoP is inversely proportional to gestational age, affecting almost all neonates born under 28 weeks' gestation and 50% of neonates between 33 and $34^6/_7$ weeks' gestation (Eichenwald et al. 2011, cited in Martin 2021b). Preterm infants have a reduced ventilatory response to elevated CO_2, which inhibits their respiratory drive, and their reduced sensitivity to hypoxia means that they first hyperventilate and then hypoventilate (and/or become apnoeic) (Erickson et al., 2021).

Prevention and management

Once other causes of apnoea have been ruled out, general measures to prevent AoP include environmental temperature control, correcting head and neck position, maintaining nasal patency, oxygen supplementation to maintain oxygen saturation within normal ranges, and nasal CPAP for infants <32 weeks' gestation (Martin, 2021b). Methylxanthines, usually caffeine, are the primary pharmacological therapy to treat AoP, and act both centrally and peripherally to stimulate breathing by activating the medullary respiratory centres, increasing sensitivity to CO_2, inducing bronchodilation, and enhancing the function of the diaphragm (Erickson et al., 2021). AoP typically resolves before 37 weeks' postmenstrual age (PMA) in neonates born after 28 weeks' gestation, but in infants born before 28 weeks the apnoea often persists until term PMA (Martin, 2021b).

In obstructive apnoea there is no air flow, but the neonate attempts to breathe throughout the pause – that is, continues to have thoracic and abdominal movement throughout the apnoeic episode (Haase et al., 2021). Purely obstructive apnoea, without a central cause, is usually associated with an anatomical or positional cause. Preterm infants have poor hypopharyngeal muscle tone resulting in airway collapse due to upper airway obstruction, especially in rapid eye movement sleep, and even more so when the neck is flexed (Martin, 2021b). The most common anatomical sites for obstruction include the upper pharynx and the entrance to the larynx, and commonly include macroglossia, micrognathia, laryngomalacia and tracheomalacia and choanal atresia (see Chapter 17).

Chronic lung disease

Aetiology

Chronic lung disease (CLD) is defined by ANZNN as an ongoing requirement for any form of respiratory support (including low-dose supplemental O_2 and/or assisted ventilation) at 36 weeks' PMA. ANZNN registrants in 2012 reported that 8.4% of neonates required respiratory support at 36 weeks' PMA. Since 2016, ANZNN has implemented a 'shift test' (performed at 35+0 to 36+6 weeks CGA to discern the neonate's physiological CL status and to provide a comparable indicator of lung disease severity regardless of the unit's practice) for all infants born at <29 weeks in order to discern their physiological CLD status and to provide a comparable indicator of lung disease severity regardless of variation in clinical practice (ANZNN, 2021).

CLD is a complication of premature lung development and the trauma of early respiratory support. CLD is also referred to as bronchopulmonary dysplasia, which describes the underlying pathological condition – these terms are frequently used interchangeably. Gestational age is the primary risk factor for CLD; other risk factors are low birthweight and male gender.

Epidemiology

The prevalence of CLD continues to be highest in neonates born at less than 27 weeks' gestation. The highest percentage is in those neonates born at 24 weeks' gestation (63.2%) (Chow et al., 2020).

Pathophysiology

According to the seminal work of Northway et al. (1967), CLD can be characterised, clinically and radiologically, by four stages:

- stage 1: radiographically indistinguishable from severe RDS (1–3 days)
- stage 2: marked radiopacity of the lungs (4–10 days)
- stage 3: clearing of the radiopacity into a cystic, bubbly pattern (10–20 days)
- stage 4: hyper expansion, linear streaks and areas of emphysema with variable cardiomegaly (>1 month) (Fig. 9.12).

While these same four factors continue to play a major role in the evolution of CLD today, increased knowledge of the processes involved in inflammation and with lung growth and a greater understanding of genetics have broadened the overall understanding of the influences that play a role in the development of CLD (Gleason & Juul, 2018).

Given its chronic nature, CLD can be diagnosed when either of the following two criteria applies: O_2 requirements beyond 28 days with abnormal X-ray (Northway et al., 1967) or the requirement of respiratory support beyond 36 weeks' post-conceptual age (Keller et al., 2017).

Management

Although O_2 and free radicals are known to be toxic to the lung, evidence that reducing O_2 exposure protects

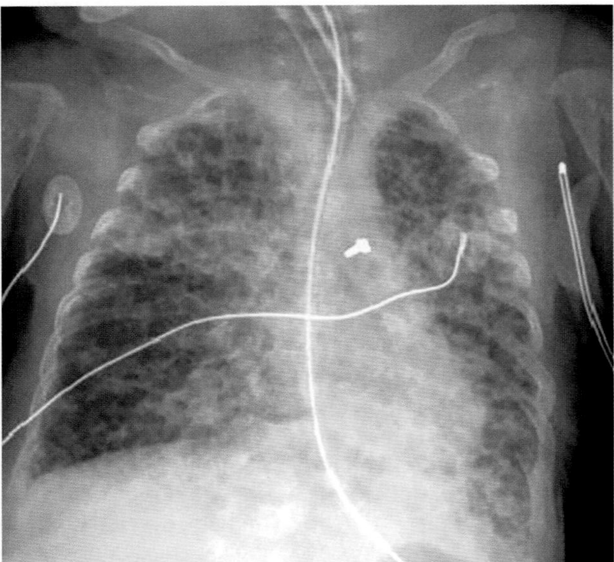

FIGURE 9.12 **A typical chest radiograph of a neonate with severe CLD demonstrating areas of over-inflation interspersed with areas of consolidation**

Source: Aly, H., and Abdel-Hady, H., eds. (2016). Respiratory management of newborns. Published: 31 August 2016 under CC BY 3.0 licence. © The Author(s). <https://www.intechopen.com/source/html/51148/media/fig1.png>.

EVIDENCE-BASED PRACTICE RESEARCH 9.5

While premature infants with respiratory failure have a surfactant deficiency, the connection between this and the development of bronchopulmonary dysplasia (BPD) (or chronic lung disease (CLD)) is unclear.

Ballard et al. (2019) took tracheal aspirates from 209 treated and untreated infants who were enrolled in the Trial of Late Surfactant at 7–14 days. In wide aggregate (active) surfactant, the content of phospholipid, surfactant protein B and total protein was determined.

Surfactant treatment increased surfactant protein B content (70%, $p < 0.01$) for 24 hours, but had no effect on recovered airway surfactant or total protein/phospholipid. The content of surfactant protein B was directly related to the level of recovered surfactant during dosing ($r = 0.50$, $p < 0.00001$) and inversely related to total protein ($r = 0.39$, $p < 0.0001$). BPD was linked to lower levels of recovered broad aggregate surfactant, higher protein content and lower SP-B levels in all babies. Small vesicle (inactive) surfactant was found in higher proportions in tracheal aspirates with lower concentrations of recovered surfactant.

According to the findings, many premature infants who have been intubated are deficient in active surfactant, which is caused in part by increased intra-alveolar metabolism, low SP-B content and protein inhibition, and the severity of this deficiency is predictive of BPD. The frequency of late surfactant treatment did not result in a sustained rise in airway surfactant.

neonates against CLD remains circumstantial. There is a body of evidence that supports early targeted surfactant administration to treat neonates with RDS, aiding in the prevention of CLD (Hentschel et al., 2020). There is some evidence to support caffeine use regarding the inflammatory response, pulmonary cell degeneration and modulation of adenosine receptor expression, providing evidence that caffeine acts as an antioxidative and anti-inflammatory drug for oxygen-mediated lung injury in animal models (Endesfelder et al., 2020). Nitric oxide therapy, however, has been associated with many positive effects in animal models of lung immaturity and lung injury, including diminution of inflammation, reduction of neutrophil infiltration and enhancement of lung growth and alveolar development (Shih-Hsin & Tsao, 2020).

The management of CLD, however, primarily concentrates on the long term. Oxygen needs to be provided for as long as necessary to maintain O_2 saturations between 90% and 95%; there is no evidence to support maintaining O_2 saturations any higher than this, and higher inspired O_2 may contribute to the disease process (Askie et al., 2017). Nebulised steroids, such as budesonide, have been found to have a beneficial effect on the risk of CLD (Tukova et al., 2020). Fluid overload needs to be avoided; yet fluid restriction is of no documented benefit. Parents of infants with CLD require extensive counselling and education, particularly when taking their baby home on O_2. See Chapter 25 for more information on this topic.

ACID–BASE HOMEOSTASIS AND BLOOD GAS INTERPRETATION

Acid–base regulation plays a vital role in all physiological processes. It influences and is influenced by the delivery of O_2 to the cells, cellular utilisation of O_2, production of energy and waste products and hormonal regulation of metabolism. Blood gas sampling can provide an accurate analysis of the metabolic and respiratory status of the neonate giving information on oxygenation, ventilation, potential hypoxia or hyperoxia and acidosis. Arterial samples provide the best indication of hypoxaemia as venous or capillary samples provide a less-accurate measure of oxygenation. In all samples, the CO_2, pH and bicarbonate readings should be accurate providing there is good peripheral circulation and the neonate is not polycythaemic.

Acid–base homeostasis is the balance between acids and bases. The pH is the measure of hydrogen ion (H^+) concentration in the blood. pH is a negative logarithm: a low concentration of H^+ results in a gradient shift and therefore a high or alkalotic pH, whereas a high concentration of H^+ will result in a low or acidotic pH.

There are various factors that create an acid–base imbalance. Acid–base disturbances can be respiratory or metabolic; in some instances, there may be a mixed metabolic and respiratory disturbance. Respiratory acidosis is caused by the accumulation of CO_2; this may occur rapidly after birth but is also promptly resolved once the neonate expels CO_2 with breathing (Patil et al., 2018). Other causes of respiratory acidosis include respiratory injuries and illness, inadequate alveolar ventilation, upper airway obstruction and significant ventilation/perfusion imbalance (Patil et al., 2018).

A metabolic acidosis is caused by a shift to anaerobic metabolism through tissue hypoxia, resulting in increased lactate and H^+ concentrations and subsequent acidosis and, if it is not corrected, it may result in irreversible organ damage (Patil et al., 2018).

The primary cause of respiratory alkalosis is most commonly iatrogenic from over-ventilation; other causes include abnormal central ventilation from a stroke or encephalopathy, or a supra-tentorial cause such as pain or stress response.

Metabolic alkalosis is caused by excessive bicarbonate (HCO_3^-) concentrations or hyperchloraemia, an electrolyte imbalance in which there are abnormally elevated levels of the chloride ion in the blood (Department of Health and Human Services, 2018).

The reference ranges for the blood gas values may vary slightly among units (Table 9.2).

The body will attempt to maintain homeostasis; when an acid–base imbalance is present the body will use compensatory mechanisms to counteract the disturbance. This is referred to as compensation; compensation occurs through buffer systems and can be either respiratory (lung) or metabolic (kidney) in nature, with one responsible for the disturbance and the alternative buffer system responsible for compensating to maintain homeostasis. Hence, for a primary respiratory disturbance, metabolic compensation will occur and, for a respiratory alkalosis or acidosis, compensation will occur through a metabolic buffer by either increasing or decreasing the levels of HCO_3^- in an attempt to normalise the pH. In contrast, for a metabolic alkalosis or acidosis, compensation will occur through the respiratory buffer by either increasing or decreasing the levels of the $PaCO_2$ in an attempt to normalise the pH. Alternatively, chemical compensation can occur externally through the administration of medications such as phosphate, bicarbonate or chloride.

In some instances, it is possible to have a mixed metabolic and respiratory disturbance. In some cases, it may be difficult to distinguish the primary acid–base disturbance from the compensatory mechanism, but it is important to remember the compensatory buffer system will never over-compensate. For example, if a neonate has a respiratory acidosis, the metabolic buffer system will never result in an alkalosis (Department of Health and Human Services, 2018).

CLINICAL PRACTICE 9.5

Step-by-step approach to blood gas interpretation

Step 1: Is the pH normal, acidotic or alkalotic?

- <7.35 = acidosis
- >7.45 = alkalosis

Step 2: Is the $PaCO_2$ within normal limits?

- Increased $PaCO_2$ = respiratory acidosis or compensation for metabolic alkalosis.
- Decreased $PaCO_2$ = respiratory alkalosis or compensation for metabolic acidosis.

Step 3: is the HCO_3^- within normal limits?

- Increased HCO_3^- = metabolic alkalosis or compensation for respiratory acidosis.
- Decreased HCO_3^- = metabolic acidosis or compensation for respiratory alkalosis.

Step 4: Determine the source of the imbalance.

- Is the source of the imbalance respiratory ($PaCO_2$ elevated or decreased)?
- Is the source of the imbalance metabolic (HCO_3^- elevated or decreased)?
- Is the source of the imbalance mixed (metabolic and respiratory cause)?

TABLE 9.2 **Reference ranges for blood gas values**

Value	Definition Normal range	
pH	The pH reflects the hydrogen concentration in the body and is represented by the acidity in the blood and the ability of the body to maintain a balance between acidotic and alkalotic substances. Less than 7.35 is referred to as acidosis and more than 7.45 is considered alkalosis	7.35–7.45
$PaCO_2$	Partial arterial pressure of CO_2 in the blood. This value is largely influenced by ventilation	35–45 mmHg
PaO_2	Partial arterial pressure of O_2 in the blood. Requires an arterial sample for accuracy and reflects the diffusion of O_2 into the blood from the alveoli	50–70 mmHg[a]
HCO_3^-	Bicarbonate is an alkaline substance that acts as a buffer to maintain/stabilise the acid–base balance	22–26 mmol/L
Base excess (BE)	Base excess refers to the amount of acid required to titrate the pH of the blood to achieve an acid–base balance	−2 to 2

[a]See World Health Organization <https://www.newbornwhocc.org/pdf/Blood-Gas-Book-workbook-2008.pdf>.

Source: Department of Health and Human Services (2018).

Step 5: Does compensation exist? If so, is it partial or complete?

- Uncompensated = HCO_3^- or $PaCO_2$ normal.
- Partial compensation = the pH remains out of range and both the primary acid–base disturbance and the compensatory buffer system values remain deranged.
- Compensated = compensation has been successful, and the pH is corrected to the normal values of 7.35–7.45.

Step 6: Are the PaO_2 and SpO_2 values within normal range? Is there evidence of hypoxaemia?

CASE STUDY 9.1

You are caring for a female neonate, born by spontaneous vaginal delivery at 39 weeks' gestation. There were no pregnancy or labour complications. The Apgar scores were 9 and 9 at 1 and 5 minutes. Over the past 2 days she has developed tachycardia, tachypnoea, substernal recession, poor feeding and decreased urine output.

Today she is 3 days old, intubated and ventilated; the following observations are documented:

- heart rate: 156 beats/minute, sinus rhythm
- respiratory rate: 60 breaths/minute
- temperature: 36.8°C per axilla.

An arterial blood gas is obtained, and the results show:

- pH: 7.5
- $PaCO_2$: 34 mmHg
- PaO_2: 76 mmHg
- HCO_3^-: 26 mEq/L
- BE: −2.6

1. What is the acid–base disturbance?
2. Does compensation exist?
3. What are the causes for this acid–base disturbance?
4. How should it be managed?

350 # RESPIRATORY MONITORING

340 One of the primary goals of the care of sick neonates is to minimise the risks associated with hypoxia and hypoxaemia. Blood gas analysis is the gold standard for assessing oxygenation and ventilation in the neonate, with the most-accurate analysis being from a sample obtained from an indwelling (umbilical or peripheral) arterial catheter. Arterial and venous puncture and capillary heel prick are other routine methods used to obtain samples for blood gas analysis.

345 Continuous monitoring of oxygen saturations (SpO_2) with pulse oximetry and partial pressure measurements of O_2 via **transcutaneous monitoring (TCM)** provide information on oxygenation only, and, to obtain reliable readings, both monitors require adequate peripheral perfusion and good contact with the neonate's skin. Transcutaneous PO_2 also plays an essential role in respiratory management to ensure there is an adequate supply of O_2 to the tissues at a cellular level for normal cell metabolism and to avoid hyperoxia and hypoxia. The non-invasive O_2- and transcutaneous CO_2-monitoring techniques do not, however, eliminate the need for blood gas sampling. Accurate blood results, including pH, serum sodium bicarbonate (HCO_3^-) and **partial arterial pressure of carbon dioxide ($PaCO_2$)**, must all be assessed to provide the necessary information to determine appropriate respiratory support and metabolic therapy. The monitors are nevertheless very useful for determining the appropriate inspired O_2 concentration.

Pulse oximetry

Pulse oximetry is the most commonly used method for monitoring oxygenation in neonates as it is non-invasive and provides a rapid reading that enables a prompt response to abnormalities in oxygenation. Emerging technologies mean that pulse oximetry is an easy and reliable point-of-care monitor in a variety of clinical settings beyond the neonatal unit, including birthing rooms, operating theatres, postnatal wards and outpatient departments. The ease of use may give rise to the view that clinicians have no difficulties using pulse oximetry monitoring in neonatal care because it is straightforward and requires simple knowledge application. It is important, however, to understand the relationship between the oxyhaemoglobin dissociation curve and pulse oximetry and the clinical factors that may affect the accuracy and reliability of pulse oximetry readings.

Pulse oximetry operates on the principle of photometric analysis based on the light-absorptive properties of haemoglobin (Hb) in pulsating arteries. The amount of O_2 bound to Hb can be measured in percentages; 100% indicates that the Hb is fully saturated.

Advantages of pulse oximetry include that it is non-invasive, requires no calibration, has a rapid response time, usually causes no tissue damage and is quite sensitive in the detection of hypoxia. Pulse oximetry requires adequate perfusion to the site and the ability to detect arterial pulsations (Gardner et al., 2020); therefore, in neonates with poor perfusion the results may be unreliable – for example, in cases of shock or hypovolaemia. It may also be limited by motion artefact and influenced by the use of phototherapy (Verklan & Walden, 2020).

When using pulse oximetry, factors such as skin maturation, correct positioning of the probe and the duration of probe attachment should all be considered.

Based on an observed increase in the risk of death associated with the lower range, the findings of Bizzarro (2018) indicate that a SpO_2 target range of 91–95% might be safer in extremely preterm infants than a range of 85–89% (Bizzarro, 2018).

Monitoring oxygenation by pulse oximetry requires the use of strict parameters of high and low alarm limits, allowing for illness state and gestation. According to the

Neonatal ehandbook (Victoria State Government, 2021), the target range for all neonates is an SpO_2 of 91–95%.

Transcutaneous monitoring

Transcutaneous monitoring (TCM) is a non-invasive method of monitoring O_2 and CO_2 tension, working on the simple principle of diffusion from the capillaries through the dermis to the skin surface. TCM involves heating the skin surface to allow continuous measurements of skin O_2 pressure (PO_2) and **partial pressure of carbon dioxide (PCO_2)** (Fig. 9.13). Although the skin PO_2 is usually low when compared with PaO_2, heating the skin surface with a transcutaneous electrode to 43°C causes vasodilation and brings the skin O_2 tension close to arterial values. This then allows for continuous non-invasive monitoring of the amount of O_2 and CO_2 being released to the tissues.

The most significant advantage of TCM monitoring is that it greatly reduces the need for frequent blood gas sampling and provides physiologically significant continuous measurement and trends (Sullivan et al., 2021). A disadvantage of TCM monitoring is that it requires frequent calibration and there may be a significant period of delay time for an accurate reading (Gardner et al., 2020). TCM monitoring is, however, not without risk and complications. As this monitoring requires the use of a heated electrode, it may cause burns in preterm infants owing to the fragility of their skin, requiring frequent re-application, and there may be inaccuracies in situations when altered perfusion, body temperature and blood pressure are an issue (Verklan & Walden, 2020).

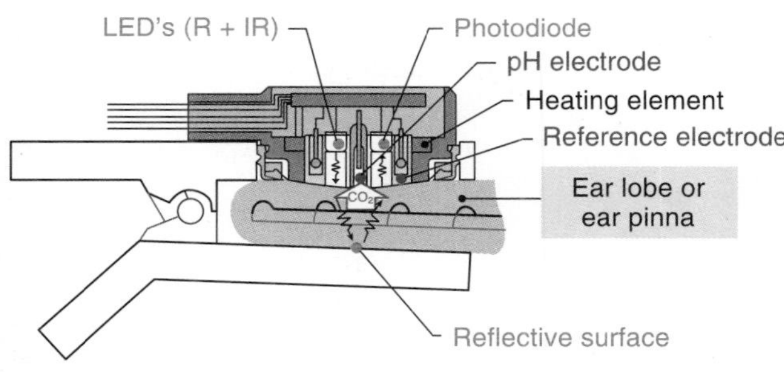

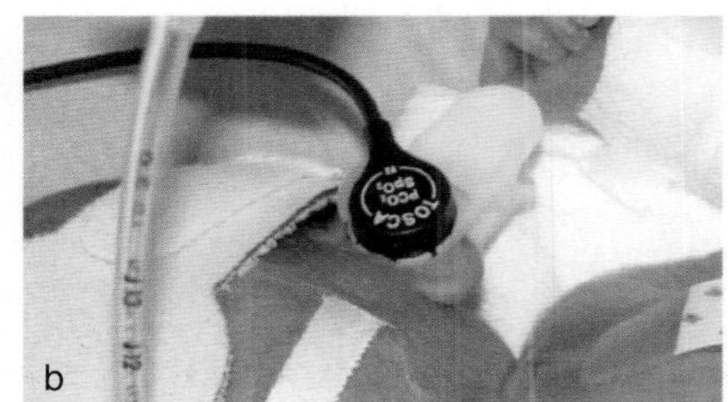

FIGURE 9.13 **Transcutaneous monitoring**

a, Elements of the apparatus; **b**, the probe attached to the neonate's ear lobe.

Source: Rubortone et al. (2012).

OXYGEN THERAPY

Oxygen is the most common drug used in the neonatal setting and can be administered to both the ventilated and non-ventilated neonate. There must, however, be clear indications for O_2 treatment and appropriate methods of delivery. When administering O_2 to a neonate, the goal is to achieve adequate delivery of O_2 to the tissues without causing harmful side effects related to oxygen toxicity such as ROP and CLD.

Oxygen free radicals have been identified as the cause of oxygen toxicity in seminal research (Saugstad, 1990). Oxygen free radicals can cause cell membrane destruction and DNA abnormalities. Mammals have an antioxidant (AO) defence to mitigate O_2 free radical injury; however, neonates are relatively AO deficient, as antioxidant enzyme levels tend to increase during the last trimester of pregnancy, similar to surfactant production, and they are thus more susceptible to lung damage.

Administration of O_2 requires precise control of the concentration, or fraction of inspired oxygen (FiO_2), relative humidity and temperature of the inspired gases. It is important to titrate O_2 therapy in increments observing for central cyanosis, heart rate and O_2 saturations. Oxygen should always be humidified and preferably warmed. Dry O_2 will irritate the airways, while cold O_2 will affect the neonate's temperature regulation. If attempts to reduce O_2 delivery through blow-by, cot or head box O_2 are unsuccessful, O_2 can be delivered via nasal cannula. Nasal cannula O_2 delivery is usually the method of choice for long-term O_2 delivery, as it allows for greater mobility, increased family interactions and easier establishment of breastfeeding. The low flow rates required are less irritating to mucosa and therefore do not usually require humidification (Martin et al., 2019).

Respiratory support

Caring for neonates requiring assisted ventilation requires neonatal nurses/midwives to be highly specialised. The two major types of assisted ventilation that will be discussed here are **intermittent positive pressure ventilation (IPPV)** and CPAP. IPPV requires an ETT to be positioned in the trachea, while CPAP can be administered via an ETT (albeit rarely) or via nasopharyngeal prongs (nasal CPAP) or mask.

Neonatal clinicians are continually exposed to emerging technologies and a plethora of research into neonatal respiratory support strategies. Understanding neonatal ventilation is challenging given the range of choice in ventilators, modes, special functions and manoeuvres. Choosing the level of respiratory support should aim to match the neonate's needs, which may vary over time, ranging from simple low- and high-flow gas therapy to nasal CPAP and mechanical ventilation via an ETT. This section will be divided into non-invasive and invasive ventilation.

Non-invasive ventilation

Continuous positive airway pressure

CPAP can be delivered via nasal masks, face masks, nasal prongs or an ETT and may be provided conventionally with a ventilator or with simpler devices. CPAP is frequently used in spontaneously breathing neonates as it does not deliver breaths, instead providing a continuous distending pressure, with the effect colloquially compared to inflating a balloon but not deflating it completely before inflating it again. The second and subsequent inflations are easier to perform because resistance is decreased.

Traditionally used to facilitate extubation and wean ventilator-dependent neonates to self-ventilation, CPAP is increasingly used for acute/early management of RDS in preterm and late preterm infants. The effectiveness of CPAP in surfactant deficient lungs lies in its ability to apply positive pressure to the airways, thereby increasing functional residual lung volume, improving oxygenation and preventing atelectasis (Noripour et al., 2017). Early and appropriate use of CPAP can avoid the need for intubation and leads to reduced rates of CLD.

'Bubble' CPAP has gained popularity, providing PEEP generated by immersion of the distal expiratory tubing into a water chamber to a desired depth to determine the CPAP level as equal to cm H_2O of pressure. Gas flow through the system creates continuous bubbling and pressure oscillations that maintain lung volumes during expiration, supporting alveolar distension and subsequent alveoli recruitment (Won et al., 2019). In some ventilator models delivering CPAP, mandatory breaths can also be applied as an alternative to intubation (Matlock et al., 2019). Referred to as nasal IPPV, this modality has demonstrated a reduction in the incidence of extubation failure and the need for re-intubation (Matlock et al., 2019). See Fig. 9.14 for a suggested set-up of a bubble CPAP circuit.

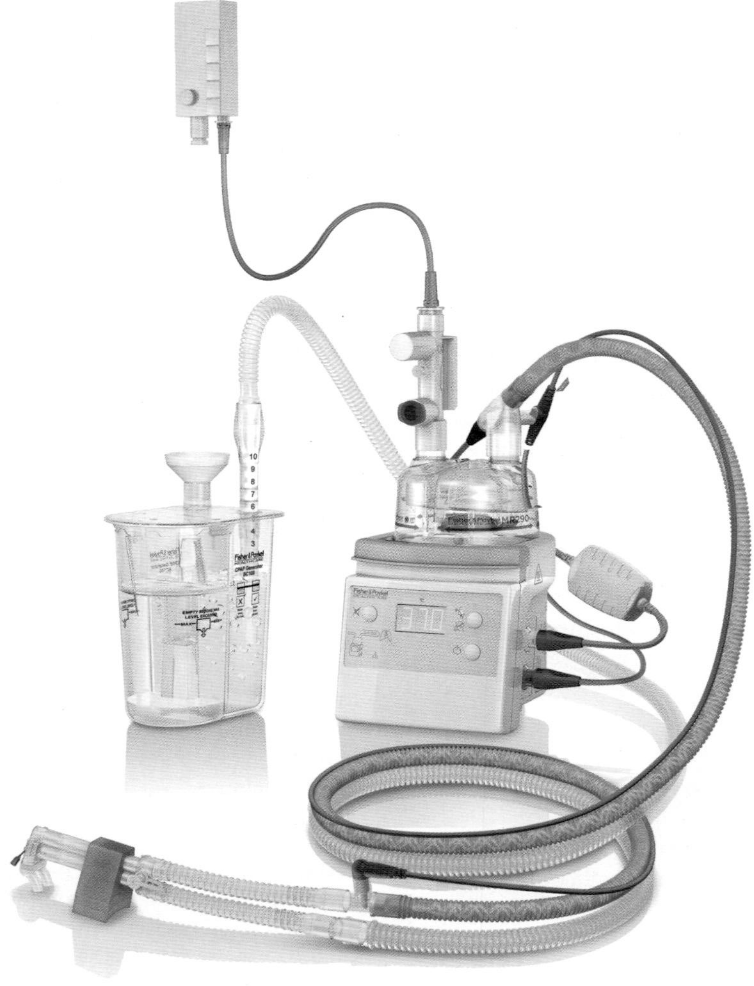

FIGURE 9.14 **Suggested set-up for delivery of bubble CPAP**

Source: © Fisher & Paykel Healthcare New Zealand.

Nursing/midwifery care of the neonate receiving nasal CPAP includes careful positioning of the binasal prongs or nasal mask in an attempt to avoid the eyes and prominent areas, a thorough assessment of the skin with care every 3 or 4 hours to prevent skin breakdown and scarring from nasal trauma and maintain a proper seal for the accurate delivery of PEEP (Haymes, 2020). Skin breakdown and nasal trauma is one of the most significant complications of nasal CPAP and in some cases the breakdown is severe, and the neonate cannot transition to nasal cannula O_2, meaning re-intubation and placement on mechanical ventilation may become necessary (Haymes, 2020).

High-flow nasal cannula oxygen delivery

High-flow nasal cannula (HFNC) O_2 and nasal high-flow therapy are synonymous terms for a form of non-invasive respiratory support for preterm neonates; this is an emerging treatment modality in neonatal units. In 2018, this therapy was administered to 32.3% of neonates enrolled in the Australian and New Zealand Neonatal Network compared with just 8.1% in 2009 (Chow et al., 2020).

Until recently, CPAP was the mainstay of non-invasive ventilator support, but there is increasing research to support the use of HFNC therapy providing humidified gases, at greater than 2 L/min, as a means of providing safe positive distending pressures (Chauvin-Kimoff & DeCaen, 2018). Liew et al. (2020) found that the airway pressures generated by HFNC therapy were influenced by the flow, the neonate's weight and whether their mouth was open or not. They concluded that the physiological effects of HFNC included a reduction in dead-space ventilation, respiratory rate and improved oxygenation. HFNC therapy appears to be better tolerated than non-invasive modes of ventilation and uses nasal cannula that are less prone to mechanical mishaps such as disconnection. Use of HFNC therapy has similar results to other non-invasive respiratory support relating to treatment failure, death and CLD as well as nasal trauma and pneumothorax (Sweet et al., 2019). There are limitations of HFNC therapy: although the nasal prongs are more convenient and less intrusive, the seal is less effective and may not prevent apnoea and stimulate spontaneous breathing.

Humidified high flow via nasal cannula is defined as a flow greater than 1 L/min (Chauvin-Kimoff & DeCaen, 2018). Air or oxygen can be given at flow rates of 2–8 L/min in spontaneously breathing neonates.

Despite HFNC being popular, with widespread use nationally and internationally, there is still a lack of evidence to support its use and the research into this treatment modality continues (National Health and Medical Research Council, 2016–2019).

HFNC have been found to have similar efficacy to CPAP in facilitating successful extubation in preterm neonates (Ferguson et al., 2016); however, treatment failure is more common when it is used as the first mode of breathing support after birth in this cohort (Roberts et al., 2016). The increased uptake of HFNC in non-tertiary settings should therefore be cautionary, as 'rescue' CPAP may be necessary.

HFNC is favoured by parents, as it enables interaction with their babies, earlier suck feeds and longer skin-to-skin contact, enhancing neurodevelopmental outcomes (Chauvin-Kimoff & DeCaen, 2018). These neonates, however, require care by appropriately skilled staff and adequate staffing ratios, with the need for comparative observations to an equivalent neonate on CPAP support.

When selecting prong size, it is important there is space around the cannula to avoid occlusion of the nares that may cause excessive airway pressure (Jabraeili et al., 2018). Like CPAP, HFNC complications include nasal trauma so the correct prong size will also reduce the risk of pressure-related tissue damage and nasal erosion from improper positioning of the tubing. In cases of nasal septum trauma, the nares may be rested by alternating gas delivery with a nasal mask. See Fig. 9.15 for the suggested set-up for HFNC delivery to a neonate.

Invasive ventilation

Mechanical ventilation is used to replace or assist spontaneous breathing, with the aim to achieve oxygenation (optimal O_2 levels) and ventilation (removal of CO_2). Ventilation may also be used to reduce the work of breathing, re-expand the collapsed lung and re-establish lung volumes. The challenge is to achieve oxygenation and optimise ventilation while protecting the lung from

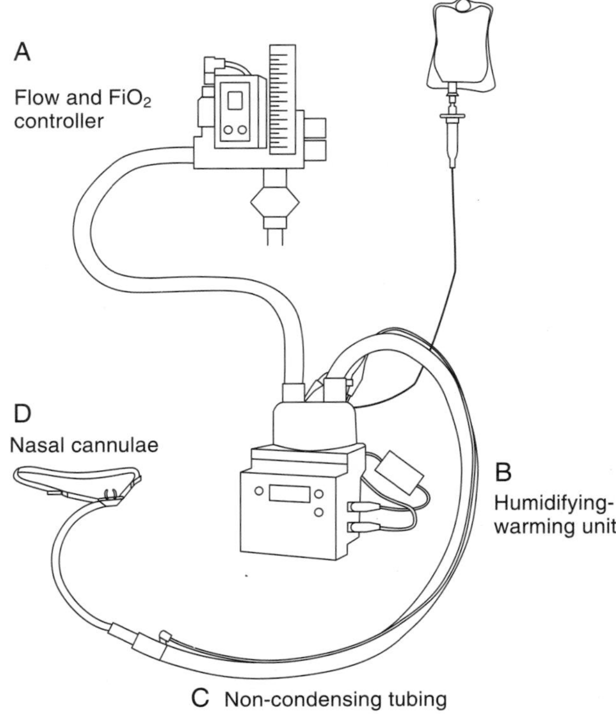

FIGURE 9.15 **Suggested set-up for high-flow nasal cannula (HFNC) oxygen delivery to a neonate**

Source: Masclans et al. (2015).

iatrogenic injury. Inadequate ventilation may result in atelectasis and sheer force injury, while over-ventilation can lead to volutrauma and barotrauma resulting in ventilator-induced lung injury. Interestingly, when neonates can select the size of their breaths, peak inspiratory pressures and tidal volumes have been found to be lower than recommended **peak inspiratory pressure (PIP)** or tidal volume ranges with pressure-limited or volume guarantee ventilation (Protain et al., 2021).

Ventilators are designed to generate either pressure or flow, depending on the ventilation mode selected. A ventilator will deliver a pressure into the lungs via a flow of gas that is either 'time limited' or 'volume limited' to move the lungs actively and passively. Volume-limited ventilation has been compared favourably with pressure-limited ventilation in reducing death/CLD, the duration of ventilation, air leak syndrome, hypocarbia and periventricular leukomalacia/severe intraventricular haemorrhage (Chen & Chen, 2019). Synchronised modes attempt to coordinate and adapt to the neonate's spontaneous breathing to maintain constant lung dynamics. The required mode and ventilator settings depend on the mechanical properties of the lung given the underlying pathophysiology. Clinicians can manipulate the inspiratory time to be appropriate for the neonate's own respiratory pattern. Peak inspiratory pressures and PEEPs are adjusted to reach appropriate target volumes (TVs) (volume delivered upon inspiration) and maintain FRC. The rate should be sufficient for adequate minute ventilation (the volume of gas inhaled or exhaled per minute) and CO_2 clearance. A minute ventilation is the total volume delivered to the patient during 1 minute of ventilation and is calculated by multiplying the frequency/respiratory rate and the TV.

When a lack of surfactant is the primary cause of the lung disease, the aim is to provide an adequate inflating pressure to distend the alveoli to ensure adequate gas exchange without causing over-distension (which may lead to air leak syndrome). Ventilation is then targeted to optimise alveolar recruitment with enough pressure to prevent atelectasis and trauma. Synchronising ventilation with neonatal breathing efforts, minimising pressures, administering the lowest O_2 concentration possible and preventing over-distension are all important considerations, as is the initiation of weaning as soon as possible.

Ventilation modes

Various ventilation modes are available in newer neonatal ventilators, and clinicians not only need to know how to manipulate the ventilator for the desired settings, but also need to understand these newer hybrid techniques and how the ventilator supports the neonate's breathing.

Intermittent mandatory ventilation

Intermittent mandatory ventilation (IMV) is a mode of ventilation that delivers a set breath rate, TV, pressure and flow via an ETT. The neonate is able to take independent breaths, but the ventilator does not synchronise with the neonate's breath. However, some IMV modes sense the neonate's intrinsic breath and synchronise; these modes are known as synchronised intermittent mandatory ventilation. IMV was the only mode that was available in early neonatal ventilation, and it can result in multiple complications. Sedation and paralysis may be required when a mandatory forced breath is given out of synchrony with the neonate's own respiratory effort; inefficient gas exchange, gas trapping, air leaks, fluctuations in arterial blood pressure and altered cerebral blood flow have been described (Martin et al., 2019). Adolescents and adults have reported discomfort during this mode of ventilation. IMV is rarely used unless a neonate is sedated and paralysed and, as such, cannot breathe spontaneously and in 'opposition' to the ventilator.

Synchronised ventilation

Innovative synchronised and/or patient triggered modes use a flow sensor usually positioned at the airway opening that detects electrical diaphragm activity at the start and/or end of the different phases of the respiratory cycle. The sensor will detect when and how the neonate is breathing and provides information on the ventilator display including graphical flow, pressure and volume waveforms as well as ventilation measurements. A synchronised mode will support either all or a set number of spontaneous patient breaths, allowing the neonate to self-regulate by reducing their breathing rate as the ventilation status improves; this subsequently reduces barotrauma (Martin et al., 2019).

Volume targeting and pressure support

Traditional pressure-limited ventilation delivers a fixed PIP above a fixed PEEP to support adequate FRC and control oxygenation and CO_2 removal. During pressure-limited ventilation the TV can fluctuate widely owing to the neonate's own breathing efforts, changes in lung mechanics and a variable ETT leak (Keszler, 2019). Too little TV will produce insufficient exchange of alveolar gases, while too much may result in alveolar over-distension and subsequent damage to the lung.

The evidence that excessive volume is the primary determinant of lung injury has led to an increasing use of volume-targeted pressure-limited ventilation. Clinicians now routinely target TV and monitor both TV and minute volume. Both TV and minute volume, or minute ventilation, are routinely measured during expiration. The rationale behind volume targeting is to avoid over-distension (Keszler, 2019).

More recently, the use of pressure-support ventilation has emerged, providing additional pressure (above PEEP) with a variable flow and inspiratory time to assist the neonate's own spontaneous breaths during weaning. The neonate completely controls the respiratory rate and TV. Pressure support can be used in conjunction with a synchronised mode or as a standalone mode and will decrease the breathing effort that is required to overcome the resistance of the ETT and the ventilator circuitry itself (Martin et al., 2019).

High-frequency oscillatory ventilation

High-frequency oscillatory ventilation (HFOV) is now a well-established mode of ventilation in neonatal intensive care settings. The use of HFOV has increased significantly over the past 20 years and, although it was initially used as a late rescue mode when conventional modes of ventilation had failed in term infants, HFOV is now used in a high proportion of very preterm and term neonates as an initial ventilation modality. It is used to treat a range of conditions such as RDS, pneumonia, MSAF aspiration, persistent pulmonary hypertension and lung hypoplasia.

There are various principles and mechanisms underlying HFOV, which enable gas exchange. These principles alternate throughout the ventilation cycle and include: Pendeluft mixing, *the mixing of gas through impedance*; Taylor dispersion, *the dispersion of molecules*; cardiogenic mixing, *molecular diffusion of the surrounding lung tissue*; turbulence; and coaxial flow patterns. In the HFOV mode, the neonate is given small, very fast, mandatory breaths at a lower airway pressure permitting gas exchange at low volumes (Lozano & Newnam, 2016). The oscillatory frequency (*rate*) (measured in units of hertz (Hz)) is calculated per second and in turn influences the oscillatory volume and the amplitude, depending on the ventilator type used. Appropriately applied HFOV can improve oxygenation and ventilation and reduce the risk of barotrauma and volutrauma compared with conventional ventilation (Lozano & Newnam, 2016).

Due to the elevated pressures utilised in HFOV and the non-compliance of lungs that often require HFOV, the technique may result in air leaks such as a pneumothorax or tension pneumothorax. The increased intrathoracic pressures may result in impaired cardiac output and subsequent hypotension; patients who experience cardiac compromise may require the use of fluid boluses and inotropic support. Observations and assessments must include chest auscultation, assessment of chest wiggle symmetry, oxygenation and CO_2 levels, blood pressure and perfusion.

High-frequency jet ventilation

High-frequency jet ventilation (HFJV) is not the same as HFOV. It releases short jets of gas into the inspiratory circuit through a pneumatic valve, and expiration is passive. The inspiratory:expiratory ratio can be changed, which is useful in cases of hypercapnoea. It is used in combination with traditional mechanical ventilation and the use of positive airway pressure (PEEP). Quick and low-volume inspirations can be combined with relatively long expirations and an inspiratory:expiratory ratio as low as 1:12 during HFJV (Carpi, 2017).

Studies comparing HFJV with traditional mechanical ventilation in preterm infants have found mixed results, ranging from a rise in air leaks with no clinical benefit compared with conventional mechanical ventilation, to a decrease in chronic lung disease incidence and home oxygen use.

It is difficult to equate these studies because of differences in research models, the absence of antenatal steroids and tracheal surfactant treatment in others, and the use of different ventilator interventions (with and without lung volume maintenance). The current evidence does not support regular use of HFJV in preterm infants with respiratory distress syndrome, and its use is severely restricted (Carpi, 2017).

Weaning ventilation

The most effective strategy to commence weaning is to plan a successful extubation at the onset of ventilation initiation and to provide ventilation that will not result in iatrogenic injury and will eventually encourage supported spontaneous breathing. Choosing the correct modality and other strategies assists in this process. Modes that allow spontaneous respiratory effort can support respiratory self-sufficiency. A back-up rate set low enough for the neonate to breathe on their own yet high enough to ensure adequate ventilation during periods of apnoea is important. Supportive strategies that reduce work of breathing, such as prone positioning and minimal handling and adequate nutrition, will promote optimal lung growth and development and pulmonary oxygenation (Martin et al., 2019).

Barriers to weaning and extubation include decreased respiratory drive (due to prematurity and sepsis, for example), muscle fatigue, lung immaturity and lung diseases affecting pulmonary perfusion and resulting ventilation/perfusion (*V/Q*) mismatch.

Nitric oxide therapy

Nitric oxide (NO) is a chemical compound and one of several oxides of nitrogen, manifesting as a colourless gas under standard conditions. Nitric oxide is a free radical – that is, its bonding structure means it has unpaired electrons, which makes it highly chemically reactive towards other substances, or even towards itself. As a clinical application, iNO is a pulmonary vasodilator that plays a major role in regulating vascular muscle tone. Over the past two decades, iNO has become a standard treatment for hypoxaemia respiratory failure in neonates who have persistent high pulmonary vascular pressure with right-to-left shunting of blood – persistent pulmonary hypertension of the newborn (PPHN) (Carey et al., 2018).

CLINICAL PRACTICE 9.6

Possible side effects of a neonate receiving nitric oxide therapy

Neonatal nurses/midwives caring for the neonate receiving iNO must understand the therapeutic effects of the gas and its basic mechanism of action as well as the inherent care, as the administration of iNO must be strictly observed because of the potential for toxic effects:

- The delivery and monitoring system for iNO consists of a cylinder of compressed iNO connected to the distal part of the inspiratory line of a ventilator circuit, which delivers the gas via an ETT. An electrochemical analyser is connected to the proximal part of the inspiratory line of the ventilator, allowing continuous monitoring of levels of iNO and the levels of nitrogen dioxide (NO_2), which is formed from the reaction of iNO with the O_2 present in the ventilatory circuit. NO_2 is potentially toxic (Angelis et al., 2021).

- The formation of nitrosyl-haemoglobin, which is converted into methaemoglobin, causes oxidative damage in terminal bronchioles and proximal alveoli. Methaemoglobin levels above 2% of total haemoglobin may impair O_2 release and worsen tissue hypoxia (Abhilash, 2019).

Extracorporeal membrane oxygenation

Extracorporeal membrane oxygenation (ECMO), also known as extracorporeal life support (ECLS), is a form of support that allows for oxygenation and the extraction of CO_2 from the blood via an extracorporeal circuit, while supporting haemodynamic function (Fig. 9.16). The administration of ECMO by a neonatal nurse/midwife requires a highly specialised skill set and the coordination of the care by cardiothoracic surgeons, perfusionists and ECLS specialists; therefore, few hospitals across Australia and New Zealand offer this service. ECMO is similar to cardiopulmonary bypass (CPB) utilised during cardiothoracic surgery but is designed for long-term use – days or weeks rather than hours. ECMO allows time for intrinsic recovery of the heart and lungs, post cardiothoracic surgery or during the transition from cardiopulmonary resuscitation directly onto ECMO (ECPR). For an individual to be a candidate for ECMO, the underlying cause of deterioration must be reversible (Barbaro et al., 2018). ECMO is not a cure and is often referred to as a 'bridge': a bridge to diagnosis, treatment, transplant or recovery.

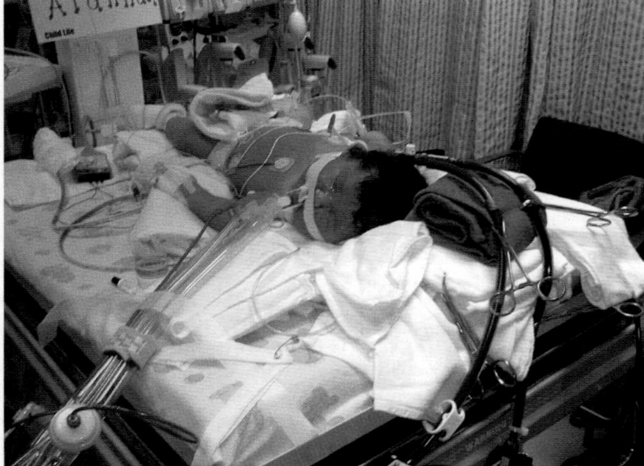

FIGURE 9.16 **A term neonate receiving ECMO**
Source: U.S. Air Force photo/Col. (Dr.) Robert Digeronimo.

ECMO can support heart and lung function, veno-arterio (VA) or lungs only, or veno-venous (VV). The choice between VA and VV ECMO is determined by the underlying diagnosis and the impact on haemodynamic function. If a neonate is commenced on VV ECMO but develops haemodynamic compromise, it may be necessary to transfer the neonate to VA ECMO. The common indications for ECMO include:

- persistent pulmonary hypertension (PPHN)
- meconium-stained amniotic fluid (MSAF) resulting in meconium aspiration
- congenital diaphragmatic hernia (CDH)
- preoperative and postoperative cardiac defects
- acute RDS
- post CPR.

With the advances in medical interventions, the prognoses and outcomes are improving; therefore, the inclusion criteria, exclusion criteria and common indicators are not definitive and may vary among institutions. There is a clear set of inclusion and exclusion criteria for the neonatal period; however, in the paediatric setting these criteria are not so conclusive and instead each case is reviewed and the decision to cannulate for ECMO is often made on a case-by-case basis (Table 9.3).

The ECMO cannula can be placed either peripherally via the neck vessels, internal jugular or common carotid artery or centrally through an open sternum. In VA ECMO,

TABLE 9.3 **Eligibility criteria indications**

Indications		
1.	Refractory cardiogenic shock	Acute myocarditis Cardiomyopathy Cardiac dysfunction in severe sepsis
2.	Postoperative refractory cardiac failure	Failure to wean from cardiopulmonary bypass Postoperative low cardiac output syndrome Refractory cardiac arrhythmias Pulmonary hypertension
3.	Cardiac arrest refractory to conventional cardiopulmonary resuscitation	
4.	Procedural support	
5.	Bridge to lung or heart transplantation or ventricular assist device	
Relative contraindications		
• End-stage primary disease with poor prognosis • Severe neurological injury or intracranial haemorrhage • Uncontrolled visceral bleeding • Prematurity (<34 weeks' gestation) • Small size (<2 kg) • Family or patient directive limiting ECMO use		

Source: Bembea et al. (2019).

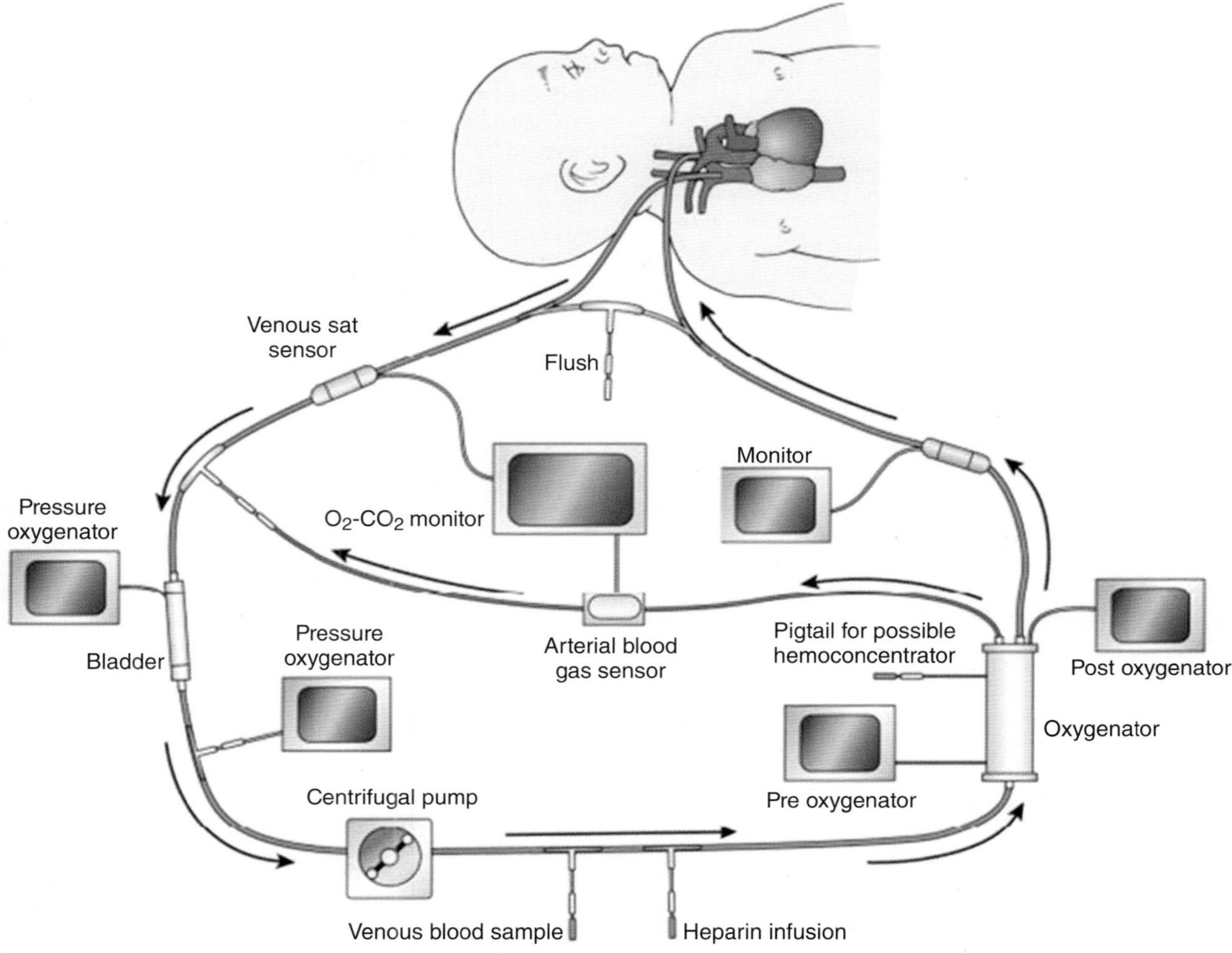

FIGURE 9.17 **Venoarterial ECMO circuit**

Source: Bembea et al. (2019).

deoxygenated blood will exit the body via the vein, through the pump head, O_2 will be collected and CO_2 extracted via the oxygenator, and oxygenated blood will return through the artery (Fig. 9.17), whereas in VV ECMO the blood exits and is returned via a vein.

Inadvertent clotting of the extracorporeal circuit may occur secondary to mechanical factors such as exposure to foreign materials activating the clotting cascade (Stocker & Horton, 2016). Therefore, it is imperative that the extracorporeal circuit is adequately anticoagulated routinely with heparin sodium (Tramarin et al., 2019). However, as there is a balance required between anticoagulation and coagulation, it is equally important to prevent the patient from bleeding. Bleeding will increase the risks associated with blood product exposure and internal haemorrhage, including intraventricular haemorrhage (IVH). The current anticoagulation strategies may slightly vary among facilities but are based upon the recommendations by the Extracorporeal Life Support Organization (ELSO) (Stocker & Horton, 2016).

Neonates receiving ECMO have an increased risk of mortality; however, it may be difficult to determine whether the risks are associated with the underlying physiology or ECMO itself. The two most common complications associated with ECMO are bleeding and clotting (Stocker & Horton, 2016). Clots occur in the circuit owing to platelets getting caught in the tubing and oxygenator, resulting in thrombocytopenia. IVH and gastrointestinal haemorrhages are of increased risk; haemorrhages may occur spontaneously throughout the body or during procedures owing to the anticoagulation requirement to prevent inadvertent clotting of the ECMO circuit. Other complications include acute renal injuries, tamponade, hypotension, hypertension, arrhythmias, cardiac stun, cerebral infarction, seizures, poor perfusion, limb ischaemia, hyperbilirubinaemia, elevated plasma haemoglobin and infection (Van Ommen et al., 2018).

CLINICAL PRACTICE 9.7

Despite the underlying respiratory diagnosis, the neonate may require VA ECMO as opposed to VV.

For example, although meconium aspiration syndrome is primarily respiratory in nature, it results in pulmonary hypertension, subsequently leading to increased pressure to the right ventricle and right ventricular dilatation. Over time this leads to heart failure and subsequent cardiac support that is offered with inotropic support and VA ECMO. However, VV ECMO may be associated with a lower rate of intracranial haemorrhage and may be the preferred first-line mode of ECMO support for primary respiratory failure (Carpenter et al., 2018).

With more than 300 ECMO centres currently recognised, there has been a recent increase in the number of centres, particularly in the last decade. The substantial increase in annual ECMO cases from less than 1800 cases per year prior to the year 2000 to more than 7000 cases per year between 2014 and 2016 represents the increase in centres providing ECMO support. Despite this increase in the number of ECMO centres, the proportion of neonatal ECMO cases has been gradually decreasing. Between 1990 and 2000, the number of neonatal cases fell from 82% to 49.3% (average for decade 65.7%), from 49.7% to 25.7% between 2001 and 2010 (average for decade 36.3%), and from 21.2% to 8.1% between 2011 and 2016. In 1990, the average number of neonatal cases per ECMO centre was 16.2, but by 2000 that number had dropped by half. Since 2010, the trend of fewer neonatal cases per ECMO centre has persisted, with an average of just 3.1 cases per centre. It was previously proposed that neonates needing ECMO care may have a greater chance of long-term survival if they were treated in hospitals with a higher ECMO case number (Mahmood et al., 2018).

Having a newborn on ECMO is challenging for the parents both visually and emotionally. Due to the administration of anticoagulation, it is common to see the neonate on ECMO bleeding or oozing from the cannula sites and other line insertion sites. This bleeding and the balance of factors in the coagulation cascade will generally require the transfusion of blood products to control the bleeding, clotting and reduce the risk of haemorrhage. Parents are unable to hold their baby; however, they should be encouraged to touch their baby and assist with care.

CONCLUSION

Given that the majority of neonates admitted to the neonatal unit will have a respiratory condition, either as the presenting problem or as a component of the presenting problem, the neonatal nurse/midwife must have exemplary skills in this area of neonatal care. The management of respiratory conditions has improved exponentially in recent decades and will continue to do so. The initiation of exogenous surfactant in the late 1980s and the transition from invasive ventilation to non-invasive ventilation in the majority of neonatal units today have changed respiratory management profoundly. The development of artificial womb technology not only raises ethical questions, but also may change the concept of ventilation in neonatal intensive care in the future (Romanis, 2018). The neonatal nurse's/midwife's proficiency in interpreting the neonate's cues, while supporting their other needs and providing support to the neonate's family, is a vital factor in the delivery of nursing/midwifery care to a neonate with respiratory distress in the neonatal unit.

Further Reading

Beke, D. M., & Imprescia, A. (2021). Nursing aspects of ECPR and ECMO training. In: L. C. Johnston & L. Su (Eds.), *Comprehensive healthcare simulation: ECMO simulation* (pp. 233–241). Champaign, IL: Springer.

Whalen, M. (2021). Basic approach to reading a radiograph in the neonate. *Neonatal Network, 40*(1), 31–37.

Online Resources

Qyeensland Clinical Guidelines: Respiratory distress and CPAP. <www.health.qld.gov.au/__data/assets/pdf_file/0012/141150/g-cpap.pdf>.

References/Acknowledgements

Abdelaal, M. A., Abushanab, D., & Al-Badriyeh, D. (2020). Surfactant therapy for meconium aspiration syndrome in neonates: a systematic overview of systematic reviews and recent clinical trials. *Journal of Comparative Effectiveness Research, 9*(8), 527–536. doi: 10.2217/cer-2020-0018.

Abdelhamid, S. M. (2017). Time to positivity and antibiotic sensitivity of neonatal blood cultures. *Journal of Global Infectious Diseases, 9*(3), 102–107. doi: 10.4103/jgid.jgid_1_17.

Abhilash, K. P. P. (2019). Methemoglobinemia: when to suspect and how to treat. *Current Medical Issues, 17*(4), 125.

Adam, A., Dixon, A., Gillard, J., Schaefer-Prokop, C., & Grainger, R. (2015). *Grainger & Allison's diagnostic radiology* (6th ed.). London: Churchill Livingstone.

Alhassen, Z., Vali, P., Guglani, L., Lakshminrusimha, S., & Ryan, R. M. (2020). Recent advances in pathophysiology and management of transient tachypnea of newborn. *Journal of Perinatology*, 41(1), 6–16.

Aly, H., & Abdel-Hady, H., eds. (2016). Respiratory management of newborns. <https://www.intechopen.com/source/html/51148/media/fig1.png>.

Angelis, D., Savani, R., & Chalak, L. (2021). Nitric oxide and the brain. Part 2: Effects following neonatal brain injury – friend or foe? *Pediatric Research, 89*(4), 746–752.

Arya, A., & Verma, A. (2017). Trans-illumination in pneumothorax: a useful bedside tool. *Indian Pediatrics, 54*(2), 149–149.

Askie, L. M., Darlow, B. A., Davis, P. G., Finer, N., Stenson, B., Vento, M., et al. (2017). Effects of targeting lower versus higher arterial oxygen saturations on death or disability in preterm infants. *Cochrane Database of Systematic Reviews, 4*, CD011190. doi: 10.1002/14651858.CD011190.pub2.

Australian and New Zealand Neonatal Network (ANZNN). (2021). *ANZNN 2020 data dictionary*. Sydney, NSW: ANZNN. <https://anznn.net/Portals/0/DataDictionaries/ANZNN_2021_Data_Dictionary.pdf> (Accessed 15 February 2022).

Ballard, P. L., Keller, R. L., Truog, W. E., Chapin, C., Horneman, H., Segal, M. R., et al. (2019). Surfactant status and respiratory outcome in premature infants receiving late surfactant treatment. *Pediatric Research, 85*(3), 305–311. doi: 10.1038/s41390-018-0144-3.

Barbaro, R. P., Xu, Y., Borasino, S., Truemper, E. J., Watson, R. S., Thiagarajan, R. R., et al. (2018). Does extracorporeal membrane oxygenation improve survival in pediatric acute respiratory failure? *American Journal of Respiratory and Critical Care Medicine, 197*(9), 1177–1186.

Barkhuff, W. D., & Soll, R. F. (2019). Novel surfactant administration techniques: will they change outcome? *Neonatology, 115*(4), 411–422.

Bembea, M. M., Goldman, A., Honjo, O., & Thiagarajan, R. R. (2019). Extracorporeal membrane oxygenation. In: R. M. Ungerleider, J. N. Meliones, K. Nelson McMillan, D. S. Cooper, & J. P. Jacobs (Eds.), *Critical heart disease in infants and children* (3rd ed., pp. 488–499.e484). Philadelphia, PA: Elsevier. doi: 10.1016/B978-1-4557-0760-7.00039-5.

Bizzarro, M. J. (2018). Optimizing oxygen saturation targets in extremely preterm infants. *Journal of the American Medical Association, 319*(21), 2173–2174.

Briceño-Pérez, C., Reyna-Villasmil, E., & Vigil-De-Gracia, P. (2019). Antenatal corticosteroid therapy: historical and scientific basis to improve preterm birth management. *European Journal of Obstetrics and Gynecology and Reproductive Biology, 234*, 32–37.

Bruschettini, M., Moresco, L., Calevo, M. G., & Romantsik, O. (2020). Postnatal corticosteroids for transient tachypnoea of the newborn. *Cochrane Database of Systematic Reviews, 3*(3), CD013222.

Bush, D., Galambos, C., Ivy, D. D., Abman, S. H., Wolter-Warmerdam, K., & Hickey, F. (2018). Clinical characteristics and risk factors for developing pulmonary hypertension in children with Down syndrome. *Journal of Pediatrics, 202*, 212–219.

Carey, W. A., Weaver, A. L., Mara, K. C., & Clark, R. H. (2018). Inhaled nitric oxide in extremely premature neonates with respiratory distress syndrome. *Pediatrics, 141*(3), e20173108. doi: 10.1542/peds.2017-3108.

Carpenter, J. L., Yangyang, R. Y., Cass, D. L., Olutoye, O. O., Thomas, J. A., Burgman, C., et al. (2018). Use of venovenous ECMO for neonatal and pediatric ECMO: a decade of experience at a tertiary children's hospital. *Pediatric Surgery International, 34*(3), 263–268.

Carpi, M. F. (2017). High-frequency jet ventilation in preterm infants: is there still room for it? *Respiratory Care, 62*(7), 997. doi: 10.4187/respcare.05647.

Chauvin-Kimoff, L., & DeCaen, A. (2018). Use of high-flow nasal cannula oxygen therapy in infants and children. *Paediatrics and Child Health, 23*(8), 555–555. doi: 10.1093/pch/pxy142.

Chen, L. J., & Chen, J. Y. (2019). Volume-targeted versus pressure-limited ventilation for preterm infants. *Journal of the Chinese Medical Association, 82*(10), 791–794.

Chow, S. S. W., Creighton, P., Chambers, G. M., & Lui, K. (2020). *Report of the Australian and New Zealand Neonatal Network 2018*. Sydney, NSW: ANZNN.

Craft, J. (2018). *Understanding pathophysiology ANZ*. [ClinicalKey Student]. <https://clinicalkeymeded.elsevier.com/> (Accessed 15 February 2022).

Cramer, S. J. E., Zanten, H. A., Boezaard, M., Hoek, P. M., Dekker, J., Hooper, S. B., et al. (2021). High variability in nurses' tactile stimulation methods in response to apnoea of prematurity – neonatal manikin study. *Acta Paediatrica, 110*(3), 799–804. doi: 10.1111/apa.15564.

Dargaville, P. A., Kamlin, C. O. F., De Paoli, A. G., Carlin, J. B., Orsini, F., Soll, R. F., et al. (2014). The OPTIMIST-A trial: evaluation of minimally-invasive surfactant therapy in preterm infants 25–28 weeks' gestation. *BMC Pediatrics, 14*(1), 213. doi: 10.1186/1471-2431-14-213.

Daskalakis, G. (2018). What are the benefits and harms of amnioinfusion for meconium-stained liquor during labor in settings with standard peripartum surveillance? *Cochrane Clinical Answers*. doi: 10.1002/cca.2208.

Dassios, T., Ali, K., Rossor, T., & Greenough, A. (2017). Ventilation/perfusion ratio and right to left shunt in healthy newborn infants. *Journal of Clinical Monitoring and Computing, 31*(6), 1229–1234.

Dassios, T., Ambulkar, H., & Greenough, A. (2020). Treatment and respiratory support modes for neonates with respiratory distress syndrome. *Expert Opinion on Orphan Drugs, 8*(5), 145–156. doi: 10.1080/21678707.2020.1769598.

Deepthi, P. B., & GiriDhar, S. (2020). Severe pulmonary air leak complicating neonatal resuscitation. *Journal of Clinical and Diagnostic Research, 14*(10), SD01–SD03.

Dehghan, K. (2019). Idiopathic chylothorax in a term neonate and successful treatment with octreotide and medium chain triglyceride-enriched formula: a case report. *International Journal of Pediatrics, 7*(6), 9535–9540.

Department of Health and Human Services. (2018). *Blood gas interpretation for neonates: 2018.*

<https://www.bettersafercare.vic.gov.au/clinical-guidance/neonatal/blood-gas-interpretation-for-neonates> (Accessed 15 February 2022).

Dilly, S. A. (1984). Scanning electron microscope study of the development of the human respiratory acinus. *Thorax, 39*(10), 733–742. doi: 10.1136/thx.39.10.733.

Endesfelder, S., Strauß, E., Bendix, I., Schmitz, T., & Bührer, C. (2020). Prevention of oxygen-induced inflammatory lung injury by caffeine in neonatal rats. *Oxidative Medicine and Cellular Longevity, 2020*, 1–19. doi: 10.1155/2020/3840124.

Erickson, G., Dobson, N. R., & Hunt, C. E. (2021). Immature control of breathing and apnea of prematurity: the known and unknown. *Journal of Perinatology, 41*, 2111–2123. doi: 10.1038/s41372-021-01010-z.

Ferguson, K. N., Roberts, C. T., Manley, B. J., & Davis, P. G. (2016). Interventions to improve rates of successful extubation in preterm infants: a systematic review and meta-analysis. *JAMA Pediatrics, 171*(2), 165–174. doi: 10.1001/jamapediatrics.2016.3015.

Fernandes, C. J. (2021). Pulmonary air leak in the newborn. In: J. A. Garcia-Pratts, G. Redding, & M. S. Kim (Eds.), *UpToDate*. Walters Kluwer. <https://www.uptodate.com/contents/pulmonary-air-leak-in-the-newborn?search> (Accessed 15 February 2022).

Gale, C., Quigley, M. A., Placzek, A., Knight, M., Ladhani, S., Draper, E. S., et al. (2021). Characteristics and outcomes of neonatal SARS-CoV-2 infection in the UK: a prospective national cohort study using active surveillance. *Lancet Child and Adolescent Health, 5*(2), 113–121. doi: 10.1016/S2352-4642(20)30342-4.

Gallacher, D. J., Hart, K., & Kotecha, S. (2016). Common respiratory conditions of the newborn. *Breathe, 12*(1), 30–42. doi: 10.1183/20734735.000716.

Garcia-Pratts, J. A. (2021). Meconium aspiration syndrome: pathophysiology, clinical manifestations and diagnosis. In: R. Martin & M. S. Kim (Eds.), *UpToDate*. Walters Kluwer. <https://www.uptodate.com/contents/meconium-aspiration-syndrome-pathophysiology-clinical-manifestations-and-diagnosis?search> (Accessed 15 February 2022).

Gardner, S., Carter, B., Enzman-Hines, M., & Niermeyer, S. (2020). *Merenstein and Gardner's handbook of neonatal intensive care* (9th ed.). St Louis, MO: Elsevier.

Gleason, C. A., & Juul, S. E. (2018). *Avery's diseases of the newborn* (10th ed.). Philadelphia, PA: Elsevier.

Goldsmith, J. P., Karotkin, E. H., Suresh, G., & Keszler, M. (2017). *Assisted ventilation of the neonate* (6th ed.). Philadelphia, PA: Elsevier.

Gregory, A., Ewer, A. K., & Singh, A. (2019). Is high-concentration oxygen therapy more effective than targeted oxygen therapy in neonatal non-tension pneumothorax? *Archives of Disease in Childhood, 104*(4), 405–406. doi: 10.1136/archdischild-2018-315659.

Gronbach, J., Ehrhardt, H., Zimmer, K. P., & Waitz, M. (2018). Early pulmonary interstitial emphysema in preterm neonates – respiratory management and case report in nonventilated very low birth weight twins. *AJP Reports, 8*(2), e99–e105. doi: 10.1055/s-0038-1648253.

Haase, B., Badinska, A. M., Poets, C. F., Koos, B., & Springer, L. (2021). An approach to define newborns' sniffing position using an angle based on reproducible facial landmarks. *Pediatric Anesthesia, 31*(4), 404–409. doi: 10.1111/pan.14154.

Haymes, E. (2020). The effects of continuous positive airway pressure (CPAP) on nasal skin breakdown. *Journal of Neonatal Nursing, 26*(1), 37–42. doi: 10.1016/j.jnn.2019.09.007.

Hentschel, R., Bohlin, K., van Kaam, A., Fuchs, H., & Danhaive, O. (2020). Surfactant replacement therapy: from biological basis to current clinical. *Pediatric Research, 88*(2), 176–183. doi: 10.1038/s41390-020-0750-8.

Hooven, T. A., & Polin, R. A. (2019). Ventilator-associated pneumonia. In: E. Bancalari (Ed.), *The Newborn Lung* (3rd ed., pp. 147–159). Philadelphia, PA: Elsevier.

Jabraeili, M., Eskandari, S., Bagher Hosseini, M., & Rahmani, P. (2018). The effect of body position on pain due to nasal continuous positive airway pressure (CPAP) in premature neonates: a cross-over clinical trial study. *International Journal of Pediatrics, 6*(1), 6861–6871.

Jackson, J. C. (2018). Respiratory disorders in the preterm infant. In: C. A. Gleason, & S. E. Juul (Eds.), *Avery's diseases of the newborn* (pp. 653–667.e652). doi: 10.1016/B978-0-323-40139-5.00046-2. Philadelphia, PA: Elsevier.

James, V., & Rajan, J. (2020). Bilateral spontaneous pneumothorax in a term newborn. *Indian Journal of Case Reports, 6*, 578–579.

Keller, R. L., Feng, R., DeMauro, S. B., Ferkol, T., Hardie, W., Rogers, E. E., et al. (2017). Bronchopulmonary dysplasia and perinatal characteristics predict 1-year respiratory outcomes in newborns born at extremely low gestational age: a prospective cohort study. *Journal of Pediatrics, 187*, 89–97.e3.

Keszler, M. (2019). Volume-targeted ventilation: one size does not fit all. Evidence-based recommendations for successful use. *Archives of Disease in Childhood-Fetal and Neonatal Edition, 104*(1), F108–F112.

Leslie, K. O., & Wick, M. R. (2018). Lung anatomy. In: K. O. Leslie, M. R. Wick, & M. L. Smith (Eds.), *Practical pulmonary pathology: a diagnostic approach* (3rd ed., pp. 1–14). Philadelphia, PA: Elsevier.

Levin, J. C., Cleveland, R. H., & Kourembanas, S. (2020). Newborn chest. In: R. H. Cleveland (Ed.), *Imaging in pediatric pulmonology* (2nd ed., pp. 51–68). New York: Springer.

Liew, Z., Fenton, A. C., Harigopal, S., Gopalakaje, S., Brodlie, M., & O'Brien, C. J. (2020). Physiological effects of high-flow nasal cannula therapy in preterm infants. *Archives of Disease in Childhood. Fetal and Neonatal Edition, 105*, 87–93.

Liu, J., Ren, X., & Li, J. (2020). POC-LUS guiding pleural puncture drainage to treat neonatal pulmonary atelectasis caused by congenital massive effusion. *Journal of Maternal–Fetal and Neonatal Medicine, 33*(1), 174–176. doi: 10.1080/14767058.2018.1526921.

Lozano, S. M., & Newnam, K. M. (2016). Modalities of mechanical ventilation: volume-targeted versus pressure-limited. *Advances in Neonatal Care, 16*(2), 99–107, quiz E101–E102. doi: 10.1097/anc.0000000000000272.

Magnani, J. E., & Donn, S. M. (2020). Persistent respiratory distress in the term neonate: genetic surfactant deficiency diseases. *Current Pediatric Reviews, 16*(1), 17–25.

Mahmood, B., Newton, D., & Pallotto, E. K. (2018). Current trends in neonatal ECMO. *Seminars in perinatology, 42*(2), 80–88.

Mandell, E., Kinsella, J. P., & Abman, S. H. (2021). Persistent pulmonary hypertension of the newborn. *Pediatric Pulmonology, 56*(3), 661–669. doi: 10.1002/ppul.25073.

Martin, R. (2021a). Overview of neonatal respiratory distress: disorders of transition. In: J. A. Garcia-Pratts, & M. S. Kim (Eds.), *UpToDate*. Walters Kluwer. <https://www.uptodate.com/contents/overview-of-neonatal-respiratory-distress-disorders-of-transition?search>. (Accessed 15 February 2022).

Martin, R. (2021b). Pathogenesis, clinical manifestations, and diagnosis of apnea of prematurity. In: J. A. Garcia-Pratts, G. B. Mallory, & M. S. Kim (Eds.), *UpToDate*. Walters Kluwer. <https://www.uptodate.com/contents/pathogenesis-clinical-manifestations-and-diagnosis-of-apnea-of-prematurity?search> (Accessed 15 February 2022).

Martin, R. J., Walsh, M. C., & Fanaroff, A. A. (2019). *Fanaroff and Martin's neonatal-perinatal medicine: diseases of the fetus and infant* (11th ed.) Philadelphia, PA: Elsevier Health Sciences.

Martinho, S., Adão, R., Leite-Moreira, A. F., & Brás-Silva, C. (2020). Persistent pulmonary hypertension of the newborn: pathophysiological mechanisms and novel therapeutic approaches. *Frontiers in Pediatrics, 8*, 342. doi: 10.3389/fped.2020.00342.

Masand, M., & Hauptfleisch, C. (2018). Severe subcutaneous emphysema in a term neonate. *Case Reports, 2018*, bcr2018226415. doi: 10.1136/bcr-2018-226415.

Masclans, J. R., Pérez-Terán, P., & Roca, O. (2015). Papel de la oxigenoterapia de alto flujo en la insuficiencia respiratoria aguda. *Medicina Intensiva, 39*, 505–515.

Mathew, B., & Lakshminrusimha, S. (2017). Persistent pulmonary hypertension in the newborn. *Children, 4*(8), 63.

Matlock, D. N., Bai, S., Weisner, M. D., Comtois, N., Beck, J., Sinderby, C., et al. (2019). Tidal volume transmission during non-synchronized nasal intermittent positive pressure ventilation via RAM® cannula. *Journal of Perinatology, 39*(5), 723–729.

McKinley, D. F., Kinney, S. B., Copnell, B., & Shann, F. (2018). Long-term effects of saline instilled during endotracheal suction in pediatric intensive care: a randomized trial. *American Journal of Critical Care, 27*(6), 486–494.

Miller, D. C., Pu, J., Kukafka, D., & Bime, C. (2020). Failure of high flow nasal cannula and subsequent intubation is associated with increased mortality as compared to failure of non-invasive ventilation and mechanical ventilation alone: a real-world retrospective analysis. *Journal of Intensive Care Medicine*, 37(1), 41–45. doi: 10.1177/0885066620968041.

Mitchell, R. N., Kumar, V., Fausto, N., Abbas, A. K., & Aster, J. C. (2017*). Pocket companion to Robbins & Cotran pathologic basis of disease* (9th ed.). Philadelphia: Elsevier.

Monica, N. F., Pamela, S., Juan, Q. L., & Li, J. (2017). Recent understanding of pathophysiology, risk factors and treatments of neonatal respiratory distress syndrome: a review. *Science Letters, 5*(1), 70–78.

Montealegre-Pomar, A., Bohorquez, A., & Charpak, N. (2020). Systematic review and meta-analysis suggest that Kangaroo position protects against apnoea of prematurity. *Acta Paediatrica, 109*(7), 1310–1316.

Nair, S., Lewis, L. E., Godinho, M. A., Murthy, S., Lakiang, T., & Venkatesh, B. T. (2018). Factors associated with neonatal pneumonia in India: protocol for a systematic review and planned meta-analysis. *BMJ Open, 8*(1), e018790. doi: 10.1136/bmjopen-2017-018790.

Nakwan, N., Jain, S., Kumar, K., Hosono, S., Hammoud, M., El-sayed, Y. Y., et al. (2020). An Asian multicentre retrospective study on persistent pulmonary hypertension of the newborn: incidence, aetiology, diagnosis, treatment and outcome. *Journal of Maternal–Fetal and Neonatal Medicine, 33*(12), 2032–2037.

Nangia, S., Thukral, A., & Chawla, D. (2017). Tracheal suction at birth in non-vigorous neonates born through meconium-stained amniotic fluid. *Cochrane Database Systemic Review, 6*(6), CD012671. doi: 10.1002/14651858.CD012671.pub2. doi: 10.1002/14651858.CD012671.

National Health and Medical Research Council (NHMRC). (2016–2019). Improving breathing support for newborn infants in non-tertiary centres: the HUNTER Trial. <https://researchdata.ands.org.au/improving-breathing-support-hunter-trial/662395> (Accessed 15 February 2022).

Noripour, S., Molaei, A., Bandari, R., Emadi, A., Farokhi Far, S. M., & Forozeshfard, M. (2017). Comparison of the results of simultaneous surfactant administration and nasal continuous positive airway pressure (INSURE) and non-administration of surfactant for the treatment of infants with respiratory distress syndrome. *Journal of Comprehensive Pediatrics, 8*(1), 37462. 10.5812/compreped.37462.

Northway, W. J., Rosan, R., & Porter, D. (1967). Pulmonary disease following respiratory therapy of hyaline membrane disease: bronchopulmonary dysplasia. *New England Journal of Medicine, 276*, 357–368.

Omansky, G. L. (2019). Pulmonary haemorrhage in the neonate. *Neonatal Network, 38*(2), 109–112.

Panza, R., Prontera, G., Ives, K. N., Zivanovic, S., Roehr, C. C., Quercia, M., et al. (2020). Pigtail catheters versus traditional chest drains for pneumothorax treatment in two NICUs. *European Journal of Pediatrics, 179*(1), 73–79.

Patil, S. S., Sukanya, Rath, S., & George, C. E. (2018). Study on umbilical cord arterial blood gas analysis and cord blood lactate levels as predictors for adverse neonatal outcome: an observational study. *International Journal of Reproduction, Contraception, Obstetrics and Gynecology, 7*(4), 1494+. <https://link.gale.com/apps/doc/A539921773/AONE?u5griffith&sid5AONE&xid52b475124> (Accessed 15 February 2022).

Perez, C. R., Romitti, M. G., Pezzotti, E., D'Andrea, V., Pezza, L., & Pittiruti, M. (2020). Subcutaneously anchored sutureless device for securement of chest tubes in neonates with pleural effusion: three case reports. *Case Reports in Pediatrics, 2020*, 5, 7480483. doi: 10.1155/2020/7480483.

Philips, J. B. (2021). Approach to the neonate with pleural effusions. In: R. Martin, & M. S. Kim (Eds.), *UpToDate*. Walters Kluwer. <https://www.uptodate.com/contents/approach-to-the-neonate-with-pleural-effusions?search> (Accessed 15 February 2022).

Protain, A. P., Firestone, K. S., McNinch, N. L., & Stein, H. M. (2021). Evaluating peak inspiratory pressures and tidal volume in premature neonates on NAVA ventilation. *European Journal of Pediatrics, 180*(1), 167–175.

Puri, P. (2020). *Pediatric surgery: general principles and newborn surgery*. Berlin/Heidelberg: Springer.

Ravikumar, C., McDaniel, D., & Quinn, A. (2019). Air leak syndrome: pneumoperitoneum in a ventilated neonate. *Case Reports in Pediatrics, 2019*, 4238601–4238604. doi: 10.1155/2019/4238601.

Roberts, C. T., Owen, L. S., Manley, B. J., Frøisland, D. H., Donath, S. M., Dalziel, K. M., et al. for the HIPSTER Trial Investigators. (2016). Nasal high-flow therapy for primary respiratory support in preterm infants. *New England Journal of Medicine, 375*, 1142–1151.

Rohrer, L., Vial, Y., Hanquinet, S., Tenisch, E., & Alamo, L. (2020). Imaging of anorectal malformations in utero. *European Journal of Radiology, 125*, 108859.

Romanis, E. C. (2018). Artificial womb technology and the frontiers of human reproduction: conceptual differences and potential implications. *Journal of Medical Ethics. 44*, 751–755.

Ruaro, B., Salton, F., Braga, L., Wade, B., Confalonieri, P., Volpe, M. C., et al. (2021). The history and mystery of alveolar epithelial type ii cells: focus on their physiologic and pathologic role in lung. *International Journal of Molecular Sciences, 22*(5), 2566.

Rubarth, L. B., & Quinn, J. (2015). Respiratory development and respiratory distress syndrome. *Neonatal Network, 34*(4), 231.

Rubortone, S. A., De Carolis, M. P., Lacerenza, S., Bersani, I., Occhipinti, F., & Romagnoli, C. (2012). Use of a combined SpO_2/$PtcCO_2$ sensor in the delivery room. *Sensors, 12*(8), 10980–10989. doi: 10.3390/s120810980.

Saugstad, O. D. (1990). Oxygen toxicity in the neonatal period. *Acta Paediatrica Scandinavica, 79*(10), 881–892. doi: 10.1111/j.1651-2227. 1990.tb11348.x.

Shih-Hsin, W., & Tsao, P. (2020). Phenotypes of bronchopulmonary dysplasia. *International Journal of Molecular Sciences, 21*(17), 6112. doi: 10.3390/ijms21176112.

Silverman, W. A., & Andersen, D. A. (1956). A controlled clinical trial of effects of water mist on obstructive respiratory signs, death rate and necropsy findings among premature infants. *Pediatrics, 17*(1), 1–10.

Stark, A. R., & Eichenwald, E. C. (2021). Persistent pulmonary hypertension of the newborn. In J. A. Garcia-Pratts, & M. S. Kim (Eds.), *UpToDate*. Walters Kluwer. <https://www.uptodate.com/contents/persistent-pulmonary-hypertension-of-the-newborn?search> (Accessed 15 February 2022).

Stocker, C. F., & Horton, S. B. (2016). Anticoagulation strategies and difficulties in neonatal and paediatric extracorporeal membrane oxygenation (ECMO). *Perfusion, 31*(2), 95–102. doi: 10.1177/0267659115590626.

Sullivan, K. P., White, H. O., Grover, L. E., Negron, J. J., Lee, A. F., & Rhein, L. M. (2021). Transcutaneous carbon dioxide pattern and trend over time in preterm infants. *Pediatric Research, 90*(4), 840–846. doi: 10.1038/s41390-020-01308-2.

Sunil K., Miall, L., Jardine, L., & Levene, M. I. (2017). *Essential neonatal medicine* (5th ed.). Chichester, UK: Wiley-Blackwell.

Sweet, D. G., Carnielli, V., Greisen, G., Hallman, M., Ozek, E., Te Pas, A., et al. (2019). European consensus guidelines on the management of respiratory distress syndrome – 2019 update. *Neonatology, 115*(4), 432–450.

Tefera, M., Assefa, N., Mengistie, B., Abrham, A., Teji, K., & Worku, T. (2020). Elective cesarean section on term pregnancies has a high risk for neonatal respiratory morbidity in developed countries: a systematic review and meta-analysis [systematic review]. *Frontiers in Pediatrics, 8*, 286. doi: 10.3389/fped.2020.00286.

Tomkins, Z. (2020). *Applied anatomy and physiology*. Chatswood, NSW: Elsevier Australia.

Tramarin, J., Cortegiani, A., Gregoretti, C., Vitale, F., Palmeri, C., Iozzo, P., et al. (2019). Regional anticoagulation with heparin of an extracorporeal CO_2 removal circuit: a case report. *Journal of Medical Case Reports, 13*(1), 1–4.

Tukova, J., Smisek, J., Zlatohlavkova, B., Plavka, R., & Markova, D. (2020). Early inhaled budesonide in extremely preterm infants decreases long-term respiratory morbidity. *Pediatric pulmonology, 55*(5), 1124–1130. doi: 10.1002/ppul.24704.

van Kaam, A. H., De Luca, D., Hentschel, R., Hutten, J., Sindelar, R., Thome, U., et al. (2021). Modes and strategies for providing conventional mechanical ventilation in neonates. *Pediatric Research, 90*(5), 957–962.

Van Ommen, C. H., Neunert, C. E., & Chitlur, M. B. (2018). Neonatal ECMO. *Frontiers in Medicine, 5*, 289.

Verklan, M. T., & Walden, M. (2020). *Core curriculum for neonatal intensive care nursing* (6th ed.). St. Louis, MO: Saunders.

Victoria State Government. (2021). *Neonatal ehandbook*. <https://www.bettersafercare.vic.gov.au/clinical-guidance/neonatal> (Accessed 15 February 2022).

Villamil, V., Fernández-Ibieta, M., Ubeda, M. A. G., García, M. J. A., Pruneda, R. R., Morote, J. M. S., et al. (2018). Correlation between pneumoperitoneum and surgical findings and morbidity and mortality in newborns with necrotising enterocolitis. *Anales de Pediatría (English Ed.), 89*(4), 205–210.

Won, A., Suarez-Rebling, D., Baker, A. L., Burke, T. F., & Nelson, B. D. (2019). Bubble CPAP devices for infants and children in resource-limited settings: review of the literature. *Paediatrics and International Child Health, 39*(3), 168–176. doi: 10.1080/20469047.2018.1534389.

CHAPTER 10

CARE OF THE NEONATE WITH A CARDIOVASCULAR DISORDER

PATRICIA BROMLEY AND GLENDA FLEMING

Learning objectives

After reading this chapter you will be able to:

- evaluate the incidence of congenital heart disease in Australia and New Zealand overall for a number of specific conditions
- recognise the early embryological development of the cardiac and circulatory system
- distinguish the various cardiac conditions and how lesions are categorised
- apply the principles of a systematic newborn physical assessment to a more focused cardiac assessment
- appraise the various management strategies required of critical cardiac conditions, including:
  - immediate and emergency management
  - surgical and non-surgical management
  - palliative management
- analyse the principles of a family-centred care approach to families and patients with cardiac conditions and synthesise these concepts into their own clinical contexts.

Key words, terms, abbreviations

acyanotic
aortic stenosis
arrhythmia
atrial septal defect (ASD)
atrioventricular septal defect (AVSD)
blood pressure (BP)
cardiac output (CO)
cardiopulmonary bypass (CPB)
coarctation of the aorta (COA)
complete heart block (CHB)
congenital heart disease (CHD)
congestive heart failure (CHF)
cyanotic
ductus arteriosus (DA)
dysrhythmias
electrocardiography (ECG)
heart rate (HR)
interrupted aortic arch (IAA)
necrotising enterocolitis (NEC)
obstructive
patent ductus arteriosus (PDA)
persistent pulmonary hypertension of the newborn (PPHN)
pulmonary atresia
shunt
supraventricular tachycardia (SVT)
tetralogy of Fallot (ToF)
total anomalous pulmonary venous return (TAPVR)
transposition of the great arteries (TGA)
ventricular septal defect (VSD)

INTRODUCTION

Cardiovascular disorders in the newborn include both structural and non-structural conditions. Congenital heart defects are structural disorders of the heart and/or related vessels. Neonates can also experience non-structural disorders that affect heart function such as myopathies and neoplasms, as well as electrophysiological disease that cause arrhythmias.

The management of **congenital heart disease (CHD)** requires the specialised services of paediatric cardiologists, paediatric cardiothoracic surgeons and a specialist cardiac nursing team as well as neonatal, paediatric and cardiac intensive care facilities. Although some neonates with CHD may be managed as outpatients, there are several congenital heart defects which require immediate transfer to a facility that offers specialised care, particularly for those neonates who require surgical or catheter-based intervention in the early newborn period. Throughout Australia and New Zealand, there are four major centres (Sydney, Melbourne, Brisbane and Auckland) which provide full neonatal cardiac surgical services. Perth offers services for some neonates requiring cardiac surgery.

This chapter will explore the more common structural and non-structural heart diseases encountered in the neonatal period. Information will include a description, pathophysiology and management of individual defects. CHD is considered a lifelong, sometimes chronic, condition and, as such, neonates with CHD develop into a very special paediatric population who will require ongoing medical and nursing/midwifery attention.

EMBRYOLOGICAL DEVELOPMENT OF THE HEART

The heart undergoes a complex transformation during early fetal life, with the development of the primitive heart tube occurring between weeks 2 and 4 of gestation (Fig. 10.1). Congenital heart defects arise at various embryological time points. Blood pumps through the primitive heart from the 4th week of gestation. Cardiac development is almost complete by week 6 of gestation, which makes the fetus vulnerable to congenital abnormalities as the pregnancy may not even be recognised (Swanson & Erickson, 2021).

Chapter 4 details fetal circulation and the transition to postnatal life.

CLINICAL PRACTICE 10.1

It is important to be familiar with the pressure gradients between the left and right sides of the heart to understand the mechanisms of the **shunt** lesions. Practise drawing the flow of blood through the heart during the fetal and then the postnatal periods.

Extrauterine circulation – normal blood flow through the heart

Deoxygenated blood returns from the systemic circulation, entering the right atrium via the inferior and superior vena cava. The deoxygenated blood is pumped from the right atrium through the tricuspid valve to the right ventricle, then through the pulmonary valve and the pulmonary artery to the pulmonary circulation, where it is oxygenated in the lungs. Oxygenated blood returns to the left atrium via four pulmonary veins (two each from the left and right lungs). The oxygenated blood then enters the left ventricle (via the bicuspid (mitral) valve) and, from there, it is pumped through the aortic valve into the aorta and on to the systemic circulation.

Fig. 10.2 shows the postnatal circulation with closed intrauterine communications.

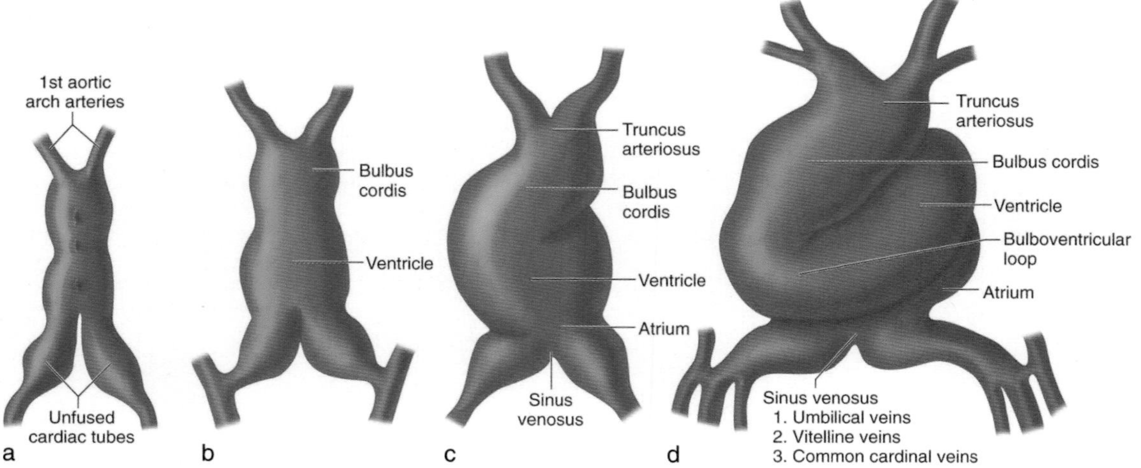

FIGURE 10.1 **Primitive heart tube development during early fetal life**

a Paired cardiac tubes fuse in head-to-toe direction (day 21 ± 1 day). **b** Fused cardiac tube with beginning of chamber differentiation (day 22 ± 1 day). **c** Bulboventricular looping to the right (day 23 ± 1 day). **d** Heart tube after completion of bulboventricular looping (day 24 ± 1 day).

Source: Gedgaudas et al. (1985).

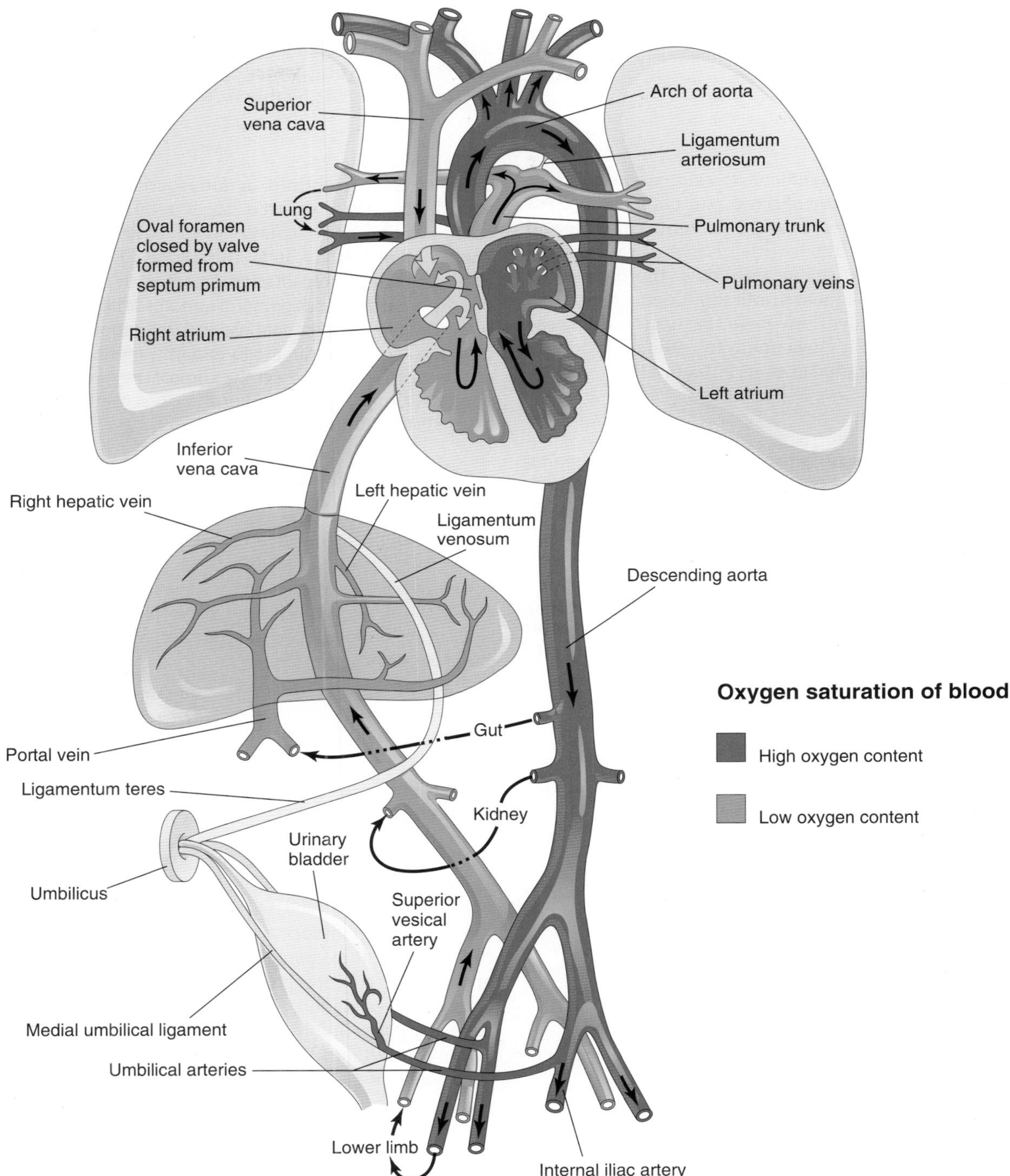

FIGURE 10.2 **Postnatal cardiovascular circulation**

The colours indicate the oxygen saturation of the blood, and the arrows demonstrate the direction of flow.
Source: Moore and Persaud (2015, Figs. 14-32, 14-33).

CLINICAL PRACTICE 10.2

An easy way to remember the valves in the heart is:

- to 'tri before you bi' (cuspid valves)
- pulmonary and aortic valves are self-explanatory.

EPIDEMIOLOGY

The incidence of CHD is difficult to estimate as different studies vary in the data collected and criteria used. For example, some defects such as a **ventricular septal defect (VSD)** may spontaneously resolve; **patent ductus arteriosus (PDA)** can significantly skew the data; some defects may not be diagnosed until adulthood; others, such as bicuspid aortic valve, may never be diagnosed. These variations can make it challenging to estimate incidence and prevalence (Mozaffarian et al., 2016, p. e235).

INCIDENCE

Congenital heart disease is the most common congenital disorder in newborns (Victor Chang Cardiac Research Institute, 2022). Current global estimates suggest up to 9 out of every 1000 live births are affected by CHD; this translates to 1.35 million neonates born with some form of CHD each year (Khasawneh et al., 2020). There is an increased incidence of CHD in preterm and extremely preterm neonates (11.6%), which is also associated with poorer outcomes and a significantly higher mortality rate (7.5-fold increased death rate) (Chu et al., 2017).

EVIDENCE-BASED PRACTICE RESEARCH 10.1

Four babies die each week from CHD in Australia (Victor Chang Cardiac Research Institute, 2022), which is the greatest cause of mortality in children under the age of 1 year (HeartKidsAustralia, 2016). Twelve neonates are born every week in New Zealand with a cardiac defect (HeartKidsNZ, n.d.).

Other factors associated with increased incidence of CHD are:

- maternal age (>35 years) (Hashim et al., 2020)
- maternal gestational diabetes (Dolk et al., 2020)
- parental consanguinity (Fazeriandy et al., 2018)
- cigarette smoking during pregnancy, particularly in the first trimester (Zhang et al., 2021).

CAUSES

Structural abnormalities of the heart arise when the heart fails to develop normally in the early weeks of gestation. Eighty-five percent of cases of CHD have no known cause (Victor Chang Cardiac Research Institute, 2022). In about 8% of infants, there is a clear genetic cause (commonly Down, cri du chat, trisomies 18 and 13 and Turner syndrome). In the remaining percentage, the causes are environmental, such as fetal exposure to teratogens through maternal drugs (e.g. antiepileptic medications and alcohol), or viral infections (e.g. rubella and cytomegalovirus) (Blackburn, 2018; Blue et al., 2012; Table 10.1).

DIAGNOSIS

Cases of CHD diagnosed by ultrasound in the antenatal period are often referred to a fetal cardiologist for confirmation and counselling. Typically, the first appointment with a fetal cardiologist is after the 18-week scan; early consultation presents an opportunity to discuss treatment pathways. Neonates who present with symptoms in the postnatal period will require transfer to a cardiac facility for diagnosis and treatment. The urgency of the transfer is based on the clinical presentation of the neonate. Generally, the earlier the presentation the more severe is the cardiac lesion.

FAMILY-CENTRED CARE 10.1

Consider the situation for parents of a newborn with a postnatal diagnosis of CHD. On hearing the provisional diagnosis of a cardiac condition, often the parents' first thought is whether their baby will survive. The family will want to know why this has happened to their baby, what treatment their baby will require and whether their baby is going to be able to lead a normal life.

Pregnancy and the birth of a baby are expected to be a joyful experience. When a child is diagnosed with CHD, this may bring fear and stress for the parents and extended family. As you read through this chapter, consider these questions and how you might address these concerns and support the family.

PHYSICAL EXAMINATION

It is important to adopt a structured systematic approach to the physical examination; a cephalo-caudal approach ensures a comprehensive assessment. Observation, inspection, palpation, percussion and auscultation are used to gather information and vital cues (Park, 2021). Table 10.2 outlines the findings on physical examination that may indicate a CHD.

FAMILY-CENTRED CARE 10.2

It is important to include parents when examining their baby. Encourage them to assist with settling and comforting their baby during examinations and procedures. Provide them with information about the examination findings and the significance of the findings.

TABLE 10.1 **Origins of cardiac defects**

Overview of causes	Genetic syndrome (chromosomal anomaly)	Proportion of patients with CHD
Chromosomal anomalies account for 8–10% of presenting cases	Edwards syndrome (trisomy 13)	90–100%
	DiGeorge (22q11.2 deletion) syndrome	75–85%
	Down syndrome (trisomy 21)	40–50%
Mendelian syndromes account for 3–5% of presenting cases	Heterotaxy syndrome	90–100%
	Alagille syndrome	85–95%
	Noonan syndrome	80–90%
	Holt–Oram syndrome	80%
Non-syndromal familial, single-gene disorders – small proportion	Familial forms of CHD	Exact numbers unknown; however, there is a recurrence risk (see below)
Non-genetic factors		Risk of CHD
Environmental factors[a] and teratogens; for many of these conditions the exact numbers are unknown	Maternal rubella	30–60%
	Maternal phenylketonuria	15–50%
	Maternal diabetes[b]	5%
Recurrence risk		Risk of CHD
Recurrence risk can be determined in a minority of cases and the risks vary considerably between the different types of CHD	One sibling with neither parent affected	1–6%
	Two siblings with neither parent affected	10%
	Mother affected	2–20%
	Father affected	1–5%
Concordance with index case		Risk of CHD
Note: an index case is defined as 'an affected individual who had prompted the referral', either the mother herself, the father, or a sibling of the current pregnancy[c]	Exact concordance – where the first recurrent case has the identical defect to the index case	37%
	Concordance with the group – where the defect belongs to the same spectrum of CHD as in the index case	47%

CHD, congenital heart disease.
[a]Environmental factors include alcohol, amphetamines, anticonvulsants, medications etc.
[b]The greatest risk for developing CHD is before the 7th week of gestation, resulting in defects of primary cardiogenesis such as atrioventricular septal defects and outflow tract abnormalities.
[c]Gill et al. (2003, p. 924).

Source: Blue et al. (2012).

CLINICAL PRACTICE 10.3

Auscultating heart sounds: it is important to maintain skills in performing a full cardiac assessment. Listening to heart sounds is challenging; however, if neonatal nurses and midwives undertake auscultation on a regular basis, they will develop the skill. The key assessment points are the same as in an adult: the second intercostal space either side of the sternum and the fourth intercostal space to the left of the sternum and the left mid-clavicular line.

Hint: to start with, listen for normal heart sounds; it will be easier when you encounter an abnormal sound. You may not know what it is, but you will recognise that it is abnormal. Sadowsky and Verklan (2021, p. 470) provide an excellent overview of heart sounds and murmurs to add to your learning in this area.

Adjunctive diagnostic tools

History

A comprehensive family history, including prenatal screenings, maternal illnesses (diabetes, rubella, teratogenic exposure and medications) is essential. For the baby, there may be a history of poor feeding and poor weight gain, coughing and cyanosis. Consider recurrence risk: a parent or sibling with CHD increases the incidence of CHD in the neonate.

Pulse oximetry

Pre- (right hand) and post- (right or left foot) ductal oxygen saturation is one of the main screening tools used in the neonatal period after the first 24 hours of life. Any difference in pre- and postductal oxygen saturations $>3\%$ on three consecutive readings, 1 hour apart, suggests a right-to-left shunt (Jullien, 2021).

TABLE 10.2 **Findings on physical examination that may indicate congenital heart disease**

System	Finding	Physiological explanation
General inspection	Dysmorphic features of genetic and congenital malformations (for example trisomy 13, 18 or 21) Congenital skeletal abnormalities – particularly hand and arm	Many congenital syndromes are associated with CHD, such as CHARGE and VACTERL associations Factors that affect the embryonic development of the heart may also impact on other structures developing concurrently
Neurological		
Inspection	Alertness – drowsy, tires easily Irritability Full fontanelle	Cerebral hypoxaemia – reduced oxygen delivery may result in changes to neurological status and even cerebral oedema Cerebral irritability can be a result of cerebral oedema A full fontanelle is a good indicator of oedema
Respiratory		
Inspection	Tachypnoea – particularly during feeding or times of exertion Intercostal/sternal recession	Normal respiratory rate is between 40 and 60 bpm Tachypnoea is associated with poor cardiac output and hypoxaemia; it is a compensatory mechanism to provide adequate oxygen to meet metabolic demands Recession – associated with a neonate's attempt to increase tidal volumes in order to maintain adequate oxygenation
	Cyanosis • Central cyanosis (chest, tongue and mucous membranes) • Differential cyanosis, compare lower limbs with upper limbs	Central cyanosis results from decreased systemic arterial oxygen saturation Mottling and cyanosis in lower limbs create suspicion of inadequate systemic circulation such as coarctation or **interrupted aortic arch (IAA)** Deoxygenated blood flows to the lower body, with oxygenated blood flowing to upper body through blood vessels proximal to the obstruction
Auscultation	Adventitious breath sounds – listen for rales (crackles) and poor air entry	Congestive heart failure and pulmonary over-circulation/pulmonary oedema
Cardiac		
Inspection	Circulation • Diaphoresis, cool, moist skin – increase during exertion such as during feeding • Pallor • Mottled • Prolonged capillary refill time (>2 seconds) • Central and differential cyanosis	Poor CO will result in blood being diverted to major organs at the expense of the peripheral perfusion Cyanosis – see Respiratory section above
	Oedema – not common initially in CHD; periorbital oedema may be seen in severe conditions Global oedema is a late sign of CHD indicated by excessive weight gain	Oedema occurs from reduced heart function and pulmonary over-circulation Peripheral oedema can also be due to renal failure or hydrops fetalis
	Visible apical (precordial) pulse	The apical pulse is normally located in the mid-clavicular line 4th or 5th intercostal space Persistent precordial pulse after first 12 hours of life is associated with volume overload and left-to-right shunt A laterally displaced apical pulse may indicate left ventricular hypertrophy
Palpation	BP on all four limbs: • decreased BP in lower limbs • widened pulse pressure Pulses: • note rhythm • palpate upper and lower limbs simultaneously; if pedal pulses are difficult to palpate try the femoral pulse	BP values depend on gestation, age and behavioural status. A pressure gradient ≥10–15 mmHg between upper and lower limbs, or weak or absent femoral pulses, may suggest left ventricular dysfunction, associated with severe coarctation of the aorta or IAA Bounding pulses and wide pulse pressure are associated with PDA[a]

TABLE 10.2 **Findings on physical examination that may indicate congenital heart disease—cont'd**

System	Finding	Physiological explanation
Auscultation	Tachycardia Murmur – most common sound S_1 and S_2 • S_1 – best heard at 4th intercostal space left sternal border and left midclavicular line • S_2 – best heard at 2nd intercostal space left sternal border	Normal sinus rhythm in the neonate is between 120 and 160 bpm HR varies with activity and whether the neonate is sleeping or awake Cardiac output is governed by stroke volume and heart rate ($CO = SV \times HR$) Neonates have limited capacity to increase SV due to the underdevelopment of the left ventricular musculature in early infancy; consequently, when the neonate requires more CO, this will increase HR rather than SV Murmurs result from abnormal turbulence or blood flow, for example through incompetent valves; physiological murmurs are often present on the first 24–48 h of life through the ductus arteriosus while circulation is transitioning from fetal circulation
Gastrointestinal		
General	Feeding difficulties Poor weight gain (failure to thrive)	Feeding is one of the most important 'stressors' for the neonate Neonates with CHD may have reduced circulating oxygen; hypoxaemia may result in lethargy and compensatory tachypnoea, which may impact on coordinating suck/swallow/breathe, making breast- or bottle-feeding difficult Neonates will often have poor nutritional intake to meet metabolic demands with poor weight gain; CHF is strongly related to poor weight gain
Inspection	Observe for distension	The risk of NEC in CHD with reduced systemic perfusion, for example coarctation of the aorta, is increased due to impaired mesenteric blood flow and gastrointestinal hypoperfusion
Palpation	Enlarged organs, particularly liver	Hepatomegaly associated with hepatic congestion Liver tip feels firm >3 cm below the right costal margin; this occurs due to back flow from the right heart to the hepatic venous circulation, particularly in left-to-right shunt defects with pulmonary over-circulation
Auscultate	Bowel sounds: • reduced or absent • sluggish	Reduced or absent bowels sounds may be an early indication of NEC Sluggish bowel sounds could indicate constipation and further compound cardiac symptoms
Renal		
Inspection	Urine output <0.5 mL/kg/h Abnormal serum electrolytes, urea, creatinine	A decreased urine output is a sign of hypoperfusion Renal function is a marker of organ perfusion

BP, blood pressure; CHARGE, coloboma, heart defects, atresia choanae (also known as choanal atresia), growth retardation, genital abnormalities, and ear abnormalities; CHD, congential heart disease; CO, cardiac output; HR, heart rate; NEC, necrotising enterocolitis; PDA, patent ductus arteriosus; SV, stroke volume; VACTERL, **v**ertebral defects, **a**nal atresia, **c**ardiac defects, **t**racheo-**o**esophageal fistula, **r**enal anomalies and **l**imb abnormalities.
[a]Park (2021).

EVIDENCE-BASED PRACTICE RESEARCH 10.2

All newborn babies should receive oxygen saturation screening for CHD between 24 and 72 hours of age (Jullien, 2021).

CLINICAL PRACTICE 10.4

Anaemia and oxygen saturation: saturation monitoring measures the amount of oxygen attached to haemoglobin. Be aware that anaemia can mask signs of hypoxaemia.

An asymptomatic anaemic neonate may record good oxygen saturations but have a decreased haemoglobin concentration, which will limit the oxygen-carrying capacity (Garcia-Prats, 2017).

Arterial blood gas values

These are used to differentiate between respiratory and heart disease. Carbon dioxide (CO_2) is quite often within normal limits in CHD, whereas it can be elevated in pulmonary disease.

CLINICAL PRACTICE 10.5

Hypoxia and hypoxaemia

The terms hypoxia and hypoxaemia are often used interchangeably; however, they are *not the same*. *Hypoxia* is a failure of oxygenation at the tissue level, whereas *hypoxaemia* is a measured value of low circulating oxygen (PaO_2). Although hypoxia and hypoxaemia may occur together, there are situations when there is hypoxaemia without hypoxia – for example, the patient can compensate for low PaO_2, primarily by increasing **cardiac output (CO)** and respiratory rate and decreasing oxygen consumption (Theodore, 2017) thereby maintaining oxygenation at cellular level.

Haematological investigations

Full blood count (FBC): avoid anaemia in **cyanotic** CHD; it is important to aim for a haemoglobin (Hb) level of 130–140 g/L. Urea and electrolytes (U&Es): it is important to evaluate baseline renal function. Neonates with CHD and reduced CO are at risk of reduced renal perfusion and impaired renal function.

Hyperoxia test

The hyperoxia test assesses the response to oxygen. The preductal (right radial) arterial oxygen tension (PaO_2) is measured while the neonate is breathing room air, and then again while breathing 100% oxygen for 10 minutes. If the cyanosis is cardiac in origin, arterial oxygen tension will remain less than 100 mmHg. Caution should be applied in infant with duct-dependent lesions as 100% oxygen is a potent pulmonary vasodilator and any sudden increase in pulmonary blood flow may result in pulmonary over-circulation (Willim & Supit, 2021). Also consider the potential effects of hyperoxygenation in the preterm population. In fact, since the advent of Doppler ultrasound, the hyperoxia test is now used very infrequently in most neonatal units.

Chest X-ray

Patients with **obstructive** CHD may develop cardiomegaly. Neonates with left-sided obstructive lesions may have cardiomegaly due to heart failure; a dilated right atrium is associated with extreme cardiomegaly. Chest X-ray can also be useful in excluding other conditions such as diaphragmatic hernia, pulmonary hypoplasia or pneumothorax. See Fig. 10.3 for more examples.

Electrocardiography

Electrocardiography (ECG) detects arrhythmias, abnormal haemodynamic structural abnormalities such as axis deviations and enlarged ventricles in the heart (Willim & Supit, 2021).

Ultrasound/echocardiogram

Antenatal ultrasounds may pick up cardiac conditions during pregnancy. After birth, a transthoracic echocardiogram will identify cardiac defects (Willim & Supit, 2021). Doppler ultrasound can determine the degree and direction of the shunt, and it will also allow for grading of obstructive lesions.

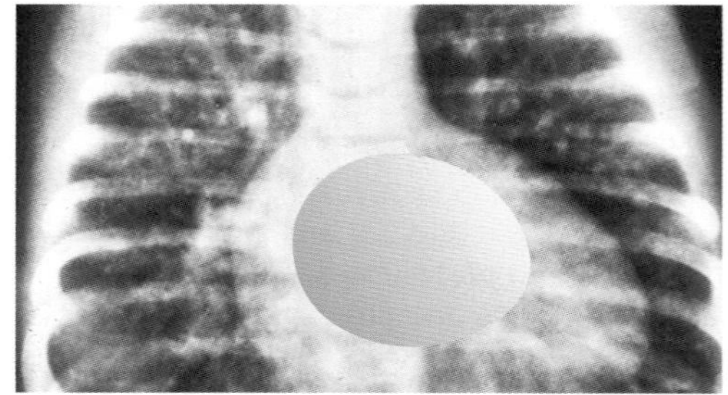

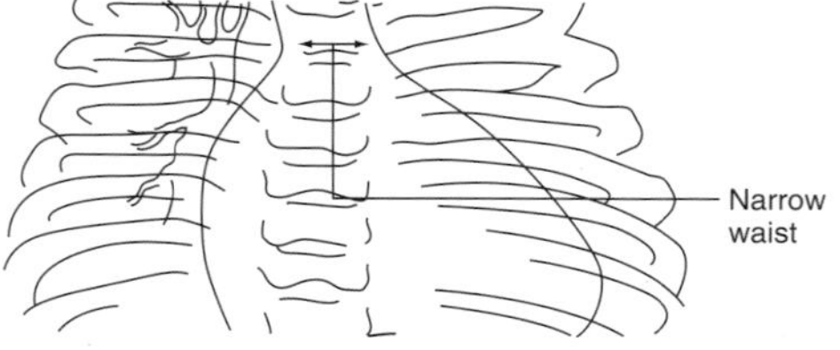

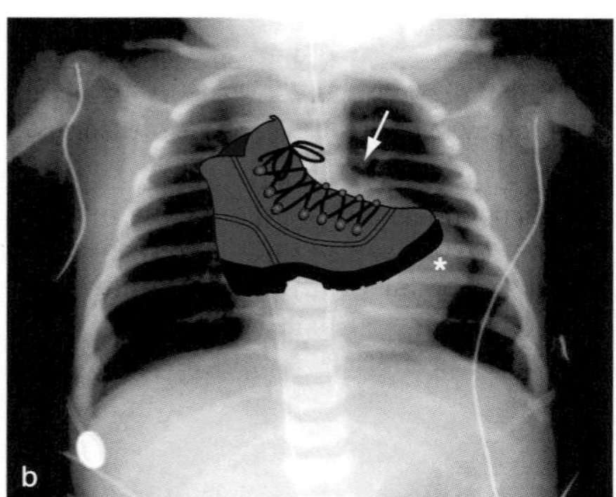

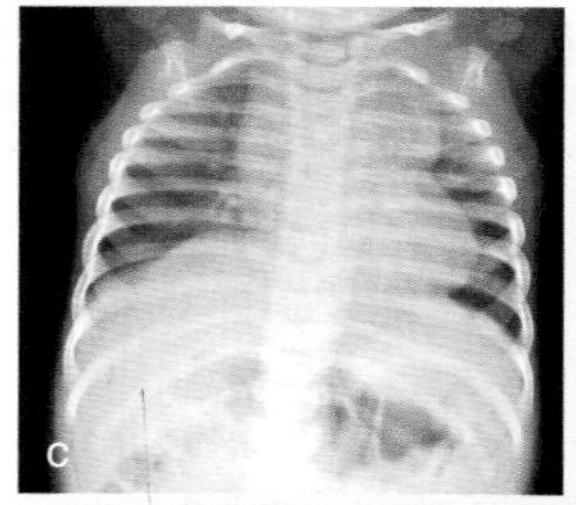

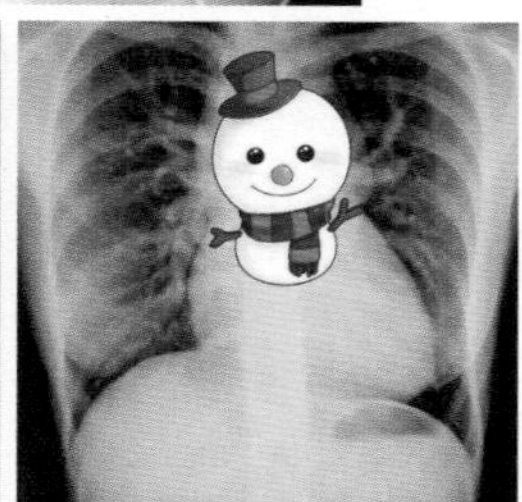

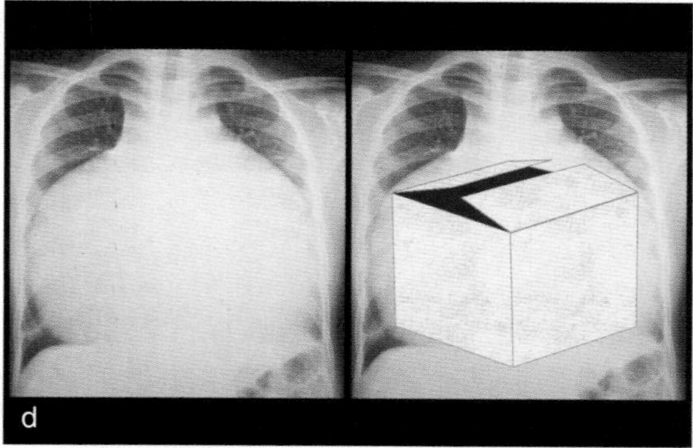

FIGURE 10.3 **Cardiac shapes on X-ray**

a Egg-on-a-string-shaped heart – transposition of the great arteries (TGA). **b** Boot-shaped heart – tetralogy of Fallot (ToF). **c** Snowman-shaped heart – total anomalous pulmonary venous return (TAPVR). **d** Ebstein's anomaly – box-shaped heart.

Images from: a Zitelli et al. (2018); ***b–d*** *Fanaroff and Fanaroff (2013). Copyright © 2013, 2001, 1993, 1986, 1979, 1973 by Saunders, an imprint of Elsevier.*

Cardiovascular magnetic resonance imaging

Cardiovascular magnetic resonance imaging (MRI) provides a 3-dimensional (3D) picture of anatomical and physiological information. More recently, 3D printing can produce a silicon model of the heart from the MRI scan. This can be used in surgical planning.

> **CLINICAL PRACTICE 10.6**
>
> In the newborn period, cardiac conditions can often present with the same signs as respiratory conditions. It is important to consider both when a neonate presents in respiratory distress. In addition to this, some neonates can have both a respiratory and a cardiac condition. Preterm neonates with cardiac conditions will also experience some degree of respiratory compromise.

Presentation

Symptoms of CHD may present within hours of delivery, within the first few days, first few months or much later in older children. Some conditions may not have clinical significance in the early neonatal period while others require emergency treatment to sustain life. Identifying which defects require immediate treatment in the postnatal period can be a challenge for the neonatal nurse/midwife.

Symptoms presenting at birth usually indicate a severe cardiac condition such as **transposition of the great arteries (TGA)** or **total anomalous pulmonary venous return (TAPVR)**. The presenting signs are usually cyanosis and respiratory distress with circulatory shock.

The clinical presentation includes poor oxygen saturations (70–75%) and respiratory distress with tachypnoea, grunting, intercostal recession, nasal flaring and cyanosis. As these signs can be similar to respiratory pathology, cardiac conditions may be misdiagnosed or missed in this early period.

Presentations within the first few days of life

These presentations are related to the closure of the **ductus arteriosus (DA)** and are referred to as 'duct-dependent' lesions. They can be further classified into two categories based upon presenting signs: cyanosis and shock.

CYANOSIS

When cyanosis is the presenting sign, it is the pulmonary circulation that is dependent on the patency of the DA. The two most likely conditions are **pulmonary atresia**, or pulmonary valve stenosis, and **tetralogy of Fallot (ToF)**.

Signs are severe cyanosis with mild respiratory distress. In fact, the mildness of the respiratory distress compared with the severity of the cyanosis is often the clue that the cause is cardiac related rather than respiratory.

SHOCK

When shock is the presenting clinical sign, it is the systemic circulation that is dependent on a patent DA. As the duct closes, systemic circulation is impaired and the neonate quickly deteriorates, developing signs of shock. This can escalate into a medical emergency. The two most likely conditions are **coarctation of the aorta (COA)** and **aortic stenosis**.

Signs are tachycardia, pallor, mottling, weak or no peripheral pulses, hypotension and no or reduced urine output; associated respiratory signs such as tachypnoea and grunting may also be apparent. One classic haemodynamic sign of COA is decreased **blood pressure (BP)** in the lower limbs; it is typically more than 10 mmHg less than that taken in a right upper extremity (Swanson & Erickson, 2021).

Conditions presenting later (in the first months of life)

In conditions presenting later (i.e. in the first months of life), there is usually a left-to-right shunt because of increased pressure in the left side of the heart. When infants present at this time, the condition tends to be less severe and related to increasing congestive heart failure (CHF). The two most common conditions are VSD and **atrioventricular septal defect (AVSD)**.

The clinical presentation includes signs of worsening cardiac failure, such as feeding difficulties with diaphoresis and mottling during and after feeds, and failure to thrive. There is also tachypnoea and tachycardia, associated with hepatomegaly and rapid weight gain due to fluid retention and oedema. These symptoms may occur during a period of rapid growth and increased activity, such as when the infant starts to crawl and the heart is unable to cope with the increased demand.

Presentations in older children

Older children presenting with defects causing left-to-right shunting are often seen when they become more active, for example, when they start school. Left-to-right shunting can occur with **atrial septal defect (ASD)** and VSD. Obstructive lesions include aortic and pulmonary stenosis.

> **CLINICAL PRACTICE 10.7**
>
> The timing and type of presentation help with the diagnosis:
> - The time of presentation relates to the severity of the condition – the earlier the presentation, the more severe is the condition.
> - Consider whether the lesion is duct dependent. If so, is it affecting the pulmonary or the systemic circulation? Is the neonate cyanosed, or shocked?
> - Obstructive or shunt lesions usually present later with increased risk of CHF.

CONGENITAL HEART DISEASE BY LESION

Acyanotic defects – left-to-right shunt

The overarching clinical feature in lesions that have a left-to-right shunt is pulmonary over-circulation, with resultant symptoms related to CHF.

Left-to-right shunts mix oxygenated blood from the left side of the heart with deoxygenated blood from the right side. The admixture does not affect the oxygen content of the blood entering the systemic circulation via the left ventricle, hence the term '**acyanotic**' heart disease.

Fig. 10.4 shows a frontal internal view of a normal heart.

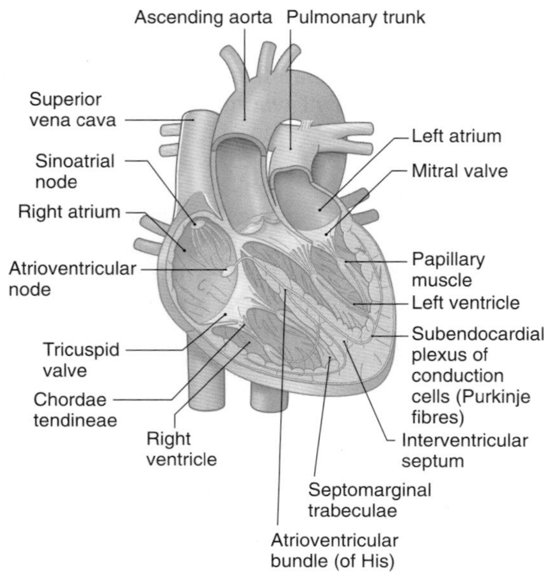

FIGURE 10.4 **Frontal internal view of a normal heart**
Source: Moses et al. (2013). Figure 30.1.

Table 10.3 describes the physiology, pathophysiology and management of the most common acyanotic defects.

CLINICAL PRACTICE 10.8

Consider whether it is a cyanotic or acyanotic disorder. One way of remembering these categories is asking: 'Where does the blood flow?'

EVIDENCE-BASED PRACTICE RESEARCH 10.3

Currently, there is some debate as to whether early closure of a PDA is essential in very low birthweight neonates. Rather than surgical or pharmacologically induced closure, interim management of the symptoms of PDA may be all that is required while the duct is allowed to close spontaneously (Park, 2021).

If early closure is indicated, ibuprofen and indomethacin are currently used for closure of PDA, with ibuprofen as the medication of choice (Ohlsson & Shah, 2020). However, the risk of pulmonary hypertension and gastrointestinal bleeding is increased with indomethacin and ibuprofen and paracetamol (acetaminophen) may be a better alternative. Trials with paracetamol have shown that the success rate on PDA closure was higher than placebo and similar to ibuprofen and indomethacin, with fewer adverse effects on kidney and liver function (Ohlsson & Shah, 2020).

TABLE 10.3 **Common acyanotic congenital heart defects**

Condition	Physiology	Pathophysiology	Management
Atrial septal defect (ASD)[a] Incidence 5–10% of CHD[b]	Communication between the right and left atrium May be at the site of the foramen ovale or another site on the septum	Only large defects will cause left-to-right shunt, pulmonary over-circulation and CHF	If symptomatic – diuretics Rarely needs repair in the neonatal period Repair via occlusive device or surgical closure when child is older[b]
Ventricular septal defect (VSD)[a] 15–20% of CHD[b]	Communication between right and left ventricles	Left-to-right shunt causes pulmonary over-circulation and CHF Signs of CHF include tachypnoea, sweating, poor weight gain and lethargy	Diuretics; may need tube feeding, increase calories and respiratory support Aim to grow neonate and delay surgery Some VSDs will close spontaneously May need pulmonary artery band to extend time to surgical repair if CHF persistent despite medical therapy Patch closure of VSD when clinically indicated[b]

TABLE 10.3 **Common acyanotic congenital heart defects—cont'd**

Condition	Physiology	Pathophysiology	Management
Atrioventricular septal defect (AVSD)[a] 2% of CHD, 30% of the defects occur in children with trisomy 21[b]	AVSDs involve the atrial septum, the ventricular septum and the atrioventricular valves; they encompass a spectrum of defects and are sub-characterised as partial or complete	Left-to-right shunt causes pulmonary over-circulation and CHF Tachypnoea, poor weight gain Usually more profound heart failure than ASD or VSD	Diuretics – may need tube feeding, increased calories and respiratory support Aim to grow neonate and delay surgery Repair via surgical procedure May need pulmonary artery band to extend time to surgical repair[b]
Patent ductus arteriosus (PDA)[a] Non-preterm 5–10% of CHD[b]; preterm 45% of neonates <1750 g, 80% of neonates <1200 g[b]	PDA is not a congenital defect in itself; rather it is a failure of the DA to close in the normal physiological extrauterine adaptation process Reasons include prematurity, raised pressure in the left side of the heart or decreased pressure in the right side of the heart Higher incidence in preterm neonates	Left-to-right shunt from aorta to pulmonary artery causes pulmonary over-circulation and CHF	May close spontaneously If not, then closure using indomethacin or ibuprofen Recent studies conclude equal efficacy between ibuprofen and paracetamol (see Evidence-based Practice 10.3) Surgical closure or device closure in catheter laboratory[b] In duct-dependent cardiac defects, the PDA is deliberately kept open using prostaglandin E_1 to provide adequate pulmonary or systemic blood flow[b]

ASD, atrial septal defect; AVSD, atrioventricular septal defect; CHD, congenital heart disease; CHF, congestive heart failure; DA, ductus arteriosus; PDA, patent ductus arteriosus; VSD, ventricular septal defect.
[a]Source: Everett & Lim (2010); images: atrial septal defect, p. 49; ventricular septal defect, p. 117; atrioventricular septal defect, p. 51; patent ductus arteriosus, p. 85.
[b]Park (2021).

Cyanotic defects – right-to-left shunt

In right-to-left shunts, poorly oxygenated blood from the right side of the heart mixes with normally oxygenated blood in the left side of the heart, reducing the oxygen content of blood being pumped to the body by the left ventricle, hence the term 'cyanotic' heart disease. Table 10.4 describes the physiology, pathophysiology and management of the most common cyanotic defects.

OBSTRUCTIVE DEFECTS

Obstruction to ventricular outflow can affect the right or left heart. Right heart obstructive defects have been included in the cyanotic defect section. Table 10.5 describes the physiology, pathophysiology and management of the most common left-sided obstructive defects.

CLINICAL PRACTICE 10.9

The five cyanotic congenital heart defects are as easy as remembering **1**, **2**, **3**, **4**, **5**:
One big trunk: truncus arteriosus
Two interchanged vessels: transposition of the great vessels
Three: tricuspid atresia
Four: tetralogy of Fallot
Five words: total anomalous pulmonary venous return

TABLE 10.4 **Common cyanotic congenital heart defects**

Condition	Physiology	Pathophysiology	Management
Pulmonary stenosis (PS) 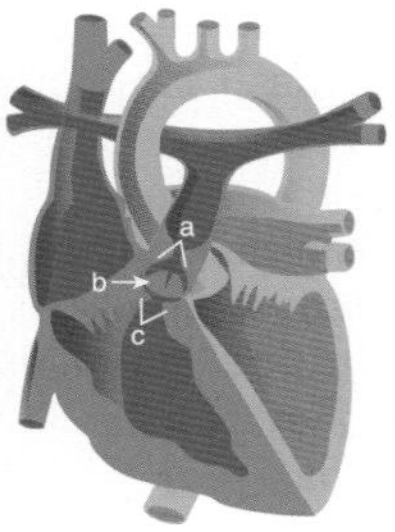 5–8% of CHD[a]	Obstruction to blood flow leaving the right ventricle Can be supravalvular (a), valvular (b) or subvalvular (c) Spectrum from mild to severe May coexist as part of ToF	Symptoms relate to the degree of obstruction to pulmonary blood flow Insufficient pulmonary blood flow results in cyanosis Right heart failure may develop Pulmonary arteries can be underdeveloped due to reduced blood flow	Balloon valvuloplasty as catheter lab procedure May need surgical correction if the pulmonary valve is dysplastic or the annulus is small[a]
Tetralogy of Fallot (ToF) 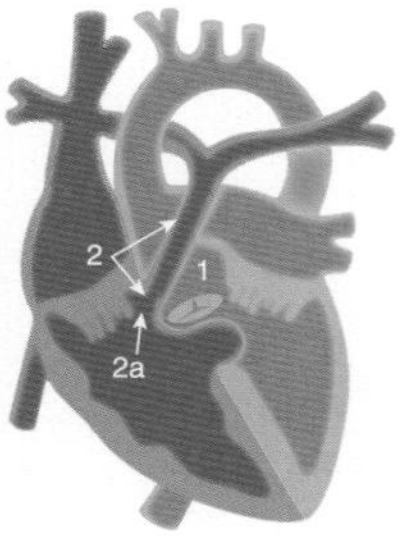 1 Aorta overriding VSD 2 Stenosis of pulmonary valve and artery 2a Infundibular stenosis 10% of CHD[a]	Four coexisting anomalies: • Large VSD • An aorta that is overriding the VSD (1) • PS with infundibular and subvalvular stenosis (2 and 2a) • Right ventricular hypertrophy	Obstruction of blood flow to the lungs causes a right-to-left shunt across the VSD with resultant cyanosis Underdevelopment of the pulmonary arteries due to reduced pulmonary blood flow Periodic infundibular spasm in the subpulmonary valve region can cause hypercyanotic spells known as 'Tet spells' Surgery	Prostaglandin E_1 infusion may be required to maintain ductal patency if severe PS For excessive cyanosis, an arterial-to-pulmonary shunt such as Blalock–Taussig (BT) shunt may be required Corrective ToF repair around 4–6 months of age[a]
Tricuspid atresia[b] 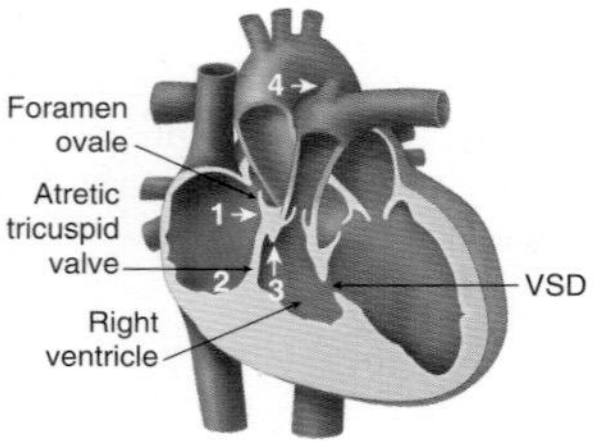 1–3% of CHD[a]	Tricuspid atresia • ASD (1) • Atretic tricuspid valve (2) • Hypoplastic right ventricle • PS (3) • Hypoplastic pulmonary arteries • PDA (4)	Variability in presentation related to accompanying defects Complete mixing of blood at atrial level If there is inadequate pulmonary blood flow, such as with PS or restrictive VSD, cyanosis will occur High pulmonary flow can occur if there is no PS with shunting left to right through the VSD	Duct-dependent circulation if PS Prostaglandin E_1 infusion to maintain duct patency Surgery follows a single ventricle physiology pathway Associated defects addressed concurrently 3-stage operative course Arterial-to-pulmonary shunt such as a BT shunt as a neonate Bidirectional Glenn shunt at 4–6 months, then a Fontan operation between 2 and 4 years later[a]
Truncus arteriosus 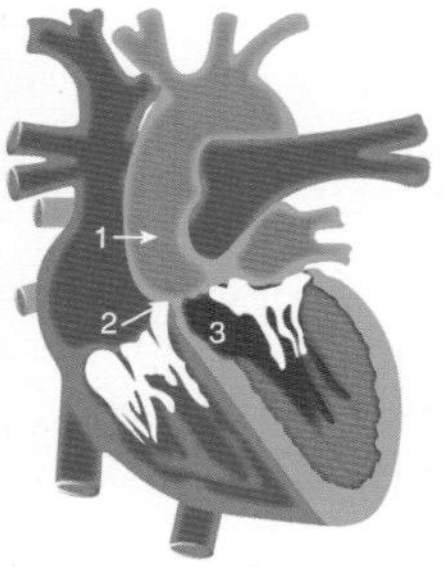 1 Truncus arteriosus type 1 2 4-leaflet truncal valve 3 VSD	Aortic and pulmonary arteries are joined together as a single common vessel with a single truncal valve Large VSD Three types classified by the way in which the pulmonary arteries arise from the truncal vessel: • Type 1 – main pulmonary artery branching off the common truncal vessel • Type 2 – pulmonary arteries positioned posteriorly • Type 3 – pulmonary arteries attached laterally from the common truncal vessel	All 3 types present with the same clinical picture of both cyanosis and congestive heart failure Complete mixing of oxygenated and deoxygenated blood at ventricular level and this will cause marked cyanosis Blood flow to the pulmonary circulation is frequently excessive, leading to symptoms of congestive heart failure	Complex surgery Common truncal vessel is committed to the systemic circulation A conduit from the right ventricle to the pulmonary artery (RV to PA conduit) to provide pulmonary blood flow The RV to PA conduit needs replacement at intervals due to the child's somatic growth Frequently, the truncal valve requires replacement later in life[a]

TABLE 10.4 **Common cyanotic congenital heart defects—cont'd**

Condition	Physiology	Pathophysiology	Management
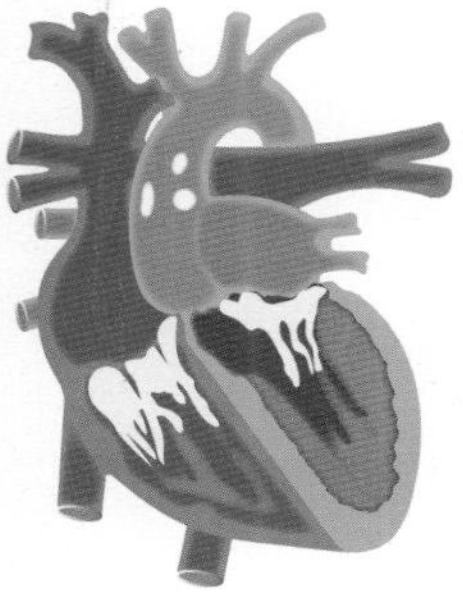 Truncus arteriosus type 2 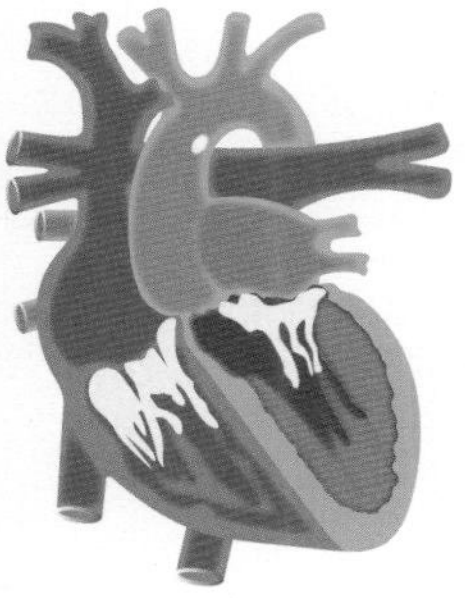 Truncus arteriosus type 3 <1% of CHD[a]			
Total anomalous pulmonary venous return (TAPVR) 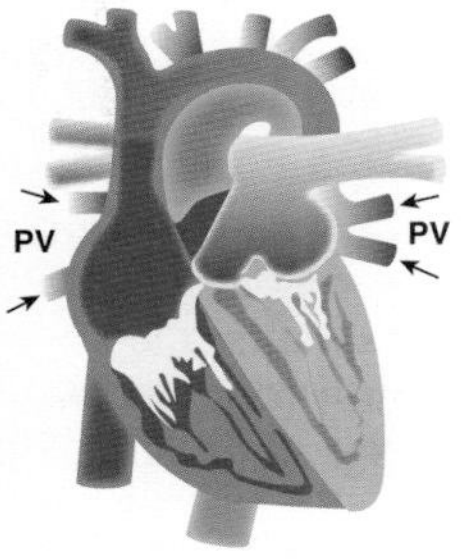 Supracardiac TAPVR 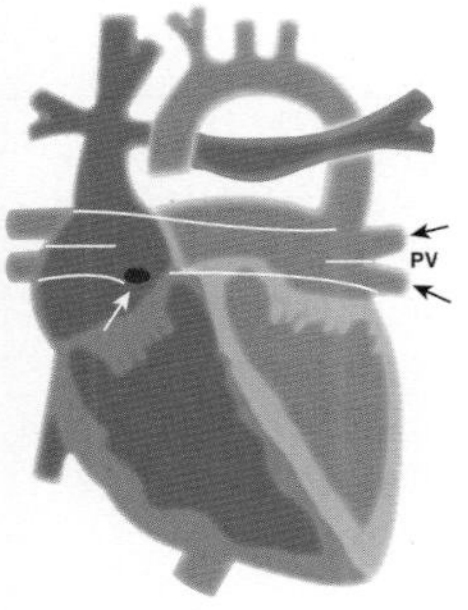 Intracardiac TAPVR	The key feature of this defect is that the pulmonary venous return goes to the right side of the heart instead of the correct left side of the heart 3 types: • Supracardiac TAPVR – the pulmonary veins enter the superior vena cava • Intracardiac TAPVR – the pulmonary veins enter the heart via the coronary sinus • Infracardiac TAPVR – the pulmonary veins connect to the portal system	In all forms of TAPVR, excessive blood flows to the right side of the heart An ASD is always present and necessary to mix the returning oxygenated blood from the lungs with deoxygenated blood returning from the body Right-to-left shunting across the ASD will result in cyanosis; if the venous return is obstructed, the degree of cyanosis will be more profound	Surgical repair is required in the neonatal period If the venous return is obstructed (more likely with infracardiac TAPVR), it is a surgical emergency to relieve the obstruction and reroute the pulmonary veins[a]

Continued

TABLE 10.4 **Common cyanotic congenital heart defects—cont'd**

Condition	Physiology	Pathophysiology	Management
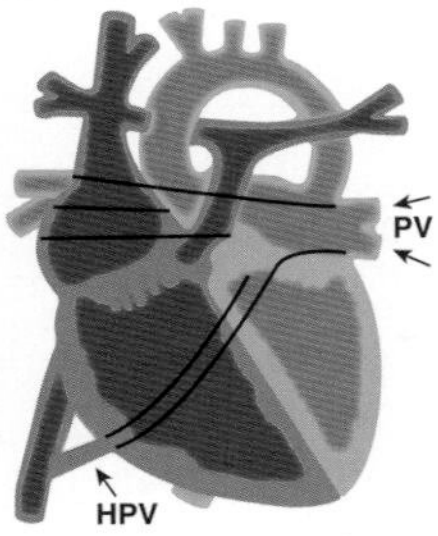 Infracardiac TAPVR 1% of CHD[a]			
Dextro-transposition of the great arteries (D-TGA)[b] 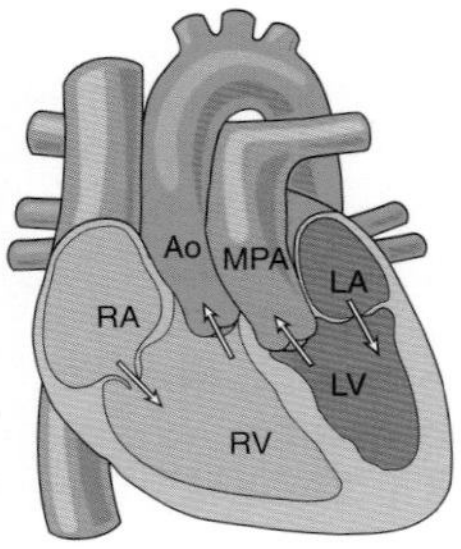 5% of CHD[a]	The aorta and main pulmonary arteries are transposed and connected to the incorrect ventricle Atrial or ventricular septal defect essential for admixture of blood Note: L-TGA (l-TGA), also known as congenitally corrected TGA, is different to D–TGA and does not need neonatal surgical correction	Deoxygenated blood will return from the body into the right atrium → right ventricle → aorta → systemic circulation causing cyanosis Oxygenated blood will return from the lungs to the left atrium → left ventricle → pulmonary artery and back to the lungs	Initially, prostaglandin E_1 to maintain ductal patency BAS if inadequate mixture of oxygenated and deoxygenated blood Surgical correction is undertaken in the first 1–2 weeks of life[a]
Ebstein's anomaly[b] 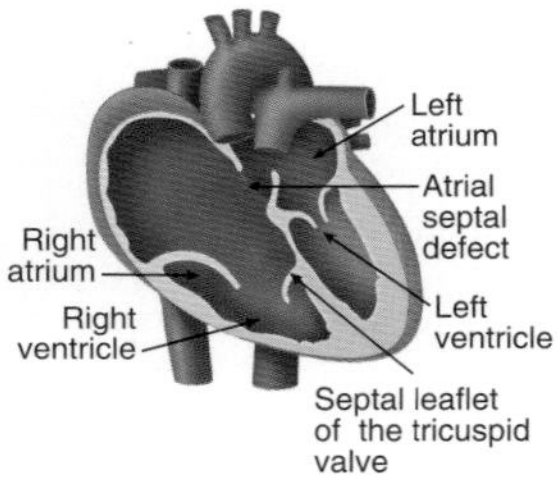 <1% of CHD[a]	Abnormal tricuspid valve with apical displacement; part of the right ventricle becomes functionally an atrial chamber Can be mild to severe	Severe cardiomegaly due to dilated right atrium Where the tricuspid valve is insufficient, the right ventricle cannot push blood forwards to the pulmonary arteries Where there is an ASD, right-to-left shunt causes cyanosis Commonly, have arrhythmia from atrial dilatation	Individually assessed Mostly a non-surgical approach in neonatal period Maintaining ductal patency may assist with pulmonary blood flow in early neonatal period Reduction of pulmonary vascular resistance using nitric oxide may be considered May require a BT shunt to augment pulmonary blood flow A Starnes procedure may be undertaken in the neonatal period for those with adequate ventricular size; may require tricuspid valve repair or replacement[a]

ASD, atrial septal defect; BAS, balloon atrial septostomy; BT, Blalock–Taussig; CHD, congenital heart disease; CHF, complete heart failure; PA, pulmonary artery; PDA, patent ductus arteriosus; PS, pulmonary stenosis; RV, right ventricle; TAPVR, total anomalous pulmonary venous return; TGA, transposition of the great arteries; ToF, tetralogy of Fallot; VSD, ventricular septal defect.
[a]Park (2021).
[b]Source: Rychik & Tian (2012).

Sources: Rao (2013a, b), Park (2021).

TABLE 10.5 **Common obstructive left heart defects**

Condition	Physiology	Pathophysiology	Management
Aortic stenosis 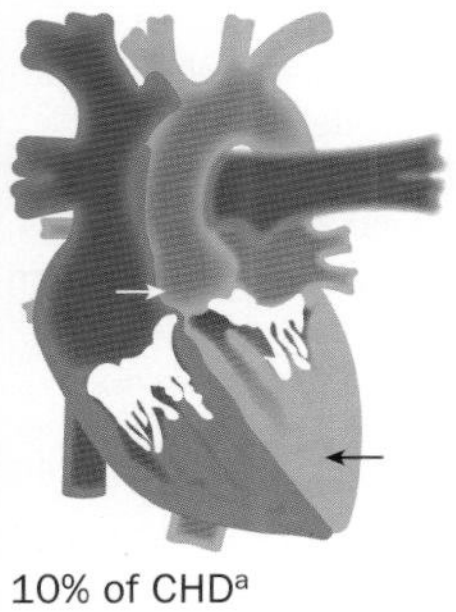 10% of CHD[a]	Obstruction of flow out of the left ventricle; can be valvular, supravalvular or subvalvular Valve may be dysplastic, bicuspid, or normal aetiology	Outflow obstruction from left ventricle may cause left ventricular hypertrophy Excessive obstruction (critical) impedes systemic blood flow and may result in extreme hypoperfusion and organ dysfunction	Initially, balloon valvotomy in cardiac catheter laboratory or surgical valvotomy Ultimately requires surgical repair or replacement of aortic valve Ross procedure considered as part of surgical planning[a]
Coarctation of the aorta[a] 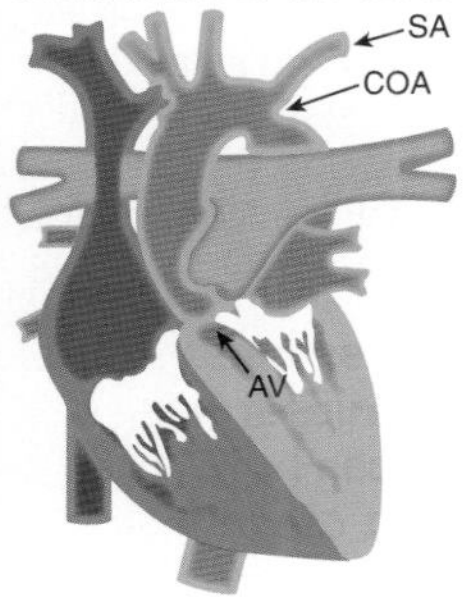 SA COA AV 8–10% of CHD[a]	Narrowing of the aortic lumen, commonly juxtaposed with the PDA	Restriction of blood flow distal to the head and neck vessels results in high blood pressure in the arms compared with the legs Obstructed left ventricular outflow leads to pulmonary venous congestion If preductal, significant systemic hypoperfusion and organ dysfunction can result as the PDA closes	PGE_1 infusion to maintain ductal patency if lower body circulation is inadequate Surgical repair is the most common treatment option when presentation is in the neonatal period May be assessed for balloon dilation and/or stent in the older child[a]
Interrupted aortic arch[a] 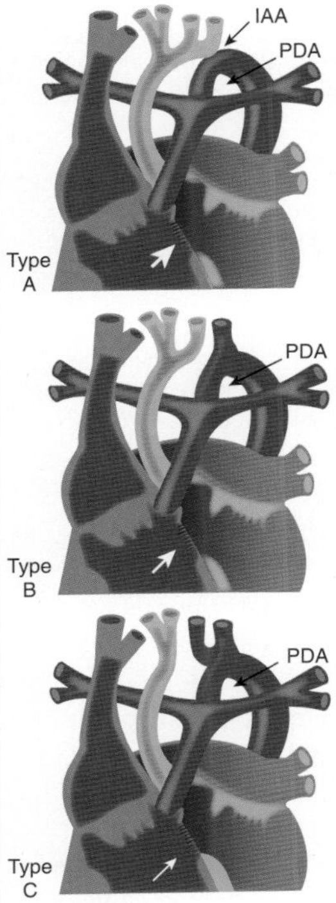 IAA PDA Type A PDA Type B PDA Type C 1% of CHD[a]	This is an extreme version of coarctation where there is no continuity between the ascending and descending aorta Immediate survival is dependent on the presence of a VSD and PDA IAA is categorised into three different types to indicate the location of the interruption: 1 Type A is distal to the left subclavian 2 Type B is between the left carotid and left subclavian arteries 3 Type C is between the in-nominate and left carotid arteries	Before duct closure blood perfusing the upper body will be oxygenated and the blood perfusing the lower body will be deoxygenated, creating a differential cyanosis between the upper and lower body After duct closure the pulmonary circulation may be excessive, potentially causing congestive cardiac failure, while the lower body may become inadequately perfused resulting in profound shock	PGE_1 infusion to maintain ductal patency Surgical correction in the first week of life[a]

Continued

TABLE 10.5 **Common obstructive left heart defects—cont'd**

Condition	Physiology	Pathophysiology	Management
Hypoplastic left heart syndrome[b] **Hypoplastic left heart syndrome** Ductus arteriosus, Aorta, Pulmonary arteries, Left atrium, Aortic atresia, Mitral atresia, Left ventricle, Right atrium, Right ventricle 1% of CHD[a]	Underdeveloped left-sided heart structures: 1 Atretic or stenotic mitral valve 2 Atretic or stenotic aortic valve 3 Hypoplastic left ventricle 4 Hypoplastic ascending aorta 5 COA 6 Atrial septal defect	If the atrial communication is unrestrictive, pulmonary over-circulation at the expense of systemic circulation will occur If the atrial communication is restrictive, both cyanosis and systemic hypoperfusion will occur Adequate mixing of blood at the atrial level is essential	PGE_1 to maintain ductal patency 3-stage operative course: 1 Norwood operation in first week of life 2 Bidirectional Glenn shunt at around 4 months 3 Fontan operation at between 2 and 4 years of age[a] An alternative to the Norwood procedure for a neonate is a hybrid procedure whereby the pulmonary arteries are banded to restrict blood flow, the atrium is opened to provide free mixing at atrial level and ductal patency is maintained with a stent The second stage for such patients requires removing the bands, reconstruction of aortic outflow, atrial septectomy and a Glenn shunt[a]

CHD, congenital heart disease; COA, coarctation of the aorta; IAA, interrupted aortic arch; PDA, patent ductus arteriosus; PGE_1, prostaglandin E_1; VSD, ventricular septal defect.
[a] Source: Park (2021).
[b] *Source: Rychik and Tian (2012).*

CASE STUDY 10.1

At 37 weeks' gestation, a neonate with a birthweight of 2900 g was born via vaginal birth with Apgar scores of 7 at 1 minute and 8 at 5 minutes.

At birth, the neonate was vigorous and crying. Concerns were raised at 30 minutes post birth when the neonate was observed to be dusky at rest, and had an episode of central cyanosis when attempting to breastfeed.

The neonate was moved to the nursery for observation. On admission to the nursery the neonate was alert, vigorous and crying. Observations were: **heart rate (HR)** 160 bpm, respiratory rate (RR) 44 breaths/min, non-invasive blood pressure 77/40 mmHg (mean 54 mmHg), SpO_2 77% in air, temperature 36.8°C and blood sugar level 3.8 mmol/L.

Oxygen administration was commenced at 2 L/min via nasal prongs, with SpO_2 remaining between 86% and 88%.

1 You are the neonatal nurse/midwife receiving the neonate into the nursery. Outline your initial comprehensive physical assessment. What information will you gather?
2 How would you determine whether this is a primary respiratory or cardiac problem?
3 What are the potential diagnoses that could present with reduced oxygen saturation?
4 When symptoms are present at birth, there is usually a severe cardiac condition. What nursing/midwifery measures could be taken to reduce physiological stress to the neonate to promote optimal oxygenation?
5 It is suspected that the neonate has a congenital cyanotic heart defect such as transposition of the great arteries.
   a What initial pharmacological agent would you anticipate being required for this neonate and why is it used?
   b What monitoring will you undertake when administering this medication?
6 The parents arrive at the nursery to be with their baby. They are concerned about the low oxygen levels and the baby's cyanosis. What information would you provide to the parents regarding a suspected cyanotic congenital heart defect?
7 The plan is to transfer the neonate to a cardiac facility for ongoing management.
   a What do you need to consider in preparation for transfer?
   b What would you explain to the parents about surgical and non-surgical management of a congenital cyanotic heart defect?
8 Many neonates with congenital cardiac defects have oxygen saturations in the range of 70–80%. Consider the difference between hypoxaemia and hypoxia and apply this to children with cyanotic forms of CHD. Plan a way in which you could discuss this with a parent if they asked you whether their child could suffer from brain damage if he or she is not reaching oxygen saturations closer to 100%.

NON-STRUCTURAL CARDIAC CONDITIONS

In addition to congenital heart defects, neonates can also present with non-structural cardiac conditions such as CHF, cardiomyopathy and alterations in electrophysiology that cause arrhythmias.

Congestive heart failure

Congestive heart failure (CHF) occurs when cardiac muscle is unable to effectively pump blood around the body, resulting in inadequate nutrition and oxygenation to meet metabolic demand. It can be the result of volume overload, pressure overload and/or ventricular dysfunction. Signs of CHF in the newborn period are diaphoresis, pallor, central cyanosis and prolonged capillary refill time. The most common presenting symptom is tachypnoea with feeding difficulties – for example, prolonged feeding times. If left untreated, this condition can lead to cardiomegaly. Management of the neonate with CHF includes decreasing their oxygen consumption by maintaining the thermal neutral environment and minimal handling, providing supplemental oxygen according to oxygen saturations, supporting nutrition and restricting fluids. Diuretics and inotropes may be needed if there is no response to these conservative measures (Sadowski & Verklan, 2021).

Persistent pulmonary hypertension of the newborn

Persistent pulmonary hypertension of the newborn (PPHN) is a respiratory condition that, if left untreated, results in acidosis and reduced CO, cardiac failure and death; Chapter 9 provides further details on this condition. Importantly, this can occur concurrently with cardiac defects and may make diagnosis of CHD difficult.

NEONATAL ARRHYTHMIAS

Arrhythmias/dysrhythmias

Arrhythmia can result in tachycardia or bradycardia and often coexist in children with CHD, but can also occur in otherwise structurally normal hearts.

Benign dysrhythmias

Benign **dysrhythmias** include sinus bradycardia, tachycardia and sinus arrhythmia. Preterm neonates may often have sinus bradycardia, where the heart rate slows below 100 bpm, but it does not last longer than 20 seconds. Preterm neonates can also experience a sinus tachycardia, where the HR can reach 200 bpm or more. This is usually associated with activities such as crying but can also occur with pain, medications (especially caffeine) and hyperthermia from an elevated environmental temperature. The HR returns to normal when the neonate settles and is nursed in a neutral thermal environment (Mazor & Mazor, 2021).

Pathological dysrhythmias

SUPRAVENTRICULAR TACHYCARDIA

Supraventricular tachycardia (SVT), as shown in Fig. 10.5, occurs where there is an accessory atrioventricular (AV) electrical pathway. The arrhythmia is sudden in onset, with sinus rates of 220–280 bpm. SVT can terminate spontaneously and return to sinus rhythm. Often SVT is well tolerated; however, it may cause symptoms of breathlessness, sweating, pallor, lethargy and reduced cardiac output. The intermittent nature of SVT can delay diagnosis until the neonate is in a healthcare facility. A 12-lead ECG is the diagnostic investigation of choice. Ambulatory ECG (Holter) monitoring can record and document the frequency of the arrhythmia over a 24-hour period (Dubin, 2017).

Infrequent, self-limiting SVT may not require treatment. However, frequent, prolonged episodes may require medical therapy with beta-blockers. Reversion of SVT can be assisted with vagal manoeuvres facilitated by placing ice slush onto the infant's face for 15–30 seconds to elicit the diving reflex. Caution must be exercised to avoid ice burns and not to impede breathing. For infants who do not revert using vagal manoeuvres, pharmacological reversion may be indicated; the first-line therapy is with adenosine. If unsuccessful, and the infant is haemodynamically compromised, cardioversion may be required (Refaat et al., 2021).

COMPLETE HEART BLOCK

Significant bradycardia can occur if there is a blockage in conduction between the atrium and the ventricle at the level of the atrioventricular (AV) node. The AV node will independently fire at a slower rate and is not synchronised with the atrial rate (Fig. 10.6), resulting in profound bradycardia with rates around 50–60 bpm. Low HR can manifest as low CO and acidosis. **Complete heart block (CHB)** will commonly be diagnosed in the antenatal period

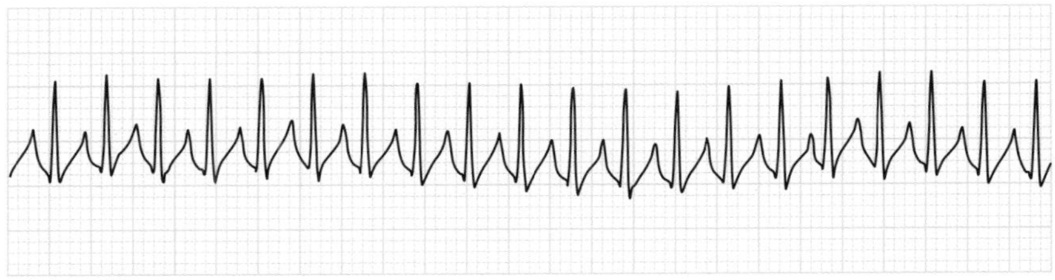

FIGURE 10.5 **Supraventricular tachycardia**
Source: Cadogan and Nickson (2017).

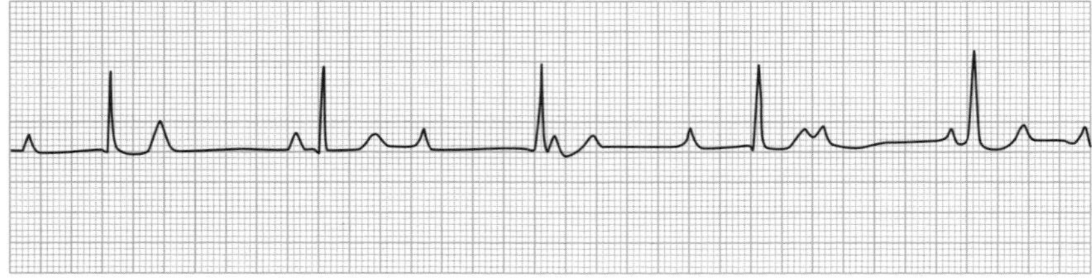

FIGURE 10.6 **Complete heart block**
Source: Cadogan and Nickson (2017).

when assessing fetal HR. Importantly, 60–90% of cases of congenital heart block are associated with neonatal lupus due to maternal antibodies (RO-SSA and LA-SSB) crossing the placenta (Zimmerman, 2017).

CHB can also present later or occur after cardiac surgery. Reversible causes of heart block, such as acidosis or electrolyte imbalance, need to be eliminated. Neonates should be transferred to a specialist centre for definitive management. An echocardiograph should be undertaken to assess for structural CHD.

The key goal of therapy is to increase HR. The initial treatment is facilitated with the use of medication and/or a pacemaker. The drug of choice is an intravenous (IV) infusion of isoprenaline. Alternatively, temporary cardiac pacing is possible using transthoracic pacing pads, such as those incorporated in modern defibrillators. Temporary transthoracic pacing can be technically difficult in the neonate owing to the relative size of the pads to the neonate. CHB will often require insertion of a permanent pacemaker to provide a secure base HR (Buyon, 2017).

SURGICAL MANAGEMENT OF CONGENITAL HEART DISEASE

Approximately 50% of Australians born with CHD will require surgery or cardiac catheter interventions, 25% within the first 12 months of life (Australian Institute of Health and Welfare (AIHW), 2019). The other 50% have minor abnormalities (minor valve lesions or very small ventricular or atrial septal defects) that have no functional impact and rarely affect wellbeing or require intervention. Approximately 30 babies undergo heart surgery in Australia every week (Victor Chang Cardiac Research Institute, 2022). Certain fetal cardiac defects may also be treated surgically before birth (e.g. aortic stenosis and hypoplastic left heart syndrome) using catheter- and balloon-based interventions. Such complex interventions are confined to a few specialised facilities around the world and, while they currently carry high levels of risk to both the fetus and the mother, it is an area that holds great promise in the future (Moon-Grady et al., 2019).

Table 10.6 outlines the major surgical procedures.

TABLE 10.6 **Surgical procedures**

Operation	Key points
Pulmonary artery band	Constrictive device placed around the pulmonary artery to restrict pulmonary blood flow and control congestive heart failure Used mainly for neonates with large VSD or AVSD Allows somatic growth and delays definitive repair until infant is older and larger
ASD repair	Stitch or patch closure of the atrial communication Requires CPB Repair rarely required as a neonate

TABLE 10.6 **Surgical procedures—cont'd**

Operation	Key points
VSD repair 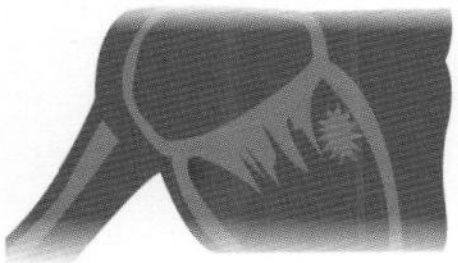	Patch closure of the ventricular communication(s) Requires CPB If a PA band had been previously placed, it will be removed at this operation
AVSD repair 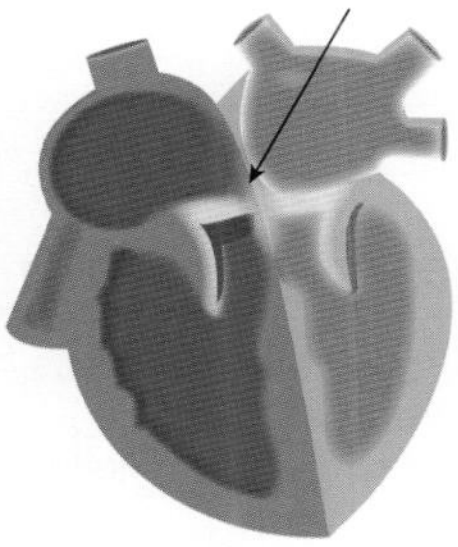 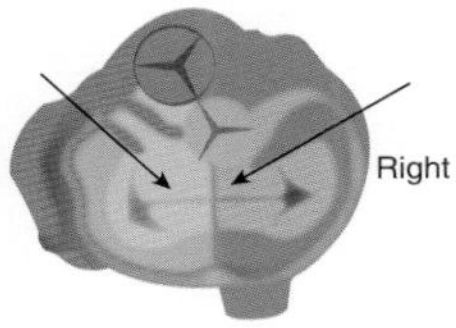 Left Right	Wide spectrum and repair individualised for patient Ultimate aim to close septal defects and repair AV valve(s) to maximise competence Can have atrial and ventricular defects closed separately or as a single patch (accompanying diagram) There is commonly incomplete valvular repair that results in various degrees of AV valve regurgitation postoperatively; this may require ongoing diuretic therapy with potential for further valve surgery in the future
PDA ligation 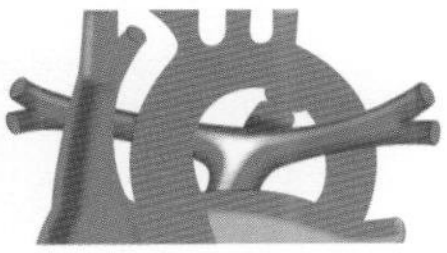	Surgical ligation of PDA involves a thoracotomy The duct is tied, then divided Does not require CPB
Tricuspid atresia staging surgery	Surgical palliation follows a 3-stage single ventricle pathway Stage 1 in a neonate is a modified BT or central shunt Stage 2 at approximately 4 months of age is a bidirectional Glenn shunt Stage 3 at approximately 4 years of age is a Fontan operation
Arterial-to-pulmonary shunts (e.g. BT shunt) 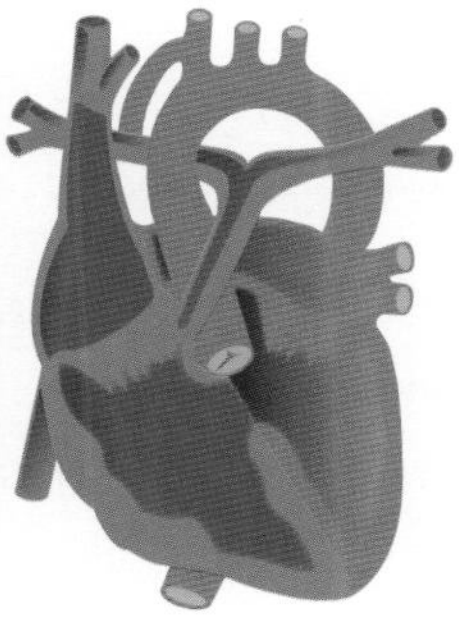	Provides pulmonary blood flow and augments pulmonary artery growth until the infant is about 4–6 months of age Most commonly this is a modified BT shunt between the subclavian artery and the pulmonary artery Other arteries can also be utilised Artificial Gore-Tex® graft material is commonly used

Continued

TABLE 10.6 **Surgical procedures—cont'd**	
Operation	Key points
Bidirectional Glenn shunt[a] 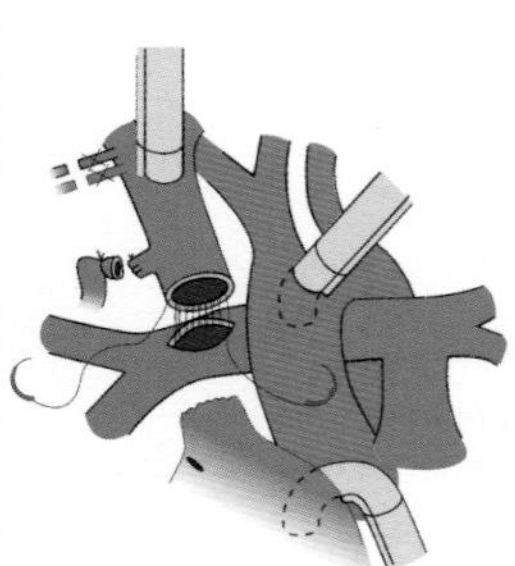	Also known as a bidirectional cavopulmonary connection. The superior vena cava is disconnected from the right atrium and connected to the pulmonary artery; some children with two superior vena cavae will have both connected to the pulmonary arteries at this stage (bilateral bidirectional Glenn) Blood flow through the main pulmonary artery is interrupted and the main pulmonary artery sutured closed Upper body blood flows directly to the pulmonary circulation Lower body blood from the inferior vena cava continues to enter the right atrium as per normal circulation This circulation requires unrestricted mixing of blood at atrial level Infant will be desaturated to around 75–85%
Fontan operation[b] 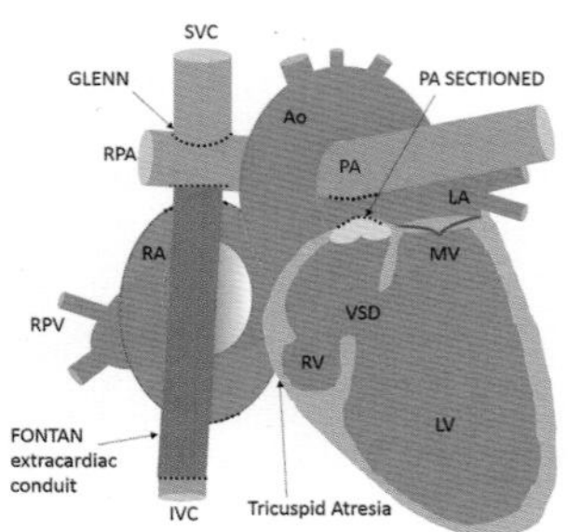	Also known as a total cavopulmonary connection (TCPC) The third stage palliative surgical procedure is performed when the child is around 4 years of age A Gore-Tex conduit joins the inferior vena cava to the pulmonary artery allowing all venous blood to return directly to the pulmonary circulation and bypass the heart altogether After this stage, the child's oxygen saturations will be in the high 90% range for the first time in their life This surgical procedure has evolved significantly over time from its initial inception
Repair tetralogy of Fallot 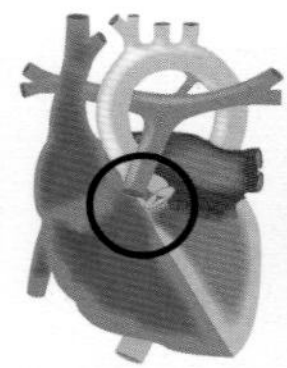 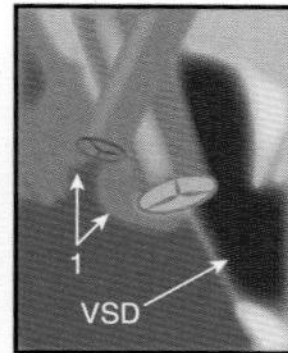 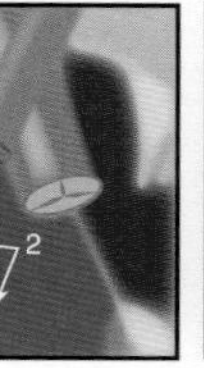 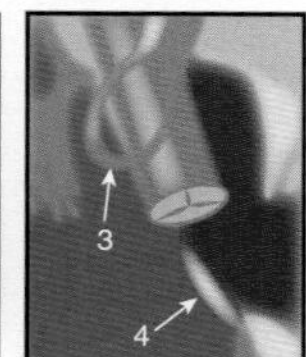	1 Shows the view of VSD and infundibular stenosis 2 The pulmonary valve is opened and enlarged; the pulmonary valve often needs to be excised. Transannular patch may be required to enlarge the pulmonary valve annulus. Hypertrophied right ventricular infundibular muscle is resected 3 The main pulmonary artery is patched to enlarge the outflow tract. Small pulmonary arteries may also be patched to enlarge 4 The VSD is patched
Truncus arteriosus repair 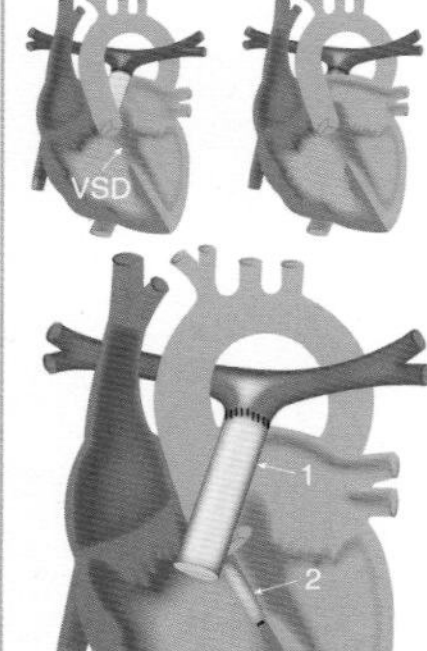	1 The pulmonary arteries are disconnected 2 Blood flow from the truncal vessel is directed to the systemic circulation by closing the VSD An RV to PA conduit is connected to enable blood flow to the pulmonary circulation This conduit requires replacement as the child grows The truncal valve can have stenosis ± regurgitation and may need replacement later in life; this is attended to at the same time as conduit replacement

TABLE 10.6 **Surgical procedures—cont'd**

Operation	Key points
Repair of TAPVR 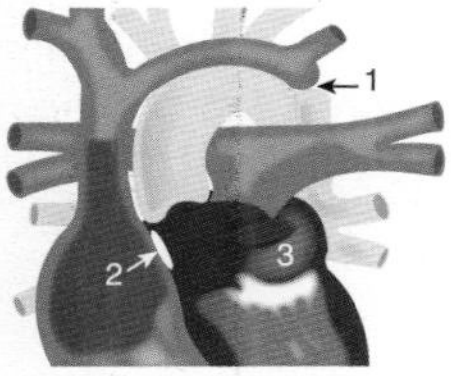	1 The vertical vein that drains the anomalous confluence is ligated 2 The anomalous veins are rerouted and joined into the posterior left atrium 3 The ASD is patched closed Normal circulation is restored Potential for narrowing of the pulmonary veins that may lead to obstruction
Arterial switch operation to repair transposition of the great arteries 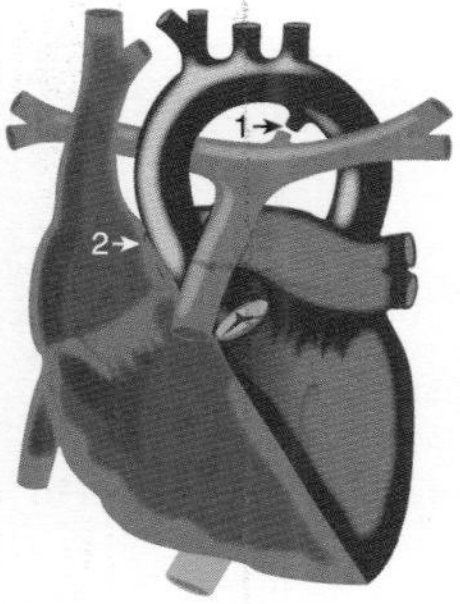	The pulmonary artery and the aorta are transected and 'switched' to the normal positions so that deoxygenated blood is sent to the lungs and oxygenated blood to the body The coronary arteries also need to be relocated to the pulmonary root (neoaorta) to enable oxygenated blood to perfuse the myocardium The PDA is ligated (1) and the atrial communication (2) closed at the time of surgery
Coarctation repair[c] 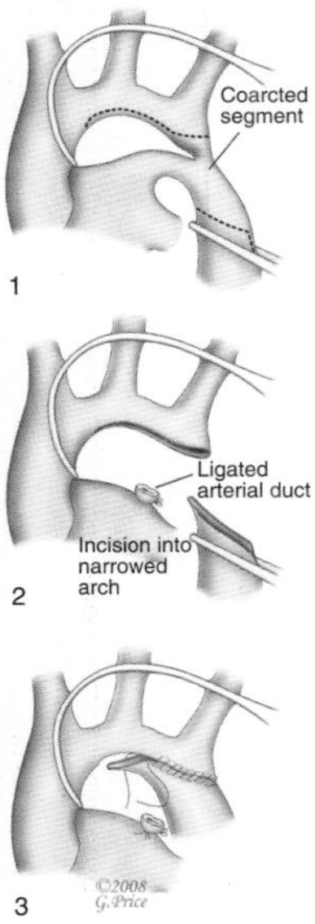 Coarcted segment 1 Ligated arterial duct Incision into narrowed arch 2 3 ©2008 G.Price	1 Coarctation of the aorta with a PDA 2 Resection and removal of the coarctation and ductus arteriosus 3 Anastomosis of the aorta Mostly an end-to-end anastomosis can be achieved Use of a subclavian flap can be considered if more comprehensive repair is required

Continued

TABLE 10.6 **Surgical procedures—cont'd**

Operation	Key points
IAA repair	Incisions are made to enable the ascending and descending aorta to be opened and joined together to form a continuous pathway The PDA is ligated (3) The VSD is closed with a patch (5) This returns the circulation to normal
Norwood stage 1 with Sano shunt[d]	The proximal main pulmonary artery is disconnected and joined to the hypoplastic aortic arch to increase its size The hypoplastic aorta is augmented (usually pulmonary homeograft tissue) to provide unobstructed systemic blood flow An atrial septectomy to ensure that pulmonary venous return can freely mix at atrial level to enter the single right ventricle Blood flow to the pulmonary system can be created as a Sano shunt (pictured); this is a conduit from the right ventricle to the pulmonary artery; both pulmonary and systemic blood flows are pumped from the single right ventricle A BT shunt can alternatively be used for pulmonary blood flow depending on surgeon preference or specific anatomical considerations; here pulmonary blood flow runs from the arterial connection and is not directly connected to the ventricle
Norwood stages 2 and 3	Stage 2 is a bidirectional Glenn procedure and removal of the Sano shunt Stage 3 is a Fontan operation

ASD, atrial septal defect; AV, atrioventricular; AVSD, atrioventricular septal defect; BT, Blalock–Taussig; CPB, cardiopulmonary bypass; IAA, interrupted aortic arch; PA, pulmonary artery; PDA, patent ductus arteriosus; RV, right ventricle; TAPVR, total anomalous pulmonary venous return; TCPC, total cavopulmonary connection; VSD, ventricular septal defect.

[a]Source: Sellke et al. (2016). Fig. 129-1.
[b]Source: Navarro-Aguilar et al. (2015). Copyright © 2014 The Royal College of Radiologists.
[c]Source: Price (2010). © Churchill Livingstone: Elsevier.
[d]Source: Yuan & Jing (2009).

CLINICAL PRACTICE 10.10

In most cases neonates will need to be transferred to a specialist cardiac centre for surgery and ongoing management. It is important to prepare the family for this by providing a full explanation about the transfer, the investigations that will be performed for diagnosis and the management strategies used.

It is good practice to arrange for at least one parent to accompany their baby to the referral facility and, if the mother is still an inpatient, to organise for her to be transferred to a nearby maternity facility as well. Taking photos and having cuddles, where possible, can ease the anxiety separation to some degree.

REFLECTION

Thinking about Clinical Practice 10.10, what else might you consider that would be helpful to ease parental anxiety?

All surgical procedures performed on neonates have associated mortality and morbidity risks, particularly those requiring **cardiopulmonary bypass (CPB)**. Simple, corrective surgery such as a VSD closure has less perioperative and long-term risk than complex defects such as hypoplastic left heart syndrome, which is life limiting and requires multiple staging operations. All neonates who undergo surgery require lifelong cardiology follow-up.

Overall, each defect has a specific risk/benefit profile that guides decision making around undertaking cardiac surgical procedures. Full disclosure of surgical risks should be undertaken during the consent process. Major morbidity includes neurological deficit, acute renal failure requiring dialysis, surgically induced AV block requiring a permanent pacemaker, unplanned reoperation and phrenic nerve injury. However, many forms of CHD are associated with far greater risk to the neonate if left unrepaired (Pasquali et al., 2020).

Cardiac catheterisation

Percutaneous cardiac catheterisation is increasingly used both diagnostically and therapeutically in neonates (Melekoglu & Baspinar, 2019). A thin hollow catheter is inserted into an artery or a vein (usually the femoral vein or artery in the groin) and threaded through the blood vessel and into the heart. This may be performed for diagnostic purposes, when contrast dye is injected into the catheter and filmed as it enters the heart, or surgical planning. Cardiac catheterisation can also be used for interventions such as a valvotomy (pulmonary or aortic), balloon atrial septostomy and balloon vessel dilation as well as the placement of stents and occlusive devices. Use of interventional cardiac procedures, both as adjunct therapy and as an alternative treatment option, has been increasing in neonatology and paediatrics with the evolution of the specialty.

NON-SURGICAL MANAGEMENT

Pharmacotherapeutic management

Table 10.7 outlines the common pharmacological preparations used in the management of heart disease in neonates. This management will most often be initiated prior to surgery to stabilise the neonate while awaiting more definitive correction or repair.

TABLE 10.7 **Pharmacotherapeutic management of congenital heart disease**

Drug class	Mode of action
Diuretics	• Primarily aimed at relieving symptoms of fluid retention in CHF Frusemide: • Most commonly used in severe CHF • IV is preferred route for rapid therapeutic onset • Narrow therapeutic window, and half-life is increased in preterm neonates • Requires further dilution and administration over time to prevent toxicity Spironolactone: • Potassium-sparing diuretic • Used in less acute stages • Important to monitor for electrolyte disturbances, cardiac arrhythmias, dehydration and hypotension
ACE inhibitors	Captopril: • Reduces systemic vascular resistance and controls pulmonary overload, decreasing PVR
Beta-blockers	Propranolol and sotalol: • Reduce HR, blood pressure and cardiac contractility • Also depress the sinus node rate and slow conduction through the AV node • Sotalol is used for tachyarrhythmias (e.g. SVT) and propranolol in tetralogy of Fallot
Sympathomimetics[a]	Isoprenaline: • Chronotrope – increases HR in complete heart block Dobutamine: • Inotrope – increases myocardial contractility Noradrenaline (norepinephrine): • Vasopressor – induces vasoconstriction, elevating the mean arterial pressure Dopamine and adrenaline (epinephrine): • Both vasopressor and inotropic actions depending on the dose administered
Antiarrhythmics	Adenosine • Depresses sinus node activity and slows conduction through the AV node • Also produces peripheral and coronary vasodilation • Rapid onset and short duration of action so must be given quickly; used in acute treatment of SVT Amiodarone: • Decreases sinus node and junctional automaticity, slows AV and bypass tract conduction, and prolongs refractory period of myocardial tissues; also has weak beta-blocker activity • Control of junctional tachycardia and ventricular tachycardia Digoxin: • Slows HR and reduces AV nodal conduction • Increases myocardial contractility and improves cardiac output • Used primarily for CHF

Continued

TABLE 10.7 **Pharmacotherapeutic management of congenital heart disease—cont'd**

Drug class	Mode of action
Anticoagulants[b]	Aspirin: • Antiplatelet to maintain patency of systemic-to-pulmonary shunt in the postoperative period; also used to reduce thrombus post stent insertion and some non-mechanical valves or patch insertion (institution and surgeon/cardiologist specific) Heparin: • Inactivates clotting factors IIa (thrombin) and Xa by binding to antithrombin III • May be used for bridging to warfarin or aspirin, central line thromboprophylaxis or thrombus treatment Warfarin: • Vitamin K antagonist; inhibits synthesis of vitamin K-dependent clotting factors (II, VII, IX, X) and the antithrombotic factors protein C and protein S • Infrequently used in the neonate; however, used for treatment of thrombus and mechanical valve thromboprophylaxis
Prostaglandin E_1 (PGE_1)	• Used to maintain patency of the DA and ensure adequate mix of oxygenated and deoxygenated blood until surgery can be performed • 50–100 ng/kg/min – titrate dose • Caution: risk of apnoea, fever and flushing; ensure facilities available to intubate and ventilate if required
Non-steroidal anti-inflammatories (NSAIDs)	Ibuprofen, indomethacin or paracetamol: • Acts as a prostaglandin inhibitor to constrict PDA
Antibiotics	Cephalosporins: • After surgery there is the potential for postoperative infection and antibiotic prophylaxis is required • Most often staphylococcal infection
Analgesics	• Pain assessment is the fifth vital sign • Neonates are non-verbal so use of a recognised pain assessment tool is essential (see Chapter 18) Sucrose: • For procedural pain Opioids and paracetamol: • Postoperative pain management

ACE, angiotensin-converting enzyme; AV, atrioventricular; CHD, congenital heart disease; CHF, congestive heart failure; DA, ductus arteriosus; HR, heart rate; IV, intravenous; PDA, patent ductus arteriosus; PVR, pulmonary vascular resistance; SVT, supraventricular tachycardia.

[a]Best administered through a large central vein.

[b]CHD has significant implications for thromboembolic prophylaxis and treatment. Refer to Giglia et al. (2013) for further reading.

Source: Australian Medicines Handbook Pty Ltd. (2021).

CLINICAL PRACTICE 10.11

One of the first-line medications used in CHD is prostaglandin E_1 (PGE_1). Side effects of this medication include hyperthermia, apnoea, tachycardia and hypotension. It is important to be aware of these side effects and meticulously monitor for them (Geggel, 2017).

Neonatal nursing/midwifery management includes a clear understanding of all prescribed medications, including the pharmacology and pharmacodynamics. It is important to understand the actions and interactions of these medications in the neonate and to monitor for therapeutic effects and side effects.

Use the resources available in your clinical area to find out important neonatal nursing/midwifery interventions for each of these medications.

Resources such as the *Australian medicine handbook*, MIMS and the *Australian injectable drugs handbook* are valuable resources.

Respiratory and ventilation management

Respiratory and ventilation management may be required to stabilise the neonate prior to corrective treatment and post surgery. The therapy required will depend on the degree of cardiopulmonary compromise.

- Position the neonate to promote maximal diaphragmatic excursion (Bahgat et al., 2021). The prone position may be utilised.
- Strive to decrease oxygen consumption by maintaining the neonate in a neutral thermal environment and limiting noxious stimulation. Occasionally, sedation may be required if the neonate is agitated.
- Assisted ventilation: neonates who are easily exhausted may benefit from non-invasive ventilation (NIV) such as nasal continuous positive airway pressure (NCPAP) to reduce the work of breathing and pulmonary oedema, and for calorie preservation.

- It is important to correct metabolic acidosis to assist with optimising cardiac function.
- Occasionally, invasive ventilation can be used to manipulate pulmonary blood flow.
- The patient should be intubated and mechanically ventilated prior to and during transport.

Nutritional management

Both CHD and CHF result in a high metabolic demand; consequently, there is a risk of hypoglycaemia in the immediate neonatal period and poor weight gain in both the pre- and postoperative periods. Initially, IV dextrose may be required and calorie supplementation may be utilised, particularly for neonates with CHF placed on diuretic therapy and/or fluid restriction. Nasogastric tube (NGT) feeding may be utilised to reduce the effort associated with suck feeds. Feeding may require fortification to allow for adequate weight gain without fluid overload, particularly in heart failure patients.

Total parenteral nutrition should be considered for neonates unable to be enterally fed, such as those with **necrotising enterocolitis (NEC)**.

PARENTING AND CONGENITAL HEART DISEASE

Parents of neonates with congenital conditions strive to normalise and preserve the quality of their family life (Govindaswamy et al., 2020). Communication and information are most vital in promoting a trusting therapeutic relationship. Being able to understand what is happening to their baby helps to alleviate some of the stress. It is important that care is focused around meeting the family's individual needs, where families stay with their infants and children as much as possible (Shackleford et al., 2021).

Incorporating the principles of family-centred care (FCC) ensures neonatal nursing and midwifery care meets individual family's needs. Parents will expect to provide care for their baby, especially in the areas of feeding, bathing, dressing, holding and providing non-pharmacological comfort measures such as skin-to-skin care and facilitated tucking. Parental presence and participation in the daily medical rounds will enhance parental engagement, confidence and competence (Lisant et al., 2019).

Providing the family with information regarding the baby's condition and supporting them to learn how to care for their baby is essential. Utilising pharmacists, dietitians and lactation consultants will ensure a comprehensive perspective in members of the multidisciplinary team.

Promotion of physical and cognitive development is important in infants with prolonged admissions to hospital. Children with CHD, particularly if associated with genetic conditions, are at risk of poor neurodevelopmental outcomes. Some studies have identified poor executive functioning in adolescents with single-ventricle-related CHD (Brosig et al., 2017).

Ultimately the goal is for families to manage at home, whether waiting for surgery or post surgery. Follow-up is essential and the intervals between appointments are individualised to the patient and family. Parental education and support services need to be geared towards promoting optimal neurodevelopment, with regular follow-up in the preschool years and adolescence (Brosig et al., 2017).

FAMILY-CENTRED CARE 10.3

The Heart Beads Program: the Children's Hospital Westmead in Sydney

Nursing staff on the cardiac ward at the Westmead Children's Hospital implemented the Heart Beads Program in 2008. The children are given a bead that represents a procedure or an event that has occurred during their hospitalisation for congenital heart conditions. The beads are small, attractive, porcelain in a variety of shapes and colours. They are threaded onto a cord that could be used as a necklace, bracelet or bookmark.

Interviews with the parents indicated the Heart Beads facilitated their ability to tell their story.

'The overriding theme was telling the child's story. The Heart Beads represented, for the families, a way of *recounting*, remembering, and explaining what the child had been through as part of their life journey that would continue into the future.' (Redshaw, 2014).

CONCLUSION

This chapter has provided information related to the care of the neonate with cardiovascular disease. The overall incidence of CHD as well as that for specific conditions has been reported. Embryological development of the cardiovascular system has been included.

It is envisaged that, after reading this chapter, the neonatal nurse/midwife will have a better understanding of cardiovascular assessment and be alert for signs and symptoms that commonly present with various congenital heart defects. It is expected that the neonatal nurse/midwife will develop an understanding of the differences between cyanotic and acyanotic cardiac defects as well as obstructive defects. This knowledge will better prepare the neonatal nurse/midwife to assist with immediate and emergency care, pharmacological therapies as well as surgical and non-surgical treatments.

Supporting the emotional needs of the family by providing information about their baby's congenital condition and psychosocial support is of paramount importance.

Online Resources

Resources for congenital heart defects

Cincinnati Children's Hospital Cardiac Centre: <https://www.cincinnatichildrens.org/patients/child/encyclopedia/defects>

Cove Point Foundation: <www.pted.org/>

HeartKids Australia: <https://www.heartkids.org.au>

HeartKids NZ: <https://heartkids.org.nz/index.php.html>

Life in the Fast Lane (ECG library): <https://www.lifeinthefastlane.com/>

Pediatric Cardiac Intensive Care Society (PCICS): <https://www.pcics.org/>

The Royal Children's Hospital Melbourne: <https://www.rch.org.au/cardiology/heart_defects/>

University of California San Francisco Medical Centre: <https://pedctsurgery.ucsf.edu/conditions—procedures.aspx>

References/Acknowledgements

Australian Institute of Health and Welfare (AIHW). (2019). *Congenital heart disease in Australia*. <https://www.aihw.gov.au/reports/heart-stroke-vascular-diseases/congenital-heart-disease-in-australia/contents/summary> (Accessed 20 February 2022).

Australian Medicines Handbook Pty Ltd. (2021). *Australian medicines handbook 2016 (online)*. Adelaide, SA: Australian Medicines Handbook Pty Ltd. <https://amhonline.amh.net.au/> (Accessed 20 February 2022).

Bahgat, E., El-Halaby, H., Abdelrahman, A., Nasef, N., & Abdel-Hady, H. (2021). Sonographic evaluation of diaphragmatic thickness and excursion as a predictor for successful extubation in mechanically ventilated preterm infants. *European Journal of Pediatrics, 180*(3), 899–908. doi: 10.1007/s00431-020-03805-2.

Blackburn, S. T. (2018). *Maternal, fetal, and neonatal physiology: a clinical perspective* (5th ed.). St Louis, MO: Elsevier.

Blue, G., Kirk, E., Sholler, G., Harvey, R., & Winlaw, D. (2012). Congenital heart disease: current knowledge about causes and inheritance. *Medical Journal of Australia, 197*(3), 155–159.

Brosig, C. L., Bear, L., Allen, S., Hoffmann, R. G., Pan, A., Frommelt, M., et al. (2017). Preschool neurodevelopmental outcomes in children with congenital heart disease. *Journal of Pediatrics, 183*, 80–86.e81.

Buyon, J. P. (2017). Neonatal lupus: management and outcomes. *UpToDate*. Waltham, MA: UpToDate Inc. <https://www.uptodate.com/contents/neonatal-lupus-management-and-outcomes> (Accessed 20 February 2022).

Cadogan, M., & Nickson, C. (2017). *Life in the fast lane*. <https://lifeinthefastlane.com/> (Accessed 20 February 2022).

Chu, P. Y., Li, J. S., Kosinski, A. S., Hornik, C. P., & Hill, K. D. (2017). Congenital heart disease in premature infants 25–32 weeks' gestational age. *Journal of Pediatrics, 181*, 37–41. doi: 10.1016/j.jpeds.2016.10.033.

Dolk, H., McCullough, N., Callaghan, S., Casey, F., Craig, B., Given, J., et al. (2020). Risk factors for congenital heart disease: the Baby Hearts Study, a population-based case-control study. *PLoS One, 15*(2), e0227908. doi: 10.1371/journal.pone.0227908.

Dubin, A. M. (2017). Management of supraventricular tachycardia in children. *UpToDate*. Waltham, MA: UpToDate Inc. <https://www.uptodate.com/contents/management-of-supraventricular-tachycardia-in-children> (Accessed 20 February 2022).

Everett, A. D., & Lim, D. S. (2010). *Illustrated field guide to congenital heart disease and repair* (3rd ed.). Charlottesville, VA: Scientific Software Solutions.

Fanaroff, A. A., & Fanaroff, J. M. (2013). *Klaus and Fanaroff's care of the high-risk neonate* (6th ed.). St Louis, MO: Saunders Elsevier.

Fazeriandy, A., Ali, M., Saing, J., Tobing, T., & Adriansyah, R. (2018). Consanguinity and congenital heart disease in offspring. *Paediatica Indonesiana, 58*(2), 75. doi: 10.14238/pi58.2.2018.75-9.

Garcia-Prats, J. A. (2017). Anaemia of prematurity. *UpToDate*. Waltham, MA: UpToDate Inc. <https://www.uptodate.com/contents/anemia-of-prematurity> (Accessed 20 February 2022).

Gedgaudas, E., Moller, J. H., Castaneda-Zuniga, W. R., & Amplatz, K. (1985). Embryology and anatomy of the heart. In: E. Gedgaudas, J. H. Moller, W. R. Castaneda-Zuniga, & K. Amplatz (Eds.), *Cardiovascular radiology* (pp. 1–23). Philadelphia, PA: WB Saunders.

Geggel, R. L. (2017). Diagnosis and initial management of cyanotic heart disease in the newborn. *UpToDate*. Waltham, MA: UpToDate Inc. <http://www.uptodate.com/contents/diagnosis-and-initial-management-of-cyanotic-heart-disease-in-the-newborn> (Accessed 20 February 2022).

Giglia, T. M., Massicotte, P., Tweddell, J. S., Barst, R. J., Bauman, M., Erickson, C. C., et al. (2013). Prevention and treatment of thrombosis in pediatric and congenital heart disease. A scientific statement from the American Heart Association. *Circulation, 128*, 2622–2703.

Gill, H. K., Splitt, M., Sharland, G. K., & Simpson, J. M. (2003). Patterns of recurrence of congenital heart disease. *Journal of the American College of Cardiology, 42*(5), 923–929.

Govindaswamy, P., Laing, S., Waters, D., Walker, K., Spence, K., & Badawi, N. (2020). Stressors of parents of infants undergoing neonatal surgery for major non-cardiac congenital anomalies in a surgical neonatal intensive care unit. *Journal of Paediatric Child Health, 56*, 512–520. doi: 10.1111/jpc.14673.

Hashim, S. T., Jr, Alamri, R. A., Bakraa, R., Rawas, R., Farahat, F., & Waggass, R. (2020). The association between maternal age and the prevalence of congenital heart disease in newborns from 2016 to 2018 in single cardiac center in Jeddah, Saudi Arabia. *Cureus, 12*(3), e7463. doi: 10.7759/cureus.7463.

HeartKidsAustralia. (2016). Crows Nest, NSW: HeartKids Australia. <https://www.heartkids.org.au> (Accessed 20 February 2022).

HeartKidsNZ. (n.d.). Auckland: HeartKidsNZ. <https://heartkids.org.nz/index.php.html> (Accessed 20 February 2022).

Jullien, S. (2021). Newborn pulse oximetry screening for critical congenital heart defects. *BMC Pediatrics, 21*, 305. doi: 10.1186/s12887-021-02520-7.

Khasawneh, W., Hakim, F., Ras, O. A., Hejazi, Y., & Abu-Aqoulah, A. (2020). Incidence and patterns of congenital heart disease among Jordanian infants, a cohort study from a university tertiary center. *Frontiers in Pediatrics, 8*, 219. doi: 10.3389/fped.2020.00219.

Lewin, M. B. (2012). *Echocardiography in congenital heart disease*. St Louis, MO: Saunders Elsevier.

Lisanti, A. J., Vittner, D., Medoff-Cooper, B., Fogel, J., Wernovsky, G., & Butler, S. (2019). Individualized family-centered developmental care: an essential model to address the unique needs of infants with congenital heart disease. *Journal of Cardiovascular Nursing*, *34*(1), 85–93. doi: 10.1097/JCN.0000000000000546.

Mazor, S., & Mazor, R. (2021). Approach to the child with tachycardia. In: G. A. Woodward, & S. M. Misra (Eds.), *UpToDate*. Walters Kluwer. <https://www.uptodate.com/contents/approach-to-the-child-with-tachycardia> (Accessed 20 February 2022).

Melekoglu, A. N., & Baspinar, O. (2019). Transcatheter cardiac interventions in neonates with congenital heart disease: a single centre experience. *Journal of International Medical Research, 47*(2), 615–625. doi: 10.1177/0300060518806111.

Moon-Grady, A. J., Ganesan, S., & Tworetzky, W. (2019). Fetal surgery for congenital heart disease. In: H. Lee (Ed.), *Medscape*. <https://emedicine.medscape.com/article/2109511-overview#a1> (Accessed 20 February 2022).

Moore, K., & Persaud, T. V. N. (2015). *Before we are born: essentials of embryology and birth defects* (9th ed.). Philadelphia, PA: Elsevier.

Moses, K., Nava, P., Banks, J., & Petersen, D. (2013). *Atlas of clinical gross anatomy* (2nd ed.). Philadelphia, PA: Saunders. Figure 30.1.

Mozaffarian, D., Benjamin, E. J., Go, A. S., Arnett, D. K., Blaha, M. J., Cushman, M., et al. (2016). Heart disease and stroke statistics – 2016 update: a report from the American Heart Association. *Circulation, 133*(4), 447.

Navarro-Aguilar, V., Flors, L., Calvillo, P., Merlos, P., Buendia, F., Igual, B., et al. (2015). Fontan procedure: imaging of normal post-surgical anatomy and the spectrum of cardiac and extracardiac complications. *Clinical Radiology, 70*(3), 295–303.

Ohlsson, A., & Shah, P. S. (2020). Paracetamol (acetaminophen) for patent ductus arteriosus in preterm or low birth weight infants. *Cochrane Database of Systematic Reviews, 1*, CD010061. doi: 10.1002/14651858.CD010061.pub4.

Park, M. K. (2021). *Park's the pediatric cardiology handbook* (6th ed.). Philadelphia, PA: Elsevier.

Pasquali, S. K., Thibault, D., O'Brien, S. M., Jacobs, J. P., Gaynor, J. W., Romano, J. C., et al. (2020). National variation in congenital heart surgery outcomes. *Circulation, 142*, 1351–1360. doi: 10.1161/CIRCULATIONAHA.120.046962.

Price, G. (2010). *Pediatric cardiology* (3rd ed.). Philadelphia, PA: Churchill Livingstone Elsevier.

Rao, P. S. (2013a). Consensus on timing of intervention for common congenital heart diseases: part I – acyanotic heart defects. *Indian Journal of Pediatrics, 80*(1), 32–38.

Rao, P. S. (2013b). Consensus on timing of intervention for common congenital heart diseases: Part II – cyanotic heart defects. *Indian Journal of Pediatrics, 80*(8), 663–674.

Redshaw, S. (2014). 'She's done two and that's harsh': the agency of infants with congenital conditions as invoked through parent narratives. *Health Sociology Review, 23*(2), 125–135. Reprinted with permission of Taylor & Francis Ltd.

Refaat, M., Abohelwa, M. M., Ahmed, M., Elgehiny, A., Ibrahim, M., Zakka, P., et al. (2021). Arrhythmias in neonates and infants at a tertiary care center. *Cureus, 13*(1), e12861. doi: 10.7759/cureus.1286.

Rychik, J., & Tian, Z. (2012). *Fetal cardiovascular imaging*. Philadelphia, PA: Elsevier Saunders.

Sadowsky, S. L. & Verklan, M. T. (2021). Cardiovascular disorders. In: M. T. Verklan, M. Walden, & S. Forest (Eds.), *Core curriculum for neonatal intensive care nursing* (6th ed., p. 470). St Louis, MO: Elsevier.

Sellke, F., del Nido, P. J., & Swanson, S. J. (2016). *Sabiston and Spencer surgery of the chest* (9th ed.). Philadelphia, PA: Elsevier.

Shackleford, J., Chambers, R., Nelson, J., Scott, M., & Brasher, S. (2021). Nurses' perceptions of rooming-in for caregivers of infants with CCHD. *Journal of Pediatric Nursing, 56*, 101–102. doi: 10.1016/j.pedn.2020.08.008.

Swanson, T., & Erickson, L. (2021). Cardiovascular diseases and surgical interventions. In: S. L. Gardner, B. S. Carter, M. I. Enzman-Hines, & J. A. Hernandez (Eds.), *Merenstein and Gardner's handbook of neonatal intensive care* (9th ed., pp. 836–885). Philadelphia, PA: Elsevier.

Theodore, C. (2017). Oxygenation and mechanisms of hypoxemia. *UpToDate*. Waltham, MA: UpToDate Inc. <https://www.uptodate.com/contents/oxygenation-and-mechanisms-of-hypoxemia> (Accessed 20 February 2022).

Victor Chang Cardiac Research Institute. (2022). Congenital heart disease. Darlinghurst, NSW: Victor Chang Cardiac Research Institute. <https://www.victorchang.edu.au/congenital-heart-disease> (Accessed 20 February 2022).

Willim, H. A., & Supit, A. I. (2021). Critical congenital heart disease in newborn: early detection, diagnosis, and management. *Bioscientia Medicina, 5*(1), 107–116.

Yuan, S.-M., & Jing, H. (2009). Palliative procedures for congenital heart defects. *Archives of Cardiovascular Diseases, 102*(6), 549–557.

Zhang, T.-N., Wu, Q.-J., Liu, Y.-S., Lv, J.-L., Sun, H., Chang, Q., et al. (2021). Environmental risk factors and congenital heart disease: an umbrella review of 165 systematic reviews and meta-analyses with more than 120 million participants. *Frontiers in Cardiovascular Medicine, 8*,137. doi: 10.3389/fcvm.2021.640729.

Zimmerman, F. (2017). Bradycardia in children. *UpToDate*. Waltham, MA: UpToDate Inc. <http://www.uptodate.com/contents/bradycardia-in-children> (Accessed 20 February 2022).

Zitelli, B. J., McIntire, S. C., Nowalk, A. J. (2018). *Zitelli and Davis' atlas of pediatric physical diagnosis* (7th ed.). Philadelphia, PA: Elsevier.

CHAPTER 11

CARE OF THE NEONATE WITH A HAEMATOLOGICAL DISORDER

VICTORIA KAIN AND TRUDI MANNIX

Learning objectives

After reading this chapter you will be able to:

- understand the unique haematopoietic profile of the neonate
- understand the aetiology, pathophysiology and clinical presentations of the common haematological disorders of the neonate
- understand the medical, nursing and pharmacological management for the different haematological disorders of the neonate
- assess, plan, implement and evaluate the relevant nursing care for the different haematological disorders of the neonate
- describe blood components, indications for use and complications.

Key words, terms and abbreviations

activated partial thromboplastin time (APTT)
breastfeeding jaundice
breast milk jaundice
direct antibody test (DAT)
disseminated intravascular coagulopathy (DIC)
erythropoiesis
erythropoietin (EPO)
fresh frozen plasma (FFP)
haematocrit (HCT)
haematological disorders
haematopoiesis
haemoglobin (Hb)
haemostasis
intravenous immunoglobulin (IVIG)
necrotising enterocolitis (NEC)
partial exchange transfusion (PET)
red blood cells (RBC)
respiratory distress syndrome (RDS)
rhesus (Rh)
serum bilirubin reading (SBR)
transcutaneous bilirubinometry (TcB)
transfusion-associated necrotising enterocolitis (TANEC)
transfusion-related acute gastrointestinal injury (TRAGI)
vitamin K deficiency bleeding (VKDB)
white blood cells (WBC)

INTRODUCTION

Haematology refers to the study of blood and the organs involved in its formation. The haematology of the newborn is unique. Given that the processes of **haematopoiesis** (*the formation of blood cellular components*) and **haemostasis** (*the body's response to blood vessel injury and bleeding*) are not fully mature until 6 months of age, a number of haematological complications may arise in the neonate, and this is particularly so in the preterm neonate. This functional and structural immaturity can lead to a variety of **haematological disorders**, including anaemia, neutropenia and thrombocytopenia. High levels of fetal erythrocytes and the subsequent breakdown of this fetal element of the neonate's blood lead to physiological jaundice, a very common neonatal condition that will also be considered in this chapter.

DEVELOPMENTAL HAEMATOLOGY

Haematopoiesis

During embryogenesis, the primary organ of haematopoiesis is not the bone marrow, as it is following birth. The process begins in the ventral aorta from an intra-embryonic source of stem cells, followed by the development of secondary centres including the spleen, liver and, finally, the bone marrow as the fetus develops (Juul & Christensen, 2018). Embryological haematopoiesis progresses at a rapid rate, stabilising at the end of gestation to be confined to the thymus (as part of the lymphatic system) and the bone marrow.

Red blood cells (erythrocytes)

Red blood cells (RBC) are also known as erythrocytes. Refer to Table 11.1 for normal laboratory values. The typical shape is a biconcave disc, and the cells do not contain a nucleus. The red blood cells contain haemoglobin, giving blood its red colour, and transport oxygen and carbon dioxide to and from the tissues. Primitive **erythropoiesis** from day 20 of embryonic life results in nucleated red blood cells. **Erythropoietin (EPO)** is produced by the fetal kidney early in fetal life and leads to the formation of red blood cells in the bone marrow. Erythropoietin levels decrease from birth, reaching levels equal to those of an adult at 4–6 weeks of life (Ohls et al., 2019). The life span of red blood cells in the preterm neonate is far shorter than that of the term neonate: 35–50 days compared with 60–90 days (Villeneuve et al., 2021) (Table 11.2), and this has implications for anaemia of prematurity, which will be discussed later in this chapter. The normal red blood cell parameters of the fetus are outlined in Table 11.3.

White blood cells

Also known as leucocytes, the life span of **white blood cells (WBC)** ranges from 13 to 20 days, after which time they are destroyed in the lymphatic system. The white blood cells are classified into two main categories: granulocytes and non-granulocytes. The granulocytes are so called because of the appearance of granules in the cell cytoplasm, and include the neutrophils, eosinophils and basophils. Non-granulocytes lack the appearance of granules and include the lymphocytes and monocytes. Refer to Table 11.1 for normal laboratory values.

Granulocyte and non-granulocyte production (granulopoiesis) begin around the eighth gestational week with the production of macrophages; these early white blood cells are produced in the yolk sac and liver (Ohls et al., 2019). At birth, a decrease in the white blood cell count is considered physiological during the first 4 hours of life and is thought to be due to a corticosteroid surge during birth (Juul & Christensen, 2018).

Platelets

Platelets, also known as thrombocytes, play a vital role in haemostasis. Platelets normally live for 10 days and then are removed by the spleen and liver. Neonatal *megakaryocytes* (the bone marrow cells responsible for producing platelets) are smaller than at other times in the life span and have lower ploidy (*a lower number of sets of chromosomes*). As a result, neonates are more prone to lower levels of platelets. Coupled with this is the fact that neonatal platelets tend to be hyporeactive (see Table 11.1).

A low platelet count (thrombocytopenia) is relatively common in the neonatal period (Wolf et al., 2020), and is seen in conditions such as disseminated intravascular coagulopathy and neonatal sepsis (Ohls et al., 2019). Platelet function in the neonate is difficult to determine, for a number of reasons. In the first instance, obtaining an adequate sample of blood to fully evaluate neonatal platelet function is difficult without compromising the newborn, especially at early gestational ages. It is also unclear how other haemostatic variables influence neonatal platelet function. The understanding of platelet function is mostly from cord blood (Sheriff et al., 2020), but generally thrombocytopenia is defined as a platelet count lower than $150/\mu L \times 10^9/L$, as it is in adults (Ohls et al., 2019).

Blood volume

Blood volume is calculated as the **haematocrit (HCT)** (the fraction of blood consisting of red blood cells) plus plasma volume. The circulating blood volume of a neonate is higher than that of adults or children. This volume is higher again in the fetus as one-third of the fetal blood volume is contained in the umbilical cord and the 'fetal side' of the placenta (Hall & Hall, 2021). At the time of birth, the term neonate will have 115 mL whole blood/kg, comprising 70 mL/kg in the neonatal circulation, with 45 mL/kg remaining in the placenta. At approximately 72 hours of age, the blood volume stabilises following plasma redistribution on the first day of life, and the total blood volume of the term neonate is estimated to be between 80 and 90 mL/kg. In the preterm neonate, the volume of circulating blood is higher at approximately 100–105 mL/kg.

TABLE 11.1 **Normal haematology values**

Age	Hemoglobin (g)	Hematocrit (%)	Mean Corpuscular Volume (fL)	Mean Corpuscular Hemoglobin Concentration (g/dL per RBC)	Reticulocytes (%)	White Blood Cells ($\times 10^3$/mcL)	Platelets ($\times 10^3$/mcL)	Red Blood Cells ($\times 10^{12}$/L)
22–25 weeks' gestation[a] (mean [SD])	12.2 (1.6)	38.59 (3.94)	125.10 (7.84)			3.73 (2.17)	247 (59)	3.09 (0.34)
26–29 weeks' gestation[a] (mean [SD])	12.91 (1.38)	40.88 (4.40)	118.50 (7.96)			4.08 (0.84)	242 (69)	3.46 (0.41)
>30 weeks' gestation[a] (mean [SD])	13.64 (2.21)	43.55 (7.20)	114.38 (9.34)			6.40 (2.99)	232 (87)	3.82 (0.64)
1–3 d[b]	M: 12.5–16.6 F: 12.7–16.4	M: 36.4–47.4 F: 36.5–47.7	M: 94.0–106.3 F: 89.7–105.4	M: 32.8–36.4 F: 31.7–36.3	M: 2.2–4.8 F: 2.1–3.7	M: 7.69–13.12 F: 7.51–15.83	M: 140–238 F: 133–255	M: 3.69–4.75 F: 3.79–4.76
4–7 d[b]	M: 12.5–16.3 F: 12.6–15.3	M: 35.9–46.6 F: 36.1–44.0	M: 87.1–96.5 F: 86.5–93.8	M: 30.9–33.4 F: 30.6–32.3	M: 0.4–2.7 F: 0.4–2.0	M: 6.54–12.32 F: 5.86–12.23	M: 129–271 F: 95–230	M: 3.98–5.08 F: 4.05–4.83
8–14 d[b]	M: 11.9–15.7 F: 12.7–14.9	M: 34.4–45.4 F: 36.6–43.2	M: 87.1–94.8 F: 87.4–92.2	M: 30.4–33.0 F: 30.5–31.9	M: 0.4–2.7 F: 0.4–2.0	M: 7.66–14.05 F: 7.46–14.55	M: 120–297 F: 106–294	M: 3.75–4.93 F: 4.01–4.73

Source: Soghier, L. M. (Ed.). (2019). Reference range values for pediatric care *(2nd ed., pp. 92-101). Itasca, IL: American Academy of Pediatrics.*

TABLE 11.2 **RBC indices**

	Preterm neonate	Term neonate	Adult
RBC life span (days)	35–50	60–90	120
Expected Hb concentration drop after birth	• 71 (65–90) g/L at 4–8 weeks of life if birthweight <1.2 kg • 90 (80–100) g/L at 8–10 weeks of life if birthweight 1.2–2.5 kg	103 g/L from 6–12 weeks of life	

Source: adapted from Villeneuve et al. (2021).

TABLE 11.3 **Normal red blood cell parameters in the fetus**

Gestational age (weeks)	Hb (g/dL)	PCV	RBC ($\times 10^{12}$/L)	MCV (fL)	MCH (pg)	MCHC (g/dL)	Nucleated RBC (% of WBC)	Reticulocytes (%)
12	8.0–10.0	0.33	1.5	180	60	34	5.0–8.0	40
16	10.0	0.35	2.0	140	45	33	2.0–4.0	10–25
20	11.0	0.37	2.5	135	44	33	1.0	10–20
24	14.0	0.40	3.5	123	38	31	1.0	5–10
28	14.5	0.45	4.0	120	40	31	0.5	5–20
34	15.0	0.47	4.4	118	38	32	0.2	3–10
Term 40 (cord)	16.8	0.53	5.25	107	34	31.7	0.01	3–7

Hb, haemoglobin; MCH, mean corpuscular haemoglobin; MCHC, mean corpuscular haemoglobin concentration; MCV, mean cell volume; PCV, packed cell volume; RBC, red blood cells count.

Source: Colombatti et al. (2016).

Haemoglobin

Haemoglobin (Hb) levels are expressed as the amount of haemoglobin in grams (g) per decilitre (dL) of whole blood, a decilitre being equivalent to 100 millilitres (see Table 11.1 for normal Hb values of the neonate). Haemoglobin is a *tetrameric* (four structural subunits) molecule consisting of two pairs of polypeptide chains and is the most abundant protein in the RBC. At the molecular level, fetal and adult haemoglobin vary significantly to accommodate the changing oxygen needs of the developing fetus. The salient difference is the higher affinity of fetal haemoglobin (HbF) for oxygen, which is necessary given the relatively hypoxic in utero environment. The normal partial pressure of oxygen in utero from the umbilical artery is 20 mmHg (with an O_2 saturation of 40%) and that of the umbilical vein is 31 mmHg (with an O_2 saturation of 72%). As the fetal circulation transitions to neonatal circulation, the oxygen saturation and PaO_2 (*partial arterial pressure of oxygen*) should start to rise over several hours. Table 11.4 shows the reference haemoglobin values in preterm neonates.

It takes a few weeks for the neonatal PaO_2 to reach adult values (Walker, 2019). The WHO recommendations on antenatal care and the US Centers for Disease Control and Prevention guidelines recommend the following trimester-specific cutoffs for anemia: first trimester: <110 g/L, second trimester: <105 g/L and third trimester: <110 g/L (Young et al., 2019). The affinity that Hb has for oxygen is mediated by a variety of factors, which include temperature, the blood pH, carbon dioxide pressure and concentration of RBC organic phosphates (Letterio et al., 2020).

TABLE 11.4 **Reference haemoglobin (Hb) values in preterm newborns**

	Hb according to birthweight	
Age (weeks)	*1000–1500 g*	*1501–2000 g*
2	16.3 (11.7–18.4)	16.8 (11.8–19.6)
4	10.9 (8.7–15.2)	11.5 (8.2–15)
8	8.8 (7.1–11.5)	9.4 (8.0–11.4)
12	9.8 (8.9–11.2)	10.2 (9.3–11.8)
16	11.3 (9.1–13.1)	11.3 (9.1–13.1)

Source: Colombatti et al. (2016).

Adult haemoglobin (HbA) appears in the fetal blood near term as minor adult globin and increases gradually in the first few months of life. See Table 11.5 for normal Hb values across the life span. As Hb molecules mature, the affinity for oxygen diminishes. The cooperative binding of oxygen to haemoglobin tetramers is well represented in the sigmoidal arc of the oxygen dissociation curve (refer to Chapter 9 for more information about the oxygen dissociation curve).

TABLE 11.5 **Normal Hb values across the life span**

Term newborns	17–22 g/dL
1 week of age	15–20 g/dL
1 month of age	11–15 g/dL
Children	11–13 g/dL
Adult males	14–18 g/dL
Adult females	12–16 g/dL

Source: Davis and Stöppler (2017).

ERYTHROCYTE DISORDERS

Anaemia – common causes and pathophysiology

Anaemia in the neonate is difficult to define; the literature offers a variety of haemoglobin values to define anaemia. *Physiological* anaemia is a normal process; all newborn infants have a physiological decline in haemoglobin levels 8–12 weeks after birth (Sharafutdinova et al., 2019). After birth, the hypoxic stimulus is removed and, as a result, fetal red cell production ceases. Erythropoietin, haemoglobin and haematocrit levels fall and reticulocytes decrease. The life spans of adult and fetal haemoglobin also reduce. There are many causes of *pathological* anaemia, with the most common being from anaemia of prematurity, haemorrhagic anaemia (blood loss), haemolytic anaemia and glucose-6-phosphate dehydrogenase (G6PD) deficiency.

Anaemia of prematurity

Whereas physiological anaemia is considered a normal process in term infants, anaemia of prematurity is a pathological anaemia occurring in preterm infants (Sharafutdinova et al., 2019). Extremely low birthweight (ELBW) neonates (those born at <1000 g) are likely to develop anaemia of prematurity because placental iron transport and fetal erythropoiesis are incomplete. Coupled with phlebotomy blood losses required for testing, and low plasma levels of erythropoietin due to both diminished production and accelerated catabolism, approximately 90% of ELBW neonates will receive at least one RBC transfusion during their clinical course (Saito-Benz et al., 2020).

Preterm neonates with anaemia are often asymptomatic, with non-specific symptoms such as tachycardia, tachypnoea, lethargy, pallor, apnoea and periods of bradycardia, poor feeding, poor growth and a persistent lactic *acidosis* (a subtype of metabolic acidosis).

Treatment is aimed at prevention, by delayed cord clamping at birth, reducing excessive blood draws, providing appropriate dietary supplementation and erythropoietin therapy. When symptoms of hypoxia are present, a blood transfusion is indicated. Indications for blood transfusion for anaemia of prematurity include a continued need for mechanical ventilation, apnoea and bradycardia, tachycardia (>180 bpm), inadequate weight gain, metabolic acidosis or anticipation of major surgery (Sharafutdinova et al., 2019). International guidelines indicating the need for transfusion considering gestational age, postnatal age, the severity of illness and Hb thresholds vary from 80–130 g/L in Australia and Canada to 70–120 g/L in France (Villeneuve et al., 2021). If the neonate has a low Hb but is stable, the reticulocyte count may indicate that an increase in Hb is imminent, and a transfusion can be avoided.

Haemorrhagic anaemia

Anaemia due to blood loss can occur before, during and after birth. Before birth, it can be caused by trauma from procedures such as amniocentesis, trauma to the maternal abdomen, gastrointestinal bleeding, twin-to-twin transfusion, placenta praevia or placental abruption (Colombatti et al., 2016). During the birthing process, anaemia due to blood loss can result from placental malformation, haematoma of the umbilical cord, rupture of the cord or accidental incision of the placenta (Colombatti et al., 2016).

After birth, anaemia can occur as a result of intracranial haemorrhage, cephalhaematoma, caput succedaneum (refer to Chapter 13 for further information about these conditions), pulmonary haemorrhage, gastrointestinal haemorrhage or subscapular liver haematoma, sepsis, inadequate nutrition and cardiorespiratory disease (Colombatti et al., 2016). Iatrogenic blood loss can occur from frequent blood sampling, failure to clamp the umbilical cord effectively or dislodged umbilical or peripheral arterial lines. Neonatal nurses/midwives play a pivotal role in ensuring blood sampling is minimised and only the required sample is removed, and lines are secure.

CLINICAL PRACTICE 11.1

The greatest contributor of anaemia of prematurity is the volume of blood lost to phlebotomy (Cibulskis et al., 2021). Four millilitres of blood in a 500-g neonate is approximately 10% of the circulating blood volume (this is equivalent to an adult losing 500 mL). For this reason, the need for blood sampling should be carefully considered, and even small aliquots of blood taken for tests need to be documented carefully and tallied.

Haemolytic anaemia

The speed of RBC destruction can be increased by certain factors, leading to profound anaemia. The most common include **rhesus (Rh)** isoimmunisation and ABO incompatibility.

Rhesus isoimmunisation leads to the most severe form of RBC destruction and can lead to significant fetal red cell haemolysis. This condition occurs when the mother is Rh negative and, in a previous pregnancy, the fetus was Rh positive. Fetal red cells enter the maternal circulation and, as a result, the mother produces antibodies against the foreign cells. In subsequent pregnancies, the maternal antibodies enter the fetal circulation and destroy the fetal red cells. In mild cases, the fetus may have mild anaemia with *reticulocytosis* (an increase in reticulocytes, or immature red blood cells). In moderate to severe cases, the fetus may have a more marked anaemia and erythroblastosis fetalis (*haemolytic disease of the newborn*). With treatment of Rh immunoglobulin (anti-D) administered by intramuscular injection to the mother, the fetal cells are destroyed before antibodies can be produced and, with the use of anti-D, the incidence can be decreased (Hamel, 2020).

ABO incompatibility is the most common form of haemolytic disease and is clinically less severe than Rh incompatibility. ABO incompatibility usually occurs only in infants with blood type A or B who are born to mothers with blood group O (to remember this, think about how there is an O in mOther). Normal anti-A and anti-B antibodies are immunoglobulin M (IgM) (*the largest antibody; produced by B cells*) and are therefore too large to cross the placenta. For reasons that are poorly understood, however, some group O women have IgG (*the smallest, most common antibody; found in all body fluids*) anti-A and anti-B, which are small enough to cross the placenta, even without prior sensitisation (Colombatti et al., 2016). Affected neonates have a positive **direct antibody test (DAT)** (sometimes referred to as a Coombs test), indicating a transfer of maternal IgG anti-A or IgG anti-B to the neonate. However, unlike anti-Rh antibodies, both anti-A and anti-B incompatibility result predominantly in hyperbilirubinaemia without significant neonatal anaemia (Pegoraro et al., 2020).

Glucose-6-phosphate dehydrogenase deficiency

Deficiency of glucose-6-phosphate dehydrogenase (G6PD) is one of the most common human enzyme disorders caused by inherited X-linked gene G6PD mutations, and therefore affects mostly males. G6PD deficiency renders red cells extremely vulnerable to haemolysis and thus susceptible to oxidative damage. There are more than 200 G6PD mutations known; about one-half are polymorphic and hence widespread in different populations. Neonates with G6PD deficiency develop jaundice in the first 24 hours of life resulting from the bilirubin produced, with the excessive destruction of RBCs and inefficient bilirubin conjugation. At the same time this destruction of RBCs leads to anaemia, pallor and splenomegaly. The newborn screening test confirms the diagnosis and treatment includes phototherapy. In extreme cases, exchange transfusion may be needed. Parental education involves avoidance of the triggers for G6PD, which include fava (broad) beans, mothballs and some medications (Wolfe & Shukla, 2020).

Signs and symptoms

The signs and symptoms of anaemia depend on the cause of the anaemia.

Chronic haemorrhagic anaemia includes signs of pallor without jaundice, compensatory reticulocytosis, hepatomegaly or hydrops fetalis (*an abnormal accumulation of fluid including ascites, pleural effusion, pericardial effusion and skin oedema* – see Fig. 11.1). The mechanism for the formation of fetal hydrops is an imbalance of interstitial fluid production and lymphatic return (Hamdan, 2017). Fluid accumulates in the fetus owing to congestive cardiac failure, obstructed lymphatic flow or decreased plasma osmotic pressure. The fetus compensates for hypoxia produced by anaemia by redirecting blood flow to the brain, heart and adrenals, causing damage to those organs, renal tubular injury, volume augmentation to increase cardiac output and marked activation of the renin–angiotensin system (Hamdan, 2017). The unique hydropic changes in the fetus result when these mechanisms also increase venous pressure, and ultimately produce interstitial fluid. By increasing capillary hydrostatic pressure and limiting lymphatic return, increased venous pressure contributes to oedema and effusion. Oliguria or anuria, as a result of impaired renal function, leads to hydrops (Hamdan, 2017). Acute haemorrhagic anaemia presents with pallor without jaundice, respiratory distress including tachypnoea and acidosis and decreased perfusion and hypotension, leading to hypovolaemic shock.

Haemolytic anaemia and G6PD present with jaundice, pallor after 48 hours, respiratory distress and hepatosplenomegaly. Anaemia of prematurity typically presents with apnoea, bradycardia, hypoxaemia, respiratory distress and poor growth/weight gain (Stark et al., 2020).

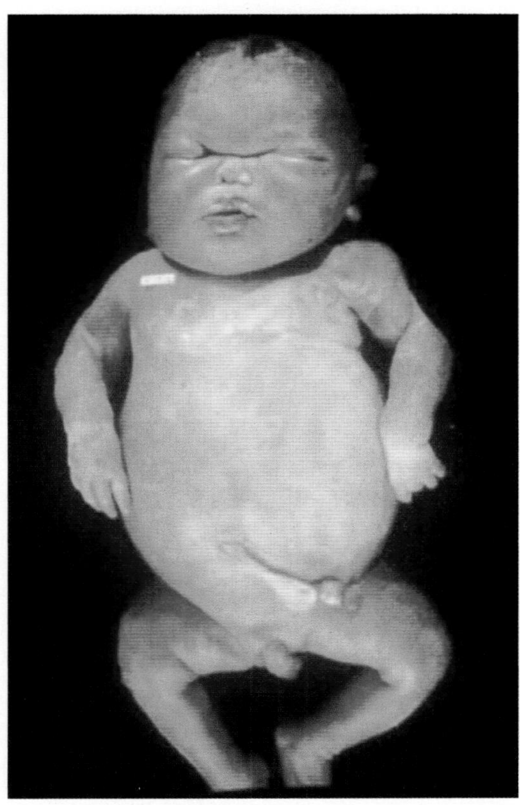

FIGURE 11.1 **Hydrops fetalis**

Source: Rodríguez-Cerdeira, C., & Silami-Lopez, V. G. (2012). © 2011 Elsevier España, S. L. and AEDV.

Diagnosis

Diagnosis of anaemia includes a full blood count (FBC) (see Tables 11.1). Further tests include a DAT, G6PD deficiency screen and a **serum bilirubin reading (SBR)**.

Management

The neonate's Hb, bodyweight, clinical condition, age and gestation need to be considered when deciding on treatments. Blood transfusions are the standard treatment for anaemia. Following the PINT study (Kirpalani et al., 2006), the recommendations shown in Table 11.6 were made to avoid unnecessary transfusion. However, thresholds for neonatal RBC transfusions are not well established, with significant factors including gestational duration, postnatal age and health status. There were contradictory findings on neurocognitive outcomes in two randomised control trials (RCTs) (Bell et al., 2005; Kirpalani et al., 2006) comparing moderate with minimal haemoglobin (Hb) transfusion levels in preterm neonates, making general guidelines difficult. This topic is now being re-examined by two RCTs (one in the United States and one in Europe) (Zerra et al., 2019). The recommendations are a guide only and careful consideration should be given in the event of poor circulation, symptomatic shock (of any form), surgery or presence of coagulopathy.

EVIDENCE-BASED PRACTICE RESEARCH 11.1

Prevention of anaemia

- The transition from fetal to postnatal life is enabled by delayed or physiological clamping of the umbilical cord. Several reports have recorded lower rates of IVH with delayed cord clamping, prompting the latest recommendations to postpone umbilical cord clamping in vigorous preterm infants for at least 30–60 seconds (Noori, 2020).
- The role of recombinant human erythropoietin (rhEPO) has been investigated for the treatment of anaemia in neonates, especially very low birthweight (VLBW) infants, because of the low physiological levels of erythropoietin in neonates. A Cochrane review reported that rhEPO is associated with a substantial decrease in the number of blood transfusions per neonate, but also a substantially increased risk of retinopathy of prematurity (Aher & Ohlssen, 2020). There were no differences in mortality or other neonatal morbidities among neonates who did or did not receive rhEPO. Because of these restricted advantages and possible significant complications of early rhEPO treatment, there is currently no clear recommendation for the systematic use of rhEPO in neonates with anaemia, but it should be considered in individual environments (Kliegman et al., 2020).

Polycythaemia/hyperviscosity

Pathophysiology

Polycythaemia is defined as a venous haematocrit greater than 65% during the first week of life. In seminal work, Nelson (1976) demonstrated that blood viscosity increases once the haematocrit rises above 65%. However, other factors can increase viscosity, including red cell number, plasma proteins and erythrocyte deformity, and less than half of neonates with polycythaemia have hyperviscocity. Table 11.7 outlines the common causes of polycythaemia.

Signs and symptoms

Neonates with polycythaemia are usually asymptomatic, or they can demonstrate a range of non-specific symptoms. Most neonates with polycythaemia will have a plethoric, sanguine appearance (Fig. 11.2). The most common symptoms are gastrointestinal (vomiting and poor

TABLE 11.6 **Comparison of BCSH, American, Australian and Canadian practice guidelines for RBC transfusion in newborn infants**

Clinical status	BCSH guideline	American Red Cross practice guideline	Australian National Blood Authority guideline	Canadian Blood Services guideline
Anaemia in the first 24 h	Hb <12 g/dL or Hct <0.36	–	No respiratory support: Hb 10–12 g/dL Respiratory support: Hb 11–13 g/dL	On ECMO and congenital cyanotic heart disease Hb <15 g/dL
Infants receiving intensive care Severe cardiopulmonary disease (FiO_2 >0.35)	Hb <12 g/dL or Hct <0.36	Hct 40–45%	Hb 11–13 g/dL	Hb <12 g/dL
Chronic oxygen dependency Moderate cardiopulmonary disease (CPAP or O_2)	Hb <11 g/dL	Hct 30–35%	Hb 8.5–11 g/dL	Hb <10 g/dL
Late anaemia, stable patient	Hb <7 g/dL	Hct 20–25%	Hb 7–10 g/dL	Hb <7 g/dL

BCSH, British Committee for Standards in Haematology; CPAP, continuous positive airway pressure; Hb, haemoglobin; Hct, haematocrit.

Source: Howarth et al. (2018).

TABLE 11.7 **Common causes of polycythaemia**

Placental hyper-transfusion (passive)	• Twin-to-twin transfusion • Maternofetal transfusion • Delayed cord clamping
Placental/maternal (active)	• Placental insufficiency • Smoking • Post maturity • Placenta praevia
Endocrine and metabolic disorders (active)	• Congenital adrenal hyperplasia • Neonatal thyrotoxicosis • Maternal diabetes
Miscellaneous (active)	• Trisomies 21, 18, 13 • Hypoxia • Beckwith–Wiedemann • Dehydration • IUGR

IUGR, intrauterine growth restriction.

Source: Carr et al. (2014).

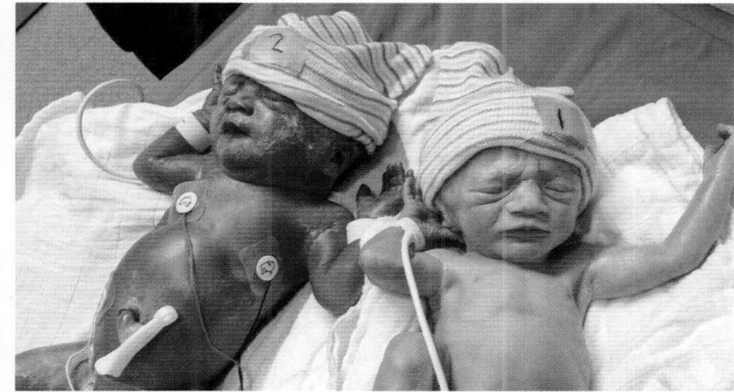

FIGURE 11.2 **Twin-to-twin transfusion: the twin on the left is polycythaemic, the twin on the right is anaemic**

Source: Wikipedia/FetalTherapyLUMC. CC BY-SA 3.0.

feeding), followed by hypoglycaemia, jaundice, cyanosis and apnoea.

Other signs may be attributed to polycythaemia, such as respiratory distress, hypocalcaemia, lethargy, irritability and seizures, but the evidence for these is not strong (Garcia-Prats, 2019).

Diagnosis

Diagnosis is made from obtaining an FBC (ideally a venous free-flowing sample, as milking – for example, from a capillary sample – can artificially increase the HCT) (Garcia-Prats, 2019) to measure the haematocrit. The HCT normally rises after birth, reaching a peak at 2 hours postpartum when the upper limit of a normal HCT can be 71%, and then slowly decreases over the next 12 hours. Further tests to detect complications include blood glucose level (BGL), serum bilirubin (SBR), blood gas analysis and serum calcium.

Management

In polycythaemic neonates with hyperviscosity, **partial exchange transfusion (PET)** significantly decreases the haematocrit and reduces total blood viscosity. Partial exchange transfusion is also effective for correcting extreme anaemia without the risk of fluid overload and cardiac failure (Jacquot et al., 2020).

The long-term advantage of early partial exchange transfusion in polycythaemic neonates is controversial, at least partially because the prognosis for such neonates depends heavily on the aetiology. As the trigger for partial exchange transfusion, a haematocrit greater than 65% is typically used because, as the haematocrit rises above this level, blood viscosity greatly increases and oxygen transfer reduces (Jacquot et al., 2020).

To normalise haematocrit levels to below 60%, partial exchange is used by extracting a percentage of the blood volume and replacing it with an equivalent amount of isotonic crystalloid solution. Crystalloid solutions are preferred to plasma to minimise plasma toxicity, as the use of plasma as a substitute solution has been correlated with **necrotising enterocolitis (NEC)** (Jacquot et al., 2020).

Complications

The hyperviscosity that can result from polycythaemia can reduce blood flow, impair tissue oxygenation and increase the tendency for microthrombus formation exacerbated by hypoxia, acidosis and/or poor perfusion. Further complications include renal venous thrombosis, adrenal insufficiency, NEC and cerebral infarction that may affect long-term neurological outcome. Severe complications are caused by the increased resistance to blood flow due to hyperviscosity, with circulation to all organs being impaired because of sluggish blood flow. These include hyperbilirubinaemia, seizures, NEC, renal failure/renal vein thrombosis, peripheral gangrene, hypoglycaemia, hypocalcaemia, congestive heart failure and motor and neurological abnormalities (Kliegman et al., 2020).

HYPERBILIRUBINAEMIA (NEONATAL JAUNDICE)

Hyperbilirubinaemia occurs when the bilirubin levels exceed the normal range for the neonate's gestation, age and weight. The term jaundice refers to the yellow discoloration of the skin and the sclera of the eyes, resulting from having too much bilirubin (hyperbilirubinaemia) (Fig. 11.3).

Jaundice is the most common clinical condition in the neonatal period, with 60% of full-term and 80% of preterm neonates having visible jaundice (Kaplan et al., 2020). As will be discussed, jaundice occurs when the level of bilirubin (*a yellow pigment produced during the normal breakdown of red blood cells*) in the blood rises. When the bilirubin level becomes elevated (*hyperbilirubinaemia*), unconjugated bilirubin can be deposited in the skin, the conjunctivae and other tissues – including the brain at toxic levels leading to a potentially lethal condition, kernicterus.

Bilirubin metabolism

Neonates normally have an elevated RBC at birth, and these cells have a shorter life span than adult RBC, leading to an increased amount of haemolysis. The ageing RBC are removed by the spleen, and Hb is broken down and recycled. The reticuloendothelial system is responsible for the breakdown of aged RBC into haem and globin. Globin is a protein, which is conserved and utilised; haem is catabolised into unconjugated bilirubin. The synthesis, pathway and metabolism of bilirubin are summarised in Fig. 11.4.

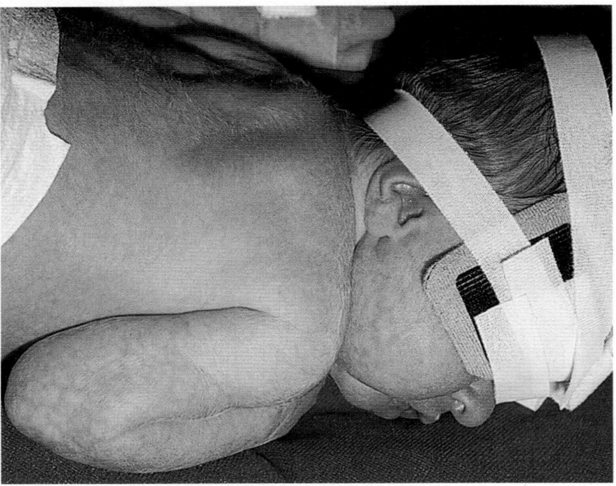

FIGURE 11.3 **The neonate with jaundice**
Source: Eichenfield et al. (2015).

Unconjugated bilirubin is *fat soluble*; therefore, it is unable to be excreted in bile or urine. In order for bilirubin to be excreted into the bile, unconjugated bilirubin must be converted into a *water-soluble* substance. Serum albumin binds bilirubin and carries it to the liver for conjugation. If there are insufficient albumin-binding sites, bilirubin can remain 'free' (*unconjugated*). It is in this state that it has a high affinity for fatty tissues, including brain cells. It is toxic to the central nervous system and may result in yellow staining of the brain – a condition referred to as *kernicterus* (Fig. 11.5). Once in the liver, glucuronic acid is added to unconjugated bilirubin facilitated by the enzyme glucuronyl transferase, which produces bilirubin diglucuronide, which is referred to as conjugated bilirubin. It is then water soluble and can be excreted in bile and urine. It poses no danger to the central nervous system. The conjugated bilirubin is deconjugated by intestinal bacteria in the colon and converted to urobilinogen. Eighty percent of this urobilinogen is further oxidised by bacteria, converted to stercobilin and then excreted in the stool. About 20% of the urobilinogen is absorbed across the intestinal mucosa, contributing, through the enterohepatic circulation, to the circulating unconjugated bilirubin pool, and then is re-presented to the liver for conjugation (Chaudhary 2020). This process is called *enterohepatic circulation* or *enterohepatic shunting* (Fig. 11.6). A small percentage of the urobilinogen reaches the kidneys and is further oxidised into urobilin and excreted into the urine (Chaudhary, 2020).

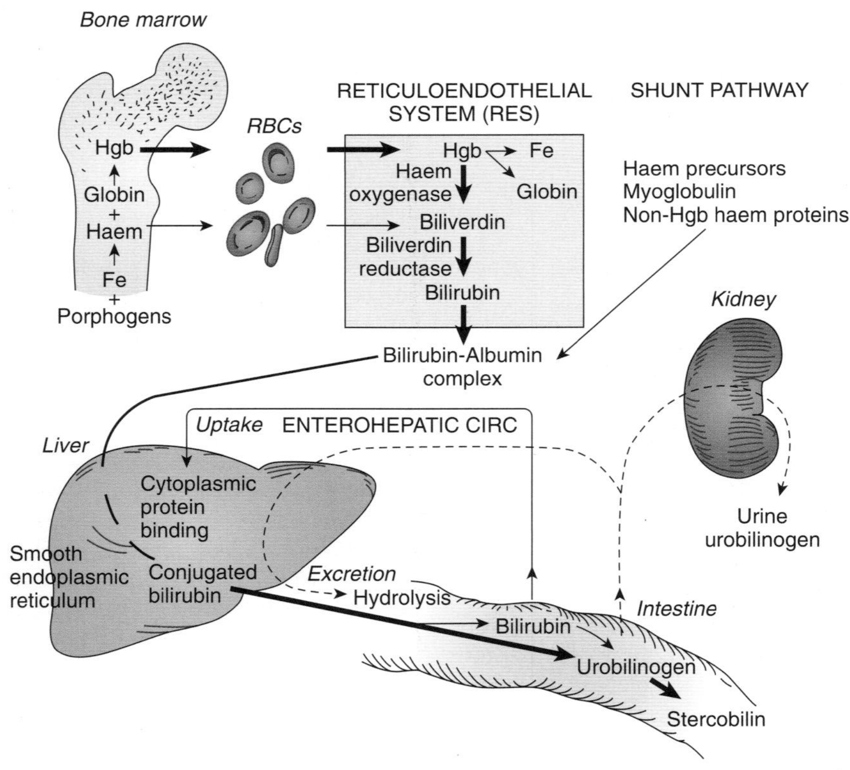

FIGURE 11.4 **Bilirubin synthesis, transport and metabolism**
Source: Assali (1972).

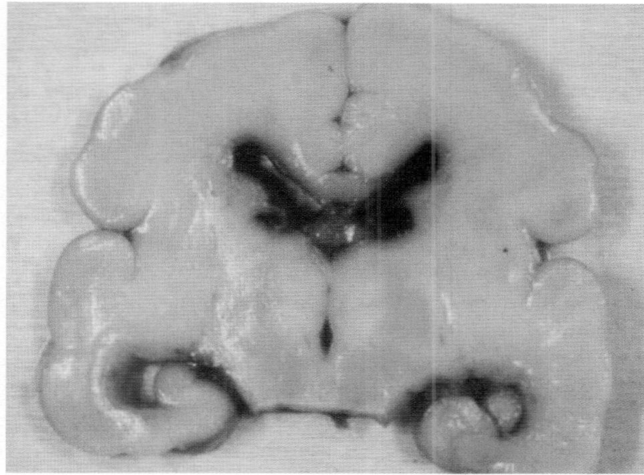

FIGURE 11.5 **Yellow staining of the brain tissue as seen in kernicterus**

Source: Rennie (2012).

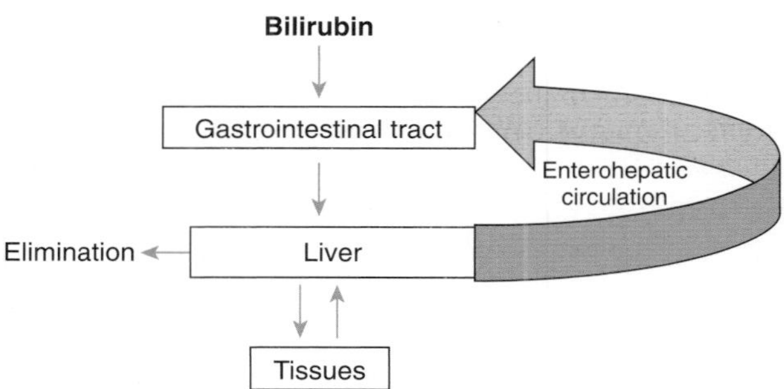

FIGURE 11.6 **Enterohepatic circulation**

Source: Wikipedia/Soladee, CC BY SA 3.0.

Physiological hyperbilirubinaemia

Physiological jaundice is an exaggerated physiological response that usually resolves within 2 weeks in a term neonate, and in up to 3 weeks in a preterm neonate. It is the most common cause of jaundice in the newborn, usually appearing on day 2–3 of life, peaking at day 6 and generally resolved by day 10.

CLINICAL PRACTICE 11.2

Jaundice is never physiological if it occurs within 24 hours of life, persists after 14 days, is associated with a sick infant or if the conjugated bilirubin is above 30 μmol/L or greater than 20% of the total serum bilirubin (Kaplan et al. 2020).

The amount of bilirubin produced is influenced by a variety of factors. Preterm infants have insufficient quantities of *glucuronyl transferase* (an enzyme that converts unconjugated to conjugated bilirubin) and take 6–7 days to produce adequate amounts. An inadequate oral intake can cause delayed bacterial colonisation of the gut and increase the enterohepatic recirculation (see Fig. 11.6). There is a vast amount of bilirubin in meconium; the longer it takes to clear the intestine, the greater the amount of bilirubin that can be absorbed. Moreover, bruising and swallowed blood can increase the bilirubin load because of the increased breakdown of these red blood cells (Kaplan et al., 2020).

Breast milk and breastfeeding jaundice

An important factor linked to neonatal jaundice is breastfeeding. For each of the first 5 days of life, breastfed infants have substantially higher serum bilirubin levels than formula-fed infants, and this type of unconjugated hyperbilirubinemia can continue for weeks to months. Research has shown that bilirubin is an effective antioxidant that is potentially of physiological benefit, as free radicals guard against cellular injury. During the first week of birth, some of the literature distinguishes this early jaundice as '**breastfeeding jaundice**' to differentiate it from the later syndrome of '**breast milk jaundice**', which develops after the first week of life, at which time the source of breast milk is well developed. The overlap between these disorders and physiological jaundice is likely to occur. In some milk samples, early findings connecting breast milk and jaundice with a steroid (pregnane-3α, 20β-diol) have not been verified by subsequent, broader research using more sensitive approaches. The presence of β-glucuronidase in human milk might promote the enterohepatic circulation of bilirubin. Caloric consumption, fluid intake, weight loss and delayed transit of meconium are other reasons probably contributing to jaundice in breastfed neonates. Breast milk jaundice has been found in stable, breastfed neonates with unconjugated hyperbilirubinemia, normal haemoglobin concentrations, normal reticulocyte counts, normal blood smears, no blood group incompatibility and no other clinical test anomalies. Since there is no clear laboratory test to validate the diagnosis of breast milk jaundice, before attributing hyperbilirubinemia to breast milk, it is important to rule out treatable causes of jaundice (Mack & Gourley, 2021).

Pathological hyperbilirubinaemia

Either over-production or under-excretion of bilirubin can result in a condition known as pathological hyperbilirubinaemia, although sometimes the condition can result from a combination of the two. This can be caused by a number of reasons, including sepsis, inborn errors of metabolism, haemolytic disease and blood type incompatibilities. Regardless of the causative factor(s), if the neonate has clinical jaundice within the first 24 hours of life, or if a term infant has clinical jaundice persisting for more than 10 days, the cause of jaundice is always regarded as pathological.

Haemolytic disease of the newborn (erythroblastosis fetalis)

Haemolytic disease of the newborn (HDN), also referred to as erythroblastosis fetalis, arises from the maternal immune system interpreting the fetal red blood cells as foreign. Maternal antibodies develop in response and attack the fetal red blood cells, causing haemolysis. The resulting haemolytic jaundice is most likely to occur within 24 hours of birth. This condition can be very dangerous as bilirubin levels rise very quickly and have the potential to be toxic to the central nervous system, resulting in kernicterus. Rhesus disease is the most severe form causing erythroblastosis fetalis.

There are two ways that the fetal blood and maternal blood may be incompatible . There are four main blood types: A, B, AB and O. If the incompatibility arises from any of these four blood types, it is referred to as an ABO incompatibility, which is the most common form of a mismatch and, in most cases, is not severe. Alternatively, if the mother is rhesus (Rh) negative and the fetus has Rh-positive cells, Rh incompatibility arises, which can cause very severe anaemia in the neonate (see the section on haemolytic anaemia). These two types of incompatibilities are described in more detail in the anaemia section of the chapter.

Clinical assessment and management of hyperbilirubinaemia

Signs and symptoms

Neonates with hyperbilirubinaemia will have yellowing of the skin and conjunctivae (jaundice) that follows a cephalocaudal progression. The neonate may be lethargic, hypotonic and have a history of poor feeding.

Diagnosis

VISUAL ASSESSMENT

Jaundice is first seen in the face and progresses caudally to the trunk and extremities (Kaplan, 2020). Visual assessment of a neonate's jaundice level can be made by blanching the skin with digital pressure to reveal the underlying skin colour. Kramer's scale is a simple, non-invasive way to determine the severity of jaundice (Fig. 11.7). Blanch the skin in each of the five zones then look at the colour of the blanched skin (it will be yellow if the baby is jaundiced) to see what the bilirubin level is. The zones depict the normal evolution of increasing levels of jaundice. Use it only as a guide, however; serum bilirubin levels should regularly be checked (Shafiq et al., 2019). Jaundice below the nipple line should be checked with transcutaneous bilirubinometry or total bilirubin. The newborn should be assessed clinically for visible jaundice with all routine vital sign checks, preferably next to a well-lit window in natural light (Khaki, 2021).

NON-INVASIVE MONITORING: TRANSCUTANEOUS BILIRUBINOMETRY

Non-invasive bilirubin measurements provide an estimate of the transcutaneous bilirubin levels. Referred to as **transcutaneous bilirubinometry (TcB)**, there are a number of benefits of using this technology as it provides a non-invasive and accurate screening for clinically significant jaundice. The readings are instant, and results can lead to a reduction in invasive blood tests. The use of TcB in jaundiced neonates has been found to be reliable and safe, resulting in a reduction of more than one-third in blood draws (Kaplan et al., 2020).

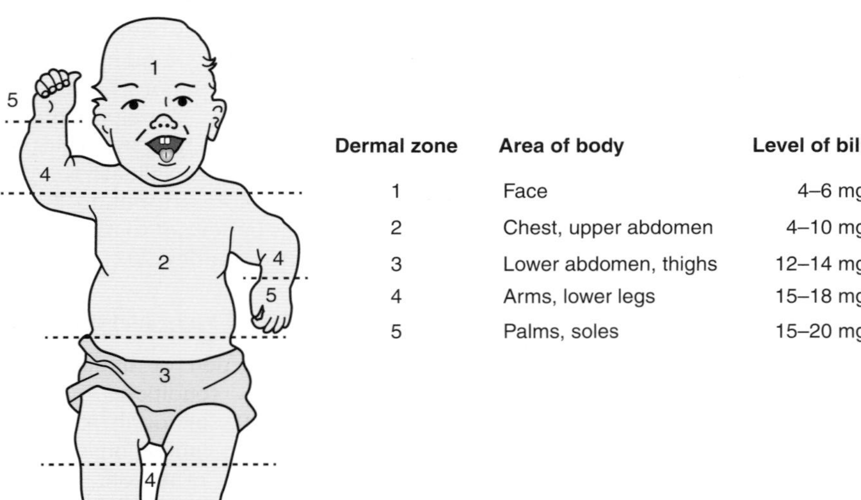

Dermal zone	Area of body	Level of bilirubin
1	Face	4–6 mg/dL
2	Chest, upper abdomen	4–10 mg/dL
3	Lower abdomen, thighs	12–14 mg/dL
4	Arms, lower legs	15–18 mg/dL
5	Palms, soles	15–20 mg/dL

FIGURE 11.7 **Modified Kramer's scale**

Source: Bhat, Sheikh and Ara (2019).

SERUM BILIRUBIN LEVELS

Serum bilirubin readings (SBR) are the most accurate way of assessing jaundice levels. SBR are usually checked again 24 hours after treatment is commenced unless the levels were particularly concerning, in which case they may be checked after 6 hours.

Tests to determine the causes of pathological jaundice may also include blood group and DAT, FBC, C-reactive protein (CRP), liver function test (LFT), albumin levels, reticulocytes, G6PD, thyroid function test, urinalysis, RBC smear, genetic screening and TORCHES CLAP screen (refer to Chapter 16 for more information on TORCHES CLAP screening).

It is important to ensure that the phototherapy unit is switched off during collection of blood for SBR levels, as both conjugated and unconjugated bilirubin are photo-oxidised when exposed to white or ultraviolet light (Achman et al., 2020).

Management

PREVENTION

The first line of management in the treatment of hyperbilirubinaemia is prevention. During pregnancy, it is recommended that women be screened for ABO, Rh (D) blood types and red cell antibodies (Minuk et al., 2020). If maternal red blood cell antibodies are detected in the antenatal period, cord blood should be analysed for blood group (including rhesus type), DAT, FBC for haemoglobin and haematocrit and total serum bilirubin and albumin. If the mother has not been screened antenatally, it is recommended that maternal blood be analysed for blood group (ABO/Rh) along with cord blood for blood group, Rh type and DAT (Queensland Health, 2019).

The risk of hyperbilirubinaemia is elevated when fluid intake is low. Zaitsu et al. (2018) found that optimal thermal control and sufficient nutrition reduced the incidence of neonatal jaundice by preventing bodyweight loss in neonates who weighed more than 2500 g. Breastfeeding can be very beneficial in the prevention of physiological jaundice. All mothers should be encouraged to breastfeed their babies 8–12 times a day in the first 2–3 days of life. Colostrum can increase stooling, which prevents resorption of bilirubin that can lead to physiological jaundice (Queensland Health, 2019).

PHOTOTHERAPY

Phototherapy guidelines for all gestational ages are included in Fig. 11.8. Phototherapy is a common treatment in the neonatal unit, and is used to convert unconjugated bilirubin to lumirubin, a water-soluble photoproduct of bilirubin formed in vivo during phototherapy and excreted in the urine. This chemical process is referred to as isomerisation. Phototherapy uses the blue light spectrum, which causes a photochemical reaction in the skin. Wavelengths in the blue–green spectrum are considered to be the more effective, with blue the most effective (Khaki, 2021). White (daylight) fluorescent tubes are less efficient than blue lamps, and white quartz lamps, though an integral part of some radiant warmers and incubators, have an energy field strongly focused on the centre, with significantly less energy delivered at the perimeter. Fibreoptic lamps are used in some phototherapy units; however, although they deliver high energy levels, they may be noisy owing to the fan in the light source and can have decreased energy delivery as the optic fibres age. 'Double' (two phototherapy units) and 'triple' phototherapy (three units) may be used to treat neonates with very high levels of serum bilirubin. A meta-analysis conducted by Nizam et al. (2020) demonstrated a considerable difference between double versus single phototherapy in the hourly decline of bilirubin levels in preterm neonates and neonates with a birthweight of >1500 grams, due to the greater body surface area of exposure and the intensity of the light.

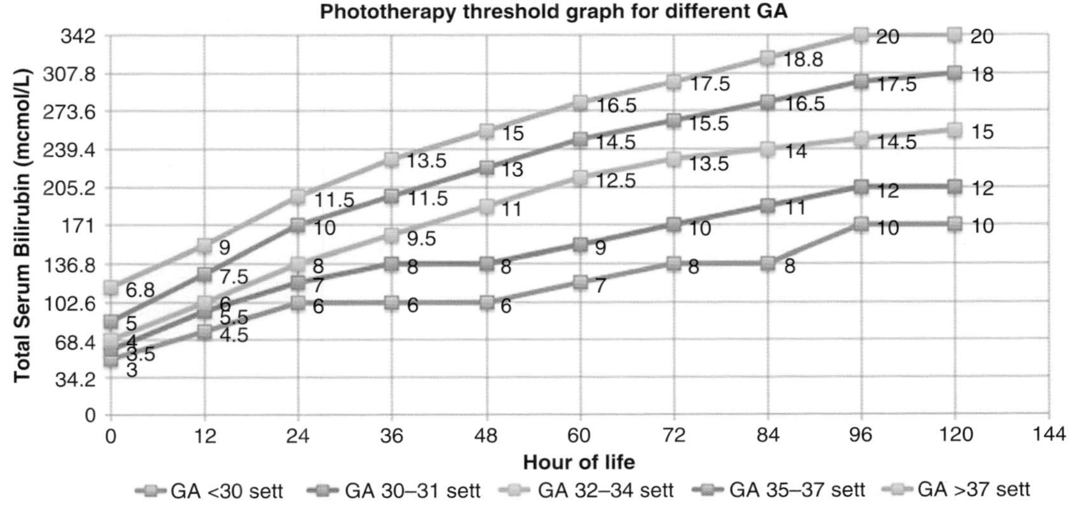

FIGURE 11.8 **Phototherapy guidelines for all gestational ages**

Adapted from: Romagnoli et al. (2014).

Fibreoptic systems are also commonly used. This system passes UV-filtered light from a tungsten–halogen bulb through a fibreoptic cable that emits from the sides and ends of the fibreoptic fibres into a plastic pad. The pad emits very low levels of heat and can be placed in direct contact with the neonate (with a disposable cover over the pad for hygiene and infection control) to deliver up to 35 mW/cm²/nm of spectral irradiation, mainly in the blue–green range. These 'blanket' systems are commonly used in postnatal wards, and even in the home, as the neonate can still be held and breastfed, which reduces infant–parent separation and the specialised care used for overhead phototherapy is not required.

Phototherapy does not treat the *cause* of hyperbilirubinaemia; it is used to *prevent bilirubin toxicity*. More recently, the effects of phototherapy have been questioned in terms of safety, especially in the ELBW population, with a large randomised controlled trial suggesting that, despite a decrease in long-term impairment, there may be an increase in mortality when aggressive phototherapy is used for neonates weighing <750 g (Khaki, 2021).

CASE STUDY 11.1 THE NEONATE WITH JAUNDICE

Baby Simon is delivered at 34 weeks' gestation. His sibling, Jessica, who is now 3 years old, was delivered at 29^4 weeks. On day 3 of life, Simon is clinically jaundiced. His total bilirubin is elevated, and treatment with phototherapy is implemented in order to prevent the neurotoxic effects of high serum levels of unconjugated bilirubin.

Simon's parents are upset and worried.

During phototherapy Simon requires ongoing monitoring of the adequacy of hydration (urine output) and nutrition (weight gain), temperature and clinical improvement in jaundice. He is also observed for signs of lethargy and poor feeding. As much of Simon's skin surface is uncovered as possible to expose him to the phototherapy light. He wears only his nappy and his protective eye covers. The neonatal nurse/midwife ensures that his eye covers are removed 4–6 hourly for eye care during his care or feeding. His eyes are observed for discharge/infection/damage. A strict fluid balance chart is maintained.

Simon's breastfeeds are limited to 20 minutes as his bilirubin level is high, and this minimises the amount of time he spends out of the lights. As a precaution, his nurse ensures that the phototherapy unit is turned off during the collection of blood for TSB/SBR levels.

1. What risk factors does Simon have for neonatal jaundice?
2. What are the neurotoxic effects of high serum levels of unconjugated bilirubin?
3. Why do you think phototherapy poses such a concern for Simon's parents?
4. Why is the phototherapy unit turned off during the collection of blood for TSB/SBR levels?

CLINICAL PRACTICE 11.3

Nursing/midwifery care of the neonate undergoing overhead phototherapy

- A clear explanation to the parents of the neonate undergoing phototherapy is paramount.
- Record the SBR on a relevant chart that takes into account the neonate's gestational age, postnatal age and risk factors such as illness severity, to ensure that phototherapy is started as soon as possible in at-risk neonates.
- Undress the neonate for overhead lights and, to ensure maximum skin exposure, use only a nappy.
- Shield the eyes with an eye mask to reduce the risk of retinal damage.
- Ensure that the phototherapy is the appropriate distance from the skin. The distance should be 30–50 cm from the neonate. Always follow the individual manufacturer's instructions.
- Hyperthermia can occur if the lights are too close.
- Monitor the temperature at least 4 hourly. The cot temperature may need to be reduced slightly once phototherapy commences.
- Observe the eyes for discharge/infection/damage and perform eye toilets with care. Assess skin integrity for rashes/pressure sores and colour, fluid input and output, and stools (it is normal for stools to go dark brown and meconium-like, or loose and explosive due to intestinal hurry-up) 4–6 hourly.
- Pulse oximetry is advisable when the neonate is under blue lights, as cyanosis can be difficult to detect.
- The neonate should be repositioned with care (at least 3–4 hourly) to ensure maximum skin exposure.
- Ensure no oils, creams or lotions are applied to the skin as these may cause burning to the skin. Water-based (as opposed to oil-based) creams can be used.
- Be aware of the interference that phototherapy causes with parental–infant interaction and the subsequent anxiety parents can feel. Unless the hyperbilirubinemia is very severe, it can be interrupted for up to 30 minutes for feeds, care and cuddling. The efficacy of intermittent phototherapy is comparable to that of continuous phototherapy (Wang et al., 2021).
- Phototherapy increases insensible water losses. While supplemental fluids are generally not required, the neonate's fluid balance and hydration should be assessed on an individual basis.
- Repeat the SBR levels daily while the neonate is under phototherapy. Turn the lights off while the sample is being taken and protect it from light until analysed.
- Rebound hyperbilirubinemia can occur after phototherapy is ceased, and the bilirubin shifts from the intravascular space to reaccumulate under the skin.

Source: adapted from Queensland Health (2019); SA Health (2019).

FAMILY-CENTRED CARE 11.1

Caring for the neonate who requires overhead phototherapy is considered 'routine practice' in the neonatal unit.

For parents and families, however, phototherapy can be traumatic. Here are some tips to involve parents and allay their anxiety:

- Remove the baby from the incubator for breastfeeding unless levels are above the phototherapy range.
- Encourage parents to talk to their baby.
- Involve parents in care wherever possible.
- Encourage parents to express their feelings and concerns.
- Provide health education about the causes of hyperbilirubinaemia resulting in jaundice.
- Explain the process of therapy and treatment.
- Give health education on how to care for the baby at home, and what to do if jaundice reappears.

EXCHANGE TRANSFUSION

Indications for exchange transfusion include hyperbilirubinaemia resulting from rhesus/ABO incompatibility, severe anaemia, hydrops fetalis, polycythaemia, hyperkalaemia, drug toxicity and disseminated intravascular coagulopathy (Letterio et al., 2020). Exchange transfusion is performed to replace antibody-coated red cells with antigen-negative red cells and remove excess bilirubin when bilirubin levels are high enough to cause concern that bilirubin toxicity may occur. With the advances in phototherapy, exchange transfusion is rare; nevertheless, on occasion it is required. Each neonatal unit will have its own policy on when and how to perform an exchange transfusion, but the following provides guidance.

The equivalent of the circulating blood volume (single volume exchange) (80 mL/kg bodyweight (BW) in a term infant or 100 mL/kg BW in a preterm infant) or two neonatal blood volumes (double volume exchange) (160 mL/kg BW in the term infant/200 mL/kg BW in the preterm infant) is replaced by aliquots of donor blood in an exchange transfusion not exceeding 10% of the total blood volume. A double volume exchange results in the replacement of around 85% of the RBC that circulate. Concentrations of bilirubin are normally decreased by 50%, although this can be expected to rebound 4 hours post transfusion to about two-thirds of the pre-exchange level. Although the procedure is relatively safe when performed in term neonates by experienced clinicians, it still carries a risk of both mortality (0.1–0.5% in term neonates) and morbidity, as well as being time-consuming and costly. Normally, the procedure takes 1–2 hours. Theoretically, slower exchanges should increase the quantity of bilirubin extracted by allowing tissue pigment equilibration, but the variations are too small to warrant the increased risk of prolonging the length of the operation. There is a need to individualise the indications for exchange transfusion, taking into account gestational age and disease severity. Exchange is recommended during acute hospitalisation if, despite intensive phototherapy, total bilirubin (TB) levels increase to the specified levels. Intensive phototherapy can be considered for readmitted infants if TB is above the exchange transfusion threshold stage, provided the infant does not show clinical symptoms of acute bilirubin encephalopathy. Serial TBs should be administered every 2–3 hours, and if TB persists at or above indicated levels, exchange after 6 hours of intense phototherapy is recommended (Kaplan et al., 2020).

PHARMACOLOGICAL MANAGEMENT

Intravenous immunoglobulin (IVIG) is a pharmacological treatment for haemolytic diseases of the newborn that reduces bilirubin concentrations in neonates with rhesus disease and other types of immune haemolytic jaundice (Patel & Josephson, 2018). Candidates for receiving IVIG include neonates with a positive DAT who, following antenatal investigation, have a risk of severe haemolytic disease, or have an elevated risk of progressing to exchange transfusion. Its use may also be recommended in circumstances such as parental refusal for exchange transfusion and where appropriate blood components for exchange transfusion are unavailable. IVIG is a relatively safe and effective means of reducing bilirubin levels in haemolytic disease of the newborn and has largely replaced exchange transfusion in neonates whose SBR rise cannot be controlled by phototherapy (Mreihil et al., 2018).

Complications

Bilirubin-induced neurotoxicity in neonates remains an area of clinical concern. Unconjugated bilirubin is neurotoxic and bilirubin encephalopathy describes the acute cerebral dysfunction that may progress to kernicterus – the histological yellow staining of the brain tissue and even death (see Fig. 11.5). Kernicterus should be used to define the chronic and permanent sequelae of bilirubin-induced neurological dysfunction. There is no absolute safe level of serum bilirubin above which toxicity occurs, and the preterm infant is known to be more susceptible to bilirubin toxicity than the term infant (Du et al., 2021). While kernicterus is rare, it results in lifelong disability and considerable costs both in handling litigation and providing for the ongoing needs of the infant. Rennie et al. (2019) recommend adherence to the NICE guidelines that advise measuring bilirubin within 6 hours in all neonates who are visibly jaundiced to avoid the devastating consequences of kernicterus.

THE HAEMOSTATIC SYSTEM (COAGULATION DISORDERS)

Coagulation protein disorders

Neonatal bleeding disorders can arise for a number of reasons, including platelet disorders, severe sepsis, coagulation protein disorders (including congenital factor deficiencies, such as X-linked recessive disorders like haemophilia A and B, and acquired deficiencies, the most common being vitamin K deficiency) and vascular integrity disorders.

Haemophilia

Haemophilia A and B are the most common inherited bleeding disorders, and both are examples of a coagulation protein disorder. Haemophilia, however, is considered a rare condition, with an incidence of 1 per 5000 male births globally (Letterio et al., 2020).

Pathophysiology

Haemophilia is a hereditary bleeding disorder linked to the X chromosome and mainly affecting male individuals, as females have two X chromosomes, one of which can protect them against the disorder. The condition is classified as either A or B depending upon whether there is a deficiency of factor VIII (type A, the most common, accounting for 85% of cases) or a deficiency of factor IX (type B). The decrease in factor VIII activity leads to an increased risk of bleeding (Letterio et al., 2020).

Signs and symptoms

Major bleeding in the neonate due to haemophilia is relatively uncommon; however, the incidence of intracranial haemorrhage is higher during the first few days of life than at any other stage in childhood. In the absence of any family history, the first sign, therefore, may be an intracranial bleed, severe gastrointestinal haemorrhage, bleeding after circumcision or bleeding from the umbilical stump (Letterio et al., 2020).

Diagnosis

Haemophilia A and B often occur in neonates with a family history, or in neonates whose mothers are known carriers, but new mutations can also occur in neonates with no known family history of the disorder (Moorehead et al., 2018) and, therefore, haemophilia may be undiagnosed during the neonatal period. In the event of an unexpected bleeding event – such as an intracranial bleed following birth, or a spontaneous gastrointestinal haemorrhage – an isolated prolonged **activated partial thromboplastin time (APTT)** on coagulation studies will be evident. The diagnosis is made on the basis of decreased plasma factor VIII or IX activity, after testing other coagulation factors (including von Willebrand factor) (Letterio et al., 2020).

Management

A multidisciplinary team including paediatric and adult haematologists, obstetricians, neonatologists and blood bank specialists is involved in the care of the newborn during the pregnancy, birth and in the neonatal period (Moorehead et al., 2018). Any carrier mothers should be referred to a tertiary centre for the birth so as to minimise the risk of complications including intracranial haemorrhage. After birth, a rapid diagnosis of haemophilia is determined, and the risk of serious bleeding is assessed and managed. Treatment for acute bleeding is paramount, with the administration of factor VIII or IX concentrates (the 'factor first' principle) before procedures or diagnostic tests (Moorehead et al., 2018). Where the bleeding is severe and persistent, general factor replacement with **fresh frozen plasma (FFP)** or cryoprecipitate may be indicated (Moorehead et al., 2018). In cases where the neonate is a known haemophilia gene carrier, cord blood should be analysed for factor VIII or IX at birth. Once the condition is known, intramuscular injections and heel prick sampling should be avoided, and vitamin K administration (orally, intramuscularly or subcutaneously) should not be delayed (Moorehead et al., 2018). Due to the risk of intracranial haemorrhage, the neonate should be carefully observed for signs of abnormal neurology.

Complications

The major haemophilia problems faced by neonates are life-threatening bleeding and inhibitor development. Inhibitors make it more difficult to arrest a bleeding episode because they prevent treatments from being effective (Letterio et al., 2020). Over the past several years, treatment strategies have increased markedly, and are centred on replacement of recombinant factors, which has led to a considerable decrease in mortality rates. Recent studies indicate that a nearly normal life expectancy is likely, even in cases of severe haemophilia (Letterio et al., 2020).

Vitamin K deficiency bleeding

Vitamin K deficiency bleeding (VKDB), historically referred to as haemorrhagic disease of the newborn, arises from transient yet serious deficits in the vitamin K–dependent coagulation factors and is characterised by haemorrhage that is most often gastrointestinal, nasal, subgaleal, intracranial or post circumcision. VKDB is classified according to the time of presentation: early (within 24 hours of birth), classic (within 1 week of birth) and late (between 2 weeks and 6 months of age) (Araki & Shirahata, 2020). Prodromal or warning signs (mild bleeding) can appear before severe intracranial haemorrhage. Laboratory research shows that both the prothrombin time (PT) and partial thromboplastin time are extended, and plasma levels of prothrombin (II) and factors VII, IX and X are significantly decreased. The pathophysiology of this acquired haemorrhagic disease results because vitamin K promotes post-transcriptional carboxylation of factors II, VII, IX and X, which is essential for its complete coagulation effect (Kliegman et al., 2020).

VKDB has been treated prophylactically with vitamin K administered intramuscularly at birth since the 1950s, which has not been without controversy. In 1992, a British study suggested a possible link between vitamin K prophylaxis via the intramuscular route and childhood cancer (Golding et al., 1992). In 2003 this link was dismissed, with no convincing evidence found that neonatal vitamin K administration, irrespective of the route by which it is given, influences the risk of childhood cancer (Fear et al., 2003). Given the compliance issue of repeated oral doses of vitamin K to achieve the same effect, the relative risk suggested by the initial British study and the later study, intramuscular vitamin K prophylaxis continues to be standard practice.

Pathophysiology

There is little transfer of vitamin K across the placenta, so neonates begin life with low stores of this fat-soluble vitamin. Clotting factors VII, IX and X and prothrombin require vitamin K to become biologically active. Neonates are at a risk for VKDB owing to in-utero and extra-utero causes (Kliegman et al., 2020). Preterm infants are at increased risk of VKDB because of delayed feeding, which delays colonisation of the gut with vitamin K-producing microflora (Ardell et al., 2018).

Breast milk provides very low quantities of vitamin K, and these combined variables place the neonate at risk of bleeding disorders. Early-onset VKDB is commonly associated with maternal malabsorption disorders and medications that inhibit the activity of vitamin K, such as antiepileptics, certain antibiotics and vitamin K antagonists such as warfarin (Araki & Shirahata, 2020). Given the administration of vitamin K prophylaxis at birth in developed countries, this risk of VKDB is very low (1 in 100,000 live births). In the absence of vitamin K prophylaxis, however, the rate of VKDB is as high as 1.7/100 (1/59).

Prevention and treatment

Since VKDB can be life threatening, all infants should receive vitamin K prophylaxis. While intramuscular prophylactic injections of vitamin K reduce the incidence of VKDB, oral administration is also effective (Araki & Shirahata, 2020), although, as previously stated, intramuscular vitamin K prophylaxis continues to be standard practice owing to compliance issues. For non-life-threatening bleeding in infants with VKDB, neonates can be treated with a slow intravenous injection of vitamin K. For cases of severe bleeding, blood products such as FFP may be needed (Araki & Shirahata, 2020).

Disseminated intravascular coagulopathy

Disseminated intravascular coagulopathy (DIC) is considered to be relatively common, and often a catastrophic condition seen in the neonatal unit. Characterised by uncontrolled bleeding, simultaneous with uncontrolled clotting, it is set into motion by an inappropriate activation and consumption of clotting factors, resulting in a haemorrhagic state due to inadequate haemostasis (Letterio et al., 2020).

Pathophysiology

It is important to note that DIC is not considered a primary diagnosis, but a secondary coagulation disorder that complicates its various primary conditions; pathologies include asphyxia, sepsis and **respiratory distress syndrome (RDS)**.

The underlying disease processes, such as those above, often result in endothelial damage, leading to the release of cytokines such as interleukins and platelet-activating factor. Through normal mechanisms of the coagulation pathway, this increased activity leads to the overproduction of thrombin. As depicted in Fig. 11.9, DIC disrupts the integrity of the haemostatic system, leading to

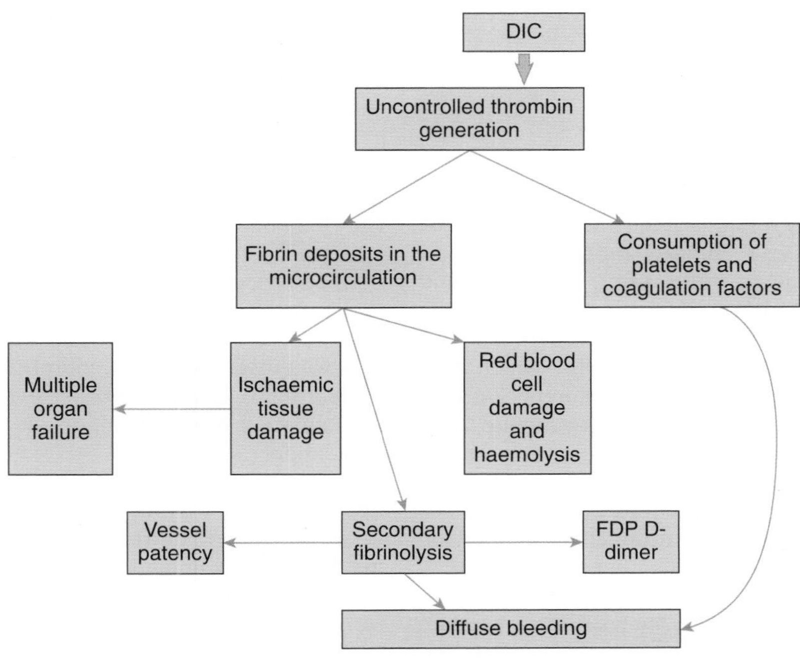

FIGURE 11.9 **Pathophysiology of disseminated intravascular coagulopathy**

a combined defect of reduced procoagulants (prothrombin converters, resulting in the consumption of fibrinogen and therefore clotting), anticoagulants (endogenous inhibitors of clotting, leading to bleeding) and components of the fibrinolytic system (Letterio et al., 2020).

Common causative factors

Sepsis is the most frequent cause of DIC in the neonate (Letterio et al., 2020). In gram-negative bacterial sepsis, endotoxins are released that trigger tissue thromboplastin, which combines with factor VII and inappropriately stimulates the coagulation pathway. This pathway is further triggered by the cardiovascular shock that often accompanies severe sepsis, which leads to further endothelial damage. Viral sepsis also inappropriately stimulates coagulation by circulating antigen–antibody complexes that activate factor XII.

DIC is often seen in neonates with perinatal asphyxia. In this instance, the initiation of coagulation (clot formation) and fibrinolysis (clot breakdown) is also due to the breakdown of RBC leading to the production of tissue plasminogen activator (tPA). Due to breakdown of the cellular endothelium caused by the hypoxic event, tissue factor (TF) – also called platelet tissue factor – combines with factor VII to form factor X and potentiates the conversion of prothrombin to thrombin and fibrinogen to fibrin. Simultaneously, tPA acts on plasminogen to convert it to plasmin to break down fibrin. This type of DIC is therefore referred to as 'consumption coagulopathy' (Letterio et al., 2020).

RDS, another cause of DIC, has similar triggering mechanisms to sepsis and asphyxia. RDS is commonly associated with hypoxia and acidosis, which lead to the increase in TF activity and endothelial destruction. RDS, however, is different in that the condition causes intra-alveolar and intravascular fibrin deposits, which are likely to contribute to severe respiratory insufficiency. These factors are responsible for inactivating considerable amounts of surfactant and worsening the disease process (Letterio et al., 2020).

Signs, symptoms and diagnosis

Clinical signs of DIC and the time of onset are variable, with the neonate first displaying signs of the underlying disease process. From there, clues to indicate impending DIC may be subtle, or there may be major signs. It is important to remember that neonates who are susceptible to DIC will already be sick, and bleeding is typically the initial presentation. The neonatal nurse/midwife may notice that the neonate continues to bleed after heel pricks for laboratory testing or following venepuncture. The beginning of haemorrhage can be subtle, ranging from oozing from an umbilical line or wound and progressing to frank blood in the mouth, nose, orogastric or endotracheal tube indicating a major gastrointestinal or pulmonary bleed. The first clinical sign may also be profound, with a sudden deterioration in vital signs. The neonatal nurse/midwife also needs to recognise that DIC may present with petechiae (Fig. 11.10), purpura, ecchymosis or haematomas.

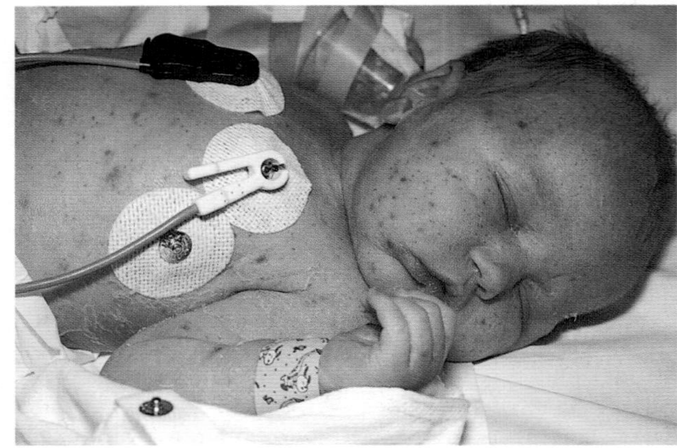

FIGURE 11.10 **Neonate with a petechial rash**
Source: Zitelli et al. (2018).

Laboratory diagnosis of DIC is complicated by the fact that sick or preterm neonates already have abnormal haematological results. The most common tests performed to evaluate coagulation and fibrinolysis include (Brennan & Leone, 2021):

- platelet count low: <100,000/mm3
- prothrombin time (PT) prolonged: >15.3 seconds in term and preterm infants
- APTT prolonged: >59.8 seconds in a term infant and >74.1 seconds in a preterm infant
- fibrinogen levels low: <150 mg/dL
- fibrin degradation product (FDP) or D-dimers: will be >10 or >0.5 mg/mL, respectively, in DIC.

Management

Management of DIC depends largely upon the underlying disease process that led to the condition. Nursing and midwifery care must be meticulous because early clinical recognition of the condition and appropriate intervention contribute to improved outcomes. However, it is emphasised that the underlying condition also needs to be addressed. If infection is identified as the precipitating factor, appropriate antibiotic treatment is vital. In neonates with RDS, exogenous surfactant may be indicated, and so forth.

Monitoring of blood gases is indicated to correct underlying hypoxia, hypercapnia and acidosis. Vital signs, sound physical assessment skills (particularly of neonatal skin to detect petechiae, purpura and ecchymosis, or haematomas), electrolyte balance and nutritional support (as tolerated) are also important when caring for this population.

Intramuscular injections, invasive procedures and any treatment that may cause trauma or bleeding should be avoided, and central access (to avoid heel sticks for the frequent examination of laboratory values such as full blood counts and coagulation studies) needs to be considered.

If the neonate is actively bleeding, replacement therapy with recommended blood components is indicated.

Platelets and FFP transfusions are most frequently used because they contain all the necessary clotting factors. Cryoprecipitate, with its high concentration of factor VIII and fibrinogen, can be used with caution, as it can also be *thrombogenic* (causing coagulation). If a specific factor deficiency is identified, concentrates can also be transfused (Brennan & Leone, 2021).

Thrombocytopenia

As previously discussed in this chapter, thrombocytopenia is described as a platelet count below 150 × 10^9/L. The established postnatal range for platelets is 150–450 × 10^9/L, with levels <60 × 10^9/L usually requiring a platelet transfusion (Scott & Flood, 2019).

Pathophysiology

Thrombocytopenia can arise during fetal life (fetal acquired thrombocytopenia), manifest at birth (early onset) or develop during the neonatal period (late onset). The most common cause of fetal acquired thrombocytopenia is from viral or bacterial infection acquired in utero. In rare cases (1 in 1000 live births in the USA), thrombocytopenia is due to maternal-mediated alloantibodies or autoantibodies (neonatal alloimmune thrombocytopenia, or NAIT) (Norton et al., 2020).

In early-onset thrombocytopenia, chronic intrauterine hypoxia is most often responsible, although perinatal infection may also be a factor. Late onset thrombocytopenia is most often caused by systemic bacterial sepsis or NEC due to platelet consumption (Scott & Flood, 2019). Table 11.8 shows the common causes of neonatal thrombocytopenia.

Signs and symptoms

Clinical signs of bleeding are often the first indicator of thrombocytopenia, particularly in severe cases. In milder cases, the condition may be found incidentally during routine blood studies. Assessment of the neonate includes close inspection of the skin for signs of petechial rashes or purpura with particular attention to the oral mucous membranes and bleeding from puncture sites where bleeding is most likely to occur (Scott & Flood, 2019). Bleeding can also occur in the intracranial space, genitourinary system, gastrointestinal system, lungs, eyes and spinal cord (Norton et al., 2020).

Diagnosis

Thrombocytopenia is diagnosed based on the platelet count and clinical signs of bleeding. If the platelets fall below 50 × 10^9/L, a cranial ultrasound to assess for intracranial haemorrhage is indicated as a matter of priority (Scott & Flood, 2019). NAIT is definitively diagnosed by platelet immunological testing on maternal and paternal blood for platelet antigen differences (Norton et al., 2020).

Management

Management is dependent upon platelet count and the underlying cause of the condition. Maternal platelets are preferred if transfusion is indicated as donor platelets do not produce a sustained increase in platelets, but maternal platelets must be washed, irradiated and leucocyte reduced to avoid transferring additional maternal alloantibodies to the neonate during the transfusion (Norton et al., 2020). Donor platelets can, however, be used as a temporary measure to reduce the risk of an intracranial haemorrhage when platelet levels are very low (Scott & Flood, 2019).

BLOOD COMPONENTS REPLACEMENT THERAPY

Transfusions can save lives, especially in neonates with haemorrhagic shock. In neonatology, as in other clinical arenas, RBC transfusions are performed to optimise oxygen

TABLE 11.8 **Causes of neonatal thrombocytopenia**

	Well-appearing, preterm		Well-appearing, full term	
Type	Early onset (<24 h)	Late onset (>72 h)	Early onset (<24 h)	Late onset (>72 h)
Common	Sepsis TORCH infection Birth asphyxia DIC NEC	Sepsis Thrombosis DIC NEC Drug-induced	Placental insufficiency Autoimmune Alloimmune (NAIT) Occult infection	Occult infection NEC
Rare	Chromosomal disorders • Trisomy 13 • Trisomy 18 • Trisomy 21 • Turner syndrome	Inborn errors of metabolism Fanconi anaemia	Inherited syndromes • Bernard–Soulier • Wiskott–Aldrich • Thrombocytopenia-absent radii • Others Vascular tumours • Kasabach–Merritt	Inborn errors of metabolism Fanconi anaemia

DIC, diffuse intravascular coagulopathy; NAIT, neonatal alloimmune thrombocytopenia; NEC, necrotising enterocolitis; TORCH, toxoplasmosis, other agents, rubella, cytomegalovirus or herpes simplex.

Source: Carr et al. (2014).

supply to tissues. In principle, increased oxygenation could increase the cardiorespiratory capacity of anaemic neonates and decrease inspired oxygen demand and apnoeic episodes. Blood transfusions are associated with both infectious (transfusion-transmitted infections) and non-infectious severe hazards of transfusion (NISHOTs), with some risks unique to preterm neonates (Villeneuve et al., 2021).

Blood products

Red cells

Red cells are obtained by removing the plasma after centrifuging whole blood. They are divided into four packs for paediatric patients so as to minimise wastage and reduce donor exposure. Each pack contains approximately 61 mL (25–100 mL) and has a haematocrit of 0.61 L/L (0.50–0.70 L/L) with a shelf life of 35 days at 2–6°C. They can be further modified (washed, CMV (cytomegalovirus) seronegative, irradiated). Washed cells are required to reduce reactions to transfused plasma proteins (e.g. IgA deficiency). CMV-seronegative cells are required for intrauterine and exchange transfusions for preterm neonates weighing <1500 g or immunocompromised neonates. Irradiated red cells should be considered for intrauterine and all subsequent neonatal exchange transfusions, or preterm neonates weighing <1300 g.

Platelets

Neonatal patients who are eligible for a platelet transfusion should initially receive 10–15 mL/kg of CMV-negative platelet suspension, prepared from a fresh unit of whole blood or by platelet pheresis. No volume-reducing processing is generally advised because of the risk of platelet loss, clumping and instability due to increased handling. The decision to provide a prophylactic platelet transfusion should be formulated on the basis of multiple considerations, including the platelet count, the cause of the thrombocytopenia, the drugs prescribed and the condition of the neonate. Typically, such judgements are organisational, 'best-guess' assessments. For infants in the first week of life at risk of haemorrhage (e.g. preterm neonates), administration of prophylactic platelet transfusions at thresholds of up to 50×10^9/L is usually thought to represent appropriate and safe clinical practice. Platelet transfusions in neonates with platelet counts of greater than 50×10^9/L should be considered only for neonates with significant bleeding, such as significant intraventricular haemorrhage or pulmonary, gastrointestinal or renal haemorrhage (Letterio et al., 2020). All platelets are leuco depleted, irradiated and tested for bacterial contamination. Platelets of identical ABO and Rh (D) group should be used; however, ABO-incompatible platelets may be used if ABO-compatible platelets are not available.

Fresh frozen plasma

Various procedures are used to prevent the incidence of haemorrhages, including the administration of platelets, vitamin K and FFP. While FFP transfusions are frequently given preventively in non-bleeding neonates, their use is not founded on robust evidence. To date, randomised trials have failed to show a positive effect of FFP transfusion on bleeding risk. Despite the lack of data, international recommendations often prescribe the use of FFP in neonates with clinically serious bleeding and those who have unusual coagulation tests, or prior to invasive interventions (Houben et al., 2020). Each unit of FFP is made from a single donation and contains all coagulation factors. It is considered a non-cellular component; therefore, leucocyte depletion, irradiation and CMV testing are not indicated. FFP must be compatible; therefore, group AB or an identical donor must be used.

Cryoprecipitate

Cryoprecipitate is an insoluble precipitate that develops from thawing of FFP between 1°C and 6°C. It comprises high concentrations of factor (F)VIII, FXIII, von Willebrand factor, fibrinogen and fibronectin. One of the most frequent reasons for using cryoprecipitate is for acquired coagulation disorders and disseminated intravascular coagulopathy, usually occurring after birth asphyxia, acidosis, respiratory distress syndrome, inflammation, necrotising enterocolitis, meconium aspiration syndrome, thrombosis and the use of therapeutic hypothermia (Tkach et al., 2018). It is derived from whole blood or via apheresis. It is considered a non-cellular component; therefore, leucocyte depletion, irradiation and CMV testing are not indicated. It takes 30 minutes to defrost and should be administered over 4 hours.

Red cell 'top-up' transfusion

Indications for transfusion

In neonatal units, RBC transfusions are most commonly performed to control anaemia of prematurity. The evidence for RBC transfusion thresholds for neonates remains suboptimal at present. In infants of any gestational age, there is no proof of an Hb or HCT threshold where insufficient tissue oxygenation (critical anaemic hypoxaemia) definitively occurs. Current transfusion guidelines, however, integrate the evidence available (and lack of evidence) and are the best source of expert practice guidance in this field (Keir et al., 2019).

Red cell requirements

Blood transfusions must be commenced within 30 minutes of receipt of the unit of red cells and completed within 4 hours of spiking the unit with an intravenous administration set. This unit should be administered via a 170–200-μm aggregate filter. The Hb content of RBCs can vary; in general, each 10–15 mL/ kg transfused is expected to increase the infant's Hb level by approximately 10–20 g/L. The usual volume of RBCs administered to neonates is 10–20 mL/kg per transfusion over 3–4 hours (Villeneuve et al., 2021). Parental informed consent is required for all blood transfusions and blood products globally (Villeneuve et al., 2021).

Nursing and midwifery management

Two registered nurses/midwives are expected to check that the three patient identifiers match on the compatibility label, compatibility report and identification band on the neonate. The ABO group, Rh (D) and unique donation number must match on the compatibility label and compatibility report. The blood must be in date and checked for signs of damage or deterioration such as an unusual colour, clots and/or signs of haemolysis. Prior to commencement, 15 minutes after commencement of the transfusion (once the red cells have entered the vein), then hourly until the transfusion is complete, and finally on completion, the neonatal nurse/midwife needs to monitor temperature, heart rate, oxygen saturation and respiration rate. If the vital signs become abnormal, the neonatal nurse/midwife needs to continue to monitor the neonate, discontinue the transfusion and immediately report the reaction to the medical officer/neonatal nurse practitioner. The remainder of any implicated blood components should be retained for further investigation.

REFLECTION

Consider the protocol for the safety checks and administration of blood products in your unit.

Best-practice statements about preparing to administer a blood component, including equipment, are available from the Red Cross website: <https://www.redcrossblood.org/content/dam/redcrossblood/hospital-page-documents/334401_compendium_v04jan2021_bookmarkedworking_rwv01.pdf>.

How do these best-practice statements compare with practice in your unit?

Complications

Complications from transfusion include **transfusion-related acute gastrointestinal injury (TRAGI)/transfusion-associated necrotising enterocolitis (TANEC)**. There is some evidence that avoiding feeding during RBC transfusion in premature babies may decrease the risk of TANEC (Hilditch & Keir, 2018). However, most of the neonates identified to be at increased risk had the following risk factors: preterm birth (<28 weeks), extremely low birthweight (<1000 g), history of patent ductus arteriosus (PDA) and significant pre-transfusion anaemia (as demonstrated by a haematocrit <30%). Another study demonstrated that it was severe anaemia among VLBW infants, rather than RBC transfusion, that was associated with increased incidence of NEC (Patel et al., 2019).

Given the lack of current scientific evidence for an association between blood transfusion and TRAGI/TANEC, the practice of withholding feeds during red cell transfusion to prevent occurrence of TRAGI/TANEC may be justified, with feeds being withheld at the discretion of the attending neonatologist based on the reported risk factors.

Other complications of the infusion of blood products include CMV, human immunodeficiency virus, hepatitis C, hepatitis B, malaria, bacterial contamination, haemolytic transfusion reactions, ABO/Rh-incompatible transfusion, allergic reactions, anaphylaxis, transfusion-related acute lung injury, transfusion-associated circulatory overload, graft versus host disease and post-transfusion purpura. Metabolic problems such as hypoglycaemia, hyperkalaemia and hypocalcaemia can also occur (Do-Hyun, 2018).

CONCLUSION

Caring for the neonate with a haematological condition is a challenging area of practice. An understanding of the normal parameters for haematological values and coagulation values assists the neonatal nurse/midwife in caring for neonates. This includes neonates with common conditions such as hyperbilirubinaemia through to more complex conditions such as bleeding disorders, including haemolytic disorders, thrombocytopenia, coagulation disorders and complex disorders of bilirubin metabolism.

Online Resources

Compendium of Transfusion Practice Guidelines (2021): <https://www.redcrossblood.org/content/dam/redcrossblood/hospital-page-documents/334401_compendium_v04jan2021_bookmarkedworking_rwv01.pdf>

References/Acknowledgements

Achman, M., Ankur, K., Gaurav, P., Madhur, P. Y., Asif Jamal, S., & Samar, K. (2020). Study of auto-inflating and deflating air bed for phototherapy treatment of infants. *International Journal of Scientific Research in Science and Technology, 4*(4), 196–203. doi: https://doi.org/10.32628/IJSRST207461.

Aher, S. M., & Ohlsson, A. (2020). Early versus late erythropoietin for preventing red blood cell transfusion in preterm and/or low birth weight infants. *Cochrane Database of Systematic Reviews*, 2(2), CD004865. doi: 10.1002/14651858.CD004865.pub4.

Araki, S., & Shirahata, A. (2020). Vitamin K deficiency bleeding in infancy. *Nutrients, 12*(3), 780–793.

Ardell, S., Offringa, M., Ovelman, C. & Soll R. (2018). Prophylactic vitamin K for the prevention of vitamin K deficiency bleeding in preterm neonates. *Cochrane Database of Systemic Reviews, 5*(2), CD008342. doi: 10.1002/14651858.CD008342.pub2.

Assali, N. (1972). *Pathophysiology of gestation*. New York: Academic Press.

Bell, E. F., Strauss, R. G., Widness, J. A., Mahoney, L. T., Mock, D. M., Seward, V. J., et al. (2005). Randomized trial of liberal versus restrictive guidelines for red blood cell transfusion in preterm infants. *Pediatrics, 115*(6), 1685–1691. doi: 10.1542/peds.2004-188.

Bhat, J. A., Sheikh, S. A., & Ara, R. (2019). Correlation of cord blood bilirubin values with neonatal jaundice in healthy newborns: A prospective observational study. *Archives of Medicine and Health Sciences, 7*(1), 48.

Brennan, K. G., & Leone, T. A. (2021). Neonatology. In: R. A. Polin & M. F. Ditmar (Eds.), *Pediatric secrets* (7th ed., pp. 394–430). Philadelphia, PA: Elsevier.

Carr, R., Kelly, A. M., & Williamson, L. M. (2014). Neonatal thrombocytopenia and platelet transfusion: a UK perspective. *Neonatology*, *107*(1), 1. doi: 10.1159/000365163.

Chaudhary, N. (2020). Bilirubin metabolism. *TeachMe Physiology*. <https://teachmephysiology.com/gastrointestinal-system/liver/bilirubin-metabolism/> (Accessed 16 February 2022).

Cibulskis, C. C., Maheshwari, A., Rao, R., & Mathur, A. M. (2021). Anemia of prematurity: how low is too low? *Journal of Perinatology, 41*(6), 1244–1257. doi: 10.1038/s41372-021-00992-0.

Colombatti, R., Sainati, L., & Trevisanuto, D. (2016). Anaemia and transfusion in the neonate. *Seminars in Fetal and Neonatal Medicine, 21*(1), 2–9. doi: 10.1016/j.siny.2015.12.001.

Davis, C. P., & Stöppler, M. C. (2017). Haemoglobin test: normal, high, low levels. *eMedicineHealth*. <https://www.emedicinehealth.com/hemoglobin_levels/article_em.htm#how_is_a_hemoglobin_test_measured> (Accessed 16 February 2022).

Do-Hyun, K. (2018). Transfusion practice in neonates. *Korean Journal of Pediatrics, 61*(9), 265–270.

Du, L., Ma, X., Shen, X., Bao, Y., Chen, L., & Bhutani, V. K. (2021). Neonatal hyperbilirubinemia management: clinical assessment of bilirubin production. *Seminars in Perinatology, 45*(1), 151351. doi: 10.1016/j.semperi.2020.151351.

Eichenfield, L. F., Frieden, I. J., Zaenglein, A. L., & Mathes, E. (2015). *Neonatal and infant dermatology* (3rd ed.). Philadelphia, PA: Elsevier.

Fear, N. T., Roman, E., Ansell, P., Simpson, J., Day, N., & Eden, O. B. (2003). Vitamin K and childhood cancer: a report from the United Kingdom Childhood Cancer Study. *British Journal of Cancer, 89*(7), 1228–1231. doi: 10.1038/sj.bjc.6601278.

Garcia-Prats, J. A. (2019). Neonatal polycythemia. *UpToDate*. Walters Kluwer. <https://www.uptodate.com/contents/neonatal-polycythemia> (Accessed 16 February 2022).

Golding, J., Greenwood, R., Birmingham, K., & Mott, M. (1992). Childhood cancer, intramuscular vitamin K and pethidine given during labour. *British Medical Journal, 305*, 341–346.

Hall, J. E., & Hall, M. E. (2021). Fetal and neonatal physiology. In: J. E. Hall & M. E. Hall (Eds.), *Guyton and Hall textbook of medical physiology*. (14th ed., pp. 1061–1070). Philadelphia, PA: Elsevier.

Hamdan, A. H. (2017). Pediatric hydrops fetalis. *Medscape*. <https://emedicine.medscape.com/article/974571-overview#a5> (Accessed 16 February 2022).

Hamel, C., Esmaeilisaraji, L., Thuku, M., Michaud, A., Sikora, L., & Fung-Kee-Fung, K. (2020). Antenatal and postpartum prevention of Rh alloimmunization: a systematic review and GRADE analysis. *PloS One, 15*(9), e0238844. doi: 10.1371/journal.pone.0238844.

Hilditch, C., & Keir, A. (2018). Do feeding practices during transfusion influence the risk of developing necrotising enterocolitis in preterm infants? *Journal of Paediatrics and Child Health, 54*(5), 582–584. doi: 10.1111/jpc.13880.

Houben, N. A. M., Heeger, L. E., Stanworth, S. J., New, H. V., van der Bom, J. G., Fustolo-Gunnink, S., et al. (2020). Changes in the use of fresh-frozen plasma transfusions in preterm neonates: a single centre experience. *Journal of Clinical Medicine, 9*(11), 3789. doi: 10.3390/jcm9113789.

Howarth, C., Banerjee, J., & Aladangady, N. (2018). Red blood cell transfusion in preterm infants: current evidence and controversies. *Neonatology, 114*(1), 7–16. doi: 10.1159/000486584.

Jacquot, C., Mo, Y. D., & Luban, N. L. C. (2020). Blood component therapy for the neonate. In: R. J. Martin, A. A. Fanaroff, & M. C. Walsh (Eds.), *Fanaroff and Martin's neonatal–perinatal medicine* (11th ed., pp. 1476–1503). Philadelphia, PA: Elsevier.

Juul, S. E., & Christensen, R. D. (2018). Developmental hematology. In: C. A. Gleason & S. E. Juul (Eds.), *Avery's diseases of the newborn* (10th ed., pp. 1113–1120.e1113). Philadelphia, PA: Elsevier.

Kaplan, M., Wong, R. J., Burgis, J. C., Sibley, E., & Stevenson, D. K. (2020). Neonatal jaundice and liver diseases. In: R. J. Martin, A. A. Fanaroff, & M. C. Walsh (Eds.), *Fanaroff and Martin's neonatal–perinatal medicine* (11th ed., pp. 1788–1852). Philadelphia, PA: Elsevier.

Keir, A. K., New, H., Robitaille, N., Crighton, G. L., Wood, E. M., & Stanworth, S. J. (2019). Approaches to understanding and interpreting the risks of red blood cell transfusion in neonates. *Transfusion Medicine (Oxford, England), 29*(4), 231–238. doi: 10.1111/tme.12575.

Khaki, S. (2021). Infant hyperbilirubinemia. In: R. D. Kellerman & D. P. Rakel (Eds.), *Conn's current therapy 2021* (pp. 1269–1273). Philadelphia, PA: Elsevier.

Kirpalani, H., Whyte, R., Asztalos, E., Heddle, N., & Blajchman, M. (2006). The premature infants in need of transfusion (PINT) study: a randomized, controlled trial of a restrictive (LOW) versus liberal (HIGH) transfusion threshold for extremely low birth weight infants. *Journal of Pediatrics, 149*(3), 301–307.e303.

Kliegman, R. M., St Geme, J. W., Blum, N. J., Shah, S. S., Tasker, R. C., & Wilson, K. M. (2020). Blood disorders. In R. M. Kliegman, J. W. St Geme, N. J. Blum, S. S. Shah, R. C. Tasker, & K. M. Wilson (Eds.), *Nelson textbook of pediatrics* (pp. 961–974.e961). Philadelphia, PA: Elsevier.

Letterio, J., Pateva, I., Petrosiute, A., & Ahuja, S. (2020). Hematologic and oncologic problems in the fetus and neonate. In: R. J. Martin, A. A. Fanaroff, & M. C. Walsh (Eds.), *Fanaroff and Martin's neonatal–perinatal medicine* (11th ed.). Philadelphia, PA: Elsevier.

Mack, C., & Gourley, G. R. (2021). Jaundice: unconjugated hyperbilirubinemia. In: R. Wyllie, J. S. Hyams, & M. Kay (Eds.), *Pediatric gastrointestinal and liver disease* (6th ed., pp. 159–167.e153). Philadelphia, PA: Elsevier.

Minuk, L., Clarke, G., & Lieberman, L. (2020). Approach to red blood cell antibody testing during pregnancy. *Canadian Family Physician, 66*, 491–498.

Moorehead, P. C., Chan, A., Lemyre, B., Winikoff, R., Scott, H., Hawes, S. A., et al. (2018). A practical guide to the management of the fetus and newborn with hemophilia. *Clinical and Applied Thrombosis/hemostasis. 24*(9_suppl), 29S–41S. doi: 10.1177/1076029618807583.

Mreihil, K., Benth, J. Š., Stensvold, H. J., Nakstad, B., & Hansen T. W. R. (2018). Norwegian NICU Phototherapy Study Group; Norwegian Neonatal Network. Phototherapy is commonly used for neonatal jaundice but greater control is needed to avoid toxicity in the most vulnerable infants. *Acta Paediatrica, 107*(4), 611–619.

Nelson, N. (1976). Respiration and circulation before birth. In: C. Smith & N. Nelson (Eds.), *Physiology of the newborn infant* (4th ed.). Springfield, IL: Charles C. Thomas.

Nizam, M. A., Alvi, A. S., Hamdani, M. M., Lalani, A. S., Sibtain, S. A., & Bhangar, N. A. (2020). Efficacy of double versus single phototherapy in treatment of neonatal jaundice: a meta-analysis. *European Journal of Pediatrics, 179*(6), 865–874. doi: 10.1007/s00431-020-03583-x.

Noori, S. (2020). Intraventricular haemorrhage. In: R. A. Polin & M. C. Yoder (Eds.), *Workbook in practical neonatology* (pp. 307–318.e301). Philadelphia, PA: Elsevier.

Norton, T., Newberry, D., & Jnah, A. (2021). Neonatal alloimmune thrombocytopenia: a concise review. *Advances in Neonatal Care,* 21(2), 115–121. doi: 10.1097/ANC.0000000000000775.

Ohls, R. K., Maheshwari, A., & Christensen, R. D. (2019). *Hematology, immunology, and genetics* (3rd ed.). Philadelphia, PA: Elsevier.

Patel, R. M., & Josephson, C. D. (2018). Neonatal transfusion. In: C. A. Gleason & S. E. Juul (Eds.), *Avery's diseases of the newborn* (pp. 1180–1186.e1183). Philadelphia, PA: Elsevier.

Patel, R. M., Knezevic, A., Yang, J., Shenvi, N., Hinkes, M., Roback, J. D., et al. (2019). Enteral iron supplementation, red blood cell transfusion, and risk of bronchopulmonary dysplasia in very-low-birth-weight infants. *Transfusion (Philadelphia, Pa.), 59*(5), 1675–1682. doi: 10.1111/trf.15216.

Pegoraro, V., Urbinati, D., Visser, G. H. A., Di Renzo, G. C., Zipursky, A., Stotler, B. A., et al. (2020). Haemolytic disease of the fetus and newborn due to Rh(D) incompatibility: a preventable disease that still produces significant morbidity and mortality in children. *PloS One, 15*(7), e0235807. doi: 10.1371/journal.pone.0235807.

Queensland Health. (2019). *Queensland maternity and neonatal clinical guideline: neonatal jaundice.* Brisbane, Qld, Australia. <https://www.health.qld.gov.au/__data/assets/pdf_file/0018/142038/g-jaundice.pdf> (Accessed 16 February 2022).

Rennie, J. M. (2012). *Rennie & Robertson's textbook of neonatology* (5th ed.). London: Churchill Livingstone.

Rennie, J. M., Beer, J., & Upton, M. (2019). Learning from claims: hyperbilirubinaemia and kernicterus. *Archives of Disease in Childhood. Fetal and Neonatal Edition, 104*(2), F202–F204.

Rodríguez-Cerdeira, C., & Silami-Lopez, V. G. (2012). Congenital syphilis in the 21st century. *Dermatology (Actas Dermo-Sifiliográficas, English Ed.), 103*(8), 679–693.

Romagnoli, C., Barone, G., Pratesi, S., Raimondi, F., Capasso, L., Zecca, E., et al. (2014). Italian guidelines for management and treatment of hyperbilirubinaemia of newborn infants ≥35 weeks' gestational age. *Italian Journal of Pediatrics, 40*, 11. doi: 10.1186/1824-7288-40-11.

SA Health (2019). *Neonatal jaundice. South Australian perinatal practice guidelines.* Adelaide, SA: SA Maternal & Neonatal Clinical Network.

Saito-Benz, M., Flanagan, P., & Berry, M. J. (2020). Management of anaemia in pre-term infants. *British Journal of Haematology, 188*(3), 354–366. doi: 10.1111/bjh.16233.

Scott, J. P., & Flood, V. H. (2019). Platelet and blood vessel disorders. In: R. M. Kliegman, J. W. St Geme, N. J. Blum, S. S. Shah, R. C. Tasker, & K. M. Wilson (Eds.), *Nelson textbook of pediatrics* (pp. 2609–2618.e2603). Philadelphia: Elsevier.

Shafiq, M. F., Ahmed, Z., & Ahmad, A. M. (2019). Validity of visual assessment of neonatal jaundice for screening significant hyperbilirubinaemia. *Pakistan Armed Forces Medical Journal, 69*(1), 212–216.

Sharafutdinova, D. R., Balashova, E. N., Ionov, O. V., Kirtbaya, A. R., Golubtsova, J. M., Zubkov, V. V., et al. (2019). The recombinant human erythropoietin therapy for extremely and very low birth weight infants. *Pediatric Hematology/Oncology and Immunopathology, Voprosy Gematologii/onkologii i Immunopatologii v Pediatrii, 18*(2), 75–82. doi: 10.24287/1726-1708-2019-18-2-75-82.

Sheriff, J., Malone, L. E., Avila, C., Zigomalas, A., Bluestein, D., & Bahou, W. F. (2020). Shear-induced platelet activation is sensitive to age and calcium availability: a comparison of adult and cord blood. *Cellular and Molecular Bioengineering, 13*(6), 575–590. doi: 10.1007/s12195-020-00628-x.

Stark, M. J., Kirpalani, H. M., & Andersen, C. C. (2020). Anemia. In: R. A. Polin & M. C. Yoder (Eds.), *Workbook in practical neonatology* (6th ed., pp. 110–128.e111). St Louis, MO: Elsevier.

Tkach, E. K., Mackley, A., Brooks, A., Kessler, J., & Paul, D. A. (2018). Cryoprecipitate transfusions in the neonatal intensive care unit: a performance improvement study to decrease donor exposure. *Transfusion (Philadelphia, Pa.), 58*(5), 1206–1209. doi: 10.1111/trf.14555.

Villeneuve, A., Arsenault, V., Lacroix, J., & Tucci, M. (2021). Neonatal red blood cell transfusion. *International Journal of Transfusion Medicine, 116*, 366–378. doi: 10.1111/vox.13036.

Walker, S. G. (2019). *Smith's anaesthesia for infants and children* (9th ed.). *Anaesthesia and Analgesia, 128*(2), e19. doi: 10.1213/ANE.0000000000003929.

Wang, J., Guo, G., Li, A., Cai, W.-Q., & Wang, X. (2021). Challenges of phototherapy for neonatal hyperbilirubinemia. *Experimental and Therapeutic Medicine, 21*(3), 231.

Wolf, M. F., Childers, J., Gray, K. D., Chivily, C., Glenn, M., Jones, L., et al. (2020). Exchange transfusion safety and outcomes in neonatal hyperbilirubinemia. *Journal of Perinatology, 40*(10), 1506–1512.

Wolfe, L. C., & Shukla, S. (2020). G6PD deficiency in the newborn. *Medscape.* <https://emedicine.medscape.com/article/119184-overview> (Accessed 16 February 2022).

Young, M. F., Oaks, B. M., Tandon, S., Martorell, R., Dewey, K. G., & Wendt, A. S. (2019). Maternal hemoglobin concentrations across pregnancy and maternal and child health: a systematic review and meta-analysis. *Annals of the New York Academy of Sciences, 1450*(1), 47–68.

Zaitsu, M., Yoshihara, T., Nakai, H., & Kubota, S. (2018). Optimal thermal control with sufficient nutrition may reduce the incidence of neonatal jaundice by preventing body-weight loss among non-low birth weight infants not admitted to neonatal intensive care unit. *Neonatology, 114*(4), 348–354.

Zerra, P. E., Hendrickson, J. E., & Josephson, C. D. (2019). Neonatal and pediatric transfusion medicine. In: B. H. Shaz, C. D. Hillyer, & M. Reyes Gil (Eds.), *Transfusion medicine and haemostasis* (3rd ed., pp. 295–299). Philadelphia, PA: Elsevier.

Zitelli, B. J., McIntire, S. C., & Nowalk, A. J. (2018). *Zitelli and Davis' atlas of pediatric physical diagnosis* (7th ed.). Philadelphia, PA: Elsevier.

CHAPTER 12

CARE OF THE NEONATE WITH A GASTROINTESTINAL DISORDER

JACQUI MCGREGOR, LINDA SWEET AND TRUDI MANNIX

Learning objectives

After reading this chapter you will be able to:

- understand the development of the gastrointestinal system
- outline the pathophysiology of gastrointestinal disorders
- identify feeding intolerance and possible causes
- discuss gastro-oesophageal reflux and its management
- identify causes of bowel obstruction
- describe the management of the neonate undergoing abdominal surgery
- identify the underlying pathogenesis of necrotising enterocolitis
- describe the management of necrotising enterocolitis.

Key words, terms and abbreviations

bowel obstruction
feeding intolerance (FI)
gastrointestinal (GI)
gastro-oesophageal reflux (GOR)
lower oesophageal sphincter (LOS)
nasogastric tube (NGT)
necrotising enterocolitis (NEC)
orogastric tube (OGT)
very low birthweight (VLBW)

INTRODUCTION

The primary role of the **gastrointestinal (GI)** system is to provide nutrition for the body, while its primary functions include ingestion, digestion, absorption and elimination. When any one of these functions is compromised, the nutritional needs of the neonate are also compromised. This chapter provides an overview of the development and function of the GI system, and describes dysfunctions including **feeding intolerance** and **gastro-oesophageal reflux (GOR)**, malformations and abdominal wall defects and pathology that often require surgical intervention, including bowel obstruction and necrotising enterocolitis (NEC). These selected conditions are by no means exhaustive of the potential GI conditions of a neonate; however, they are the more common conditions seen globally that require neonatal nursing/midwifery interventions.

EMBRYOLOGICAL AND FETAL DEVELOPMENT OF THE GASTROINTESTINAL SYSTEM

Embryological development of the gut commences during the fourth week, when the primitive gut is formed. Progressing in a cephalocaudal direction, the primitive gut develops into four sections: the pharyngeal gut, foregut, midgut and hindgut (Singh, 2020) (Fig. 12.1).

The pharyngeal gut forms the pharynx, the lower respiratory tract and the upper oesophagus. This process involves the development of indentations or pouches in the mesenchymal tissue. Congenital malformations of the pharyngeal gut include cleft lip and palate (Singh, 2020).

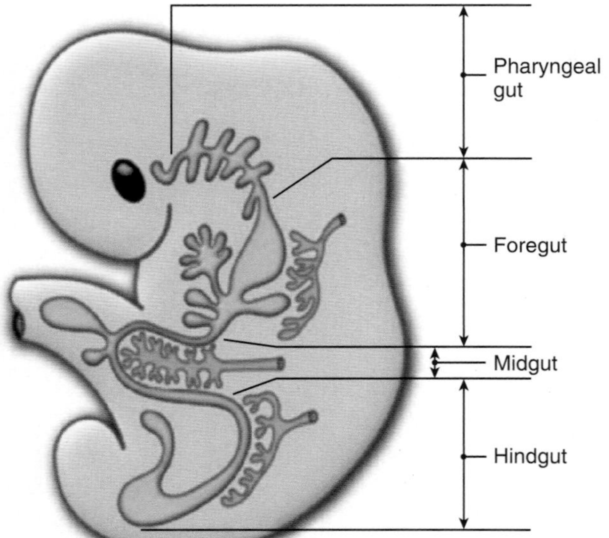

Pharyngeal gut
Foregut
Midgut
Hindgut

FIGURE 12.1 **Initial differentiation of the gut tube**

Source: Rubarth and Van Woudenberg (2016, p. 157). With permission of Springer Publishing Company.

The foregut forms the lower oesophagus, stomach, liver, pancreas and upper duodenum. This section develops through division from the respiratory system, followed by elongation, recanalisation of tubal structures and dilation and rotation of the stomach and pancreas. Congenital malformations of the foregut include abnormalities connected with the lungs and airways, including oesophageal atresia and tracheo-oesophageal fistulas, with other differentiation-related malformations including pyloric stenosis, annular pancreas and atresia of the gallbladder (Singh, 2020). The midgut includes the lower duodenum and small intestines, caecum, appendix, ascending colon and the transverse colon. The midgut forms through herniation, rotation, retraction and fixation processes, processes that are completed by the tenth week of gestation. Development of the hindgut is associated with the developing urogenital system. The hindgut forms from the distal colon to the anus. Congenital malformations of the hindgut include imperforate anus (Moore et al., 2018).

REFLECTION

Fetal development is dependent on maternal factors such as genetics, exposure to chemicals and drugs, infectious diseases and the environment. Consider how you would respond to a woman who gave birth to an infant with a congenital abnormality, such as cleft lip/palate or tracheo-oesophageal fistula, if she raised concerns about genetics.

Reflecting on and reviewing one's own practice is a key clinical practice competency for neonatal nurses and midwives (Jones, 2019).

Anatomy and physiology

The gross anatomy of the GI tract is anatomically complete by 20–22 weeks' gestation, with functional maturity continuing to develop long after birth. Organised peristalsis is established by 28–30 weeks' gestation, and coordinated sucking and swallowing develops at 32–34 weeks' gestation (Moore et al., 2018). By 40 weeks' gestation, the fetus swallows about 150 mL/kg/d of amniotic fluid, containing carbohydrates, proteins, fat, electrolytes, immunoglobulins and growth factors, all of which play an important role in the development of GI function (Brown et al., 2020). The mature neonate born at term can coordinate sucking and swallowing for ingestion with respiration. However, after birth the GI tract must further adapt for mucosal growth and differentiation, peristalsis, digestion of food and absorption of nutrients (Brown et al., 2020).

Adaptations of the gastrointestinal tract at birth

The fetal GI system is involved with ingestion and excretion of amniotic fluid, while the nutritional needs of the fetus are provided by the mother via the placenta (Blackburn, 2017). Following birth, the neonate's GI system commences primary responsibility for ingestion, digestion, absorption and excretion. The capacity at which the neonate can do this depends on gestational age and functional maturity, and any underlying malformations or pathophysiology. The intestines are sterile at birth, but rapidly colonise after birth, with the method of feeding having a significant impact on this process. However, the intestinal mucosal barrier remains immature for 4–6 months because of pancreatic lipase levels (Blackburn, 2017). Maturation of the GI system after birth relies on hormone regulatory mechanisms and gut trophic factors (Blackburn, 2017).

CLINICAL PRACTICE 12.1

Every newborn requires a brief physical examination within the first few minutes after birth, followed by a thorough head-to-toe physical examination prior to discharge from hospital. Newborn assessment is an important mechanism of screening for major congenital malformations. Newborn assessment must always include inspection of the mouth, abdomen and anus for any signs of congenital malformations related to the GI tract. Having the capacity to undertake a thorough newborn assessment is a key clinical practice competency for neonatal nurses and midwives (Jones, 2019).

Preterm birth interrupts normal GI development, resulting in both anatomical and functional limitations to its primary functions, leading to a 'nutritional emergency' (Roggero et al., 2020, p. 2). Even if nutrients are provided parenterally, lack of enteric intake leads to decreased circulating gut peptides, slower enterocyte (cells that absorb water and nutrients from the digestive tract) turnover and nutrient transport, and decreased bile acid secretion (Blackburn, 2017). Furthermore, there is an increased susceptibility to infection, owing to impaired barrier function of the intestinal epithelium, lack of colonisation by normal commensal flora and colonisation by pathogenic organisms (Blackburn, 2017).

FEEDING INTOLERANCE

There is no universal definition of feeding intolerance (FI) in the neonate, but there is agreement that it is manifest as an inability to digest enteral feeds, and is associated with increased gastric residuals, abdominal distension, vomiting and a disruption to the enteral feeding plan (Hu et al., 2021). Feeding intolerance is one of the most significant contributors to growth failure in **very low birthweight (VLBW)** neonates (Ahammad et al., 2018). It is common in preterm or sick term neonates, but can still occur in otherwise healthy term neonates, and it has been reported in as many as two-thirds of VLBW infants (Dubey et al., 2018). This discussion focuses on feeding intolerance due to functional immaturity in the preterm neonate. Most preterm neonates will be fed via a **nasogastric tube (NGT)** or **orogastric tube (OGT)**, until they are able to coordinate sucking, swallowing and breathing adequately (Hair, 2021). A neonate's intolerance of enteral feeding is a common factor in the decision to either temporarily discontinue feeds or delay an advancement in feeds (Hair, 2021). Although most episodes resolve spontaneously and without sequelae, any signs of feeding intolerance should be regarded as potentially serious. The neonatal nurse/midwife should be prompted to reassess the neonate and evaluate the possibility of FI or an underlying pathology (Hair, 2021).

CLINICAL PRACTICE 12.2

Immediate parenteral support and early enteral feedings are fundamental in the management of the compromised neonate, as they promote ongoing maturation and development of the GI tract. Having the capacity to develop and implement individualised care plans is a key clinical practice competency for neonatal nurses (Jones, 2019).

Pathophysiology

While feeding intolerance can occur in neonates of all gestational ages, preterm neonates have anatomical, neurological and functional immaturity limits to the digestion and tolerance of enteral feedings (Basu & Smith, 2021). Those limitations include reduced digestive and absorptive capacities caused by delayed gastric emptying, limited intestinal motility leading to prolonged intestinal transit times compared with the term neonate, and a reduced capacity to absorb fat (Neal-Kluever et al., 2019).

Epidemiology

Feeding intolerance is a common problem in preterm infants and low birthweight infants, and a major contributor to poor weight gain and increased lengths of stay (Seiiedi-Biarag & Mirghafourvand, 2020). Ahammad et al. (2018) reported a rate of FI at 36% in preterm infants, with those under 32 weeks' gestation at an even higher risk because of immature gastric motility, slow gastric emptying and immature hormonal control of their gastrointestinal system. Intra-uterine growth-restricted infants are also at greater risk of feeding intolerance (Brown et al., 2020). There is a scarcity of evidence about FI in the literature, with most authors agreeing that more research needs to be done in this area, especially considering the impact on costs of care, both financial and psychosocial.

EVIDENCE-BASED PRACTICE RESEARCH 12.1

Symptoms of feeding intolerance may be an early warning sign of other illnesses, so any infant who presents with indicators of FI, which may include cardiorespiratory events (apnoea, bradycardia and desaturation) should have a full examination for potential comorbidities (Hasenstab et al., 2019). Prompt assessment and providing evidence-based neonatal nursing care is a key clinical practice competency for neonatal nurses (Jones, 2019).

Clinical assessment and findings

Assessment for signs of feeding intolerance is a core neonatal nursing/midwifery skill (Jones, 2019), and important for early identification of illness and prevention of serious sequelae. Nurses/midwives should be constantly aware of any change in the neonate's overall condition and feed tolerance. Symptoms of feeding intolerance include regurgitation, spilling or vomiting, a gastric residual volume of more than 50% of the previous feed volume (2–4 mL/kg), or a 1-hour volume if on continuous feeds, and abdominal distension (Brown et al., 2020; Mohamed & Ahmed, 2018). The preterm neonate's capacity to adapt to bolus feed volume and flow can also impact on their suck–swallow–breathe coordination, contributing to feeding difficulties and swallowing dysfunction. This can cause cardiorespiratory compromise resulting in apnoea and bradycardia (Hasenstab et al., 2019).

Diagnostic markers of feeding intolerance remain undefined (Yuan et al., 2019). Given the aforementioned symptoms of FI, clinical assessment would include gastric residual measurement, girth measurement or observation to detect abdominal distension, and presence of emesis (Basu & Smith, 2021). Yuan et al. (2019) found that the gut microbiota of preterm infants changes significantly with feeding intolerance, with an abundance of *Klebsiella*, and that the finding of *Klebsiella* in the gut could be a potential diagnostic biomarker for feeding intolerance in these neonates.

EVIDENCE-BASED PRACTICE RESEARCH 12.2

Kennedy et al. (2020) conducted a literature review of the evidence surrounding routine gastric aspiration in preterm infants and found a paucity of data to support the practice. They concluded that the evidence failed to make the case for routine gastric aspiration prior to feeds in preterm infants, and that it was a 'time and equipment consuming procedure, with a potential to irritate gastric mucosa and remove precious orogastric secretions' (p. 1152). Incorporating research into practice is a key competency for neonatal nurses and midwives (Jones, 2019).

Management

Assessment of the feeding tube placement is an important first step in ensuring enteral feeds are being delivered accurately into the stomach. The most accurate method of determining placement of a nasogastric tube has not been determined. In a survey of 60 neonatal nurses, Parker et al. (2018) found that 63% utilised the nose–ear–midway to the umbilicus (NEMU) method, which was included in 50% of protocols and was up to 90% accurate. The nose-to-ear-to-xiphoid method was used by 32% of nurses and recommended in 30% of protocols. Ninety-eight percent of nurses verified the placement of the tube by auscultation of a whoosh sound, and 83% used aspiration of gastric contents. More research is needed to accurately determine the placement of these tubes.

EVIDENCE-BASED PRACTICE RESEARCH 12.3

Kato et al. (2020) used radiography to determine the optimal placement of nasogastric tubes and recommended the following formula: (5 × weight (kg) + 10 (in infants with a BW <1.0 kg)) or (3 × weight (kg) + 12.5 (in infants with a BW between 1.0 and 2.5 kg)). However, gastric aspiration and pH testing is often routinely used to determine NGT/OGT placement in clinical settings because of cost, convenience, time and resource availability (Lyman & Guenter, 2019). Complying with local policy and practice based on available resources is a key professional practice competency for neonatal nurses and midwives (Jones, 2019).

Modifying the enteral feeding plan is usually the first line of management. Depending on the severity of symptoms, the neonate's gestational age and existing feeding plan, this may necessitate a reduction in feed volume, a change in feeding frequency or a change in enteral feed type. An exclusive human milk diet (mother's milk or donor milk) is associated with better feeding tolerance in preterm infants compared with formula (Eibensteiner et al., 2019), so neonatal nurses and midwives must encourage early and regular breast milk expression and breast feeding as the infant's capacity increases.

Minimal enteral feeding has been shown to reduce the incidence of feeding intolerance in preterm neonates (Eibensteiner et al., 2019) and is protective against other serious comorbidities. Early enteral feeding with human milk, as small as 1-mL bolus feeds, will 'prime' the gut, preparing it for feeding, and aid the transition to enteral feeds. Over time, neonates will tolerate increased feeds by either slow, continuous infusion or slow bolus feeds (Brown et al., 2020). In the event of intolerance, these feeds may be reduced in volume or frequency until the neonate is able to tolerate them. (See Chapter 5 for more detail about feeding practices.)

Simple measures such as changing the neonate's position from supine to prone have been shown to decrease gastric residuals (Brown et al., 2020) and promote feeding tolerance. Placing the neonate in the right lateral recumbent position also aids in gastric emptying owing to the positioning of the intestine (Brown et al., 2020). Abdominal massage stimulates the digestive system and the vagus nerve in preterm infants, contributing to parasympathetic nerve stimulation. This increases gastric motility and reduces gastric residual volumes and vomiting, but more studies with larger sample sizes are needed to confirm an effect on feeding intolerance (Seiiedi-Biarag & Mirghafourvand, 2020). A systematic review conducted by Basu and Smith (2021) found that macrolides such as erythromycin are beneficial in the prevention and treatment of feeding intolerance as they increase gastric tone and the magnitude of gastro-antral and small bowel contractions. Prebiotic and probiotic supplementation also improves feeding tolerance in preterm infants by early colonisation of the gut (Chi et al., 2019).

FAMILY-CENTRED CARE 12.1

Feeding is an excellent way to involve parents in their baby's care. Parents should be involved in discussions of feeding practices and milk choices. Scheduling feeds to coincide with parents' visits enables them to actively participate in providing care. During gavage feeds, parents should be encouraged to hold their baby and support the pacifier/dummy to encourage non-nutritive sucking. Parents may like to hold their baby skin to skin and allow the baby to nuzzle at the breast while the gavage is in progress. Neonatal nurses/midwives in some neonatal units teach parents how to administer feeds via the gavage tube. Provision of infant–family-centred developmental care is a key clinical practice competency for neonatal nurses (Jones, 2019). Finding ways to involve and promote participation of families in neonatal care is paramount for optimal outcomes.

Outcomes

As feeding intolerance generally leads to an interruption of the enteral-feeding plan, it prolongs the time to reach full enteral feeding and increases length of stay (Basu & Smith, 2021). Feeding intolerance is usually a feature of GI immaturity in the preterm neonate and, therefore, as postnatal weight increases and the neonate matures, the incidence of feeding intolerance reduces. Although feeding intolerance is usually a benign condition in the neonate, it may also be a symptom of a multitude of conditions that can range from mild, self-limited diseases to severe, life-threatening disorders (Brown et al., 2020).

GASTRO-OESOPHAGEAL REFLUX

Gastro-oesophageal reflux (GOR) describes the normal movement of acidic gastric contents from the stomach into the oesophagus, and is most commonly due to the transient relaxation of the lower oesophageal sphincter (Lenfestey & Neu, 2018). GOR is a developmental process related to functional immaturity and is almost universal in healthy preterm neonates, in whom gastric fluids reflux into the oesophagus dozens of times daily (Eichenwald & AAP, 2018). On the other hand, gastro-oesophageal reflux disease (GORD) is accompanied by complications such as oesophageal inflammation or narrowing, pulmonary or upper airway aspiration, or other problematic symptoms (Lopez & Lemberg, 2020). This discussion focuses on GOR.

FAMILY-CENTRED CARE 12.2

Although it can be very distressing to parents, neonates normally regurgitate their feeds and have episodic vomiting, and the problem usually resolves by itself (Lopez & Lemberg, 2020). Changing formula or changing from breastfeeding to formula is unlikely to have any positive effect on GOR and is not recommended. While most GOR is non-pathological and requires no treatment, explanations and reassurance to parents are important as they will be anxious about the effect on their baby. The provision of effective communication is a key professional practice competency for neonatal nurses and midwives (Jones, 2019).

Pathophysiology

The primary mechanism of GOR in the preterm infant is transient relaxation of the lower oesophageal sphincter (LOS) muscle, which reduces the pressures in the LO to less than that of the intragastric space (Eichenwald & AAP, 2018). The reflux is mediated by the vagus nerve, which is triggered by distention of the stomach, which activates inhibitory neurons in the lining of the LOS. Nitric oxide is then released in the intramural lining, which relaxes the LOS (Lenfestey & Neu, 2018). The LOS resting pressure is only 4 mmHg at 28 weeks' gestation, compared with 18 mmHg in term infants (the same as in adults) (Lenfestey & Neu, 2018). The presence of a nasogastric tube exacerbates the condition as it impairs closure of the LOS. It appears that delayed gastric emptying does not contribute to GOR, but gastric distension immediately after a feed does precipitate episodes (Eichenwald & AAP, 2018). The estimated incidence of gastro-oesophageal reflux in infants born at less than 34 weeks' gestation is approximately 22% (Leung & Hon, 2019).

Diagnosis

Rossor et al. (2018a) have shown that a diagnosis based on clinical suspicion is frequently incorrect, and that pH probe monitoring is more accurate. Monitoring with a pH probe can detect the total number of reflux episodes, their duration and the reflux index (RI: the percentage of total recording time with an oesophageal pH less than 4; an RI >7% is considered abnormal) (Eichenwald & AAP, 2018). While multi-channel intraoesophageal impedance (MII) testing detects all oesophageal bolus movements, and can detect reflux, it is not as accurate as the pH probe. However, the MII test can also assess mucosal integrity, which can help clinicians target acid suppression therapy (Rossor et al., 2018b). Most neonatal units, however, do not have access to pH probe monitoring or MII testing, and therefore rely on the results of a detailed feeding history and physical examination of the neonate. More than half (58%) of the neonatal units in the UK who responded to a survey conducted by Rossor et al. (2018b) used a trial of therapy to help establish the diagnosis.

Clinical assessment and findings

Regurgitation, posseting or spilling with occasional episodes of vomiting are the most common presenting symptoms of neonatal GOR. GOR should be suspected in a neonate who is unsettled or irritable, with cyanotic or desaturation episodes, apnoea and bradycardia. The neonate with GOR may experience poor growth and failure to thrive (Eichenwald & AAP, 2018).

CLINICAL PRACTICE 12.3

During infancy, GOR is common, and generally resolves spontaneously with no investigations required. As clinicians, it is important to explore differential diagnoses, while taking a history and performing an examination (Leung & Hon, 2019). This will often involve the multidisciplinary team. The incorporation of collaborative practice is a key leadership and teamwork competency for neonatal nurses (Jones, 2019).

EVIDENCE-BASED PRACTICE RESEARCH 12.5

Wallenstein et al. (2019) reviewed the evidence and found that, among preterm infants with suspected gastro-oesophageal reflux, transpyloric tube feeding reduced episodes of apnoea and bradycardia, compared with gastric feeding. However, they recommended that further randomised controlled trials were required to confirm this outcome.

Management

The initial management of GOR is conservative, so non-pharmacological strategies are implemented in the first instance, and then medication is administrated to neonates who are unresponsive to conservative measures, or who suffer severe symptoms that are strongly suspicious of GORD. Even though there is increased use of pharmacological management of GOR in neonatal units in recent years, there are not enough data about their effectiveness and on their short- and long-term outcomes (Eichenwald & AAP, 2018).

Parents should be reassured that GOR is especially common in preterm infants and is a developmental process that resolves with maturation. Although the evidence is not strong, positioning in the left-side-down lateral position or prone position after a feed does have some effect on reducing the symptoms of GOR (Eichenwald & AAP, 2018). Reducing the feed volume and/or frequency, and slowing the rate of feeding, has also been shown to reduce GOR episodes. Antacid medications such as ranitidine and omeprazole are over-prescribed in the neonatal unit, and have a limited role in infants with uncomplicated GOR (Martin & Hibbs, 2020). Prokinetic agents such as metoclopramide or cisapride improve gastric emptying and/or oesophageal tone, but are not recommended for the management of GOR infants because of the safety concerns and low efficacy (Martin & Hibbs, 2020). The American Academy of Pediatrics (AAP) determined that the routine use of anti-reflux medications for symptomatic GOR in preterm infants had questionable value (Eichenwald & AAP, 2018). Transpyloric tube feeds may be useful in the interim in neonates with other problems who cannot tolerate feeds owing to significant GOR; however, the procedure is technically difficult and benefits are inconclusive (Martin & Hibbs, 2020).

EVIDENCE-BASED PRACTICE RESEARCH 12.4

Positioning in the right-side-down lateral position after a feed worsens GOR symptoms compared with either the left-side-down lateral position or prone position (Eichenwald & AAP, 2018). There is also not enough evidence to show that elevating the head of the cot improves GOR symptoms. This practice is also not in line with safe-sleeping guidelines, and is not a model for teaching parents about safe sleeping after discharge (Eichenwald & AAP, 2018). Maintaining a safe and secure environment for neonates is a key professional practice competency for neonatal nurses (Jones, 2019).

Management strategies **not** recommended include the following:

- *Thickening feeds:* clinical and pH study data do not demonstrate consensus for thickening feeds; this strategy appears to reduce vomiting episodes, but not reflux episodes (Lopez & Lemberg, 2020). Thickening feeds can also reduce intestinal absorption and gastric-emptying time.
- *Prokinetic agents:* studies of prokinetic agents that improve gastric emptying and/or oesophageal sphincter tone have failed to demonstrate any clear benefit in the neonatal population. These drugs are associated with rare but significant side effects (e.g. prolonged QT interval with the use of cisapride and extrapyramidal neurological effects with the use of metoclopramide) (Martin & Hibbs, 2020).
- *Gastric irritants:* gastric irritants such as caffeine citrate should be avoided if possible as they increase the risk of GOR. Some antibiotics can also increase GOR (e.g. Augmentin© and Flucloxacillin©). Cow's milk protein intolerance can also cause significant vomiting that settles only with a change of formula (e.g. soya).

Outcomes

Eichenwald and the AAP (2018) found that GOR is a common diagnosis in neonatal units and contributes to length of stay and higher hospital costs. Many infants who are treated for GOR continue to be treated after they are discharged from hospital, despite the fact that there is scant evidence that GOR actually causes harm to the preterm infant. Physiological GOR is typically a developmental process that resolves with maturation. GOR generally resolves by itself by 1 year of age (Martin & Hibbs, 2020).

CHOLESTASIS

Neonatal cholestasis is generally defined as conjugated hyperbilirubinaemia (when the conjugated bilirubin is more than 20% of the total serum bilirubin,) that is present at birth or develops in the first few months of life (Pandita et al., 2018). Cholestasis results from diminished bile formation and/or excretion, which can be caused by several disorders. Neonates are susceptible to cholestasis for several reasons, including a smaller circulating bile acid pool size, a lower rate of synthesis, recirculation of bile acids and immature function of the canalicular bile acid transporting system. The aetiology remains unclear, and it may result from either extrahepatic or intrahepatic disorders. The most common cause of neonatal obstructive cholestasis is biliary atresia, accounting for 25–45% of cases (Feldman & Sokol, 2020). Neonatal cholestasis has a reported prevalence of 1 in 2500 neonates (Mandato et al., 2019) and is common in VLBW neonates where the normal immaturity of biliary excretion is exaggerated.

Pathophysiology

Bile is formed in the liver and is primarily composed of bile acids, bilirubin and fats. Bile flows into biliary ducts, from where it is ultimately secreted into the intestine. A disruption in production or excretion may result in cholestasis, causing the abnormal accumulation of bile salts, bilirubin and lipids in the liver and the blood (Pandita et al., 2018).

The primary failure in cholestasis is of bilirubin excretion, resulting in excess conjugated bilirubin in the bloodstream and decreased bile salts in the GI tract. This results in malabsorption of fat and fat-soluble vitamins, and therefore leads to vitamin deficiency, inadequate nutrition and growth failure (Feldman & Sokol, 2020). Prolonged use of parenteral nutrition can increase the risk of cholestasis as it is toxic to the liver and causes biliary stasis, portal inflammation, bile duct proliferation and portal fibrosis (Bae et al., 2019).

CLINICAL PRACTICE 12.4

Causes of neonatal cholestasis can be divided into the following categories:

- anatomical obstruction
- infections
- inborn errors of metabolism/genetic
- toxins
- immune
- endocrine
- other.

Although there are multiple causes of neonatal cholestasis, biliary atresia must be differentiated from other causes of cholestasis promptly, as early surgical intervention (i.e. in the first 30–45 days of life) results in better patient outcomes (Feldman & Sokol, 2020).

Diagnosis

An elevated level of conjugated bilirubin (when direct bilirubin levels are >20% of the total bilirubin, and >1 mg/dL (= 17 μmol/L) implies impairment of biliary excretion and requires investigation (Feldman & Sokol, 2020). Laboratory data such as the high conjugated bilirubin levels, high serum bile acids, low albumin levels, prolonged prothrombin time and deranged liver function tests are also suggestive of liver failure (Mandato et al., 2019). Other diagnostic investigations may be required to rule out underlying metabolic, genetic or septic causes of conjugated hyperbilirubinaemia, such as septic screening, abdominal ultrasound, gene sequencing and liver biopsy (Feldman & Sokol, 2020).

Clinical assessment

Prolonged jaundice and a history of dark yellow urine and pale (acholic) stools due to malabsorption of fat should alert the neonatal nurse/midwife to a potential for cholestasis. Examination reveals hepatomegaly in most cases and splenomegaly in some and, depending on the cause of the cholestasis, other symptoms may include irritability, lethargy, poor feeding, hypotonia, coagulopathy and poor weight gain (Pandita et al., 2018). Delayed passage of meconium may also indicate cystic fibrosis.

FAMILY-CENTRED CARE 12.3

Jaundice is a common condition in neonates, especially preterm neonates, and is generally self-limiting. Parents whose baby is jaundiced due to causes that are not self-limiting will require information and support during the period of investigation and management. While there are many causes of cholestasis, neonates with biliary atresia (the most common cause) tend to be healthy at birth and develop progressive jaundice within the first 8 weeks of life. This compounds the need for parental support during the period of diagnosis and treatment.

Management

Once cholestasis is confirmed, referral to a paediatric gastroenterologist is recommended in order to assist in diagnostic and therapeutic interventions to optimise the neonate's clinical outcome. Management is specific to the aetiology; for example, infection is treated according to the causative organism (see Chapter 16). Bae et al. (2019) found that the cyclic use of parenteral nutrition (PN), where there was a 1–2-hour break in the daily administration time of PN, may be effective in the prevention and management of PN-associated cholestasis. Expedient diagnosis of obstruction due to biliary atresia facilitates early surgery before 45 days of age to improve clinical outcomes. The Kasai hepatic portoenterostomy restores bile flow and slows the progression of the disease until a liver transplant can be performed. Targeted pharmacological, dietary or surgical treatments are available for some genetic causes of cholestasis, such as the use of nitisinone in tyrosinaemia type 1 (Feldman & Sokol, 2020). Scottoni and Davenport (2020) believe that the evidence to support the use of current adjuvant therapies, such as steroids or ursodeoxycholic acid, is limited.

Maximising nutrition is an essential component of treatment in all neonates with cholestasis as they fail to absorb fat and fat-soluble vitamins. Some infant formulas contain larger amounts of medium-chain triglycerides and essential fatty acids along with added calories to support the neonate waiting for liver transplantation (Feldman & Sokol, 2020).

Outcomes

The outcomes of cholestasis are dependent on the specific disorders (e.g. metabolic disease or infection) and are therefore variable, ranging from a completely benign course to a progressive disease resulting in cirrhosis. Early recognition is fundamental to attain better outcomes, which includes an awareness by neonatal nurses and midwives of the importance of the pale stool colour in the screening for biliary atresia. Infants who undergo portoenterostomy before 10 weeks of age are less likely to require early liver transplantation (Schwarz, 2021).

Biliary atresia, if untreated, may result in liver failure, cirrhosis and death; however, the diagnosis and management of this disorder has not advanced significantly in the past decade (Wehrman et al., 2019).

BOWEL OBSTRUCTION

Bowel obstruction in the neonate is one of the most common and potentially dire neonatal surgical emergencies (Desoky et al., 2018). The incidence of bowel obstruction is not precisely known, but is estimated to be approximately 1 in 2500 live births (Tullie & Stanton, 2019). According to Desoky et al. (2018), the causes of obstruction are diverse, with varied embryological origins, and the aetiology of most neonatal bowel obstructions is not known; however, they are linked to both genetic and environmental factors. Proximal obstructions are commonly associated with maternal polyhydramnios (Bradshaw, 2020).

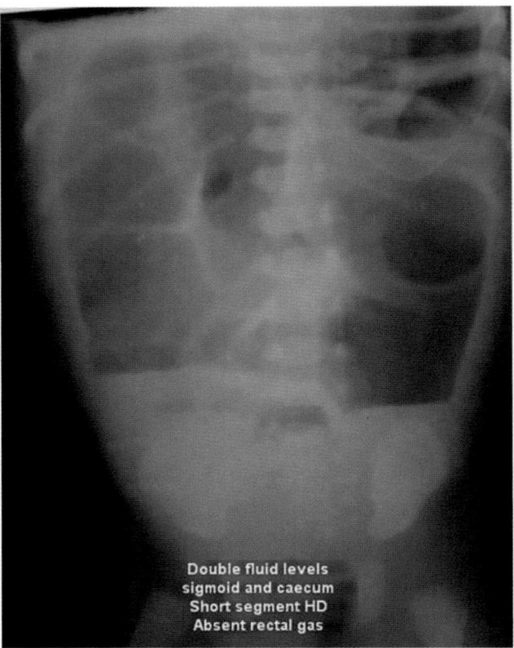

FIGURE 12.2 **X-ray showing absent gas in the pelvis/aganglionosis of the distal colon typical of Hirschsprung disease**

Source: Prasad and Aziz (2017).

Pathophysiology

There are many causes of bowel obstruction, including duodenal, jejunal or ileal atresia, meconium ileus, Hirschsprung disease and anorectal malformations, but the most potentially dangerous is volvulus related to malrotation of the midgut (Wesson, 2021). An atresia is the absence or narrowing of a portion of the GI tract. Obstructions caused by atresia of the pylorus, duodenum, jejunum, ileum and colon collectively are the most common causes of neonatal bowel obstruction (Wesson, 2021). Meconium ileus occurs when insufficient pancreatic enzymes are produced to digest intestinal contents (as in cystic fibrosis), and thick secretions from the intestinal glands create tenacious, viscous meconium which obstructs the bowel lumen, causing a blockage (Gallagher et al., 2021). Hirschsprung disease is a developmental disorder that leads to large intestine obstruction due to the absence of ganglia in the distal colon, which disrupts effective peristalsis (Gallagher et al., 2021). Fig. 12.2 shows a typical X-ray of Hirschsprung disease where there is no gas visible in the rectum (Prasad & Aziz, 2017).

Neonates with anorectal malformations such as imperforate anus will not pass meconium unless there is a fistula to the perineum or urogenital tract. Unless a careful examination is performed, an imperforate anus may be overlooked until symptoms of distal intestinal obstruction, such as abdominal distension and vomiting, raise concerns. In neonatal unit settings, rectal thermometry has been replaced by the axillary method so as to minimise discomfort and the potential risk of perforation (Gardner & Niermeyer, 2021), reinforcing the need for a careful examination of the anus of the newborn for patency after birth (Gallagher et al., 2021). This can be done on routine inspection of the genital region by gently parting the buttocks and checking for the anal opening.

The return of the herniated gut to the abdominal cavity and its counterclockwise rotation are complete by the 12th week of gestation (Singh, 2020). Malrotation covers a spectrum of rotational anomalies, ranging from type 1 (non-rotation) to types 3A–D (various levels of rotation and abnormal fixation of the duodenum and jejunum) (da Costa & Saxena, 2020). In complete malrotation, the entire small bowel sits in the upper right quadrant, with the colon on the left. In this case, the bowel is loosely suspended by the superior mesenteric artery and vein, which predisposes the midgut and its tenuous blood supply to twisting (also known as volvulus), which then leads to ischaemia and bowel infarction (Gallagher et al., 2021). Ladd's bands may form, which are bands of fibrous tissue that compress and obstruct the duodenum.

Clinical assessment and findings

Wesson (2021) writes that the type and timing of the signs of intestinal obstruction in newborns depends on the location of the obstruction, and whether the obstruction is partial or complete, but may include:

- bilious vomiting in the first 24–48 hours of life
- failure to pass meconium in the first day of life
- abdominal distension (more common in distal obstructions), visible loops of bowel and abdominal tenderness

- respiratory compromise due to massive abdominal distension causing elevation of the diaphragm
- signs of volume depletion (i.e. oliguria, dry mucous membranes and poor skin turgor) due to vomiting
- jaundice.

Presentation may vary from subtle and easily overlooked findings on physical examination to massive abdominal distension with respiratory distress and cardiovascular collapse. A careful history (including maternal and prenatal) and physical examination often identify the diagnosis. In acute cases of obstruction, the clinical manifestations include bilious vomits, abdominal distension, rectal bleeding, abdominal pain, signs of shock and sepsis. In less-acute cases, the symptoms include failure to thrive, intermittent bilious vomiting and abdominal tenderness (Wesson, 2021).

EVIDENCE-BASED PRACTICE RESEARCH 12.6

Almost all healthy term neonates should pass meconium in the first 24 hours of life. Any delay in the passage of meconium beyond 24 hours should raise the suspicion of obstruction or meconium ileus (Messina et al., 2018).

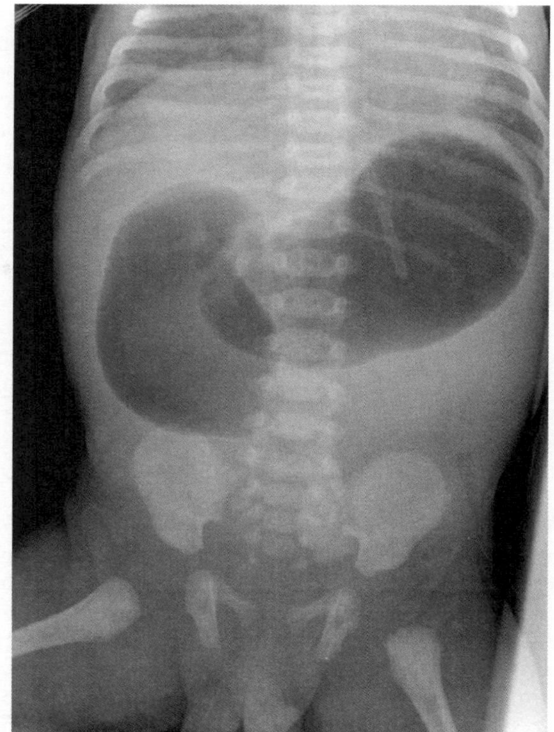

FIGURE 12.3 **Abdominal X-ray showing the 'double bubble' sign with gastric and proximal duodenum distension and no distal air**

Source: Ballesteros et al. (2015).

Diagnosis

Many causes of bowel obstruction in the newborn can be readily diagnosed with physical examination and radiographic examination. The presence of symptoms, with evidence of duodenal obstruction and scanty gas distributed throughout the remainder of the bowel on abdominal X-ray, is diagnostic. An airless abdomen is an obvious sign and an upper GI contrast X-ray film will show a distended stomach and a beak-like narrowing at the pylorus. When the intestinal loops become twisted and volvulus occurs, a 'double-bubble' sign on X-ray is seen, with gastric and proximal duodenum distension and no distal air (Fig. 12.3). A radiograph diagnostic for pyloric stenosis due to a single large gastric bubble without distal intestinal air, in a neonate with a maternal history of polyhydramnios, is shown in Fig. 12.4. A barium enema will locate the position of the caecum under fluoroscopy. If the duodenum fails to cross the midline, the diagnosis of malrotation is confirmed (Tullie & Stanton, 2019).

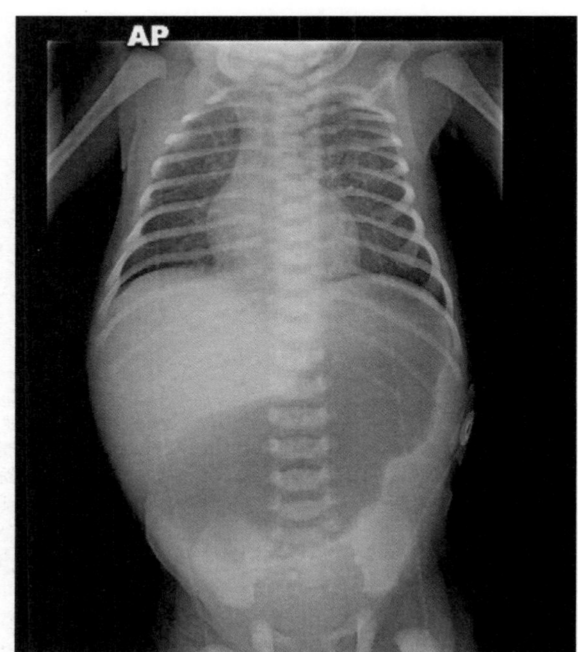

FIGURE 12.4 **Abdominal radiograph of an infant with pyloric stenosis**

Source: Juang and Snyder (2012, p. 687).

REFLECTION

Consider the information and advice given to mothers who are discharged within 12 hours of giving birth.

- How might you respond to maternal concerns about a delay in passage of her baby's stools?
- At what point would you encourage further assessment and investigation of the absence of passing meconium?

Management

Successful management of a neonate with a bowel obstruction depends upon timely diagnosis and prompt therapy. Workup usually involves abdominal X-ray, which may direct further evaluation with fluoroscopic radiography (Desoky et al., 2018). Urgent resuscitation and support of both the cardiovascular and the respiratory systems with fluids, inotropes, supplemental oxygen and mechanical ventilation may be necessary. Enteral feeds will be ceased, and gastric decompression achieved with a nasogastric tube. The neonate's vital signs should be continuously assessed. A neonatal pain assessment tool should be used to assess for and guide pain management, and analgesia provided accordingly. Further management will depend on the cause of the bowel obstruction, but surgical intervention is often necessary, with a laparotomy to divide the Ladd's bands and correct the malrotation. If volvulus is present, the bowel is untwisted and allowed to reperfuse, then the necrotic segments are resected and a stoma created as indicated (Gallagher et al., 2021).

Outcomes

The overall mortality rate after surgery for malrotation is 3–9%, and increases in neonates with volvulus, intestinal necrosis, prematurity and associated anomalies (Wesson, 2021). Postoperative complications include short gut syndrome and adhesions resulting in small bowel obstruction (Wesson, 2021).

NECROTISING ENTEROCOLITIS

Necrotising enterocolitis (NEC) is one of the most common gastrointestinal emergencies in the neonatal unit. Despite early recognition and aggressive management, it still accounts for substantial long-term morbidity in survivors, especially in preterm and low birthweight infants (Kim & Seo, 2020). NEC is an inflammatory disease of the bowel, with or without necrosis, and occurs at a rate of 1 in 1000 live births, and in 5% of infants born weighing less than 1500 g (Gallagher et al., 2021). Any portion of the bowel can be affected, but damage is mainly seen in the terminal ileum, caecum and ascending colon. The bowel appears purple and discoloured, and is often distended with areas of serosal damage (i.e. necrosis and ischaemia). Perforation is a late sign and will often require urgent surgery in order to avoid further damage. Despite recent advances in neonatal intensive care, NEC remains a major health concern in the neonatal unit and a significant cause of neonatal morbidity and mortality (Kim & Seo, 2020).

Pathophysiology

While there has been great debate regarding the causes of NEC, the pathogenesis is still largely unknown. For about 90% of preterm infants, available evidence supports a multifactorial mechanism that includes an immature intestinal tract and immune system, and disruption to the normal intestinal microbiome allowing bacterial colonisation of the gut (Kim & Seo, 2020). Perinatal stress leading to hypoxic–ischaemic injury and nutritional substrate in the gut lumen have also been implicated in the development of NEC (Gallagher et al., 2021). Over the past several years, increasing evidence has suggested that the risk factors of NEC, namely bacterial colonisation, intestinal ischaemia and/or necrosis and formula feeding, stimulate pro-inflammatory mediators, which in turn activate a series of events at the cellular level leading to necrosis of the bowel (Kim & Seo, 2020). A compensatory mechanism, commonly referred to as the 'diving reflex', is activated so that a neonate in stress will redirect its blood supply away from non-essential organs to maintain the vital organs. (This redistribution of cardiac output shunts blood away from the mesenteric, renal and peripheral vascular beds to protect the brain and heart from ischaemia.) This relative circulatory insufficiency to the bowel may result in intestinal ischaemia (Godek & Freeman, 2020). Thus, there is an increased incidence of NEC in neonates who experience a significant hypoxic or asphyxial event.

Asphyxiated neonates and those suffering respiratory distress syndrome, apnoeic episodes or cyanosis, hypotension, congenital heart disease, patent ductus arteriosus, heart failure, anaemia or polycythaemia are most commonly affected (Kim & Seo, 2020). Hypoxic injury associated with inflammation has been identified as an important factor in NEC pathogenesis (Gallagher et al., 2021). Any procedure that has a potential for causing haemodynamic change, such as umbilical catheterisation or exchange transfusion, may be a contributing factor in developing NEC.

It is understood that bacterial overgrowth and increased intestinal permeability cause bacterial translocation from the intestinal lumen into tissues, thereby producing inflammatory responses activating cytokines (Schanler, 2017). Most of the defences that would normally prevent passage of bacteria across the mucosal barrier, such as a well-functioning immune system, intact mechanical defences and normal intestinal microflora, are impaired in neonates with NEC.

Although the mechanism is not well understood, enteral feeding has been reported to promote NEC, by providing an avenue for increased proliferation of potentially pathogenic bacteria that may then go on to invade the bowel wall. Preterm neonates are most at risk because of their immature local host defences, with diminished concentrations of secretory IgA, mucosal enzymes and other protective agents, and increased gastric pH that promotes bacterial overgrowth. Preterm neonates also have immature mucosal barriers, with increased permeability and bacterial penetration into the intestinal wall. They have decreased small bowel motility, resulting in delayed transit time, which further increases bacterial proliferation and overgrowth (Macdonald & Green, 2018).

EVIDENCE-BASED PRACTICE RESEARCH 12.7

Enteral feeding is implicated as an important contributor to the development of NEC, as studies have shown that the introduction of enteral feeding causes a disruption of the mucosal lining of the gut and disrupts blood flow (Gallagher et al., 2021).

In comparison to formula-fed neonates, neonates who receive expressed breast milk (EBM) or are breastfed are rarely affected by NEC, presumably because of the protective secretory immunoglobulin and anti-inflammatory components that breast milk provides (Kim & Seo, 2020). Incomplete digestion of formula can supply substrate for bacterial growth. Also, it is believed that formula intake may provide a substance on which bacteria can feed and flourish.

Anaemia and transfusion with packed red blood cells have also been cited as risk factors for NEC, but a systematic review conducted by Yeo et al. (2019) found that cessation of feeding during blood transfusion made no difference in the development of NEC, although the evidence was of a very low quality. Rina et al. (2020) investigated whether antibiotic exposure increased the risk of NEC by conducting a meta-analysis of 13 studies on the topic. They found that the empirical use of antibiotics for more than 5 days was associated with an increased risk of NEC.

Epidemiology

About 90% of NEC cases occur in preterm neonates (Macdonald & Green, 2018). It is suggested that the incidence of NEC is inversely proportional to gestational age and birthweight, with VLBW neonates and those born preterm and growth restricted making up the higher percentage (Jin et al., 2019). With improving survival of preterm infants, the number of infants at risk of NEC is rising. Battersby et al. (2018) conducted a systematic review of NEC rates in high-income countries and found wide variations in the reported incidence of NEC owing to a lack of standard data-collecting procedures. They reported a 2–7% incidence of NEC in neonates born less than 32 weeks' gestation, and a 5–22% incidence of NEC in neonates born under 1000 grams. Of the Australia and New Zealand Neonatal Network database registrants in 2018, the percentage of neonates with confirmed NEC was 1.4%. Of these, 62.3% were born before 28 weeks' gestation, 55.2% of whom underwent surgery; 18.2% were born between 28 and 31 weeks' gestation, and 42.9% required surgery (Chow et al., 2020, p. 29). Internationally, regardless of gestation, NEC incidence is reported as lowest in Japan, and highest in Australia, Canada, USA, Poland and Italy (Alganabi et al., 2019).

CLINICAL PRACTICE 12.5

The risk of NEC and mortality decreases with increasing birthweight (BW) as follows (Kim & Seo, 2020):

- BW 501–750 g: 12% risk, 42% mortality with NEC
- BW 751–1000 g: 9% risk, 29% mortality with NEC
- BW 1001–1250 g: 6% risk, 21% mortality with NEC
- BW 1251–1500 g: 3% risk, 16% mortality with NEC.

Therefore, preventing preterm birth is a major health priority.

Prevention

Prevention of NEC is a multidisciplinary effort involving neonatal nurses/midwives, neonatal nurse practitioners, medical staff and parents. Having a standardised approach to feeding at-risk neonates reduces the risk of NEC (Jin et al., 2019). Such an approach should include:

- use of human breast milk, including pasteurised human donor milk (Jin et al., 2019) and human milk-based fortifier (Gallagher et al., 2021)
- allowing adequate time for gut maturation by starting trophic feeds slowly, with small volumes of breast milk, and increasing feeds daily by 10–20 mL/kg/day if tolerated (Jin et al., 2019)
- avoidance of hyperosmolar feeds and medications such as caffeine
- timely correction of contributing factors such as hypoxia, acidosis, hypovolaemia and polycythaemia
- use of probiotics, although the effect is of low certainty (Sharif et al., 2020).

REFLECTION

Breastfeeding is a crucial factor in the prevention of NEC in preterm neonates. Maastrup et al. (2021) conducted a large multi-centred intervention study in Denmark to examine the effects of a training program for neonatal nurses on the facilitation of breastfeeding in preterm infants. They measured the rates of exclusive breastfeeding at discharge between a control group of 420 mothers and their preterm neonates, and an intervention group of 494 preterm mother–infant dyads. They found that significantly more preterm infants in the intervention group were exclusively breastfed at discharge (66.6%) than in the control group (58.1%; $p < 0.008$). They found that breastfeeding rates improved if the mother began breast milk expression within 6 hours of birth, had daily skin-to-skin contact with her baby and did not use a nipple shield.

- How can neonatal nurses and midwives in your setting use these findings to facilitate breastfeeding?

EVIDENCE-BASED PRACTICE RESEARCH 12.8

Sharif et al. (2020) conducted a systematic review of 56 trials comparing probiotic supplementation with placebo or no probiotics to reduce the risk of NEC in very preterm or low birthweight infants. Most of the trials were small and some had design flaws, resulting in the inability to be certain about the results. They concluded that there was a 'low certainty' of possibility that probiotics reduced the risk of NEC, death and serious infection, and that more randomised placebo-controlled studies were needed to ensure more-meaningful results.

Clinical assessment and findings

Neonatal nurses/midwives caring for the preterm neonate are in a unique position to detect and respond to the early signs of NEC. On average, symptoms generally present within 23 days of birth; however, it has been shown that 25% of cases present later than 30 days after birth (Schanler, 2017). The early signs are highly variable, but generally include non-specific signs of GIT compromise (mild abdominal distension, increasing gastric residuals, vomiting that may or may not be bilious and bloody stools) or non-specific signs of infection (lethargy, temperature instability, apnoea and bradycardia), or both (van Druten et al., 2019). Abdominal distension occurs as gas builds up in the bowel as a result of the fermentation of carbohydrate by intestinal flora that yields hydrogen and carbon dioxide. Peritonitis is evidenced by erythema, oedema and marked tenderness of the abdomen. As the disease progresses, hypovolaemia occurs, due to third spacing of fluids in the interstitial compartments of the damaged intestines, and blood pressure falls. Urine output may decrease and poor perfusion is evident, with the septic neonate appearing pale and mottled (Kim & Seo, 2020).

Bell's staging criteria have traditionally been the standard in assigning severity of disease to NEC cases, but they have been modified as our understanding of NEC has evolved (Kim & Seo, 2020). Table 12.1 outlines the characteristics of the staging of NEC according to Bell's modified criteria (Gregory et al., 2011).

Diagnosis

Abdominal X-rays confirm the diagnosis of NEC and are used to follow the progression of the disease. However, when there are equivocal X-ray findings, treatment decisions should be based upon clinical suspicion (Kim, 2020). Abdominal X-rays can be taken in the supine position, but in neonates with more-advanced illness in whom pneumoperitoneum is suspected the neonate can be positioned in the lateral decubitus position with the left side down, when free air can then be detected in the abdomen (Schanler, 2017).

Pneumatosis intestinalis is considered a hallmark of NEC in stages II and III, when bubbles of gas appear as a characteristic train-track lucency configuration within the bowel wall on X-ray (Kim & Seo, 2020). Bacterial gas may enter the portal system and outline the branching segments of the vascular tree. A large distended immobile intestinal loop on repeated X-ray suggests a gangrenous loop of bowel, and a gasless abdomen may indicate perforation and peritonitis. Air within the portal vein system is frequently seen with near-total intestinal necrosis. Fig. 12.5 depicts an abdominal radiograph in a neonate with NEC demonstrating pneumatosis intestinalis (intramural air) and gut perforation (evidenced by gas situated anterior to the liver in this supine film). Van Druten et al. (2019) believe that abdominal ultrasound can lead to earlier diagnosis of preterm NEC and therefore improve outcomes.

Laboratory findings are often non-specific and include abnormal blood gas results, caused by apnoea and acidosis, and abnormal blood count results resulting from sepsis. A full blood examination may reveal thrombocytopenia, a frequent finding that can result in significant bleeding or disseminated intravascular coagulopathy (DIC) (Macdonald & Green, 2018). In the early course of NEC, declining platelets correlate with necrotic bowel and worsening disease, whereas a subsequent rise often signals improvement (Schanler, 2017). Typical sepsis findings include an increase in the immature-to-mature neutrophil ratio, an elevated C-reactive protein and positive blood cultures. Electrolyte imbalances may result from feeding intolerance and vomiting. Hyponatraemia and metabolic acidosis may

TABLE 12.1 **Modified Bell's staging criteria for NEC**

Stage	Classification	Systemic signs	Intestinal signs	Radiological signs
IA	Suspected NEC	Temperature instability, apnoea, bradycardia, lethargy	Increased pre-gavage residuals, mild abdominal distension, emesis, blood-positive stool	Normal or intestinal dilation, mild ileus
IB	Suspected NEC	Same as above	Bright red blood from rectum	Same as above
IIA	Proven NEC – mildly ill	Same as above	Same as above, plus absent bowel sounds, with or without abdominal tenderness	Intestinal dilation, ileus, pneumatosis intestinalis
IIB	Proven NEC – moderately ill	Same as above, plus mild metabolic acidosis, mild thrombocytopenia	Same as above, plus absent bowel sounds, definite abdominal tenderness, with or without abdominal cellulitis or right lower quadrant mass	Same as IIA, plus portal venous gas, with or without ascites
IIIA	Advanced NEC – severely ill, bowel intact	Same as IIB, plus hypotension, bradycardia, severe apnoea, combined respiratory and metabolic acidosis, disseminated intravascular coagulation and neutropenia	Same as above, plus signs of generalised peritonitis, marked tenderness and distension of abdomen	Same as IIB, plus definite ascites
IIIB	Advanced NEC – severely ill, bowel perforated	Same as IIIA	Same as IIIA	Same as IIB, plus pneumoperitoneum

Source: adapted from Lee, J. S. & Polin, R. A. (2003). Treatment and prevention of necrotizing enterocolitis. Seminars in Neonatology, *8, 449–459.*

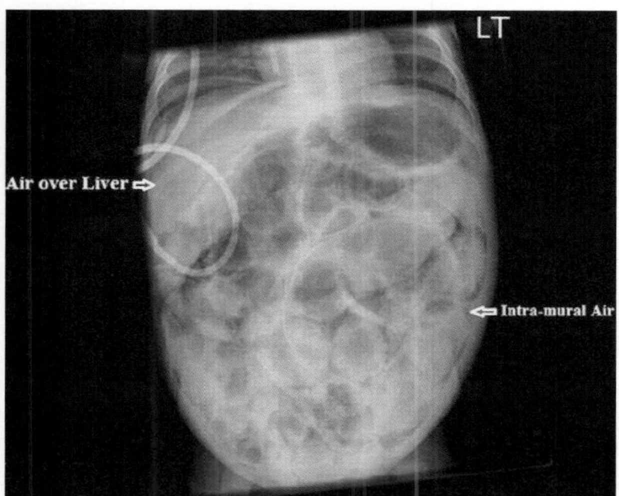

FIGURE 12.5 **Abdominal radiograph in a neonate with NEC**
Source: Sodhi and Fiset (2012).

indicate necrotic bowel or sepsis (Schanler, 2017). Acid–base studies will show respiratory and metabolic acidosis and hypoxaemia. Platelet count and coagulation factors may indicate DIC, an acquired haemorrhagic disorder associated with underlying disease that is manifested as an uncontrolled activation of coagulation and fibrinolysis (Schanler, 2017).

Management

The management of NEC is dependent on the stage of disease. The recognition and prompt treatment of early signs is best practice. The overall aim of treatment is to rest the bowel, control infection, restore metabolic equilibrium and maintain the neonate in an optimal condition until the bowel heals (Kim & Seo, 2020). Bowel rest is achieved with the cessation of enteral feedings, typically for the duration of antibiotic therapy (10–14 days), and GI decompression with a nasogastric tube on free drainage. A central venous catheter is usually sited to administer total parenteral nutrition, and enteral feeds can be gradually resumed as the neonate's clinical condition improves (Kim & Seo, 2020).

Assessment and support of both the cardiovascular and the respiratory systems with fluids, inotropes, supplemental oxygen and mechanical ventilation may be needed (Kim & Seo, 2020). Broad-spectrum antibiotic combinations are administered for 10–14 days. Australian and New Zealand approaches to antimicrobials for the treatment of suspected NEC are similar, with 89% using an aminoglycoside, metronidazole, and a penicillin (Carr et al., 2017). Serial X-rays are taken every 6–12 hours during the first few days, or until the neonate improves, to track the course of the disease (Kim & Seo, 2020). Surgery is indicated if intestinal perforation occurs, or if the infant is at high risk of perforation; however, it is difficult to identify those high-risk infants accurately (Kim & Seo, 2020).

Complications and outcomes

NEC is the primary cause of loss of life among hospitalised neonates, with risks of infectious complications, DIC, and respiratory, cardiovascular and metabolic complications (Kim & Seo, 2020). Long-term complications include wound infections, intestinal strictures, malabsorption conditions (i.e. short bowel syndrome) due to the reduced functional small bowel and neurodevelopmental delay (Gallagher et al., 2021). The overall survival rate for infants weighing more than 1000 grams is approximately 50–80% (Gallagher et al., 2021).

EVIDENCE-BASED PRACTICE RESEARCH 12.9

The economic burden of NEC is substantial. Cheah (2019) found that neonatal intensive care was expensive, especially for infants with NEC and even more so if they needed surgery. She believed that costs could be significantly reduced by reducing the rate of admission to NICU of moderate to late preterm infants, providing high-quality care in NICU and improving antenatal, perinatal and essential newborn care in low- and middle-income countries.

CONCLUSION

The GI system is integral for normal body function. This chapter has provided an overview of the development and function of the GI system, and described common disorders including feeding intolerance and GOR, malformations and abdominal wall defects and pathology that often requires surgical intervention, including cholestasis, bowel obstruction and NEC. These are by no means exhaustive of the variety of GI disorders that may present in the neonatal period.

Neonatal nurses/midwives have a vital role in assessment and management of a neonate's gastrointestinal status and nutrition management. A thorough physical assessment at birth is vital to detect congenital abnormalities. Furthermore, early detection of signs of feeding intolerance or abnormal physical symptoms can be life saving. Nurses/midwives have an important role in supporting infant–family-centred developmental care and health promotion to maximise neonatal outcomes.

Neonatal nurses/midwives need to be able to anticipate and recognise conditions early and, therefore, minimise the effects of GI disorders to avoid long-term disability. Conditions need to be treated promptly and appropriately, while encouraging and promoting positive interaction between parents and their baby.

Further Reading

Eichenwald, E. C. and the AAP Committee on Fetus and Newborn. (2018). Diagnosis and management of gastro-esophageal reflux in preterm infants. *Pediatrics, 142*(1), e2018061.

Hair, A. B. (2021). Approach to enteral nutrition in the premature infant. In: *UpToDate*. Walters Kluwer. <https://www.uptodate.com/contents/approach-to-enteral-nutrition-in-the-premature-infant?search> (Accessed 17 February 2022).

Mohamed, F. Z., & Ahmed, E. S. (2018). Efficacy of abdominal massage on feeding intolerance of preterm neonates. *American Journal of Nursing Research, 6*(6), 371–379.

Online Resources

Australia and New Zealand Neonatal Network (lists articles on clinical outcomes for neonates whose data appear on the Australia and New Zealand Neonatal Network (ANZNN) database): < https://www.anznn.net/research/articles>

Kids Health for Parents (provides overviews on many of the GI disorders addressed in this chapter, written for parents): <https://www.kidshealth.org/en/parents>

MSD Manual Professional Version (provides an overview of GI disorders in neonates and infants): <https://www.msdmanuals.com/professional/pediatrics/gastrointestinal-disorders-in-neonates-and-infants/overview-of-gastrointestinal-disorders-in-neonates-and-infants?query=overview%20of%20GI%20disorders%20in%20neonates%20and%20infants>

Neonatal eHandbook (provides a structured approach to the clinical management of conditions regularly encountered by health professionals caring for newborns): <https://www.bettersafercare.vic.gov.au/clinical-guidance/neonatal>

NICE: National Institute for Health and Care Excellence, population group infant and neonate: <https://www.nice.org.uk/guidance/population-groups/infants-and-neonates/products?Status5Published>

References/Acknowledgements

Ahammad, F., Begum, T., & Nasrin, E. (2018). Comparison of feeding intolerance between very preterm and moderate preterm neonates – a prospective cohort study. *Journal of Pediatrics and Neonatal Care, 8*(4), 6–10.

Alganabi, M., Lee, C., Bindi, E., Li, B., & Pierro, A. (2019). Recent advances in understanding necrotizing enterocolitis. *F1000Research, 8*, F1000 Faculty Rev-107. doi: 10.12688/f1000research.17228.1.

Bae, H. J., Shin, S. H., Kim, E-K., Kim, H-S. Cho, Y. S., & Gwak, H. S. (2019). Effects of cyclic parenteral nutrition on parenteral nutrition-associated cholestasis in newborns. *Asia Pacific Journal of Clinical Nutrition, 28*(1), 42–48. doi: 10.6133/apjcn.201903_28(1).0007.

Ballesteros, G. E., Torremadé, A. A., Durán, F. C., Martín, M. C., & Caro, T. A. (2015). Intestinal malrotation – volvulus: imaging findings. *Radiologia, 57*(1), 9–21.

Basu, S., & Smith, S. (2021). Macrolides for the prevention and treatment of feeding intolerance in preterm low birth weight infants: a systematic review and meta-analysis. *European Journal of Pediatrics, 180*(2), 353–378. doi: 10.1007/s00431-020-03814-1.

Battersby, C., Santhalingam, T., Costeloe, K. & Modi, N. (2018). Incidence of neonatal necrotising enterocolitis in high-income countries: a systematic review. *Archives of Disease in Childhood. Fetal and Neonatal Edition, 103*(2), F182–F189.

Blackburn, S. T. (2017). *Maternal, fetal, and neonatal physiology: a clinical perspective* (5th ed.). St Louis, MO: Elsevier Saunders.

Bradshaw, W. T. (2020). Gastrointestinal disorders. In: T. Verklan & M. Walden (Eds.), *Core curriculum for neonatal intensive care nursing* (6th ed., Ch. 29, pp. 504–542). St Louis, MO: Elsevier Saunders.

Brown, L. D., Hendrickson, K., Evans, R., Davis, J., William, W., & Hay, W. W. (2020). Enteral nutrition. In: S. L. Gardner, B. S. Carter, M. I. Enzman-Hines, & S. Niermeyer (Eds.), *Merenstein & Gardner's handbook of neonatal intensive care: an interprofessional approach* (9th ed., p. 377). St Louis, MO: Elsevier.

Carr, J. P., Burgner, D. P., Hardikar, R. S., & Buttery, J. P. (2017). Empiric antibiotic regimens for neonatal sepsis in Australian and New Zealand neonatal intensive care units. *Journal of Paediatrics and Child Health, 53*(7), 680–684. doi: 10.1111/jpc.13540.

Cheah, I. G. S. (2019). Economic assessment of neonatal intensive care. *Translational Pediatrics, 8*(3), 246–256.

Chi, C., Buys, N., Li, C., Sun, J., & Yin, C. (2019). Effects of prebiotics on sepsis, necrotizing enterocolitis, mortality, feeding intolerance, time to full enteral feeding, length of hospital stay, and stool frequency in preterm infants: a meta-analysis. *European Journal of Clinical Nutrition, 73*, 657–670.

Chow, S. S. W., Creighton, P., Chambers, G. M., & Lui, K. (2020). *Report of the Australian and New Zealand Neonatal Network 2018*. Sydney, NSW: ANZNN. <https://www.anznn.net/> (Accessed 2 March 2022).

da Costa, K. M., & Saxena, A. K. (2020). Laparoscopic Ladd procedure for malrotation in newborns and infants. *American Surgeon, 87*(2), 253–258.

Desoky, S., Kylat, R., Udayasankar, U., & Gilbertson-Dahdal, D. (2018). Managing neonatal bowel obstruction: clinical perspectives. *Research and Reports in Neonatalogy, 8*, 19–32.

Dubey, S. P., Jain, A., Kumari, N., Bhatnagar, A., & Devgan, V. (2018). Pre feed aspirates versus abdominal girth monitoring for detection of feed intolerance in VLBW babies. *Indian Journal of Neonatal Medicine and Research, 6*(2) 6–12. doi: 107860/IJNMR/2035573.2229.

Eibensteiner, F., Auer-Hackenberg, L., Jilma, B., Thanhaeuser, M., Wald, M., & Haiden, N. (2019). Growth, feeding tolerance and metabolism in extreme preterm infants under an exclusive human milk diet. *Nutrients, 11*(7), 1443. doi: 10.3390/nu11071443.

Eichenwald, E. C. & AAP Committee on Fetus and Newborn. (2018). Diagnosis and management of gastroesophageal reflux in preterm infants. *Pediatrics, 142*(1), e2018061.

Feldman, A. G., & Sokol, R. J. (2020). Recent developments in diagnostics and treatment of neonatal cholestasis. *Seminars in Pediatric Surgery, 29*(4), 150945, doi: 10.1016/j.sempedsurg.2020.150945.

Gallagher, M. E., Pacetti, A. S., Lovvorn III, H. N., & Carter, B. S. (2021). Neonatal surgery. In: S. L. Gardner, B. S. Carter, M. I. Enzman-Hines, & S. Niermeyer (Eds.), *Merenstein & Gardner's handbook of neonatal intensive care: an interprofessional approach* (9th ed., pp. 996–1038). St Louis, MO: Elsevier.

Gardner, S. L., & Niermeyer, S. (2021). Immediate newborn care after birth. In: S. L. Gardner, B. S. Carter, M. I. Enzman-Hines, & S. Niermeyer (Eds.), *Merenstein & Gardner's handbook of neonatal intensive care: an interprofessional approach* (9th ed., pp. 93–136). St Louis, MO: Elsevier.

Godek, D., & Freeman, A. M. (2020). Physiology, diving reflex. In: *StatPearls*. Treasure Island, FL: StatPearls Publishing. <https://www.ncbi.nlm.nih.gov/books/NBK538245/> (Accessed 2 March 2022).

Gregory, K., DeForge, C., Natale, K., Phillips, M., & Van Marter, L. (2011). Necrotizing enterocolitis in the premature infant. *Advances in Neonatal Care, 11*(3), 155–164. doi: 10.1097/anc.0b013e31821baaf4.

Hair, A. B. (2021). Approach to enteral nutrition in the premature infant. In: *UpToDate*. Walters Kluwer. <https://www.uptodate.com/contents/approach-to-enteral-nutrition-in-the-premature-infant> (Accessed 2 March 2022).

Hasenstab, K. A., Nawaz, S., Lang, I. M., Shaker, R., & Jadcherla S. R. (2019). Pharyngoesophageal and cardiorespiratory interactions: potential implications for premature infants at risk of clinically significant cardiorespiratory events. *American Journal of Physiology – Gastrointestinal and Liver Physiology, 316*, G304–G312.

Holcomb, G. W., Murphy, J. P., & Ostie, D. J. (2014). *Ashcraft's pediatric surgery* (6th ed.). Philadelphia, PA: Elsevier.

Hu, X., Chang, Y., Wang, Z., Bao, W., & Li, Z. (2021). Altered gut microbiota is associated with feeding intolerance in preterm infants. *Turkish Journal of Pediatrics, 63*(2), 206–217.

Jin, Y. T., Duan, Y., Deng, X. K., & Lin, J. (2019). Prevention of necrotizing enterocolitis in premature infants – an updated review. *World Journal of Clinical Pediatrics, 8*(2), 23–32. doi: 10.5409/wjcp.v8.i2.23.

Jones, T., on behalf of Council of International Neonatal Nurses, Inc. (COINN) Working Group. (2019). International neonatal nursing competency framework. *Journal of Neonatal Nursing, 25*, 258–264. doi: 10.1016/j.jnn.2019.07.007.

Juang, D., & Snyder, C. L. (2012). Neonatal bowel obstruction. *Surgical Clinics of North America, 92*(3), 685–711, ix–x. doi: 10.1016/j.suc.2012.03.008.

Kato, Y., Hirata, K., Oshima, Y., & Wada, K. (2020). Weight-based estimation of insertion length of the nasogastric tube in extremely low birth-weight infants. *Advances in Neonatal Care, 20*(2), E31–E34 doi: 10.1097/ANC.0000000000000692.

Kennedy , L., Rogerson , T., & Keir , A. K. (2020). Does selective evaluation of gastric aspirates in preterm infants influence time to full enteral feeding? *Journal of Paediatric Child Health*, 56(7), 1150–1154. doi: 10.1111/jpc.14993.

Kim, W., & Seo, J. M. (2020). Necrotizing enterocolitis. *New England Journal of Medicine, 383*(25), 2461. doi: 10.1056/NEJMicm2020782.

Lenfestey, M. W., & Neu, J. N. (2018). Gastrointestinal development implications for management of preterm and term infants. *Gastroenterology Clinics of North America, 47*, 773–791.

Leung, A. K., & Hon, K. L. (2019). Gastroesophageal reflux in children: an updated review. *Drugs in Context, 8*, 212591. doi: 10.7573/dic.212591.

Lopez, R. N., & Lemberg, D. A. (2020). Gastro-oesophageal reflux disease in infancy: a review based on international guidelines. *Medical Journal of Australia, 212*(1), 40–44.

Lyman, B., & Guenter, P. (2019). Feeding tube placement and verification: best practices needed now. *Advances in Neonatal Care, 19*(2), 82–82.

Maastrup, R., Rom, A. L., Walloee, S., Sandfeld, H. B., & Kronborg, H. (2021). Improved exclusive breastfeeding rates in preterm infants after a neonatal nurse training program focusing on six breastfeeding-supportive clinical practices. *PLoS One, 16*(2), e0245273. doi: 10.1371/journal.pone.0245273.

Macdonald, A., & Green, J. (2018). Necrotising enterocolitis and neonatal sepsis: a literature review. *Journal of Neonatal Nursing, 24*(2), 80–85. doi: 10.1016/j.jnn.2017.08.001.

Mandato, C., Zollo, G., & Vajro, P. (2019). Cholestatic jaundice in infancy: struggling with many old and new phenotypes. *Italian Journal of Pediatrics*, 45(1), 83. doi: 10.1186/s13052-019-0679-x.

Martin, R., & Hibbs, A. M. (2020). Gastroesophageal reflux in premature infants. In: *UpToDate*. Walters Kluwer. <https://www.uptodate.com/contents/gastroesophageal-reflux-in-premature-infants> (Accessed 2 March 2022).

Messina, M., Angotti, R., & Molinaro, F. (2018). Meconium plug syndrome. In: G. Buonocore, R. Bracci, & M. Weindling (Eds.), *Neonatology: a practical approach to neonatal diseases*. (pp 133–134). Champaign, IL: Springer.

Mohamed, F. Z., & Ahmed, E. S. (2018). Efficacy of abdominal massage on feeding intolerance of preterm neonates. *American Journal of Nursing Research, 6*(6), 371–379.

Moore, K. L., Persaud, T. V. N., & Torchia, M. G. (2018). *The developing human: clinically oriented embryology* (11th ed.). Philadelphia, PA: Saunders Elsevier.

Neal-Kluever, A., Fisher, J., Grylack, L., Kakiuchi-Kiyota, S., & Halpern, W. (2019). Physiology of the neonatal gastrointestinal system. *Drug Metabolism and Disposition, 47*(3), 296–313.

Pandita, A., Gupta, V., & Gupta, G. (2018). Neonatal cholestasis: a Pandora's box. *Clinical Medicine Insights: Pediatrics, 12*, 1179556518805412. doi: 10.1177/1179556518805412.

Parker, L. A., Withers, J. H., & Talaga, E. (2018). Comparison of neonatal nursing practices for determining feeding tube insertion length and verifying gastric placement with current best evidence. *Advances in Neonatal Care, 18*(4), 307–317.

Prasad, G. R., & Aziz, A. (2017). Abdominal plain radiograph in neonatal intestinal obstruction. *Journal of Neonatal Surgery, 6*(1), 6. doi: 10.21699/jns.v6i1.483.

Rina, P., Zeng, Y., Ying, J., Qu, Y., & Mu, D. (2020). Association of initial empirical antibiotic therapy with increased risk of necrotizing enterocolitis. *European Journal of Pediatrics, 179*(7), 1047.

Roggero, P., Liotto, N., Menis, C., & Mosca, F. (2020). New insights in preterm nutrition. *Nutrients, 12*(6),1857. doi: 10.3390/nu12061857.

Rossor, T., Lingham, I., Douiri, A., Bhat, R., & Greenough, A. (2018a). Detection of gastro-oesophageal reflux in the neonatal unit. *Acta Paediatrica, 107*, 1535–1540.

Rossor, T., Andradi, G., Bhat, R., & Greenough, A. (2018b). Investigation and management of gastro-oesophageal reflux in United Kingdom neonatal intensive care units. *Acta Paediatrica, 107*, 48–51.

Rubarth, L. B., & Van Woudenberg, C. D. (2016). Development of the gastrointestinal system: an embryonic and fetal review. *Neonatal Network, 35*(3), 156–158. doi: 10.1891/0730-0832.35.3.156.

Schanler, R. J. (2017). Clinical features and diagnosis of necrotizing enterocolitis in newborns. <https://www.semanticscholar.org/paper/Clinical-features-and-diagnosis-of-necrotizing-in-Schanler-Abrams/5411b72c1f6d4055745a6e634284a097bcd4a252> (Accessed 2 March 2022).

Schwarz, S. M. (2021). Pediatric biliary atresia. *Medscape.* <https://emedicine.medscape.com/article/927029-overview#a2> (Accessed 2 March 2022).

Scottoni, F., & Davenport, M. (2020). Biliary atresia: potential for a new decade. *Seminars in Pediatric Surgery, 29*(4), 150940. doi: 10.1016/j.sempedsurg.2020.150940.

Seiiedi-Biarag, L., & Mirghafourvand, M. (2020). The effect of massage on feeding intolerance in preterm infants: a systematic review and meta-analysis study. *Italian Journal of Pediatrics, 46*(1), 52.

Sharif, S., Meader, N., Oddie, S. J., Rojas-Reyes, M. X., & McGuire, W. (2020). Probiotics to prevent necrotising enterocolitis in very preterm or very low birth weight infants. *Cochrane Database of Systematic Reviews, 10*, CD005496. doi: 10.1002/14651858.CD005496.pub5.

Singh, V. (2020). *Textbook of clinical embryology* (2nd ed.). New Delhi: Elsevier.

Sodhi, P., & Fiset, P. (2012). Necrotizing enterocolitis. *Continuing Education in Anaesthesia, Critical Care and Pain, 12*(1), 1–4. doi: https:// doi.org/10.1093/bjaceaccp/mkr043.

Tullie, L. G. C. & Stanton, M. P. (2019). Bilious vomiting in the newborn. *Surgery (Oxford), 37*(11), 614–619. doi: 10.1016/j.mpsur.2019.09.008.

van Druten, J., Khashu, M., Chan, S. S., Sharif, S., & Abdalla, H. (2019). Abdominal ultrasound should become part of standard care for early diagnosis and management of necrotising enterocolitis: a narrative review. *Archives of Disease in Childhood. Fetal and Neonatal Edition, 104*(5), F551–F559. doi: 10.1136/archdischild-2018-316263.

Wallenstein, M. B., Brooks, C., Kline, T. A., Beck, R. O., Yang, W., Shaw, G. M., et al. (2019). Early transpyloric vs gastric feeding in preterm infants: a retrospective cohort study. *Journal of Perinatology, 39*, 837–841. doi: 10.1038/s41372-019-0372-3.

Wehrman, A., Waisbourd-Zinman, O., & Wells, R. G. (2019). Recent advances in understanding biliary atresia. Version 1. *F1000Research, 8*, F1000 Faculty Rev-218. doi: 10.12688/f1000research.16732.1.

Wesson, D. E. (2021). Intestinal atresia. In: *UpToDate*. Walters Kluwer. <https://www.uptodate.com/contents/intestinal-atresia?search> (Accessed 3 March 2022).

Yeo, K. T., Kong, J. Y., Sasi, A., Tan, K., Lai, N. M., & Schindler, T. (2019). Stopping enteral feeds for prevention of transfusion-associated necrotising enterocolitis in preterm infants. *Cochrane Database of Systematic Reviews, 10*, CD012888. doi: 10.1002/14651858.CD012888.pub2.

Yuan, Z., Yan, J., Wen, H., Deng, X., Li, X., & Su, S. (2019). Feeding intolerance alters the gut microbiota of preterm infants. *PLoS One, 14*(1), e0210609. doi: 10.1371/journal. pone.0210609.

CHAPTER 13

CARE OF THE NEONATE WITH A NEUROLOGICAL DISORDER

KIM FLETCHER AND KAREN WALKER

Learning objectives

After reading this chapter you will be able to:

- describe the embryological and fetal development of the neurological system
- describe the anatomy and physiology of the neonatal neurological system
- discuss the pathophysiology, aetiology, epidemiology, prevention, clinical presentation, diagnosis, management, prognosis and complications of common neonatal neurological conditions
- describe the neonatal nursing/midwifery care of a neonate with a neurological condition
- understand the use of assessment tools and the importance of early diagnosis of cerebral palsy and neurodevelopmental delay
- understand the importance of, and facilitate, family-centred care for a neonate with a neurological condition.

Key words, terms and abbreviations

cerebral blood flow (CBF)
cerebral palsy (CP)
cerebrospinal fluid (CSF)
computed tomography (CT)
electroencephalogram (EEG)
hypoxic ischaemic encephalopathy (HIE)
intraventricular haemorrhage (IVH)
magnetic resonance imaging (MRI)
neural tube defects (NTDs)
periventricular leucomalacia (PVL)
post-haemorrhagic hydrocephalus (PHH)

INTRODUCTION

This chapter will discuss the embryological and fetal development of the central nervous system (CNS) and the anatomy and physiology of the neonatal brain. Specific neurological conditions affecting the neonate and the skilled neonatal nursing/midwifery care required will be discussed, highlighting the importance of the family, its needs and the involvement and support essential from a multidisciplinary team.

Data on the incidence of neurological disorders in Australia and New Zealand are difficult to ascertain, with no central data repository specifically for them. From the literature, it is clear there have been many advances in imaging techniques, both medical and surgical interventions and treatment of neonates with neurological conditions. With increasing survival, the focus is to decrease long-term morbidity.

EMBRYOLOGICAL AND FETAL DEVELOPMENT OF THE CENTRAL NERVOUS SYSTEM

Neural development begins early in embryogenesis and continues after birth. The complexity of this structure leaves it susceptible to injury throughout pregnancy, birth and the postnatal period, especially when birth occurs prematurely. Its development progresses through six characteristic stages (Blackburn, 2016).

1. Neurulation (development of the neural tube) occurs in three stages from weeks 3 to 4:
   stage 1: development of the neural plate from a thickened area of the ectoderm (outermost layer of cells/tissues), becomes the CNS
   stage 2: neural groove and folds develop when the lateral edges of the neural plate rise (~day 18)
   stage 3: development of the neural tube occurs when the neural folds fuse together (~week 3) (Fig. 13.1). This is an open-ended tube, with failure to close contributing to a major class of neural abnormalities (neural tube defects (NTDs)). This takes place near the future cervical region.
2. Development of the prosencephalon (forebrain) occurs from weeks 5 to 6, forming the forebrain, midbrain and hindbrain structures, as well as the ventricles (Fig. 13.2).
3. Neuronal proliferation and differentiation (~8 to 16 weeks) involve:
   a. formation of neurons and glial cells, which occurs in the germinal matrix (Fig. 13.3)
      i. neurons:
      - classified as multipolar, bipolar, pseudo-unipolar or unipolar

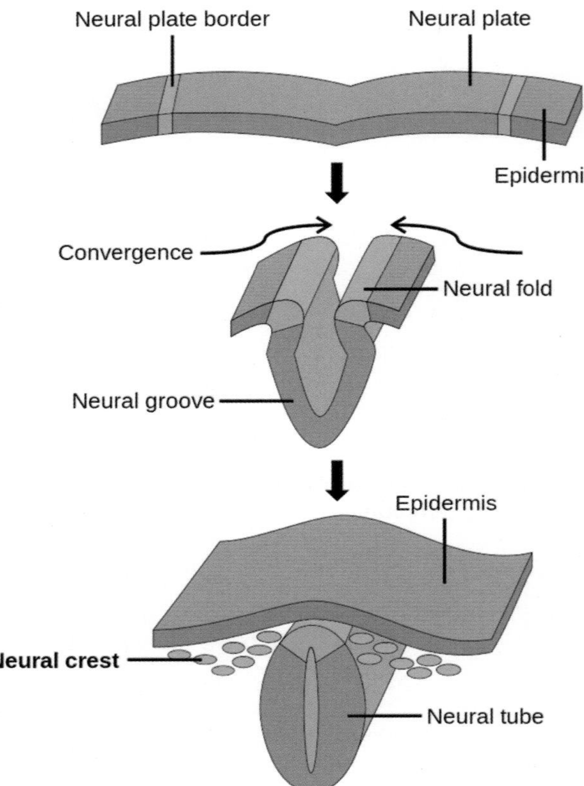

FIGURE 13.1 **Neural tube development**
Source: Wikipedia/NikNaks.

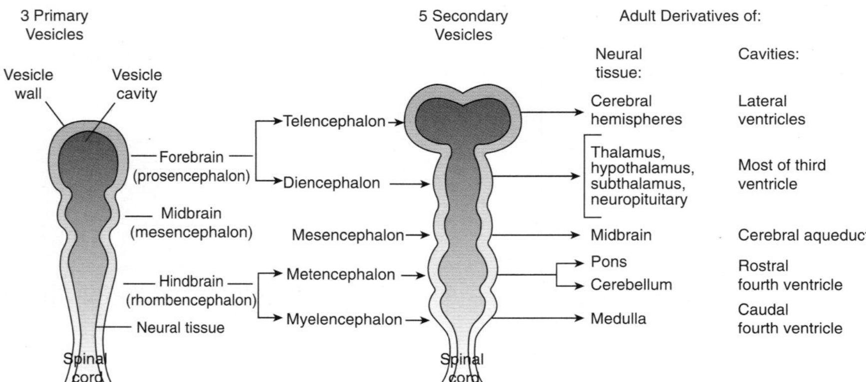

FIGURE 13.2 **Development of the prosencephalon**

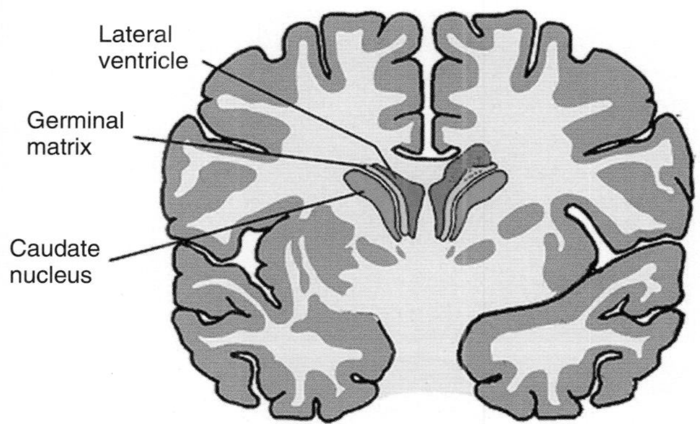

FIGURE 13.3 **Location of the germinal matrix**
Source: Talbert (2016).

- responsible for the conduction or inhibition of nerve impulses

ii. glial cells:
- supporting cells
- responsible for maintaining the optimum environment for normal neural function

b thickening of the germinal matrix, which begins to decrease from 24 weeks through to term.

4 Migration (neuronal complete by ~20 weeks; glial by ~36 weeks):
a of neurons and glial cells from the germinal matrix to the cerebrum
b neuronal migration in the cerebellum continues into the postnatal period.

5 Organisation (~20 weeks until the first 1–2 years, but continues to adulthood):
a CNS develops the capacity to act as an integrated whole, with different parts of the brain and body communicating
b development of the neocortex: axons and dendrites linking nerve cells, synapses, balancing of both excitatory and inhibitory processes and removing excess elements, with the total numbers of neurons halving between 24 weeks' gestation and 4 weeks' postnatally. This process results in rapidly increasing sulcation and gyration (Fig. 13.4).

6 Myelination occurs from ~29 weeks to early adulthood. Myelin is a protective sheath that surrounds the axons of the neural cell to improve transmission of nerve impulses. Myelination begins with the brain stem and generally proceeds inferior→superior, posterior→anterior, with most major tracts significantly myelinated by early childhood. Peripherally, this process is completed by Schwann cells, whereas in the CNS it is performed by oligodendrocytes. These glial cells are particularly vulnerable to injury (van Tilborg et al., 2018).

The entirety of this process is a continuum that is not complete at birth but occurs throughout the lifetime (Fig. 13.5).

Early in development, the CNS is essentially avascular. The blood vessels form in the meninges before growing

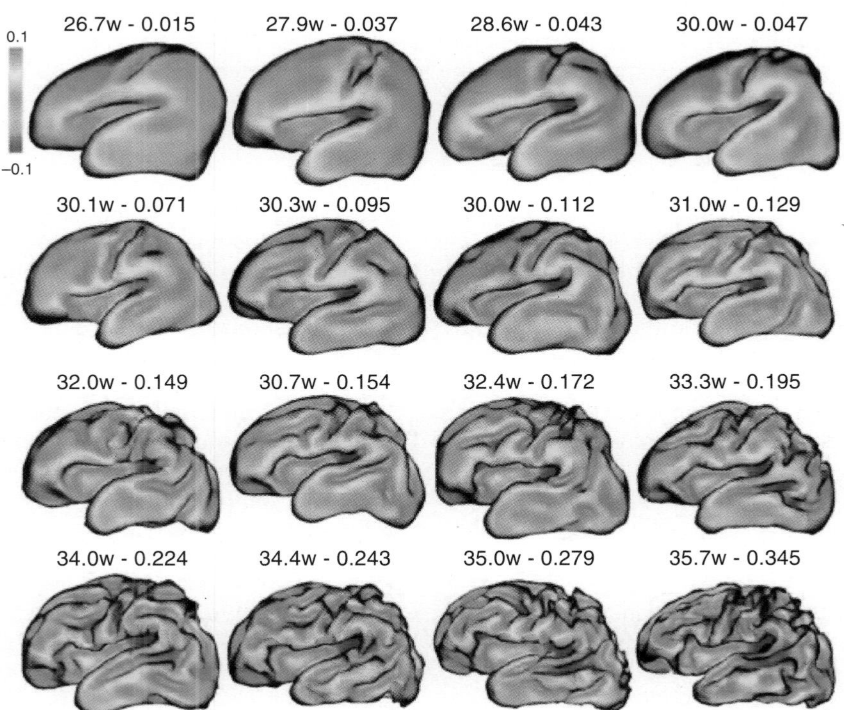

FIGURE 13.4 **Increase in cortical sulcation with age**
Source: Dubois et al. (2008), with permission of Oxford University Press.

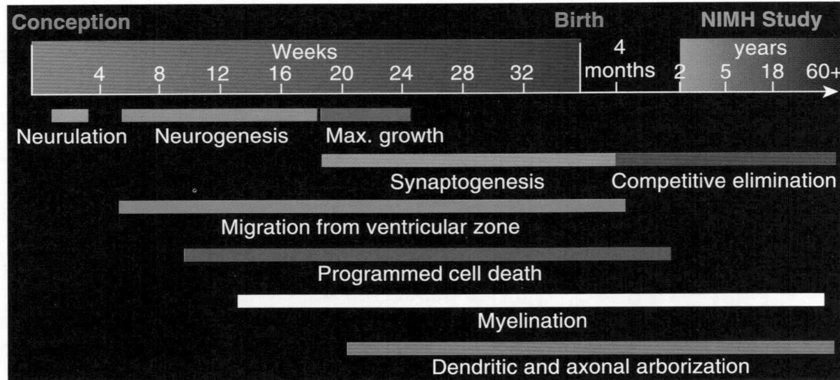

FIGURE 13.5 **Sequence of events in brain maturation**
Source: Lenroot and Giedd (2006).

into the CNS, developing into the blood–brain barrier. The blood–brain barrier is a collection of capillary–endothelial cell junctions that filter passage of substances between the bloodstream and **cerebrospinal fluid (CSF)**. This barrier is immature in the neonate, consequently allowing more potential toxins and harmful substances (teratogens) to reach the CNS.

ANATOMY AND PHYSIOLOGY OF THE NEONATAL CENTRAL NERVOUS SYSTEM

The CNS is made up of two major structures: the brain, protected by the skull, and the spinal cord. The rapid brain growth throughout gestation is accommodated by the bony plates of the skull that are held together by fibrous material called sutures. There is one occipital, two frontal and two parietal bones. The major sutures of the skull include the metopic, coronal, sagittal and lambdoid sutures. There are two fontanelles where suture lines intersect: the anterior and posterior fontanelles. These structures also allow the head to pass through the birth canal. The posterior fontanelle fuses within months of birth, while the anterior fontanelle does not close until 6–24 months. The brain is a mass of neurons that communicate with one another via synapses. The major structures include the brain stem, cerebellum and cerebrum. Communication between the brain and spinal cord occurs via the brain stem, which acts as a relay centre.

Cerebral blood flow (CBF) is regulated to maintain adequate oxygen and substrate delivery to the brain by systemic and local factors, including arterial blood pressure, intracranial pressure, arterial O_2 content, haematocrit and arterial CO_2 tension. Autoregulation refers to the maintenance of constant CBF over a range of changes in arterial blood pressure or cerebral perfusion pressure. Immaturity of the autonomic system means that prematurity, severe perinatal asphyxia, hypoxia, birth trauma and hypercapnia, even if mild, can alter the functioning of autoregulation and CBF (Kooi et al., 2017). The implications of each of these changes will be discussed throughout the chapter.

NEONATAL SEIZURES

Neonatal seizures are those that occur at ≤28 days of age. They are, in essence, paroxysmal alterations in neurological function (Abend et al., 2018) that result from abnormal electrical discharge of neurons. Neonatal seizures can be subtle and difficult to differentiate from normal neonatal reflexes, such as the startle reflex, 'jitteriness', tremors and benign sleep myoclonus (Abend et al., 2018). The majority of seizures (~90%) in term neonates have identifiable causes. These include (Ramantani et al., 2019):

- hypoxic ischaemic encephalopathy (46–49%)
- CNS infection (5–17%)
- cerebral infarction (6–12%)
- cerebral trauma (7–15%)
- metabolic abnormalities, including hypoglycaemia (3–9%)
- drug withdrawal (4%)
- congenital intracranial anomalies (4%).

Seizures in neonates can be categorised as subtle, clonic, tonic or myoclonic (Table 13.1), though a modification to this classification has been proposed (Pressler et al., 2021).

Neonatal seizures can be difficult to identify, as up to 50% are subtle in clinical presentation. Unlike in adults, they often do not manifest as generalised tonic–clonic activity, owing to the immaturity of the neonatal nervous systems and pattern of myelination. Common features include ocular movements, lip smacking, bicycling movements, apnoea, hypertension, tachycardia, bradycardia and oxygen desaturation. Typically, neonatal seizures do not occur in response to stimuli, and cannot be halted by holding the affected limb in a flexed position.

Appropriate diagnosis is critical to management. The history and timing of the seizures will guide the next steps. Pathology investigations include septic workup, CSF, electrolyte analysis, blood gas analysis and additional metabolic workup as indicated. Neurological imaging techniques for potential intracranial pathologies such as haemorrhage or congenital anomalies include

TABLE 13.1 **Neonatal seizure classification**

Subtle	Clonic	Tonic	Myoclonic
Most common Described as subtle because clinical manifestations are often overlooked as they imitate normal behaviours and reactions	Most commonly associated with electrographic seizures Involve one extremity or one side of the body The rhythm is usually slow, at 1–3 movements per second	May involve one extremity or whole body *Focal* tonic seizures involving one extremity often associated with electrographic seizures Often involve tonic extension of the upper and lower limbs; may involve the trunk and head in an opisthotonic fashion May mimic decorticate posturing; the majority are not associated with electrographic seizures	May occur focally in one extremity or in several areas (described as 'multifocal myoclonic seizures') Focal and multifocal myoclonic seizures not usually associated with electrographic seizures Most likely non-epileptic in nature and a reflection of severe encephalopathy

Source: Anand and Nair (2014).

TABLE 13.2 **Clinical management of neonatal seizures**

Initial	First-line medication	Second-line medication	Breakthrough medication	Ongoing medication
Airway, breathing, circulation	Phenobarbitone	Phenytoin	Clonazepam	Levetiracetam
Treat reversible causes: • hypoglycaemia • hypocalcaemia • meningitis • electrolyte disturbances		Midazolam		Pyridoxine (if deficiency identified)

cranial ultrasound, **magnetic resonance imaging (MRI)** and, rarely, **computed tomography (CT)** scans. Cranial ultrasound is the least invasive and identifies intraventricular or parenchymal haemorrhage, while MRI is superior in identifying the extent of intracranial haemorrhage, cortical lesions, subarachnoid blood and other pathologies (Ibrahim et al., 2018). Bedside amplitude-integrated electroencephalogram (aEEG) monitoring is routinely used to assess for electrical seizure activity and correlation with clinical signs, whereas formal **electroencephalogram (EEG)** is indicated if the seizures are difficult to control or require the use of multiple anticonvulsants (Kadivar et al., 2019).

Clinical management is summarised in Table 13.2.

Neonatal seizures are rarely idiopathic and are a major predictor of adverse outcomes in the neonate (Glass et al., 2018). Outcome is dependent on the underlying cause and associated long-term prognosis.

NEURAL TUBE DEFECTS

Neural tube defects (NTDs) occur at around 3–4 weeks' gestation, caused by abnormal development of the spinal cord, meninges and vertebral arches resulting in failure of the neural tube to close. There has been a continued downward trend in the overall prevalence of all NTDs and they fell by 14% in Australia following mandatory folic acid fortification of bread (Australian Institute of Health and Welfare (AIHW), 2016).

Although there is a range of defects, as depicted in Fig. 13.6, myelomeningocele is seen most commonly. Myelomeningocele occurs when a sac containing the meninges, spinal fluid and elements of the spinal cord protrudes through an open vertebral lesion. It may be covered with skin or a thin membrane. The cause is unclear; however, risk factors include maternal folate deficiency, some epileptic medications, diabetes, obesity and exposure to alcohol. The use of folic acid in pregnancy reduces the risk of NTD (Murphy & Westmark, 2020), and many countries now have mandatory folic acid fortification (van Gool et al., 2018; Viswanathan et al., 2017). Mandatory folic acid fortification of all wheat flour for bread making commenced in Australia from 2009, with the primary benefit being prevention of NTDs. In New Zealand, the voluntary addition of folic acid to certain foods has been permitted since 1996. Europe is yet to implement such an approach, and a recent study has suggested that a much higher incidence exists in these countries. In countries with mandatory fortification, the prevalence was approximately 5 per 10,000 live births; however, in countries without fortification it was more than double that figure (Murphy et al., 2020).

EVIDENCE-BASED PRACTICE RESEARCH 13.1

In 2014, mandatory fortification of foodstuffs with folic acid was recommended (D'Antoine & Bower, 2019; Shlobin et al., 2020). Food Standards Australia New Zealand (FSANZ) and the USA Food and Drug Administration have implemented mandatory folic acid fortification for the prevention of neural tube defects; however, much of the world still has not (Blencowe et al., 2018).

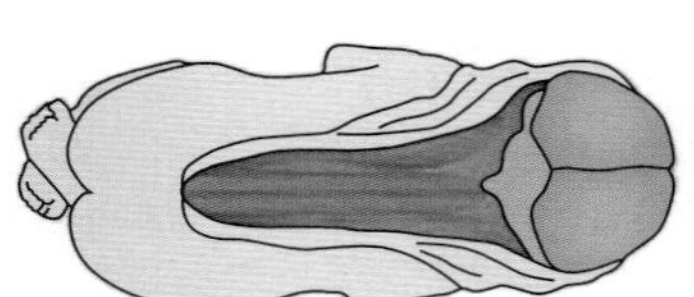

Craniorachischisis
Completely open brain and spinal cord

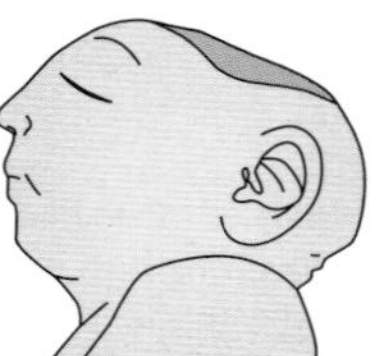

Anencephaly
Open brain and lack of skull vault

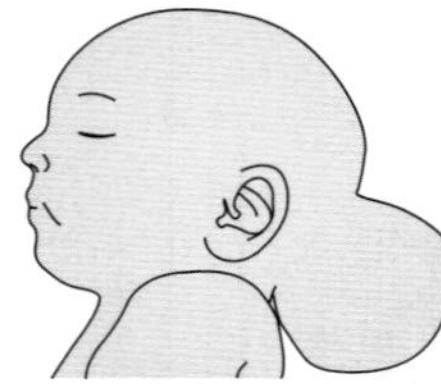

Encephalocele
Herniation of the meninges (and brain)

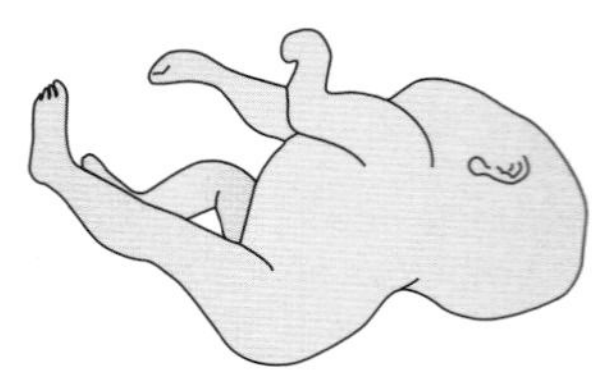

Iniencephaly
Occipital skull and spine defects with extreme retroflexion of the head

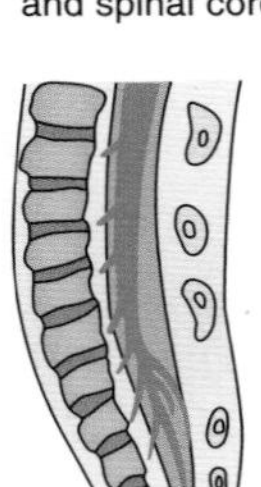

Spina bifida occulta
Closed asymptomatic NTD in which some of the vertebrae are not completely closed

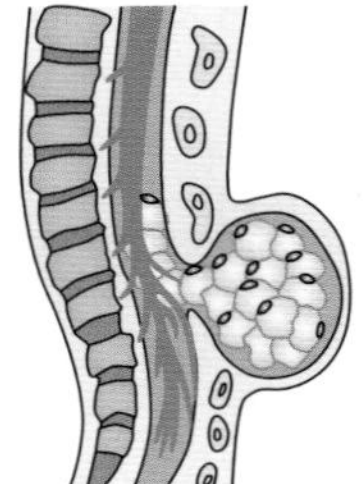

Closed spinal dysraphism
Deficiency of at least two vertebral arches, here covered with a lipoma

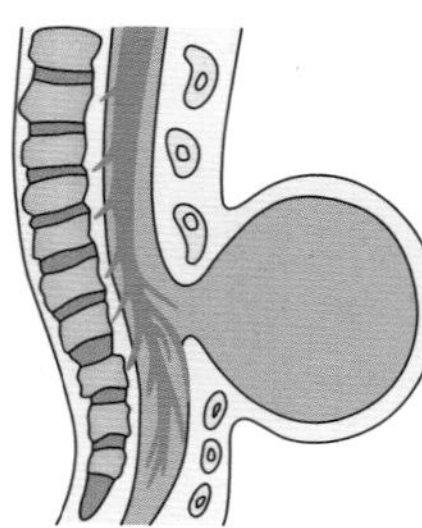

Meningocele
Protrusion of the meninges (filled with CSF) through a defect in the skull or spine

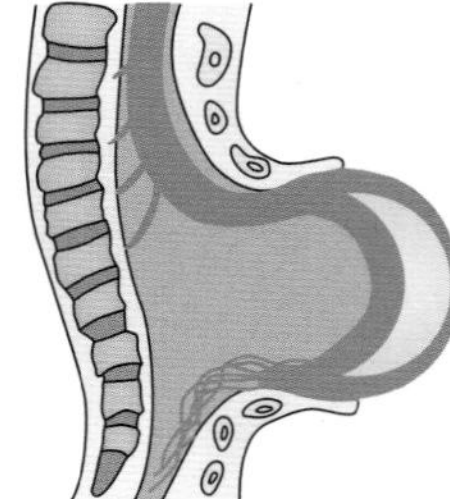

Myelomeningocele
Open spinal cord (with a meningeal cyst)

FIGURE 13.6 **Neural tube defects**

Source: reprinted from: Copp et al. (2015). Spina bifida. Nature Reviews Disease Primers, *1, 15007. 10.1038, Figure 1. <https://www.nature.com/articles/nrdp20157>, with permission of Macmillan Publishers Ltd.*

The lesions can vary in size and diameter and can be found anywhere along the spine, but are most commonly located between the lower thoracic and sacral region of the spine. The location and presence of neural tissues will determine the severity of the subsequent physical impairments, with higher spinal lesions causing more disability. Associated diagnoses include neurogenic bladder (lack of bladder control due to a neurological condition), orthopaedic and limb complications, hydrocephalus and Arnold–Chiari malformation (herniation of the cerebellum and medulla down into the spinal canal and up into the middle fossa) (Volpe, 2008).

Affected neonates require surgery within the first 72 hours of life; however, CSF leak warrants more immediate surgery, usually within the first 24 hours. Surgical neonatal nursing/midwifery care is detailed in Chapter 17.

Arnold–Chiari II malformations are the major cause of mortality. Infants who require a shunt for hydrocephalus have an increased risk of mortality due to malfunction of the shunt, frequent revisions of the shunt and shunt-related infections (Ranalli et al., 2020). Other complications include respiratory impairment, swallowing dysfunction and renal complications. Mobility depends on the site of the lesion: lower lesions can result in independent mobility, while neonates with lesions above lumbar II are likely to require a wheelchair as they grow (Kellogg et al., 2018). Children with a myelomeningocele are also at risk of developmental delay, and parents require early involvement and support from the multidisciplinary team, including social workers, physiotherapists and rehabilitation consultants.

FAMILY-CENTRED CARE 13.1

Family functioning and spina bifida (myelomeningocele)

It may be thought that having a child with meningomyelocele or spina bifida (SB) could disrupt normal family functioning but, in reality, many families adapt and demonstrate considerable resilience in the face of adversity.

It is acknowledged that youths with SB, and particularly those from lower socioeconomic homes, may be at risk for psychosocial difficulties. These include the development of internalising symptoms, attention deficit problems, educational difficulties, social maladjustment and delays in the development of independent functioning (Peterson et al., 2020).

MICROCEPHALY

Microcephaly is defined as a head circumference greater than three standard deviations below the mean (Kalmin et al., 2019). Its two main classifications are based on the presence of a genetic aetiology: primary (genetic) and secondary (non-genetic). Genetic causes include familial and autosomal dominant conditions, such as chromosomal syndromes (trisomies 21 and 18, Cornelia de Lange syndrome, Smith–Lemli–Opitz syndrome and cri du chat syndrome). Non-genetic causes include congenital infections (cytomegalovirus (CMV), Zika, rubella, toxoplasmosis, herpes), radiation, maternal drugs (alcohol or phenytoin), maternal metabolic conditions (diabetes mellitus, hyperphenylalaninaemia), postnatal infections (meningitis, encephalitis), malnutrition and hypoxic ischaemic encephalopathy.

Microcephaly presents as a small head circumference that developed in utero and persisted, because either the brain has not developed properly or it has stopped growing. In any case, intellectual impairment due to reduced brain size is a common side effect. Diagnosis includes a thorough family history and serial head measurements, compared with the parents' head circumferences. Laboratory and diagnostic investigations are based on the history and physical examination, and may include:

- chromosomal – karyotype and microarray
- metabolic – plasma amino acids, urine organic acids, serum ammonia, lactate and pyruvate
- infective – torch titres, HIV virus testing, urine or buccal CMV polymerase chain reaction (PCR), Zika virus serology
- imaging – MRI can identify structural brain abnormalities, and cranial ultrasound can detect intracerebral calcifications seen with congenital infections (Devakumar et al., 2018).

Treatment is limited and diagnosis dependent. Care begins with initial evaluation, further investigations as indicated and referral to a geneticist and/or subspecialist as needed. Prognosis is also diagnosis dependent, but can be associated with developmental delay and deficits.

CRANIOSYNOSTOSIS

Craniosynostosis occurs when there is premature closure of one or more of the sagittal, metopic, coronal or lambdoid sutures (Fig. 13.7). The most common form is sagittal synostosis, with a birth prevalence of 190 in 1,000,000 (Jung et al., 2018). Neonates with this condition require surgery to repair the defect, which is normally performed within the first years of life. Children with single-suture craniosynostosis are at risk of developmental delay (Jung et al., 2018).

BIRTH TRAUMA

Risk factors for neurological trauma include vaginal breech, instrumental deliveries and neonates born weighing more than 4500 g (Ojumah et al., 2017). It is important for all neonates to have haematological investigations to identify underlying diseases and causes of haemorrhage, such as clotting disorders.

NEONATAL INTRACRANIAL HAEMORRHAGE

The neonatal scalp has five layers, as depicted in Fig. 13.8, and is particularly vulnerable to trauma:

1. skin – the outermost layer
2. dense subcutaneous connective tissue
3. galea aponeurotica
4. loose connective tissue
5. dense periosteum.

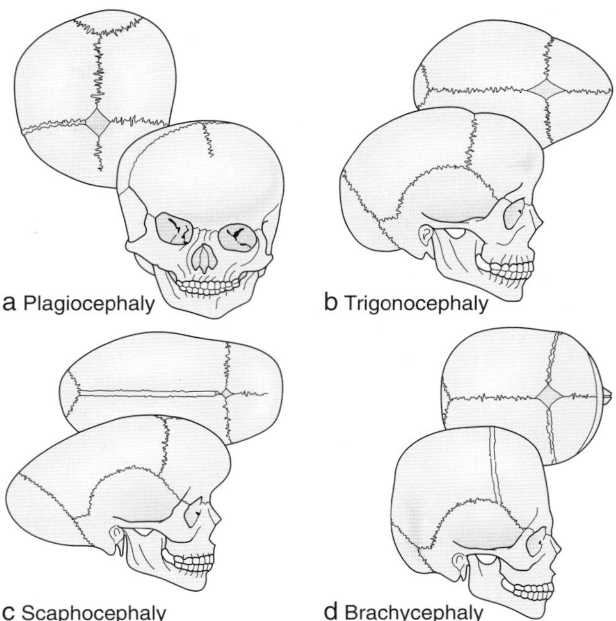

FIGURE 13.7 **Infant skull deformities caused by synostosis**
Source: Seruya et al. (2012).

Caput succedaneum

Caput succedaneum (Fig. 13.9) is oedema of the scalp, usually over the presenting part of the neonate's head and crossing the suture lines. It occurs as a result of pressure during the birth process and self-resolves within a few days.

Cephalhaematoma

A cephalhaematoma is a collection of blood located between the skull and the periosteum, caused by trauma, prolonged labour and, more commonly, following an instrumental birth. They are usually unilateral and do not cross suture lines. Generally, the haematoma resolves over a few weeks without intervention; however, cases of infected haematoma have been reported. Other complications include hyperbilirubinaemia (Aygün et al., 2020).

Subgaleal haemorrhage

In the normal scalp, the tissues adhere to each other with no space between them. With a subgaleal haemorrhage (also called subaponeurotic haemorrhage), blood creates a space between the galea aponeurotica and the periosteum. Subgaleal haemorrhages can occur spontaneously; however, most are caused by traction on the scalp. Their incidence is reported to range from 4 per 10,000 births, following a normal vaginal birth, to 59 per 10,000 births, following a vacuum-assisted birth (Ojumah et al., 2017). Neonatal nurses/midwives should be aware of the increased need for observations (including scalp observations) following instrumental birth.

Subgaleal haemorrhage is often not diagnosed quickly but is a potentially fatal condition. In Australia, coronial

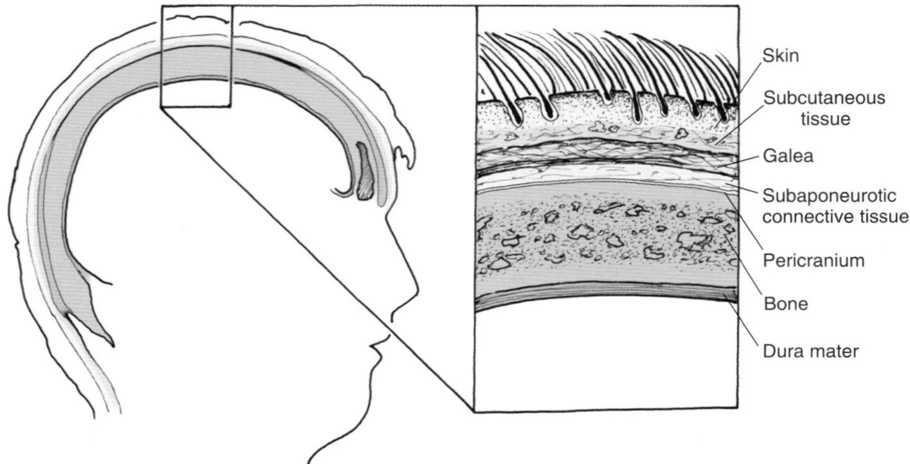

FIGURE 13.8 **Anatomy of the scalp**
Source: Baker (2014).

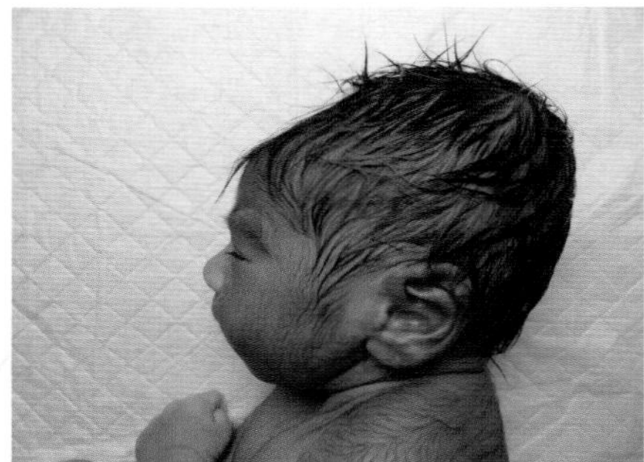

FIGURE 13.9 **Caput succedaneum**
Source: © Manish Bhalla.

inquiries into three deaths from subgaleal haemorrhage in 2015 highlighted the importance of early diagnosis and aggressive management and resuscitation (Colditz et al., 2015). Early diagnosis is easier when the onset is rapid; however, it can be challenging when the onset of haemorrhage is insidious.

CLINICAL PRACTICE 13.1

Classical signs of subgaleal haemorrhage are:

- diffuse, 'boggy' gravity-dependent swelling of the scalp, which increases in size and becomes tense
- increase in head circumference
- signs of early shock such as hypotension, narrow pulse pressure, tachycardia progressing to bradycardia, tachypnoea, apnoea and hypothermia.

Observe for a change in head shape, change in colour and displacement of the ears:

- monitor fluid output
- assess perfusion
- coagulation studies
- management includes inotropes/vasopressors
- perform ongoing assessment for jaundice.

Management is focused on aggressively treating shock and ensuring normal fluid and electrolyte balance, while controlling the haemorrhage with clotting factors such as fresh frozen plasma, cryoprecipitate and platelet transfusions. The mortality associated with this condition ranges from 2.8% to 14%; however, there is improved survival when there is increased surveillance following vacuum deliveries. Long-term outcomes are generally good for infants who survive the neonatal period; however, more-severe haemorrhages are associated with neurodevelopmental impairment (Ojumah et al., 2017).

CLINICAL PRACTICE 13.2

Extra-axial haemorrhage

- Extradural haemorrhage
- Subdural haemorrhage
- Subarachnoid haemorrhage

Intra-axial haemorrhage

- Intracerebral haemorrhage
- Intraventricular haemorrhage (IVH)

Extradural haemorrhage

An extradural haemorrhage is a type of extra-axial haemorrhage and is a collection of blood between the skull and the dura. The majority are supratentorial and usually caused by a skull fracture with tearing of the middle meningeal artery. Skull fractures can occur during instrumental deliveries. Both CT scans and MRI will demonstrate the haematoma. Surgical treatment is required to evacuate a larger clot.

Subdural haemorrhage

Subdural haemorrhages are a collection of blood between the dura and the arachnoid mater. Seizures, hyperbilirubinaemia, a rapidly enlarging head, poor

Moro reflex or extensive retinal haemorrhages can occur with this type of haemorrhage (Hong & Lee, 2018). The usual presentation is either a thin film over the occipital poles or a small infratentorial bleed and is not an unusual finding in post-mortem inspection following intrauterine, perinatal or neonatal deaths (Högberg et al., 2018).

Subarachnoid haemorrhage

A subarachnoid haemorrhage occurs when blood is located in the subarachnoid space, between the pia mater and the arachnoid. Although this type of haemorrhage can occur in various clinical contexts, the most common reason in the neonate is head trauma during the birthing process. This haemorrhage type usually occurs in full-term neonates and presents as seizure activity, lethargy and apnoea. Subarachnoid haemorrhages can also lead to hydrocephalus, **periventricular leucomalacia (PVL)**, **cerebral palsy (CP)** and permanent brain damage (Inder et al., 2018).

CLINICAL PRACTICE 13.3

Signs and symptoms of neurological impairment include (Novak et al., 2018):

- focal and generalised seizures
- apnoea
- lethargy
- vomiting
- irritability
- poor feeding
- abnormal neurological exam
- bulging fontanelles
- increasing head circumference.

SKULL FRACTURES

Neonatal skull fractures may be caused by trauma during birth, instrumental deliveries or accidental or non-accidental falls and, when present, can be associated with serious intracranial haemorrhage (Högberg et al., 2020). Imaging is vital to identify their extent, which often involves an MRI or CT scan to provide more information than conventional skull X-rays. A linear skull fracture (Fig. 13.10) refers to a fracture that is non-depressed and is most commonly located in the parietal region. This is considered a relatively common skull fracture and is often associated with extracranial (cephalhaematoma) and intracranial (epidural and subdural haemorrhage and cerebral contusion) complications. Treatment is not usually indicated for linear skull fracture (Volpe, 2018). Conversely, a depressed skull fracture (see Fig. 13.10) may be more serious – especially if related to a forceps-facilitated birth. The most common site of a depressed skull fracture is the parietal bone, and has a characteristic 'ping-pong' appearance, given the inward buckling of the unusually resilient neonatal bone without loss of bony continuity. Radiological assessment of the lesion is the most common approach, often in conjunction with CT scan, to rule out an extradural or subdural clot or bone fragments. The treatment approach is usually non-surgical unless otherwise indicated (Volpe, 2018).

NERVE INJURIES

The most common nerve injuries associated with birth trauma are facial nerve palsy and brachial plexus injury.

The facial nerve is the seventh cranial nerve (C7) and is at risk of trauma because of its proximity to the surface. Australian and New Zealand data are not available, but facial nerve palsy occurs in approximately 0.8–7.5 per 1000 births globally. Instrumental birth (leading to nerve damage if encountered by a forceps blade), prolonged labour, primigravida, heavier birthweight and prematurity are the major risk factors (Ojumah et al., 2017). Neonates most often present with facial asymmetry because of the involvement of the nerve after it exits the stylomastoid foramen (Ojumah et al., 2017). Usually no treatment is required, with spontaneous recovery within weeks. Care must be taken to lubricate the eye to prevent corneal abrasions if the eye cannot close, and feeding may be challenging if the neonate is unable to close the mouth because of palsy and will often require lactation support to successfully latch and feed.

The brachial plexus, from cervical 5 (C5) to thoracic spinal 1 (T1), is a bundle of nerves that innervate the upper limbs and the diaphragm. A brachial plexus injury is thought to result from stretching of the brachial plexus by extreme lateral traction, with its roots anchored to the

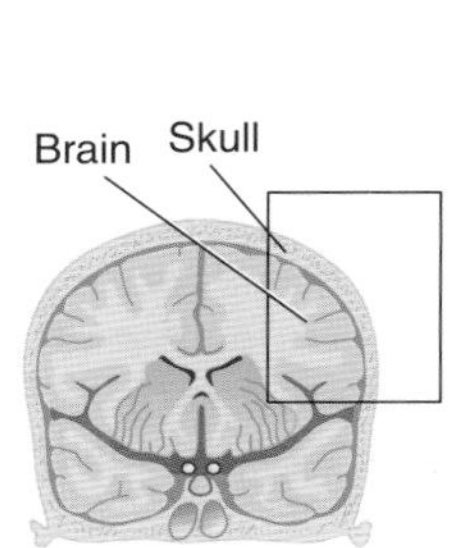

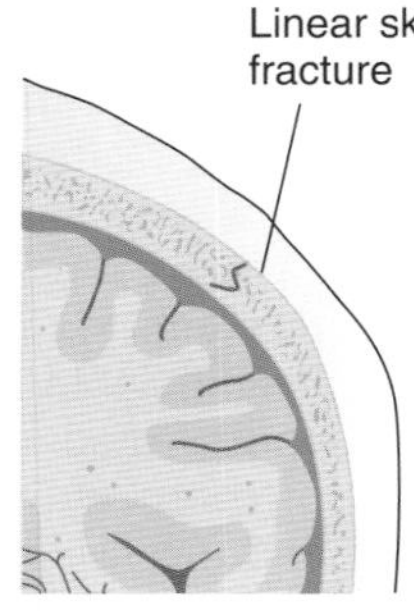

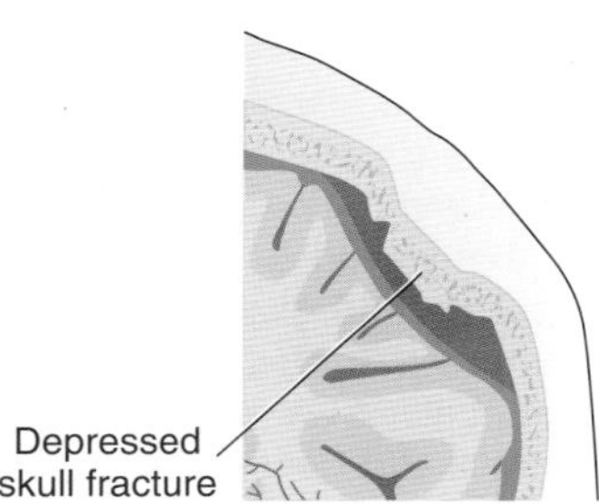

FIGURE 13.10 **Skull fractures**

Source: adapted from University of Miami (2017).

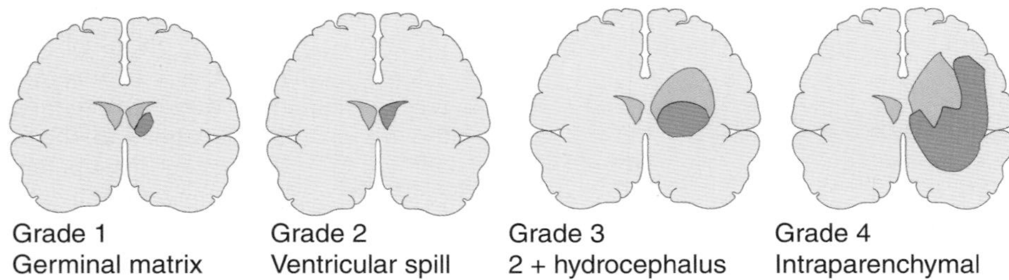

FIGURE 13.11 **Classification of IVH grades 1–4**

Source: Pilu et al. (2013).

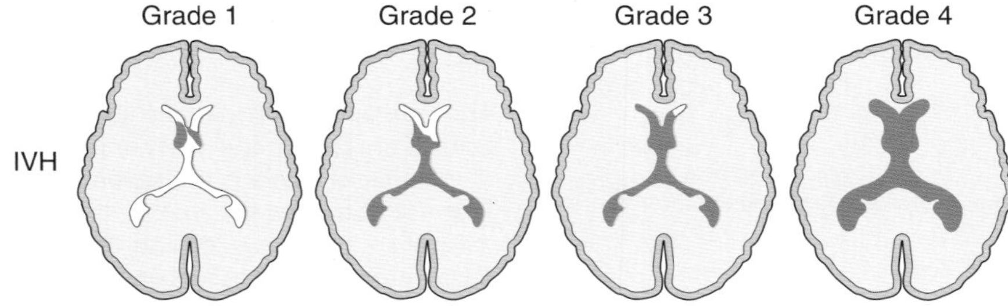

FIGURE 13.12 **Radiographic imaging of IVH**

cervical cord, and is more commonly right-sided than left, and rarely bilateral (Volpe, 2018). Australian and New Zealand data are not available, but the condition has an incidence ranging from 0.3 to 0.8 per 100 live births. Instrumental deliveries, increased birthweight and shoulder dystocia are risk factors. Erb's palsy occurs when there is damage to C5, C6 or C7. Although most neonates recover from a brachial plexus injury with physiotherapy over time, surgical repair may be necessary to optimise function (Ojumah et al., 2017; Smith et al., 2018).

Intraventricular haemorrhage

An **intraventricular haemorrhage (IVH)** is a bleed into the germinal matrix of the developing brain and is graded on the Papile classification system developed in 1978 (Sandoval et al., 2019) (Figs 13.11 and 13.12):

grade 1: germinal matrix haemorrhage
grade 2: IVH, with no ventricular dilation
grade 3: IVH with ventricular dilation
grade 4: IVH, ventricular dilation and extension of haemorrhage into the brain parenchyma.

The germinal matrix is a layer of tissue under the lining of the ventricles rich with thin-walled, fragile blood vessels that actively produces neurons and glial cells until 34–35 weeks, which explains why it is the usual site of IVH in preterm neonates (Tortora et al., 2018).

According to the Australia and New Zealand Neonatal Network (ANZNN) data, a normal cerebral ultrasound was recorded for 81.4% of registrants (Yeo et al., 2020). Of babies born at <32 weeks, 3.2% had a grade 3 or 4 IVH. The highest percentage of babies who had severe IVH (grade 4) were born before 26 weeks' gestation, with the majority (55.3%) of babies born before 25 weeks. The risk factors for IVH are related to birth history and clinical events, as listed in Table 13.3.

TABLE 13.3 **Risk factors for IVH**

Birth history	Clinical
Extreme prematurity Low birthweight History of asphyxia Birthing in a non-tertiary centre	Patent ductus arteriosus Severe respiratory distress syndrome Pneumothorax Labile blood pressure Hyper- or hypocapnia Seizures Infections Coagulopathies

Sources: Murthy et al. (2020); Wilson et al. (2020).

Clinical presentation can vary from an acute collapse through to a silent occurrence. Signs include falling haemoglobin/haematocrit, deterioration including apnoeic and/or bradycardic episodes, hypotension, altered level of consciousness and tone, seizures, bulging fontanelles and increasing head circumference. Prevention of IVH is the primary goal of management, and therefore the care provided by the astute neonatal nurse/midwife is pivotal in reducing the risk of IVH (see Clinical Practice 13.4).

CLINICAL PRACTICE 13.4

Neonatal nursing/midwifery care that can minimise the development of an IVH includes:

- slow administration of volume expansion
- minimisation of endotracheal suctioning, performed only as clinically indicated
- positioning the neonate to avoid neck flexion or lifting the lower body above the head
- avoiding constricting headbands (Murthy et al., 2020)
- avoiding episodes of crying by providing comfort, analgesia, etc.
- ensuring that all neonates are handled gently and developmentally appropriately.

White matter injury

White matter injury (WMI) is classically termed periventricular leucomalacia involving macroscopic cysts; however, it also includes both focal and diffuse non-cystic lesions that result in myelination disturbances due to oligodendrocyte degeneration (Ballabh & de Vries., 2021). This spectrum of damage is thought to occur as a result of immature vascular supply and cerebral autoregulation, and vulnerable pre-myelinating oligodendrocytes, with subsequent release of extracellular glutamate (excitotoxicity), reactive oxygen and nitrogen species (oxidative stress) and pro-inflammatory cytokines (inflammation) (Ballabh & de Vries, 2021). The resulting neuronal/axonal damage, degeneration and cystic development can involve cerebral white matter, thalamus, basal ganglia, cerebral cortex, cerebellum and brain stem. This damage is known to affect nerve pathways involved in motor control, increasing the risk for CP, learning difficulties and poorer neurodevelopmental outcomes.

Impairment of cerebrospinal fluid flow

When the CSF flow is obstructed, ventricular dilation can develop. IVH can result in **post-haemorrhagic hydrocephalus (PHH)** due to multiple small blood clots partially occluding the channels of CSF circulation, and blood-induced inflammation within subarachnoid spaces, which reduces CSF resorption (Spaull et al., 2019). The venous drainage system at the level of the foramen of Monro and caudate nucleus has a U-shaped turn, making it highly susceptible to obstruction. PHH also results in WMI by disturbing periventricular fibres, increasing intracranial pressure, introducing iron-induced hydroxyl free radicals and eliciting cytokine responses (Ballabh & de Vries, 2021). Depending on IVH severity, 25–80% of affected neonates can develop PHH, with 15% requiring intervention (Ballabh & de Vries, 2021; Gilard et al., 2018).

When neonates develop PHH, temporary CSF diversion may be established by a ventricular access device (VAD; Fig. 13.13), commonly known as a Rickham's reservoir (Bock et al., 2018). This subcutaneous reservoir is accessed to aspirate CSF at regular intervals in order to maintain

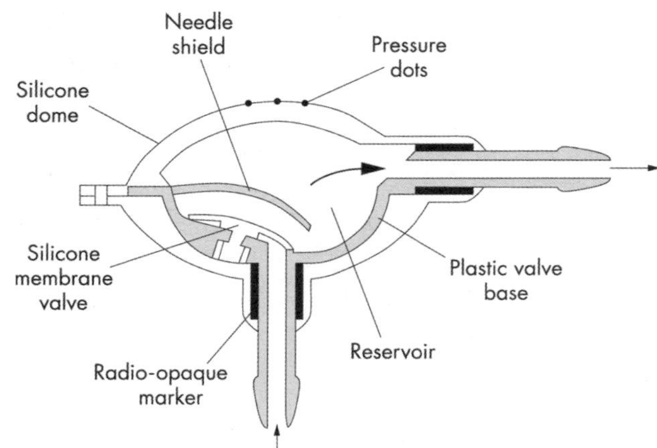

FIGURE 13.13 **Ventricular access device**

Source: Pople (2002), with permission from BMJ Publishing Group Ltd.

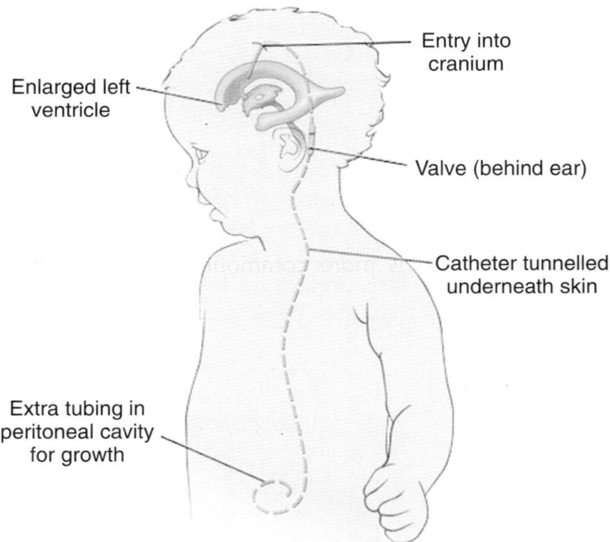

FIGURE 13.14 **Ventriculoperitoneal shunt**

Source: Horton et al. (2012).

head circumference and ventricular stability on ultrasound imaging. Definitive treatment for CSF diversion requires a ventriculoperitoneal shunt (VPS; Fig. 13.14) if the PHH does not resolve over time and requires ongoing drainage, but is usually not performed in neonates <2 kg (Bock et al., 2018).

Diagnosis of intraventricular haemorrhage, white matter injury and hydrocephalus

Diagnosis is made on serial cranial ultrasound scans (CrUSS), with MRI at term equivalent age (TEA) to assess for both brain injury and growth. Ultrasound is the established method for initial evaluation and follow-up; however, research has demonstrated that MRI can identify more-subtle forms of injury previously undetectable (Ballabh & de Vries, 2021).

CLINICAL PRACTICE 13.5

Rather than treatment, the focus for preterm brain injury is prevention while maximising normal brain growth. Prevention considers the impact of the ex-utero environment on the vulnerable developing brain, with care being provided in an approach that is neuroprotective. Neonatal nurses/midwives are in the optimal position to ensure that neuroprotective strategies are standard of care in neonatal intensive care units (NICUs), incorporating the domains:

- healing environment
- partner with families
- protect sleep
- pain and stress assessment and management
- optimal positioning and handling
- skin protection
- optimise nutrition.

Evidence for the impact of this type of care-giving approach has been the focus of much research and incorporation into clinical practice (Altimier & Phillips, 2018; Givrad et al., 2020; Murthy et al., 2020).

Outcomes are related to the site and complexity of the haemorrhage(s) and damage. Mortality is a major consequence of severe IVH/PHH: 30% for grade 3 IVH and 60% for grade 4 IVH (Ballabh & de Vries, 2021). Neonates with more-severe IVHs and white matter changes have increased risk of cognitive, behavioural, attentional and socialisation problems, along with motor deficits such as CP and epilepsy, whereas neonates with grades 1–2 IVH have been shown to have similar neurodevelopmental outcomes to those without haemorrhage. The risk of impairment increases for those with PHH. Significant differences between unilateral and bilateral grade 4 IVHs and PVL have been demonstrated regarding rates of CP, intellectual disability (ID), strabismus and visual impairment, and the development of seizure disorders. Poor brain growth (demonstrated by reduced brain volume at TEA) without specific injury (IVH/PVL/PHH) has also been shown to independently affect later cognitive function (Ballabh & de Vries, 2021).

PERINATAL STROKE

Strokes occur far more often during the perinatal period than at any other time in childhood. Perinatal stroke is caused by an acute vascular event that interrupts the blood supply to the brain. It can occur at any age from fetal life through to the 28th postnatal day and can be focal or multifocal. The incidence of perinatal stroke has been estimated to be 1 per 2300 births (Dunbar & Kirton, 2019); however, there is limited available epidemiological information regarding perinatal stroke in Australia and New Zealand. The type of stroke depends on the vessel affected and the aetiology of the vascular event (Fig. 13.15) (Dunbar & Kirton, 2019). The aetiology of perinatal stroke is outlined in Table 13.4.

Seizures are the most common clinical presentation, with other non-specific symptoms including poor feeding, cyanosis and unexplained tachypnoea or apnoea. Later

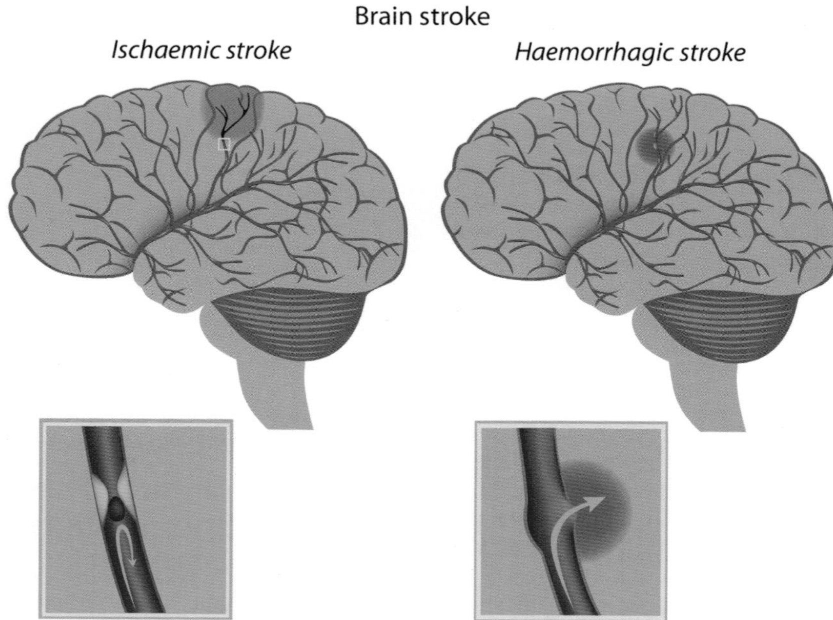

FIGURE 13.15 **Haemorrhagic and ischaemic stroke**
Source: Shutterstock/Alila Medical Media.

TABLE 13.4 **Aetiology of perinatal stroke**

Maternal causes	Placental causes	Neonatal causes
Autoimmune disorders Anticardiolipin antibodies Medications Coagulation disorders Cocaine usage Twin-to-twin transfusion syndrome	Placental thrombosis Placental abruption Fetomaternal haemorrhage Chorioamnionitis	Congenital heart disease AV malformation Homocysteine defect Blood disorders Hypoxia Organic acidaemias

AV, arteriovenous.

signs involve motor deficits or CP. Diagnosis is confirmed by MRI or CT scan (Dunbar & Kirton, 2019). Treatment of perinatal stroke in the acute setting is largely supportive and is aimed at managing symptoms. Anticoagulation or antiplatelet therapy should be considered only in the rare neonate at high risk of recurrence due to complex congenital heart disease or thrombophilia. There is no evidence of benefit from thrombolytics after stroke in neonates (Ferriero et al., 2019).

HYPOXIC ISCHAEMIC ENCEPHALOPATHY

Hypoxic ischaemic encephalopathy (HIE) is the result of any condition leading to decreased oxygen supply (hypoxia) and decreased blood supply (ischaemia), with resulting neural tissue destruction (Lee et al., 2017). This process evolves from the initial insult through to the recovery period.

HIE usually occurs following an acute episode that results in perinatal asphyxia: placental abruption, prolapsed cord, uterine rupture, acute blood loss or obstructed labour. It can also occur secondary to chronic or episodic conditions (e.g. placental insufficiency or cord compression) (Lee et al., 2017).

The areas of impact are gestation dependent: ischaemic events are more likely to involve the white matter between 26 and 34 weeks' gestation whereas for the term neonate the cortex, including the paracentral gyrus and motor cortex, known as the 'watershed areas', is the region affected (Lee et al., 2017).

Injury results from the initial insult, with both a primary and a secondary phase (Fig. 13.16). A window for neuroprotection exists between these two phases and will be discussed later in the chapter.

A standardised clinical descriptor of the stages of HIE, called the Sarnat staging system, has been in existence since the 1970s (Mrelashvili et al., 2020).

The clinical presentation of HIE is usually preceded by a history of severe depression and/or need for resuscitation, with respiratory and metabolic acidosis, low Apgar scores, abnormal neurological examination and abnormal cerebral function on EEG. Neurological symptoms follow with early and often refractory seizures, hypotonia, respiratory depression and apnoea and a decreased level of consciousness. The subsequent multiorgan dysfunction occurs as a result of the 'diving reflex', where blood is redirected to protect vital organs (brain, heart, lungs), at the expense of less-vital organs (kidneys, gastrointestinal tract, liver). This can present

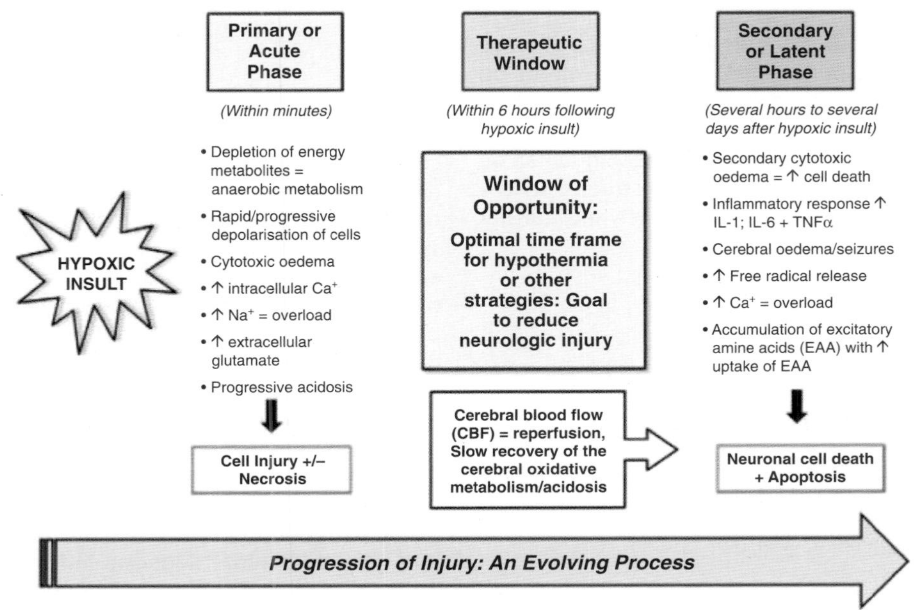

FIGURE 13.16 **Pathophysiology of hypoxic ischaemic encephalopathy**

Source: Newnam and DeLoach (2011).

as a combination of renal failure, decreased cardiac function and hypotension, disseminated intravascular coagulation and clotting abnormalities and liver dysfunction. Definitive diagnosis is made following the clinical presentation, with a combination of cranial ultrasound, EEG and MRI including diffusion-weighted imaging (a technique that uses the diffusion of water molecules), which is considered the gold standard at 5–7 days following the initial insult (Ouwehand et al., 2020).

Goals for management involve adequate ventilation; supporting perfusion; preventing hypotension, hypoxia and acidosis; avoiding rapid alterations in systemic blood pressure (therefore CBF); minimising severe apnoeic and bradycardic events; neurological observation; fluid restriction for limiting cerebral oedema and alterations in renal function; and treatment of seizure activity.

Therapeutic hypothermia has become the standard of care for term neonates with HIE stage 2 and above (Sarnat staging). The mechanism for neuroprotection using hypothermia includes decreased rate of cellular death, decreased cellular metabolism, conservation of adenosine triphosphate (ATP) stores and limitation of free radical release in the recovery phase. Cooling is provided to any neonate of >35 weeks' gestational age (GA), who meets several predefined criteria related to HIE (Mietzsch et al., 2020):

- within 6 hours of birth
- severe acidosis (ph <7.15, base excess <−10)
- 10-minute Apgar ≤5
- assisted ventilator support continued until 10 minutes of age
- acute perinatal event.

Cooling was originally applied to either the whole body or selectively just the head; however, whole-body cooling is more effective and is now standard clinical practice. Core body temperatures are reduced to a predetermined range (usually ≈33–34°C) for 48–72 hours, followed by a gradual, controlled rewarming period of 12–24 hours (Montaldo et al., 2019). Passive cooling, with down-regulating or turning off the radiant warmer and ensuring the neonate's core temperature does not fall below the set range, can be commenced in a non-tertiary setting as instructed by the retrieval team where cooling criteria are met, and transfer to the tertiary setting is in progress.

CLINICAL PRACTICE 13.6

Active cooling is applied by local preference with either:

- cooling mat
- cold fridge packs to the neonate's head/torso.

Monitoring required includes:

- cardiorespiratory and pulse oximetry
- continuous rectal temperature
- skin temperature probe may also be utilised.

Possible complications of cooling involve haemodynamic changes (decreased heart rate, stroke volume and, therefore, cardiac output), pulmonary hypertension, renal impairment, acid–base and electrolyte imbalances and coagulation abnormalities, although these are reversible following temperature normalisation.

HIE has a high burden of mortality and morbidity. It accounts for 23–25% of all neonatal deaths, is the leading cause of all brain injury in the perinatal period and is a major contributor to neonatal seizures in term neonates. HIE has a high mortality and morbidity rate, with outcomes largely dependent on the severity and length of the initial insult, postnatal management and other contributing factors, including fetal maturity (Greco et al., 2020). Cerebral palsy is the most common complication (10–15% of survivors) because of the motor cortex involvement, along with the risk of cognitive dysfunction, memory impairments, developmental delay, behavioural problems, autism and epilepsy (Schreglmann et al., 2020).

EVIDENCE-BASED PRACTICE RESEARCH 13.2

A Cochrane systematic review of therapeutic hypothermia in the neonate (Jacobs et al., 2013), including 11 randomised controlled trials (RCTs), demonstrated a reduction in mortality with no increase in major disability in those with moderate to severe HIE.

EVIDENCE-BASED PRACTICE RESEARCH 13.3

Potential neuroprotective therapies currently under investigation in clinical trials include erythropoietin, hyperbaric oxygen therapy, topiramate, caffeine, magnesium sulfate, xenon, allopurinol and stem cell transplantation (Ahmed et al., 2021; Juul et al., 2018; Rüegger et al., 2018; Tsuji et al., 2020).

MENINGITIS

Meningitis is infection of the meninges (dura, arachnoid and pia mater) that protect and cover the brain and spinal cord. The infective organism can be bacterial, viral or fungal (Bundy & Noor, 2020). Infection begins by colonisation of the nasopharyngeal mucosa or bacteraemia from a systemic infection. This can spread via physical barriers and through the blood–brain barrier. Bacteria invade the meninges through the endothelium of the choroid plexus and meningeal capillaries, resulting in hyperaemia of blood vessels, which increases the permeability of the blood–brain barrier (Bundy & Noor, 2020). Alternatively, following neurosurgical procedures, nosocomial infections can directly enter the subarachnoid space. The infective organisms can then proliferate, as CSF contains low levels of immunoglobulins and complement components, which results in poor opsonisation and phagocytosis. Replication and lysis of bacteria trigger an inflammation cascade in both the CSF and the subarachnoid space, resulting in meningeal inflammation. The inflammation and breakdown products lead to neuronal injury and hydrocephalus, vasculitis, abscess formation and/or increased intracranial pressure (ICP), which causes decreased cerebral perfusion pressure and ischaemia. Prognosis is dependent upon the severity of disease at presentation, plus time to treatment. Mortality is dependent on age, with potential neurological sequelae in up to 50% of survivors (Bundy & Noor, 2020; Xu et al., 2019) including:

- sensorineural hearing loss
- seizures
- hydrocephalus
- developmental disorders
- neuropsychological impairment.

CASE STUDY

13.1

Part 1

A male neonate was born via a normal vaginal birth at 31^4 weeks' gestation to a primigravida G1P0. The pregnancy had been unremarkable and was considered low risk; therefore, management was provided through a non-tertiary hospital.

The mother presented in spontaneous labour, with preterm rupture of membranes, retrospectively identified as occurring up to 1 week prior to the birth. A dose of steroids was administered, but the neonate was delivered via NVD within a few hours. He was in good condition at birth, with Apgar scores of 8–9, and required CPAP only. His birthweight was 1900 g.

He was intubated by the transfer team for desaturations and apnoeic episodes. His initial blood gas demonstrated a mixed acidosis, with pH 7.15, $PaCo_2$ 72, HCO^{3-} 23, base excess −4.2 and lactate 6.6. He received ×1 dose of surfactant and was loaded with caffeine citrate. A normal saline 0.9% bolus, 10 mL/kg, was administered. Blood cultures and inflammatory markers were taken, and he was given IV antibiotics (benzylpenicillin and gentamicin). He received his birth injections (vitamin K and hepatitis B vaccine). He was transferred to a tertiary NICU for ongoing management.

1 What would your list of differential diagnoses be at this stage?

Placental histology was subsequently found to be consistent with chorioamnionitis, and initial blood cultures grew *E. coli*. He developed generalised tonic–clonic clinical seizures on day 1, with associated electrical seizure activity on EEG monitoring. He required phenobarbitone, phenytoin and midazolam to control his seizure activity, which was no longer evident by day 3 of life.

2 Consider how you would expect this presentation to affect treatment decisions.

He was treated with intravenous (IV) cefotaxime for 3 weeks, despite a negative culture on lumbar puncture, but elevated white cell counts in the CSF. He was successfully extubated to CPAP by day 8 of life, and was self-ventilating in room air by day 10 of life. He was also treated for hypotension, coagulopathy and hyperglycaemia, thought to be secondary to the sepsis/meningitis.

An MRI was performed by 2 weeks of age, demonstrating abnormal periventricular white matter changes in the frontal and parieto-occipital regions, bilaterally consistent with areas of gliosis, which held unknown clinical significance. There were also abnormal signals within the basal ganglia bilaterally and evidence of a previous IVH, without ventricular dilation. His head circumferences were tracking appropriately, and his neurological presentation was normal.

Enteral feeds were slowly introduced, and he was tolerating 3-hourly nasogastric tube feeds of fortified EBM, when he was transferred back to a level 2 special care nursery for ongoing establishment of oral feeds and growth at approximately 35 weeks' corrected gestational age (CGA). He had no retinopathy of prematurity (ROP) and no osteopenia of prematurity. He was ready for discharge home at 36 weeks' CGA.

3 Consider the discharge education for this family.

CEREBRAL PALSY

Cerebral palsy (CP), the most common physical disability in childhood, is an umbrella term describing a group of motor disorders that occur as a result of injury to the developing brain. The majority of brain injuries occur in the perinatal period (94%); however, CP can occur in early childhood. Recently published data report the prevalence of CP has decreased in Australia from 2 per 1000 live births to 1.4 per 1000 live births, and the severity of cerebral palsy has also decreased (Australian Cerebral Palsy Register, 2018). Prematurity and low birthweight are known risk factors for CP; within an ANZNN report (Chow et al., 2021), 7.4% of infants assessed at 18 months of age had this condition. For many neonates, the complete causal pathway to CP is unclear, but it is often associated with factors including birth asphyxia, congenital infections, birth defects, sentinel events such as acute and sustained fetal bradycardia, head trauma or cerebral infarctions. Associated impairments include epilepsy, speech, vision, hearing impairments and intellectual impairment (Australian Cerebral Palsy Register, 2018).

Cerebral palsy is classified into four predominant types: spastic (85%), dyskinetic (6%), ataxic (5%) and hypotonic (3%).

The average age of diagnosis of CP is 18 months; however, earlier identification is desirable, as the optimal time for neuroplasticity and early intervention is in the young infant. Recently, there has been a shift in focus from a referral for early intervention with a confirmed diagnosis of CP to 'at risk' of CP. This has been related to the implementation of the general movements (GMs) assessment into clinical practice in neonatal units. The

GMs assessment evaluates the quality of movement in infants to approximately 5 months' post-term age and is a strong predictor of CP in the preterm neonate. Increasing evidence supports the value of this in improving outcomes.

EVIDENCE-BASED PRACTICE RESEARCH 13.4

A study on early intervention using a motor-learning environmental enrichment program for children with CP has shown significant improvement compared with control infants (Novak et al., 2017).

Cerebral palsy is a lifelong condition and parents require candid information regarding the outcomes, support available and the future for their children. Families should be referred to CP-specific services such as the Cerebral Palsy Alliance.

CLINICAL PRACTICE 13.7

All neonates in the neonatal unit should have a GM assessment, and those with a suspected brain injury should have an MRI.

If identified as 'at high risk of CP', immediate referral for early intervention is recommended.

NEONATAL NURSING/ MIDWIFERY CONSIDERATIONS

Specific neonatal nursing/midwifery care related to the neonate with neurological disorders includes the monitoring of treatment efficacy and therapy complications and evaluating of abnormal neurological signs, levels of consciousness and/or seizure activity (see Chapter 3). This includes neurological observations and careful monitoring of vital signs, oxygen saturations, blood gases, blood pressure, tone and activity. It is important to reduce environmental stressors, such as noise and light, as these neonates may have heightened sensitivity (see Chapter 22). Low levels of consciousness and reduced activity also place these neonates at high risk of pressure areas and skin breakdown, so careful management is required (see Chapter 19). Assessing pain in a neonate with a neurological condition is particularly challenging to both staff and parents, as the neonate's perception of pain and ability to communicate that experience may be severely altered, but it is imperative that adequate analgesia and non-pharmacological support, such as positioning, are maintained (see Chapter 18).

Family involvement is central to neonatal nursing/midwifery care, and detailed strategies are outlined in Chapter 21. However, the neonate with an abnormal neurological state, and often in a critical medical condition, can be extremely challenging for parents to cope with. Involving parents in the care of their infant as much as possible may require intense neonatal nursing/midwifery support and education to teach and enable parents to appropriately handle and interact with their baby. Ensuring that parents understand their infant's condition and prognosis on a day-to-day basis and identifying the family that has not been adequately counselled by members of the multidisciplinary team are valuable elements of the bedside neonatal nurse's/midwife's role. Parents need to have questions answered in a timely, sensitive and understandable manner, and recognition of parental concerns about their often very unwell, and sometimes palliative, infant's immediate and long-term prognosis is a key element of the neonatal nursing/midwifery role.

REFLECTION

Every neonate is at risk of abnormal neurological sequelae, regardless of gestation and risk factors. Abnormal findings on clinical presentation can be subtle and difficult to identify, but their identification is imperative for prompt management and appropriate treatment.

Care of the parents is also vital to support and achieve best outcomes for every neonatal patient, especially those whose prognosis is likely to be poor and needs are complex.

What can neonatal nurses/midwives teach parents about optimising their infant's neurodevelopment while in the neonatal unit and following discharge?

CASE STUDY 13.1

Part 2

The male infant re-presented to the local emergency department 2 days later with irritability, hypothermia, tachycardia and a 1-day history of poor feeding with weight loss. He was commenced on broad-spectrum IV antibiotics (flucloxacillin and gentamicin) with mildly elevated inflammatory markers, and transfer to a tertiary NICU was organised. He deteriorated quickly throughout the transfer and presented to the receiving NICU in septic shock. He required intubation for respiratory acidosis, hypoxia and apnoea. He received several normal saline 0.9% boluses, 10 mL/kg, and inotropic support for hypotension. He received packed red blood cells (PRBC) for volume expansion and both fresh frozen plasma (FFP) and platelets for a coagulopathy and thrombocytopenia. Metronidazole was also added to his antibiotic regimen, until serial abdominal X-rays (AXR) ruled out necrotising enterocolitis (NEC), and his remaining cover was initially changed to vancomycin and cefotaxime. His blood and CSF cultures were positive for *E. coli*, and he received a 6-week course of IV cefotaxime. He also required morphine and paracetamol for analgesia throughout the acute phase of this deterioration.

1 Reflect on your priorities of care (don't forget the family!).

He was again successfully extubated to CPAP and then self-ventilating in air within 10 days of this acute episode. Enteral feeds were able to be reintroduced, and he quickly tolerated full feeds; however, oral feeds were not initially tolerated. Serial CrUSS and MRI imaging demonstrated development of ventriculitis and abscess formation, as well as bilateral watershed infarcts due to ischaemia. There was no evidence of ventricular obstruction or development of hydrocephalus. Formal EEG also found abnormal tracing, consistent with his clinical presentation. He also began to demonstrate poor head growth. He now presented with abnormal increased tone and movements in all limbs and back arching, but not thought to be seizures. He also had ongoing difficulty with maintenance of normal temperatures.

Significant concerns throughout his inpatient stay were raised because of poor attendance and contact from family. There was considerable distress expressed by the parents, and development of anxiety and depression. Discharge planning was complicated by concerns regarding the parents' ability to care for him and his increased medical needs.

2 What long-term concerns would you have for this infant?

3 What interventions could be provided?

CONCLUSION

This chapter provides a synopsis of some neonatal neurological conditions. Caring for neonates with a neurological condition requires great skill and knowledge, with clinical care based on the best evidence and neonatal nursing/midwifery practice as outlined in the Australian College of Neonatal Nurses (ACNN), the Neonatal Nurses College of Aotearoa (NNCA) *Standards for neonatal nursing practice* and the Council of International Neonatal Nurses (COINN) competency framework (ACNN, 2019; Jones & COINN Working Group, 2019; NNCA, 2015).

The neurodevelopmental outcomes for neonates with neurological conditions are a great source of concern for parents, and neonatal nurses/midwives are integral in providing support and accurate information to parents.

Online Resources

Australian and New Zealand Neonatal Network: <https://www.anznn.net/>

Cerebral Palsy Alliance: <https://www.cerebralpalsy.org.au>

Cerebral Palsy Society: <https://www.cerebralpalsy.org.nz>

Neonatal encephalopathy consensus statement from the Newborn Clinical Network: <https://www.starship.org.nz/guidelines/neonatal-encephalopathy-consensus-statement-from-the-newborn-clinical/>

References/Acknowledgements

Abend, N. S., Jensen, F. E., Inder, T. E., & Volpe, J. J. (2018). Neonatal seizures. In: J. J. Volpe, T. E. Inder, B. T. Darras, A. J. du Plessis, J. J. Neil, & J. M. Perlman (Eds.), *Volpe's neurology of the newborn* (6th ed., pp. 275–321). Philadelphia, PA: Elsevier.

Ahmed, J., Ak, P. S., Robertson, N. J., & More, K. (2021). Melatonin for neuroprotection in neonatal encephalopathy: a systematic review & meta-analysis of clinical trials. *European Journal of Paediatric Neurology, 31*, 38–45. doi: 10.1016/j.ejpn.2021.02.003.

Altimier, L., & Phillips, R. (2018). Neuroprotective care of extremely preterm infants in the first 72 hours after birth. *Critical Care Nursing Clinics, 30*(4), 563–583.

Anand, V., & Nair, P. M. C. (2014). Neonatal seizures: predictors of adverse outcome. *Journal of Pediatric Neurosciences, 9*(2), 97–99. doi: 10.4103/1817-1745.139261.

Australian Cerebral Palsy Register. (2018). *Report of the Australian Cerebral Palsy Register birth years 1995–2012.* <https://cpregister.com/wp-content/uploads/2019/02/Report-of-the-Australian-Cerebral-Palsy-Register-Birth-Years-1995-2012.pdf> (Accessed 3 March 2022).

Australian College of Neonatal Nursing (ACNN). (2019). *Australian standards for neonatal nurses* (4th ed.). Camperdown, NSW: ACNN. <https://www.acnn.org.au/resources/resources/ACNN-Standards-for-Practice-4th-Ed.pdf> (Accessed 3 March 2022).

Australian Institute of Health and Welfare (AIHW) National Perinatal Statistics Unit. (2016). *Monitoring the health impacts of mandatory folic acid and iodine fortification 2016.* <https://www.aihw.gov.au/reports/food-nutrition/monitoring-health-impacts-of-mandatory-folic-acid/contents/table-of-contents> (Accessed 3 March 2022).

Aygün, E., Ertürk, E. Y., Sayman, Ö. A., & Tiryaki, F. K. (2020). Evaluation of etiological, clinical and laboratory findings in infants with prolonged jaundice. *Biomedical Journal of Scientific & Technical Research, 31*. doi: 10.26717/BJSTR.2020.31.005151.

Baker, S. R. (2014). *Local flaps in facial reconstruction* (3rd ed.). Philadelphia, PA: Saunders Elsevier.

Ballabh, P., & de Vries, L. S. (2021). White matter injury in infants with intraventricular haemorrhage: mechanisms and therapies. *Nature Reviews: Neurology, 27*, 1–6.

Blackburn, S. (2016). Brain injury in preterm infants: pathogenesis and nursing implications. *Newborn and Infant Nursing Reviews*, *16*(1), 8–12.

Blencowe, H., Kancherla, V., Moorthie, S., Darlison, M. W., & Modell, B. (2018). Estimates of global and regional prevalence of neural tube defects for 2015: a systematic analysis. *Annals of the New York Academy of Sciences, 1414*(1), 31–46.

Bock, H. C., Feldmann, J., & Ludwig, H. C. (2018). Early surgical management and long-term surgical outcome for intraventricular hemorrhage–related posthemorrhagic hydrocephalus in shunt-treated premature infants. *Journal of Neurosurgery: Pediatrics, 22*(1), 61–67.

Bundy, L. M., & Noor, A. (2020). Neonatal meningitis. In: *StatPearls*. Treasure Island, FL: StatPearls Publishing. <https://www.statpearls.com/articlelibrary/viewarticle/25670/> (Accessed 3 March 2022).

Colditz, M. J., Lai, M. M., Cartwright, D. W., & Colditz, P. B. (2015). Subgaleal haemorrhage in the newborn: a call for early diagnosis and aggressive management. *Journal of Paediatrics and Child Health, 51*(2), 140–146.

Chow, S. S. W., Creighton, P., Chambers, G. M., & Lui, K. (2021). *Report of the Australian and New Zealand Neonatal Network 2019*. Sydney, NSW: ANZNN.

Copp, A. J., Adzick, N. S., Chitty, L. S., Fletcher, J. M., Holmbeck, G. N., & Shaw, G. M. (2015). *Nature Reviews. Disease Primers, 1*, 15007, Figure 1.

D'Antoine, H., & Bower, C. (2019). Folate status and neural tube defects in Aboriginal Australians: the success of mandatory fortification in reducing a health disparity. *Current Developments in Nutrition, 3*(8), nzz071.

Devakumar, D., Bamford, A., Ferreira, M. U., Broad, J., Rosch, R. E., Groce, N., et al. (2018). Infectious causes of microcephaly: epidemiology, pathogenesis, diagnosis, and management. *Lancet – Infectious Diseases, 18*(1), e1–e3.

Dubois, J., Benders, M., Cachia, A., Lazeyras, F., Ha-Vinh Leuchter, R., Sizonenko, S. V., et al. (2008). Mapping the early cortical folding process in the preterm newborn brain. *Cerebral Cortex, 18*, 1444–1454.

Dunbar, M., & Kirton, A. (2019). Perinatal stroke. *Seminars in Pediatric Neurology, 32*, 100767. doi: 10.1016/j.spen.2019.08.003.

Ferriero, D. M., Fullerton, H. J., Bernard, T. J., Billinghurst, L., Daniels, S. R., DeBaun, M. R., et al. (2019). Management of stroke in neonates and children: a scientific statement from the American Heart Association/American Stroke Association. *Stroke, 50*(3), e51–e96.

Gilard, V., Chadie, A., Ferracci, F. X., Brasseur-Daudruy, M., Proust, F., Marret, S., et al. (2018). Post hemorrhagic hydrocephalus and neurodevelopmental outcomes in a context of neonatal intraventricular hemorrhage: an institutional experience in 122 preterm children. *BMC Pediatrics, 18*(1), 1–8.

Givrad, S., Hartzell, G., & Scala, M. (2021). Promoting infant mental health in the neonatal intensive care unit (NICU): a review of nurturing factors and interventions for NICU infant-parent relationships. *Early Human Development,* 154, 105281. doi: 10.1016/j.earlhumdev.2020.105281.

Glass, H. C., Grinspan, Z. M., & Shellhaas, R. A. (2018). Outcomes after acute symptomatic seizures in neonates. *Seminars in Fetal and Neonatal Medicine, 23*(3), 218–222.

Greco, P., Nencini, G., Piva, I., Scioscia, M., Volta, C. A., Spadaro, S., et al. (2020). Pathophysiology of hypoxic–ischemic encephalopathy: a review of the past and a view on the future. *Acta Neurologica Belgica, 120*(2), 277–288.

Högberg, U., Andersson, J., Squier, W., Högberg, G., Fellman, V., Thiblin, I., et al. (2018). Epidemiology of subdural haemorrhage during infancy: a population-based register study. *PLoS One, 13*(10), e0206340.

Högberg, U., Fellman, V., Thiblin, I., Karlsson, R., & Wester, K. (2020). Difficult birth is the main contributor to birth-related fracture and accidents to other neonatal fractures. *Acta Paediatrica, 109*(10), 2040–2048.

Hong, H. S., & Lee, J. Y. (2018). Intracranial hemorrhage in term neonates. *Child's Nervous System, 34*(6), 1135–1143.

Horton, C., Byrd, L., Lucht, H., & Higby, N. (2012). Emergency care of children with high-technology neurologic disorders. *Clinical Pediatric Emergency Medicine, 13*(2), 114–124.

Ibrahim, J., Mir, I., & Chalak, L. (2018). Brain imaging in preterm infants <32 weeks gestation: a clinical review and algorithm for the use of cranial ultrasound and qualitative brain MRI. *Pediatric Research, 84*(6), 799–806.

Inder, T. E., Perlman, J. M., & Volpe, J. J. (2018). Intracranial hemorrhage: subdural, subarachnoid, intraventricular (term infant), miscellaneous. In: J. J. Volpe, T. E. Inder, B. T. Darras, A. J. du Plessis, J. J. Neil, & J. M. Perlman (Eds.), *Volpe's neurology of the newborn* (6th ed., pp. 593–622). Philadelphia, PA: Elsevier.

Jacobs, S. E., Berg, M., Hunt, R., Tarnow-Mordi, W. O., Inder, T. E., & Davis, P. G. (2013). Cooling for newborns with hypoxic ischaemic encephalopathy. *Cochrane Database of Systematic Reviews, 1*, CD003311. doi: 10.1002/14651858.CD003311.pub3.

Jones, T., & COINN Working Group. (2019). International neonatal nursing competency framework. *Journal of Neonatal Nursing*, 25(5), 258–264. <https://www.healthynewbornnetwork.org/hnn-content/uploads/International-Neonatal-Nursing-Competency-Framework.pdf> (Accessed 16 March 2022).

Jung, J., Lam, J., deSouza, R. M., Anderson, I., & Chumas, P. (2018). Craniosynostosis. *Advances in Clinical Neuroscience and Rehabilitation, 18*(2), 5–11.

Juul, S. E., Comstock, B. A., Heagerty, P. J., Mayock, D. E., Goodman, A. M., Hauge, S., et al. (2018). High-dose erythropoietin for asphyxia and encephalopathy (HEAL): a randomized controlled trial – background, aims, and study protocol. *Neonatology, 113*(4), 331–338.

Kadivar, M., Moghadam, E. M., Badv, R. S., Sangsari, R., & Saeedy, M. (2019). A comparison of conventional electroencephalography with amplitude-integrated EEG in detection of neonatal seizures. *Medical Devices (Auckland, NZ), 12*, 489.

Kalmin, M. M., Gower, E. W., Stringer, E. M., Bowman, N. M., Rogawski McQuade, E. T., & Westreich, D. (2019). Misclassification in defining and diagnosing microcephaly. *Paediatric and Perinatal Eepidemiology, 33*(4), 286–290.

Kellogg, R., Lee, P., Deibert, C. P., Tempel, Z., Zwagerman, N. T., Bonfield, C. M., et al. (2018). Twenty years' experience with myelomeningocele management at a single institution: lessons learned. *Journal of Neurosurgery: Pediatrics, 13*, 22(4), 439–443.

Kooi, E. M., Verhagen, E. A., Elting, J. W., Czosnyka, M., Austin, T., Wong, F. Y., et al. (2017). Measuring cerebrovascular autoregulation in preterm infants using near-infrared spectroscopy: an overview of the literature. *Expert Review of Neurotherapeutics, 17*(8), 801–818.

Lee, W. L., Michael-Titus, A. T., & Shah, D. K. (2017). Hypoxic–ischaemic encephalopathy and the blood–brain barrier in neonates. *Developmental Neuroscience, 39*(1–4), 49–58.

Lenroot, R. K., & Giedd, J. N. (2006). Brain development in children and adolescents: insights from anatomical magnetic resonance imaging. *Neuroscience and Biobehavioural Reviews, 30*, 718–729.

Mietzsch, U., Radhakrishnan, R., Boyle, F. A., Juul, S., & Wood, T. R. (2020). Active cooling temperature required to achieve therapeutic hypothermia correlates with short-term outcome in neonatal hypoxic–ischaemic encephalopathy. *Journal of Physiology, 598*(2), 415–424.

Montaldo, P., Lally, P. J., Oliveira, V., Swamy, R., Mendoza, J., Atreja, G., et al. (2019). Therapeutic hypothermia initiated within 6 hours of birth is associated with reduced brain injury on MR biomarkers in mild hypoxic–ischaemic encephalopathy: a non-randomised cohort study. *Archives of Disease in Childhood. Fetal and Neonatal Edition, 104*(5), F515–F520.

Mrelashvili, A., Russ, J. B., Ferriero, D. M., & Wusthoff, C. J. (2020). The Sarnat score for neonatal encephalopathy: looking back and moving forward. *Pediatric Research, 88*, 824–825.

Murphy, M. E., & Westmark, C. J. (2020). Folic acid fortification and neural tube defect risk: analysis of the Food Fortification Initiative Dataset. *Nutrients, 12*(1), 247.

Murthy, P., Zein, H., Thomas, S., Scott, J. N., Abou Mehrem, A., Esser, M. J., et al. (2020). Neuroprotection care bundle implementation to decrease acute brain injury in preterm infants. *Pediatric Neurology, 110*, 42–48.

Neonatal Nurses College of Aotearoa (NNCA). (2015). *NNCA standards for neonatal nursing practice*. Wellington: New Zealand Nurses Organisation. <https://www.nzno.org.nz/Portals/0/Files/Documents/Groups/Neonatal%20Nurses/2016-05-11%20Final%20draft%20Neonatal%20Nursing%20Standards%202015.pdf> (Accessed 3 March 2022).

Newnam, K., & DeLoach, D. (2011). Neonatal hypothermia, newborn and infant. *Nursing Reviews, 11*(3), 113–124.

Novak, C. M., Ozen, M., & Burd, I. (2018). Perinatal brain injury: mechanisms, prevention, and outcomes. *Clinics in Perinatology, 45*(2), 357–375.

Novak, I., Morgan, C., Adde, L., Blackman, J., Boyd, R. N., Brunstrom-Hernandez, J., et al. (2017). Early, accurate diagnosis and early intervention in cerebral palsy: advances in diagnosis and treatment. *Journal of the American Medical Association: Pediatrics, 171*(9), 897–907.

Ojumah, N., Ramdhan, R. C., Wilson, C., Loukas, M., Oskouian, R. J., & Tubbs, R. S. (2017). Neurological neonatal birth injuries: a literature review. *Cureus, 9*(12), e1938. doi: 10.7759/cureus.1938.

Ouwehand, S., Smidt, L. C., Dudink, J., Benders, M. J., de Vries, L. S., Groenendaal, F., et al. (2020). Predictors of outcomes in hypoxic-ischemic encephalopathy following hypothermia: a meta-analysis. *Neonatology, 117*(3), 271–287.

Peterson, M. D., Lin, P., Kamdar, N., Mahmoudi, E., Marsack-Topolewski, C. N., Haapala, H., et al. (2020). Psychological morbidity among adults with cerebral palsy and spina bifida. *Psychological Medicine, 27*, 1–8.

Pilu, G., Malinger, G., & Buyukkurt, S. (2013). Intracranial hemorrage. *Visual encyclopedia of ultrasound in obstetrics and gynecology*. <https://www.isuog.org/education/visuog.html> (Accessed 3 March 2022).

Pople, I. K. (2002). Hydrocephalus and shunts: what the neurologist should know. *Journal of Neurology, Neurosurgery, and Psychiatry, 73*, i17–i22.

Pressler, R. M., Cilio, M. R., Mizrahi, E. M., Moshé, S. L., Nunes, M. L., Plouin, P., et al. (2021). The ILAE classification of seizures and the epilepsies: modification for seizures in the neonate. Position paper by the ILAE Task Force on Neonatal Seizures. *Epilepsia, 62*(3), 615–628.

Ramantani, G., Schmitt, B., Plecko, B., Pressler, R. M., Wohlrab, G., Klebermass-Schrehof, K., et al. (2019). Neonatal seizures – are we there yet? *Neuropediatrics, 50*(5), 280–293.

Ranalli, N. J., Limbrick, D. D., & Park, T. S. (2020). Outcomes for the surgical management of Chiari I and Chiari II malformations. In: R. S. Tubbs, M. Turgut, & W. J. Oakes (Eds.), *The Chiari malformations* (pp. 515–525). Champaign, IL: Springer.

Rüegger, C. M., Davis, P. G., & Cheong, J. L. (2018). Xenon as an adjuvant to therapeutic hypothermia in near-term and term newborns with hypoxic–ischaemic encephalopathy. *Cochrane Database of Systematic Reviews, 8*(8), CD012753. doi: 10.1002/14651858.CD012753.pub2.

Sandoval, P. V., Rosales, P. H., Hernández, D. G., Naranjo, E. A., & Navarro, V. G. (2019). Intraventricular hemorrhage and posthemorrhagic hydrocephalus in preterm infants: diagnosis, classification, and treatment options. *Child's Nervous System, 35*(6), 917–927.

Schreglmann, M., Ground, A., Vollmer, B., & Johnson, M. J. (2020). Systematic review: long-term cognitive and behavioural outcomes of neonatal hypoxic–ischaemic encephalopathy in children without cerebral palsy. *Acta Paediatrica, 109*(1), 20–30.

Seruya, M., Magge, S., & Keating, R. (2012). Diagnosis and surgical options for craniosynostosis. In: R. G. Ellenbogen, S. Abdulrauf, & L. Sekhar (Eds.), *Principles of neurologic surgery* (3rd ed., p. 138). St Louis, MO: Saunders.

Shlobin, N. A., LoPresti, M. A., Du, R. Y., & Lam, S. (2020). Folate fortification and supplementation in prevention of folate-sensitive neural tube defects: a systematic review of policy. *Journal of Neurosurgery: Pediatrics, 27*(3), 294–310.

Smith, B. W., Daunter, A. K., Yang, L. J., & Wilson, T. J. (2018). An update on the management of neonatal brachial plexus palsy – replacing old paradigms: a review. *Journal of the American Medical Association: Pediatrics, 172*(6), 585–591.

Spaull, R., McPherson, B., Gialeli, A., Clayton, A., Uney, J., Heep, A., et al. (2019). Exosomes populate the cerebrospinal fluid of preterm infants with post-haemorrhagic hydrocephalus. *International Journal of Developmental Neuroscience, 73*, 59–65.

Talbert, D. (2016). Cerebral venous malformation as a cause of neonatal intra-ventricular haemorrhage and unexplained infant subdural haemorrhage. *Anatomy and Physiology, 6*, 202.

Tortora, D., Martinetti, C., Severino, M., Uccella, S., Malova, M., Parodi, A., et al. (2018). The effects of mild germinal matrix-intraventricular haemorrhage on the developmental white matter microstructure of preterm neonates: a DTI study. *European Radiology, 28*(3), 1157–1166.

Tsuji, M., Sawada, M., Watabe, S., Sano, H., Kanai, M., Tanaka, E., et al. (2020). Autologous cord blood cell therapy for neonatal hypoxic–ischaemic encephalopathy: a pilot study for feasibility and safety. *Scientific Reports, 10*(1), 1–10.

van Gool, J. D., Hirche, H., Lax, H., & De Schaepdrijver, L. (2018). Folic acid and primary prevention of neural tube defects: a review. *Reproductive Toxicology, 80*, 73–84.

van Tilborg, E., de Theije, C. G., van Hal, M., Wagenaar, N., de Vries, L. S., Benders, M. J., et al. (2018). Origin and dynamics of oligodendrocytes in the developing brain: implications for perinatal white matter injury. *Glia, 66*(2), 221–238.

Viswanathan, M., Treiman, K. A., Kish-Doto, J., Middleton, J. C., Coker-Schwimmer, E. J., & Nicholson, W. K. (2017). Folic acid supplementation for the prevention of neural tube defects: an updated evidence report and systematic review for the US Preventive Services Task Force. *Journal of the American Medical Association, 317*(2), 190–203.

Volpe, J. (2008). *Neurology of the newborn* (vol. 5). Philadelphia, PA: Saunders Elsevier.

Volpe, J. J. (2018). Injuries of extracranial, cranial, intracranial, spinal cord, and peripheral nervous system structures. In: J. J. Volpe, T. E. Inder, B. T. Darras, A. J. du Plessis, J. J. Neil, & J. M. Perlman (Eds.), *Volpe's neurology of the newborn* (6th ed., pp. 1093–1123). Philadelphia, PA: Elsevier.

Wilson, D., Kim, D., & Breibart, S. (2020). Intraventricular hemorrhage and posthemorrhagic ventricular dilation: current approaches to improve outcomes. *Neonatal Network, 39*(3), 158–169.

Xu, M., Hu, L., Huang, H., Wang, L., Tan, J., Zhang, Y., et al. (2019). Etiology and clinical features of full-term neonatal bacterial meningitis: a multicenter retrospective cohort study. *Frontiers in Pediatrics, 13*, 7, 31.

Yeo, K. T., Thomas, R., Chow, S. S., Bolisetty, S., Haslam, R., Tarnow-Mordi, W., et al. (2020). Improving incidence trends of severe intraventricular haemorrhages in preterm infants < 32 weeks gestation: a cohort study. *Archives of Disease in Childhood. Fetal and Neonatal Edition, 105*(2), 145–150.

CHAPTER 14

CARE OF THE NEONATE WITH A RENAL OR GENITOURINARY DISORDER

VICTORIA KAIN[a]

Learning objectives

After reading this chapter you will be able to:

- explain embryological development of the renal and genitourinary systems
- understand normal anatomy and physiology of the neonatal renal and genitourinary systems, including renal haemodynamic factors, factors influencing glomerular filtration rate and the kidney's role in acid–base homeostasis
- define the aetiology, pathophysiology, diagnosis, clinical presentation, medical, pharmacological and neonatal nursing/midwifery management and complications of common disorders of the neonatal renal and genitourinary systems
- undertake a systematic approach to a neonatal renal and genitourinary assessment
- understand the causes, manifestations and management of acute renal failure in the neonate
- explain the long-term outcome of the selected disorders.

Key words, terms and abbreviations

acute kidney injury (AKI)
acute renal failure (ARF)
dimercaptosuccinic acid scan (DMSA)
extracellular fluid (ECF)
glomerular filtration rate (GFR)
intracellular fluid (ICF)
low birthweight (LBW)
oliguria
renal blood flow (RBF)
urinary tract infection (UTI)

[a]The authors would like to acknowledge Kristen James Nunez and Kaye Spence, co-authors of this chapter in the 1st edition of this book.

INTRODUCTION

The fetal kidney is not required in utero for fluid and electrolyte homeostasis or toxin removal, as this is primarily the role of the placenta. However, postnatally the kidney must assume this role. Due to the relative immaturity of the renal system in the early neonatal period, renal function can be erratic and often difficult to manage. The delicate balance to maintain homeostasis is an essential component of the effective management of the neonate. Congenital abnormalities of the renal and genitourinary system can lead to further implications for this balance. Diligent diagnosis, assessment and management are crucial to prevent long-term sequelae and complications.

The aim of this chapter is to present information on some common disorders of the renal and genitourinary system that can affect fluid and electrolyte homeostasis, focusing on the renal and genitourinary system from embryonic development to neonatal presentation, assessment and diagnosis, through to treatment and long-term outcomes.

EMBRYOLOGICAL DEVELOPMENT

The development of the renal and genitourinary system begins in the second week of gestation, reaching functionality by 34 weeks' gestation. It is derived from the intermediate mesoderm ridge (intermediate mesoderm) in the posterior wall of the abdominal cavity. During the development of the embryo, three sets of excretory organs develop, the final set forming the permanent kidneys. The three sets are the:

1. *pronephros* (the rudimentary kidney) – a non-functioning structure that plays a primary role in normal organogenesis, appearing during the third week of gestation and degenerating by the fifth week, leaving a duct that is used by the next structure
2. *mesonephros* – originating during the fifth week of gestation (prior to degeneration of the pronephros) and contributing to urine production (consisting of 30 to 40 glomerulotubular units) but degenerating by the 11th to 12th week of gestation in females, and leaving only its caudal tubules to develop into the genital system in males, where these embryonic structures persist and develop into the epididymis, vas deferens, seminal vesicles and the ejaculatory duct
3. *metanephros* – (the permanent kidney) appearing in the fifth week of gestation and developing into the ureteric bud including the metanephric duct, which progresses to form the ureters, renal pelvis, the major and minor calyces and the collecting tubules, and the metanephric blastemal, which forms the nephrons (Rehman & Ahmed, 2021).

The definitive kidney develops in the sacral region, and ascends along the dorsal aorta up into the renal fossa in the lumbar region before rotating medially. By 9 weeks' gestation, the kidneys have taken up the adult, retroperitoneal position in the abdomen (Nicolaou et al., 2015).

Initial functionality of the kidneys develops by the 12th week of gestation, contributing urine to the amniotic fluid from the 14th week. They do not play a major excretory role in this early gestational period with the placenta functioning as the excretory organ. The kidney continues to develop forming nephrons (nephrogenesis) up to term, with approximately 1 million nephrons appearing by 34 to 36 weeks' gestation. After a preterm neonate is born, nephrogenesis continues at the same rate as it would in utero (Baum, 2020).

Development of the urinary tract occurs synchronously with the early stages of metanephric development, with the urinary bladder developing at approximately 6 weeks' gestation. Formation of the urethra is completed by the end of the first trimester, with the fetal ureter opening functionally into the bladder at the ninth week of gestation. The vascular pattern of the fetal kidney resembles that of the mature kidney by the 14th to 15th week of gestation; however, **renal blood flow (RBF)** in the fetus is low owing to high vascular resistance and low systemic blood pressure (Nicolaou et al., 2015).

RENAL ANATOMY

Kidneys

The kidneys, normally located between the transverse processes of the T12–L3 vertebrae, serve three main functions, including filtration and excretion of metabolic waste products (urea and ammonium); regulation of electrolytes, fluid and acid–base balance; and stimulation of red blood cell production. They also serve intermediate functions including regulation of blood pressure via the renin–angiotensin–aldosterone system and control of reabsorption of water to maintain intravascular volume. In addition, the kidneys reabsorb glucose and amino acids, and have hormonal functions via erythropoietin, calcitriol and vitamin D activation (Baum, 2016).

Structures of the kidney

The major structures of the kidney are shown in Fig. 14.1 and include the following:

- *Renal cortex*: the outermost portion of the kidney, the renal cortex contains the glomeruli, proximal and distal convoluted tubules and collecting ducts of the nephron.
- *Renal medulla*: located in the mid-section of the kidney, the medulla is formed by the straight segments of the proximal and distal tubules and the collecting ducts. It contains the renal pyramids, loops of Henle, vasa recta and terminal collecting ducts.
- *Renal sinus and pelvis*: the innermost part of the kidney, the renal sinus contains the uppermost part of the renal pelvis and calyces. It is surrounded by fat in which branches of the renal vessels and nerves are embedded (Dias et al., 2014).

NEPHRONS

The nephron is a tubular structure with subunits that include the renal corpuscle, proximal convoluted tubule,

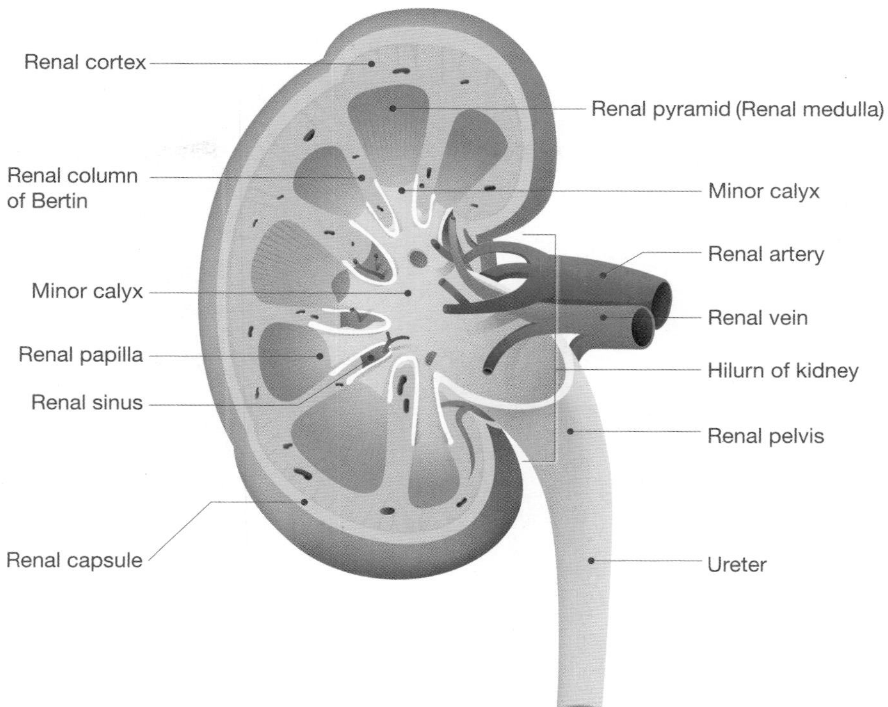

FIGURE 14.1 **Longitudinal section showing the internal structure of the kidney**
Source: iStock photo/solar22.

loop of Henle, distal convoluted tubule and the collecting ducts, all of which contribute to the formation of the final urine. Fig. 14.2 is a magnified wedge cut from a renal pyramid showing the nephron's structures and a schematic of the nephron including the blood supply and the tubules down to the collecting tubule. The kidney has three types of nephrons:

1. *superficial cortical nephrons* (85%), which extend only partially into the medulla
2. *mid-cortical nephrons*, with short or long loops
3. *juxtamedullary nephrons*, which lie close to and extend deep into the medulla and are important in the process of concentrating urine (Nicolaou et al., 2015).

Ureters

The urine produced by the nephrons flows from the distal tubules and collecting ducts through the duct of Bellini, the renal papillae and into the calyces and is collected in the renal pelvis. From the renal pelvis, urine is funnelled into the ureters. The lower ends of the ureters pass obliquely through the posterior aspect of the bladder wall. The close approximation of muscle cells permits the direct transmission of electrical stimulation with resulting peristaltic activity to propel the urine into the bladder (Boubred & Simeoni, 2018).

Bladder and urethra

The bladder is comprised of a weave of smooth muscle fibres that distend as the bladder fills with urine. In neonates, the bladder rises above the symphysis pubis before it settles in the adult position in the true pelvis. The urethra extends from the inferior side of the bladder to the outside of the body. Two muscles (sphincters) control the expulsion of urine from the bladder through the urethra (Ogobuiro & Tuma, 2021).

NEONATAL RENAL PHYSIOLOGY

During late gestation, the fetal kidneys are responsible for the maintenance of amniotic fluid volume. Urine output is approximately 10 mL/kg/h and the urine is high in sodium. At birth, dramatic and rapid physiological changes occur to ensure a successful transition from intrauterine to extrauterine physiology. While changes occurring in the respiratory and cardiovascular systems are immediate, slower adaptations occur within the renal system. The neonatal renal system responds slowly and erratically to the physiological demands placed on it, and transition to adult renal function evolves over a period of months to years (Boubred & Simeoni, 2018).

For successful transition to extrauterine life, homeostasis regulation transfers from the placenta to the neonatal kidney. Homeostasis is regulated through three fundamental functions: tubular function and water shifts, glomerular filtration rate and creatinine clearance, and is dependent on the development of RBF (Ogobuiro & Tuma, 2021).

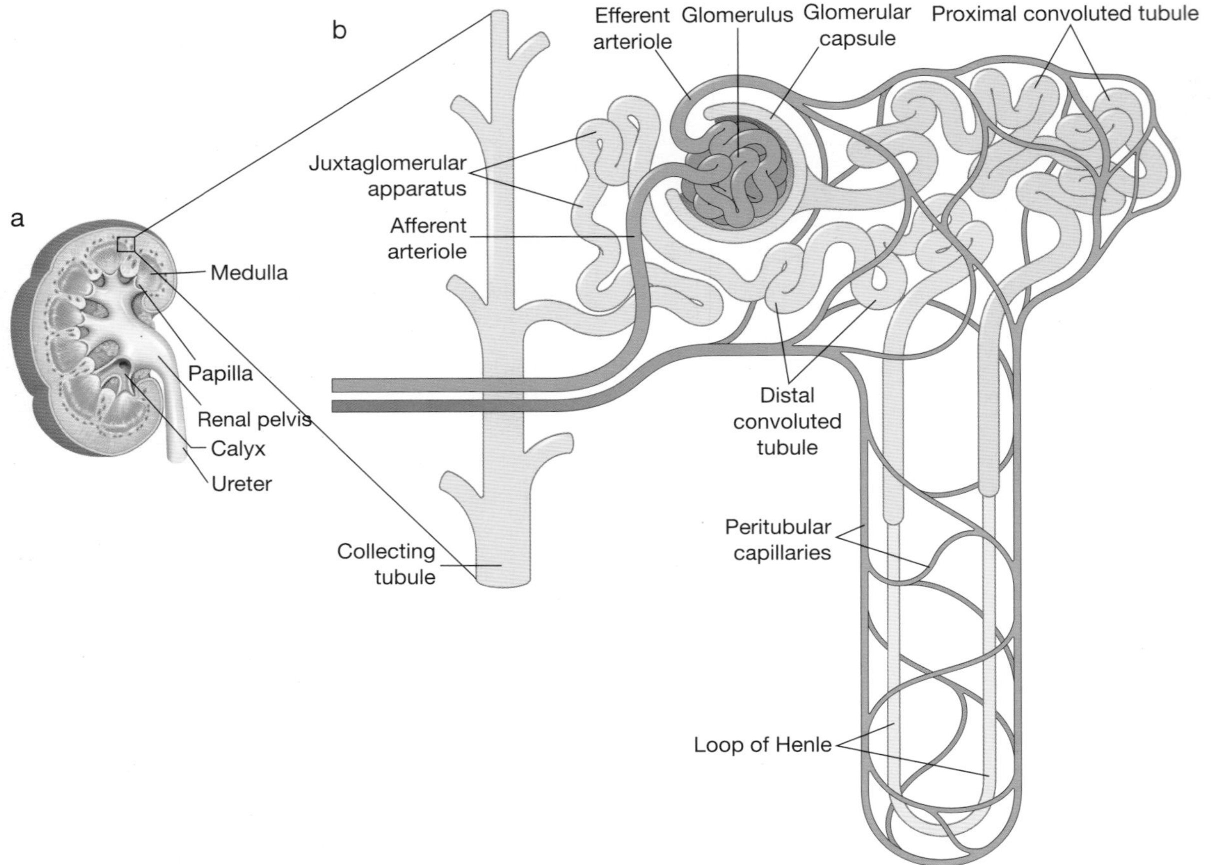

FIGURE 14.2 **a Magnified wedge cut from a renal pyramid showing the nephron's structures. b Schematic of the nephron including the blood supply and the tubules down to the collecting tubule**

Source: Craft, Gordon, Huether et al. (2019).

Tubular function and water shift

A physiological redistribution in body water occurs during the transition from intrauterine to extrauterine life. At birth, there is a shift of water and electrolytes from the **intracellular fluid (ICF)** to **extracellular fluid (ECF)** compartments, which causes the ECF compartment to become even more expanded. This fluid is then subsequently lost as the neonate experiences a physiological diuresis with subsequent weight loss. This redistribution of body water is referred to as 'contraction'. At term, 75% of bodyweight is water, and in the preterm neonate the water content is even higher at 85%. After this transition, the kidney's concentrating capacity increases and water loss is reduced (Filler et al., 2016).

In the immediate postnatal period, urine output may be less than 1 mL/kg/h; however, due to increased cardiac output and renal blood flow, output increases during the first 24 hours and peaks on day 3 to 5–7 mL/kg/h, decreasing to 1–3 mL/kg/h thereafter (Boubred & Simeoni, 2018).

Tubular reabsorption is the movement of substance from the filtrate into the tubule lumen as it moves back into the capillary system (Filler et al., 2016). Tubular function is altered in the newborn and matures more slowly than GFR. This process is even more delayed in preterm neonates, owing to combined tubular immaturity and reduced GFR, and contributes to impaired reabsorption of electrolytes, in particular sodium and potassium (Boubred, 2018).

Glomerular filtration rate

The **glomerular filtration rate (GFR)** refers to the flow rate of filtered fluid through the kidney. It is determined by the balance of Starling forces across the capillary wall, rate of plasma flow, permeability of the glomerular wall and total surface area of the capillaries (Ogobuiro & Tuma 2021).

A local mechanism in the kidney tends to keep the rate of glomerular perfusion and hence the GFR reasonably consistent over a range of arterial pressures between 80 and 180 mmHg. Afferent arteriolar pressure and resistance both change in the same direction. As a result, regardless of renal perfusion pressure, intrarenal blood flow and GFR are largely constant, a relationship maintained by an intrinsic autoregulatory myogenic process of contraction when blood vessels are stretched. The goal of autoregulation of intrarenal blood flow is to maintain RBF and GFR constant as systemic blood pressure rises or falls. Despite fluctuations in arterial pressure, solute and water excretion, and therefore blood volume, are regulated, and barotrauma is avoided in situations of high systemic blood pressure (McCance & Huether, 2018).

Tubuloglomerular feedback is a second mechanism of RBF and GFR autoregulation. Because the glomerular filtration rate in a single nephron changes in response to changes in arterial pressure, the macula densa cells of the juxtaglomerular apparatus in the distal tubule detect changes in the amount of filtered sodium. When GFR and salt concentrations fall, the macula densa cells improve GFR by stimulating afferent arteriolar vasodilation. Simultaneously, juxtaglomerular cells secrete renin, which causes angiotensin II release, resulting in vasoconstriction of the efferent arterioles and an increase in glomerular hydrostatic pressure and GFR. Increases in GFR and salt content at the macula densa have the opposite effect (see Fig. 14.3). This system keeps the body's water and salt levels stable (McCance & Huether, 2018).

Glomerular filtration is established during intrauterine life, but remains insignificant until birth when the kidney takes over function. The GFR is established immediately after birth, and variations in GFR are clinically relevant because they affect fluid and electrolyte homeostasis as well as excretion of drugs (Allegaert et al., 2020). Preterm neonates born before 34 weeks' gestation have a low GFR until nephrogenesis is complete at their equivalent to term gestation (Boubred & Simeoni, 2018).

Term neonates' GFR increases from approximately 5 mL/min/1.73 m^2 to 40 mL/min/1.73 m^2 in the first week of life. In the preterm infant of less than 34 weeks' gestation, the GFR remains constant at 0.5–1 mL/min/1.73 m^2, increasing by four to five times within a 1-week period once over 35 weeks' gestation, correlating with the completion of nephrogenesis (Nicolaou et al., 2015).

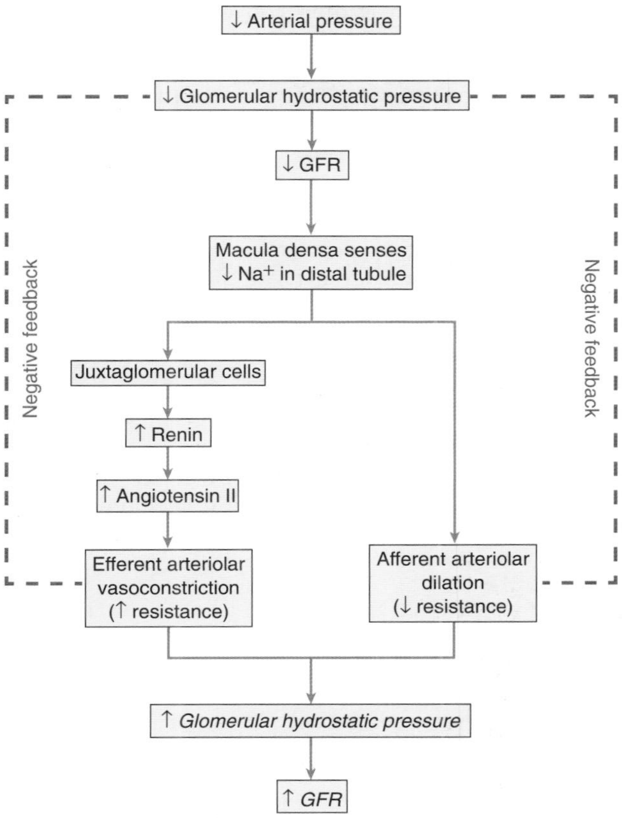

↓ Arterial pressure

↓ Glomerular hydrostatic pressure

↓ GFR

Macula densa senses ↓ Na^+ in distal tubule

Juxtaglomerular cells

↑ Renin

↑ Angiotensin II

Efferent arteriolar vasoconstriction (↑ resistance)

Afferent arteriolar dilation (↓ resistance)

↑ *Glomerular hydrostatic pressure*

↑ *GFR*

Negative feedback

Negative feedback

FIGURE 14.3 **Tubuloglomerular feedback**

GFR, glomerular filtration rate.

Source: McCance and Huether (2019).

EVIDENCE-BASED PRACTICE RESEARCH 14.1

The most common clinical factors for altered nephron numbers are **low birthweight (LBW)** (2500 g), intrauterine growth restriction (IUGR) and preterm birth (<37 weeks' gestational age), all of which are associated with an increased risk of hypertension, proteinuria and kidney disease later in life. The most-relevant strategy for evaluating the risk of future kidney diseases in newborn children with LBW, IUGR or premature birth is an indirect estimate of total nephron number based on postnatal indicators. However, according to current research, IUGR and preterm can both affect nephrogenesis and kidney function, and their effects tend to be cumulative if they occur concurrently (Grandi, 2021).

Creatinine clearance

Creatinine is a metabolic by-product that is freely filtered in the Bowman's space. Creatinine clearance is the volume of blood plasma that is cleared of creatinine per unit of time and is a useful measure, approximating the GFR. It is another important marker of renal function in the neonatal period (Filler et al., 2021). In term neonates, plasma creatinine falls over the first few days, from maternal creatinine to neonatal levels. The rate of this decrease can be quite variable depending on the neonate's hydration and clinical status. Preterm neonates under 34 weeks' gestation have little increase in creatinine clearance, which can be related to the immaturity of their renal system; however, this improves at 34 weeks' gestation with completion of nephrogenesis (Filler et al., 2021). It is important to note that a rising creatinine level is never normal when the neonate reaches 1 week of age or more and may be an important early clinical indicator of the presence of congenital disease (Filler et al., 2021).

Neonatal renal haemodynamic factors

Renal blood flow comprises 4–6% of the cardiac output during the first 12 hours of postnatal life and 8–10% of cardiac output during the first week of postnatal life. The rate of RBF is determined by the cardiac output and the ratio of renal to systemic vascular resistance. Developmental changes in these parameters contribute to the postnatal increase in renal blood flow. The primary factor responsible for this change is decreased renal vascular resistance (Khan et al., 2015).

Regulation of RBF is maintained by autoregulation through myogenic mechanisms (dilation and constriction of afferent arterioles in response to changes in vascular wall tension) and hormonal regulation through the renin–angiotensin–aldosterone system and prostaglandins (Khan et al., 2015).

Fluid and electrolyte balance

Water and electrolytes are vital components of physiological stability and are particularly pertinent in the newborn. Regulation of water and electrolytes in a neonate can be impaired owing to immaturity and/or lack of function, and can lead to significant morbidity if not detected and treated early (Boubred & Simeoni, 2018).

SODIUM BALANCE

Sodium is the major cation in ECF and is vital for the regulation of circulating blood volume, as well as weight gain and tissue growth, with sodium exchange predominantly completed in the distal tubules. The term neonate can filter and reabsorb sodium reasonably efficiently. The preterm neonate is less efficient at both filtering a delivered sodium load and reabsorbing filtered sodium, and this places them at greater risk of sodium imbalance (Boubred & Simeoni, 2019).

POTASSIUM BALANCE

Potassium is the principal intracellular cation and is required for the maintenance of the ICF volume. Potassium is freely filtered by the glomerulus and reabsorption occurs in the proximal tubules with the final concentration determined by its secretion in the distal tubules (Boubred & Simeoni, 2018).

CALCIUM BALANCE

Calcium balance in the body is maintained by a well-coordinated mechanism between the gastrointestinal tract, bone and the kidney. The kidney maintains calcium homeostasis by regulating its reabsorption throughout the nephron via various active and passive processes (Boubred & Simeoni, 2018).

PHOSPHORUS BALANCE

Phosphorus is regulated with calcium concordantly. It has an important role in bone structure and various metabolic processes. Renal excretion is the primary mechanism by which phosphorus is regulated in the body, which is controlled through the parathyroid hormone (Boubred & Simeoni, 2018).

GLUCOSE BALANCE

The kidneys play an important role in glucose homeostasis through gluconeogenesis, glucose uptake and utilisation and glucose reabsorption in the proximal renal tubules (Boubred & Simeoni, 2018).

Acid–base balance

Acid–base balance is regulated by a combination of the respiratory, buffer and renal systems. The buffer systems are the primary mechanism for maintaining acid–base balance in the newborn; however, the kidney is involved in regulating the plasma bicarbonate balance by reabsorbing filtered bicarbonate and affecting hydrogen ion secretion through the formation of titratable acids and ammonium (Boubred & Simeoni, 2018). (See Chapter 9 for more information about acid–base balance.)

Maintenance of the renin–angiotensin–aldosterone axis

The renin–angiotensin system is responsible for blood pressure regulation, renal haemodynamic parameters and fluid and electrolyte balance. Renin is a crucial component of the system that is produced in the kidney by juxtaglomerular cells and stimulates the synthesis of angiotensin I, which is then converted to angiotensin II (ATII) by angiotensin-converting enzyme (Boubred & Simeoni, 2018). Intrarenal effects of ATII include regulation of renal function through primary vasoconstriction of renal vasculature, which, in conjunction with aldosterone, can modulate reabsorption of sodium and water by the kidney.

COMMON DISORDERS

This chapter focuses on postnatal renal and genitourinary disorders – congenital disorders are covered in Chapter 17. See Table 14.1 for a summary of presentation and investigation pathways.

Urinary tract infection

Urinary tract infection (UTI) is the most common bacterial infection in febrile neonates, and is defined as an infection of the kidney and/or bladder. The overall occurrence of UTI is higher in preterm newborns than in term infants. The incidence of UTI increases with postnatal

TABLE 14.1 **Summary of presentation and investigation pathways**

Condition	Postnatal presentation	Renal function (↑ creatinine)	Electrolyte disturbance	Outflow obstruction	Investigations
Acute renal failure	✓	✓	✓	–	Ultrasonography
Renal vein thrombosis	✓	✓	✓	✓	Doppler ultrasonography
Urinary tract infection	✓	✓	✓	✓	Ultrasonography DMSA

DMSA, dimercaptosuccinic acid scan

age in both groups, ranging from 1–2% in the first 72 hours after birth to 25% thereafter. As a result, urine cultures are not routinely performed in newborns with early-onset sepsis. UTI in preterm newborns can occur as a result of bacteraemia, but it can also occur as a result of a primary infection in the urinary tract, leading to bacteraemia. Data on urine cultures in the evaluation of late-onset sepsis in preterm infants admitted to the NICU are scarce (Mohseny et al., 2018). However, because the overall risk of UTI increases with decreasing gestational age, low birthweight and postnatal age greater than 72 hours after birth, urine should be examined when late-onset sepsis is suspected. However, the existence of other infection risk factors may cause clinicians to be hesitant to collect urine cultures during the basic sepsis evaluation. The use of central arterial or venous lines in these newborns, which provides a direct source of bacteraemia, is a significant risk factor and is frequently the cause of systemic infection (Mohseny et al., 2018).

Jaundice is one of the most prevalent signs of neonatal UTIs and may be the only sign. UTIs are well known to cause prolonged jaundice and are routinely investigated. In the newborn period, UTI manifests as a variety of symptoms. Non-specific symptoms (e.g. low weight gain, vomiting, diarrhoea, fever, irritability, lethargy, jaundice) may be the only ones present, with jaundice being one of the most common. UTIs are well known to cause long-term jaundice. Along with prolonged jaundice, UTIs may be the cause of unexplained pathological jaundice in the first 2 weeks of life. However, testing for UTI in patients with unexplained jaundice in the first 2 weeks of life remains controversial (Bahat Ozdogan et al., 2018).

Epidemiology

Occurrence of UTI in the neonatal unit has been suggested to be as high as 6.3%, with preterm and LBW neonates having an increased incidence to approximately 20%. This higher rate may be secondary to hospital-acquired infections and increased susceptibility due to immaturity (Zhang et al., 2020).

A strong male predominance is seen mainly because the likelihood of UTI in uncircumcised males is known to increase the risk by 10 times (Moore et al., 2015). However, the debate is controversial, with many believing that the risks of circumcision outweigh any reduction in UTI. Breastfeeding and rooming-in (to colonise the neonate with maternal bacteria) are recommended to reduce the incidence of UTI in infancy. Repeated episodes of acute UTI are distressing to neonates and their parents or carers, and can lead to extended and repeated hospitalisation.

Clinical presentation

Symptoms of UTI are non-specific and can be similar to the clinical presentation of other sepsis. Clinical symptoms of UTI may include (Arshad & Seed, 2015):

- fever (39°C or more), seen more commonly with UTI, although not all neonates presenting with UTI will have febrile episodes
- poor feeding
- lethargy
- failure to thrive (late presentation)
- vomiting
- diarrhoea
- prolonged jaundice
- irritability
- respiratory symptoms such as apnoea, hypoxia and tachypnoea (in 50% of preterm neonates)
- offensive-smelling urine
- haematuria.

Risk factors

Risk factors for UTI include:

- maternal history of UTI during pregnancy, which increases the risk 5.9-fold
- prematurity (under 34 weeks' gestation)
- prolonged hospitalisation
- renal and urinary tract abnormalities.

Diagnosis

The gold standard for diagnosis of UTI is a positive urine culture for a single organism. A positive culture is defined as a growth of 10,000 or more colony-forming units (CFUs). The most common bacterial aetiology for neonatal UTI is *Escherichia coli* (*E. coli*), accounting for 80–88%, with other causative pathogens including other gram-negative organisms such as *Klebsiella* and *Enterobacter*. Gram-positive organisms account for a very small percentage of neonatal UTIs (Arshad & Seed, 2015). Fungal UTI is predominantly seen in nosocomial UTI infection and is mainly caused by *Candida* (Zhang et al., 2020).

Urinalysis findings including nitrites (presence of nitrate reductase) and leucocyte esterase (which is released by white blood cells and indicates the presence of pyuria) are diagnostically as useful as microscopy and culture (National Institute for Health and Care Excellence (NICE), 2018).

A raised C-reactive protein (CRP) and procalcitonin have been found to have low sensitivity in predicting UTI in the neonatal population (Zhang et al., 2020).

Investigations

The NICE guidelines (2018) suggest the following initial investigations and follow-up assessment for a UTI in the neonatal period:

- Neonates should have an ultrasound of the urinary tract during the acute infection to rule out structural abnormalities of the urinary tract such as obstruction.
- For infants younger than 6 months, including neonates with a first-time UTI that responds to treatment, follow-up ultrasound should be carried out within 6 weeks of the UTI.
- A **dimercaptosuccinic acid scan (DMSA)** scan 4–6 months following the acute infection should be used to detect renal parenchymal defects.
- Routine imaging to identify vesicoureteral reflux (VUR) with micturating cystourethrogram (MCUG) is not recommended for neonates, infants and children who have had a UTI but should be considered in atypical UTI with poor urine flow, abdominal or bladder mass, raised creatinine, septicaemia, failure to respond to treatment

with suitable antibiotics within 48 hours, or infection with non-*E. coli* organisms.
- Neonatal nurses/midwives should ensure that parents or carers are given information about the need for treatment, the importance of completing any course of treatment and advice about prevention and possible long-term management.
- Neonatal nurses/midwives should ensure that parents or carers are aware of the possibility of a UTI recurring and understand the need for vigilance and to seek prompt treatment from a healthcare professional for any suspected re-infection.

Management

Once a UTI is diagnosed and culture and sensitivities are available, antibiotic treatment should be tailored according to these results (Baracco & Mattoo, 2014). Limited data to guide the duration of parenteral antibiotic treatment are available in the neonatal population. Neonates with bacteraemia are usually treated for 10–14 days. The use of oral antibiotic treatment has not been studied. Prompt and effective treatment is essential not only to treat bacteraemia but also to prevent complications of UTI, which include renal scarring. The risk of renal scarring in infants younger than 1 year with first-time UTI is 43% (Zhang et al., 2020). Antibiotic prophylaxis is not routinely recommended in infants and children following first-time UTI, but should be considered in recurrent UTI or when MCUG shows evidence of VUR. If indicated, prophylaxis is recommended using cephalexin at a dosage of 10 mg/kg/dose as a single daily dose (Moore et al., 2015).

Prognosis/complications

The long-term outcome following UTI is dependent on renal investigations at the time of and following acute infection. As discussed, renal scarring is a common complication post infection that can lead to renal hypertension and chronic kidney disease (Zhang et al., 2020).

CASE STUDY 14.1

Billy, a 2-week-old male term infant, is being treated in the neonatal unit for a febrile UTI. His urine contained nitrites, 2+ leucocyte esterase and 50 white blood cells per high-power field. Intravenous antibiotics are administered. Forty-eight hours after hospitalisation, his urine culture revealed *E. coli* with >100,000 CFU/mL that were pan-resistant to antibiotics. Blood and cerebrospinal fluid cultures obtained upon admission were negative. A renal ultrasound was conducted during his admission, and the results were normal.

Acute renal failure

Acute renal failure (ARF) in a neonate is a serious condition with a rapid onset, and results from the loss of the kidney's ability to maintain water and electrolyte homeostasis. It is associated with a decline in GFR, an elevation in creatinine and potential anuria. Prompt evaluation and treatment are required to avoid additional complications (Filler et al., 2021).

There are varying aetiologies for ARF, which are typically divided into three subsets: pre-renal, renal (or intrinsic) and post-renal. Each subset is associated with varying causes:

- *Pre-renal ARF* is characterised by renal hypoperfusion with preserved parenchymal integrity, occurs in 55–60% of cases and is caused by hypoxia, dehydration, haemorrhage, necrotising enterocolitis, respiratory distress syndrome, decreased cardiac output or hypoalbuminaemia. Pre-renal ARF is associated with **oliguria**, low urinary sodium and highly concentrated urine. The goal of treatment for pre-renal ARF is to establish renal perfusion, usually by increasing intravascular volume.
- *Post-renal ARF* is less common in neonates and accounts for less than 5% of ARF cases. Post-renal aetiologies are primarily urinary tract obstructive pathologies, which include PUVs, prune belly syndrome and bilateral pelvic–ureteric junction (PUJ) obstruction. Post-renal ARF is usually resolved by relieving the obstruction.
- *Renal or intrinsic ARF* accounts for 35–45% of cases. Causes include pyelonephritis, acute tubular necrosis, acute interstitial nephritis, toxic nephropathy, renal artery thrombosis or renal vein thrombosis. It is associated with high urinary sodium, normal concentration of urine and poor response to fluids. Intrinsic or renal ARF is most often treated medically with diuretics, electrolyte correction and fluid restriction (Khan et al., 2015).

Aetiology

In critically ill neonates, ARF is secondary to hypovolaemia, hypotension and ischaemia, commonly arising from asphyxia, sepsis, necrotising enterocolitis and major surgery, but it should be considered in any neonate whose urine output falls abruptly (under 1 mL/kg/h) following the first few days of postnatal age (Gallo et al., 2021).

Epidemiology

Acute renal failure is said to occur in as many as 8% of neonates admitted to the neonatal intensive care unit (NICU) (Filler et al., 2021). NICU admissions have extended hospital stays with a variety of exposures covering several phases of kidney development, which increase the risk for acute kidney injury (AKI). Because of antenatal, intrapartum and early postnatal transition events, the first week after birth is a sensitive phase for the development of neonatal AKI. Specifically, the typical neonatal kidney physiology (with a fundamentally low GFR) predisposes the immature kidney to AKI during the transition into the extrauterine environment. Because the neonate's blood creatinine will reflect maternal levels at delivery before evolving over the next several postnatal days to achieve a new 'steady state', the definition of neonatal AKI in the first week may differ from other time points (Charlton et al., 2019).

Clinical assessment/diagnosis

- Evaluation of urine output, in particular defining oliguria (urine output below 0.5 mL/kg/h).

- Palpation of the bladder, which should be performed with caution, will eliminate acute urinary retention.
- Assessment of circulation (blood pressure and capillary refill time) is important to determine perfusion as a reflection of the adequacy of renal perfusion.
- Diagnosis depends on renal ultrasound to clearly identify any anatomical abnormality, obstructive problem, congenital malformation or renal vein thrombosis.

Management

Management should be directed to correcting the underlying cause.

- All nephrotoxic medications should be ceased where possible.
- Low-dose dopamine may aid in renal perfusion; however, in higher doses it leads to renal vasoconstriction.
- ARF may also necessitate dialysis in a neonate until the underlying aetiology is corrected or previous measures have been unsuccessful. Reasons to initiate dialysis include recalcitrant electrolyte abnormalities, worsening uraemia, fluid overload and persistent acid–base abnormalities.
- Peritoneal dialysis (PD) is considered the optimal dialysis modality in neonates because of its slow removal of fluid and solutes while avoiding haemodynamic instability (Khan et al., 2015).

CLINICAL PRACTICE 14.1

Peritoneal dialysis is the optimal dialysis modality for neonates. Through PD there is a slow removal of fluid and solutes. Technically, it is simple and can be undertaken in the neonatal unit.

Silicone catheters are used, with side perforations. They are inserted either laterally or through the rectus muscle directly into the peritoneum.

The dialysis procedure has four components:

1. composition of the dialysis fluid (dialysate), usually dextrose 2.5–4.25%
2. volume of fluid per exchange
3. frequency and duration of exchanges, including the fill, dwell and drain times
4. monitoring of the neonate's weight and the fluid for signs of peritonitis.

Nutrition is particularly important and a goal of 100–140 kcal is required to maintain growth.

Peritoneal fluid leakage around the PD catheter and along the tunnel is a serious problem that can increase the risk of bacterial and fungal peritonitis. This can be an issue in neonates of lower birthweights. Management strategies include discontinuation of PD in favour of haemodialysis, placement of a new PD catheter (rare), temporary discontinuation of PD for 2–7 days or substantially decreasing the PD fill volume (Kara et al., 2018).

Prognosis/complications

The key to reducing complications in neonates who have suffered ARF is prompt and effective management, with evidence suggesting preservation of renal function. However, ARF remains a significant cause of mortality in the neonatal unit, ranging from 14% to 73%. Further complications can include chronic renal failure, decreased GFR, impaired tubular function, chronic hypertension, nephrocalcinosis and impaired renal growth (Filler et al., 2021).

Renal vein thrombosis

Renal vein thrombosis (RVT) refers to the formation of a clot in the veins leading to the kidney. It is the most common non-catheter-related vascular condition affecting the neonatal kidney and can result in severe renal damage (Ouellette et al., 2020).

Pathophysiology

Neonates, particularly preterm neonates, are more susceptible to renal vein thrombosis owing to immaturity of the haemostatic system, slow perfusion through the kidneys' double capillary network, small vessel diameters and underlying disease (Boubred & Simeoni, 2018). About 90% of cases of renal vein thrombosis in the neonate are caused by the placement of central venous catheters (Ouellette et al., 2020).

Epidemiology

The incidence of symptomatic RVT is 2.2 per 100,000 births, and it is present in 0.5 per 1000 admissions to the neonatal unit. Risk factors for RVT include maternal diabetes, perinatal asphyxia, hypertonic dehydration, congenital heart disease, acute blood loss, presence of an indwelling catheter, sepsis and hereditary prothrombotic factors (Ouellette et al., 2020). The aetiology remains unclear in the majority of cases and probably occurs before birth (Chan & Bhatt, 2018).

Clinical assessment

Clinical assessment of a neonate with RVT should consider the following:

- the typical triad of features associated with RVT is macroscopic haematuria, palpable abdominal mass and thrombocytopenia
- additional symptoms include hypertension, oliguria and gross haematuria.

Clinical assessment therefore is focused on:

- urinalysis, in particular monitoring for haematuria
- physical abdominal assessment assessing for an abdominal mass
- full blood count evaluation focusing on platelets, prothrombin time and activated partial thromboplastin time and haemoglobin
- blood pressure monitoring
- strict fluid balance including input and output
- urine output monitoring for oliguria
- serum electrolyte, urea and creatinine monitoring (Saxonhouse, 2015).

Diagnosis

The gold standard for diagnosis of RVT is contrast angiography, but the less invasive and more cost-effective diagnostic tool is Doppler ultrasonography (Khan et al., 2015). A full coagulation profile and thrombophilia screen are also recommended to identify antithrombin, protein C and S deficiencies and factor V Leiden and prothrombin gene defects (Chan & Bhatt, 2018).

Management

Management of renal vein thrombosis is determined by the degree of, or the extension of, the thrombosis to the inferior vena cava and renal compromise. Treatment with low-molecular-weight heparin is the most common management recommendation (Chan & Bhatt, 2018), with additional treatment to correct the underlying condition, including correction of electrolyte imbalance and fluid balance and treating the renal insufficiency and the coagulation disorders (Khan et al., 2015).

Prognosis/complications

The long-term outcome of RVT includes impairment of renal function, hypoplasia of the kidney, hypertension and tubular defects (Chan & Bhatt, 2018); however, these complications are limited when prompt effective treatment is provided (Khan et al., 2015).

CONCLUSION

Prompt and effective management of congenital renal and genitourinary disorders is critical in improving the outcome and preserving renal function for the affected newborn. The delicate balance to maintain homeostasis in these neonates poses significant clinical challenges. The skilled neonatal nurse/midwife must understand these disorders and the implications for renal function, and implement effective management techniques to ensure the best outcomes for this cohort of neonates.

Recommended Reading

Management of fetal renal tract dilation: https://media.starship.org.nz/renal-tract-dilation-flow-chart/renal-tract-dilation-flow-chart.pdf.

References/Acknowledgements

Allegaert, K., Smits, A., van Donge, T., van den Anker, J., Sarafidis, K., Levtchenko, E., et al. (2020). Renal precision medicine in neonates and acute kidney injury: how to convert a cloud of creatinine observations to support clinical decisions. *Frontiers in Pediatrics, 8*, 366. doi: 10.3389/fped.2020.00366.

Arshad, M., & Seed, P. C. (2015). Urinary tract infections in the infant. *Clinics in Perinatology, 42*, 17–28. doi: 10.1016/j.clp.2014.10.003.

Bahat Ozdogan, E., Mutlu, M., Camlar, S. A., Bayramoglu, G., Kader, S., & Aslan, Y. (2018). Urinary tract infections in neonates with unexplained pathological indirect hyperbilirubinemia: prevalence and significance. *Pediatrics and Neonatology, 59*(3), 305–309. doi: 10.1016/j.pedneo.2017.10.010.

Baracco, R., & Mattoo, T. K. (2014). Diagnosis and management of urinary tract infection and vesicoureteral reflux in the neonate. *Clinics in Perinatology, 41*, 633–642. doi: 10.1016/j.clp.2014.05.011.

Baum, M. (2016). Neonatal nephrology. *Current Opinion in Pediatrics, 28*(2), 170–172. doi: 10.1097/MOP.0000000000000325.

Boubred, F., & Simeoni, U. (2018). Pathophysiology of fetal and neonatal kidneys. In: G. Buonocore, R. Bracci, & M. Weindling (Eds.) *Neonatology: a practical approach to neonatal diseases* (2nd ed., pp. 1018–1026). Cham. IL: Springer. doi: 10.1007/978-3-319-18159-2_261-2.

Chan, A. K. C., & Bhatt, M. D. (2018). Neonatal thrombosis: management and outcome. In: D. H. Mahoney, J. A. Garcia-Prats & C. Armsby (Eds.). *UpToDate*. Wolters Kluwer. <https://www.uptodate.com/contents/neonatal-thrombosis-management-and-outcome?search5Chan%202018%20Management%20of%20thrombosis%20in%20the%20newborn&source=search_result&selectedTitle=1~150&usage_type=default&display_rank=1> (Accessed 20 February 2022).

Charlton, J. R., Boohaker, L., Askenazi, D., Brophy, P. D., D'Angio, C., Fuloria, M., et al. (2019). Incidence and risk factors of early onset neonatal AKI. *Clinical Journal of the American Society of Nephrology, 14*(2), 184–195. doi: 10.2215/CJN.03670318.

Craft, J., Gordon, C., Huether S. et al (2019). The structure and function of the urinary system. *Understanding Pathophysiology ANZ*, 857–881, Sydney, Elsevier Australia.

Dias, T., Sairam, S., & Kumarasiri, S. (2014). Ultrasound diagnosis of foetal renal abnormalities. *Best Practice and Research Clinical Obstetrics and Gynaecology, 28*, 403–415. doi: 10.1016/j.bpobgyn.2014.01.009.

Filler, G., Guerrero-Kanan, R., & Alvarez-Elias, A. C. (2016). Assessment of glomerular filtration rate in the neonate: is creatinine the best tool? *Current Opinion in Pediatrics, 28*(2), 173–179. doi: 10.1097/MOP.0000000000000318.

Filler, G., Bhayana, V., Schott, C., & Diaz-Gonzalez de Ferris, M. (2021). How should we assess renal function in neonates and infants? *Acta Paediatrica*. 110(3), 773–780. doi: 10.1111/apa.15557.

Gallo, D., de Bijl-Marcus, K. A., Alderliesten, T., Lilien, M., & Groenendaal, F. (2021). Early Acute kidney injury in preterm and term neonates: incidence, outcome, and associated clinical features. *Neonatology, 118*, 174–179. doi: 10.1159/000513666.

Grandi, C. (2021). Alterations in fetal kidney development and increased risk for adult diseases. *Archives of Argentinian Pediatrics, 119*(5), e480–e486. doi: 10.5546/aap.2021.eng.e480.

Kara, A., Gurgoze, M. K., Aydin, M., Taskin, E., Bakal, U., & Orman, A. (2018). Acute peritoneal dialysis in neonatal intensive care unit: an 8-year experience of a referral hospital. *Science Direct, 59*, 375–379. doi: 10.1016/j.pedneo.2017.11.008.

Khan, O. A., Hageman, J. A., & Clardy, C. (2015). Acute renal failure in the neonate. *Pediatric Annals, 44*(10), 251–253. doi: 10.3928/00904481-20151012-10.

McCance, K. L., & Huether, S. E. (2018). *Pathophysiology: the biologic basis for disease in adults and children*. Amsterdam: Elsevier Health Sciences. [E-book]

McCance, K. L., & Huether, S. E. (2019). *Pathophysiology: Structure and Function of the Renal and Urologic Systems*. Amsterdam: Elsevier Health Sciences. [E-book]

Mohseny, A. B., van Velze, V., Steggerda, S. J., Smits-Wintjens, V. E., Bekker, V., & Lopriore, E. (2018). Late-onset sepsis due to urinary tract infection in very preterm neonates is not uncommon. *European Journal of Pediatrics, 177*(1), 33–38. doi: 10.1007/s00431-017-3030-9.

Moore, S. S., Bahat, H., Rachmiel, M., Ziv-Baran, T., Youngster, I., & Goldman, M. (2015). Guidelines for urinary tract infections and antenatal hydronephrosis should be gender specific. *Acta Paediatrica, 164*, e512–e517. doi: 10.1111/apa.13129.

National Institute for Health and Care Excellence (NICE). (2018). *Urinary tract infection in under 16s: diagnosis and management*. (NICE Clinical Guidelines, No. 54.) London: NICE. <https://www.ncbi.nlm.nih.gov/books/NBK553083/> (Accessed 20 February 2022).

Nicolaou, N., Renkema, K. Y., Bongers, E., Giles, R. H., & Knoers, N. A. (2015). Genetic, environmental, and epigenetic factors involved in CAKUT. *Nature Reviews. Nephrology, 11*, 720–731. doi: 10.1038/nrneph.2015.140.

Ogobuiro, I., & Tuma F. (2021). Physiology, renal. In: *StatPearls*. Treasure Island, FL: StatPearls Publishing. <https://www.ncbi.nlm.nih.gov/books/NBK538339/> (Accessed 20 February 2022).

Ouellette, A. C., Darling, E. K., Sivapathasundaram, B., Babe, G., Perez, R., Chan A. K., et al. (2020). Incidence, risk factors, and outcomes of neonatal renal vein thrombosis in Ontario: population-based cohort study. *Kidney, 360, 1*(7), 640–647. doi: 10.34067/KID.0000912019.

Rehman S., & Ahmed D. (2021). Embryology, kidney, bladder, and ureter. In: *StatPearls*. Treasure Island, FL: StatPearls Publishing. <https://www.ncbi.nlm.nih.gov/books/NBK547747/> (Accessed 20 February 2022).

Saxonhouse, M. A. (2015). Thrombosis in the neonatal intensive care unit. *Clinics in Perinatology, 42*, 651–673. doi: 10.1016/j.clp.2015.04.010.

Zhang, H., Zhang, L., & Guo, N. (2020). Validation of "urinary tract dilatation" classification system; correlation between fetal hydronephrosis and postnatal urological abnormalities. *Medicine, 99*(2), e18707. doi: 10.1097/md.0000000000018707.

CHAPTER 15

CARE OF THE NEONATE WITH A METABOLIC OR ENDOCRINE DISORDER

DEBORAH HARRIS AND VICTORIA KAIN

Learning objectives

After reading this chapter you will be able to:

- define the relationship between glucose and insulin for the fetus
- list the metabolic changes that occur during transition to extrauterine life
- identify those neonates at risk of transient hypoglycaemia
- identify normal glucose levels for neonates and gold standard equipment for accurate diagnosis of hypoglycaemia
- discuss treatment options for hypoglycaemia
- define the endocrine system and its primary functions
- discuss the aetiology, pathophysiology and clinical presentations of common neonatal endocrine disorders
- assess, plan, implement and evaluate the care of neonates and their families with metabolic and endocrine disorders.

Key words, terms, abbreviations

adenosine triphosphate (ATP)
adipose tissue
dextrose gel
endocrine
gluconeogenesis
glucose
glycogen
glycogenolysis
homeostasis
hyperglycaemia
hyperinsulinism
hypoglycaemia
inborn errors of metabolism (IEM)
insulin
ketogenesis
large for gestational age (LGA)
lipolysis
metabolic
newborn screening (NBS)
Newborn Screening Card
point-of-care testing (PoCT)
tandem mass spectrometry (TMS)
thyroid-stimulating hormone (TSH)
total parenteral nutrition (TPN)

INTRODUCTION

The human **metabolic** and **endocrine** systems are intricate networks of organs, hormones and genes that interact and influence one another to maintain the body in a state of **homeostasis**. As science and technology provide new methods to diagnose and analyse metabolic and endocrine disorders in both the prenatal and postnatal periods, our understanding of these systems is constantly evolving. This chapter will look at what is currently known about the fetal and neonatal metabolic and endocrine systems, with a focus on **glucose** homeostasis and **inborn errors of metabolism (IEM)**. Understanding glucose homeostasis and the necessity of early identification and management of the most prevalent endocrine and IEM disorders enables neonatal nurses and midwives to improve both short- and long-term neonatal outcomes while also providing appropriate support and education to families. Table 15.1 defines the terms commonly used in metabolic pathways.

METABOLIC ADAPTATION

Before birth

The fetus is fully dependent on the transport of nutrients from the maternal circulation prior to birth. Glucose is the primary fetal oxidative substrate. Glucose concentrations in the mother and the fetus have a direct link. In humans, fetal blood glucose concentrations are 60–70% of maternal concentrations. Glucose reaches the placenta via facilitated diffusion along a concentration gradient (Harding et al., 2017).

TABLE 15.1 **Terms related to metabolic pathways**

Term	Definition
Glucagon	A hormone secreted by pancreatic alpha cells when glucose levels are low causing the liver to convert stored glycogen into glucose. Also a drug used to treat protracted hypoglycaemia in neonates with adequate glycogen stores
Gluconeogenesis (*also known as 'endogenous glucose production'*)	Metabolic pathway resulting in the generation of glucose from substrates such as lactate, glycerol and glucogenic amino acids
Glycogen	Stored in the liver and skeletal muscle, can be transformed into glucose
Glycogenesis	Formation of glycogen from glucose
Glycogenolysis	Process where glycogen is broken down into glucose providing immediate energy and maintaining glucose levels during fasting. Occurs primarily in the liver, stimulated by the hormones glucagon and adrenaline (epinephrine)
Glycolysis (*also known as 'oxidation'*)	Process where glucose is broken down to carbon dioxide, water and energy in the form of **adenosine triphosphate (ATP)**
Ketogenesis	Biochemical process that produces ketone bodies by breaking down fatty acids and ketogenic amino acids. Supplies energy to certain organs (e.g. the brain)
Lipolysis	Biochemical process where lipids are broken down to generate the energy substrates of glycerol and free fatty acids

With advancing gestation, uterine blood flow increases to meet the rising metabolic demands of the growing fetus. In the third trimester, the fetus converts some of the glucose to **adipose tissue** and **glycogen** in preparation for the metabolic changes that will occur at birth. Lactate is also an important oxidative fuel prior to birth. Other fuels such as amino acids are also actively transported to the fetus against a transplacental gradient. The human placenta is also permeable to small amounts of triglycerides, fatty acids and glycerol. The fetus produces **insulin** early in gestation as the fetal pancreatic cells begin to develop between 10 and 12 weeks' gestation, with the structures being fully developed by 22 weeks' gestation. Insulin does not cross the placenta; the fetus must produce this hormone independently.

At birth

At birth the blood glucose concentration of the neonate is approximately 70% of the maternal concentration. Once the umbilical cord is severed, the neonate must adapt from a continuous glucose supply to intermittent feeding and fasting. There is a transient decrease in blood glucose concentrations (referred to as the 'nadir') during the first 1–2 hours after birth until glucose is mobilised. This occurs through **glycogenolysis** (breakdown of glycogen molecules into glucose) and **gluconeogenesis** (a process leading to the generation of glucose from sources other than glycogen, including pyruvate, lactate, glycerol and some amino acids) (Hatting et al., 2018), which provides the only glucose fuel source until feeding is established. Glycogenolysis accounts for approximately 50% of total endogenous glucose production and gluconeogenesis is responsible for 30–40%.

Neonates have a larger brain-to-body weight ratio than adults and children (Dani & Corsini, 2020), and 80% of the total glucose utilisation in the neonate occurs in the brain. Despite this demand during the first few hours of life, alternative cerebral fuels, primarily lactate, meet the energy demands of the brain.

The normal metabolic and hormonal transition is complex. The production of glucose from gluconeogenesis has been estimated to be 4–5 mg/kg/min in the first hours after birth, and glucose production and mobilisation then gradually increases during the first few days. By 72 hours of age, the blood glucose concentrations are the same as those considered normal in the adult (Harris et al., 2020).

NEONATAL ENERGY SOURCES AND GLUCOSE HOMEOSTASIS

Glycogenolysis

Glycogenolysis is the breakdown of glycogen stored in the liver. This breakdown results in the production of glucose-6-phosphate, which can be converted to free glucose by the action of glucose-6-phosphatase (Fig. 15.1). Glycogen is also stored in muscle, but this glycogen cannot be released into the circulation because muscle cells lack glucose-6-phosphatase (Feher, 2017a). Conditions that encourage glycogenolysis include suppressed insulin concentrations and elevated concentrations of glucagon and adrenaline.

Gluconeogenesis

Gluconeogenesis ensures the continued supply of glucose. Gluconeogenesis is the production of glucose from precursors such as lactate, alanine, glutamine and glycerol. The conversion mostly occurs in the liver, with a small amount in the kidneys (see Fig. 15.1).

Fig. 15.2 shows the complex pathways that maintain glucose balance and energy production. As hepatic and muscle glycogen stores are depleted, the neonate synthesises ketone bodies and uses its fat stores, with the release of free fatty acids (**lipolysis**) to maintain glucose homeostasis.

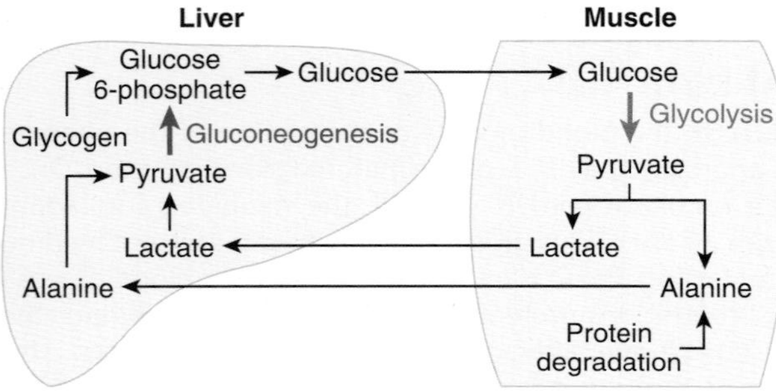

FIGURE 15.1 **Gluconeogenesis pathways**

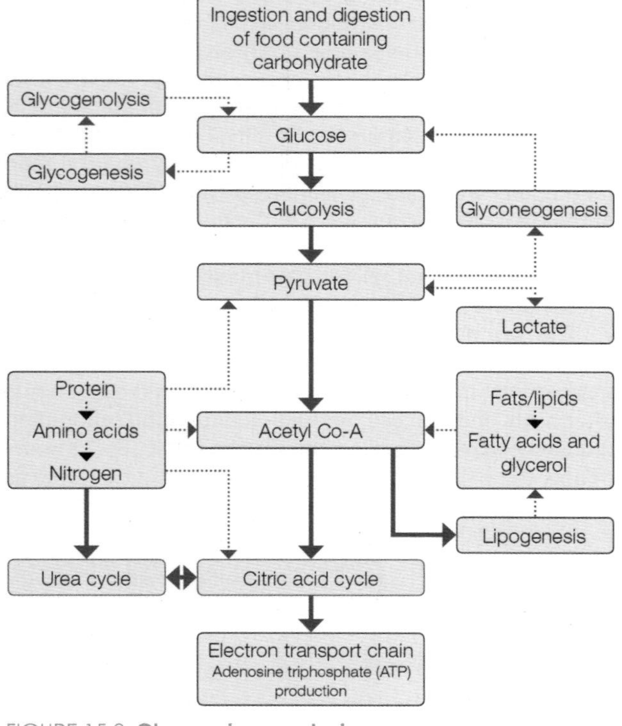

FIGURE 15.2 **Glucose homeostasis**

Ketogenesis

Ketogenesis is the production of ketones, β-hydroxybutyrate and acetoacetate from fatty acid oxidation. In both animal and human studies, these substrates are used as alternative cerebral oxidative fuels (Qian et al., 2020). The neonatal brain can extract and utilise ketones at a rate that is four to five times faster than that of an adult. The availability and usage of ketones and lactate in the brain are related to plasma concentrations. Factors including gestation, postnatal age, the type of milk received and feeding intervals all influence plasma concentrations of both fuels. Ketogenesis is also dependent on the inhibition of insulin secretion, which allows fatty acid mobilisation for ketogenesis (Harris et al., 2021). Ketones provide an important cerebral fuel source. The cerebral utilisation of ketones is directly related to the plasma concentrations. In healthy, regularly fed neonates, ketones supply up to 12% of the cerebral oxygen consumption following a 6-hour fast (Aliefendioğlu et al., 2018).

Blood ketone concentrations increase hours after birth and peak on day 3 before falling. During the first few days after birth, when **hypoglycaemia** is more common, term breastfed neonates have been reported to have lower blood glucose and higher ketone concentrations than those who have been formula fed. It has been postulated that formula feeding may suppress ketogenesis. The exact mechanism for this is not clear but it is speculated that a factor in breast milk, which is absent in infant formula, augments ketogenesis (de Rooy & Hawdon, 2002).

Formula feeding has been linked to faster weight gain during the first few months of life, as well as variations in metabolism and the faecal microbiome compared with breastfeeding. When compared with breastfed infants, infants fed formula had increased protein degradation products such as amino acids, creatinine and urea in the serum. Breastfed infants, it was found, have fat-based metabolism, resulting in higher ketone bodies in the blood that is irrespective of blood glucose levels and neonatal anthropometry. Increased ketone bodies have significant implications for the developing infant brain, as the brain has a high energy requirement, and ketones contribute around 30% of the overall energy requirement. Ketone bodies also serve as carbon skeletons for brain lipids, including fatty acids and sterols (H. Lee et al., 2021).

Paradoxically, neonates who are not feeding well also have higher blood ketone concentrations and lower blood glucose concentrations, which is similar to the starving adult or child. If practicable to measure ketones in the clinical environment, it is important to determine that a neonate with high ketone concentrations is feeding well (Futatani et al., 2017). Furthermore, ketogenesis is suppressed by insulin, which also increases glucose utilisation. Many hypoglycaemic neonates have high concentrations of insulin and very low or un-recordable blood ketone concentrations and are therefore unlikely to be provided with the neuroprotective fuel source afforded by ketone bodies (Harris et al., 2015).

Lipolysis

Lipolysis is the breakdown of fat, which results in the formation of free fatty acids. In the healthy neonate, there is a surge of glycerol and free fatty acids following birth, in response to the elevated plasma adrenaline and growth hormone (GH) concentrations and the suppression of insulin. Fatty acids cannot be used as a cerebral energy source but can be converted in the liver to lactate and ketones (Feher, 2017b) (see Fig. 15.2).

Lactate

Lactate is an important energy source during the first few hours of life. The healthy neonate also produces lactate within the brain parenchyma, via glutamate-activated glycolysis in the astrocytes (Harris et al., 2015).

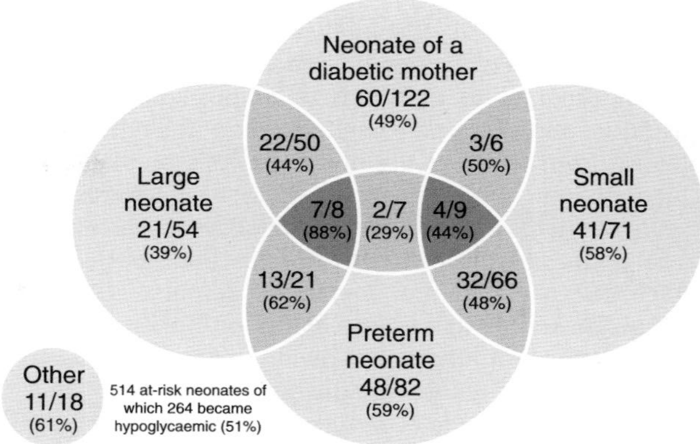

FIGURE 15.3 **Incidence of neonatal hypoglycaemia**
Source: adapted from: Harris et al. (2012).

HYPOGLYCAEMIA

Neonatal hypoglycaemia results from either normal metabolic demand for glucose in the presence of decreased availability of substrate, or normal substrate availability in the presence of excessive metabolic demands. The period following birth is a transition period when hypoglycaemia is most common and is usually transient, resulting from delayed or impaired metabolic adaptation. Persistent hypoglycaemia is often the result of complex endocrine disorders. It is important for neonatal nurses and midwives to recognise neonates at risk of hypoglycaemia and prevent its occurrence, as long-term neurological impairment is possible, even when there are no symptoms. Magnetic resonance studies on the brains of newborns with hypoglycaemia have shown that it leads to oedema in the posterior occipital and cortex regions, which impacts on cognitive skills, adaptability and visual skills (Qiao et al., 2019).

Definition

Hypoglycaemia can be defined physiologically as the blood glucose level at which cerebral energy needs fail to be met. There is no widely accepted definition of hypoglycaemic levels because of the complex metabolic and hormonal adaptations at birth. Variations range from a blood glucose level of less than 2.6 mmol/L (American Academy of Pediatrics (AAP) cited in Chappe, 2020; Harris et al., 2014), to less than 2.7 mmol/L in the first 48 hours and less than 3.33 mmol/L after the first 48 hours (Pediatric Endocrine Society cited in Chappe, 2020). The extent, duration and frequency of hypoglycaemia necessary to induce neurodevelopmental damage are unknown. Statistical, metabolic, neurophysical and neurodevelopmental approaches have all been used to define newborn hypoglycaemia, and each has limitations. Since there are few studies in healthy term neonates, particularly those who are low risk and exclusively breastfed, the diagnosis of neonatal hypoglycaemia remains elusive.

Incidence

The incidence of hypoglycaemia in the first 48 hours of life in infants greater than 35 weeks' gestation is approximately 25% of all deliveries; of those at-risk infants, 51% will experience at least one episode of hypoglycaemia (Abramowski et al., 2021). Fig. 15.3 demonstrates the incidence of neonatal hypoglycaemia within the first 48 postnatal hours within identified at-risk groups.

Neonates at risk due to limited glucose and alternative cerebral fuels

Preterm neonates

There are multiple factors that predispose the preterm neonate to hypoglycaemia. In the last trimester of pregnancy, the fetus accumulates both glycogen and adipose tissue. Preterm neonates are born with significantly less glycogen and adipose tissue (Sharma et al., 2017) and therefore have limited ability to release glucose from the liver via glycogenolysis or to produce gluconeogenic precursors via lipolysis. In addition, preterm neonates have low concentrations of glucose-6-phosphatase, which is essential for both glycogenolysis and gluconeogenesis. The production of glucose-6-phosphatase may remain low in these neonates for some months following birth. Therefore, with advancing postnatal age as the feeding interval increases, preterm neonates may remain at risk of developing intermittent hypoglycaemia (De Angelis et al., 2021). In addition, preterm infants have increased cerebral metabolic demands because of their relatively large brain size (Abramowski et al., 2021), and may have increased general metabolic demands due to conditions such as respiratory distress or hypothermia.

Preterm neonates may be at a higher risk for neurological damage when hypoglycaemic as they are less able to mobilise alternative cerebral fuels such as ketones from fat stores and have an immature counter-regulatory hormone response to hypoglycaemia (Sharma et al., 2017).

Growth-restricted neonates

Similar to the preterm neonate, growth-restricted neonates do not accumulate glycogen or adipose tissue in late gestation, and therefore there is limited ability to release glucose from the liver via glycogenolysis or to produce gluconeogenic precursors via lipolysis. Asymmetrically grown neonates with growth restriction also have relatively large brain sizes in comparison with their birthweight, which increases cerebral metabolic demands (Rozance, 2021a). These infants are also at risk of higher metabolic demands than term neonates owing to conditions such as hypothermia and respiratory distress.

The regulation of fetal growth is determined not only by the nutrients available to the fetus, but also by the insulin–IGF/IGF-binding protein 3 (IGFBP-3) axes. IGF factors I and II collaborate to control fetal growth via changes in placental size and function. IGF-II promotes placental growth and development, allowing more nutrients to reach the fetus. IGF-I functions as a 'nutrient sensor', fine-tuning nutrition flow across the placenta in response to both the maternal environment and fetal demand. IGF-I production, which is especially vulnerable to maternal malnutrition and parental imprinting, modulates signalling via its receptor. Growth disorders caused by disruption of this imprinting include Beckwith–Wiedemann syndrome, which is linked with fetal overgrowth, and Silver-Russell syndrome, which is associated with intrauterine growth restriction (IUGR). Several studies have found that neonates born with growth restriction have lower levels of IGF-I, IGFBP-3 and insulin than appropriately grown infants of the same gestational age. The IGF system, specifically IGF-I and IGF-II, is essential for fetal and placental growth. IGF-I, IGF-II or IGF-IR gene disruption causes IUGR, whereas IGF-IIR gene disruption or IGF-II over-expression promotes fetal growth (Baud & Berkane, 2019).

See Chapter 3 for more information about the definitions and causes of growth restriction.

Neonates with poor feeding

Decreased substrate availability to the tissues can be due to either inadequate delivery or inadequate production. An inadequate caloric intake due to poor feeding or inadequate parenteral nutrition increases the risk of neonatal hypoglycaemia when the stored substrates are exhausted. It is not uncommon for late preterm neonates to be re-admitted to the hospital for treatment of hypoglycaemia caused by poor feeding after being discharged (Huff et al., 2019).

Hypothermic neonates

Hypothermia is common following birth and is associated with hypoglycaemia and poor neurodevelopmental outcome (Pinchefsky et al., 2021). Hypothermia increases metabolic demands, which depletes substrate owing to rapid lipolysis of brown fat stores for thermogenesis, in addition to exhaustion of glycogen stores.

Neonates with perinatal asphyxia

An increased metabolic demand commonly occurs in neonates who are unwell. Neonates suffering from perinatal asphyxia have rapid depletion of substrate stores during the period of anaerobic metabolism. In addition, these neonates frequently have hypoxic liver damage, resulting in impaired gluconeogenesis and glycogenolysis. It is particularly important to maintain blood glucose concentrations within normal ranges for neonates suffering from perinatal asphyxia, as the combined insult of either hypo- or hyperglycaemia is associated with poorer neurodevelopmental outcomes (Qiao et al., 2019).

Neonates with systemic conditions

Any condition that increases metabolic demand, such as sepsis or viral illnesses, will affect feeding, alter perfusion, compromise the gastrointestinal tract or liver and places the neonate at risk for decreased availability of glucose and alternative fuels and, therefore, at risk of hypoglycaemia.

Maternal medication

Some commonly used maternal medications can put the neonate at risk of neonatal hypoglycaemia, including beta-blockers, calcium channel blockers, beta sympathomimetics and oral hypoglycaemic agents (Dassios et al., 2017). If in doubt about the risk of a maternal medication to the neonate, it is important to review the available evidence.

Inborn errors of metabolism or endocrine insufficiency

Inborn errors of metabolism and disorders of the endocrine system are rare and frequently present with hypoglycaemia. The most common inborn errors of metabolism presenting in the neonatal period are defects of fatty acid oxidation, and the most common congenital endocrine disorders are defects related to cortisol production; these are discussed later in the chapter.

Neonatal hyperinsulinism

Hyperinsulinism is the term given when hypoglycaemia results from inadequate suppression of plasma insulin. This can be transient, as in the infant of a diabetic mother, or when perinatal stress may be part of an underlying condition. However, when it is associated with an underlying condition, this is most commonly a congenital defect in the regulation of insulin secretion.

Hyperinsulinism contributes to hypoglycaemia by increasing cellular glucose uptake and by suppressing hepatic glycogenolysis, gluconeogenesis, adipose tissue lipolysis and hepatic ketogenesis. Insulin also diminishes the counter-regulatory response to hypoglycaemia. Hence, affected neonates have a limited ability to produce alternative cerebral fuels such as ketones and, therefore, may be at greater risk for neurological damage from hypoglycaemia than those from non-diabetic pregnancies, although the data on neurodevelopmental outcomes in this cohort is limited (Riskin & Garcia-Prats, 2020).

Infants of diabetic mothers

The prevalence of maternal diabetes is dramatically increasing in both developed and developing countries, with a quadrupling of rates in Australia over the last decade (Laurie & McIntyre, 2020). Therefore, the incidence of neonates affected by a diabetic pregnancy is also increasing. Neonates born following a diabetic pregnancy have differing body compositions compared with those from non-diabetic pregnancies and are frequently macrosomic and at increased risk for developing hypoglycaemia (Peters et al., 2020). The mechanism for fetal overgrowth remains unclear. Pederson was the first to hypothesise that the increased transfer of maternal glucose across the placenta stimulated the release of insulin by the fetal pancreatic beta cells (Pedersen et al., 1954). Because insulin is a major fetal growth factor, macrosomia occurs. Other factors in the maternal metabolic environment, including free fatty acids, triglycerides, insulin resistance and inflammation, are now also thought to contribute to neonatal macrosomia (Abramowicz & Ahn, 2020).

During a diabetic pregnancy, the fetus is exposed to episodic periods of excess glucose from the mother. Insulin does not cross the placenta. From approximately 16 weeks' gestation the fetus produces insulin in response to the excess glucose in order to normalise its own blood glucose concentrations. After birth, when the umbilical cord is cut and the source of glucose is removed, the neonate continues to produce excess insulin for several days, resulting in the risk of hypoglycaemia (Peters et al., 2020).

Macrosomic neonates

Neonates from both diabetic and non-diabetic pregnancies can be born **large for gestational age (LGA)**. The term 'macrosomic' is frequently used to describe a neonate with a birthweight >4000 g or with a weight over the 90th percentile; the latter is preferred as it accounts for gestational age and therefore allows for the identification of LGA preterm neonates. The prevalence of macrosomia is increasing in developed countries and may in part be due to the increasing prevalence of diabetes, excessive gestational weight gain (GWG) and obesity. Macrosomia increases the risk for neonatal hypoglycaemia (Peters et al., 2020).

Neonates born to women with high body mass index

Maternal obesity is increasingly common. In Australia it has been estimated that one in five women has a body mass index (BMI) greater than 30 kg/m^2 and in New Zealand over half of pregnant women are either overweight (BMI between 25 and 29 kg/m^2) or obese at their initial antenatal visit (Ministry of Health, 2017). In Europe, 7–25% of expectant mothers are overweight, and in the United States only 45% of mothers are of healthy weight when they become pregnant (Helle & Priest, 2020). Maternal obesity is linked to poor maternal and perinatal outcomes including neonatal hypoglycaemia. These neonates are at increased risk of hypoglycaemia because they have been exposed to excess glucose, glycerol, fatty acids and triglycerides in utero. Additionally, obese mothers can have more difficulty establishing and maintaining breastfeeding (Ballesta-Castillejos et al., 2020).

Neonates with Beckwith–Wiedemann syndrome

This condition is frequently diagnosed antenatally as such neonates have congenital abnormalities including exomphalos, macroglossia, visceromegaly and ear lobe abnormalities. Hyperinsulinism is common and screening should continue until normal blood glucose concentrations have been demonstrated for 48 hours (Wang et al., 2020).

Neonates with congenital hyperinsulinism

Congenital hyperinsulinism (CHI) is the most common cause of neonatal hypoglycaemia that persists for longer than the first week after birth (Huerta-Saenz et al., 2018). There are two major types of disease: diffuse changes to the pancreas, characterised by beta-cell hypertrophy and hyperplasia known as nesidioblastosis, and confined focal lesions known as insulinoma.

In Western populations, the incidence of CHI is estimated to be 1:50,000. The incidence of recessively inherited genetic mutations can be as high as 1:2500 in consanguineous populations. However, these incidence rates do not account for resolving/transient CHI and are skewed towards the severe end of the spectrum, where children may be unresponsive to conservative medical treatment. Despite its rarity, CHI is one of the most common causes of recurrent and persistent hypoglycaemia in infancy (Banerjee et al., 2019).

THE INSULIN PATHWAY

The insulin pathway starts with the pancreatic beta cells acting as highly responsive sensors, allowing insulin to be released by the K_{ATP} channels as required. To maintain a physiological glucose balance at rest, the K_{ATP} channels on the beta cells are open. When the blood glucose concentration increases, glucose is transported into the beta cells by the glucose transporter GLUT2 and undergoes rapid phosphorylation to glucose-6-phosphate catalysed by the enzyme glucokinase. This increases the ATP/ADP ratio causing the K_{ATP} channel to close, resulting in depolarisation of the cell membrane and allowing the influx of calcium through voltage-gated calcium channels. This influx of calcium into the beta cells triggers exocytosis of insulin-containing granules, and insulin is secreted (Gupta, 2022) (Fig. 15.4).

Prevention of hypoglycaemia

Neonatal hypoglycaemia is common, with approximately 30% of all neonates born being at risk. Half of these neonates will become hypoglycaemic. It is essential that preventing hypoglycaemia is a priority, with the aim to protect the neonate from a potentially damaging neurological insult.

Early feeding (within the first hour), skin-to-skin care (Chiruvolu et al., 2017) and **dextrose gel** (Hegarty et al., 2016) have been shown to prevent hypoglycaemia within the first 48 hours after birth. It remains unclear whether prophylactic treatment for neonatal hypoglycaemia will reduce admission to the neonatal unit and/or improve breastfeeding rates (Hegarty et al., 2016). If the neonate is unable to feed, prompt attention to glucose administration is essential.

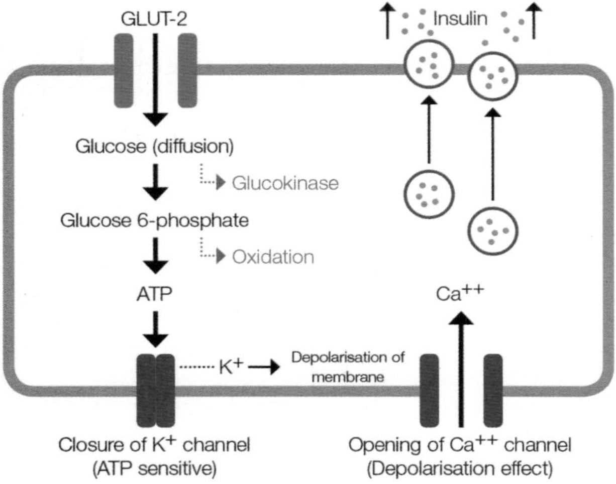

FIGURE 15.4 **Insulin pathway**

Blood glucose screening

As the clinical signs of neonatal hypoglycaemia are non-specific, blood glucose screening is recommended in developed countries (Alsweiler et al., 2021). Only those at risk of neonatal hypoglycaemia should be screened (see the section about at-risk neonates). The initial screening is recommended between 1 and 2 hours after birth as the blood glucose concentrations are known to fall rapidly following birth, reaching a nadir at approximately 2 hours. Regular blood glucose measurements are recommended over the next 12–48 hours until there is no longer a risk for low blood glucose concentrations. The screening samples are usually taken before the neonate is fed. However, there is no evidence that the blood glucose concentration is lowest before a feed or that the timing of the blood glucose measurement has an impact on neurodevelopmental outcomes (Harding et al., 2017).

CLINICAL PRACTICE 15.1

Identify the target thresholds and recommendations for treatment of hypoglycaemia in your area of practice.

Do the protocols in your work setting align with the recommended guidelines for treatment for neonates at risk of neonatal hypoglycaemia?

Many centres screen for hypoglycaemia using **point-of-care testing (PoCT)** rather than sending blood samples to the laboratory (Nichols et al., 2021). This is an attractive option because only a small sample is required, the result is immediately available and, therefore, treatment is provided promptly. However, most PoCT instruments do not use the gold standard of enzymatic analysis, and the results are inaccurate compared with analysis using a laboratory glucose oxidase method (Ba et al., 2018). The rationale for screening is to identify those neonates at risk of hypoglycaemia and treat them to avoid neurosensory damage; it is ethically questionable that PoCT instruments continue to be used.

CLINICAL PRACTICE 15.2

Historically, it has been demonstrated that point-of-care blood glucose analysers designed for the assessment of diabetes in adults and children are *not* useful for the diagnosis of hypoglycaemia in neonates (Beardsall et al., 2011).

Ba et al. (2018) devised a three-step validation procedure to determine the clinical accuracy risk of blood glucose-monitoring devices (BGMs). The three-step approach included: (1) validation of the laboratory reference method's accuracy and isotope dilution mass spectrometry (IDMS) traceability with international reference, (2) an analytical risk assessment including method correlation, precision and specificity studies performed on two BGMs, and (3) a clinical accuracy risk assessment performed with the BGMs demonstrating better specificity and the lowest analytical risk.

Identify the analyser used for measuring blood glucose concentrations in your work setting. Is the instrument a reliable analyser for the assessment of blood glucose concentrations in neonates?

Accuracy of blood glucose measurements

Taking blood via a heel-prick lance is difficult in the neonate. Errors are common. The procedure is painful and observing the test can cause distress to parents. It is useful to prewarm the heel and important to use pain-relieving strategies (Fig. 15.5). Blood samples taken from a poorly perfused heel will cause misleading findings. Importantly, there is variation in the results depending on whether the sample taken is arterial or venous. Arterial results have slightly higher glucose levels than venous samples by 10–15%, with capillary samples (from heel-prick lances) being somewhere in between. Red blood cells use glucose as their primary energy source and, therefore, a neonate with a high haematocrit will have a lower blood glucose concentration (Kallem et al., 2017).

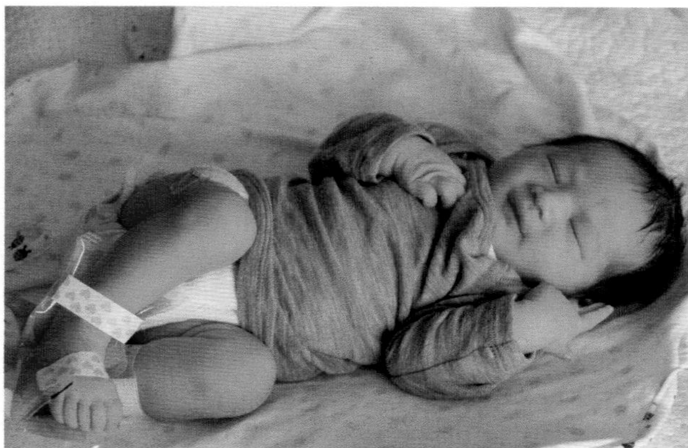

FIGURE 15.5 **Warming a neonate's heel prior to a capillary blood test (note the continuous glucose monitor in the thigh)**

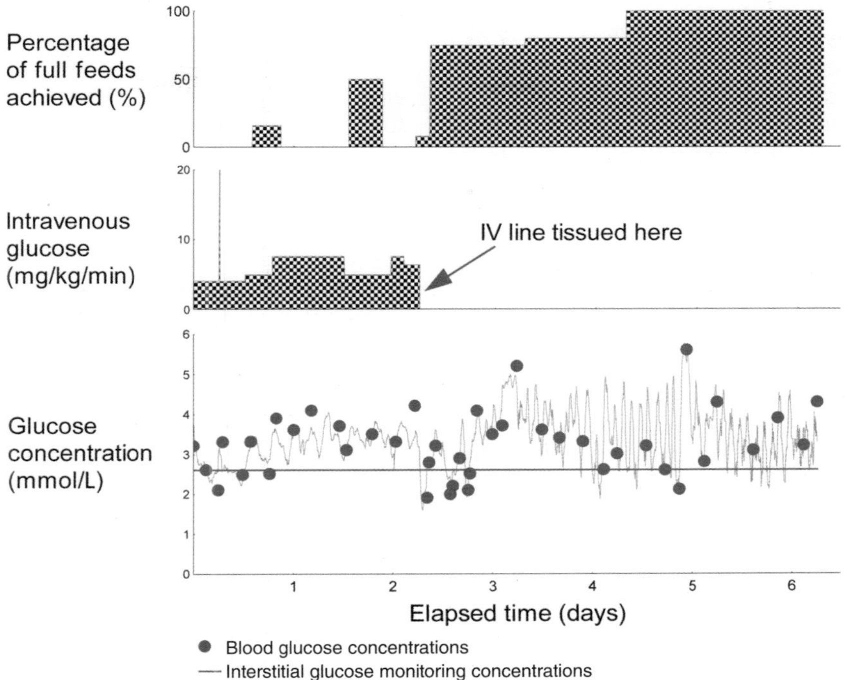

FIGURE 15.6 **Blood and interstitial glucose concentrations related to treatment and feeding**

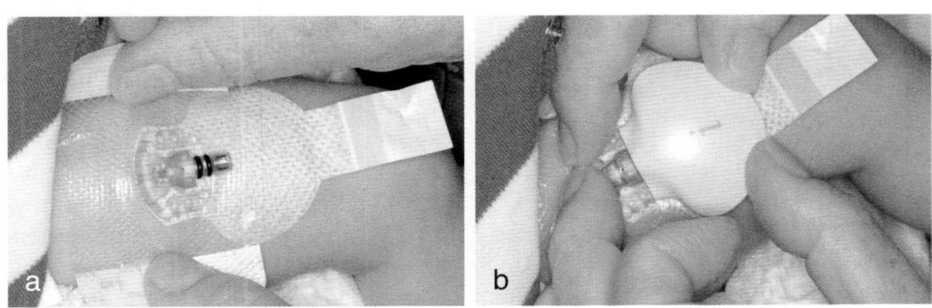

FIGURE 15.7 **Continuous glucose monitoring**

a Insertion of the continuous glucose sensor. **b** Attachment of the continuous glucose monitor.

Source: McKinlay et al. (2017a).

Real-time continuous glucose monitoring

Continuous glucose monitoring measures interstitial glucose concentrations and has been shown to be reliable and accurate in at-risk neonates in a research setting (Harris et al., 2010) (Fig. 15.6). However, this technology is not yet ready for routine clinical use. The advantages of continuous glucose monitoring include providing data about the duration, severity and frequency of glucose fluctuations, detecting undiagnosed episodes of both hypo- and hyperglycaemia and evaluating the neonate's response to treatment, coupled with decreasing the repetitive painful stimulation caused by heel-prick lances (Fig. 15.7). However, further research is required before this less-invasive monitoring can become the norm (McKinlay et al., 2017a).

Signs, symptoms and management of hypoglycaemic neonates

Clinical signs and symptoms

Early documented reports on neonatal hypoglycaemia identified most subjects as having no clinical signs or symptoms (Pildes et al., 1967), and later reports confirmed these findings (Rozance, 2021a). However, neonates may also demonstrate any of the following: jitteriness, poor feeding, apnoea, cyanosis, hypothermia, poor body tone, lethargy, coma or seizures.

Treatment

The aim of treatment is to improve the blood glucose concentrations, hence providing adequate cerebral fuel and decreasing the risk of brain injury. The most-common treatment for asymptomatic hypoglycaemia is to increase the frequency of feeding (Kallem et al., 2017). In the neonate who can feed, milk is the preferred treatment rather than glucose-containing solutions. This is because lactose (milk sugar) contains 50% galactose. Galactose is initially cleared by the liver after absorption from the intestine into the portal vein for glycogen production and does not stimulate the pancreas to secrete insulin, which can be counterproductive. However, if feeding does not improve the blood glucose concentration or the neonate is not feeding, admission to a neonatal unit is required for intravenous glucose.

Breastfeeding

The advantages of breastfeeding are well recognised. Unfortunately, hypoglycaemia is most common in the first 48 hours after birth at a time when breastfeeding is being established, the volume of breast milk is low, and the milk content is high in protein but considerably lower in carbohydrate and fat than mature milk. The neonate's energy expenditure is also likely to exceed energy input at this time. In addition, a neonate with hypoglycaemia can often require considerable encouragement to feed because of lethargy and poor tone. Coupled with this, the diagnosis of neonatal hypoglycaemia can cause considerable anxiety for mothers, all of which can contribute to difficulties with early breastfeeding. These mothers require considerable support and expert neonatal nursing and midwifery care during this time. There are few reports about breastfeeding as a treatment for neonatal hypoglycaemia. However, assessment of pre-feed alertness and scoring of the quality of the breastfeed have been shown not to be reliable predictors for improved blood glucose concentrations in hypoglycaemic neonates within the first 48 hours after birth (Harris et al., 2016a).

Expressed breast milk

Antenatal expression of breast milk is often encouraged for a mother with gestational diabetes, largely on the assumption that feeding expressed breast milk to neonates at risk will help improve blood glucose concentrations or treat hypoglycaemia, although there is no evidence that this actually occurs (Harris et al., 2017). Furthermore, findings from the Diabetes and Antenatal Milk Expressing (DAME) randomised trial showed that advising women with diabetes to antenatally express breast milk from 36 weeks' gestation did not alter the incidence of neonatal hypoglycaemia, requirement for intravenous dextrose or admission to the neonatal unit, but did reduce the use of formula (Forster et al., 2017).

Infant formula

Infant formula has been the most commonly used treatment for neonatal hypoglycaemia (Harris et al., 2014). The carbohydrate content of infant formula is significantly higher than that of breast milk, and formula is relatively inexpensive and easy to administer. However, feeding with infant formula risks disrupting the establishment and duration of breastfeeding, alters the microbiome and increases the risk of infections and allergies compared with exclusively breastfed neonates. Whether these disadvantages outweigh the disadvantages of admission to the neonatal unit and intravenous glucose as the alternative treatment for hypoglycaemia is strongly debated.

Dextrose gel

Dextrose gel 200 mg/kg massaged into the buccal mucosa before a feed is effective in improving blood glucose concentrations in hypoglycaemic late preterm and term neonates in the first 48 hours after birth (Harding et al., 2021). Treatment with dextrose gel also reduces admissions to the neonatal unit for treatment of hypoglycaemia, is well tolerated, is acceptable to staff and parents, accords with the Baby Friendly Hospital Initiative (BFHI) and is inexpensive. Recurrent and rebound episodes of hypoglycaemia are uncommon and hyperglycaemia following dextrose gel treatment has never been described. At follow-up at 2 years of age, dextrose gel appeared safe, with no effects on neurosensory impairment, processing difficulties or developmental and growth outcomes (Harris et al., 2016b).

Dextrose gel in conjunction with breastfeeding provides an attractive non-invasive alternative to infant formula and is increasingly being used as first-line treatment (Edwards et al., 2021), without any apparent harm to breastfeeding (Meneghin et al., 2021). The procedure for the administration of dextrose gel is demonstrated in Fig. 15.8.

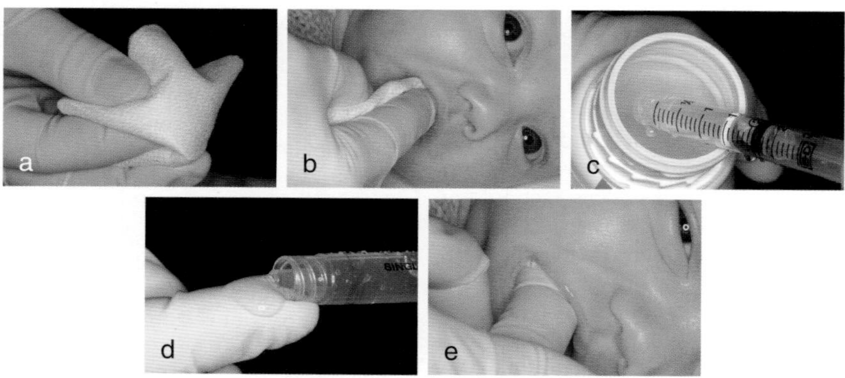

FIGURE 15.8 **How to give dextrose gel**

a Apply gloves and obtain a dry gauze square. **b** Dry the buccal mucosa with the gauze square. **c** Ensure the correct dose (200 mg/kg) is in the syringe. **d** Place a small amount of dextrose gel on a gloved finger. **e** Massage the dextrose gel into the buccal mucosa (the inside of the cheek) and repeat until the full dose is administered.

CASE STUDY

15.1

Alana G1, P0 was diagnosed with gestational diabetes at 28 weeks' gestation, at which time she received counselling regarding diet and exercise from her midwife. However, diet and exercise alone did not control her blood glucose concentrations and she required oral hypoglycaemic medication. Alana had until now enjoyed good health, and she and her husband were eagerly anticipating the birth of their first baby. Both attended antenatal classes and learned about the multiple health advantages associated with breastfeeding and were determined to exclusively breastfeed.

Alana presented to the hospital at 39 weeks' gestation in established labour. During her labour, she required an insulin infusion to maintain her blood glucose concentrations, which were stable, ranging from 5 to 8 mmol/L. Her daughter was born at 21:37 hours with Apgar scores of 8^1 and 9^5 minutes, respectively. She weighed 3210 grams (average for gestational age) and was placed skin to skin. Breastfeeding was established within 30 minutes of the birth. At 2 hours of age, the neonate had a blood glucose concentration of 2.1 mmol/L, which was measured on a glucose oxidase analyser in the postnatal area. Alana's midwife reassured her that treatment with dextrose gel massaged into the inside of her baby's cheek was safe and most likely to increase her baby's blood glucose concentration, and not interfere with breastfeeding. The midwife dried and massaged 200 mg/kg of the dextrose gel into the buccal mucosa at the bedside in the postnatal area. The blood glucose concentration was checked 30 minutes after treatment and another breastfeeding attempt and found to be 2.5 mmol/L and, therefore, the treatment was repeated. When the blood glucose concentration was repeated at 30 minutes, it was 3.2 mmol/L.

Alana's baby continued to have routine blood glucose screening according to the hospital protocols for the management of neonatal hypoglycaemia and had no further episodes of hypoglycaemia. Alana's baby was treated promptly, and her breastfeeding experience was supported.

1. List the maternal risk factors for gestational diabetes.
2. Explain the mechanism of how dextrose gel assists in glucose homeostasis.

Intravenous glucose

For neonates who remain hypoglycaemic after initial treatment or whose blood glucose concentrations are very low, admission to the neonatal unit for treatment with intravenous glucose is recommended. There are only two reports about the use of intravenous glucose in neonates and these reports underpin current clinical practice (Lilien et al., 1977, 1980); updated research is necessary in this area of practice. Hypoglycaemic neonates are usually given an intravenous bolus dose of 10% glucose at 2 mL/kg followed by a continuous infusion of 10% glucose at a rate of 5–8 mg/kg of glucose per minute. Blood sugar levels should be checked 30–45 minutes after the intravenous infusion commences to allow for early adjustments to therapy (Rozance, 2021b). Frequently, this treatment will restore the blood glucose concentration within 1 minute. There is a paucity of evidence about the rate of blood glucose concentration correction and neurosensory outcomes (Harding et al., 2017).

Other medications

Persistent hypoglycaemia that does not resolve is a medical emergency and can be difficult to manage. Treatment options include medications such as glucagon, glucocorticoid steroids, diazoxide and octreotide. In cases where venous access is difficult, or impossible, glucagon can be given intramuscularly in neonates with adequate glycogen stores (Smolkin et al., 2019).

Neurosensory outcomes of hypoglycaemia

There is no doubt that severe, persistent hypoglycaemia can cause seizures and brain injury in neonates. However, the long-term significance of early, asymptomatic or transitional low glucose concentrations is less clear. Population-based studies suggest that exposure to even brief, mild-to-moderate asymptomatic hypoglycaemia may permanently impair brain development and later learning (McKinlay et al., 2017b). Understanding of the long-term effects of neonatal hypoglycaemia has been limited by a paucity of studies that are adequately powered and involve detailed assessment of neonatal blood glucose concentrations and later neurocognitive function. There are no studies comparing total primary cerebral fuels (glucose, ketones and lactate) and later neurocognitive function.

However, the CHYLD (**c**hildren with **hy**poglycaemia and their **l**ater **d**evelopment) Study (McKinlay et al., 2015) followed up those neonates in the Sugar Babies (Harris et al., 2013) and Babies Study cohorts (Harris et al., 2011) and aimed to prospectively evaluate the long-term effects of neonatal hypoglycaemia in term and late preterm neonates born at risk. The findings from the 2- and 4.5-year-old follow-up assessments showed that there were no differences between at-risk children who were and were not exposed to neonatal hypoglycaemia. However, the overall rate of neurosensory impairment was high: 38% at 2 years (McKinlay et al., 2015) and 4.5 years. Hypoglycaemia was associated with a dose-dependent increased risk of poor executive function and visual motor function, even if not detected clinically (blinded continuous glucose monitoring), and this is likely to influence later learning (McKinlay et al., 2017b).

HYPERGLYCAEMIA

The prevalence of **hyperglycaemia** in preterm infants is 25–75% (Lemelman et al., 2018). Hyperglycaemia is also common in unwell, stressed and post-surgery neonates, regardless of gestational age or weight, and is reported as a considerable risk to both morbidity and mortality. Historically, excessive glucose administration was considered to be the cause of hyperglycaemia. However, more recently studies have demonstrated that the condition is complex and related to excess glucose production and insulin resistance, and/or glucose intolerance, and inflammatory markers leading to an inability of the preterm neonate to maintain normal glycaemia (Zamir et al., 2018).

Pathophysiology

The fetus produces insulin as early as 11 weeks' gestation. However, it may not be released into the bloodstream in response to hyperglycaemia until 16–20 weeks' gestation. Once released, the fetus can remain unresponsive to insulin. The rationale for poor insulin sensitivity in the preterm neonate is complex and poorly understood. Possible mechanisms included a poorly controlled stress and counter-regulatory hormonal response. In addition, the glucose transporters and enzyme activities that regulate the glycogenolysis and gluconeogenic pathways are poorly developed, leading to an inability to maintain normal blood glucose concentrations.

Hyperglycaemia can be a marker of a neonate becoming unwell, as the neonate experiencing stress can increase plasma cortisol concentrations. The relationship between increased cortisol and hyperglycaemia is unclear. However, post-surgical hyperglycaemia may be linked to the increased cortisol release during surgery. Increased parenteral glucose administration, sepsis, increased counter-regulatory hormones due to stress, and medications such as steroids are common causes of hyperglycaemia in this population (Lemelman et al., 2018).

Diagnosis

Similarly to hypoglycaemia, the diagnosis must be made on a reliable neonatal glucose analyser (Ba et al., 2018). Regardless of gestational or postmenstrual age, neonatal hyperglycaemia is defined as serum glucose greater than 150 mg/dL (8.3 mmol/L) or whole blood glucose greater than 125 mg/dL (6.9 mmol/L) (Balasundaram & Dumpa, 2021).

Clinical signs and symptoms

Similarly to hypoglycaemia, most neonates with hyperglycaemia will have no clinical signs or symptoms. However, features may include dehydration due to osmotic diuresis, weight loss, failure to thrive, fever, glycosuria, ketosis and metabolic acidosis.

Treatment and management

There remains considerable variation in the management of neonates with hyperglycaemia, which in part may be due to the lack of evidence-based guidelines for management. Insulin is the mainstay of treatment yet, due to the potential for hypoglycaemia in the preterm population, there has been substantial controversy about the safety of insulin use in this population (Thomson et al., 2019). There are few randomised controlled trials and findings are difficult to compare owing to the differing methodologies used. Findings from the 7-year follow-up after randomisation as preterm neonates to either a tight control (4–6 mmol/L) or standard treatment (8–10 mmol/L) showed that, although mortality was high, the use of insulin in preterm babies did not alter the rates of mortality. However, at 7 years of age the children that were randomised to the tightly controlled group were shorter and had altered body compositions (Tottman et al., 2018).

Feeding has been shown to promote pancreatic function and the secretion of insulin (Moullé & Parnet, 2019). Small amounts of milk encourage the production of gastric hormones including gastric inhibitory polypeptides and pancreatic polypeptides. These hormones increase the secretion of insulin from the pancreas. Therefore, continuing to feed the hyperglycaemic neonate may be helpful. If hyperglycaemia persists, it is important to exclude neonatal diabetes, and further blood tests should include levels of insulin, C-peptide and ketone bodies.

Prognosis and complications

Hyperglycaemia has been linked to significant neonatal morbidity including retinopathy of prematurity and increased mortality. It is unclear whether the hyperglycaemia is the cause or the consequence of the mortality. Hyperglycaemia has been reported to cause an increase in serum osmolality; each increase of 1 mmol/L in blood glucose concentration increases the serum osmolality by 1 mOsm/L (Najem et al., 2021). Increased osmolality can lead to osmotic diuresis that may result in polyuria, dehydration and intraventricular haemorrhage.

THE ENDOCRINE SYSTEM

The endocrine system is complex. The glands of the endocrine system include the hypothalamus, pituitary, adrenal, thyroid, pancreas, parathyroid and pineal glands and the gonads (ovaries and testes). These glands release hormones into the bloodstream and lymphatic system (Table 15.2). The hormones regulate growth and development; tissue function; metabolism and energy balance; mobilisation of body defences; maintenance of fluid, electrolyte and nutrient balance; sexual function and reproductive processes; and mood and sleep cycles. Hormone release is coordinated in response to changing blood concentrations (humoral), the influence of other hormones (hormonal) and interactions from the nervous system (neural) (Fig. 15.9).

To develop and successfully maintain a healthy pregnancy, a coordinated sequence of actions must occur. Human pregnancy endocrinology is concerned with endocrine and metabolic changes caused by physiological changes at the mother–fetus border. This interface, known as the feto-placental unit (FPU), is a significant location of protein and steroid hormone production and secretion. It also functions as an endocrine, respiratory, alimentary and excretory organ, allowing nutrients and metabolic products to be exchanged between the mother and fetus.

TABLE 15.2 **Endocrine glands and their hormones**

Endocrine gland		Hormones produced
Hypothalamus		Corticotrophin-releasing hormones (CRH) Dopamine Growth-hormone-releasing hormone (GHRH) Somatostatin Gonadotrophin-releasing hormone (GnRH) Thyrotrophin-releasing hormone (TRH) Oxytocin Vasopressin (antidiuretic hormone, ADH)
Pituitary	Anterior	Adrenocorticotrophic hormone (ACTH) Follicle-stimulating hormone (FSH) Luteinising hormone (LH) Prolactin (PRL) Thyrotrophin (thyroid-stimulating hormone, TSH) Growth hormone (GH)
	Posterior	Oxytocin Vasopressin (antidiuretic hormone, ADH)
Thyroid		Thyroxine (T4) Triiodothyronine (T3) Calcitonin
Parathyroid		Parathyroid hormone (PTH)
Adrenal	Cortex	Glucocorticoids (i.e. cortisol) Mineralocorticoids (i.e. aldosterone) Androgens (i.e. testosterone)
	Medulla	Adrenaline (epinephrine) Noradrenaline (norepinephrine) Dopamine
Pancreas		Insulin Glucagon Somatostatin Pancreatic polypeptide
Gonads	Ovaries	Oestrogens Progesterone Relaxin Inhibin
	Testis	Testosterone Inhibin Mullerian inhibiting hormone (MIH)
Pineal		Melatonin

Source: Greenstein and Wood (2011).

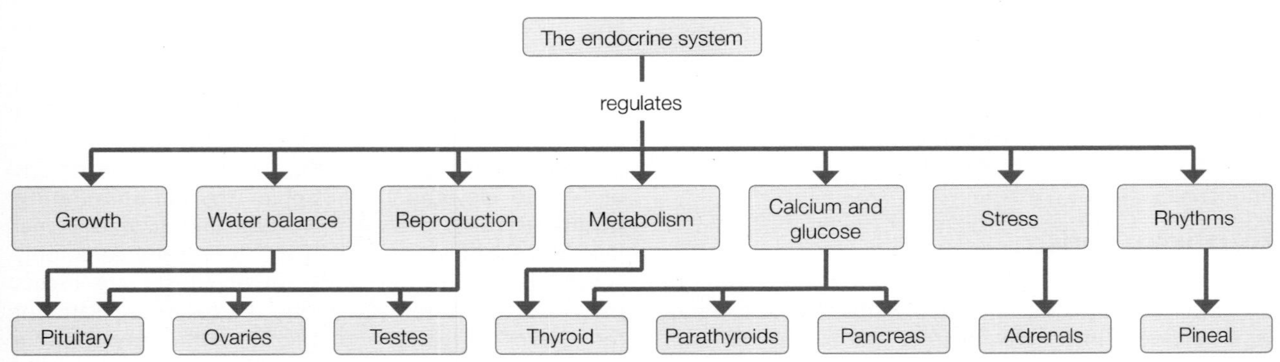

FIGURE 15.9 **Overview of the endocrine system**

For appropriate intrauterine growth and development, the fetus is dependent on this successful interaction with the mother. As a result, it is unsurprising that the fetus initiates and influences maternal modifications to enhance this exchange through complicated hormonal pathways. Many of the endocrine and metabolic alterations that occur during pregnancy can be directly linked to FPU-derived hormonal signals. Pregnancy initiation and maintenance are essentially determined by the interplay of neural and hormonal variables. The proper timing of these neuroendocrine activities within and between the placental, fetal and maternal compartments is crucial for regulating fetal growth and development and synchronising parturition timing. Maternal adaptations to hormonal changes during pregnancy have a direct impact on the development of the fetus and placenta. The establishment of a receptive endometrium, implantation and the maintenance of early pregnancy, modification of the maternal system to provide adequate nutritional support for the developing fetus, and preparation for parturition and subsequent lactation are all examples of gestational adaptations that occur during pregnancy (Tal & Taylor, 2021).

Adaptation at birth

The endocrine system has a significant influence on the fetus in the preparation for birth and postnatal life and this adaptation is multifaceted and complex. During fetal development, the concentrations of cortisol, from the adrenal glands, and T3 (triiodothyronine), from the thyroid gland, steadily increase. This results in enhanced sensitivity of epithelial cells, particularly within the airways, which peaks during labour and delivery leading to a reduction in fetal lung fluid and the release of surfactant. Catecholamines are also involved in increasing myocardial contractility and systemic vascular resistance, as well as triggering the onset of thermogenesis through the mobilisation of energy substrates. Without these pathways, successful adaptation to extrauterine life is impossible.

DISORDERS OF THE ENDOCRINE SYSTEM

Endocrine organ developmental disorders commonly manifest during the neonatal period. In neonates, endocrine organ function is influenced by organ development as well as the maternal, placental and fetal hormone milieu. Fetal adaptation or maladaptation to the hormonal environment may play a role in neonatal disease. The following sections discuss disorders of the neonatal endocrine system.

Hypopituitarism

The pituitary gland is pea sized and sits at the base of the brain connecting directly to the hypothalamus. It is divided into two distinct parts: the anterior (adenohypophysis) and posterior (neurohypophysis). By 7 weeks' gestation, the anterior pituitary is capable of secreting hormones.

The hypothalamus and anterior pituitary form a neuroendocrine unit that mediates between the central nervous system and the peripheral tissues and produces hormones for growth and development. It receives signalling factors from the hypothalamus through the hypothalamic–pituitary portal system. Hypopituitarism results from a deficiency in any or all of the hormones secreted by the pituitary gland.

Clinical features

These include:

- symptomatic hypoglycaemia
- asymptomatic hypoglycaemia
- prolonged jaundice
- dysmorphic neonate with midline anomalies including septo-optic dysplasia and optic nerve hypoplasia
- micropenis.

Neonatal hypopituitarism can occur because of pituitary gland developmental problems, genetic mutations and perinatal and neonatal events. Congenital hypopituitarism is estimated to affect 1 in 4000 to 1 in 10,000 people.

Hypopituitarism is uncommon, and symptoms may not be evident in the neonatal period and may manifest with a variety of non-specific clinical features. Furthermore, the sensitivity of laboratory procedures may not be appropriate for neonates (Kurtoğlu et al., 2019).

Hypothyroidism

The first gland of the endocrine system to develop is the thyroid gland, as early as the 24th day of gestation. This gland uses iodine to produce fundamental hormones for metabolism, growth, maturation and regulation of many functions of the body. By 12 weeks' gestation, the fetal thyroid is capable of storing iodine, and by 20 weeks the fetus is able to implement feedback mechanisms for the production of thyroid hormones.

Thyroxine (T4) and T3 are fundamental to fetal growth and development and have an effect on nearly every cell. The neonatal brain is dependent on thyroid hormones for development, and this dependence continues until the child is at least 2–3 years old. They also play an important role in maintenance of blood pressure, regulation of tissue growth and development, development of the skeletal and nervous systems and maturation of reproductive capabilities.

Congenital hypothyroidism (CH) is defined as a deficiency of thyroid hormones, which can be transient or permanent. Transient congenital hypothyroidism is identified when the neonate has low concentrations of T4 and elevated thyrotrophin **(thyroid-stimulating hormone (TSH)**) levels, which eventually return to normal over the first few months of life. It is most commonly caused by iodine deficiency; other causes are excess maternal anti-thyroid medications (maternal treatment for Graves' disease) and transplacental thyrotrophin receptor-blocking antibodies. Permanent congenital hypothyroidism results from a primary dysfunction of the thyroid gland itself, in conditions such as ectopic thyroid gland, or a secondary (or central) dysfunction of the pituitary and/or hypothalamus, most commonly hypopituitarism (Kanike et al., 2017).

Clinical features

These include:

- low baseline heart rate
- hypothermia or cold intolerance
- slowed gastrointestinal tract
- reduced sensitivity to catecholamines
- decreased glucose metabolism
- oedema
- prolonged physiological jaundice
- slowed brain development and growth.

Severe hypothyroidism, also known as cretinism, is associated with severe developmental delay. These neonates may also have a short disproportionate body and a thick tongue and neck (Kanike et al., 2017).

Diagnosis and treatment

If hypothyroidism is suspected from the clinical signs, thyroid function tests are required. The diagnosis will be made on a finding of low T4 and elevated TSH. T3 concentrations are variable and may be within the normal range initially. Thyroid function tests are normally performed on day 5 after birth, as early sampling may reflect the maternal concentrations. Newborn screening programs have also significantly contributed to the diagnosis of hypothyroidism. Treatment includes administration of thyroxine and must commence without delay to avoid delayed brain growth and development of neuro-impairment (Kanike et al., 2017).

REFLECTION

Consider the burden of endocrine disease, with a substantial proportion of children with lifelong neurodevelopmental compromise or even dying without proper diagnosis and/or access to early appropriate treatment.

What are the implications for the neonate, family and the community?

Hyperthyroidism

Hyperthyroidism in the neonatal period is rare. The most common cause is maternal Graves' disease, which is an autoimmune disease where antibodies that mimic TSH continuously stimulate the release of thyroid hormones. The maternal TSH receptor-stimulating antibodies cross the placenta and stimulate the neonate's own thyroid to increase hormone production (Cheetham & Lane, 2017). The disease is normally transient and improves as the maternal antibodies clear, which is usually between 3 and 12 weeks (Segni, 2019).

Clinical features

These may be present at birth or can be delayed for several days, and include:

- tachycardia
- hyperthermia
- irritability
- hypertension
- proptosis
- diarrhoea
- muscle atrophy and weakness.

Hypoparathyroidism

The parathyroid glands secrete parathyroid hormone, which is most important for controlling calcium balance. The parathyroid glands begin to develop at 4 weeks' gestation and are required to produce parathyroid hormone by the seventh week when the fetal bones start ossifying. Complete physiological functioning is normally established at the beginning of the second trimester. Plasma calcium ion homeostasis is essential for transmission of nerve impulses, muscle contraction and blood clotting. During pregnancy the mother provides calcium and phosphorus to the fetus, promoting skeletal development and tissue growth.

After birth the neonate is responsible for their own calcium homeostasis through calcium intake, mobilisation of stores, parathyroid hormone, vitamin D and calcitonin. In the first few days after birth there is a drop in calcium concentrations followed by a critical increase in parathyroid hormone, which then increases calcium concentrations (Datye & Bremer, 2013). The parathyroid hormone is released in response to falling concentrations of ionised calcium in the blood, causing a release of calcium from the cells within the bones. Parathyroid hormone activates the synthesis of calcitriol in the kidney and increases calcium reabsorption from the distal tubule and phosphate excretion from the proximal tubule of the kidneys. Vitamin D (calciferol) is particularly necessary for the absorption of calcium from food via the intestine.

The presentation of hypoparathyroidism can be divided into early (within the first 4 days) and late (after day 5) (Thomas et al., 2012). Early onset is often associated with prematurity, perinatal asphyxia, neonates of diabetic mothers and maternal hyperparathyroidism. Late hyperparathyroidism is usually iatrogenic and caused by excessive intake of phosphate. Elevated blood concentrations of parathyroid hormone are associated with hypercalcaemia, indicating neonatal hyperparathyroidism.

The diagnosis of parathyroid dysfunction is made using both blood and urine samples, and treatment is aimed at normalising calcium concentrations and managing symptoms (Capozza et al., 2018).

Diabetes insipidus

Diabetes insipidus (DI) arises in the neonate either when there is deficient secretion of arginine vasopressin (AVP) – also known as antidiuretic hormone (ADH) – from the pituitary or when the renal tubules are unresponsive to ADH (Roth, 2017). In the neonatal period, diabetes insipidus can be secondary to underlying genetic conditions, such as septo-optic dysplasia, agenesis of the corpus callosum and holoprosencephaly, or a consequence of intraventricular haemorrhage or sepsis (Patti et al., 2020).

Clinical features

These include:

- inappropriate water loss
- large quantities of dilute urine.

Congenital adrenal hyperplasia

Congenital adrenal hyperplasia (CAH) is the most common cause of adrenal hypofunction and ambiguous genitalia. It is caused by an autosomal recessive disorder of steroidogenesis resulting in a cortisol deficiency and excessive secretion of ACTH from the pituitary (Badeghiesh et al., 2020).

CAH is the most common cause of over-virilisation, the masculinisation of the human body. This is due to defects in the gene encoding the 21-hydroxylase enzyme (P450c21) and results in decreased cortisol synthesis, increased androgen production and, hence, virilisation of the external genitalia. An example of decreased androgen metabolism is placental–fetal aromatase deficiency, which results in an increase in testosterone concentrations for the female fetus. This can be due to exposure to maternal androgen-secreting adrenal or ovarian tumours; after birth, fetal exposure to the hormone ceases (Datye & Bremer, 2013).

Clinical features

These can be seen in the neonatal period, and are more common in preterm neonates than in term neonates:

- hypoglycaemia
- hyponatraemia
- hypotension
- ambiguous genitalia
- skin pigmentation, particularly around the scrotum.

Diagnosis

Diagnosis includes:

- cortisol levels: up to three random blood tests as it is secreted in a pulsatile manner
- adrenocorticotrophic hormone levels: expected to be elevated
- synacthen test: cortisol levels following administration of synacthen to examine adrenal gland response
- long-chain fatty acids: if the synacthen test shows poor cortisol response
- urine screening: for analysis of steroids
- adrenal ultrasound scan: to assess haemorrhage or hypertrophy
- genetic analysis
- brain MRI scan: to determine any abnormalities.

Treatment will be individualised to the needs of the neonate and family. However, it is likely to include steroid replacement and blood glucose monitoring.

Ambiguous genitalia

Differentiation of the female ovaries and male gonads begins during the seventh week of gestation. After primitive gonad development, the fetal hormonal profile then directs the development of the female or male reproductive structures. Unless the expression of certain genes and hormones occurs at precise times, a female embryo will develop. In females the primordial follicles are observed at 18 weeks, and oocytes progressively decline from 3–6 million at 5 months' gestation to 2 million at term. For males the testes begin to descend at 8 weeks' gestation and continue until 6 weeks postnatally until they have fully descended into the inguinal canal.

Disorders of sexual differentiation include pure gonadal dysgenesis (46, XY), when the testicles fail to differentiate and the neonate has female internal genitalia; mixed gonadal dysgenesis (45, XO/46, XY), when the neonate's ambiguous genitalia are asymmetric; and Klinefelter syndrome (usually 47, XXY) and Turner syndrome (45, X or a variation of this). True hermaphroditism refers to neonates with both ovarian and testicular tissues. Most are 46 XX and may have ovotestes containing both tissues or they may have an ovary on one side and testis on the other. It is also possible to have complex congenital internal reproductive organs and external ambiguous genitalia or to have entirely female external genitalia. Diagnosis is performed through biopsy. Treatment was once considered to be urgent, requiring immediate gender assignment. However, more recently treatment is individualised to the family and can involve removing dysgenetic testicular tissue and gender assignment (B. R. Lee et al., 2021).

Ambiguous genitalia occur in approximately one in 4500 births. Because the situation is rarely anticipated, neonatal nurses and midwives have a significant role in the support of parents who will most likely be confused, distressed and saddened. It is not useful to rush to decide on a gender for the neonate; a decision is made once test results become available.

FAMILY-CENTRED CARE 15.1

There have been many cases where neonates with ambiguous genitalia were unable to be diagnosed antenatally and clinicians have unknowingly identified the incorrect gender at birth.

On further assessment, an incorrect gender assignment was found. Consider how this might affect the family and the neonate. What are the tools available to the multidisciplinary team to assist families in this situation in your area of practice? As the neonatal nurse/midwife caring for this neonate and family, how do you help them understand and cope with the diagnosis?

Inborn errors of metabolism

Inborn errors of metabolism (IEMs) are rare genetic disorders, usually autosomal recessive, that develop when there is an enzyme defect in the body, leading to either an accumulation or a deficiency in a particular metabolite (Jeanmonod et al., 2022). This can occur through exogenous exposure, for example dietary intake, or through endogenous pathways of protein, carbohydrate or fat metabolism. The presentation of an IEM in the neonatal period is varied and depends on the individual condition. Often by the time symptoms are evident there could already be significant irreversible effects for the neonate. Early diagnosis and treatment at or near birth can counter the adverse effects of some IEMs, resulting in normal or near-normal health outcomes. In many cases, simple nutritional interventions are used to manage these disorders. However, if left untreated, serious adverse health outcomes including intellectual disability, behavioural dysfunction, inadequate growth, abnormal development, nutrient deficiencies and sequelae that require complex hospital care will be experienced (Saudubray & Garcia-Cazorla, 2018). The five most common diseases screened including IEMs are described in Table 15.3.

While IEMs in neonates are rare, this group of disorders can be life changing and/or threatening. Most disorders are treatable and, therefore, prompt diagnosis and intervention can alter the life trajectory of a neonate and their family. Clinical presentation can be subtle and interpretation of endocrine function in the neonatal period can be difficult, particularly during transition following birth. Identification of disorders can be further complicated when presented in a preterm neonate.

Clinical features

These are subtle with non-specific signs and symptoms appearing as the by-products of metabolism accumulate to toxic levels:

- vomiting
- poor weight gain
- growth abnormalities
- encephalopathy.

FAMILY-CENTRED CARE 15.2

Parents whose neonates have a metabolic or endocrine disorder can be anxious and distressed and require considerable support as they manage the uncertainty of the future for their baby.

Providing positive caring and clear communication will help parents to manage the stress associated with the loss of the expected healthy neonate and the reality of a neonate who may have significant long-term health issues.

TABLE 15.3 **The five most common inborn errors of metabolism**

Disease	Date screening available	Rates	Cause	Outcome
Phenylketonuria (PKU)	1960s	1:13,000	The body cannot break down amino acids, phenylalanine found in foods high in protein	Neurological damage
Congenital hypothyroidism (CH)	1970s	1:4000	Inadequate iodine intake during fetal development, hypopituitarism, genetic disorders or agenesis of the thyroid	Intellectual impairment and dwarfism May be transient or develop within first year of life
Cystic fibrosis (CF)	1980s	1:2500 European descent	Defect in the *CFTR* gene	May present in the neonatal period with meconium ileus
Galactosaemia	1980s	1:30,000 European descent	A complete absence of galactose-1-phosphate uridyltransferase	Sepsis, hypoglycaemia, liver damage, brain damage and cataracts, all usually occurring in the neonatal period Early treatment avoids the neonatal complications; however, neurological defects may still develop later in life
Congenital adrenal hyperplasia (CAH)	1980s	1:10,000–20,000	Deficiency of 21-hydroxylase	Hyponatraemia, hyperkalaemia and hypoglycaemia. Virilisation in females Prompt diagnosis at birth can avoid adrenal crises after the first week of life

Source: Clague and Thomas (2002).

Newborn screening

Dr Robert Guthrie was an American microbiologist who developed the seminal work on **newborn screening (NBS)**. Guthrie developed a technique in the 1960s that enabled the identification of neonates with phenylketonuria (PKU) through analysis of a dried blood spot (Guthrie, 1992). NBS is now an accepted part of routine neonatal healthcare in many countries and was established in Australasia in the late 1960s.

Guthrie also developed the filter paper on which the blood specimen is collected. Originally known as the Guthrie Screening Card, it is now known as the **Newborn Screening Card**. The neonate's blood is collected between 48 and 72 hours after birth by a heel prick and blotted onto the filter paper, then sent to a specialised laboratory for analysis. The Newborn Screening Card is made to strict specifications so that the blood can be collected and analysed correctly. In Australia and New Zealand, NBS for metabolic disorders is offered at no cost to families. NBS in some form is now present in every European country, except in Albania, Kosovo and Tajikistan, where lack of financial resources has been cited to explain the absence of NBS in those countries (Koracin et al., 2021).

Low birthweight, preterm and unwell neonates pose a special problem for NBS programs. The results of screening for neonates who are nil by mouth, receiving **total parenteral nutrition (TPN)** or certain medications, or who have had blood transfusions can be inaccurate. Though there is a section on the Newborn Screening Card where information on the neonate's feeding history, age at time of collection and use of TPN can be documented, increasing the accuracy of the results, work continues to investigate ways to make the screening as accurate as possible. Morris et al. (2014) developed a protocol for interrupting TPN infusions 3 hours before the NBS is taken. This process resulted in a 74% reduction in false positives in their neonatal unit.

Newborn screening protocol

Fig. 15.10 shows an example of collection of a sample for newborn screening. The protocol involves the following steps (Morris et al., 2014):

- First screening, 48–72 hours. If the neonate is to receive a blood transfusion, consider collecting the NBS prior and then repeating the collection 48 hours afterwards.
- Second screening, 14 days for neonates born weighing less than 1.5 kg.
- Third screening, 28 days for neonates born weighing less than 1 kg.

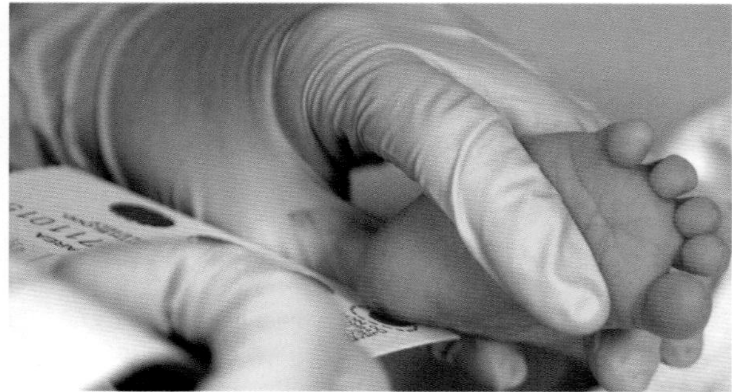

FIGURE 15.10 **Newborn screening sample collection**
Source: U.S. Air Force photo/Staff Sgt Eric T. Sheler.

EVIDENCE-BASED PRACTICE RESEARCH 15.1

Inborn errors of metabolism frequently manifest in infancy as life-threatening episodes of metabolic decompensation. Prior to metabolic screening for these disorders, studies suggested that they were responsible for 1–6% of sudden unexpected death in infancy (SUDI). However, a study of a cohort that had undergone extensive neonatal screening for inborn errors of metabolism revealed that the prevalence of these diseases was not increased among infants who died suddenly. These data imply that integrating comprehensive metabolic disease screening in NBS has effectively reduced or eliminated the contribution of undetected metabolic disorders presenting as SUDI (Crown & McClain, 2018). See Chapter 2 for more information regarding SUDI.

Tandem mass spectrometry

Tandem mass spectrometry (TMS) has enabled the growth of NBS programs during the 1990s. Because of its sensitive, specific nature and ability to analyse dozens of metabolites at the same time, it can aid in the detection of more inborn errors of metabolism. NBS has progressed from a basic blood or urine screening test to a comprehensive and complicated screening system that can detect over 50 different IEM diseases. TMS technology was then used to increase neonatal screening in the United Kingdom, Germany, Australia, South Korea, Japan and other nations.

IEM is well known to have an autosomal recessive inheritance pattern (i.e. the gene variants are mostly inherited from the parents). Furthermore, the clinical symptoms of IEM are complex and diverse. It is also challenging for physicians to understand IEM screening results because there are so many signs and ratios to consider. As a result, additional TMS diagnosis of potentially positive children is critical. The detection of disease-caused gene variants may aid in the diagnosis of IEM. NGS (next-generation sequencing) technology has gradually gained prominence in the field of genetic diagnosis. It can sequence millions of DNA molecules at the same time and can be used in a variety of biomedical research applications. NGS has been increasingly and widely used in clinical practice in recent years, and has dramatically transformed the diagnosis, prognosis and therapy of many human diseases (Wang et al., 2020).

REFLECTION

As screening protocols may differ among organisations, identify your local NBS program and what testing is included for the neonates. Consider the implications of early discharge on the outcomes of a successful NBS program.
Does your organisation audit its program and who contacts those parents whose neonates have missed being screened prior to discharge?

Ethical considerations

The available technology has undoubtedly provided significant improvements to NBS programs. However, experts in this field highlight concerns that, with the emphasis on technology, the direct benefit to the neonate may have been lost (Ross & Waggoner, 2012) and that the clinical value of expanding screening may be in conflict with the evidence-based public health approach (Ross & Waggoner, 2012). Problems facing NBS worldwide include over-diagnosis, expensive testing, lack of available follow-up and lack of robust evidence regarding which new screening tests to include. Screening neonates for rare diseases that may not develop and for which there are not yet simple, effective treatments is ethically fraught. The major driving force behind NBS programs is not only the development of the screening tools but also that of effective treatments. It is recommended that future translational research includes ways to access affordable medical foods and remove barriers to treatments. The choices made around which diseases to add to a screening program should be through analysis of the:

- positive predictive value of the test
- financial and social costs of screening
- cost and success of treatments
- benefit of early diagnosis and commencement of treatment prior to symptoms becoming evident
- advantage to quality of life (Goldenberg et al., 2016).

CLINICAL PRACTICE 15.3

The World Health Organization (WHO) developed guiding principles on population screening outlining that the disease must have a clear test and an acceptable treatment and that the cost of diagnosis should be weighed against the expense of treatment. Over the past 50 years with the advent of new technologies, a vast array of diseases has been added to NBS programs worldwide. Through these programs, thousands of neonates born with potentially devastating diseases have been identified and treated.

However, there is still a significant amount of variability among the screening profiles of countries and even of regions, particularly in the developing world. Australia's nearest neighbour Papua New Guinea is currently without an NBS program.

Consent

Evidence shows conflicting opinions on whether parental consent is required prior to blood being collected for NBS. The Human Genetics Society of Australasia *Policy PL02 for newborn bloodspot testing* (2011, p. 3) states: 'Participation in a NBS program should not be mandatory. Parents should be informed of the availability of testing. If after discussion the parents refuse to have their newborn tested, they should sign a statement that they are fully informed about the test and the consequences of not testing.' Screening in 48 states of the USA is mandatory and, therefore, parental consent is not required, though parents are 'allowed' to opt out in certain circumstances (Ross & Waggoner, 2012).

In some states the Newborn Screening Card may be returned to families after analysis is complete. This is facilitated through the individual laboratory that performed the screening. There are also local policies and ethics committees that identify the process for informing and gaining consent from families when the samples are to be used for purposes other than NBS. Parents have filed lawsuits in the USA, British Columbia, Ireland and New Zealand when they have learned that their neonate's blood spots were used for research purposes without their consent (Ross & Waggoner, 2012), leading to the consideration expressed by Esquerda et al. (2021) that the sample and non-useful information obtained from it should be destroyed after genetic screening.

CLINICAL PRACTICE 15.4

Consider what you have read about parent-informed consent and the NBS.

1. In your workplace, how does this discussion with parents take place?
2. Do neonatal nurses and midwives provide written material about the NBS?
3. Do parents have time to consider their response before agreeing and can they opt out?
4. Is there a difference in this practice between the neonatal and maternity unit?

Follow-up

All NBS programs are required to have follow-up processes for positive results, including notification to the doctor and/or midwife and the family, recommendations of further diagnostic testing and referral for ongoing treatment. Depending on the diagnosis, consideration will be given to the need for relevant paediatric specialists such as endocrine, genetic and palliative care teams to become involved in the neonate's care. Parents may also require testing; this will be used to assess the risk in future pregnancies and engagement with maternal–fetal medicine services.

Maternity and neonatal unit early-discharge programs can introduce some practical difficulties for local NBS programs. When families are discharged from hospital prior to the neonate being 48 hours of age, they will not have had their first screen taken. Local processes around parent education prior to discharge, linking with extended midwifery and child health services and local blood-collecting services, are important. An established audit process between maternity hospitals and the NBS laboratory to identify those neonates who were born but did not have an NBS collected for analysis is imperative for the neonates' wellbeing.

CONCLUSION

The diagnosis of an endocrine disorder or inborn error of metabolism can be devastating. These diseases are often lifelong and can be life limiting, and the diagnosis can be complicated. However, early diagnosis and prompt treatment can considerably improve the outcome for the neonate and the family. It is imperative that maternity and neonatal units have processes in place for screening and follow-up. Families with a positive diagnosis need the support of the multidisciplinary team including neonatology, paediatric subspecialties, allied health and community-based family supports. Neonatal nurses/midwives are pivotal in not only caring for the neonate's health and wellbeing but also supporting the family through education, empathy and coordination of the healthcare team.

Online Resources

Centres for Disease Control and Prevention, Newborn Screening Quality Assurance Program (NSQAP): <https://www.cdc.gov/labstandards/nsqap.html>

Ministry of Health, New Zealand Government, Newborn metabolic screening programme: <https://www.health.govt.nz/your-health/pregnancy-and-kids/first-year/first-6-weeks/health-checks-first-6-weeks/newborn-screening-tests/newborn-metabolic-screening>

Queensland Health Clinical Guidelines for neonatal hypoglycaemia: <https://www.health.qld.gov.au/__data/assets/pdf_file/0043/881899/g-hypogly.pdf>

University of Auckland, Faculty of Medical and Health Sciences oral dextrose gel to treat neonatal hypoglycaemia: clinical practice guidelines: <https://www.fmhs.auckland.ac.nz/clinicalpracticeguidelines>

NBS programs

Australasia: <https://www.hgsa.org.au/about/hgsa-committees/joint-hgsaracp-newborn-screening-committee>

Centers for Disease Control and Prevention, Newborn screening portal: <https://www.cdc.gov/newbornscreening/index.html>

New Zealand National Screening Unit, Newborn Metabolic Screening Programme – heel prick test: <https://www.nsu.govt.nz/pregnancy-newborn-screening/newborn-metabolic-screening-programme-heel-prick-test>

Organisations supporting families affected by rare disorders

National Organisation for Rare Disorders: <https://rarediseases.org/>

New Zealand Organisation for Rare Disorders (NZORD): <https://www.nzord.org.nz/>

Rare Voices Australia: < https://www.rarevoices.org.au/>

Superpower Baby Project book: <https://www.superpowerbabyproject.org>

Further Reading

Eng, L., & Lam, L. (2020). Thyroid function during the fetal and neonatal periods. *NeoReviews, 21*(1), e30–e36.

Nicolaides, N. C., Kanaka-Gantenbein, C., Papadopoulou-Marketou, N., Sertedaki, A., Chrousos, G. P., & Papassotiriou, J. (2020). Emerging technologies in pediatrics: the paradigm of neonatal diabetes mellitus. *Critical Reviews in Clinical Laboratory Sciences, 57*(8), 522–531. doi: 10.1080/10408363.2020.1752141.

References/Acknowledgements

Abramowicz, J. S., & Ahn, J. T. (2020). Fetal macrosomia. In: D. Levine (Ed.), *UpToDate*. Walters Kluwer. <https://www.uptodate.com/contents/fetal-macrosomia?search> (Accessed 16 February 2022).

Abramowski, A., Ward, R., & Hamdan, A. (2021). *Neonatal hypoglycaemia*. *StatPearls*. Treasure Island, FL: StatPearls Publishing. <https://www.ncbi.nlm.nih.gov/books/NBK537105/> (Accessed 16 February 2022).

Aliefendioğlu, D., Çoban, A., Hatipoğlu, N., Ecevit, A., Arısoy, A. E., Yeşiltepe, G., et al. (2018). Management of hypoglycaemia in newborn: Turkish Neonatal and Pediatric Endocrinology and Diabetes Societies consensus report. *Turkish Archives of Pediatrics/Türk Pediatri Arşivi, 53*(suppl 1), S224.

Alsweiler, J. M., Harris, D. L., Harding, J. E., & McKinlay, C. J. (2021). Strategies to improve neurodevelopmental outcomes in babies at risk of neonatal hypoglycaemia. *Lancet Child and Adolescent Health, 5*(7), 513–523. doi: 10.1016/S2352-4642(20)30387-4.

Ba, Y., Xu, J., Yuan, L., Zhu, H., Yang, Y., Lam, M. M., et al. (2018). Assessment of the performance of blood glucose monitoring systems for monitoring dysglycaemia in neonatal patients. *BMJ Paediatrics Open, 2*(1), e000339. doi: 10.1136/bmjpo-2018-000339.

Badeghiesh, A., Ismail, S., Baghlaf, H., Suarthana, E., & Dahan, M. H. (2020). Pregnancy, delivery and neonatal outcomes among women with congenital adrenal hyperplasia: a study of a large US database. *Reproductive BioMedicine Online, 41*(6), 1093–1099.

Balasundaram, P., & Dumpa, V. (2021). Neonatal hyperglycaemia. *StatPearls*. Treasure Island, FL: StatPearls Publishing. <https://www.uptodate.com/contents/neonatal-hyperglycemia?search> (Accessed 16 February 2022).

Ballesta-Castillejos, A., Gomez-Salgado, J., Rodriguez-Almagro, J., Ortiz-Esquinas, I., & Hernandez-Martinez, A. (2020). Relationship between maternal body mass index with the onset of breastfeeding and its associated problems: an online survey. *International Breastfeeding Journal, 15*, 55. doi: 10.1186/s13006-020-00298-5.

Banerjee, I., Salomon-Estebanez, M., Shah, P., Nicholson, J., Cosgrove, K. E., & Dunne, M. J. (2019). Therapies and outcomes of congenital hyperinsulinism-induced hypoglycaemia. *Diabetic Medicine, 36*(1), 9–21.

Baud, O., & Berkane, N. (2019). Hormonal changes associated with intra-uterine growth restriction: impact on the developing brain and future neurodevelopment [review]. *Frontiers in Endocrinology,* 10, 179. doi: 10.3389/fendo.2019.00179.

Beardsall, K., Pesterfield, C. L., & Acerini, C. L. (2011). Neonatal diabetes and insulin pump therapy. *Archives of Disease in Childhood. Fetal and Neonatal Edition, 96*(3), F223–F224.

Capozza, M., Chinellato, I., Guarnieri, V., Di Lorgi, N., Accadia, M., Traggiai, C., et al. (2018). Case report: acute clinical presentation and neonatal management of primary hyperparathyroidism due to a novel CaSR mutation. *BMC Pediatrics, 18*(1), 340. doi: 10.1186/s12887-018-1319-0.

Chappe, M. K. (2020). Hypoglycaemia in high-risk infants within the immediate postnatal period. *Neonatal Network, 39*(5), 263–267. doi: 10.1891/0730-0832.39.5.263.

Cheetham, T., & Lane, L. C. (2017). Who needs thyroid function testing at birth? *Archives of Disease in Childhood, 102*(3), 212–215.

Chiruvolu, A., Miklis, K., Stanzo, K., Petrey, B., Groves, C., & McCord, K. (2017). Effects of skin-to-skin care on late preterm and term infants at-risk for neonatal hypoglycaemia. *Pediatric Quality and Safety, 2*, e030.

Clague, A., & Thomas, A. (2002). Neonatal biochemical screening for disease. *Clinica Chimica Acta, 315*(1–2), 99–110.

Crown, M. J., & McClain, M. (2018). Sudden unexpected infant death including SIDS: initial management. In: G. B. Mallory, T. K. Duryea, & A. G. Randolph (Eds.), *UpToDate*. Walters Kluwer. <https://www.uptodate.com/contents/sudden-unexpected-infant-death-including-sids-initial-management?search> (Accessed 16 February 2022).

Dani, C., & Corsini, I. (2020). Guidelines for management of neonatal hypoglycaemia: are they actually applicable? *JAMA Pediatrics, 174*(7), 638–639.

Dassios, T., Greenough, A., Leontiadi, S., Hickey, A., & Kametas, N. (2017). Admissions for hypoglycaemia after 35 weeks of gestation: perinatal predictors of cost of stay. *Journal of Maternal–Fetal and Neonatal Medicine, 2*(3), 448–454. doi: 10.1080/14767058.2017.1381905.

Datye, K. A., & Bremer, A. A. (2013). Endocrine disorders in the neonatal period. *Pediatric Annals, 42*(5), 67–73.

De Angelis, L. C., Brigati, G., Polleri, G., Malova, M., Parodi, A., Minghetti, D., et al. (2021). Neonatal hypoglycaemia and brain vulnerability. *Frontiers in Endocrinology, 12*, 195.

de Rooy, L., & Hawdon, J. (2002). Nutritional factors that affect the postnatal metabolic adaptation of full-term small- and large-for-gestational-age infants. *Pediatrics, 109*(3), e42.

Edwards, T., Liu, G., Hegarty, J. E., Crowther, C. A., Alsweiler, J., & Harding, J. E. (2021). Oral dextrose gel to prevent hypoglycaemia in at-risk neonates. *Cochrane Database of Systematic Reviews, 5*, CD012152. doi: 10.1002/14651858.CD012152.pub3.

Esquerda, M., Palau, F., Lorenzo, D., Cambra, F. J., Bofaruli, M., & Cusi, V.; Grup Interdisciplinar En Bioetica. (2021). Ethical questions concerning newborn genetic screening. *Clinical Genetics*, 99, 93–98. doi: 10.1111/cge.13828.

Feher, J. (2017a). *2.9 – ATP production I: glycolysis quantitative human physiology* (2nd ed., pp. 218–226). Boston, MA: Academic Press.

Feher, J. (2017b). *2.11 – ATP production III: fatty acid oxidation and amino acid oxidation quantitative human physiology* (2nd ed., pp. 241–252). Boston, MA: Academic Press.

Forster, D. A., Moorhead, A. M., Jacobs, S. E., Davis, P. G., Walker, S. P., McEgan, K. M., et al. (2017). Advising women with diabetes in pregnancy to express breastmilk in late pregnancy (Diabetes and Antenatal Milk Expressing [DAME]): a multicentre, unblinded, randomised controlled trial. *Lancet, 389*(10085), 2204–2213.

Futatani, T., Shimao, A., Ina, S., Higashiyama, H., Fujita, S., Ueno, K., et al. (2017). Capillary blood ketone levels as an indicator of inadequate breast milk intake in the early neonatal period. *Journal of Pediatrics, 191*, 76–81.

Goldenberg, A. J., Comeau, A. M., Grosse, S. D., Tanksley, S., Prosser, L. A., Ojodu, J., et al. (2016). Evaluating harms in the assessment of net benefit: a framework for newborn screening condition review. *Maternal and Child Health Journal, 20*(3), 693–700.

Greenstein, B., & Wood, D. (2011). T*he endocrine system at a glance* (3rd ed.). Oxford: John Wiley.

Gupta, A. (2022). Regulation of insulin secretion. In: A. Gupta (Ed.), *Understanding insulin and insulin resistance* (Ch 5, pp. 159–178). Amsterdam: Elsevier. doi: 10.1016/B978-0-12-820234-0.00001-9.

Guthrie, R. (1992). The origin of newborn screening. *Screening, 1*, 5–15.

Harding, J. E., Harris, D. L., Hegarty, J. E., Alsweiler, J. M., & McKinlay, C. J. (2017). An emerging evidence base for the management of neonatal hypoglycaemia. *Early Human Development, 104*, 51–56.

Harding, J. E., Hegarty, J. E., Crowther, C. A., Edlin, R. P., Gamble, G. D., Alsweiler, J. M., et al. (2021). Evaluation of oral dextrose gel for prevention of neonatal hypoglycaemia (hPOD): a multicentre, double-blind randomized controlled trial. *PLoS Medicine, 18*(1), e1003411. doi: 10.1371/journal.pmed.1003411.

Harris, D. L., Weston, P. J., Battin, M. R., & Harding, J. E. (2010). Continuous glucose monitoring in newborn babies at risk of neonatal hypoglycaemia. *Journal of Pediatrics, 157*(2), 198–202.

Harris, D. L., Weston, P. J., Williams, C. E., Pleasants, A. B., Battin, M. R., Spooner, C. G., et al. (2011). Cot-side electroencephalography monitoring is not clinically useful in the detection of mild neonatal hypoglycaemia. *Journal of Pediatrics, 159*(5), 755–760, e751.

Harris, D. L., Weston, P. J., & Harding, J. E. (2012). Incidence of neonatal hypoglycaemia in babies identified as at risk. *Journal of Pediatrics, 161*(5), 787–791.

Harris, D. L., Weston, P. J., Signal, M., Chase, J. G., & Harding, J. E. (2013). Dextrose gel for neonatal hypoglycaemia (the Sugar Babies Study): a randomised, double-blind, placebo-controlled trial. *Lancet, 382*(9910), 2077–2083.

Harris, D. L., Weston, P. J., Battin, M. R., & Harding, J. E. (2014). A survey of the management of neonatal hypoglycaemia within the Australian and New Zealand Neonatal Network. *Journal of Paediatrics and Child Health, 50*(10), E55–E62. doi: 10.1111/j.1440-1754.2009.01599.x.

Harris, D. L., Weston, P. J., & Harding, J. E. (2015). Lactate, rather than ketones, may provide alternative cerebral fuel in hypoglycaemic newborns. *Archives of Disease in Childhood. Fetal and Neonatal Edition, 100*(2), F161–F164.

Harris, D. L., Weston, P. J., & Harding, J. E. (2016a). A good breastfeed does not always result in an increase in blood glucose concentrations, in hypoglycaemic babies. *Journal of Paediatrics and Child Health Supplement, 52*(S2), 3–124.

Harris, D. L., Alsweiler, J. M., Ansell, J. M., Gamble, G. D., Thompson, B., Wouldes, T. A., et al.; Children with Hypoglycaemia and their Later Development Study Team. (2016b). Outcome at 2 years after dextrose gel treatment for neonatal hypoglycaemia: follow-up of a randomized trial. *Journal of Pediatrics, 170*, 54–59, e52.

Harris, D. L., Gamble, G. D., Weston, P. J., & Harding, J. E. (2017). What happens to blood glucose concentrations after oral treatment for neonatal hypoglycaemia? *Journal of Pediatrics, 190*, 136–141.

Harris, D. L., Weston, P. J., Gamble, G. D., & Harding, J. E. (2020). Glucose profiles in healthy term infants in the first 5 days: the Glucose in Well Babies (GLOW) study. *Journal of Pediatrics, 223*, 34–41.e34. doi: 10.1016/j.jpeds.2020.02.079.

Harris, D. L., Weston, P. J., & Harding, J. E. (2021). Alternative cerebral fuels in the first five days in healthy term infants: the Glucose in Well Babies (GLOW) study. *Journal of Pediatrics, 231*, 81–86.

Hatting, M., Tavares, C. D., Sharabi, K., Rines, A. K., & Puigserver, P. (2018). Insulin regulation of gluconeogenesis. *Annals of the New York Academy of Sciences, 1411*(1), 21.

Hegarty, J. E., Harding, J. E., Gamble, G. D., Crowther, C. A., Edlin, R., & Alsweiler, J. M. (2016). Prophylactic oral dextrose gel for newborn babies at risk of neonatal hypoglycaemia: a randomised controlled dose-finding trial (the Pre-hPOD Study). *PLoS Medicine, 13*(10), e1002155.

Helle, E., & Priest, J. R. (2020). Maternal obesity and diabetes mellitus as risk factors for congenital heart disease in the offspring. *Journal of the American Heart Association, 9*(8), e011541. doi: 10.1161/JAHA.119.011541.

Huerta-Saenz, L., Saunders, C., & Yan, Y. (2018). Challenging diagnosis of congenital hyperinsulinism in two infants of diabetic mothers with rare pathogenic KCNJ11 and HNF4A gene variants. *International Journal of Pediatric Endocrinology, 2018*(1), 1–6.

Huff, K., Rose, R. S., & Engle, W. A. (2019). Late preterm infants: morbidities, mortality, and management recommendations. *Pediatric Clinics, 66*(2), 387–402.

Human Genetics Society of Australasia. (2011). Policy. Newborn bloodspot testing. <https://www.hgsa.org.au/documents/item/8693> (Accessed 16 February 2022).

Jeanmonod, R., Asuka, E., & Jeanmonod, D. (2022). Inborn errors of metabolism. In: *StatPearls*. Treasure Island, FL: StatPearls Publishing. <https://www.ncbi.nlm.nih.gov/books/NBK459183/> (Accessed 16 February 2022).

Kallem, V. R., Pandita, A., & Gupta, G. (2017). Hypoglycaemia: when to treat? *Clinical Medicine Insights: Pediatrics*, 11, 1179556517748913.

Kanike, N., Davis, A., & Shekhawat, P. S. (2017). Transient hypothyroidism in the newborn: to treat or not to treat. *Translational Pediatrics, 6*(4), 349–358.

Koracin, V., Mlinaric, M., Baric, I., Brincet, I., Djordjevic, M., Torkar, A. D., et al. (2021). Current status of newborn screening in South-eastern Europe. *Frontiers in Pediatrics, 9*, 391. doi: 10.3389/fped.2021.648939.

Kurtoğlu, S., Özdemir, A., & Hatipoğlu, N. (2019). Neonatal hypopituitarism: approaches to diagnosis and treatment. *Journal of Clinical Research in Pediatric Endocrinology, 11*(1), 4–12. doi: 10.4274/jcrpe.galenos.2018.2018.0036.

Laurie, J. G., & McIntyre, H. D. (2020). A review of the current status of gestational diabetes mellitus in Australia – the clinical impact of changing population demographics and diagnostic criteria on prevalence. *International Journal of Environmental Research and Public Health*, *17*(24), 9387. doi: 10.3390/ijerph17249387.

Lee, B. R., Strobel, K. M., & Chu, A. (2021). The neonate with ambiguous genitalia. *NeoReviews, 22*(4), e241–e249.

Lee, H., Slupsky, C. M., Heckmann, A. B., Christensen, B., Peng, Y., Li, X., et al. (2021). Milk fat globule membrane as a modulator of infant metabolism and gut microbiota: a formula supplement narrowing the metabolic differences between breastfed and formula-fed infants. *Molecular Nutrition and Food Research, 65*(3), 2000603.

Lemelman, M. B., Letourneau, L., & Greeley, S. (2018). Neonatal diabetes mellitus: an update on diagnosis and management. *Clinics in Perinatology, 45*(1), 41–59. doi: 10.1016/j.clp.2017.10.006.

Lilien, L. D., Grajwer, L. A., & Pildes, R. S. (1977). Treatment of neonatal hypoglycaemia with continuous intravenous glucose infusion. *Journal of Pediatrics, 91*(5), 779–782.

Lilien, L. D., Pildes, R. S., Srinivasan, G., Voora, S., & Yeh, T. (1980). Treatment of neonatal hypoglycaemia with minibolus and intravenous glucose infusion. *Journal of Pediatrics, 97*(2), 295–298.

McKinlay, C. J., Alsweiler, J. M., Ansell, J. M., Anstice, N. S., Chase, J. G., Gamble, G. D., et al. (2015). Neonatal glycemia and neurodevelopmental outcomes at 2 years. *New England Journal of Medicine, 373*(16), 1507–1518.

McKinlay, C. J. D., Chase, J. G., Dickson, J., Harris, D. L., Alsweiler, J. M., & Harding, J. E. (2017a). Continuous glucose monitoring in neonates: a review. *Maternal Health, Neonatology and Perinatology, 3*, 18.

McKinlay, C. J. D., Alsweiler, J. M., Anstice, N. S., Burakevych, N., Chakraborty, A., Chase, J. G., et al.; Children with Hypoglycaemia & their Later Development Study Team. (2017b). Association of neonatal glycemia with neurodevelopmental outcomes at 4.5 years. *Journal of the American Medical Association. Pediatrics, 171*(10), 972–983. doi: 10.1001/jamapediatrics.2017.1579.

Meneghin, F., Manzalini, M., Acunzo, M., Daniele, I., Bastrenta, P., Castoldi, F., et al. (2021). Management of asymptomatic hypoglycaemia with 40% oral dextrose gel in near term at-risk infants to reduce intensive care need and promote breastfeeding. *Italian Journal of Pediatrics, 47*, 20. doi: 10.1186/s13052-021-01149-7.

Ministry of Health. (2017). *Report of maternity 2015*. <https://www.health.govt.nz/publication/report-maternity-2015> (Accessed 16 February 2022).

Morris, M., Fischer, K., Leydiker, K., Elliott, L., Newby, J., & Abdenur, J. E. (2014). Reduction in newborn screening metabolic false-positive results following a new collection protocol. *Genetics in Medicine, 16*(6), 477–483.

Moullé, V. S., & Parnet, P. (2019). Effects of nutrient intake during pregnancy and lactation on the endocrine pancreas of the offspring. *Nutrients, 11*(11), 2708. doi: 10.3390/nu11112708.

Najem, O., Shah, M. M., & De Jesus, O. (2021) Serum osmolality. In: *StatPearls*. Treasure Island, FL: StatPearls Publishing. <https://www.ncbi.nlm.nih.gov/books/NBK567764/> (Accessed 16 February 2022).

Nichols, J. H., Brandler, E. S., Fantz, C. R., Fisher, K., Goodman, M. D., Headden, G., et al. (2021). A multicentre evaluation of a point-of-care blood glucose meter system in critically ill patients. *Journal of Applied Laboratory Medicine, 6*(4), 820–833. doi: 10.1093/jalm/jfab005.

Patti, G., Ibba, A., Morana, G., Napoli, F., Fava, D., di Iorgi, N., et al. (2020). Central diabetes insipidus in children: diagnosis and management. *Best Practice and Research Clinical Endocrinology and Metabolism, 34*(5), 101440.

Pedersen, J., Bojsen-Moller, B., & Poulsen, H. (1954). Blood sugar in newborn infants of diabetic mothers. *Acta Endocrinologica (Copenhagen), 15*, 33–52.

Peters, S., Andrews, C., & Sen, S. (2020). Care of infants born to women with diabetes. *Current Diabetes Reports, 20*(8), 39. doi: 10.1007/s11892-020-01331-x.

Pildes, R. S., Forbes, A. E., & Cornblath, M. (1967). The incidence of neonatal hypoglycaemia: a completed survey. *Journal of Pediatrics, 70*(1), 76–80.

Pinchefsky, E. F., Schneider, J., Basu, S., Tam, E. W. Y., & Gale, C. (2021). Nutrition and management of glycemia in neonates with neonatal encephalopathy treated with hypothermia. *Seminars in Fetal and Neonatal Medicine, 26*(4), 101268. doi: 10.1016/j.siny.2021.101268.

Qian, M., Wu, N., Li, L., Yu, W., Ouyang, H., Liu, X., et al. (2020). Effect of elevated ketone body on maternal and infant outcome of pregnant women with abnormal glucose metabolism during pregnancy. *Diabetes, Metabolic Syndrome and Obesity: Targets and Therapy, 13*, 4581–4588. doi: 10.2147/DMSO.S280851.

Qiao, L-X., Wang, J., Yan, J. H., Xu, S-X., Wang, H., Zhu, W-Y., et al. (2019). Follow-up study of neurodevelopment in 2-year-old infants who had suffered from neonatal hypoglycaemia. *BMC Pediatrics, 19*, 133. doi: 10.1186/s12887-019-1509-4.

Riskin, A., & Garcia-Prats, J. A. (2020). Infants of women with diabetes. In: L. E. Weisman, & J. I. Wolfsdorf (Eds.). *UpToDate*. Walters Kluwer. <https://www.uptodate.com/contents/infants-of-women-with-diabetes?search> (Accessed 16 February 2022).

Ross, L. F., & Waggoner, D. J. (2012). Parents: critical stakeholders in expanding newborn screening. *Journal of Pediatrics, 161*(3), 385–389.

Roth, K. A. (2017). Pediatric diabetes insipidus. *Emedicine*. <https://emedicine.medscape.com/article/919886-overview> (Accessed 16 February 2022).

Rozance, P. J. (2021a). Pathogenesis, screening, and diagnosis of neonatal hypoglycaemia. In: J. A. Garcia-Pratts & J. I. Wolfsdorf (Eds.), *UpToDate*. Walters Kluwer. <https://www.uptodate.com/contents/pathogenesis-screening-and-diagnosis-of-neonatal-hypoglycemia?search> (Accessed 16 February 2022).

Rozance, P. J. (2021b). Management and outcome of neonatal hypoglycaemia. In: J. A. Garcia-Pratts & J. I. Wolfsdorf (Eds.), *UpToDate*. Walters Kluwer. <https://www.uptodate.com/contents/management-and-outcome-of-neonatal-hypoglycemia?search> (Accessed 16 February 2022).

Saudubray, J. M., & Garcia-Cazorla, A. (2018). An overview of inborn errors of metabolism affecting the brain: from neurodevelopment to neurodegenerative disorders. *Dialogues in Clinical Neuroscience, 20*(4), 301–325. doi: 10.31887/DCNS.2018.20.4/jmsaudubray.

Segni, M. (2019). Neonatal hyperthyroidism. In: K. R. Feingold, B. Anawalt, A. Boyce, et al. (Eds.), *Endotext*. South Dartmouth, MA: MDText.com. <https://www.ncbi.nlm.nih.gov/books/NBK279019/> (Accessed 16 February 2022).

Sharma, A., Davis, A., & Shekhawat, P. S. (2017). Hypoglycaemia in the preterm neonate: etiopathogenesis, diagnosis, management and long-term outcomes. *Translational Pediatrics, 6*(4), 335–348.

Smolkin, T., Makhoul, J., Elias, R., Farah, F., Kugelman, A., Dallashi, M., et al. (2019). Experience with intramuscular glucagon for infants with early neonatal hypoglycaemia. *Journal of Pediatric Endocrinology and Metabolism, 32*(9), 1023–1026. doi: 10.1515/jpem-2018-0562.

Tal, R., & Taylor, H. S. (2021). Endocrinology of pregnancy. In: K. R. Feingold, B. Anawalt, A. Boyce, et al. (Eds.), *Endotext*. South Dartmouth, MA: MDText.com. <https://www.ncbi.nlm.nih.gov/books/NBK278962/> (Accessed 16 February 2022).

Thomas, T. C., Smith, J. M., White, P. C., & Adhikari, S. (2012). Transient neonatal hypocalcaemia: presentation and outcomes. *Pediatrics, 129*(6), e1461–e1467.

Thomson, L., Elleri, D., Bond, S., Howlett, J., Dunger, D. B., & Beardsall, K. (2019). Targeting glucose control in preterm infants: pilot studies of continuous glucose monitoring. *Archives of Disease in Childhood. Fetal and Neonatal Edition, 104*(4), F353. doi: 10.1136/archdischild-2018-314814.

Tottman, A. C., Alsweiler, J. M., Bloomfield, F. H., Gamble, G., Jiang, Y., Leung, M., et al. (2018). Long-term outcomes of hyperglycaemic preterm infants randomized to tight glycaemic control. *Journal of Pediatrics, 193*, 68–75, e1.

Wang, K. H., Kupa, J., Duffy, K. A., & Kalish, J. M. (2020). Diagnosis and management of Beckwith-Wiedemann syndrome [review]. *Frontiers in Pediatrics, 7*(562). doi: 10.3389/fped.2019.00562.

Zamir, I., Tornevi, A., Abrahamsson, T., Ahlsson, F., Engström, E., Hallberg, B., et al. (2018). Hyperglycaemia in extremely preterm infants – insulin treatment, mortality and nutrient intakes. *Journal of Pediatrics, 200*, 104–110.

CHAPTER 16

CARE OF THE NEONATE WITH AN INFECTION

LAURENE AYDON AND TRUDI MANNIX

Learning objectives

After reading this chapter you will be able to:

- describe the embryological development, functions, components and responses of the neonatal immune system
- outline the history and epidemiology of neonatal infections
- explain how infections are transmitted to the neonate
- outline the maternal, neonatal and environmental factors that place the neonate at risk of acquiring an infection
- describe how a diagnosis of neonatal infection is made, including clinical assessment, laboratory evaluation and other diagnostic screening tools
- outline the prevention, presentation, diagnosis, treatment and prognosis of specific neonatal infections (bacterial, viral and fungal)
- describe the nursing care provided to a neonate with sepsis
- describe the evidence-based principles, procedures and protocols associated with infection control in a neonatal unit.

Key words, terms and abbreviations

blood culture (BC)
bundle approach
central line-associated bloodstream infection (CLABSI)
cerebrospinal fluid (CSF)
early-onset sepsis (EOS)
full blood count (FBC)
hand hygiene
healthcare workers (HCWs)
hospital-acquired infection (HAI)
immunity
infection
infection control
late-onset sepsis (LOS)
micro-culture and specificity (MCS)
nosocomial infection
personal protective equipment (PPE)
sepsis
standard precautions
transmission precautions
ventilator-associated pneumonia (VAP)

INTRODUCTION

Neonatal **sepsis** continues to be a leading cause of neonatal morbidity and mortality worldwide, being responsible for approximately one-quarter of all neonatal deaths, with estimates of 1.3 million annual cases of neonatal sepsis and other infections and 203,000 deaths attributed to sepsis annually (Fleischmann et al., 2021). In the USA, neonatal sepsis is responsible for 4 infections per 1000 live births/year (Shane et al., 2017). In the United Kingdom, Cailes et al. (2018) reported that neonatal infections occurred in 6.1/1000 live births annually, accounting for 48.8/1000 of neonatal admissions. While the availability of data on rates of neonatal sepsis in Australia and New Zealand is limited, the Australian and New Zealand Neonatal Network (ANZNN) found rates of symptomatic, **blood culture (BC)** positive septicaemia in 4.9% of ANZNN registrants in 2018 (Chow et al., 2020). The most susceptible neonates at risk of sepsis are those born preterm, specifically those less than 28 weeks' gestation. In a recently published systematic review of 21 studies examining length of stay and costs of healthcare-acquired bloodstream infections, sepsis increases the length of stay, and as such represents a significant financial cost, especially in low- and middle-income countries (Odabasi & Bulbul, 2020). In their role at the cot-side caring for neonates around the clock, neonatal nurses/midwives are the first to recognise the subtle signs of **infection** in a newborn. This chapter provides a comprehensive review of common infections that affect the neonate and the immune response. You will read about how to identify the neonate with an infection and how sepsis is diagnosed and treated. There is an emphasis on **infection control** measures and the nursing and midwifery care that a neonate with an infection requires. Comprehensive tables explain the causative factors, preventative measures, clinical signs, diagnostic tests, treatment and prognosis for the most prevalent neonatal infections.

EPIDEMIOLOGY

The causative organisms associated with neonatal sepsis have changed over the past 50–60 years. In the 1950s, the most prevalent organisms were *Staphylococcus aureus* and *Escherichia coli*. Over the next few decades, group B streptococcus (GBS) overtook *S. aureus* as the most common gram-positive organism to lead to **early-onset sepsis (EOS)**. During the 1990s, GBS and *E. coli* continued to contribute significantly to neonatal sepsis, but coagulase-negative *Staphylococcus epidermis* was more frequently observed. Other organisms such as *Listeria monocytogenes*, *Chlamydia pneumoniae*, *Haemophilus influenzae*, *Enterobacter aerogenes* and *Clostridium* were identified. The incidence of EOS in the newborn has decreased over the past decade; however, it remains a major causative factor of mortality and morbidity in the newborn worldwide (Johansson Gudjónsdóttir et al., 2019). Most cases are due to GBS and gram-negative bacteria (Goel et al., 2020). GBS continues as one of the most frequent contributors to EOS and occurs more commonly in term neonates. Although *E. coli* is the second most common causative factor of EOS in the preterm neonate, there has been a decrease in EOS due to *E. coli* globally, predominantly in developed countries. This has been attributed to the implementation of screening programs during the antenatal period and adherence to treatment protocols for women with GBS-positive vaginal swabs. This global acceptance of general screening programs and the use of antibiotic therapy for pregnant women during labour has seen a shift in epidemiology related to GBS, with the USA Centers for Disease Control and Prevention (CDC) reporting the likely incidence of infection reduced to 1 in 4000 in those who received antibiotic therapy (CDC, 2020). Similarly, GBS epidemiology within the Australian population has also changed, with the implementation of a national recommendation to adopt screening policies antenatally. However, within the ANZNN group there are some neonatal units that have not adopted the national guidelines. *L. monocytogenes* is also a causative factor of EOS in the preterm group and is frequently associated with maternal illness. There are marked differences in the incidence of EOS among developing countries, which is attributable to socioeconomics, health prevention and strategies utilised for screening pregnant women (Amare et al., 2019).

Late-onset sepsis (LOS) is predominantly acquired from the hospital environment in both the neonatal intensive care unit (NICU)/special care baby unit (SCBU) and postnatal areas, and may result in bacteraemia and meningitis. Similarly, these conditions cause increased incidence of morbidity and increasing length of hospital stay. Epidemiological data on very preterm and low birthweight neonates show that the predominant pathogens of neonatal LOS are coagulase-negative staphylococci, accounting for 53.2–77.9% of LOS in industrialised countries and 35.5–47.4% in some developing regions (Grassham et al., 2021), followed by gram-negative bacilli and fungi. To a lesser degree, respiratory viral infections are commonly transmitted from staff or visitors occurring within the hospital setting or soon after discharge.

FUNCTIONS AND COMPONENTS OF THE IMMUNE SYSTEM

The immune system is a complex system of structures and processes in the body that defends against infection and foreign agents, and is able to distinguish between the individual's own cells and those of harmful invading organisms while promoting protective responses (Male et al., 2021). Front-line barriers to infection include the skin, the digestive tract and the respiratory tract. In the newborn, the vernix provides an antimicrobial layer of proteins and peptides that form a protective barrier on the skin. Protective mucus coats the nose and mouth, and a sneeze or a cough can expel microbes out of the respiratory tract. Acids in the stomach can destroy any pathogens that may be swallowed (Collins et al., 2018).

The lymphoid organs of the immune system include: the thymus, where T lymphocytes ('T cells') develop; the bone marrow, where white blood cells such as B lymphocytes ('B cells') or phagocytes develop from immature stem cells; and the spleen, tonsils, adenoids, appendix and lymph nodes, where *non-specific* immune cells congregate and confront pathogens, or antigens (innate **immunity**). Granulocytes (such as neutrophils, eosinophils, basophils and mast cells) migrate to the sites of inflammation to perform phagocytosis, ingesting and digesting foreign particles, or releasing chemicals when they encounter harmful cells or microbes (Male et al., 2021).

B cells are responsible for the production of antibodies (immunoglobulins) into the body's fluids; they confront matched antigens in the bloodstream (*specific* immunity) but cannot penetrate cells. T cells, on the other hand, can directly attack infected cells, but do not recognise antigens (cell-mediated immunity). Tightly packed epithelial cells line the digestive, respiratory and urogenital tracts and block entry to pathogens and, under them, macrophages and B and T cells lie in wait for any germs that might bypass the surface barriers. With increasing postnatal age, some T and B cells become memory cells and afford the body *acquired* immunity after exposure to a certain antigen (Collins et al., 2018). Natural killer (NK) T cells also mature in the thymus and are cytotoxic to viruses. They directly attack cells carrying foreign or abnormal molecules, or antigen fragments, on their surfaces. The granules inside NK cells contain potent chemicals that are released on contact with a foreign cell (Male et al., 2021).

Communication among the components of the immune system occurs by chemical messengers, in the form of proteins called cytokines. The *complement* system is made up of about 25 proteins that work together to complement the action of antibodies in destroying bacteria (*non-specific* immunity). Complement proteins circulate in the blood in an inactive form and, when the first substance of the cascade is triggered by an antibody interlocked with an antigen, a ripple effect is set in motion (Male et al., 2021).

CLINICAL PRACTICE 16.1

Gram-positive bacteria have a very thick outer covering and, even though the cell membrane of gram-negative bacteria is much thinner, it is much more difficult to penetrate. This means that gram-negative bacteria are more dangerous than gram-positive bacteria as disease organisms. They are often more resistant to antibiotics and other antibacterial interventions. In addition, their outer membrane is often hidden by a capsule or slime layer, which camouflages the antigens of the cell, making it difficult for antibodies to recognise and attack them (Oliveira & Reygaert, 2021).

EMBRYOLOGY AND LIMITATIONS OF THE NEONATAL IMMUNE SYSTEM

To understand the limitations of the neonatal immune system, it is important to understand its development. In the fourth week of gestation, the thymus forms, and with it the production of leucocytes begins. By the eighth week of gestation, T cells, B cells and NK cells differentiate in the thymus. Although the term neonate is considered 'mature', the immune system is considerably immature; the non-specific immune function has reduced inflammatory markers and the adaptive immune system has only 10–80% of the complement proteins of an adult (Glaser et al., 2020). As it takes 5–7 days after exposure to a pathogen for immunological memory to develop T and B cells, neonates rely mainly on the non-specific/innate response, such as physical barriers (such as the skin and the mucosa of the respiratory and gastrointestinal systems), antimicrobial proteins and peptides, and passively acquired immunoglobulin from the mother (Collins et al., 2018).

Circulating neutrophils in the newborn peak at around 12 hours of life and then decline to normal levels. The bone marrow storage pool of neutrophils at birth is only 20–30% of the circulating pool in adults. Both term and preterm neonates have a significant number of neutrophils that migrate out of the capillaries into an infected site to destroy a pathogen. Neutrophils in the newborn have reduced capacity for chemotaxis, adhesion, phagocytosis and bacterial killing. Neutropenia rather than neutrophilia is typical in infection of the newborn owing to the poor bone marrow response to acute infectious stress. The bone marrow initially responds to bacterial infection by releasing neutrophils from the marrow storage pool. This increased activity in cell proliferation in the bone marrow is accompanied by a reduction in the length of time that neutrophils are stored, and enhances the release of both immature and mature neutrophils into the circulation. The percentage of immature neutrophils is usually about 15% of the total count of neutrophils; however, with the onset of bacterial infection, neutrophil concentration increases, and the immature-to-total (I:T) neutrophil ratio also increases above 20% (Odabasi & Bulbul, 2020).

In the newborn, complement levels are reduced, as maternal complement is not transferred. These decreased levels can be 50–80% lower than adult levels, and even lower in the preterm neonate. B cells are precursors of antibody-producing cells, first produced in the liver; then, by 12 weeks' gestation, production transfers to the bone marrow. NK cells are found in greater concentrations in the peripheral blood of newborns at birth, but their numbers diminish rapidly after birth. In the newborn, there is a delay in the development of cytotoxic T lymphocytes, which increases the risk of viral infections (Glaser et al., 2020).

Immunoglobulin G (IgG) is the major immunoglobulin of the serum and interstitial fluid and is maternally derived. IgG provides immunity against bacterial and viral pathogens, crossing the placenta from 6 weeks of gestation and peaking at term; therefore, IgG levels are lower in preterm neonates. Levels may be decreased in intrauterine growth-restricted neonates or small for gestation and post-term neonates.

Immunoglobulin M (IgM) does not cross the placenta, which increases fetal and neonatal susceptibility to gram-negative infections. IgM synthesis occurs early in fetal life, and levels have been detected at 30 weeks of gestation; however, they are higher in the fetus in the presence of infection.

Immunoglobulin A (IgA), a mucosal immunoglobulin, is commonly found in the gastrointestinal and respiratory tracts and, importantly for protection of the preterm and/or sick neonate, in human colostrum and breast milk (Collins et al., 2018). IgA does not cross the placenta and levels are very low in the fetus or neonate without infection.

Immunoglobulin E (IgE) is present in small amounts in serum and secretions and has a major role to play in allergic reactions.

The chemical and physical barriers to infection in the newborn are functionally deficient. Skin and mucous membranes are easily broken down, and the invasive procedures that preterm and/or sick neonates often undergo also breach physical barriers and create additional risks. In addition to the reduction in immunity with lessening gestation, the neonate's immune system has no experience with microbes, and there is a lack of resident and balanced flora (Glaser et al., 2020). These factors lead to an overall reduced capacity for the immune system to react, causing concern in the immediate period after birth, especially for the extremely preterm neonate (Singh et al., 2021). Of concern to neonatal nurses/midwives, the neonate's inability to mount an effective inflammatory response results in a diffuse, rather than localised, response to infection. Consequently, clinical signs of systemic infection may be difficult to recognise (Crocker et al., 2021).

RISK FACTORS FOR NEONATAL INFECTION

Identifying risk factors for neonatal sepsis is an essential component of neonatal nursing care. Grouping these into three categories (maternal, neonatal and environmental (also known as nosocomial or hospital-acquired)) aids in understanding the importance of prevention and identification of sepsis in the prenatal and immediate neonatal period. Table 16.1 lists the risk factors under those three categories. Even though risk factors can often be determined, 60% of EOS cases in term neonates have no identifiable risk factors.

Breastfeeding is protective against infection in the neonatal period. Granger et al. (2021, p. 450) conducted a narrative review to summarise the benefits of breast milk and found that maternal breast milk is 'the single most important factor in modifying the infant gut microbiome', reducing the risk of necrotising enterocolitis (NEC) in preterm infants. Chapter 2 provides more detail about its specific advantages, and it is important that neonatal nurses/midwives caring for neonates communicate to the mother that her breast milk is a precious medicine that she alone can provide.

TABLE 16.1 **Risk factors for neonatal sepsis**

Categories	Risk factors
Maternal	Preterm labour at <37 weeks' gestation Prolonged ROM >18 h Maternal pyrexia in labour <38°C Maternal GBS colonisation Chorioamnionitis Induction of labour Instrumental birth Meconium-stained liquor Maternal urinary tract infection Multiple vaginal examinations in labour (>6) Lifestyle factors (poor nutrition, inadequate antenatal care, low SES, substance abuse)
Neonatal	Preterm birth Low birthweight Prolonged LOS of VLBW and LBW neonates Invasive procedures such as insertion of central lines, IV cannulas and ETTs Exposure to antibiotics Prolonged parenteral nutrition Resuscitation at birth Male neonate
Environmental (nosocomial, or hospital-acquired); Pittet (2017)	Contact with HCWs Contact with inanimate objects Contact with parents and extended family Staff and visitors who have poor compliance with infection control techniques Overcrowding Inadequate staffing Sharing equipment Prolonged hospitalisation

ETTs, endotracheal tubes; GBS, group B streptococcus; HCWs, healthcare workers; IV, intravenous; LBW, low birthweight; LOS, late-onset sepsis; ROM, rupture of membranes; SES, socioeconomic status; VLBW, very low birthweight.

Source: Wilson et al. (2016)

EVIDENCE-BASED PRACTICE RESEARCH 16.1

Lactoferrin is a naturally occurring protein in breast milk. In a recently published systematic review on the use of lactoferrin to prevent sepsis or NEC in preterm infants, Pammi and Gautham (2020) conducted a meta-analysis of 12 randomised controlled trials and concluded that lactoferrin decreases late-onset sepsis but not NEC.

TRANSMISSION OF INFECTION TO THE NEONATE

The timing of the transmission of infection has led to definitions of 'early-onset' and 'late-onset' neonatal sepsis by the Australian and New Zealand Neonatal Network (Chow et al., 2020 , p. 24) as follows:

- Early-onset sepsis is the presence of at least one episode of systemic sepsis where the initial symptoms occurred within the first 48 hours after birth – that is, in babies aged from 0 to 47 hours.
- Late-onset sepsis is the presence of at least one episode of systemic sepsis, with the initial symptoms occurring among babies aged 48 or more hours. Episodes of sepsis involving the same organism separated by at least 14 days are new episodes of infection.

In addition to these definitions, further descriptions in Table 16.2 outline the possible progression of sepsis in the newborn, from sepsis through severe sepsis to septic shock. Early-onset sepsis predominantly results from transplacental or, more often, vertical (ascending) transmission from the maternal birth canal and is acquired during the intrapartum period. With the exception of *L. monocytogenes*, it is usually associated with pneumonia and/or septicaemia, and the mortality risk is high (10–30%). Late-onset sepsis is associated with the acquisition of infections from the postnatal nosocomial (hospital-acquired) or community environment, with the peak incidence reported to be between the 10th and 22nd day of life. The incidence of neonatal late-onset sepsis is inversely related to gestational age and birthweight (Grassham et al., 2021).

Viral infections are known to be transmitted via the placenta during pregnancy, vertically during labour and via the birth canal. They are well-described causes of stillbirth or increased neonatal morbidity and mortality.

The list of acquired congenital viral infections was previously known as ToRCH infections. This list has been expanded and the infections are now known as the ToRCHES CLAP infections (***To****xoplasma gondii* – **r**ubella virus – **c**ytomegalovirus – **h**erpes simplex virus – **e**nteroviruses – **s**yphilis – **c**hickenpox (varicella zoster virus) – **L**yme disease – **A**IDS – **p**arvovirus B19) (Maldonado et al., 2016, p. 6). Maternal history and assessment should alert the clinician to potential specific problems if these infections are acquired. Poorly grown fetuses in the absence of other maternal factors may be indicative of growth restriction secondary to these infections (Koet al., 2020). This group of infections presents as mild flu-like illnesses within the general population and, if acquired antenatally, may go undiagnosed. Severe infection during pregnancy potentially results in poor outcomes for the neonate with clinical signs of non-immune hydrops fetalis (see the comprehensive lists of diseases in Tables 16.3–16.5).

Community-acquired viral infections such as those causing respiratory and enteral pathology should be considered in the newborn period if the neonate becomes unwell and has symptoms of generalised signs of infection on examination 48 hours after birth (Australian and New Zealand Neonatal Network (ANZNN), 2020). These viruses are typically responsible for episodes of LOS in the neonatal unit. When considering LOS, awareness of current community circulation of viruses such as influenza strains, respiratory syncytial viruses (RSV) or coronaviruses (SARS-2) should be considered. Transmission occurs from infected personnel including parents, families and **healthcare workers (HCWs)**.

TABLE 16.2 **Useful definitions**

Term	Definition
Bacteraemia	The presence of viable bacteria in the blood
Systemic inflammatory response syndrome (SIRS)	Systemic inflammatory response triggered by infectious or non-infectious conditions
Sepsis	The presence of both infection and a systemic inflammatory response accompanied by more than one of the following: (1) temperature >38°C or <36°C, (2) tachycardia >90 bpm, (3) tachypnoea, (4) alteration in white blood cell count >12,000/mm^3 or <4000/mm^3, or >10% immature neutrophils
Severe sepsis	Sepsis complicated by organ dysfunction
Septic shock	Acute circulatory failure characterised by persistent hypotension despite adequate fluid resuscitation

CLINICAL ASSESSMENT

Early recognition and awareness of sepsis risk factors arising during the ante- and intrapartum periods are pivotal in the prevention and management of neonatal sepsis. As clinical manifestations of sepsis in the newborn are frequently non-specific, the neonatal nurse/midwife must be aware of the risk factors present in the maternal and neonatal history for each individual neonate in their care (Puopolo et al., 2018).

CLINICAL PRACTICE 16.2

Obtaining a thorough history of the immediate prenatal period and birth, along with physical examination, is essential to diagnose EOS and alert the neonatal nurse/midwife to the risk factors, signs and symptoms of possible developing sepsis (Glaser et al., 2020). Any neonate who is unwell must be considered at risk of sepsis.

Treating suspected sepsis in the newborn is not without risk. Discomfort to the newborn, stress to the parents and cost to the organisation should be considered. Furthermore, there are emerging concerns about a link between newborn antibiotic therapy, alteration of the newborn's microbiome, allergic reactions, asthma and autoimmune disease (Uzan-Yulzari et al., 2021). Algorithms to assist in defining when treatment is required and

TABLE 16.3 **Bacterial diseases responsible for early- and late-onset sepsis**

Organism	EOS/LOS	History/causative factor/epidemiology	Prevention	Clinical signs	Diagnosis	Treatment	Prognosis
Group B streptococcus (GBS) Group B haemolytic streptococci Gram-positive cocci	EOS more prevalent LOS	Predominant cause of neonatal sepsis in the 1970–1980s • Source: Genitourinary tract • PROM • Chorioamnionitis • LOS may be attributable to breast milk colonisation	Antenatal screening programs Women routinely screened on more than one occasion Regimen of antibiotic therapy intrapartum when culture positive	Presents as a multisystem disease Collapsed unwell newborn Early respiratory distress Hypothermia LOS may present as acute episode	BC CRP FBC Relevant radiological exam Breast milk culture	Penicillin course specific to site culture for 7–21 days LOS: specific course of penicillin per site culture and clinical picture	Meningitis and congenital pneumonia Morbidity and mortality high if not recognised early
Group A streptococcus Gram-positive cocci	EOS more prevalent	Causes: • Puerperal infection • PROM • Chorioamnionitis • Toxic shock syndrome	Attention to maternal history Precautionary measures with obstetric antisepsis if ROM No specific prevention program	Similar presentation to GBS Skin abscess/es	BC CRP FBC Relevant radiological exam Relevant surface swabs and/or culture	Penicillin course specific to site culture	Meningitis and congenital pneumonia Morbidity and mortality high if not recognised early
Streptococcus pneumonia Gram-positive cocci	EOS	Unusual occurrences		EOS similar to GBS Severe symptoms of sepsis	BC CRP FBC Radiological exam CSF if indicated	Penicillin and cephalosporin/ ceftriaxone (resistance known to occur)	Associated morbidity and mortality Severe pneumonia and/or meningitis
Listeria *Listeria monocytogenes* Gram-positive cocci	EOS LOS	Maternal ingestion of contaminated foods (*Listeria* habitat in decaying plant matter) First identified in 1929 Transmission occurs in utero via infected amniotic fluid or maternal circulation Occurs after day 7 of life	Maternal consumption of unpasteurised raw dairy products, processed cheese or foods contaminated with the organism from the soil	Similar presentation to GBS with respiratory distress, sepsis, acute collapse, meningitis, bacteraemia, pneumonia Granulomatous rash may be evident if severe Granulomatosis infantisepticum	BC CRP FBC CSF Radiological exam	Ampicillin in combination with aminoglycoside	Infections in pregnancy associated with spontaneous abortion, still birth, early neonatal death, preterm birth Mortality high when infection is a result of maternal illness and preterm birth Morbidity is reported, however, associated with those of the preterm or unwell term newborn Reported long-term sequelae uncommon
Haemophilus influenzae Gram-positive organism	EOS/LOS	Colonises the maternal genital tract Incidence is significantly higher in neonates born preterm	*H. influenzae* type b (Hib) conjugate vaccine	Presents as overwhelmingly septic with signs of pneumonia and meningitis	FBC CRP Consider coagulation profiles BCs Lumbar puncture CSF for MCS	Ceftriaxone and azithromycin	• High mortality and morbidity rates in the preterm • Chronic lung disease • Intraventricular haemorrhage • Cerebral palsy

Continued

TABLE 16.3 **Bacterial diseases responsible for early- and late-onset sepsis—cont'd**

Organism	EOS/LOS	History/causative factor/epidemiology	Prevention	Clinical signs	Diagnosis	Treatment	Prognosis
Enterococcus sp. *Enterococcus faecalis/ faecium* Gram-positive cocci	EOS/LOS	Formerly classified as strep D in the 1980s Most infections and colonisations with *Enterococcus* are due to patient's endogenous flora that can spread directly from the patient, or indirectly through contaminated surfaces, shared equipment, or hands of HCWs	Infection control practices Cohort neonates with resistant *Enterococcus*	EOS: mild disease LOS: presents as a respiratory illness and associated diarrhoea	BC Stool culture	Ampicillin (specific treatment for site culture)	Enterococcus is susceptible to resistance to vancomycin and gentamicin (GRE VRE)
Escherichia coli Gram-negative bacilli	EOS/LOS	Colonises the maternal genital tract Colonises the lower intestine in the first few days of life There are 6 recognised enteric pathotypes of *E. coli*	Acquired prior to birth through antenatal and intrapartum transmission Breastfeeding thought to provide some protection Outbreaks in the newborn nursery due to cross infection	Mild illness: reluctance to feed, spitting up, mild abdominal distension, weight loss, loose watery stools Severe illness: bacteraemia, meningeal signs, septic shock	BC FBC CRP Throat and rectal swabs (to determine if resistance is present) Urine culture	Ampicillin or cefotaxime and gentamicin	Severe dehydration High mortality rates in the preterm
Staphylococci species *Staphylococcus aureus* Coagulase-negative staphylococci (CONS) Gram-positive organism	May present as EOS, however predominantly LOS	Related to HAI, VAP and CLABSI The bacterial capsule polysaccharide of CONS adheres well to the plastic polymers of intravascular catheters and intraventricular shunts	Hand hygiene and procedure compliance by HCWs Bundle approach to ventilator care Bundle approach to central line care The use of specific checklists, inclusive of daily review of line status	LOS symptoms vary from a subtle increase in apnoea and bradycardia requiring respiratory support to major collapse and haemodynamic/ respiratory instability	BC CRP FBC Radiological exam Additional CSF and urine culture for LOS If ventilated: tracheal aspirates for MCS CONS is normal skin flora and therefore a frequent contaminant of blood and CSF cultures, leading to false positive or contaminated specimens	LOS: second intervention broad spectrum antibiotics related to local practice guidelines (generally vancomycin and gentamicin); however, empirical therapy within per the local environment is necessary Central line sepsis suspected: catheter removal is imperative EOS treated with penicillin and gentamicin until specific sensitivities reported	Depending on severity of the infection early antibiotic therapy and supportive treatment prognosis favourable BC positive with CONS infection is a contributor to increased length of stay as prolonged treatment is required This is similar if CSF is culture positive and treatment is required for weeks to eradicate causative organism May increase length of stay CONS sepsis is a causative factor in worsening of lung disease and neurological sequelae

Enterobacter Gram-negative cocci	EOS	*Enterobacter* are common commensals of the human gastrointestinal tract Nosocomial spread occurs directly from the patient, or indirectly through contaminated surfaces, shared equipment, or hands of healthcare workers	Cot spacing Hand hygiene Infection control practices	May present as a multisystem disease Collapsed unwell newborn Hypothermia	BCs FBC CRP	Ampicillin	
Acinetobacter	LOS	Risk factors associated with **nosocomial infection** include mechanical ventilation, surgery and trauma Septicaemia is common in babies with predisposing factors such as intravascular catheterisation, endotracheal intubation, parenteral nutrition, broad spectrum antibiotic therapy and artificial ventilation	Cot spacing Hand hygiene Infection control practices	LOS symptoms vary from a subtle increase in apnoea and bradycardia requiring respiratory support to major collapse and haemodynamic/ respiratory instability	FBC CRP Consider coagulation profiles BCs Lumbar puncture CSF for MCS	Potential multi-drug resistance	Associated brain abscesses Dissemination to other organs Multi-drug resistant nosocomial *Acinetobacter* septicaemia may cause severe clinical disease in neonates that is associated with a high mortality
Serratia Gram-negative organism *Serratia marcescens*	Potential EOS LOS	Maternal colonisation and transmission can occur at ToB LOS attributable to HAI; survives well in soil and moist environments Environmental source of spread may include colonised hand wash soap or breast pumps, NICU sinks or taps, medical devices, medical charts, computer keyboards and mouses, linen Contamination of these surfaces demonstrates non-compliance with hand hygiene by HCWs	Cot spacing Hand hygiene Infection control practices Environmental cleaning Ocular and rectal colonisation play an important role in spread of infections	Moist eyes Symptoms associated with neonatal sepsis Hypothermia	Eye, rectal and throat swabs BCs CSF FBC Coagulation studies Urine culture	Third generation cephalosporin and/ or aminoglycosides	Poor neurological outcome if meningitis evident High risk of brain abscess

Continued

TABLE 16.3 **Bacterial diseases responsible for early- and late-onset sepsis—cont'd**

Organism	EOS/LOS	History/causative factor/epidemiology	Prevention	Clinical signs	Diagnosis	Treatment	Prognosis
Pseudomonas Gram-negative organism *Pseudomonas aeruginosa*	LOS	LOS attributable to HAI; survives well in moist environments Soil and water are environmental source of spread Additional risk factors for preterm neonates are associated with preterm birth and long-term hospitalisation: • antimicrobial drugs • transfusion of blood products • intravenous delivery of nutrients/electrolytes • exposure to umbilical venous catheter • increasing age • use of artificial finger-nails are risk factors for colonisation of hands of HCWs	Cot spacing Hand hygiene Infection control practices Environmental cleaning	Clinical signs of respiratory distress Bloodstream infection Meningitis VAP	BCs CSF FBC Coagulation studies ETT aspirates CXR (resembles HMD) Urine culture Eye swabs	Aminoglycosides	Gangrenous areas around nose, lips and mouth have been associated with *Pseudomonas* Conjunctivitis destroys eye tissue Worsening lung disease
Klebsiella sp. Gram-negative organism *Klebsiella pneumonia/ oxytocia*	LOS	Nosocomial pathogen Most common infection is the urinary tract or bloodstream Soft tissues Lungs Environmental source of spread	Cot spacing Hand hygiene Infection control practices Environmental cleaning	Clinical signs associated with bloodstream infection Meningitis VAP	BCs CSF FBC Coagulation studies ETT aspirates Urine culture	Potential resistance to antimicrobials	High mortality
Gonococcal infections *Neisseria gonorrhoeae* Gram-negative diplococcus	EOS/LOS	Maternal infection	Targeted treatment campaigns amongst at-risk groups are recommended	Purulent conjunctivitis appearing 2–5 days after birth Neonatal sepsis, arthritis and skin abscesses may be evident	Surface swabs of any purulent areas, eyes, abscesses for gram stain and identification are necessary	Penicillin resistance is documented Ceftriaxone is known to be effective in different dosing regimens for types of associated infection	Ophthalmia neonatorum Meningitis Sepsis Arthritis Scalp lesions Risk of long-term sequelae and corneal damage if untreated

Note: Although the table provides information on the antibiotics that may be used to treat each infection, each worksite may use alternatives.
BC, blood culture; CLABSI, central line-associated bloodstream infection; CRP, C reactive protein; CSF, cerebrospinal fluid; EOS, early-onset sepsis; FBC, full blood count; HAI, hospital-acquired infection; HCWs, healthcare workers; LOS, late-onset sepsis; MCS, micro-culture and specificity; PROM, premature rupture of membranes; ROM, rupture of membranes; ToB, time of birth; VAP, ventilator-associated pneumonia.

Source: Wilson et al. (2016).

TABLE 16.4 **Viral diseases responsible for early- and late-onset sepsis**

Organism	EOS/LOS	History/causative factor/epidemiology	Prevention	Clinical signs	Diagnosis	Treatment	Prognosis
Human immunodeficiency virus	EOS acquired LOS (prolonged breast feeding)	Antenatal infection (PROM, amniocentesis, invasive monitoring, chorioamnionitis) Intrapartum From breast milk if there is prolonged breastfeeding in at-risk populations	HIV-exposed neonates recommended to receive prophylaxis soon after birth, usually for 6 weeks duration	Interstitial lung disease Cardiovascular complications Gastrointestinal disease Haematological problems Skin disease Malignancies	Surface swabs: ear, eyes, throat, rectum Serology Immunological status	Nucleoside reverse transcriptase inhibitors (antiretroviral drug) e.g. zidovudine	Variable clinical course and duration of survival depending on the country they are treated in
Toxoplasmosis *Toxoplasma gondii* was first described in a rodent (*Ctenodactylus* gundi) by Charles Nicolle in Tunisia in 1908 Parasite	EOS congenital	Primary maternal infection, gestational age at which the maternal infection occurs is relevant and associated with parasitic load in the amniotic fluid Potential for severe damage at the embryological stage The risk of vertical transmission increases as the gestation increases; however the risk of organ damage decreases Associated with preterm birth when maternal seroconversion has occurred before 20 weeks of gestation	Maternal education (the promotion of improved hand and food hygiene and recommendations not to eat undercooked meat would also help to preclude contact with other pathogens)	Clinical examination is most often normal, with 80–90% of neonates with congenital toxoplasmosis having no symptoms at birth The complete classic triad of hydrocephalus, intracerebral calcifications and retinochoroiditis occurs in a small proportion of newborns Signs of progressive generalised fetal disease may be evident: hepatomegaly, splenomegaly jaundice, skin rash myocarditis, thrombocytopenic purpura, anaemia, myocarditis, respiratory distress or CNS sequelae (microcephaly, hydrocephalus, seizures)	PCR serology	Regimens may vary; however, continuous use of pyrimethamine and a sulfonamide are recommended Associated use of corticosteroids may also be recommended	Evaluation of *T. gondii* concentration in amniotic fluid by quantitative PCR assay is also a good indicator of risk of severe fetal outcome in humans Toxoplasma affects all organs/ systems: known causes of deafness and blindness

Continued

TABLE 16.4 **Viral diseases responsible for early- and late-onset sepsis—cont'd**

Organism	EOS/LOS	History/causative factor/epidemiology	Prevention	Clinical signs	Diagnosis	Treatment	Prognosis
Cytomegalovirus (CMV)	EOS congenital. LOS = maternal or HAI	Maternal transmission (intrauterine) Vertical transmission (from mother to neonate) Intrauterine transfusion with blood infected with CMV	Nosocomial infection in the postnatal period due to blood transfusion (strict screening for blood products administered to newborn) Nosocomial transmission is possible in the nursery setting, which suggests that workers' hands or contaminated fomites might be involved; however, this is considered a rare occurrence	IUGR Rash and petechiae Pneumonitis Hepatosplenomegaly Microcephaly Ocular defects	Urine or saliva sample for viruses Antibody titre to diagnose in utero transmission PCR for systemic infection	Chemotherapy (ganciclovir)	Hearing loss Psychomotor impairment Ocular lesions Delayed neurological development Language delays
Enterovirus Parechovirus	LOS	Vertical transmission from an index case	Infection control practices HAI Hand hygiene Isolation procedures Risk of horizontal transmission	Mild gastroenteritis Sepsis-like syndrome with septicaemia or meningitis/ encephalitis Seizures Apnoea Temperature instability Vomiting Abdominal distension	Swabs – nose, throat and rectum Stool specimen Blood and CSF cultures if acute sepsis	Antiviral medication	Poor outcome if acute sepsis
Herpes simplex virus (HSV 1, HSV 2) Human herpes virus family inclusive of CMV varicella zoster	EOS/LOS	Maternal infection via vertical transmission Person-to-person contact (mucosal surfaces or abraded skin)	Prevent exposure of neonates to active maternal infection	Localised infection, e.g. eyes and mouth Disseminated infection = symptoms of viraemia Symptoms of multi-organ dysfunction and haemorrhagic necrosis	Blood for viral PCR Surface swabs – eyes, nose, throat, rectum	Antiviral/ acyclovir	Life-threatening disease in the newborn May require long-term management by infectious diseases specialist
Respiratory viruses Parainfluenza Coronavirus (SARS 1, MERS, SARS 2, Covid 19) Respiratory syncytial virus (RSV) Influenza A Adenovirus	LOS	Contact, droplet and aerosol transmission from infected personnel, family, HCWs	Infection control practices Transmission base precautions HAI – isolation procedures Risk of horizontal transmission Rapid diagnosis and cohorting of infected patients and assigned staff	Rhinorrhoea Tachypnoea Retractions Nasal flaring Rales Wheezing Sepsis-like symptoms Apnoea Gastrointestinal symptoms	Secretions and swabs for MCS Viral culture and PCR	Non-specific – supportive	Variable

Note: Although the table provides information on the medicines that may be used to treat each infection, each worksite may use alternatives.
CMV, cytomegalovirus; CNS, central nervous system; CSF, cerebrospinal fluid; EOS, early-onset sepsis; HAI, hospital-acquired infection; HCWs, healthcare workers; HIV, human immunodeficiency virus; IUGR, intrauterine growth restriction; LOS, late-onset sepsis; MCS, micro-culture and specificity; MERS, Middle East respiratory syndrome; PCR, polymerase chain reaction; PROM, premature rupture of membranes; RSV, respiratory syncytial virus; SARS, severe acute respiratory syndrome.

Source: Wilson et al. (2016)

TABLE 16.5 **Fungal and spore diseases responsible for early- and late-onset sepsis**

Organism	EOS/LOS	History/causative factor/epidemiology	Prevention	Clinical signs	Diagnosis	Treatment	Prognosis
Syphilis *Treponema pallidum* *Spirochaetales*	EOS	Maternal infection Transmission is vertical prior to birth	Targeted and treatment campaigns amongst at-risk groups are recommended Prenatal screening	If fetal infection occurs, signs after birth are indicative of overwhelming sepsis with multisystem infection (IUGR, hepatosplenomegaly, non-immune hydrops fetalis, lymphadenopathy, periostitis, external blistered lesions)	Surface swabs of lesions Serology Immunological status	Standard precautions/ contact isolation (at least for first 24 h of treatment) Antibiotic of choice is crystalline penicillin Ceftriaxone may be used in times of penicillin shortage	If untreated spontaneous abortion may occur or late-term stillbirth Premature or neonatal death
Chlamydia	EOS	Maternal infection	Targeted treatment campaigns amongst at-risk groups are recommended	Clinical signs of respiratory distress Feeding problems Apnoea Mucopurulent eye discharge	Radiological exam CXR Eye swabs Specific respiratory secretion assay by tracheal aspirate PCR	Erythromycin orally to treat conjunctivitis and pneumonia If poorly tolerated azithromycin may be used	
Candida species	Predominantly LOS	Risk factors for candida or disseminated candidiasis are: • Preterm <28 weeks • VLBW • Apgar score <5 at 5 minutes • Prolonged broad spectrum antibiotic therapy • Parenteral nutrition • Central catheters • Surgery • NEC • Prolonged hospitalisation • Neutropenia • Hyperglycaemia	Prophylactic antifungal treatment regimens Fluconazole Nystatin regimens for all newborns in an NICU with invasive devices or receiving antibiotic therapy Prevention of HAI	Mild irritation thrush Nappy dermatitis Skin lesions Non-specific signs of sepsis Feeding problems Hyperglycaemia Temperature instability	Culture of lesions Gram stain of vesicular contents Cultures of blood, CSF and urine Invasive disease may require further investigation with ultrasound to determine any deposits in organs such as kidneys and heart	Systemic or topical treatment according to severity Systemic – amphotericin regimen Fluconazole Micafungin (severe disseminated infection)	If dissemination does not occur treatment is effective CNS – poor prognosis Renal – good prognosis ROP risk in VLBW

Note: Although the table provides information on the medicines that may be used to treat each infection, each worksite may use alternatives.
CNS, central nervous system; CSF, cerebrospinal fluid; CXR, chest X-ray; EOS, early-onset sepsis; HAI, hospital-acquired infection; IUGR, intrauterine growth restriction; LOS, late-onset sepsis; NEC, necrotising enterocolitis; NICU, neonatal intensive care unit; PCR, polymerase chain reaction; ROP, retinopathy of prematurity; VLBW, very low birthweight.

Source: Wilson et al. (2016).

TABLE 16.6 **Signs of neonatal infection according to body system**

System	Sign
Central nervous system	Behaviour – not tolerating handling; 'not quite right' Lethargy or irritability (may or may not indicate CNS involvement) Poor feeding Tremors Twitching Seizures Hypotonia or hypertonia Bulging fontanelles High-pitched cry
Thermoregulation	Unstable temperature (especially in gram-negative sepsis) Hyperthermia/hypothermia Cool peripheries
Respiratory	Use of accessory muscles (rib retractions/sternal recession) Grunting Nasal flaring Tachypnoea Apnoea Increasing oxygen requirements/desaturations
Cardiac	Tachycardia Bradycardic episodes Arrhythmia Murmur Hypotension or hypertension (hypotension most likely)
Gastrointestinal	Poor feeding Abdominal distension Vomiting Bile or abnormal aspirates Loose stools/diarrhoea/blood in stools Glucose instability (hyperglycaemia is a response to early infection, then hypoglycaemia is most likely) Hepatomegaly and splenomegaly
Skin	Mottling Rash/pustules Petechiae Jaundice Umbilical stump redness/moist/smelly Cold, clammy skin
Haemodynamics/haematology	Capillary refill time >2 seconds Pallor Cyanosis Hypotension Abnormal full blood count/coagulation profile Thrombocytopenia Acidosis Metabolic acidosis

Source: adapted from: Crocker et al. (2021); Glaser et al. (2020).

steps to take have been used in clinical practice for many years, with success. Evaluation of the newborn with risk factors for EOS using an algorithm developed in 2012 and modified in 2014 to develop a web-based tool (sepsis indicator tool) has aided clinicians in the decision to treat or not to treat for suspected sepsis. Results of a subsequent quality improvement activity published by Akangire et al. (2020) have improved on the original tools, decreasing the use of antibiotics in infants at risk of sepsis.

The use of a sepsis indicator tool assists with identification of those at considerable risk for EOS, and works to support the judicial use of antibiotics; however, this instrument is not recommended for use in newborns of less than 34 weeks' gestation. The provision of risk evaluation tools such as these guides clinicians to prescribe antibiotic therapies when the risk of sepsis is high, and to observe the neonate when the risk is considered low (Bridges et al., 2019). The use of a septic calculator tool in the case of a newborn who is symptomatic of sepsis soon after birth will place the newborn in the high-risk category. This neonate will require proactive management to treat the suspected infection, prior to a confirmation of the diagnosis, owing to the potential for rapid deterioration. Newborns display very subtle, non-specific signs of sepsis that are difficult to define, and therefore a comprehensive approach to their physical assessment involves a systematic approach to detecting those signs, as shown in Table 16.6.

DIAGNOSTIC SCREENING

Diagnosis of neonatal sepsis has proven to be difficult owing to the fact there is not a single definitive or sensitive test that can confirm the diagnosis within a timely manner and no clinical sign that is specific (Hincu et al., 2020). A universal approach used to investigate suspected sepsis consists of a **full blood count (FBC)**, C-reactive protein (CRP), BCs and either chest X-rays (CXR) or abdominal X-rays (AXR) (Table 16.7). If the newborn is severely compromised and has neurological symptoms, a lumbar puncture with **cerebrospinal fluid (CSF)** microscopy and culture is required. Coagulation profiles should be considered as the risk of developing septic-related coagulopathy is increased with overwhelming sepsis. Assessment of the general wellbeing of the neonate is also important, including blood gases, serum electrolytes and blood glucose.

CLINICAL PRACTICE 16.3

In an unwell neonate, treatment with antibiotics should not be delayed if blood cultures cannot be obtained in a timely manner (Singh et al., 2021).

Where potential sepsis is considered a risk factor soon after birth, a comprehensive maternal and neonatal history is required. If specific risk factors in the maternal history indicate the potential for chorioamnionitis, placental histology and/or review of maternal vaginal swabs is indicated. Neonatal early investigations may

TABLE 16.7 **Diagnostic tests used in sepsis**

Diagnostic test	Component/use	Normal findings	Result indicating sepsis	Notes
FBC (full blood count)	Total white blood cell (WBC) count	9000–30,000 × 10^6/L	Total WBC <5000 × 10^6/L	Elevated WBC (>20,000) is not predictive of infection in newborn neonates
	Neutrophils	Neutrophil count varies with gestation, age in hours or days	>40,000/mm^3 or <7500	Total count may not be indicative of sepsis The predictive value varies with neonatal maturity, mode of birth, hours of age and associated clinical factors
	Immature to total neutrophil count (I:T ratio)	0.16	>0.2	85% sensitive and specific, particularly for early-onset sepsis (EOS)
	Polymorphonucleocyte (PMN) count	Can be normal in a third of cases of confirmed sepsis	PMN count often grouped with neutrophils	Can be elevated in the absence of infection
	Platelets	100,000–150,000/mm^3	<50,000/mm^3	Unexplained thrombocytopenia may be associated with sepsis and is not recommended to be used as a diagnostic test However, it is often a latent indicator of bacterial sepsis Thrombocytopenia is also associated with intrauterine pathology such as intrauterine congenital infections, birth asphyxia, umbilical catheter placement, mechanical ventilation, meconium aspiration, multiple exchange transfusions and necrotising enterocolitis
C-reactive protein (CRP)	A non-specific marker of inflammation or tissue necrosis Raised in 85% of episodes of confirmed sepsis with a specificity of 90% High sensitivity and negative predictive value for both early-onset and late-onset sepsis	The upper limit of normal for the neonate is 10 mmol/L There is an increase within 4–6 hours after the onset of sepsis, with a peak at 36–50 hours; remains high with ongoing infection Quickly decreases with resolution of infection because of short half-life (4–7 hours)	CRP rise >10 mmol/L	Elevated in bacterial sepsis and meningitis A single normal value cannot rule out infection as sampling may have preceded the CRP rise CRP levels are helpful in combination with other sepsis screening tests Caution should be taken not to use one single test alone as an assumption; this could result in 10% of cases being missed and 5% of cases being wrongly treated
Blood culture (0.5–1 mL of blood in culture bottle/s as per unit policy); aim for 1 mL if possible to increase potential to identify causative organism	Primary sepsis investigation	Negative growth	Positive within 24–48 hours of incubation	Blood cultures do not reach 100% sensitivity for the diagnosis of neonatal infection Sterile collection of blood cultures should be undertaken; however results are often indicative of contamination when weakly positive and do not necessarily indicate bloodstream infection Small volumes of blood aspirated from VLBW infants may affect the overall result of the blood culture if too little is inoculated into the culture bottle

Continued

TABLE 16.7 **Diagnostic tests used in sepsis—cont'd**				
Diagnostic test	Component/use	Normal findings	Result indicating sepsis	Notes
Lumbar puncture (LP)	Performed when the index of suspicion of meningitis is high (abnormal conscious state or seizures) LP is indicated in LOS if there is significant risk of bloodstream infection and the rise in CRP is exaggerated	Lymphocytes: ≤5–20 × 10^6/L Protein: ≤0.4–1.0 g/L Glucose: 38–179 mg/dL (mean 67 mg/dL); 2.1–9.9 mmol/L (mean 3.7 mmol/L) RBC: traumatic puncture may increase RBC up to 500/mm^3, and interferes with CSF analysis, changing its parameters	Raised lymphocytes, protein and glucose	May need to be delayed until the neonate can tolerate the procedure and coagulopathy status is normal
Urine cultures	Urine cultures performed when infection is suspected after 72 h of age Sterile specimen obtained from suprapubic urine tap or alternatively clean catch from a sterile urine bag may suffice	Negative culture when micro-culture and specificity (MCS) performed in laboratory setting	Positive culture when MCS performed Microscopy may reveal leucocytes	May be helpful in LOS when other laboratory investigations are negative, or CRP rise insignificant (low grade)
Postnasal aspirates (PNA) Endotracheal (ETT) aspirate	Investigation of LOS HAI when neonate ventilated, i.e. suspected bacterial or viral infections. Sterile aspirate of ETT and clean aspirate of postnasal spaces in non-ventilated neonates	Negative growth	Positive culture of bacteria or viruses on MCS or PCA	Results from MCS if positive usually reported in <48 h. Availability of PCA results for viruses vary in timeframe. Rapid screening is available in some laboratory settings
Swabs	Swabs of nose, throat and rectum for suspected bacterial or viral infection			

CSF, cerebrospinal fluid; HAI, hospital-acquired infection; LOS, late-onset sepsis; PCA, plate count agar; RBC, red blood cells; VLBW, very low birthweight.

include surface swabs such as ear swabs and gastric aspirates for **micro-culture and specificity (MCS)**. Ear swabs should be taken soon after birth prior to bathing and, similarly, gastric aspirate prior to feeding. When pustules or vesicles are present at birth, surface swabs should be taken prior to bathing. These swabs inform the clinician about the circulating and potentially infective organisms acquired in utero or during the birth process, enabling the appropriate treatment to be initiated. Should respiratory infections be considered as a cause of the infection, collection of secretions via endotracheal aspirate or postnasal aspirate should be considered, along with nose, throat and rectal swabs sent for microscopy or polymerase chain reaction (PCR) analysis (Odabasi & Bulbul, 2020).

Episodes of suspected LOS may require additional screening of the CSF even when neurological symptoms are not present. Blood cultures should be drawn if a central line is in place to screen for **central line-associated bloodstream infection (CLABSI)**, or endotracheal aspirates for suspected ventilation-associated pneumonia. Further diagnostic tests are taken to determine the need for empirical antibiotics and identification of causative organisms. Radiological evaluation (CXR or AXR) is of value either to contribute to the diagnosis of infection, such as pneumonia or necrotising enterocolitis, or to further exclude ongoing chest or gut pathology contributing to the septic episode (Singh et al., 2021). More information about illnesses such as pneumonia (see Chapter 9) and necrotising enterocolitis (see Chapter 12) is found in detail elsewhere in this text. Where there is no known history to assist with the diagnosis, or there is a history of contact with viruses, viral infection should always be considered (e.g. in cases of herpes simplex contact or varicella).

EVIDENCE-BASED PRACTICE RESEARCH 16.2

Use of clinical pathways for the screening and management of women and neonates with sepsis is necessary to guide best practice. The Royal Australian and New Zealand College of Obstetricians and Gynaecologists (RANZCOG, 2019) developed a pathway to screen all pregnant women for GBS at 35–37 weeks' gestation, and to treat them with intrapartum antibiotics if they were at increased risk of early-onset GBS sepsis (EOGBS). Following these pathways, after birth the term neonate with identified risk factors may be able to be cared for in the postnatal ward under observation, and receive intravenous antibiotics if the FBC is abnormal. The antibiotics can be ceased after 24 hours if the neonate remains asymptomatic, blood cultures are normal and the FBC at 24 hours is normal. A symptomatic neonate born to a mother with suspected chorioamnionitis should be transferred to a tertiary level neonatal unit for investigation and intravenous antibiotics.

MEDICAL AND PHARMACOLOGICAL TREATMENT OF NEONATAL INFECTION

Acute onset of sepsis, especially in the preterm neonate, requires supportive therapy coupled with investigations and broad-spectrum antibiotics such as aminoglycosides and penicillin, with the aim of preventing an overwhelming septic event leading to morbidity. As causative organisms are identified, antibiotics are tailored to specific culture sensitivities. The recommended length of antibiotic treatment is determined by identification of the causative organisms and site cultures (Puopolo et al., 2018). Consideration should be given to false-positive results with potentially contaminated specimens or to negative results due to maternal antibiotics delivered in the intrapartum period. Early treatment with antibiotics should also consider any known colonisation of the neonate – for example, endotracheal colonisation or current infective organisms circulating within the neonatal unit (Glaser et al., 2020). The course of therapy is 7–10 days for culture-positive results, and up to 21 days for CSF-positive newborns, with consideration given to repeat cultures of CSF and blood part way through the antibiotic/antiviral course, depending on the response of the newborn or the organism identified. Aminoglycosides are used to treat bacterial infections in neonates. Adverse effects on auditory and renal functions have been known to occur and this is directly related to the dosage, interval and, in turn, the drug levels in plasma.

EVIDENCE-BASED PRACTICE RESEARCH 16.3

In a Cochrane review published in 2016, Rao et al. found that safer and potentially more effective levels of aminoglycosides could be maintained using a one dose per day treatment schedule. Subsequently, Bergenwall et al. (2019) studied steady-state gentamicin concentration data in 60 infants without renal impairment, and recommended dosing intervals varying from every 48 hours to every 72 hours, depending on the infant's weight.

Antibiotics are generally ceased when the regimen is complete, the clinical condition of the neonate improves and infective indices are negative. Local policies regarding the administration of antimicrobials are important to minimise their exposure in sick and/or preterm neonates and the risk of subsequent resistance (Mukhopadhyay et al., 2019). As antibiotic overuse in neonates is associated with adverse outcomes, such as their effect on the intestinal microbiome, including the development of atopic diseases, broad-spectrum therapy should be reserved for neonates with risk factors, and their administration should be de-escalated promptly once culture results become available (Gkentzi & Dimitriou, 2019).

EVIDENCE-BASED PRACTICE RESEARCH 16.4

Intravenous immunoglobulin (IVIG) provides IgG that has a variety of actions that potentially reduce mortality and morbidity associated with neonatal infection. However, a recent Cochrane review found that its use to treat suspected or proven infection in neonates made no difference to outcomes (Ohlsson & Lacy, 2020).

Along with treating the suspected or known sepsis with appropriate antibiotic therapy, supporting normal haemodynamic status for the unstable neonate may require the implementation of normotensive agents/strategies such as plasma volume expanders (normal saline bolus infusions of 10–20 mL/kg). Corticosteroid therapy during this period is worth considering to assist with the stabilisation of the neonate's blood pressure (Schwarz & Dempsey, 2020). Consideration should be given to correcting imbalances in biochemistry (i.e. electrolytes and glucose) and in the neonate's haematological status.

EVIDENCE-BASED PRACTICE RESEARCH 16.5

Probiotics administered to preterm neonates are thought to reduce the incidence and effect of NEC and do not appear to have any adverse effects (Deshpande et al., 2018). A recent Cochrane review reported a 'low certainty' of efficacy due to small trials and possible biased methods. While the review acknowledged the efficacy in reducing the risk of NEC and probably a reduction in serious infection and death, the administration of probiotics requires further in-depth investigation (Sharif et al., 2020).

CLINICAL PRACTICE 16.4

Appropriate hand hygiene before and after handling patients, before and after procedures, and before and after handling body fluids and touching patient surroundings leads to less cross-contamination of microorganisms between healthcare workers, inanimate objects and patients (Hillier, 2020).

However, inappropriate use of non-sterile gloves can be more detrimental, leading to contamination of surfaces and inanimate objects, patients and healthcare workers (Pittet, 2017).

In addition to this intervention, there has been an increase in evidence that creating a bundled and checklist approach to infection control for specific procedures and interventions has reduced the degree of **hospital-acquired infection (HAI)**. A bundle is defined as 'a small, straight-forward set of evidence-based practices that, when performed collectively and reliably, are proven to improve patient outcomes' (Pogorzelska-Maziarz, 2016, p. 148). Hand hygiene is a **bundle approach** to decontaminating and preventing the spread of microorganisms (Balla et al., 2018). Neonates requiring intensive care are exposed to numerous invasive medical devices to support their wellbeing. Device-related infections are hospital acquired. Bloodstream infections or CLABSI account for a large percentage of these infections, and those that are ventilator associated, like **ventilator-associated pneumonia (VAP)**, are among the second most significant (Balla et al., 2018).

EVIDENCE-BASED PRACTICE RESEARCH 16.6

The use of central venous catheters and indwelling intravenous devices to deliver parenteral nutrition, and exposure to healthcare workers utilising these lines for medications and fluid administration, further increases the risk for HAI (Cho & Cho, 2019).

Reducing HAI due to these devices by utilising the bundle care and checklist approach to management has been successful (Cho & Cho, 2019). Infection surveillance is monitored at unit level throughout the globe, with larger collaborative units collating results, enabling trends to be observed and evidence-based practices to be monitored and improved. This practice has continued during the past few decades, resulting in strategies to tackle HAI by providing benchmarking figures for quality improvement activities at a neonatal unit level (ANZNN, 2020).

CLINICAL PRACTICE 16.5

At least daily routine cleaning of the neonate's immediate environment, floors, sinks, doors and windows, trolleys and work surfaces reduces the number of inanimate objects that are potential vehicles for transport of harmful bacteria (National Health and Medical Research Council (NHMRC), 2019; Rutala & Weber, 2019).

Infection control practices are embedded within clinical guidelines at hospital and unit levels. Isolation and infection control procedures are aimed at controlling and preventing the spread of infection. Understanding the role of both standard and transmission-based precautions is essential for neonatal nurses/midwives because patients in their care are extremely vulnerable to infection, as discussed previously in this chapter. '**Standard precautions**' are guidelines for health professionals to use in daily point-to-point care to prevent transmission of infection from one patient to another. '**Transmission precautions**' are used in conjunction with standard precautions when there is suspected or confirmed infection that is able to be transmitted to other patients via contact, droplet or airborne routes (Table 16.8). Within these guidelines is a framework for environmental care and cleaning specifically to minimise the risk of HAI.

The current novel coronavirus pandemic has highlighted the need for standardised protocols to mitigate the spread of infection to vulnerable neonatal patients and among essential healthcare workers. As the main mechanism of spread of coronavirus is via person-to-person contact by respiratory droplets, procedures such as the provision of high-flow oxygen and endotracheal intubation pose high risk of infection for healthcare workers such as neonatal nurses and midwives. The correct use of **personal protective equipment (PPE)**, such as face shields or goggles, gowns, gloves and masks, to protect HCWs from transmissible pathogens is essential (McCarthy et al., 2020). Meticulous donning and doffing of PPE is vital to reduce contamination of HCWs (see Clinical Practice 16.6).

TABLE 16.8 **Standard and transmission precautions**

Standard precautions	Transmission precautions
Hand hygiene Personal protective equipment (PPE) The safe use and disposal of sharps Environmental cleaning Reprocessing of reusable medical equipment and instruments Respiratory hygiene and cough etiquette Aseptic technique Waste management Appropriate handling of linen	Contact precautions: • most common transmission • blood or body substances • direct or indirect Droplet precautions: • respiratory droplets transmitted over short distances from the infected person to another contact • indirectly via hands Airborne precautions: • dissemination occurs via aerosols over long distances by air currents (air-conditioning/ventilation systems) • small particles created by breathing, talking, coughing, sneezing • evaporation of droplets in low humidity

CLINICAL PRACTICE 16.6 Sequence for donning (putting on) and doffing (taking off) personal protective equipment

Donning PPE	Doffing PPE
1 PERFORM HAND HYGIENE Wash hands or use alcohol-based hand rub. **2 PUT ON GOWN** Ensure the gown fully covers the torso and neck to knees, arms to end of wrist, and wraps around the back. Fasten/tie at the back of neck and waist. **3 PUT ON MASK** Surgical mask or P2/N95. Surgical mask: secure ties or ear loops. Mould nose piece into the mask and position over nose and mouth, then chin. Position according to training and manufacturers' instruction. Perform fit check. **4 PUT ON EYE PROTECTION** Place over face and eyes. Adjust to fit. **5 PUT ON GLOVES** Fit gloves over the cuffs ensuring the gown and sleeves are covered by the glove. **6 PPE CHECK** Check all items of PPE are correctly in place. Check integrity of PPE.	**1 REMOVE GLOVES** Grasp outside with opposite gloved hand, peel off. Hold removed glove in the gloved hand. Slide fingers of ungloved hand under the remaining glove at the wrist. Peel gloves off over the first gloves. Discard gloves in waste container. **2 PERFORM HAND HYGIENE** Wash hands or use alcohol-based hand rub. **3 REMOVE GOWN** Undo fasteners or ties. Pull away from neck or shoulders touching the inside of the gown only. Turn gown inside out, away from clothing. Fold or roll into a bundle and discard in waste container. **4 PERFORM HAND HYGIENE** Wash hands or use alcohol-based hand rub. **5 REMOVE EYE PROTECTION** Do not touch the front surfaces. Handle by headband or side arms. Place in designated container for reprocessing or in waste container. **6 PERFORM HAND HYGIENE** Wash hands or use alcohol-based hand rub. **7 REMOVE MASK** Do not touch the front of the mask. Grasp lower, then top ties or elastics and remove as per training and manufacturers' guidelines to avoid self-contamination. Discard in waste container. **8 PERFORM HAND HYGIENE** Wash hands or use alcohol-based hand rub immediately after removing all PPE.

Source: SA Health (2019).

FAMILY-CENTRED CARE 16.1

Family members can be enlisted to help with infection control measures in the neonatal unit. Neonatal nurses/midwives should demonstrate and teach appropriate hand hygiene to parents to use before and after handling their baby, before and after handling body fluids and when touching their baby's surroundings so as to minimise transmission of infection in the neonatal unit. Parents and extended family should be informed that they should not visit the neonatal unit if they do not feel well. They need to be shown how to dispose of dirty linen or equipment. Mothers should be shown how to express breast milk with clean hands and equipment, and how to handle expressed breast milk so as to reduce the possibility of the transmission of infection.

Isolation procedures are also embedded within the hospital guidelines. Methods to reduce the spread of infection throughout the population in the NICU and SCBU include immediate isolation in specific isolation areas or cohorting or grouping together of potentially infected patients to reduce spread by contact with HCWs to other patients (University of Notre Dame, 2019).

NURSING CARE OF THE SEPTIC NEONATE

A neonate with confirmed sepsis should be cared for in a neonatal intensive or special care unit where they can be observed closely. However, if the neonate is clinically well and the septic markers are benign – for example, where antibiotics have been commenced while waiting to rule out sepsis – the neonate may be cared for in a postnatal ward to promote bonding and attachment and to facilitate breastfeeding. Where possible, neonates should be cared for in the postnatal ward with an intravenous cannula in place and receive intravenous antibiotics as ordered. In these circumstances, the neonate is best cared for by nurses/midwives who have experience in a special care neonatal unit setting, facilitating regular reviewing and evaluation of changes in vital signs, and providing skilled cue-based care to the sick neonate (Council of International Neonatal Nurses (COINN), 2019).

Whether in the postnatal ward, SCBU or NICU, the neonate will require special attention to thermoregulation (refer to Chapter 8). As respiratory distress is a common symptom of sepsis, ensuring that the neonate is positioned in such a way to support the airway and has adequate respiratory support, including oxygen therapy, is an important role of the neonatal nurse/midwife (refer to Chapter 9). The neonatal nurse/midwife must also ensure adequate caloric intake for the neonate to meet the added metabolic demands of sepsis. Support for the mother during this time with assistance in breast milk expression is essential if the neonate is unable to feed at the breast. Furthermore, an unwell neonate is often irritable and unable to tolerate the handling that may be required with breastfeeding. Both term and preterm neonates may require supplemental or full feeds enterally via gavage tubes. Output, including urine and stool, should also be monitored closely and documented. The neonate's comfort needs must be met, including positioning in comfort, preferably one of flexion, where limbs are contained and boundaries nestle the neonate. The neonatal nurse/midwife is also responsible for the administration of antibiotics, analgesia and other medications, intravenous fluids including parenteral nutrition and the maintenance of intravenous lines and sites, monitoring of vital signs and taking specimens for laboratory investigations. Importantly, high standards of infection control, as outlined in the previous section, are crucial when caring for these neonates. This includes diligent **hand hygiene**, cleaning and a reduction in the amount of equipment shared.

Family-centred care is important in the context of a neonate with sepsis, especially with EOS, as mothers may feel guilty about the maternal transmission of the infective organism, and this may affect attachment and bonding. You can read about the reactions that parents may experience when their baby is admitted to the neonatal unit, and how to support them, in Chapter 21. With the onset of sepsis, neonates can become very physiologically unstable, and parents feel less confident in their ability to participate in the care of their sick neonate (Pineda et al., 2018). Previously well term neonates may be transferred to the neonatal unit and be further separated from their parents in an isolette, exacerbating the parents' stress. Neonatal nurses/midwives caring for the family should focus on promoting positively what parents can do to support their baby during this period – for example, hand holding, skin-to-skin cuddles if tolerated and providing breast milk to protect their infant. They should be shown how to perform hand hygiene. Information about not visiting if they are unwell is also essential. When facilitating family-centred care for neonates with sepsis, it is crucial that the neonatal nurse/midwife involves parents in the regular care of the neonate, provides continual updates, uses appropriate language, educates the parents and provides breastfeeding support to the mother (Oude Maatman et al., 2020) (refer to Chapter 21).

FAMILY-CENTRED CARE 16.2

How can you make families more aware of the infection risks to their baby in a sensitive and useful way?

CASE STUDY 16.1

Joshua was born at term by normal vaginal birth to Jessica after a normal pregnancy and labour. Jessica was GBS negative on her 36-week high vaginal swab. However, Joshua was noted to be lethargic and not interested in feeding just 6 hours after being born. He was transferred to the special care unit and found to be tachypnoeic and tachycardic, with a per axilla temperature of 37.8°C. Blood cultures were taken, and he was treated with prophylactic antibiotics.

The next day Joshua developed jaundice and was placed under phototherapy. That evening, he was lethargic and his breathing was increasingly laboured. He was transferred to intensive care and required mechanical ventilation. His condition continued to deteriorate, and at midnight he had a seizure. The next afternoon the family was told he had GBS.

Joshua remained in intensive care for just over a week, and then in the special care unit until he was 4 weeks old. His cranial ultrasounds and MRI showed changes to the brain, including cysts and loss of white matter. The family was told that he would most likely have problems with his movement and possibly some form of cerebral palsy.

1. After being admitted to the neonatal care unit, what further laboratory investigations could be recommended for Joshua?
2. How often does the CRP need to be monitored during treatment, and why?
3. What other investigations could Joshua have to evaluate neurological function and assist with prognosis?
4. If meningitis is considered in this case, how long would antibiotics be administered and by what route?
5. What further follow-up may be required for Joshua?

CONCLUSION

Sepsis in the newborn can be a devastating event. Term newborns who suffer from EOS are exposed to an increased length of hospital stay, invasive procedures and the risk of long-term complications. Mortality in this group of newborns is less than in the preterm infant group; however, serious infections can lead to increased morbidity in these neonates. Preterm and small for gestational age infants are at increased risk of infection for a multitude of reasons that have been addressed throughout this chapter. In preterm infants, the effects of sepsis are exacerbated by their inexperience with infection, reducing the effectiveness of the immune system. The symptoms are often subtle and generalised, and deterioration can be rapid. Morbidity varies with the intensity of the infection, from mild to severe neurological impairment and related complications. Mortality rates for LOS are lower than for EOS, with higher rates in very low birthweight (VLBW) and extremely low birthweight (ELBW) neonates. While gram-positive infections have a 10% mortality rate, gram-negative sepsis has a worse prognosis with a 45% mortality rate (Glaser et al., 2020). The neonatal nurse/midwife caring for the neonate is the most likely clinician to detect the subtle signs of infection. With well-developed assessment skills and the capacity to provide holistic care based on the best available evidence, the neonatal nurse/midwife can make a positive difference to the outcomes for the septic infant and his/her family.

Recommended Reading / Online Resources

Wilson, C. B., Nizet, V., Maldonado, Y. A., Remington, J. S., & Klein, J. O. (2016). *Remington and Klein's infectious diseases of the fetus and newborn infant* (8th ed.). Philadelphia, PA: Elsevier Saunders. <www.clinicalkey.com.au/#!/browse/book/3-s2.0-C20120035843>.

References/Acknowledgements

Akangire, G., Simpson, E., Weiner, J., Noel-MacDonnell, J., Petrikin, J., & Sheehan, M. (2020). Implementation of the neonatal sepsis calculator in early-onset sepsis and maternal chorioamnionitis. *Advances in Neonatal Care, 20*(1), 25–32. doi: 10.1097/ANC.0000000000000668.

Amare, D., Mela, M., & Dessie, G. (2019). Unfinished agenda of the neonates in developing countries: magnitude of neonatal sepsis: systematic review and meta-analysis. *Heliyon, 5*(9), e02519. doi: 10.1016/j.heliyon.2019.e02519.

Australian and New Zealand Neonatal Network (ANZNN). (2020). *ANZNN data dictionary*. Sydney, NSW: ANZNN.

Balla, K. C., Rao, S. P., Arul, C., Shashidhar, A., Prashantha, Y. N., Nagaraj, S., et al. (2018). Decreasing central line-associated bloodstream infections through quality improvement initiative. *Indian Pediatrics, 55*(9), 753–756.

Bergenwall, M., Walker, S. A. N., Elligsen, M., Iaboni, D. C., Findlater, C., Seto, W., et al. (2019). Optimizing gentamicin conventional and extended interval dosing in neonates using Monte Carlo simulation – a retrospective study. *BMC Pediatrics, 19*(1), 318. doi: 10.1186/s12887-019-1676-3.

Bridges, M., Pesek, E., McRae, M., & Chabra, S. (2019). Use of an early onset-sepsis calculator to decrease unnecessary NICU admissions and increase exclusive breastfeeding. *Journal of Obstetric, Gynecologic and Neonatal Nursing, 48*, 372–382.

Cailes, B., Kortsalioudaki, C., Buttery, J., Pattnayak, S., Greenough, A., Matthes, J., et al. (2018). Epidemiology of UK neonatal infections: the neonIN infection surveillance network. *Archives of Disease in Childhood. Fetal and Neonatal Edition, 103*(6), F547–553.

Centers for Disease Control and Prevention (CDC). (2020). Group B strep (GBS): fast facts. Atlanta, GA: US Department of Health and Human Services, CDC. <https://www.cdc.gov/groupbstrep/about/fast-facts.html> (Accessed 20 February 2022).

Cho, H. J., & Cho, H. K. (2019). Central line-associated bloodstream infections in neonates. *Korean Journal of Pediatrics, 62*(3), 79–84. doi: 10.3345/kjp.2018.07003.

Chow, S. S. W., Creighton, P., Chambers, G. M., & Lui, K. 2020. *Report of the Australian and New Zealand Neonatal Network 2018*. Sydney, NSW: ANZNN.

COINN (Council of International Neonatal Nurses). (2019). International neonatal competency framework. *Journal of Neonatal Nursing, 25*, 258–264.

Collins, A., Weitkamp, J-H., & Wynn, J. L. (2018). Why are preterm newborns at increased risk of infection? *Archives of Disease in Childhood. Fetal and Neonatal Edition, 103*(4), F391–F394. doi: 10.1136/ archdischild-2017-313595.

Crocker, L. W., White, A., Heaton, P. A., Horta, D. P., & Paul, S. P. (2021). Recognition and management of neonatal sepsis. *British Journal of Nursing, 30*(7), 410–415.

Deshpande, G., Athalye-Jape, G., & Patole, S. (2018). Para-probiotics for preterm neonates – the next frontier. *Nutrients, 10*(7), 871. doi: 10.3390/nu10070871.

Fleischmann, C., Reichert, F., Cassini, A., Horner, R., Harder. T., Markwart R., et al. (2021). Global incidence and mortality of neonatal sepsis: a systematic review and meta-analysis. *Archives of Disease in Childhood, 106*(8), 745–752.

Gkentzi, D., & Dimitriou, G. (2019). Antimicrobial stewardship in the neonatal intensive care unit: an update. *Current Pediatric Reviews, 15*(1), 47–52. doi: 10.2174/1573396315666190118101953.

Glaser, M. A., Hughes, L. M., Jnah, A., & Newberry, D. (2020). Neonatal sepsis. *Advances in Neonatal Care, 21*(1), 49–60.

Goel, N., Shrestha, S., Smith, R., Mehta, A., Ketty, M., Muxworthy, H., et al. (2020). Screening for early onset neonatal sepsis: NICE guidance-based practice versus projected application of the Kaiser Permanente sepsis risk calculator in the UK population. *Archives of Disease in Childhood. Fetal and Neonatal Edition, 105*(2), 118–122. doi: 10.1136/archdischild-2018-316777.

Granger, C. L., Embleton, N. D., Palmer, J. M., Lamb, C. A., Berrington, J. E., & Stewart, C. J. (2021). Maternal breast-milk, infant gut microbiome and the impact on preterm infant health. *Acta Paediatrica, 110*, 450–457.

Grassham, C. D., Kamm, C., Pao aroon, C. N., McGuire, K. N., & Maxwell, J. R. (2021). Improving outcomes in neonatal late onset sepsis: where every second matters. *Journal of Neonatal Nursing, 27*, 100–105.

Hillier, M. D. (2020). Using effective hand hygiene practice to prevent and control infection. *Nursing Standard, 35*(5), 45–50. doi: 10.7748/ns.2020.e11552.

Hincu, M-A., Zonda, G-I., Stanciu, G. D., Nemescu, D., & Paduraru, L. (2020). Relevance of biomarkers currently in use or research for practical diagnosis approach of neonatal early-onset sepsis. *Children, 7*(309), 1–25.

Johansson Gudjónsdóttir, M., Elfvin, A., Hentz, E., Adlerberth, I., Tessin, I., & Trollfors, B. (2019). Changes in incidence and aetiology of early-onset neonatal infections 1997–2017 – a retrospective cohort study in western Sweden. *BMC Pediatrics, 19*, 490. doi: 10.1186/s12887-019-1866-z.

Ko, H., Dehority W., & Maxwell J. R. (2020). The impact of maternal infection on the neonate. *Online First*. <https://www.intechopen.com/online-first/the-impact-of-maternal-infection-on-the-neonate> (Accessed 20 February 2022).

Maldonado, Y. A., Nizet, V., Klein, J. O., Remington, J. S., & Wilson, C. B. (2016). Current concepts of infections of the fetus and newborn infant. In: C. B. Wilson, V. Nizet, Y. Maldonado, J. S. Remington, & J. O. Klein (Eds.), *Remington and Klein's infections diseases of the fetus and newborn infant* (8th ed., pp. 3–23). Philadelphia, PA: Elsevier Saunders.

Male, D., Stokes Peebles Jr, R. & Male, V. (2021). *Immunology* (9th ed.). Edinburgh: Churchill Livingstone Elsevier.

McCarthy, R., Gino, B., d'Entremont, P., Barari, A., & Renouf, T. S. (2020). The importance of personal protective equipment design and donning and doffing technique in mitigating infectious disease spread: a technical report. *Cureus, 12*(12), e12084. doi: 10.7759/cureus.12084.

Mukhopadhyay, S., Wade, K. C., & Puopolo, K. M. (2019). Drugs for the prevention and treatment of sepsis in the newborn. *Clinics in Perinatology, 46*(2), 327–347. doi: 10.1016/j.clp.2019.02.012.

National Health and Medical Research Council (NHMRC). (2019). *Australian guidelines for the prevention and control of infection in healthcare*. <https://www.nhmrc.gov.au/about-us/publications/australian-guidelines-prevention-and-control-infection-healthcare-2019> (Accessed 20 February 2022).

Odabasi, I. O., & Bulbul, A. (2020). Neonatal sepsis. *Sisli Etfal Hastanesi tip Bulteni, 54*(2), 142–158. doi: 10.14744/SEMB.2020.00236.

Ohlsson, A., & Lacy, J. B. (2020). Intravenous immunoglobulin for suspected or proven infection in neonates. *Cochrane Database of Systematic Reviews, 3*, CD001239. doi: 10.1002/14651858.CD001239.pub56.

Oliveira, J., & Reygaert, W. C. (2021). Gram negative bacteria. *StatPearls*. Treasure Island, FL: StatPearls Publishing. <https://www.ncbi.nlm.nih.gov/books/NBK538213/> (Accessed 20 February 2022).

Oude Maatman, S. M., Bohlin, K., Lilliesköld, S., Garberg, H. T., Uitewaal-Poslawky, I., Kars, M. C., et al. (2020). Factors influencing implementation of family-centred care in a neonatal intensive care unit. *Frontiers in Pediatrics, 8*, 222. doi: 10.3389/fped.2020.00222.

Pammi, M., & Gautham, K. S. (2020). Enteral lactoferrin supplementation for prevention of sepsis and necrotizing enterocolitis in preterm infants. *Cochrane Database of Systematic Reviews, 3*, CD007137. doi: 10.1002/14651858.CD007137.pub6.

Pineda, R., Bender, J., Hall, B., Shabosky, L., Annecca, A., & Smith, J. (2018). Parent participation in the Neonatal Intensive Care Unit: predictors and relationships to neurobehavior and developmental outcomes. *Early Human Development, 117*, 32–38.

Pittet, D. (2017). Hand hygiene: from research to action. *Journal of Infection Prevention, 18*(3), 100–102. doi: 10.1177/1757177417705191.

Pogorzelska-Maziarz, M. (2016). The use and effectiveness of bundles for prevention of central line-associated bloodstream infections in neonates: a review of the literature. *Journal of Perinatal and Neonatal Nursing, 30*(2), 148–159.

Puopolo, K. M., Benitz, W. E., & Zaoutis, T. E. (2018). Management of neonates born at ≤34 6/7 weeks' gestation with suspected or proven early-onset bacterial sepsis. *Pediatrics, 142*(6), e20182896. doi: 10.1542/peds.2018-2896.

Rao, S. C., Srinivasjois, R., Moon, K., & Cochrane Neonatal Group. (2016). One dose per day compared to multiple doses per day of gentamicin for treatment of suspected or proven sepsis in neonates. *Cochrane Database Systemic Review,* 2016(12), CD005091. doi: 10.1002/14651858.CD005091.pub4.

Royal Australian and New Zealand College of Obstetricians and Gynaecologists (RANZCOG). (2019). *Maternal group B streptococcus in pregnancy: screening and management*. St Leonards, NSW: RANZCOG. <https://ranzcog.edu.au/RANZCOG_SITE/media/RANZCOG-MEDIA/Women%27s%20Health/Statement%20and%20guidelines/Clinical-Obstetrics/Maternal-Group-B-Streptococcus-in-pregnancy-screening-and-management-(C-Obs-19).pdf?ext=.pdf> (Accessed 20 February 2022).

Rutala, W. A., & Weber, D. J. (2019). Best practices for disinfection of noncritical environmental surfaces and equipment in health care facilities: a bundle approach. *American Journal of Infection Control, 47S*, A96–A105. doi: 10.1016/j.ajic.2019.01.014.

SA Health. (2019). *Sequence for donning and doffing PPE*, <https://www.sahealth.sa.gov.au/wps/wcm/connect/759d0d97-e9a4-480d-949a-a8316027e028/20015.18+PPE+Sequencing+A3+Poster-online.pdf > (Accessed 20 February 2022).

Schwarz, C. E., & Dempsey, E. M. (2020). Management of neonatal hypotension and shock. *Seminars in Fetal and Neonatal Medicine, 25*, 101121.

Shane, A. L., Sánchez, P. J., & Stoll, B. J. (2017). Neonatal sepsis. *Lancet, 390*, 10104, 1770–1780. doi: 10.1016/S0140-6736(17)31002-4.

Sharif, S., Meader, N., Oddie, S. J., Rojas-Reyes, M. X., & McGuire, W. (2020). Probiotics to prevent necrotising enterocolitis in very preterm or very low birth weight infants. *Cochrane Database of Systematic Reviews, 10*, CD005496. doi: 10.1002/14651858.CD005496.pub5.

Singh, M., Alsaleem, M. & Gray, C. P. (2021). Neonatal sepsis. *StatPearls*. Treasure Island, FL: StatPearls Publishing. <https://www.ncbi.nlm.nih.gov/books/NBK531478/> (Accessed 20 February 2022).

University of Notre Dame. (2019). NICU design standards. <https://nicudesign.nd.edu/nicu-standards/> (Accessed 20 February 2022).

Uzan-Yulzari, A., Turta, O., Belogolovski, A., Ziv, O., Kunz, C., Perschbacher, S., et al. (2021). Neonatal antibiotic exposure impairs child growth during the first six years of life by perturbing intestinal microbial colonization. *Nature Communications, 12*(443), 1–12. doi: 10.1038/s41467-020-20495-4.

Wilson, C. B., Nizet, V., Maldonado, Y. A., Remington, J. S., & Klein, J. O. (2016). *Remington and Klein's infectious diseases of the fetus and newborn infant* (8th ed.). Philadelphia, PA: Elsevier Saunders.

CHAPTER 17

CARE OF THE NEONATE WITH A CONGENITAL ABNORMALITY

VICTORIA KAIN AND TRUDI MANNIX

Learning objectives

After reading this chapter you will be able to:

- describe common congenital disorders that are apparent in the newborn period and care management for each
- undertake a systematic approach to assessment of the neonate with a congenital abnormality
- analyse the principles of a family-centred care approach to families and patients with congenital abnormalities and synthesise these concepts into their own clinical contexts.

Key words, terms and abbreviations

abdominal wall defects (AWDs)
achondroplasia
anencephaly
anorectal malformations
antenatal hydronephrosis (ANH)
bladder exstrophy
choanal atresia
cleft lip and/or palate
closed spinal dysraphisms
congenital abnormalities of the kidney and urinary tract (CAKUT)
congenital abnormality
congenital cardiac defects
congenital diaphragmatic hernia (CDH)
congenital hypertrophic pyloric stenosis (CHPS)
craniorachischisis
cryptorchidism
duodenal atresia/stenosis
encephalocele
epidermolysis bullosa
gastroschisis
haemangioma
Hirschsprung disease
hydrocephaly
hydronephrosis
hypospadias
imperforate anus
indirect inguinal hernia
laryngomalacia
lipomyelomeningocele
macroglossia
malrotation
meconium ileus
meningocele
microcephaly
micrognathia
multi-cystic dysplastic kidney disease (MCDKD)
myelomeningocele
neural tube defects (NTDs)
oesophageal atresia (OA)
omphalocele
patent urachus
pelvic–ureteric junction (PUJ) obstruction
polydactyly
spina bifida occulta
Sturge–Weber syndrome
syndactyly
tracheoesophageal fistula (TOF)
tracheomalacia
trisomy 13
trisomy 18
trisomy 21
Turner syndrome
undescended testes (UDT)
VACTERL association
vesico-ureteric junction (VUJ) obstruction
vesico-ureteric reflux (VUR)
volvulus

INTRODUCTION

A **congenital abnormality** is a structural or functional abnormality that develops during intrauterine life and is diagnosed prenatally, at birth, postnatally, during infancy or later. It is sometimes referred to as a congenital defect, congenital anomaly, congenital disease or congenital deformity. Despite the fact that several genetic and environmental factors are known to cause congenital abnormalities, up to 50% do not have a known aetiology (World Health Organization (WHO), 2016). According to the WHO, 7.9 million newborns worldwide were born with congenital abnormalities in 2015, with 303,000 dying during the first month of life (WHO, 2016). Congenital abnormalities and chromosomal abnormalities are the primary causes of death in infants under 1 year of age in the United States, accounting for 20.8% of all neonatal deaths (Heron, 2018). In Australia, congenital abnormality is the most common cause of perinatal death, accounting for 31% of stillbirths and 33% of neonatal deaths (Australian Institute of Health and Welfare (AIHW), 2021), while in New Zealand all congenital and chromosomal anomalies account for 88.08 in 1000 live births (Environmental Health Intelligence New Zealand, 2020).

This chapter begins with a systems approach to the description of some of the more common congenital abnormalities reported globally and then describes common chromosomal disorders.

CONGENITAL ABNORMALITIES OF THE RESPIRATORY SYSTEM

Congenital lung malformations are a diverse group of fetal lung abnormalities and can be classified into bronchopulmonary anomalies, vascular or combined lung and vascular anomalies, where lung development is interrupted in various stages of embryogenesis (Mehta & Sharma, 2021). The most common types are congenital pulmonary adenomatoid malformation (CPAM) and pulmonary sequestrations, with an incidence between 1 in 10,000 and 1 in 35,000 births. Of the five major subtypes, the most common is type 1 (70% of all CPAM), which originates in the bronchi with multiloculated cysts forming in one lobe. The prognosis is generally excellent after resection (Mehta & Sharma, 2021). Many conditions are asymptomatic and hence the option of early surgical treatment versus active surveillance remains controversial. In recent years, thoracoscopic surgery has become more commonly used and is shown to decrease the length of stay in hospital by up to a half (Xie et al., 2020).

Obstructive disorders

Macroglossia

Macroglossia, or an abnormally enlarged tongue (Fig. 17.1), is a congenital condition that is usually associated with another congenital disorder, such as Down syndrome, Apert syndrome or Beckwith–Wiedemann syndrome (Schendel, 2019). The tongue will often protrude from the mouth and interfere with feeding. The neonate with macroglossia may present with stridor and snoring. In the absence of any other disorder, a family history may reveal the autosomal dominant genotype associated with idiopathic macroglossia. Treatment focuses on reducing alterations to the face, airway, feeding and speech, and can include radiation, steroids, cryotherapy, electrocautery and embolisation, depending on the cause. Surgery in the form of a midline or peripheral reduction glossectomy is indicated in about 10% of cases when the airway is at risk of obstruction, but there is no consensus on the best surgical technique for this complex problem (Kutti Sridharan & Rokkam, 2021; Núñez-Martínez et al., 2016).

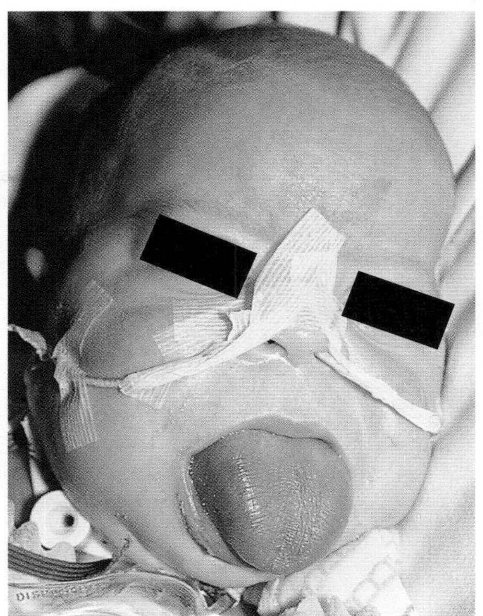

FIGURE 17.1 **Macroglossia**
Source: Eichenfeld et al. (2015).

Micrognathia

Micrognathia (Fig. 17.2) refers to a condition whereby the lower jaw is smaller than normal. Micrognathia is most commonly initially diagnosed on routine ultrasound scans in the second trimester of pregnancy. Positional obstruction leading to apnoea may occur in the neonatal period as the tongue is more posteriorly situated in the oropharynx, and feeding problems requiring specialised teats are often necessary. Micrognathia is frequently a part of other genetic syndromes, including Marfan syndrome, Pierre Robin syndrome, Treacher–Collins syndrome, trisomy 13 and 18 and XO syndrome (Turner syndrome) (Evans et al., 2018). Prone positioning is useful to prevent airway obstruction. Generally, mandibular growth 'catches up' by 6–12 months of age, but surgery may be needed for infants with significant respiratory or feeding issues (Fraser, 2021, p. 413).

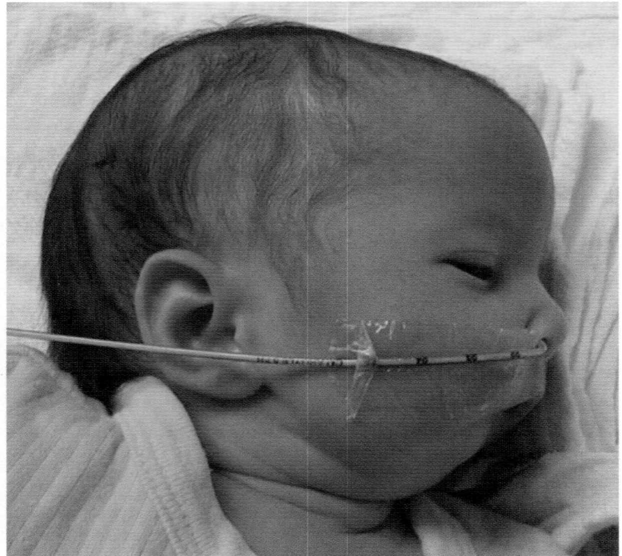

FIGURE 17.2 **Micrognathia**

Source: Bio23/CC BY SA 3.0.

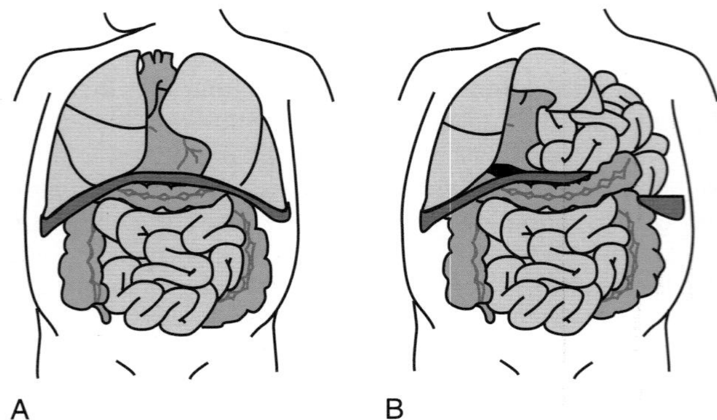

FIGURE 17.3 **Congenital diaphragmatic hernia**

a Normal positioning of the bowel contents in the abdominal cavity. **b** Herniation of the abdominal contents through the defect in the diaphragm, into the thorax, causing pulmonary hypoplasia.

Source: From Maheshwari and Carlo (2018).

Laryngomalacia and tracheomalacia

Laryngomalacia and **tracheomalacia** are conditions where there is a collapse of either the laryngeal or the tracheal structures, respectively, owing to a loss of structural integrity. Laryngomalacia is the most common of these disorders, but tracheobronchomalacia and bronchomalacia are also seen. The term 'malacia' essentially means 'softening' and the condition causes the airway to collapse in on itself, particularly during expiration. This explains why inspiratory stridor is the most common feature, although increased work of breathing, swallowing dysfunction (i.e. coughing, choking, gagging, vomiting, poor feeding) and aspiration are also recurring symptoms (Irace et al., 2019). Although presentation is most common in the neonatal period, it can take up to 2–3 months to become clinically evident (Wallis et al., 2019). A multidisciplinary approach to management will allow consideration of nasogastric or gastrostomy feeding, diet modification, feeding strategies, counselling of families and supraglottoplasty (Irace et al., 2019).

Choanal atresia

Choanal atresia is a congenital condition defined as the developmental absence of the normal communication between the posterior nasal cavity and the nasopharynx (Shute et al., 2021), resulting in either a narrowing or a complete blockage of the nasal airway by tissue. The condition is potentially serious, as complete nasal obstruction may result in death from asphyxia. The obstruction is momentarily relieved when the neonate cries as they breathe in via the mouth with crying, but, given that neonates are obligatory nose breathers, once crying ceases the airway occlusion results in obstructive apnoea. Unilateral atresia occurs more frequently on the right side, with a ratio of unilateral to bilateral cases of 2:1. The average rate of choanal atresia is 1 in 5000–8000 children (Attya et al., 2021). A diagnosis can be made if a size 8F catheter cannot be passed through the nares/s. The neonate can be managed with an oral airway, or even intubated, until surgical intervention can be undertaken.

Diaphragmatic hernia

A **congenital diaphragmatic hernia (CDH)** is an abnormality in the muscle of the diaphragm which allows herniation of the abdominal contents through the defect into the thorax, causing severe respiratory distress due to pulmonary hypoplasia (Fig. 17.3). Most CDHs are diagnosed antenatally, but some are diagnosed in symptomatic newborns, and even asymptomatic or mildly symptomatic children, teens and adults (Longoni et al., 2020, p. 4). CDH occurs in approximately 1 in 2200–4000 live births; a left-sided hernia is the most commonly sited abnormality, with 80% on this side (Longoni et al., 2020). At birth, neonates with a CDH present with severe respiratory distress, reduced breath sounds on the affected side, pulmonary hypertension, a barrel-shaped chest and a scaphoid abdomen. The survival of neonates with CDH has increased over the last few decades with the instigation of comprehensive principles of resuscitation, stabilisation and management. Neonates with a right-sided abnormality have an increased mortality rate and, although extremely rare, a bilateral CDH is usually fatal. With increasing survival to over 90% in some centres, long-term respiratory, neurodevelopmental and nutritional complications are becoming more apparent (Gerall et al., 2021).

Preoperative management strategies include avoiding high airway pressures, the establishment of a satisfactory (>85%) pre-ductal arterial saturation (SaO_2), avoiding bag and mask ventilation to prevent over-distension of the intestines, the management of pulmonary hypertension, and optimising haemodynamic and respiratory status prior to surgery. A large-bore nasogastric tube (NG) is essential to decompress the abdomen, as are arterial and central venous lines. Infants receive low-dose sedation via continuous intravenous infusion rather than neuromuscular block/paralysis (Duncan et al., 2021). Ventilation strategies are aimed at preventing lung injury, with the preferred mode being volume-targeted ventilation with low tidal volumes and peak pressure limits to minimise lung injury. Initial tidal volume targets of 3–4 mL/kg are set, with peak inspiratory pressure (PIP) <25 mmHg (Duncan et al., 2021). Inhaled nitric oxide is a powerful pulmonary vasodilator and is widely used in neonates with CDH (Hedrick & Adzick, 2021). (See Chapter 9 for more information about ventilation.)

The delay of surgical repair until physiological stabilisation is achieved is now considered best practice. Surgical repair (closure of the diaphragmatic defect and reduction of the viscera into the abdominal cavity) is individualised for each neonate and depends on the available diaphragm muscle available for closure, the amount of bowel in the thorax and surgical preference. The repair of the diaphragm can either be primary, involving direct closure of the abnormality, or, if there is insufficient diaphragm muscle available, a synthetic patch is used. The abdominal wall may be difficult to close following reduction of the hernia, and the use of a temporary wall silo may be helpful to gradually return the organs to the abdominal cavity (Hedrick & Adzick, 2021).

Outcomes are improved when there is no liver involvement in the herniation ('liver down') and the neonate has access to very intensive support after birth in a specialist centre that can offer extracorporeal membrane oxygenation (ECMO). Survival rates of 70–92% are reported at tertiary centres, but there are significant morbidities such as gastroesophageal reflux, hearing loss, growth failure, respiratory complications and neurodevelopmental delay (Hedrick & Adzick, 2021).

EVIDENCE-BASED PRACTICE 17.1

Gerall et al. (2021) conducted a retrospective review of 193 neonates who underwent CDH repair, and found that long-term outcomes included 'gastroesophageal reflux disease (42.0%), diaphragmatic hernia recurrence (10.9%), asthma (23.6%), neurodevelopmental delay (28.6%), attention deficit hyperactivity disorder (7.3%), autism (1.6%), chest wall deformity (15.5%), scoliosis (11.4%) and inguinal hernia (6.7%)'. They concluded that neonates discharged after CDH repair should be followed up by a multidisciplinary team in a long-term follow-up clinic using best-practice surveillance strategies.

For all neonates who undergo surgery for CDH, enrolment in long-term multidisciplinary follow-up clinics is recommended.

Oesophageal atresia (+/− fistula)

Oesophageal atresia (OA) is a rare congenital anomaly in which there is an interruption of the oesophagus, with or without communication with the trachea. It is commonly associated with a tracheal–oesophageal fistula as depicted in Fig. 17.4, the most common type (85% of cases) being a proximal atresia with a distal fistula (Aumar et al., 2021). It has an incidence of 2.4 per 100,000. In 1941, Cameron Haight completed the first successful repair of OA and **tracheoesophageal fistula (TOF)** and, 70 years later, survival is now over 90%. In the majority of cases, OA is associated with a TOF, a fistula between the trachea and the oesophagus; however, it can be isolated. Associated

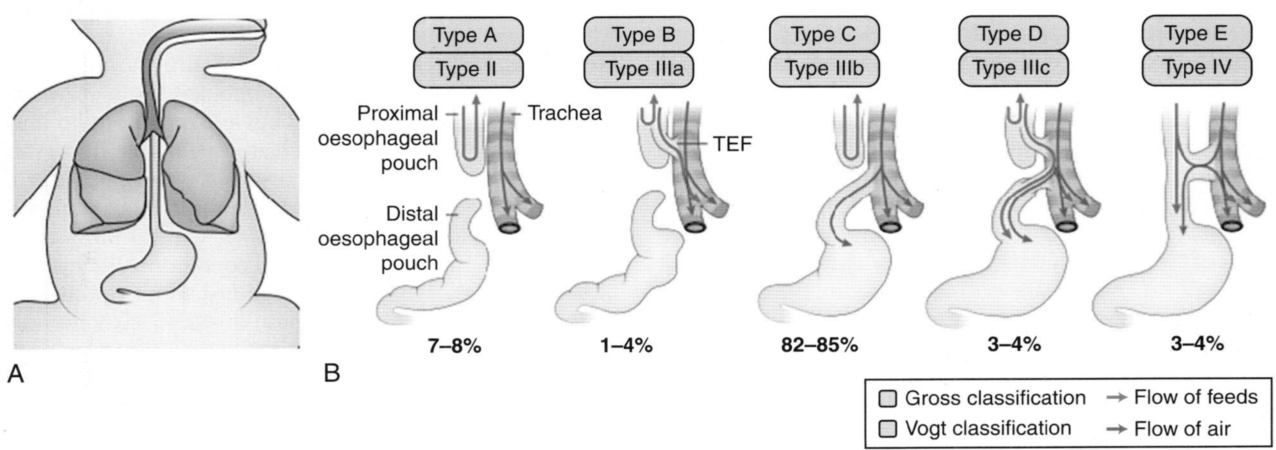

FIGURE 17.4 **Oesophageal atresia**

a Normal oesophageal anatomy, with the trachea and oesophagus anatomically distinct. **b** Oesophageal atresia (EA) is classified as follows: EA without trachea-oesophageal fistula (TEF), (Gross type A, Vogt type II), EA with proximal TEF (Gross type B, Vogt type IIIa), EA with distal TEF (Gross type C, Vogt type IIIb), EA with distal and proximal TEF (Gross type D, Vogt type IIIc) and TEF without EA (Gross type E, Vogt type IV). The frequency of each subtype is indicated by the percentages below each one.

Source: van Lennep et al. (2019).

anomalies including chromosomal anomalies are found in up to 60% of affected neonates, and it is also included as part of the **VACTERL association** (**V**ertebral anomalies, **A**norectal, **C**ardiac defects **T**racheo**e**sophageal, **R**enal and **L**imb anomalies) (Aumar et al., 2021; Haight, 1944). Symptoms occur when saliva and oral feeds cannot pass through to the oesophagus and, in the case of the proximal TOF, reach the lungs, and include excessive bubbly oral secretions and respiratory distress during the first feed.

Oesophageal atresia is not normally a surgical emergency. Preoperative management is aimed at stabilising the neonate, confirming the diagnosis, identifying other anomalies and preparing for surgery. Preoperatively, neonates should be nil by mouth, with a Replogle tube inserted to allow for continuous aspiration of the blind oesophageal pouch, thereby reducing the risk of aspiration pneumonia. A Replogle tube is a double-lumen tube that is inserted through the nostril and into the blind-ending oesophageal pouch to drain the excess build-up of saliva by continuous suction. The second lumen allows the tube to be flushed, reducing the risk of blockage and the accumulation of thick, viscous secretions. Nursing the neonate with the head of the cot elevated by 30–40 degrees also reduces the risk of aspiration pneumonia. The use of mechanical ventilation should be avoided whenever possible; however, if it is required, care should be taken to use the lowest pressures possible to avoid preferential ventilation of the fistula leading to over-distension of the stomach and subsequent perforation (Thompson et al., 2019). Preoperative management also includes an echocardiogram and chest and abdominal radiographs, routine preoperative bloods and bloods for genetic analysis. Postoperatively the neonate should be screened for associated anomalies (Brosens et al., 2021).

A primary repair of OA and TOF requires a surgical incision, ligation and division of the TOF, and an end-to-end anastomosis of the upper and lower ends of oesophagus is performed. There is an increasing trend for a thoracoscopic approach for this operation. If a staged repair is required (i.e. if the gap is too wide between the upper and lower end of the oesophagus) then the fistula is ligated and a gastrostomy inserted to allow for gastric decompression and feeding. Continuous drainage of the oesophageal pouch continues with the use of a Replogle tube. A delayed primary repair will then occur within the next few weeks. If the length of the gap between the two ends of the oesophagus is too large for a repair, a number of different techniques are available to restore oesophageal continuity, including using a 'gastric tube' or a colonic interposition. The preferred technique in long-gap cases is to wait until the oesophageal pouches grow until they are close enough for repair (van Lennep et al., 2019). Three early postoperative complications are an anastomotic leak, stricture and recurrent TOF (van Lennep et al., 2019). Other complications include gastro-oesophageal reflux and chylothorax. See Chapter 12 for more information about these conditions. Outcomes for children with OA in early childhood include dysphagia (in 35% of children at age 6), anastomotic strictures (8–60%) and gastro-oesophageal reflux (26–70%) (Aumar et al., 2021). Children are also at risk for cognitive and motor delay (IJsselstijn et al., 2016).

CONGENITAL ABNORMALITIES OF THE GASTROINTESTINAL SYSTEM

The most common congenital disorders of the gastrointestinal system involve the abdominal wall, namely **gastroschisis** and **omphalocele**. The incidence of gastroschisis is rising, and it now affects 3–4 out of every 10,000 infants (Allin et al., 2021).

FAMILY-CENTRED CARE 17.1

Identification of an abdominal wall defect most often occurs during pregnancy through routine morphological ultrasound. Hence, parents should be counselled about the prognosis and management well before the birth. The role of the neonatal nurse/midwife is therefore to educate parents on basic information regarding the environment, equipment, treatment, prognosis and process of recovery for their neonate. It is important that such information is realistic and presented in a supportive and caring manner. If a novice neonatal nurse/midwife does not feel adequately prepared to provide education for families of neonates with significant abdominal wall defects, it would be appropriate to seek advice and assistance from a more-expert neonatal nurse/midwife (Jones, 2019).

Gastroschisis

Gastroschisis (and omphalocele) are two of the most prevalent congenital abdominal wall abnormalities (Bielicki et al., 2021). Gastroschisis is a full-thickness abdominal wall defect where the intestines protrude from the abdomen without a protective barrier shielding the umbilical cord (Stephenson et al., 2021). During fetal development, the abdominal wall fails to seal properly, and the intestines protrude via this abdominal wall opening. Amniotic fluid exposes prolapsed organs and bowel loops in utero and the organs are exposed to the environment after birth. The stomach, intestine, liver, biliary system, pancreas, spleen, kidneys, ureters and suprarenal glands can all herniate along with the gut (Fig. 17.5).

Gastroschisis is not a hereditary condition. Anticipatory ultrasonography at the end of the first trimester or high maternal serum alpha fetoprotein level (Stephenson et al., 2021) can detect gastroschisis. In the prenatal period, serial ultrasonography should be conducted to detect gut and stomach dilation, thickness or oedema (Stephenson et al., 2021). The risk of preterm birth must be evaluated, and most centres deliver at 37 weeks' gestation (Bielicki et al., 2021). No evidence exists to justify caesarean birth over vaginal birth (Bielicki et al., 2021).

The neonate should be born in a tertiary hospital where experienced staff can provide resuscitation and stabilisation (Anyanwu et al., 2020). A doughnut-shaped

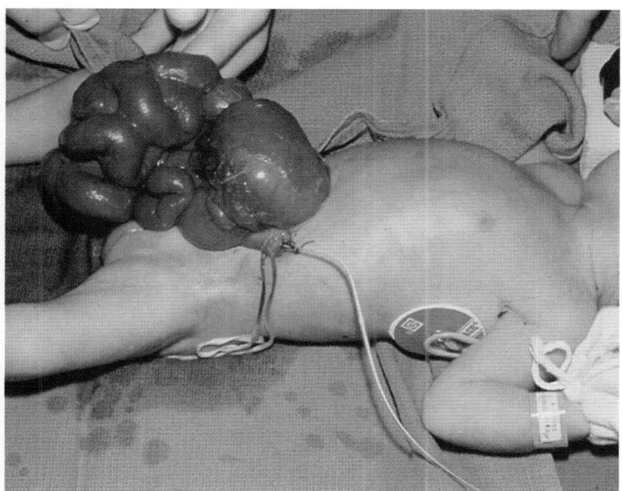

FIGURE 17.5 **Gastroschisis**

Source: Courtesy Albert E. Chudley, MD, FRCPC, FCCMG, Medical Director, Program in Genetics and Metabolism, Professor, Department of Paediatrics and Child Health, Department of Biochemistry and Medical Genetics, University of Manitoba.

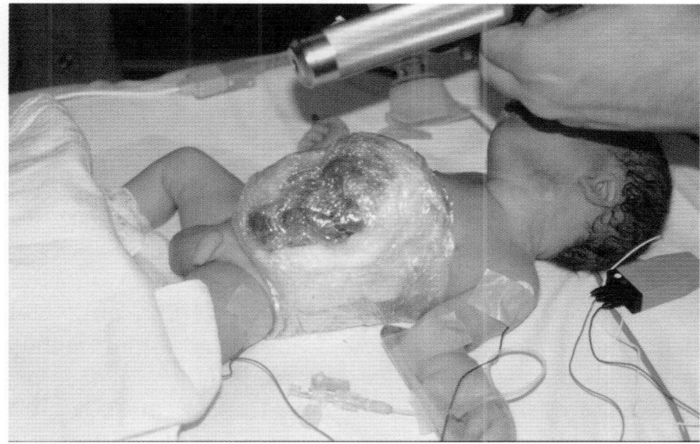

FIGURE 17.6 **Gastroschisis – neonate with cling wrap doughnut and cling film wrap around the abdomen**

Source: From https://www.safercare.vic.gov.au/clinical-guidance/neonatal/gastroschisis-in-neonates (accessed on 27 June 2022).

roll is made from a cloth nappy covered in transparent and latex-free cling wrap. A large piece of cling film is also slid under the neonate's buttocks and back. Once the cardiorespiratory stability of the neonate is managed as per usual practice, any obvious twists in the bowel and pedicle are corrected (Bhat et al., 2020), and it is supported in place in the doughnut roll in the centre of the abdomen wall. The cling wrap under the neonate is then gently wrapped around the abdomen and exposed organs, ensuring that no bowel is exposed to the air (Vic Health, 2022) to protect it from fluid and heat losses (Fig. 17.6). The exposed bowel should be handled with sterile latex-free gloves and great care, as it is susceptible to atresia and infarction caused by over-handling and malrotation. A wide-bore NG tube (Replogle) is inserted to aspirate the stomach and left in situ on free drainage to decompress the stomach and avoid distension of the gastrointestinal tract (Bhat et al., 2020). Although fluids are administered via either a peripherally inserted central catheter and/or a peripheral intravenous line to replace the high fluid losses, Bhat et al. (2020) warn against intensive fluid resuscitation because it raises the risk of adverse outcomes. Baseline laboratory results include a complete blood count, blood cultures and blood glucose levels to evaluate for infection and monitor blood glucose levels (Ferguson, 2017). Broad-spectrum antibiotics are commenced, and nursing/midwifery care related to thermoregulation, continuous pulse oximetry and cardiorespiratory monitoring, along with comfort measures, will support the neonate in the preoperative period. While the neonate is nil by mouth, total parenteral nutrition will support their nutritional requirements (Ferguson, 2017).

Once the neonate is stable, surgery to restore the bowel to the abdominal cavity is planned (Bischoff, 2021). When the abnormality is minor, the bowel is returned to the abdominal cavity in a primary one-step repair under general anaesthesia within a day of birth. If the abnormality is too large for a primary repair, a staged closure without anaesthesia is performed over several days to weeks, by suspending the bowel in a silastic silo (Allin et al., 2021). This permits gravity and daily gentle manual decompression by the surgeon to gradually reduce the size of the intestines, and slowly return them to the abdominal cavity. After the bowel is returned to the abdomen, the skin and muscle are closed under general anaesthesia (Dekonenko & Fraser, 2020). The least common form of closure is the sutureless abdominal wall closure method, where the viscera are reduced at the bedside without anaesthetic and the fascia left open to allow the defect to contract circumferentially. This procedure avoids intubation and anaesthesia, leads to less ventilator use/time, less antibiotics use, is more cost effective and is more cosmetically pleasing (Dekonenko & Fraser, 2020; Dekonenko et al., 2021).

In the postoperative period, the infant will most likely be supported by mechanical ventilation and require antibiotics, sedation and analgesia. Abdominal compartment syndrome due to increased intra-abdominal pressure can occur after primary closure and compromise respiratory function and renal output. Total parenteral nourishment, accurate fluid balance records and continuous NG free drainage with replacement of NGT losses will continue for 1–2 weeks until enteral feeds can be slowly introduced (Bhat et al., 2020). Breast milk is slowly introduced and advanced once NG drainage has reduced and bowel function has returned (Bhat et al., 2020). While early initiation of trophic feeds can improve peristalsis and reduce bacterial growth, feeding intolerance is common owing to intestinal dysmotility (Bhat et al., 2020).

Outcomes for neonates with gastroschisis largely depend on the condition of bowel at birth, with a mortality rate for infants with a simple gastroschisis at 3.4%, and for those with a complex gastroschisis at 9.3% (Bhat et al., 2020). Bowel obstruction occurs in about 25% of neonates with a simple gastroschisis and in over 70% of neonates with a complex gastroschisis. Preterm and out-born infants, sepsis, intestinal disease (such as ischaemia or perforation) and hypothermia all increase mortality (Anyanwu et al., 2020). Intestinal dysmotility in the postoperative period increases the risks of feeding intolerance, necrotising enterocolitis, stricture and short gut syndrome.

CLINICAL PRACTICE 17.1

In view of the fact that **abdominal wall defects (AWDs)** are uncommon, neonatal nurses/midwives may not have enough exposure to them to feel confident with their immediate care at birth. Bischoff (2021) developed simulation scenarios and created mannequins with simulated gastroschisis and omphalocele to allow nurses/midwives to develop and practise stabilisation techniques. The simulation sessions were held in the birthing unit and lasted 90 minutes, including the debrief. All nurses/midwives felt empowered after the training and subsequently cared for three infants with AWD whose outcomes were favourable.

Nursing/midwifery actions at birth should aim to:

1. reduce evaporative heat and fluid loss from the exposed intestine by covering with cling wrap and placing the lower half of the infant in a plastic bag
2. prevent kinking of the mesenteric vessels by positioning the infant on their side, in the right lateral decubitus position (Bhat et al., 2020)
3. enable gastric decompression to avoid distension by insertion of a large-bore gastric tube
4. obtain intravenous access to maintain hydration and to administer antibiotics and sedation
5. obtain baseline blood tests and monitor glucose level for homeostasis
6. prevent contamination of the exposed intestine
7. prepare for and/or transfer the neonate for surgical repair (Bielicki et al., 2021).

Omphalocele

An omphalocele (also known as an exomphalos) is a congenital abdominal wall defect that affects 3.38 out of every 10,000 infants (Hijkoop et al., 2018). Unlike gastroschisis, an omphalocele causes abdominal viscera herniation through the umbilical cord, which is protected by the peritoneum and amniotic membrane sac.

The pathophysiology is unknown; however, it is thought to be linked to inadequate closure of the ventral abdominal wall before the ninth week of pregnancy (Bielicki et al., 2021). This causes herniation of the abdominal viscera through the abdominal wall at the base of the umbilicus (Fig. 17.7), with peritoneum, Wharton's jelly and amnion covering the abnormality (Anyanwu et al., 2020). The abnormality ranges in size from 2 to 10 cm, and the sac may contain the omentum and some intestine if it is small, and more intestine, spleen, bladder and liver if it is large (more than 5 cm), also referred to as a giant omphalocele (Cubo et al., 2020).

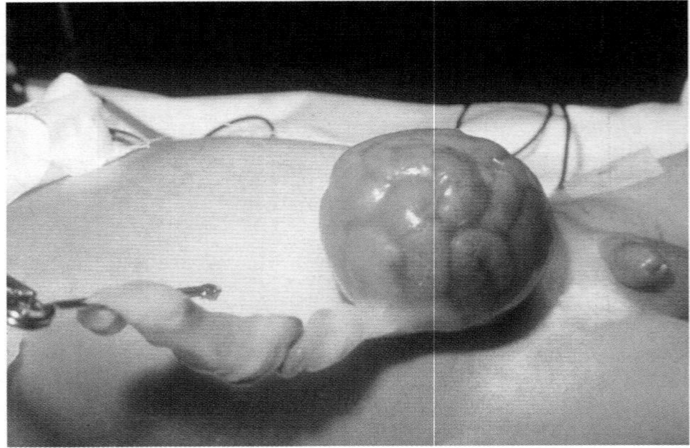

FIGURE 17.7 **Omphalocele**

Source: From Rodgers (2018).

An omphalocele is typically associated with chromosomal or structural abnormalities, with 50% of cases having trisomy 13, 14, 15, 18 or 21, and 30–50% having a cardiac anomaly (Anyanwu et al., 2020). Omphalocele, like gastroschisis, has no known environmental cause, yet it is linked to advanced maternal age, obesity, Afro-American ethnicity, poor maternal glycaemic management and multiple births (Bielicki et al., 2021).

Prenatal ultrasound deems an umbilical herniation physiological unless it is equivalent to or greater than the size of the abdomen. It is consequently risky to diagnose omphalocele in the first trimester. However, 20-week morphological scans are diagnostic. Detailed ultrasonography, karyotyping, DNA screening and fetal echography are used to detect additional abnormalities related to omphalocele (Bielicki et al., 2021).

Neonates should be birthed in a tertiary centre and be attended by a multidisciplinary team. Vaginal birthing is safe for minor abnormalities; however, caesarean birthing is indicated for major deformities or where the liver is herniated (Bielicki et al., 2021). The sac should be covered with clear plastic film or placed in a plastic bag, and the stomach decompressed with a Replogle/NG tube, as with infants born with gastroschisis (Anyanwu et al., 2020).

Primary closure of a minor omphalocele (less than 5 cm) occurs shortly after birth under general anaesthesia to restore the organs to the abdomen and close the abdominal wall opening (Bielicki et al., 2021). The abdominal and thoracic cavities are small and underdeveloped in giant omphaloceles. A phased closure is suggested in situations of pulmonary hypoplasia in order to avoid haemodynamic and respiratory problems (Bielicki et al., 2021). This method uses a silo, as with a gastroschisis. The return of normal bowel function can take from around 6 weeks to several months. When a newborn's respiratory system is compromised, ventilator support is required (Gallagher et al., 2021). Large omphaloceles can place a metabolic burden on the body, and poor nutrition increases the risk of sepsis.

The critical factor for survival with large omphaloceles is the size of the thoracic cavity and associated pulmonary hypoplasia with chronic respiratory failure. However, pulmonary growth and development does continue into childhood, which encourages optimism regarding the ultimate prognosis of these neonates. Complications often seen after omphalocele repair include gastroesophageal reflux, failure to thrive and chronic lung disease (Bielicki et al., 2021). Survival rates are influenced by other structural and chromosomal abnormalities, and was 75% at 2 years of age in a study by Hijkoop et al. (2018).

CASE STUDY

17.1

An 18-year-old Caucasian gravida 1 woman presented for a targeted anatomy ultrasound in the setting of an elevated maternal serum alpha fetoprotein (MSAFP) obtained from routine prenatal screening. An antenatal abdominal ultrasound revealed a full-thickness abdominal wall defect (AWD) to the right of the umbilical cord insertion, with herniation of abdominal contents. Free-floating loops of bowel were seen in the amniotic fluid without evidence of a covering membrane. The woman underwent serial ultrasounds to assess fetal growth and wellbeing. At 38 weeks' gestation, fetal testing revealed a biophysical profile (BPP) that was abnormal. The woman was subsequently admitted for induction of labour. She proceeded to have an uncomplicated vaginal birth. At birth, the neonate's exposed intestine was wrapped in plastic. The neonate was transferred to the neonatal intensive care unit where she underwent a successful reduction of abnormality.

1. Outline the differences between a gastroschisis and an omphalocele.
2. What is the most likely diagnosis for this neonate? Why?
3. What are the associated problems that this neonate may have?
4. What postnatal work-up may be done prior to surgical intervention?
5. What is the management of gastroschisis and omphalocele?

Indirect inguinal hernia

An **indirect inguinal hernia** is a congenital type of inguinal hernia. It is a ventral hernia that results when an intra-abdominal structure protrudes through an abnormality in the inguinal canal (Hammoud & Gerken, 2021).

Gonads descend from the urogenital ridge, in the upper abdomen near the developing kidneys, to the internal ring at 12 weeks' gestation. The processus vaginalis then develops from the peritoneal lining. At 24–28 weeks' gestation, descent of the gonads continues through the inguinal canal and by 32–36 weeks' gestation the testes come to rest in the scrotum. Gradual obliteration of the processus vaginalis then occurs, which subsequently becomes the tunica vaginalis. Incomplete obliteration of the processus vaginalis is the underlying feature of inguinal hernia and hydrocele (Hammoud & Gerken, 2021).

The incidence of inguinal hernia in males is nearly 10 times than in females, and it is more common in preterm neonates. Preterm neonates under 32 weeks' gestation have a 13% incidence, with a 30% incidence in neonates weighing less than 1000 g. Inguinal hernias are more common on the right side (75%), primarily because of the later descent of the right testicle. Nearly one-third of cases present before 6 months of age, and bilateral herniation occurs in 15–20% of cases (Hammoud & Gerken, 2021).

Clinical assessment and diagnosis of inguinal hernia includes:

- examination of the groin assessing for intermittent bulges in the groin, scrotum or labia made worse by activities that increase intra-abdominal pressure (crying or straining)
- in males, examination of the testicles and scrotum, with the absence of a testicle suggestive of undescended or retractile testicle
- in females, the ovary is the most common structure to be palpated in a hernia.

Incarcerated hernia involves the following:

- if the hernia is complicated by incarceration (cannot be returned by manipulation), presentation will include pain, abdominal distension and emesis
- an incarcerated hernia becomes a surgical emergency to prevent bowel strangulation (Hammoud & Gerken, 2021).

Congenital hypertrophic pyloric stenosis

Hypertrophic pyloric stenosis is one of the common surgical conditions in early infancy (Ramji & Joshi, 2021), and the disorder is titled **congenital hypertrophic pyloric stenosis (CHPS)** when genetic factors are involved in the aetiology (Jawade et al., 2017). CHPS causes severe pyloric canal stenosis due to the thickening of the smooth muscle of the pylorus. Gastric emptying is significantly reduced, which usually results in projectile vomiting after a feeding. The condition is more prevalent in male infants and clinical manifestations generally do not appear until 3–8 weeks after birth. Diagnosis is confirmed by palpating a pyloric mass in the right upper quadrant (RUQ) during a test feeding (Netter, 2019).

Typically, infants with CHPS are hungry after vomiting and demand to be fed again. As the vomiting persists, a gradual loss of fluid, hydrogen ions and chloride results in hypochloraemic metabolic alkalosis. Because of increased awareness of CHPS, there are fewer occurrences of infants with chronic malnutrition and severe dehydration as these infants are identified sooner.

The most common clinical association with CHPS is hyperbilirubinemia, commonly known as icteropyloric syndrome. Unconjugated hyperbilirubinemia is more common than conjugated hyperbilirubinemia and usually resolves with surgical repair of the pyloric stenosis. It may be connected with a lower level of glucuronyl transferase, as seen in approximately 5% of affected babies; mutations in the bilirubin uridine diphosphate glucuronosyltransferase gene (*UGT1A1*) have also been implicated. If conjugated hyperbilirubinemia is present, alternative aetiologies must be investigated (Kliegman et al., 2020). For further information about conjugated hyperbilirubinaemia, see Chapter 11.

Small bowel atresia

Intestinal atresia and stenosis refers to the congenital occlusion or narrowing of the lumen of any section of the small intestine, including the pylorus, duodenum, jejunum or ileum. The reported incidence of intestinal atresia ranges from 1.3 to 3.5 per 10,000 live births, of which about 20% are associated with a chromosomal abnormality, typically trisomy 21 (Wesson, 2021).

The most common atretic problem is **duodenal atresia/stenosis**; 30% of neonates with duodenal atresia also have other anomalies, primarily trisomy 21. A classic sign of duodenal atresia is the 'double bubble' where there is dilated bowel and fluid in the stomach and part of the duodenum, but no fluid beyond that point on the radiograph. Dilated bowel prior to the blockage can also be detected on antenatal ultrasound, and small bowel atresia is often associated with polyhydramnios.

Abdominal distension is a common feature of intestinal obstruction, and may cause splinting of the diaphragm, compromise respiratory function and increase the risk of aspiration. Vomiting, usually bilious, most often occurs in the first 24–48 hours (Wesson, 2021). Feeds are withheld in these neonates, and a large-bore NG tube should be inserted, left on free drainage and aspirated hourly to decompress the stomach. Fluid and electrolyte balance is maintained with intravenous fluids. Surgical repair involves major abdominal surgery, with resection of the atresia, end-to-end or side-to-side duodenoduodenostomy and commonly formation of a stoma. The prognosis is very good (Wesson, 2021). A classification of atresia is outlined in Fig. 17.8.

In type I, a membrane or web causes the obstruction; type II shows a blind-ending proximal loop connected by a fibrous cord; in type IIIA, the atresia ends blindly with no fibrous connecting with a mesenteric abnormality; type IIIB, 'apple peel-type' atresia, consists of a proximal jejunal atresia and the absence of the superior mesenteric artery; type IV has multiple-segment atresia (Okuyama, 2016).

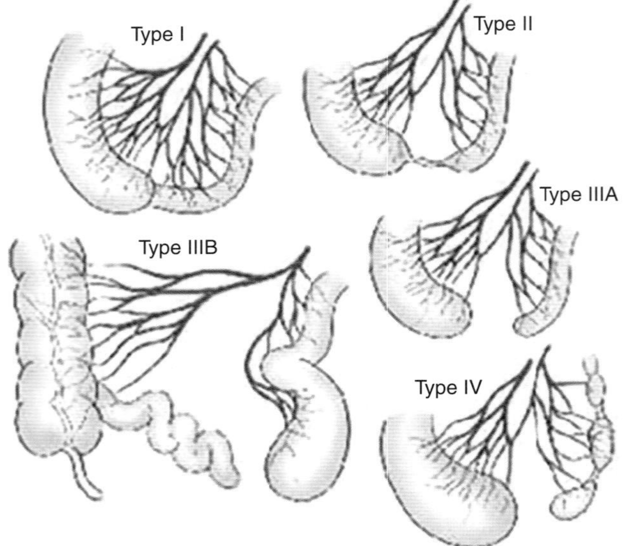

FIGURE 17.8 **Classification of atresia**

Source: From https://www.cincinnatichildrens.org/health/i/obstructions (accessed on 27 June 2022).

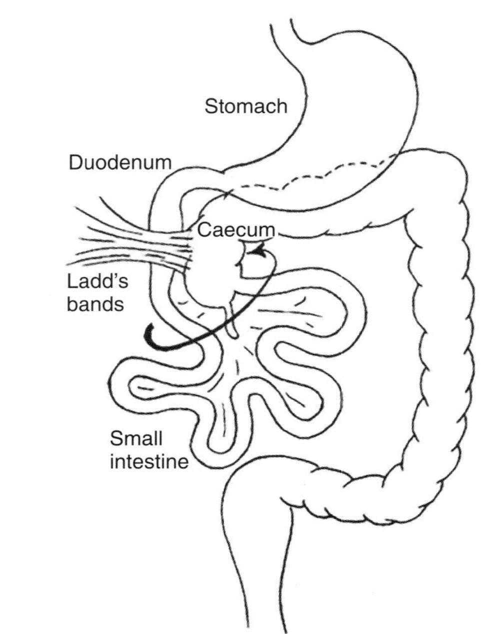

FIGURE 17.9 **Malrotation**

Source: From https://embryology.med.unsw.edu.au/embryology/images/0/03/Intestinal_malrotation.jpg (accessed on 27 June 2022).

Malrotation and volvulus

Malrotation occurs when the intestine does not rotate, or rotates incompletely, during fetal development, and can lead to a potentially fatal volvulus (Fig. 17.9). **Volvulus** comes from the Latin word 'volvere' and refers to when the bowel twists on itself, leading to disruption of the blood supply and obstruction. Bilious vomiting in the neonate is considered a sign of a surgical emergency until malrotation and volvulus can be excluded. Other symptoms include abdominal distension, abdominal tenderness and haemodynamic instability (Brandt, 2021). The incidence of malrotation has been reported as 1 in 500 live births, with symptomatic malrotation occurring in approximately 1 in 6000 live births (Brandt, 2021). Abdominal radiograph is not usually useful in the diagnosis of malrotation, with an upper gastrointestinal contrast study being the gold standard for diagnosis in infants (Brandt, 2021). Surgery usually involves the open Ladd procedure, where the bowel is untwisted into a position of non-rotation (small bowel on the right and colon on the left). Although the procedure can be performed laparoscopically, it is a controversial approach in neonates owing to the high risk of volvulus after the surgery (Brandt, 2021).

Hirschsprung disease

Hirschsprung disease (also known as congenital aganglionic megacolon) is a disorder in which ganglion cells fail to develop in a portion of the large intestine during fetal development. In the majority of cases (80%) the ganglion cells are absent in the sigmoid portion or in the rectum; however, the condition can affect the entire large intestine and rectum (5%) (Fig. 17.10). There is a higher incidence of Hirschsprung disease in females, and it is also associated with genetic syndromes such as trisomy 21. The prevalence has recently been reported as approximately 1 per 5000 births (Wesson & Lopez, 2021).

Clinically, neonates present with failure to pass meconium within 48 hours of birth, abdominal distension, bilious vomiting and signs of a bowel obstruction. Investigations include abdominal radiographs and contrast studies; however, a suction rectal biopsy is the gold standard for diagnosis, confirming the absence of ganglia on the sample, and the neonate will require rectal washouts until surgery. Surgery is either open or laparoscopic, with the goal to resect the affected segment and re-anastomose the two healthy segments. Most centres now perform a transanal 'pull-through' procedure in one stage, laparoscopically assisted (Wesson & Lopez, 2021). If a two-stage procedure is used, an interim colostomy is formed until the definitive pull-through. Long-term multidisciplinary follow-up is required, as these children are at risk of constipation, further obstruction, faecal incontinence and enterocolitis (Wesson & Lopez, 2021).

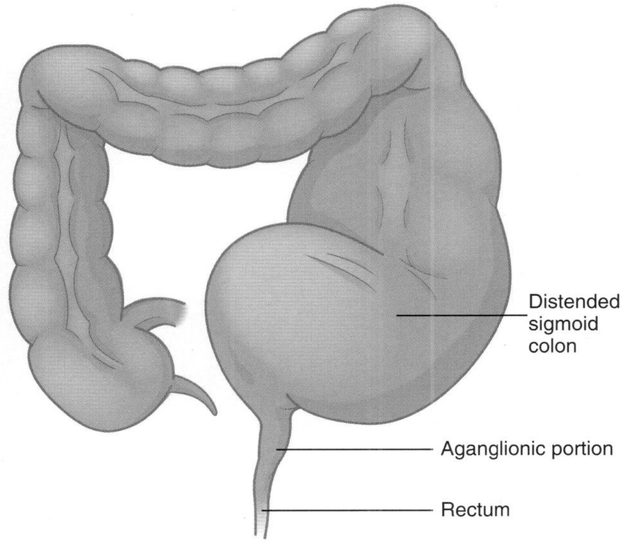

FIGURE 17.10 **Hirschsprung disease**
Source: From Sables-Baus and Fidanza (2020).

Meconium ileus/plug

Meconium ileus occurs in 10–20% of babies with cystic fibrosis. Mutations in the gene encoding the cystic fibrosis transmembrane conductance regulator (CFTR) are the cause of cystic fibrosis. A secondary obstruction of the luminal lumen lining these cells – mucus-secreting glands of the intestinal wall and exocrine pancreatic ductal cells – results in dehydration and hyperviscosity (Dingeldein, 2020).

The hyperviscosity of mucosal cell secretion causes thick, tar-like meconium to develop, which becomes inspissated further down the small bowel lumen, culminating in small, dense meconium pellets and a microcolon. Small intestinal blockage is usually present at birth and can be detected via antenatal ultrasound. Postnatal bowel blockage symptoms include abdominal distension, inability to defecate and bilious vomiting. Abdominal examination often reveals pliant, dough-like bowel loops. Air bubbles in the meconium can cause granular, soap bubble-like abdominal radiographs. This clinical picture depicts uncomplicated meconium ileus. This type of luminal bowel obstruction can lead to volvulus, necrosis and perforation, which is referred to as complex meconium ileus (Dingeldein, 2020).

If intestinal necrosis and perforation occur in utero, a pseudocyst may emerge and be palpable at birth. In addition to dilated bowel loops, abdominal radiography may reveal a huge mass of calcified material (pseudocyst) or calcifications spread throughout the peritoneal cavity (meconium peritonitis). There may be ascites, free air, or granular, soap bubble-like meconium generated by air bubbles. This does not rule out meconium ileus. The microcolon is nearly always accompanied with little 'rabbit-pellet' meconium concretions detected proximally in contrast enema. Congenital hypothyroidism and meconium plug syndrome are among the differential diagnoses (Dingeldein, 2020).

Presenting symptoms include abdominal distension and failure to pass meconium, with or without vomiting (Sabharwal & Schwarzenberg, 2021). Treatment options for meconium ileus vary depending on the symptoms. Gastric decompression with a Replogle tube, correction of fluid and electrolyte balance and antibiotic treatment are always general management concepts.

Simple meconium ileus (MI) might be non-operative or surgical. Before attempting non-operative intervention, additional reasons of distal bowel blockage (volvulus, necrosis, perforation, pseudocyst or peritonitis) must be excluded. An enema of hyperosmolar solution (usually Gastrografin®) is given to reflux into the ileum. The hypertonic solution creates a concentration gradient across the intestinal wall, drawing fluid into the lumen, breaking down the meconium mass and promoting meconium passage (Dingeldein, 2020). Surgical procedures for cases of MI that do not clear with non-operative intervention include resection with ileostomy, simple enterotomy with lavage and double enterostomy. Close monitoring of growth and nutrition is needed for neonates with MI to avoid the long-term effects of poor growth (Sabharwal & Schwarzenberg, 2021).

ANORECTAL MALFORMATIONS

Anorectal malformations are a rare group of conditions which affect the rectum and anus, with an incidence of around 1–2 in 5000 live births. They range from mild to severe, and may have many associated anomalies including malformations of the genitourinary tract and the spine (Fig. 17.11). Children and adults with these conditions can also have lifelong psychological effects and long-term follow-up is essential.

Imperforate anus occurs in 1 in 5000 live births, with a 58% male predominance. Anorectal abnormalities range from simple anal stenosis to persistence of a cloaca. Normally the anal membrane ruptures between 8 and 9 weeks of gestation, but in imperforate anus the anal canal ends at the membrane (Ditzenberger, 2018). Imperforate anus with a fistula occurs between the distal colon and urethra in boys and the vaginal vestibule in girls. It divides the cloaca into the anterior urogenital sinus and the posterior anorectal canal by the sixth week of pregnancy.

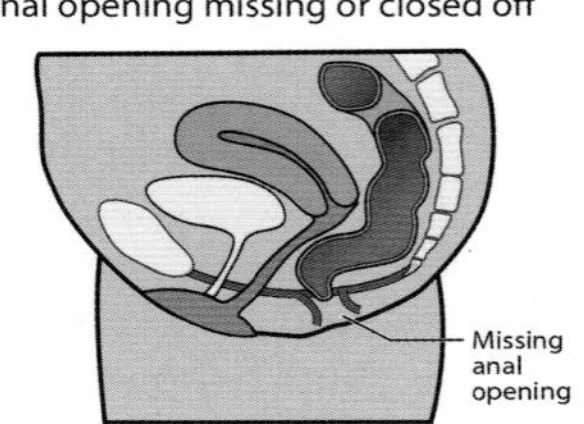

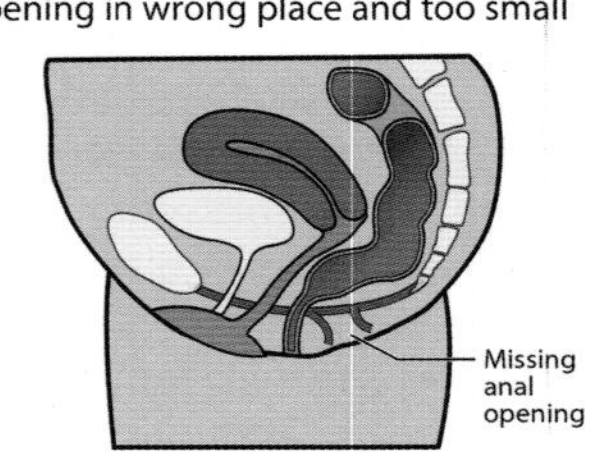

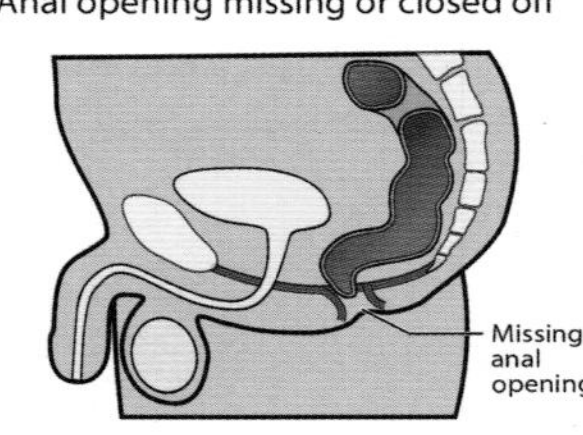

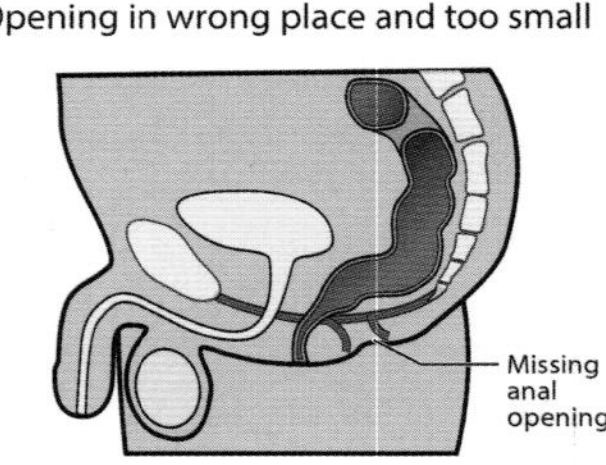

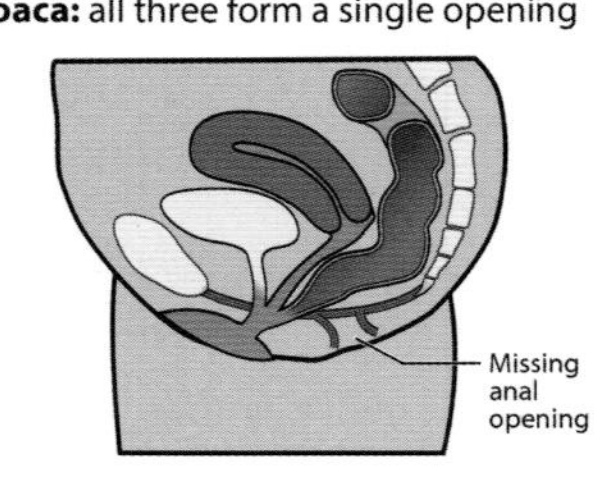

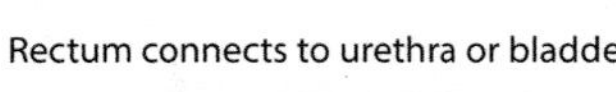

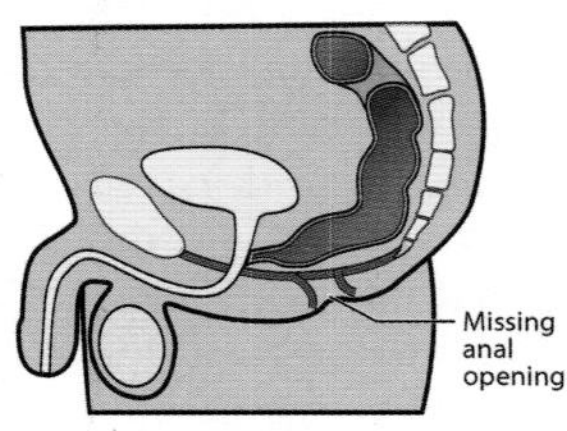

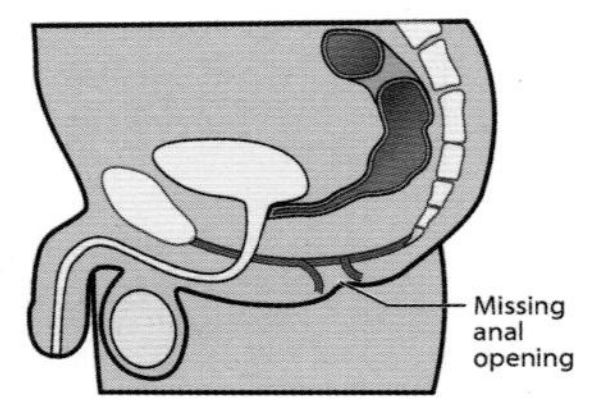

FIGURE 17.11 **Anorectal malformations**

Source: From http://pedsurg.ucsf.edu/media/6452442/anorectal-malformation-v4-all.gif.

This results in a fistula between the bowel and urinary tract (in boys) or vagina (in girls). An anal membrane or stenosis occurs when the anal membrane fails to resorb completely. Cloacal folds, which run from the anterior genital tubercle to the anus, are formed by the perineum. These folds fuse to form the perineal body. The external anal opening is anterior to the external sphincter when the cloacal membrane breaks down (i.e. anteriorly displaced anus) (Chung, 2022). The neonate with anal stenosis or imperforate anal membrane may have a normal-looking rectum and the condition may be detected only after failure to pass meconium (Bradshaw, 2021), highlighting the importance of the first physical examination by the neonatal nurse/midwife and documentation of the first meconium. Surgical repair depends on the level of the anorectal pouch; high pouches are treated with a colostomy and then a pull-through procedure at around 8 months of age, and an anoplasty can be performed on neonates with a low pouch (Wood & Levitt, 2020).

CONGENITAL ABNORMALITIES OF THE CARDIOVASCULAR SYSTEM

Congenital cardiac defects are structural heart or intrathoracic vascular abnormalities that are evident at birth and impact cardiac function. They are the most prevalent type of congenital abnormality and the major cause of congenital anomaly death. Other extracardiac anomalies, including renal agenesis, omphalocele, tracheoesophageal fistula and diaphragmatic hernia, are frequently associated with congenital cardiac defects. Most congenital cardiac defects have an unknown cause. The vast majority of malformations are assumed to be multifactorial, caused by a complex combination of genetic and environmental factors. Certain maternal variables have been linked to an increased risk of congenital cardiac defects. A parent or sibling with a history of congenital cardiac defects is a known risk factor. If one child has a congenital cardiac defect, it is very likely that other children will also have a congenital cardiac defect. See Chapter 10 for content regarding these congenital disorders.

CONGENITAL ABNORMALITIES OF THE ORAL AND CRANIOFACIAL REGIONS

Orofacial abnormalities are comprised of a number of distinct disorders. The oral, craniofacial and dental regions are among those most commonly affected by congenital malformations, which can affect up to 15% of newborns. It is possible that the discovery of a single craniofacial abnormality at birth will signal the presence of a complicated condition. Most of these syndromes have an occurrence rate ranging between 1 in 5600 and 1 in 100,000 individuals (Iannetti et al., 2018). Given the number of disorders, this chapter will describe cleft lip and/or palate only.

Cleft lip and/or palate

Cleft lip and/or palate are common congenital malformations defined by abnormalities and displaced orofacial soft tissue, muscle, bone and cartilage involving the soft palate, hard palate, lip and nasal sill. The incidence of orofacial cleft is 1 in 500–550 births (Tolarova et al., 2020). Orofacial abnormalities are classified into two types: cleft lip with or without palatal clefting, and cleft palate alone. Lip clefts can manifest as unilateral, bilateral or, in rare cases, midline abnormalities, and occur when medial and lateral nasal processes fail to fuse with the maxillary process before the seventh week of gestation (Ditzenberger, 2018). Cleft lip and palate are more prevalent than cleft palate alone, and they are less likely to be associated with a congenital condition.

Palate clefts can range from a malformation affecting only the posterior soft palate to a malformation including the entire length of the soft and hard palates. Occult submucous cleft may develop later in life with signs of velopharyngeal insufficiency (e.g. feeding problems, speech impairment, eustachian tube dysfunction) in the absence of any evident malformation in the palate.

Cleft lip and palate, as well as cleft palate alone, may be coupled with the existence of other serious congenital abnormalities. Different major congenital anomalies involving other organ systems can be found in up to 21% of individuals with orofacial clefting.

The majority of orofacial clefting is detected in the neonate through physical examination; around 25% of cleft lips with or without cleft palate are diagnosed antenatally through normal prenatal ultrasonography.

Basic anatomy misalignment, feeding challenges, dental problems, speech impairments, eustachian tube dysfunction and insufficient maxillofacial growth can all be concerns for neonates with orofacial clefting. A multidisciplinary team with competence in the treatment of neonates with cleft lip and/or palate is necessary to support the neonate and family. The ability to maintain airway patency and the newborn's ability to feed are the primary issues for infants with cleft palate with or without cleft lip. Aspiration is a risk because of the communication between the oral and nasal cavities. Most infants with cleft palate are unable to breastfeed because they cannot generate enough negative pressure to apply suction to the breast. Neonates with a unilateral cleft lip may be able to breastfeed when positioned such that the cleft is obstructed by the breast. Various squeezable bottles with special teats have been designed for neonates with clefts, as have palatal obturators. Feeding in an upright or seated position prevents leakage of milk to the nose and subsequent choking. Preventing aspiration and ear infections and gaining weight are important goals for neonates in the first few days and weeks of life (Ditzenberger, 2018; Tolarova et al., 2020).

The primary treatment is surgery to restore normal face morphology and feeding function, as well as to eliminate hearing and speech difficulties. Surgery for cleft lips is generally performed at 3 months of age, while cleft palates are repaired between 9 and 12 months. Orthodontic treatment may continue for many years (Tolarova et al., 2020). To monitor and manage any problems, long-term interdisciplinary care is required, including by speech therapists, orthodontists, dentists, plastic surgeons, nurse practitioners, paediatricians and genetic counsellors.

The occurrence of additional associated congenital malformations or syndromes affects the prognosis, which is mainly dependent on the type and degree of orofacial cleft. Surgery has a high success rate as the primary treatment for restoring normal face structure and feeding capacity, as well as reducing hearing and speech impairment (Dhar, 2020). Parents of infants with clefts are at increased risk of depression and stress, and early psychological support has been shown to reduce their stress scores at 4 months (Grollemund et al., 2020). In addition, parents who received a prenatal diagnosis are much better prepared to accept the waiting period until the first surgery.

CONGENITAL ABNORMALITIES OF THE NEUROLOGICAL SYSTEM

The majority of congenital CNS malformations are caused by errors in neural tube closure during fetal development. Though the cause of **neural tube defects (NTDs)** (Fig. 17.12) is unknown, they are thought to result from the interaction of many genes that can be impacted by fetal environment factors. Factors such as maternal anticonvulsant treatment (e.g. valproic acid or carbamazepine), methotrexate (a chemotherapeutic medicine), opiate use during the first trimester, maternal obesity and maternal diabetes have all been implicated. Excessive maternal body heat exposure during the early first trimester, severe febrile sickness and a lower socioeconomic status can all raise the chance of an NTD. Maternal folic acid shortage has a direct impact on neural tube closure failure. Folic acid supplementation (0.4 mg/day) is therefore recommended as a prophylactic measure for women of reproductive age; those with a history of NTDs should take 400 mg daily. Folic acid dosage should last at least until the first trimester of pregnancy (Prasad et al., 2021).

NTDs are among the most common congenital abnormalities worldwide; however, their frequency varies greatly. The global prevalence is projected to be 18.6 per 10,000 births (including stillbirths and elective terminations of pregnancy); NTDs occur in 5.5 per 10,000 live births in the Americas (Dukhovny & Wilkins-Haug, 2021). Because of increased folic acid intake before and during pregnancy, and its fortification in commonly consumed foods such as bread, flour and pasta, the incidence of NTDs has reduced over the last 20 years.

NTDs occur when there is disruption to the closure of the neural tube between 24 and 26 days of embryological life (Blackburn, 2018) and include anencephaly, encephalocele and myelomeningocele. A meningomyelocele sac contains spinal cord or nerve roots, meninges and cerebrospinal fluid (CSF) and, because of the impaired differentiation of nerve fibres, these neonates have a neurological deficit below the level of the sac (Blackburn, 2018). Abnormalities can be either open, where there is exposure of the spinal cord and brain, or closed, where the skin covers the abnormality (see Fig. 17.12). In some centres, in utero surgical repair is

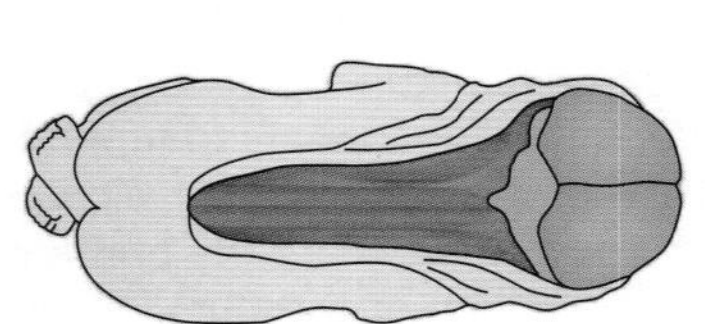

Craniorachischisis
Completely open brain and spinal cord

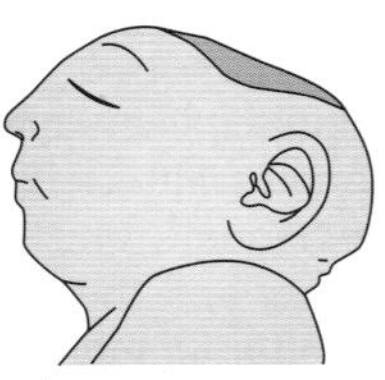

Anencephaly
Open brain and lack of skull vault

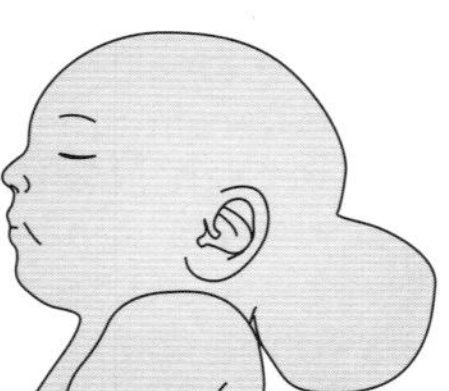

Encephalocele
Herniation of the meninges (and brain)

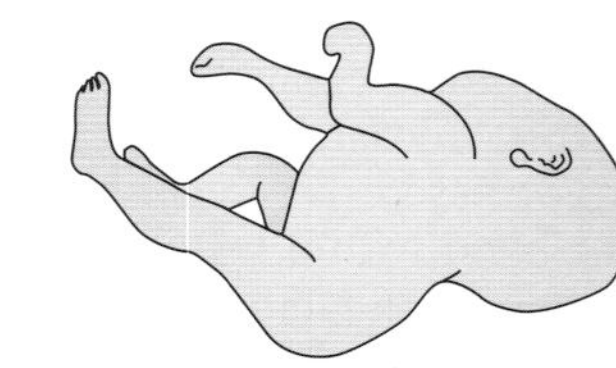

Iniencephaly
Occipital skull and spine defects with extreme retroflexion of the head

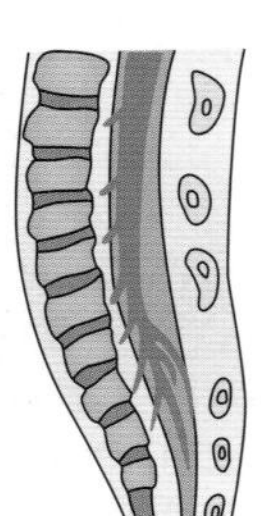

Spina bifida occulta
Closed asymptomatic NTD in which some of the vertebrae are not completely closed

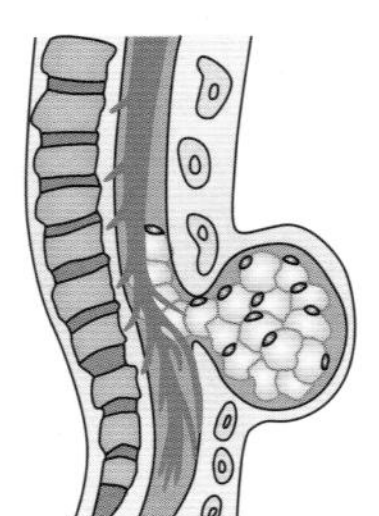

Closed spinal dysraphism
Deficiency of at least two vertebral arches, here covered with a lipoma

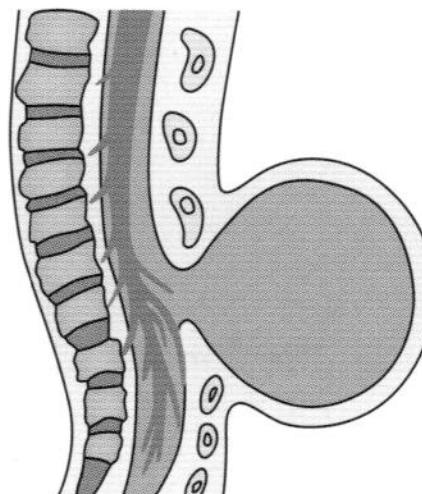

Meningocele
Protrusion of the meninges (filled with CSF) through a defect in the skull or spine

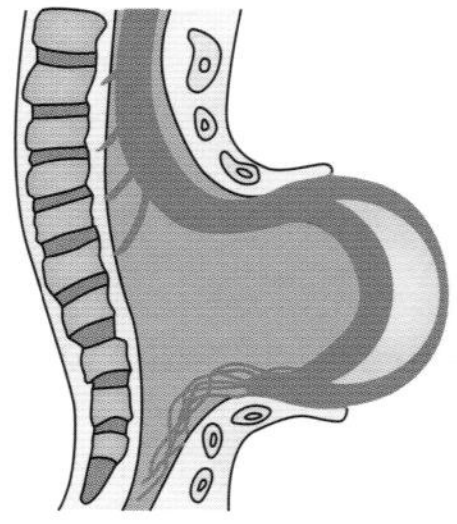

Myelomeningocele
Open spinal cord (with a meningeal cyst)

FIGURE 17.12 **Neural tube defects**

Source: Copp et al. (2015). Spina bifida. Nature Reviews Disease Primers, 1, 15007. 10.1038. <https://www.nature.com/ articles/ nrdp20157>. @ Macmillan Publishers Ltd.

performed to arrest the leakage of spinal fluid, to prevent or reverse herniation of the hindbrain, and to reduce the development of hydrocephalus and the need for shunting postnatally, although this poses considerable risk to both the mother and the fetus (Bowman, 2021). There is no evidence to support either vaginal or caesarean delivery for neonates with myelomeningocele. At the delivery, non-latex gloves should be worn to reduce the risk of latex sensitisation, and the defect should be covered with a transparent, latex-free cling wrap to prevent heat loss. The neonate is then maintained in the prone or lateral recumbent position with intravenous therapy initiated, feeds withheld and antibiotics commenced (Ellenbogen, 2019). A thorough physical examination and then head ultrasound and MRI will aid understanding of the extent of the lesion before surgery to replace the neural placode in the spinal cord (Ellenbogen, 2019). Hydrocephalus is common after surgery, and active surveillance of head circumference and serial neuroimaging will determine whether a ventriculoperitoneal shunt is needed. Outcomes range from normal intelligence to learning disabilities, seizures, neurogenic bladder, faecal incontinence, pressure ulcers and scoliosis (Bowman, 2021).

Encephalocele

An **encephalocele** occurs as a result of small defects in the skull through which meninges and/or brain tissue herniate. Depending upon severity, the encephalocele is divided into three types: meningocele, meningoencephalocele and meningohydroencephalocele (Singh, 2020, p. 105). The prevalence of encephalocele worldwide is 0.8–4 per 10,000 live births (Nagy & Saleh, 2021). The encephalocele may be fully covered by skin, or thin, malformed meningeal membranes may be revealed. Hydrocephalus arises when the ventricular system is also ruptured into the encephalocele sac. Infection spreads quickly when CSF leaks. Some encephaloceles, particularly those in the occipital midline, can grow to the size of the infant's head. Although nasopharyngeal encephaloceles are uncommon, they can cause meningitis owing to CSF leakage through the nose. Visceral organ malformations frequently coincide with encephaloceles and other congenital abnormalities of the eyes and face; cleft palate and polydactyly are also common. The brain as a whole may be significantly hypoplastic.

The majority of encephaloceles are parietal or occipital in nature and contain supratentorial or cerebellar tissue, or both. Frontal encephaloceles are less common in North America and Europe, but they are the most common type in Thailand, Vietnam and neighbouring countries. They frequently contain olfactory tissue. Encephaloceles caused by Agent Orange (a pesticide containing the herbicides 2,4-dichlorophenoxyacetic acid (2,4-D) and 2,4,5-trichlorophenoxyacetic acid (2,4,5-T)) have been documented in Cambodia.

Frontal and nasal encephaloceles protrude via bony foramina that ordinarily close in the fetus: the fonticulus frontalis for frontal (forehead midline) encephaloceles and the foramen cecum for intranasal encephaloceles. Clinically, nasal encephaloceles and nasal polyps can be mistaken, and CSF leak in the nose can be misdiagnosed with benign nasal secretions. Because of deficient prosencephalic neural crest tissue, which migrates from the dorsal section of the lamina terminalis as a vertical sheet of cells in the frontal midline, both of these foramina fail to close (Tomita & Ogiwara, 2021). Outcomes for neonates with encephalocele are poor, and most children suffer intellectual impairment, seizures, ataxia and visual disturbances (Nagy & Saleh, 2021).

Congenital hydrocephaly

Infancy is the most common age group for the onset of **hydrocephaly**. Hydrocephalus is a disorder where excessive amounts of CSF build up in the cerebral ventricles and/or the subarachnoid spaces, causing dilation of the ventricles and raised intracranial pressure (Haridas & Tomita, 2020), and is a common symptom of a variety of congenital and acquired neurological conditions. The majority of children with a hydrocephalus are diagnosed at or shortly after birth. Obstructive (non-communicating) hydrocephalus is the most common and occurs when there is a structural blockage to the flow of CSF in the ventricles, whereas communicating hydrocephalus occurs when CSF accumulates because its absorption is impaired in the subarachnoid spaces (Haridas & Tomita, 2020). Post-haemorrhagic hydrocephalus occurs commonly in preterm infants with intraventricular haemorrhage, and can be obstructive, communicating, or both (Haridas & Tomita, 2020). Neonates with hydrocephalus present with a large head, widened sutures, bulging fontanelles, vomiting, lethargy or irritability and 'sun-setting' eyes (Ditzenberger, 2018, p. 637). Temporary measures to control hydrocephaly include acetazolamide, frusemide and serial lumbar punctures, whereas the usual surgical treatment to divert the CSF in neonates is a ventriculoperitoneal (VP) shunt (Haridas & Tomita, 2020). Mortality is high in untreated hydrocephalus. Epilepsy rates were reported to be 32% in children treated with a VP shunt, and seizures are associated with poor cognitive outcome. Motor deficits are common, as are visual and auditory defects. Adverse neurodevelopmental outcomes are experienced by extremely low birthweight infants who were shunted for hydrocephalus after an intraventricular haemorrhage (Haridas & Tomita, 2020).

Microcephaly

Microcephaly is defined as a skull that is disproportionately small for the fetal age and body size. It is difficult to define microcephaly precisely, but, in general, it is diagnosed when the head circumference, measured across the occipitofrontal circumference, is fewer than three standard deviations below the predicted mean and intrauterine growth restriction (IUGR) has been ruled out. It has been recommended that two standard deviations be used, although this would encompass too many otherwise normal individuals (Boom, 2020). The prevalence of microcephaly varies around the world: 0.2 in 1000 live births in Europe and 0.87 in 1000 live births in the US (Shen et al., 2021). The diagnosis implies that brain development has stalled (micrencephaly). The aetiology is complex and can be linked to a wide range of prenatal causes, including genetic factors, environmental issues, asphyxia, infections (e.g. Zika virus), maternal conditions (e.g. phenylketonuria), drugs (e.g. fetal alcohol syndrome), various syndromes (e.g. Smith–Lemli–Opitz, Cornelia de Lange) and radiation exposure. Pathological examination may reveal that the brain is small but normal in appearance, or that it has a variety of findings, such as simplified gyri, porencephaly and a missing corpus callosum. It is common to have both CNS and non-CNS problems. Brain abnormalities, an abnormal head-to-abdomen circumference ratio, a sloping forehead and a reduced frontal lobe size are among the other findings (Toi & Levine, 2018). After a careful history and physical examination, investigations may include neuroimaging (MRI), genetic testing, TORCH (**TO**xoplasmosis, **R**ubella, **C**ytomegalovirus, **H**erpes simplex and HIV) screening and evaluation for metabolic disorders. The severity of the microcephaly generally indicates the level of cognitive impairment (Boom, 2020).

Neural tube defects (see Fig. 17.12)

Anencephaly

The cranial section of the neural tube fails to close in this condition, resulting in exencephaly (with a large amount of protruding brain tissue and absence of calvarium). As a result, the neural tissue is exposed to a destructive intra-amniotic environment, transforming exencephaly into **anencephaly** (Singh, 2020). Anencephaly identified during early pregnancy may result in a legal termination of the pregnancy because the condition is incompatible with survival. The vast majority of anencephalic neonates die within the first 24 hours of life. Surgical intervention is not advised (Chubarova, 2019).

Spina bifida occulta

Spina bifida occulta is a common abnormality characterised by a midline lesion of the vertebral bodies with no spinal cord or meningeal protrusion. The majority of cases are asymptomatic and have no neurological symptoms, and the condition is usually of no consequence. There is no accompanying spinal cord deformity with this minor abnormality. The majority of these cases include cutaneous symptoms such as a haemangioma, skin discoloration, pit, lump, dermal sinus or a hairy patch (Kinsman & Johnston, 2020).

Closed spinal dysraphism

Closed spinal dysraphisms are classified based on the presence of a subcutaneous mass. Spina bifida occulta (as described), **lipomyelomeningocele**, dorsal dermal sinus, split cord malformation, neuroenteric cyst and several other disorders are examples of closed spinal dysraphisms. They are frequently grouped together under the umbrella phrase 'tethered cord syndrome', which more accurately represents the constellation of symptoms that might be linked with these conditions.

Lipomyelomeningocele is a complex closed spinal dysraphism that most commonly affects the lumbar or sacral area. It is distinguished by a subcutaneous lipoma that spreads through the lumbosacral fascia, vertebral arches and dura to form a tethering mass to the spinal cord. If left untreated, it can cause significant neurological degeneration due to its relationship with spinal cord tethering. Neonates with lipomyelomeningocele have a congenital spinal cord malformation as well as a risk of re-tethering the spinal cord following release owing to scarring. As a result of the tethered cord, these newborns may have a neurogenic bladder or bowel, orthopaedic abnormalities, scoliosis and spasticity (Hills & Tomei, 2020).

Meningocele and myelomeningocele

When the meninges herniate through an abnormality in the posterior vertebral arches or the anterior sacrum, a **meningocele** forms. Although there may be cord tethering, syringomyelia (where a fluid-filled cyst – a syrinx – forms within the spinal cord) or diastematomyelia (a split cord malformation), the spinal cord is usually normal and assumes a normal position in the spinal canal. A fluctuant midline mass, which may transilluminate, develops along the vertebral column, most commonly in the lower back. Most meningoceles are skin covered and provide no immediate danger to the neonate. A thorough neurological evaluation is required. Orthopaedic and urological investigations should also be performed. Surgery may be delayed or not performed in asymptomatic children with normal neurological results and full-thickness skin covering the meningocele.

Myelomeningocele is the most severe form of dysraphism. It involves an aperta, referred to as open form, involving the vertebral column and spinal cord; it affects around 1 in every 4000 live births.

The aetiology of myelomeningocele is unknown, but, as with many neural tube closure disorders, including anencephaly, there is a hereditary predisposition; the risk of recurrence after one affected child is 3–4%, and escalates to 10% with two prior affected children. Both epidemiological evidence and the occurrence of considerable familial aggregation of anencephaly, myelomeningocele and **craniorachischisis** indicate heredity as a significant component to the aetiology of NTDs on a polygenic foundation. The aetiology of myelomeningocele is also influenced by nutritional and environmental variables (Kinsman & Johnston, 2020).

CONGENITAL ABNORMALITIES OF THE KIDNEY AND URINARY TRACT

Congenital abnormalities of the kidney and urinary tract (CAKUT) collectively refer to a diverse group of structural malformations that are characterised by abnormalities in embryonic kidney development.

These anomalies constitute approximately 20–30% of all congenital malformations, and their prevalence is estimated to range between 0.3 and 1.6 per 1000 in live- and stillborn infants (Rosenblum, 2021). Successful detection of CAKUT in utero has dramatically improved, which can be related to the increased availability and use of prenatal ultrasound. However, many cases remain undetected (Boubred & Simeoni, 2018). See Table 17.1 for a summary of presentation and investigation pathways in CAKUT. Table 17.2 outlines the diagnostic investigations of congenital uropathies.

Vesico-ureteric reflux

Vesico-ureteric reflux (VUR) is defined as the back-flow of urine from the urinary bladder into one or both ureters, the renal pelvises, or both. The most widely cited classifications are defined by the International Reflux Study, in which grade I indicates reflux of urine into part of the ureter, and grade V indicates gross dilation and tortuosity of the ureter, renal pelvis and calyces (Fig. 17.13). Each ureter is graded separately and the classification is usually based on the grade of the more affected side. VUR is a common finding in most urinary outflow tract obstructions or malformations (Läckgren et al., 2021).

Hydronephrosis detected on prenatal ultrasound suggests a finding of VUR in the newborn, with a VUR prevalence rate of 16.2% after prenatal hydronephrosis was diagnosed (Mattoo & Greenfield, 2021). The gold standard for diagnosing VUR is a radiological cystourethrogram (MCUG), but it is an invasive procedure requiring catheterisation and radiation exposure and should be performed only if there is bilateral **antenatal hydronephrosis (ANH)** in a male, or if the postnatal ultrasound shows persistent moderate to severe hydronephrosis (Mattoo & Greenfield, 2021). This procedure produces images of the bladder and urethra, allowing reflux to be graded using the International Reflux Study in Children criteria (Nelson & Koo, 2020). Grading of antenatal hydronephrosis is outlined in Table 17.3.

The major goals of treating VUR are to reduce recurrent febrile urinary tract infections (UTIs) and kidney scarring. Treatment of the VUR itself is not recommended because sterile VUR is not linked to renal scarring. The severity of reflux, history of UTIs, coexisting urogenital abnormalities and urologist preference all factor into treatment considerations (Läckgren et al., 2021). Prophylactic antibiotics are used to prevent recurring UTIs and maintain renal function; however, antibiotic resistance makes this strategy unsustainable (Läckgren et al., 2021).

TABLE 17.1 **Summary of presentation and investigation pathways in CAKUT**

Condition	Antenatal presentation	Renal function (↑creatinine)	Electrolyte disturbance	Outflow obstruction	Investigations
Hydronephrosis	Fetal hydronephrosis	✓	✓	—	Ultrasonography MCUG
Pelvic–ureteric junction obstruction	Fetal hydronephrosis	✓	✓	✓	Ultrasonography MCUG MAG3 MRI
Vesico–ureteric junction obstruction	Fetal hydronephrosis	✓	✓	✓	Ultrasonography MCUG MAG3 MRI
Posterior urethral valve	Fetal hydronephrosis	✓	✓	✓	Ultrasonography MCUG
Multi-cystic dysplastic kidney disease	Fetal hydronephrosis	✓	✓	✓	Ultrasonography MCUG MAG3
Hypospadias	—	—	—	—	Clinical examination
Cryptorchidism	—	—	—	—	Clinical examination Ultrasonography
Inguinal hernia	—	—	—	—	Clinical examination Ultrasonography
Bladder exstrophy	Fetal ultrasonography	—	—	—	Clinical examination Ultrasonography
Patent urachus	—	—	—	—	Ultrasonography MCUG

DMSA, dimercaptosuccinic acid; MAG3, mercaptoacetyltriglycine or renal scan; MCUG, micturating cystourethrogram; MRI, magnetic resonance imaging.

TABLE 17.2 **Diagnostic investigations of congenital uropathies**

Test	Indication	Practice points
Ultrasound	Hydronephrosis	• Timing dependent on severity of fetal hydronephrosis and whether there is bilateral or single kidney involvement • Further investigations may be required to ascertain definitive diagnoses • Can detect most congenital anomalies of the kidney and urinary tract associated with fetal hydronephrosis • Should be avoided in first 2–3 days after birth as hydronephrosis may not be detected due to ECF shifts (underestimation of hydronephrosis) (Baskin, 2020b)
Micturating cystourethrogram MCUG	Persistent postnatal hydronephrosis (>10 mm) to identify bladder outlet obstruction, most commonly caused by PUV and to detect VUR	• A urinary catheter is inserted into the bladder and contrast material instilled • Fluoroscopic monitoring is performed while the bladder is filling and emptying (Nepple & Cooper, 2021)
DTPA/MAG3 scan	To diagnose urinary tract obstruction in neonates with persistent hydronephrosis, usually ordered after an MCUG has demonstrated no renal reflux	• Measures drainage time from renal pelvis, and assesses relative contribution of each kidney to overall renal function • Requires insertion of a bladder catheter to relieve pressure • Radioisotope (technetium-99m-mercaptoacetyltriglycine) is administered intravenously and taken up by the renal cortex, filtered across the glomerular basement membrane to the renal tubules and excreted into the renal pelvis and urinary tract (Baskin, 2020b)
DMSA scan	Measures individual kidney function	• A nuclear medicine scan involving injection of (DMSA) • DMSA attaches only to functioning kidney tissue, measuring function of each kidney • When performed regularly, provides information on changes of the kidney over time (Guarino et al., 2020)
MRI	Diagnosis and management of congenital uropathies including PUJ obstruction, rotation or ascent anomalies or single kidney anomalies	• Clearly defines anatomy and delineates most appropriate surgical approach • The disadvantage is the potential requirement for general anaesthesia or heavy sedation (Zhang et al., 2020)

DMSA, dimercaptosuccinic acid; DTPA, diethylenetriamine pentaacetic acid; ECF, extracellular fluid; MAG3, mercaptoacetyltriglycine or renal scan; MCUG, micturating cystourethrogram; MRI, magnetic resonance imaging; PUJ, pelvic–ureteric junction; PUV, posterior urethral valve; VUJ, vesico-ureteric junction; VUR, vesico-ureteric reflux.

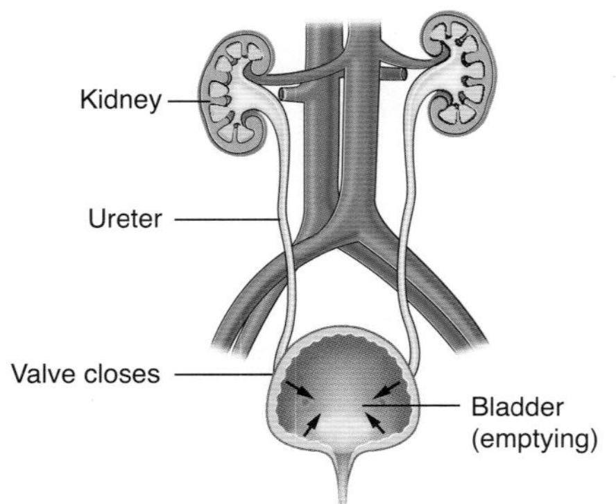

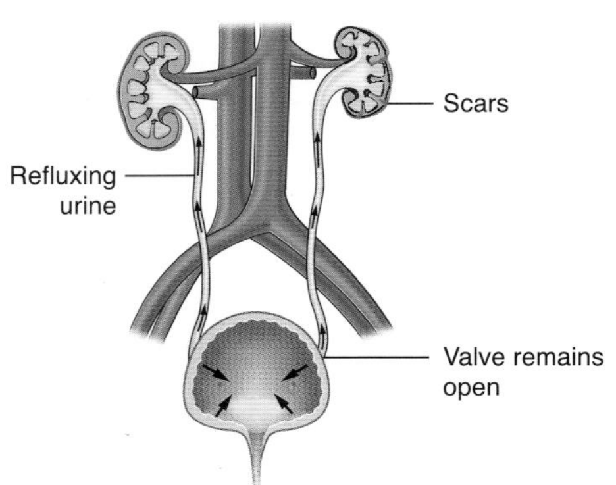

FIGURE 17.13 **Vesico-ureteric reflux**

TABLE 17.3 **Grading antenatal hydronephrosis (renal pelvis dilation[a])**

Degree of ANH	Second trimester (mm)	Third trimester (mm)	Postnatal (mm)
Normal	<5	<7	<5
Mild	4–7	7–9	5–10 Normal calyces
Moderate	7–10	9–15	10–15
Severe	>10	>15	>15 Calyceal dilation

[a]As measured in millimetres using the anteroposterior diameter of the renal pelvis in the transverse plane.

Source: adapted from Nguyen et al. (2010).

Pelvic–ureteric junction and vesico-ureteric junction obstruction

The **pelvic–ureteric junction (PUJ) obstruction** and **vesico-ureteric junction (VUJ) obstruction** develop in week 5 of embryogenesis and are canalised in weeks 10–12 of gestation. The PUJ area is the last to canalise, correlating with the increased incidence of PUJ obstruction over VUJ. Inadequate canalisation of this area leads to PUJ and VUJ blockages. Obstructed urinary tract anomalies, such as PUJ obstruction, VUJ obstruction and posterior urethral valves (PUVs), represent a challenge to clinicians. One in 500 live births have PUJ blockage. Males are affected more than females, and left-sided lesions are more common than right-sided. Around 10% of cases have bilateral involvement (Baskin, 2020a). Obstruction of the VUJ occurs in 1 in 1500–2000 newborns. It generally occurs in isolation.

Obstruction of the PUJ or VUJ is detected postnatally and should be explored in both unilateral and bilateral ANH. Hydronephrosis occurs when anatomical or functional obstruction restricts urine flow across the ureteropelvic junction (Baskin, 2020b). The enlarged and obstructed kidney causes a palpable mass in most cases. If the neonate is symptomatic, surgery can be performed to remove the blockage (Baskin, 2020b).

The next treatment goal is to balance fluid and electrolytes. Acute renal tubule dysfunction (especially proximal renal tubule dysfunction) can result in sodium and bicarbonate losses (Bandari et al., 2015).

PUJ obstruction is a partial or intermittent blockage of urine flow at the renal pelvis–proximal ureter junction (Baskin, 2020b). A VUJ obstruction restricts urine flow at the ureter–bladder junction. The obstruction prevents urine from reaching the bladder, causing ureters and kidneys to enlarge (mega-ureter and hydronephrosis) (Baskin, 2020a).

There are several causes of PUJ and VUJ obstruction that affect urine flow from the kidneys to the ureter. These include insertional anomalies, functional abnormalities, peristaltic anomalies of the bladder or ureter and ureteral polyps. The management of PUJ blockage is classified into three categories: (1) observation, (2) urgent repair and (3) repair following observation. Guidelines state that, rather than a single test, management decisions should be based on serial tests performed at the same institution. Intervention aims to maintain renal function and relieve symptoms. Until VUR is ruled out, all newborns with antenatally diagnosed hydronephrosis require antibiotic prophylaxis (such as trimethoprim 1–2 mg/kg and cephalexin 5 mg/kg) (Gunawardena et al., 2019).

The renal pelvis is rebuilt or revised during laparoscopic or open surgery to drain and decompress the kidneys (Gunawardena et al., 2019). There are limited longitudinal data on the outcomes of newborns treated surgically versus conservatively. Approximately 5% of infants who had surgery developed recurring blockage (Baskin, 2020a). The goal of treating VUJ blockage is to preserve renal function. Approximately 50% of infants with improved dilation can be monitored without intervention. Renal dysfunction or recurrent UTIs necessitate surgery in 10–20% of babies.

CASE STUDY **17.2**

Megan is a 32-year-old G4P3. Routine antenatal ultrasound at 20 weeks' gestation noted fetal hydronephrosis graded as mild (5–7 mm).

1 What further assessment needs to be considered?

Further assessment in the third trimester noted persistent hydronephrosis, now graded as moderate (10–15 mm).

2 What postnatal investigations would you anticipate?

Postnatal ultrasound on day 4 noted unilateral hydronephrosis (predominantly on the right).

3 What conditions do you suspect, given this history?

4 What further information would you require?

5 What clinical assessment would be undertaken on this newborn?

6 What monitoring would you undertake on this neonate?

Multi-cystic dysplastic kidney disease

Multi-cystic dysplastic kidney disease (MCDKD) is a condition that results in the development of cysts in the kidneys, resulting in non-functioning, dysplastic kidneys and urethral atresia. It is the most severe form of renal dysplasia, with bilateral involvement considered incompatible with life (Psooy, 2016). It is postulated that multi-cystic dysplastic kidneys result from an abnormal induction of the metanephric mesenchyme by the ureteral bud. The final structure of the dysplastic kidney depends on the timing of the injury to the ureteric bud and on the effect of the injury on the ureteric bud branching (Sugimoto et al., 2021).

Multi-cystic dysplastic kidneys usually develop as a sporadic problem, although familial occurrence has been reported. Causes of MCDKD have been reported to include in utero exposure to viral infection: cytomegalovirus (CMV), enterovirus and adenovirus. Teratogens may also play a role in abnormal renal development, although their association is not clear (Sugimoto et al., 2021).

MCDKD is the most common form of renal cystic disease in neonates. It is reported in as many as 1 in every 4300 live births. It is seen in males and females equally and the most common presentation is unilateral (Sugimoto et al., 2021).

Multi-cystic dysplastic kidney disease presents in the newborn period following an antenatal history of oligohydramnios and fetal hydronephrosis detected on ultrasound as early as 15 weeks' gestation. The postnatal physical examination may reveal:

- a palpable abdominal mass (seen in approximately 13–22% of cases)
- raised creatinine on blood chemistry
- reduced urine output (below 1 mL/kg/h after the first 24 hours of life).

Postnatal investigations include:

- a renal ultrasound that shows communicating cysts of varying sizes and a lack of normal renal parenchyma
- an MCUG that shows the degree of VUR
- a mercaptoacetyltriglycine (MAG3) scan to demonstrate the function of the kidneys, in particular the cystic kidney.

Management of MCDKD can take two approaches, non-surgical and surgical, and is dependent on the degree of renal complications.

The non-surgical approach includes:

- serial monitoring of hydronephrosis through regular ultrasound examination
- monitoring of renal function focusing on creatinine levels
- close monitoring for urinary infection with prompt treatment
- assessment for signs and symptoms of renal failure including decreased urine output, and rising creatinine levels.

In 60% of MCDKD cases, there is natural involution of the affected kidney within the first 5 years of life without intervention, and the contralateral kidney grows to compensate, negating the need for surgery (Niaudet, 2021).

Prognosis depends on whether the involvement is unilateral or bilateral, and on the presence and severity of associated anomalies. Most individuals with an isolated unilateral multi-cystic dysplastic kidney do not experience any problems or complications as a consequence of this congenital abnormality (Sugimoto et al., 2021).

Hypospadias

Hypospadias refers to a urogenital congenital anomaly characterised by an abnormal ventral opening of the urethral meatus between the distal glans of the penis and perineum (Fig. 17.14).

Hypospadias occurs as a result of an abnormal closure of the urethral folds at approximately 8–14 weeks' gestation.

There are three types of hypospadias depending on the location of the opening of the urethra:

1. *subcoronal* – the opening of the urethra is located somewhere near the head of the penis
2. *midshaft* – the opening of the urethra is located along the shaft of the penis
3. *penoscrotal* – the opening of the urethra is located where the penis and scrotum meet.

Although hypospadias is common, a definitive incidence is not well defined. There may be a multifactorial inheritance. Several studies have suggested that LBW and increasing maternal age are associated with hypospadias. The reported incidence is 1 in 250 male newborns (Hassan et al., 2021).

The diagnosis of hypospadias is made from clinical examination and assessment including:

- a physical examination noting the urinary meatus located on the under-surface of the penis
- deviation of the urinary stream
- the presence of chordee (downward curving of the penis; there is an association between the degree of chordee and the degree of hypospadias)
- a physical examination to detect the presence of **undescended testes (UDT)** and an inguinal hernia, as these are also common associations
- evaluation of urinary and renal function, which should be normal.

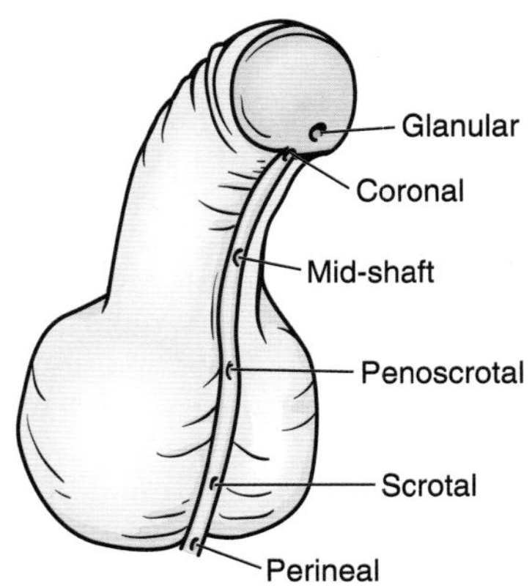

FIGURE 17.14 **Hypospadias**
Source: From Sawyer (2020).

The main treatment for hypospadias is surgical repair, aiming to correct the functionality of the penile urethra and improve the cosmetic appearance. International guidelines recommend repair between 6 and 12 months of age (Gatti & Kirsch, 2021).

Complications without repair can include difficulty in voiding while standing, and the presence of chordee, which may cause painful erections. Postsurgical complications can include urethro-cutaneous fistula, meatal stenosis, urethral stricture and urethral diverticulum; however, complication rates remain low with surgical repair (Gatti & Kirsch, 2021).

Cryptorchidism

The word '**cryptorchidism**' implies a hidden testis and is the most common congenital disorder of the genitourinary system affecting male neonates. The testis may prove to be absent, truly undescended, in an ectopic location or ascended. The term serves as a broad clinical category and includes a variety of conditions. Therefore, the use of precise terminology to characterise specific physical findings on examination is critical for accurate diagnosis and treatment planning (Rodprasert et al., 2020).

Testicular descent from the abdomen to the scrotum normally occurs at 28 weeks' gestation, following a pattern of descent over three phases (Rodprasert et al., 2020). The first phase (the transabdominal phase) begins at 10–15 weeks' gestation and is usually completed by 22–25 weeks' gestation. The second phase of descent (the transinguinal phase) occurs at 25–30 weeks' gestation and is a rapid process in which the testes migrate through the short inguinal canal to the external inguinal ring. The third phase of descent (the scrotal phase) occurs as the pregnancy approaches term, from 30–35 weeks' gestation. Governed in part by androgen production, in 97% of males the testes travel from the external inguinal ring to the final position in the scrotum near term, and in the remaining cases the descent occurs postnatally in the first 3 months of life (Singh, 2020, p. 281).

The staged nature of testicular descent demonstrates why the prevalence of cryptorchidism is so much higher among preterm neonates because preterm birth interrupts the natural progression of the testes (Rodprasert et al., 2020). The true pathophysiology of UDT is not fully understood, although several theories exist. Identified risk factors for UDT include preterm birth, LBW, twinning, maternal exposure to oestrogen in the first trimester, a family history of UDT and maternal alcohol or tobacco use (Sumfest et al., 2020).

The incidence in term neonates is reported to be 3–5%, with an increased risk in preterm neonates to be as much as 20–25%, and with risk increasing as gestational age decreases (Rodprasert et al., 2020).

Competent clinical examination is essential for evaluation and to differentiate the category of cryptorchidism. Examination is best performed with the neonate relaxed, in a supine, partially frog-legged position. Visual inspection to demonstrate the resting position of the testis and the movement of the testis with palpation are key for assessment. Visual inspection may demonstrate the testis residing in the middle to lower scrotum, with subsequent palpation along the inner thigh or scrotum stimulating a cremasteric reflex (contraction of the ipsilateral cremaster muscle) that retracts the testis to the upper scrotum/lower inguinal canal.

Neonates with symmetric scrota are much more likely to have retractile testes than UDT, whereas most patients with asymmetry have UDT. Additionally, the term 'ascended testis' describes a testis, often a previously retractile testis, once documented in a scrotal position, that has subsequently ascended to a suprascrotal position spontaneously, and may be due to abnormal gubernaculum attachment (Alchoikani & Ashour, 2021).

Diagnosis of cryptorchidism includes the following:

- a clinical examination by an experienced clinician, as a careful physical examination is key to establishing the most accurate diagnosis as well as appropriate therapy
- diagnostic laparoscopy, as it is the current gold standard to locate an intra-abdominal testis
- ultrasound, as a relatively inexpensive, non-invasive and accessible form of imaging, and therefore commonly used in evaluation of cryptorchidism, although it is not cost effective and may delay referral and surgical treatment (Sumfest et al., 2020).

Most UDT migrate into the lower scrotum in the first 3 months of life, presumably as a consequence of a postnatal testosterone surge, with 1% remaining undescended by 1 year of age. Surgical management with orchiopexy (a surgical procedure that alters the course of the spermatic artery and creates a direct line from the renal pedicle to the scrotum) is required if the testis remains undescended by 1 year of age (Rodprasert et al., 2020).

Possible sequelae include infertility and testicular cancer. The presence of bilateral non-palpable UDT is an indication for evaluation for a disorder of sexual development (DSD) (Rodprasert et al., 2020).

Bladder exstrophy

Bladder exstrophy is a rare yet complicated disorder that poses a number of management challenges, which occurs when the bladder is exposed and protrudes through a defect in the abdominal wall (Fig. 17.15) (Promm & Roesch, 2019).

Bladder exstrophy occurs when the anterior abdominal wall fails to close at the point of the bladder. During the fourth week of gestation, the abdominal wall begins to fuse. Exstrophy results when the mesenchymal cells fail to migrate over the abdomen, and a thin membrane forms over the abdominal contents. This membrane later ruptures and leaves the bladder exposed. Exstrophy of the bladder is a rare condition that occurs in 1 in 10,000 births (Singh, 2020, p. 261).

Clinical presentation includes (Promm & Roesch, 2019):

- exposed bladder on the abdominal wall
- umbilicus displaced downwards
- pubic rami (bony projections of the pubic bone) widely separated in the midline
- separation of the rectus muscles.

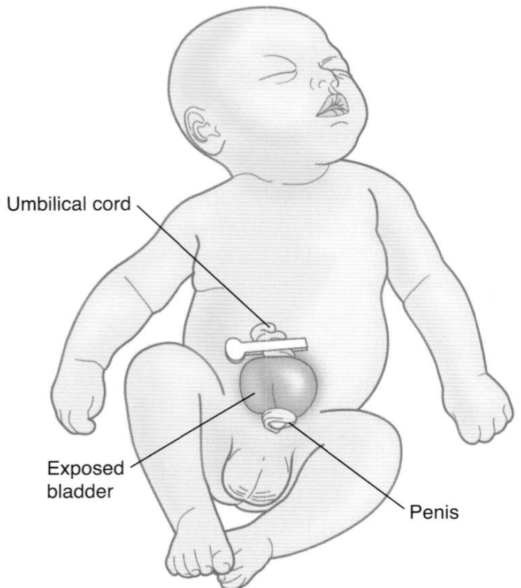

FIGURE 17.15 **Bladder exstrophy**

The incidence of bladder exstrophy has been estimated at 2–3.3 per 100,000 births, with the rate in males being double that of females (Borer, 2020).

Clinical assessment includes:

- observation of the externally presented bladder
- assessment of associated anomalies, including epispadias in males, bifid clitoris and anteriorly placed vagina in females, and anteriorly located anus
- palpation of the testes to assess descent, and of the groin to assess the presence of inguinal hernia
- examination of the symphysis pubis to assess widening and the need for orthopaedic surgical repair.

Clinical investigations include (Promm & Roesch, 2019):

- X-ray including abdomen and pubic bones
- renal ultrasound to determine the presence or absence of upper tract abnormalities.

Bladder exstrophy can be diagnosed antenatally with ultrasound between the 15th and 32nd weeks of gestation. In the fetus, absence of bladder filling, a low-set umbilicus, widened pubic rami, small genitalia and a lower abdominal mass that increases throughout gestation are all indicative of the condition. Fetal MRI is a conclusive diagnostic tool when bladder exstrophy is suspected on fetal ultrasound. Postnatal diagnosis is made on clinical assessment that differentiates bladder exstrophy from other congenital abnormalities involving abdominal wall defects such as omphalocele and cloacal exstrophy (Borer, 2020).

Preoperative management includes:

- managing neonates with bladder exstrophy at a tertiary centre with availability of experienced paediatric urologists and orthopaedic surgery teams
- covering the exposed bladder with a non-adherent film of plastic wrap to prevent trauma to the exposed bladder and prevent insensible water losses through the exposed viscera
- considering prophylactic antibiotic treatment
- assessing fluid balance and urine output diligently.

Surgical correction is the definitive management. Two approaches have been considered (complete versus staged approach) with the ultimate aim of primary bladder closure.

Pelvic osteotomies (cutting of the pubic bone to allow for medial realignment) reduce the distance between the pelvic symphysis bones, allowing for adequate bladder closure.

Initial postoperative management includes (Promm & Roesch, 2019):

- diligent fluid balance and urine output assessment, with bladder drainage from suprapubic and ureteral stents to prevent ureteral obstruction hypertension
- monitoring of electrolyte balance and initiation of supplementation when required
- monitoring of urine function, in particular creatinine levels
- antispasmodics, analgesics and sedation, which may be required to prevent bladder spasm and disruption of the surgical closure
- assessment for sepsis, including septic screen in the presence of a febrile episode
- prophylactic antibiotic coverage using treatment dosage for 5–7 days' post closure
- gallows traction for pelvic immobilisation in the immediate postoperative period following osteotomy, allowing for adequate bony ossification.

The most important predictor of long-term bladder development and continence is successful primary closure. The long-term prognosis of classic bladder exstrophy is good, with preservation of renal and sexual function, the achievement of normal-appearing abdominal wall and genitalia and urinary continence rates approaching 70%. Parents experience a significant amount of stress and require medical, nursing, social and emotional support from a multidisciplinary team (Borer, 2020).

Patent urachus

The urachus is a tubular structure that is patent during gestation. It connects the allantois (a small sausage-shaped out-pouching from the caudal wall of the yolk sac of the early embryo) at the umbilicus to the dome of the bladder during fetal development. The lumen normally closes at about the 12th week of gestation and obliterates completely. Following obliteration, all that typically remains is a fibrous cord running from the inferior aspect of the umbilicus to the dome of the bladder. The urachus is accompanied by umbilical arteries on either side, which undergo fibrosis and become the medial umbilical ligaments (Tatekawa, 2019).

Failure of the epithelial-lined urachal canal to completely obliterate results in a urachal remnant, including a **patent urachus** (Tatekawa, 2019) (Fig. 17.16).

- A patent urachus is suspected with the presence of urine draining from the umbilicus and an abnormal-appearing umbilicus in the neonatal period.
- Additional presentation findings may include an oedematous umbilicus, granuloma and delayed healing of the cord stump.

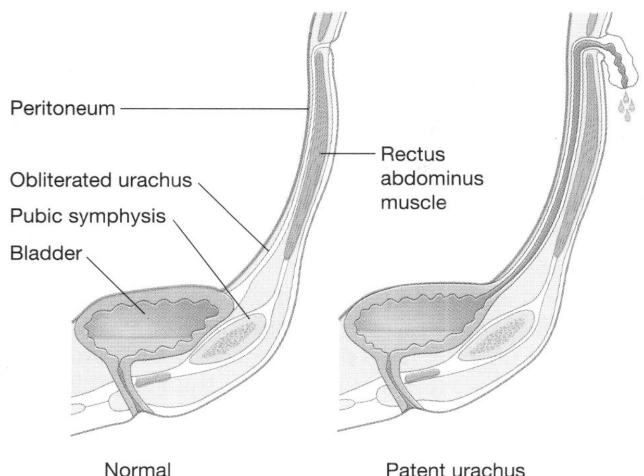

FIGURE 17.16 **Normal and patent urachus**

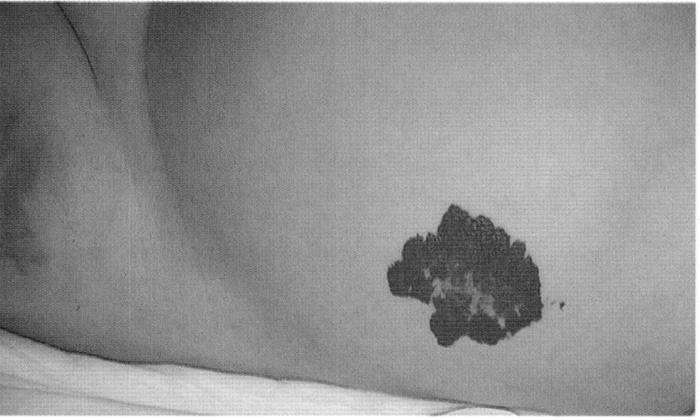

FIGURE 17.17 **Capillary haemangioma**

Source: From Callen et al (2000).

- A patent urachus must be distinguished from omphalitis, which typically presents as a superficial cellulitis; and a patent omphalomesenteric duct remnant, which can present with feculent umbilical drainage (Soliman et al., 2015).

The diagnosis is confirmed by demonstration of a fluid-filled cystic structure on an ultrasound scan extending from the dome of the bladder to the umbilicus. The passage of contrast at the umbilicus is seen on voiding cystourethrogram (Tatekawa, 2019).

Urachal remnants in infants younger than 6 months of age are likely to spontaneously resolve and, therefore, surgical excision should be considered only in cases of a persistent urachal remnant. Short-term urethral catheter drainage has been reported to facilitate spontaneous closure (Soliman et al., 2015).

Common complications with patent urachus can include UTIs and excoriation to the skin around the umbilicus (Tatekawa, 2019).

CONGENITAL ABNORMALITIES OF THE INTEGUMENTARY SYSTEM

Various skin conditions and lesions present themselves during the neonatal period. Some are more prevalent in the preterm neonates (such as **haemangioma** or erythema toxicum) whereas others (such as **Sturge–Weber syndrome** or **epidermolysis bullosa**) need immediate specialist care.

Infantile haemangioma

Infantile haemangiomas are caused by a proliferation of capillaries in the dermal and subdermal layers of the skin (Kowalska et al., 2021), and are the most frequent benign tumours in infancy, with a prevalence of 4.5% (Fig. 17.17). They appear in the first few weeks of life and follow a predictable growth and involution pattern (Léauté-Labrèze et al., 2017). They are more prevalent in the preterm and low birthweight neonatal population compared with other newborns (Metry, 2021). After birth the haemangioma may not be very obvious, but it then enlarges, with the maximum increase in size occurring around 5–7 weeks of age, and then a spontaneous involution phase typically starts closer to 12 months of age, before regression by the age of 4 years in 90% of cases (Kowalska et al., 2021). Infantile haemangiomas are classified as focal, segmental or indeterminate (Chan & Goodyear, 2015) and occur most commonly in the upper extremities (Reimer et al., 2016).

Treatment is required if the haemangioma causes a physical obstruction to the airway or the eye, if it is ulcerated or if the size of the haemangioma may cause disfigurement or scarring. Beta-blockers such as propranolol and timolol may be prescribed for their vasoconstrictive effects. Oral propranolol doses range from 1 to 3 mg/kg, or 1–2 drops of a 5 mg/mL topical timolol maleate (Léauté-Labrèze et al., 2017). Occasionally, laser or excisional surgery is recommended if the lesions have inadequate involution by age 4 and are in cosmetically concerning locations; however, cautery, irradiation and cryotherapy are not recommended because of safety concerns and scarring (Metry, 2021). Treatment and intervention of infantile haemangioma are based on the features presented in Table 17.4; low-risk cases would usually not require treatment.

Sturge–Weber syndrome

Sturge–Weber syndrome (SWS) is a rare congenital vascular condition first described in 1879 by William Sturge. SWS is characterised by a port wine-stained appearance of the face, scalp and the trunk. While uncommon, the condition is associated with brain abnormalities, seizures and vascular abnormalities involving the trigeminal nerve and vision complications (Zallmann et al., 2018). No specific treatment exists for SWS, and the cutaneous, ocular and neurological manifestations are treated with mixed success. Observational data suggests that low-dose aspirin may be beneficial, beginning in infancy (Patterson, 2021).

TABLE 17.4 **Intervention assessment for infantile haemangioma**

Risk	Location, size, type
High	• Segmental >5 cm – face, lumbosacral/perineal area • Bulky lesion – face • Central face (periorbital, perinasal, perioral)
Intermediate	• Lateral face, scalp, hands, feet • Body folds, neck, perineum, axilla • Segmental >5 cm – trunk, arms, legs
Low	• Trunk, arms, legs

Source: adapted from Luu and Frieden (2013).

Epidermolysis bullosa

Epidermolysis bullosa (EB) is a rare inheritable disorder where blistering and erosion in the skin occur with any handling. There are four subtypes, with a spectrum of presentation that relates to gene mutations (Bardhan et al., 2020). An antenatal diagnosis with family history is important, as it can be confused with scalded skin syndrome or thermal/chemical burns if undiagnosed. The best-practice care for an infant with EB is summarised in Table 17.5.

MISCELLANEOUS CONGENITAL ABNORMALITIES

Polydactyly presents with an extra non-functional digit on the hand or foot attached by a skin bridge, or a small bump on the ulnar aspect of the hand/foot (Fig. 17.18). Minor forms that do not involve bone or nerves can be tied off with a non-absorbable suture, although this practice is called into question by Chopan et al. (2020) who report acute and long-term complications. Surgical excision involves an elliptical incision at the base of the duplicated digit, excision of the digit with high ligation/excision of the accessory nerve and then skin closure, which is usually performed around 1 year of age. More research is needed to determine the optimal approach (Chopan et al., 2020).

Syndactyly occurs when there is webbing of fingers or toes, and can be simple (when the web is constructed of skin and connective tissue) or complex (when there is a degree of bone or nail fusion) (Sullivan & Adkinson, 2017). Surgical correction is recommended when the infant is 12–18 months of age, and is important to preserve hand function and to reduce the psychological impact on the patient's life (Chouairi et al., 2020). Surgical approaches include release of the digit and then either a skin flap, skin grafting or bone osteotomies, depending on the complexity of the syndactyly (Chouairi et al., 2020).

TABLE 17.5 **Best-practice guidelines for skin and wound care in epidermolysis bullosa**

Procedure(s)	Action	Rationale
Care at birth	• Minimise trauma at birth and resuscitation • Commercial plastic cling film (or bag) to optimise skin protection	Avoid skin injury
Ongoing care	• Silicone dressing to skin before the application of leads	Avoid skin injury
Blood sampling	• Avoid tourniquets, shearing and rubbing (firm hold) • Gauze around skin, before applying pressure or milking for sample • Environmental factors: avoid ID tags, consider cord tie or suture instead of clamp, minimise time in incubator (may exacerbate blistering)	Minimise trauma
General care (birth and hospital stay)	• Hand hygiene • Avoid applying any adhesive dressings or tape • Avoid bathing in first week of life (until trauma healed) • Attachment-free clothing (e.g. Velcro and press studs) • Silk and satin sheets may prevent friction injuries	Prevent infections
Dressings and blister care	• Wet glove tips with paraffin and apply 50% soft paraffin to gloves (to prevent fingers sticking) • Warm saline to irrigate old dressings to remove them • One limb at a time • Lance blisters with sterile needles • Compress with gauze and expel the liquid • Leave the roof of the blister intact	Avoid trauma; blisters will get larger if left intact
Nappy care	• 50% liquid paraffin, 50% white soft paraffin to clean area • Line nappy with polar fleece • Hydrogel-impregnated dressing to raw groin or nappy area	Cleansing without trauma; reduce pain and friction
ANALGESIA: adequate pain relief prior to skin care, dressing changes and interventions as can be painful and traumatic		

Source: adapted from Denyer and Pillay (2012).

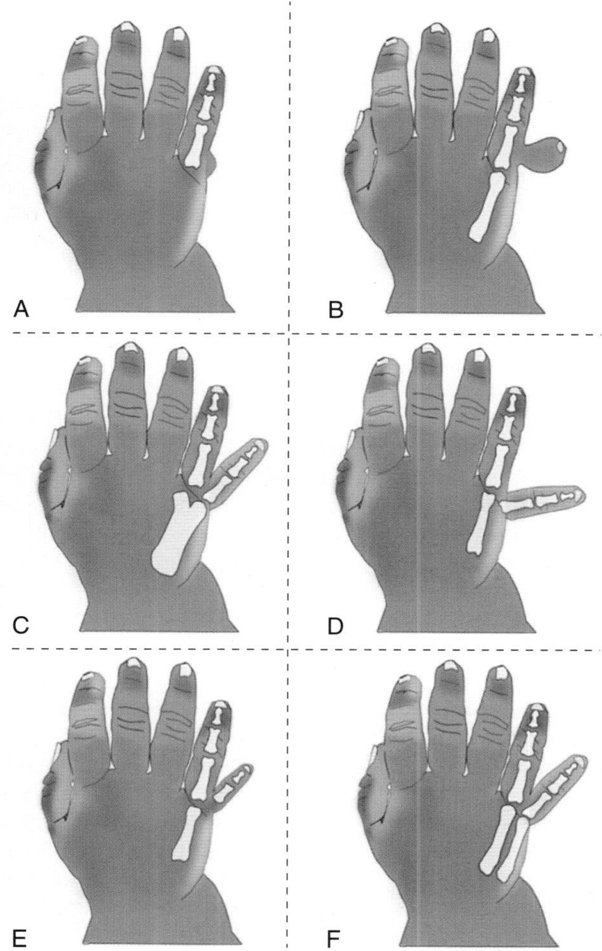

FIGURE 17.18 **Polydactyly types**

a Soft tissue nub/remnant. **b** Pedunculated non-functioning digit. **c** Well-formed functioning digit that is articulating with a bifid fifth metacarpal head. **d** Well-formed digit that is fused at a right angle to the fifth metacarpal. **e** Well-formed digit that has a hypoplastic/absent proximal phalanx. **f** Complete duplication with a separate sixth metacarpal.

Source: Chopan et al. (2020).

Achondroplasia is a short-limb (as opposed to short-trunk) dwarfing condition apparent at birth which affects arms and thighs in particular, and is due to abnormal endochondral ossification (Parikh & Batra, 2022). It is transmitted as an autosomal dominant trait; however, at least 80% of cases are due to a random new mutation. Morbidity associated with achondroplasia includes recurrent otitis media, respiratory insufficiency, hydrocephalus, cervicomedullary compression leading to hypotonia, sleep apnoea and feeding problems. Parents benefit from support groups and the coordinated care from a multidisciplinary team including paediatricians, psychologists, dietitians, physiotherapists, occupational therapists, ear, nose and throat specialists, and orthopaedic and neurological surgeons to ensure good outcomes (Bacino, 2021).

COMMON CHROMOSOMAL DISORDERS

Chromosomes can have a normal number (diploid) but an aberrant structure. Structural chromosomal abnormalities include inversions, deletions and translocations of genetic material. These can occur as new (sporadic) mutations in the egg or sperm from which the embryo was produced, in which case the parents' probability of having another child with a chromosomal abnormality is 1–2%. On the other hand, the anomaly could be inherited from a phenotypically normal parent who is a 'carrier' of a structural chromosomal aberration. A chromosomal translocation is a balanced but architecturally aberrant collection of chromosomes that affects about 1 in 520 normal individuals (Madan-Khetarpal & Arnold, 2018).

Trisomy 13

Trisomy 13 (Patau syndrome) is a relatively uncommon (1 in 5000) genetic disorder characterised by the presence of extra chromosomal material from all or a significant portion of chromosome 13. The great majority of embryos with complete 13th chromosome trisomy abort spontaneously, although about 5% survive to be live born. They have a severe, recognised pattern of malformations that allows clinicians to immediately suspect its aetiology. The distinguishing hallmarks are forebrain developmental anomalies similar to those observed in holoprosencephaly, aplasia cutis congenita, polydactyly (most commonly of the postaxial kind) and narrow hyperconvex nails. Trisomy 13 and trisomy 18 share structural abnormalities, as do many syndromes; nevertheless, they are usually distinctly based on the pattern of anomalies present. Trisomy 13 infants born alive have the least-severe structural abnormalities in major organs. Only approximately 5% of these survive the first 6 months of life (Madan-Khetarpal & Arnold, 2018).

Trisomy 18

Trisomy 18 (Edwards syndrome) occurs in approximately 1 in every 8000 live births. Stillbirth is a common occurrence. Fetal movement is minimal, and approximately 50% have a non-reassuring fetal status during labour. Mean survival is estimated in months for live births, and significant developmental and growth restriction is evident. Around 80% of trisomy 18 cases are the result of primary non-disjunction (47 + 18). Typically, errors occur during maternal meiosis, most frequently during meiosis II. The chance of recurrence is about 1% (Driscoll & Simpson, 2021). The most common anatomical malformations in trisomy 18 neonates and fetuses include congenital heart problems, central nervous system anomalies, hydrocephalus, diaphragmatic hernia, omphalocele (70% of which only contain bowel) and abnormally clenched fists (with overlapping index fingers) (Bromley & Benacerraf, 2018).

Trisomy 21

Trisomy 21 (Down syndrome) is the most frequent chromosomal abnormality and the most common form of inherited intellectual disability, with the universally recognised features of upslanting palpebral fissures, epicanthic folds and brachycephaly (Ostermaier, 2020). Trisomy 21 is a genetic abnormality that produces developmental delays, cognitive impairment, short stature, ophthalmological disorders, hearing loss, thyroid disorders, craniofacial abnormalities, hypotonia and a number of other disorders (e.g. congenital heart defects, haematological abnormalities, endocrine abnormalities, atlantoaxial instability, early-onset dementia) (Ostermaier, 2020). There are numerous congenital abnormalities that are related with this condition, as follows.

Cardiac

Congenital cardiac problems affect up to 50% of patients; the most common abnormalities involve the endocardial cushion:

- Forty-five percent of newborns have an atrioventricular septal defect (with or without additional congenital cardiac abnormalities).
- Thirty-five percent of patients have a ventricular septal defect (with or without other congenital cardiac abnormalities).
- Eight percent of cases have an isolated secundum atrial septal defect.
- Seven percent of patients have isolated chronic patent ductus arteriosus.
- Four percent of cases have an isolated tetralogy of Fallot present (Ostermaier, 2020).

Otolaryngeal

Congenital deafness is prevalent when compared with the overall neonatal population, occurring in up to 15% of babies (0.25% prevalence). Conditions include:

- auditory canal enlargement or stenosis
- stenotic canals in many newborns, which make it difficult to visualise the tympanic membranes
- lower airway problems affecting approximately 25% of children
- tracheobronchomalacia
- subglottic stenosis
- tracheal stenosis
- cataracts (in approximately 15%)
- stenosis of the lacrimal duct (Ostermaier, 2020).

Gastrointestinal

Anomalies in structural design are seen in approximately 12% of newborns. Conditions include:

- atresia of the duodenum (occasionally associated with annular pancreas)
- atresia or stenosis of the anorectum
- atresia of the oesophagus with tracheoesophageal fistula
- Hirschsprung disease (Ostermaier, 2020).

Haematological

Conditions include:

- transient myeloproliferative disorder (4–10% of newborns) – spontaneous resolution is prevalent within the first 3 months of infancy and is associated with an increased chance of developing acute myelogenous leukaemia later in life
- polycythaemia (18–64% of newborns)
- musculoskeletal
- dislocation of the hip (up to 6%)
- atlantoaxial instability (Ostermaier, 2020).

Endocrine

Conditions include:

- hypothyroidism from birth (approximately 1%) (Ostermaier, 2020).

Urogenital

Conditions include:

- hypoplasia of the kidneys
- obstructive uropathy and posterior urethral valves
- cryptorchidism
- hypospadias.

Counselling parents expecting a baby with Down syndrome should commence as soon as the prenatal diagnosis is suspected, and include the wide range of variability in outcomes and prognosis. The discussion should include medical and educational interventions, parent groups and advocacy groups (Ostermaier, 2020).

Turner syndrome

Turner syndrome is a disorder described by a combination of clinical traits and is characterised by complete or partial monosomy of the X chromosome, leading to short stature and ovarian insufficiency in females. Half of Turner syndrome patients have a 45,X chromosome complement. The other half exhibit mosaicism, which is defined as the presence of two or more cell lineages with different genotypes arising from a single zygote in a single individual (Queremel Milani & Chauhan, 2021, p. 1), with various associated structural X or Y chromosomal abnormalities. Maternal age is not a risk factor for children who have 45,X. Turner syndrome affects about 1 in every 5000 female live births. The missing sex chromosome is of paternal origin in 75% of individuals (whether an X or a Y). 45, X is one of the most common chromosomal abnormalities associated with spontaneous abortion. It is estimated that 95–99% of 45,X conceptions end in miscarriage.

Although many neonates are phenotypically normal, clinical abnormalities in newborns can include being small for gestational age, webbing of the neck, nail dysplasia, narrow and arched palate, protruding ears and lymphoedema of the hands and feet (Backeljauw, 2021). Older children and adults are low in stature and have a variety of dysmorphic characteristics. Congenital cardiac abnormalities (40%) and structural renal malformations (60%) are both prevalent. Bicuspid aortic valves, coarctation of the aorta, aortic stenosis and mitral valve prolapse are the most common cardiac abnormalities. The gonads are typically fibrous tissue streaks (gonadal dysgenesis). Primary amenorrhea and a lack of secondary sex characteristics are present (Bacino & Lee, 2020). Intelligence is usually normal in patients with Turner syndrome, but they may have deficits in social and verbal function (Backeljauw, 2021). Parents should be offered support of a multidisciplinary team and relevant Turner syndrome support groups.

CONCLUSION

Many congenital abnormalities necessitate early intervention following birth. A collaborative interprofessional team approach is required, which should include medical specialists from maternal–fetal medicine, neonatology, paediatric subspecialties (e.g. surgery), nursing, midwifery and social work, as well as many others as necessary to meet the unique requirements of each newborn and family. Surgical intervention during the neonatal period may be necessary if the infant requires rapid correction or a palliative operation to alleviate the anomaly's symptoms before final correction can be performed.

To meet the needs of these high-risk infants, the healthcare team must be highly skilled. Nurses and midwives play a critical role in stabilising the infant (oxygenation and perfusion of tissues), performing preoperative interventions such as placing an orogastric tube for abdominal decompression, monitoring temperature and pain, maintaining fluid and electrolyte balance, and supporting and educating the family.

Further Reading

Bischoff, M. (2021). Prepare for the rare: innovation simulation for managing abdominal wall defects. *Neonatal Network, 40*(2), 98–102.

References/Acknowledgements

Alchoikani, N., & Ashour, K. (2021). Ascending testis: a congenital predetermined condition. *Journal of Pediatric Urology, 17*(2), 192.e1–192.e3. doi: 10.1016/j.jpurol.2020.12.016.

Allin, B. S., Opondo, C., Kurinczuk, J. J., Baird, R., Puligandla, P., Skarsgard, E., et al. (2021). Management of gastroschisis: results from the NETS2G study, a joint British, Irish, and Canadian prospective cohort study of 1268 infants. *Annals of Surgery, 273*(6), 1207–1214. doi: 10.1097/SLA.0000000000004217. PMID: 33201118.

Anyanwu, L. C., Ade-Ajayi, N., & Rolle, U. (2020). Major abdominal wall defects in the low- and middle-income setting: current status and priorities. *Pediatric Surgery International, 36*(5), 579–590. doi: 10.1007/s00383-020-04638-8.

Attya, H., Callaby, M., & Thevasagayam, R. (2021). Choanal atresia surgery: outcomes in 42 patients over 20 years and a review of the literature. *European Archives of Oto-Rhino-Laryngology, 278*(7), 2347–2356.

Aumar, M., Nicolas, N., Sfeir, R., Seguy, D., & Gottrand, F. (2021). Long term digestive outcome of oesophageal atresia. *Best Practice and Research Clinical Gastroenterology*, 101771. doi: 10.1016/j.bpg.2021.101771.

Australian Institute of Health and Welfare (AIHW). (2021). Stillbirths and neonatal deaths. <https://www.aihw.gov.au/reports/mothers-babies/stillbirths-and-neonatal-deaths> (Accessed 3 March 2022).

Bacino, C. A. (2021). Achondroplasia. In: S. Hahn (Ed.), *UpToDate*. Walters Kluwer. <https://www.uptodate.com/contents/achondroplasia#!> (Accessed 3 March 2022).

Bacino, C. A., & Lee, B. (2020). Cytogenetics. In: R. M. Kliegman, J. W. St Geme, N. J. Blum, S. S. Shah, R. C. Tasker, & K. M. Wilson (Eds.), *Nelson textbook of pediatrics* (21st ed., pp. 652–676.e651). Philadelphia, PA: Elsevier.

Backeljauw, P. (2021). Clinical manifestations and diagnosis of Turner syndrome. In: P. J. Snyder, H. V. Firth, & M. E. Geffner (Eds.), *UpToDate*. Walters Kluwer. <https://www.uptodate.com/contents/clinical-manifestations-and-diagnosis-of-turner-syndrome?search> (Accessed 3 March 2022).

Bandari, J., Dangle, P. P., Tennyson, L. E., Correa, A. F., & Cannon, G. M. (2015). Large bladder clot: an unusual presentation of neonatal bilateral renal vein thrombosis – case report and review of literature. *Urology, 86*, 811–813.

Bardhan, A., Bruckner-Tuderman, L., Chapple, I. L., Fine, J. D., Harper, N., Has, C., et al. (2020). Epidermolysis bullosa. *Nature Reviews Disease Primers, 6*(1), 1–27.

Baskin, L. S. (2020a). Congenital ureteropelvic junction obstruction. In: D. Wilcox, & M. S. Kim (Eds.), *UpToDate*. Walters Kluwer. <https://www.uptodate.com/contents/congenital-ureteropelvic-junction-obstruction?search> (Accessed 3 March 2022).

Baskin, L. S. (2020b). Fetal hydronephrosis: postnatal management. In: D. Wilcox, & M. S. Kim (Eds.), *UpToDate*. Walters Kluwer. <https://www.uptodate.com/contents/fetal-hydronephrosis-postnatal-management?search> (Accessed 3 March 2022).

Bhat, V., Moront, M., & Bhandari, V. (2020). Gastroschisis: a state-of-the-art review. *Children (Basel, Switzerland), 7*(12), 302. doi: 10.3390/children7120302.

Bielicki, I. N., Somme, S., Frongia, G., Holland-Cunz, S. G., & Vuille-Dit-Bille, R. N. (2021). Abdominal wall defects – current treatments. *Children, 23*, 8(2), 170. doi: 10.3390/children8020170.

Bischoff, M. (2021). Prepare for the rare: innovation simulation for managing abdominal wall defects. *Neonatal Network, 40*(2), 98–102.

Blackburn, S. T. (2018). *Maternal, fetal, and neonatal physiology: a clinical perspective* (5th ed.). St Louis, MO: Elsevier Saunders.

Boom, J. A. (2020). Microcephaly in infants and children: etiology and evaluation. In: J. E. Drutz, H. V. Firth, & M. C. Patterson (Eds.), *UpToDate*. Walters Kluwer. <https://www.uptodate.com/contents/microcephaly-in-infants-and-children-etiology-and-evaluation?search> (Accessed 3 March 2022).

Borer, J. G. (2020). Surgical management and postoperative outcomes of children with bladder exstrophy. In: L. S. Baskin (Ed.), *UpToDate*. Walters Kluwer. <https://www.uptodate.com/contents/surgical-management-and-postoperative-outcome-of-children-with-bladder-exstrophy?search> (Accessed 3 March 2022).

Boubred, F., & Simeoni, U. (2018). Pathophysiology of fetal and neonatal kidneys. In: G. Buonocore, R. Bracci, & M. Weindling (Eds.), *Neonatology: a practical approach to neonatal diseases* (pp. 1016–1026). Champaign, IL: Springer. doi: 10.1007/978-3-319-18159-2_261-2.

Bowman, R. M. (2021). Myelomeningocele (spina bifida): management and outcome. In: M. C. Patterson, L. E. Weisman, & T. K. Duryea (Eds.), *UpToDate*. Walters Kluwer. <https://www.uptodate.com/contents/myelomeningocele-spina-bifida-management-and-outcome?search> (Accessed 3 March 2022).

Bradshaw, W. T. (2021). Gastrointestinal disorders. In: M. T. Verklan, M. Walden, & S. Forest (Eds.), *Core curriculum for neonatal intensive care nursing* (6th ed., pp. 504–542). St Louis, MO: Elsevier.

Brandt, M. L. (2021). Intestinal malrotation in children. In: J. I. Singer, & M. B. Heyman (Eds.), *UpToDate*. Walters Kluwer. <https://www.uptodate.com/contents/intestinal-malrotation-in-children?search> (Accessed 3 March 2022).

Bromley, B., & Benacerraf, B. (2018). Chromosomal abnormalities. In: C. M. Rumack & D. Levine (Eds.), *Diagnostic ultrasound* (pp. 1088–1114).

Brosens, E., Brouwer, R. W. W., Douben, H., Yolande, V. B., Brooks, A. S., Wijnen, R. M. H., et al. (2021). Heritability and de novo mutations in oesophageal atresia and tracheoesophageal fistula aetiology. *Genes, 12*(10), 1595. doi: 10.3390/genes12101595.

Callen J et al (2000): *Color Atlas of Dermatology*, 2nd ed, Saunders.

Chan, S. A., & Goodyear, H. M. (2015). Infantile haemangioma: their presentation and management. *British Journal of Hospital Medicine, 76*(9), 523–527.

Chopan, M., Sayadi, L., Chim, H., & Buchanan, P. J. (2020). To tie or not to tie: a systematic review of postaxial polydactyly and outcomes of suture ligation versus surgical excision. *Hand (New York, N.Y.), 15*(3), 303–310. doi: 10.1177/1558944718810885.

Chouairi, F., Mercier, M. R., Persing, J. S., Gabrick, K. S., Clune, J., & Alperovich, M. (2020). National patterns in surgical management of syndactyly: a review of 956 cases. *Hand (New York, N.Y.), 15*(5), 666–673. doi: 10.1177/1558944719828003.

Chubarova, A. I. (2019). Neonatal medicine. *IntechOpen*. doi: 10.5772/intechopen.76552.

Chung, D. H. (2022). Pediatric surgery. In: C. M. Townsend, R. D. Beauchamp, B. M. Evers, & K. L. Mattox (Eds.), *Sabiston textbook of surgery* (20th ed., pp. 1844–1882). Philadelphia, PA: Elsevier.

Copp, A. J., Adzick, N. S., Chitty, L. S., Fletcher, J. M., Holmbeck, G. N., & Shaw, G. M. (2015). Spina bifida. *Nature Reviews Disease Primers, 1*, 15007, Figure 1.

Cubo, A. M., Lapresa Alcalde, M. V., Gastaca, I., Rodríguez-Martín, M. O., Martín Seisdedos, M., Velasco Ayuso, M. V. R., et al. (2020). Giant isolated omphalocele: role of prenatal diagnosis in prognostic assessment and perinatal management. *Case Reports in Medicine,* 2020, 4578912. doi: 10.1155/2020/4578912.

Dekonenko, C., & Fraser, J. D. (2020). Approaches for closing gastroschisis. *Advances in Pediatrics, 67*, 123–129. doi: 10.1016/j.yapd.2020.03.005.

Dekonenko, C., Fraser, J. D., Deans, K. J., Fallat, M. E., Helmrath, M., Kabre, R., et al. (2021). Outcomes in gastroschisis: expectations in the postnatal period for simple vs complex gastroschisis. *Journal of Perinatology, 41*(7), 1755–1759. doi: 10.1038/s41372-021-01093-8.

Denyer, J., & Pillay, E. (2012). *Best practice guidelines for skin and wound care in epidermolysis bullosa*. International Consensus, DEBRA. <https://www.wcs-belgie.be/wp-content/uploads/2015/03/Guideline-Wound_Care_-_DEBRA_UK.pdf > (Accessed 3 March 2022).

Dhar, V. (2020). Cleft lip and palate. In: R. M. Kliegman, J. W. St Geme, N. J. Blum, S. S. Shah, R. C. Tasker, & K. M. Wilson (Eds.), *Nelson textbook of pediatrics* (21st ed., pp. 1915–1917. e1911). Philadelphia, PA: Elsevier.

Dingeldein, M. (2020). Selected gastrointestinal anomalies in the neonate. In: R. J. Martin, A. A. Fanaroff, & M. C. Walsh (Eds.), *Fanaroff and Martin's neonatal–perinatal medicine* (pp. 1541–1570). St Louis, MO: Mosby Elsevier.

Ditzenberger, G. R. (2018). Gastrointestinal and hepatic systems and perinatal nutrition. In: S. T. Blackburn (Ed.), *Maternal, fetal, and neonatal physiology: a clinical perspective* (5th ed., pp. 387–420). Philadelphia, PA: Elsevier.

Driscoll, D. A., & Simpson, J. L. (2021). Genetic screening and diagnosis. In: M. B. Landon, H. L. Galan, E. R. M. Jauniaux, D. A. Driscoll, V. Berghella, W. A. Grobman, et al. (Eds.), *Gabbe's obstetrics: normal and problem pregnancies* (8th ed., pp. 180–201). Philadelphia, PA: Elsevier.

Dukhovny, S., & Wilkins-Haug, L. (2021). Open neural tube defects: risk factors, prenatal screening and diagnosis, and pregnancy management. In: D. Levine, & L. L. Simpson (Eds.), *UpToDate*. Walters Kluwer. <https://www.uptodate.com/contents/open-neural-tube-defects-risk-factors-prenatal-screening-and-diagnosis-and-pregnancy-management?search> (Accessed 3 March 2022).

Duncan, K., Polites, S., Krishnaswami, S., & Scottoline, B. (2021). Congenital diaphragmatic hernia management: a systematic review and care pathway description including volume-targeted ventilation. *Advances in Neonatal Care, 21*, E138–E143. doi: 10.1097/ANC.0000000000000863.

Eichenfield, L. F., Frieden, I. J., Zaenglein, A. L., & Mathes, E. (2015). *Neonatal and infant dermatology* (3rd ed.). Philadelphia, PA: Elsevier Saunders.

Ellenbogen, R. G. (2019). Neural tube defects in the neonatal period: treatment and management. In: T. Rosenkrantz (Ed.), *Medscape*. <https://emedicine.medscape.com/article/1825866-treatment#d12>. (Accessed 3 March 2022).

Environmental Health Intelligence New Zealand. (2020). Birth defects ascertained among livebirths, 2012–2019. <https://www.ehinz.ac.nz/projects/new-zealand-congenital-anomalies-registry/data-2/>. (Accessed 3 March 2022).

Evans, K. N., Hing, A. V., & Cunningham, M. L. (2018). Craniofacial malformations. In: C. A. Gleason & S. E. Juul (Eds.), *Avery's diseases of the newborn* (10th ed., pp. 1417–1437. e1412). Philadelphia, PA: Elsevier.

Ferguson, M. (2017). Nursing management of gastroschisis in the newborn. *Journal of Neonatal Nursing, 23*(1), 40–45. doi: 10.1016/j.jnn.2016.08.004.

Fraser, D. (2021). Respiratory distress. In: M. T. Verklan, M. Walden, & S. Forest (Eds.), *Core curriculum for neonatal intensive care nursing* (6th ed., pp. 394–416). St Louis, MO: Elsevier.

Gallagher, M. E., Pacetti, A. S., Lovvorn, H. N., & Carter, B. S. (2021). Neonatal surgery. In: *Merenstein & Gardner's handbook of neonatal intensive care nursing: an interprofessional approach* (9th ed., pp. 996–1038). St Louis, MO: Elsevier.

Gatti, J. M., & Kirsch, A. J. (2021). Hypospadias. In: M. Cendron (Ed.), *Medscape*. <https://emedicine.medscape.com/article/1015227-overview> (Accessed 3 March 2022).

Gerall, C. D., Stewart, L. A., Price, J., Kabagambe, S., Sferra, S. R., Schmaedick, M. J., et al. (2021). Long-term outcomes of congenital diaphragmatic hernia: a single institution experience. *Journal of Pediatric Surgery*, S0022-3468(21) 00473-5. doi: 10.1016/j.jpedsurg.2021.06.007.

Grollemund, B., Dissaux, C., Gavelle, P., Martínez, C. P., Mullaert, J., Alfaiate, P., et al. (2020). The impact of having a baby with cleft lip and palate on parents and on parent–baby relationship: the first French prospective multicentre study. *BMC Pediatrics, 20*, 230. doi: 10.1186/s12887-020-02118-5.

Guarino, S., Capalbo, D., Martin, N., Campana, G., Rambaldi, P. F., Del Giudice, E. M., et al. (2020). In children with urinary tract infection reduced kidney length and vesicoureteric reflux predict abnormal DMSA scan. *Pediatric Research, 87*(4), 779–784.

Gunawardena, R. M. T. M., Weerawardhana, P. A. Y. P., & Lamahewage, A. K. (2019). Paediatric pelvi-ureteric junction obstruction. *Sri Lanka Journal of Child Health, 48*(2), 100–104.

Haight, C. (1944). Congenital atresia of the oesophagus with tracheoesophageal fistula: reconstruction of oesophageal continuity by primary anastomosis. *Annals of Surgery, 120*, 623–652.

Hammoud, M., & Gerken, J. (2021). Inguinal hernia. In: *StatPearls*. Treasure Island, FL: StatPearls Publishing. <https://www.ncbi.nlm.nih.gov/books/NBK513332/> (Accessed 3 March 2022).

Haridas, A., & Tomita, T. (2020). Hydrocephalus in children: management and prognosis. In: M. C. Patterson (Ed.), *UpToDate*. Walters Kluwer. <https://www.uptodate.com/contents/hydrocephalus-in-children-management-and-prognosis?search> (Accessed 3 March 2022).

Hassan, A. A., Mahmoud, N. A. S., Sabry, A. H., & Nashed, D. S. S. (2021). Meta analysis study of complications following repair of mid penile hypospadius using different surgical techniques. *Quarterly Journal of Medicine, 114*(suppl 1), hcab105.006. doi: 10.1093/qjmed/hcab105.006.

Hedrick, H. L., & Adzick, N. S. (2021). Congenital diaphragmatic hernia in the neonate. In: L. E. Weisman (Ed.), *UpToDate*. Walters Kluwer. <https://www.uptodate.com/contents/congenital-diaphragmatic-hernia-in-the-neonate?search> (Accessed 3 March 2022).

Heron, M. (2018). Deaths: leading causes for 2016. *National Vital Statistics Reports, 67*, 1–76.

Hijkoop, A., Peters, N. C. J., Lechner, R. L., van Bever, Y., van Gils-Frijters, A. P. J. M., Tibboel, D., et al. (2018). Omphalocele: from diagnosis to growth and development at 2 years of age. *Archives of Disease in Childhood – Fetal–Neonatal Edition, 104*(1), F18–F23. doi: 10.1136/archdischild-2017-314700.

Hills, B., & Tomei, K. (2020). Spinal dysraphisms. In: R. J. Martin, A. A. Fanaroff, & M. C. Walsh (Eds.), *Fanaroff and Martin's neonatal–perinatal medicine* (pp. 1073–1080). St Louis, MO: Mosby Elsevier.

Iannetti, G., Fadda, M. T., Della Monaca, M., & Bosco G. (2018). Orofacial malformations. In: G. Buonocore, R. Bracci, & M. Weindling (Eds.), *Neonatology: a practical approach to neonatal diseases* (pp. 664–674). Champaign, IL: Springer.

IJsselstijn, H., Gischler, S. J., Toussaint, L., Spoel, M., van der Cammen-van Zijp, M. H. M., & Tibboel, D. (2016). Growth and development after oesophageal atresia surgery: need for long-term multidisciplinary follow-up. *Paediatric Respiratory Reviews, 19*, 34–38.

Irace, A. L., Dombrowski, N. D., Kawai, K., Watters, K., Chou, S., Perez, J., et al. (2019). Evaluation of aspiration in infants with laryngomalacia and recurrent respiratory and feeding difficulties. *JAMA Otolaryngology Head and Neck Surgery, 145*(2), 146–151. doi: 10.1001/jamaoto.2018.3642.

Jawade, K. S., Muqtadir, A. M., Jadhav, S. P., & Raut, A. B. (2017). Congenital hypertrophic pyloric stenosis at a tertiary care hospital: a surgical experience with 30 infants. *Journal of Medical Science and Clinical Research, 5*, 9. doi: 0.18535/jmscr/v5i9.99.

Jones, T., on behalf of Council of International Neonatal Nurses, Inc. (COINN) Working Group. (2019). International neonatal nursing competency framework. *Journal of Neonatal Nursing, 25*, 258–264. doi: 10.1016/j.jnn.2019.07.007.

Kinsman, S. L., & Johnston, M. V. (2020). Congenital anomalies of the central nervous system. In R. Kliegman, J. W. St Geme, N. J. Blum, S. S. Shah, R. C. Tasker, & K. M. Wilson (Eds.), *Nelson textbook of pediatrics* (21st ed., pp. 3063–3082. e3061). Philadelphia, PA: Elsevier.

Kliegman, R. M., St Geme, J. W., Blum, N. J., Shah, S. S., Tasker, R. C., & Wilson, K. M. (2020). Pyloric stenosis and other congenital anomalies of the stomach. In: R. M. Kliegman, J. W. St Geme, N. J. Blum, S. S. Shah, R. C. Tasker, & K. M. Wilson (Eds.), *Nelson textbook of pediatrics* (21st ed., pp. 1946–1950.e1941). Philadelphia, PA: Elsevier.

Kowalska, M., Dębek, W., & Matuszczak, E. (2021). Infantile hemangiomas: an update on pathogenesis and treatment. *Journal of Clinical Medicine, 10*(20), 4631. doi: 10.3390/jcm10204631.

Kutti Sridharan, G., & Rokkam, V. R. (2021). Macroglossia. In: *StatPearls*. Treasure Island, FL: StatPearls Publishing. <https://www.ncbi.nlm.nih.gov/books/NBK560545/>. (Accessed 3 March 2022).

Läckgren, G., Cooper, C. S., Neveus, T. & Kirsch, A. J. (2021). Management of vesicoureteral reflux: what have we learned over the last 20 years? *Frontiers in Pediatrics, 9*, 228.

Léauté-Labrèze, C., Harper, J. I., & Hoeger, P. H. (2017). Infantile haemangioma. *Lancet, 390*(10089), 85–94.

Longoni, M., Pober, B. R., & High, F. A. (2020). Congenital diaphragmatic hernia overview. In: M. P. Adam, H. H. Ardinger, R. A. Pagon, et al. (Eds.), *GeneReviews@*. Seattle, WA: University of Washington, Seattle. <https://www.ncbi.nlm.nih.gov/books/NBK1359> (Accessed 3 March 2022).

Luu, M., & Frieden, I. J. (2013). Haemangioma: clinical course, complications, and management. *British Journal of Dermatology, 169*(1), 20–30.

Madan-Khetarpal, S., & Arnold, G. (2018). Genetic disorders and dysmorphic conditions. In: B. J. Zitelli, S. C. McIntire, & A. J. Nowalk (Eds.), *Zitelli and Davis' atlas of pediatric physical diagnosis* (8th ed., pp. 1–43). Philadelphia, PA: Elsevier.

Maheshwari, A., & Carlo, W. A. (2018). Diaphragmatic hernia. In R. M. Kliegman, B. F. Stanton, J. W. St Geme III, et al. [Eds.], *Nelson textbook of pediatrics* [20th ed.]. Philadelphia: Elsevier.

Mattoo, T. K., & Greenfield, S. P. (2021). Clinical presentation, diagnosis, and course of primary vesicoureteral reflux. In: L. S. Baskin, & F. B. Stapleton (Eds.), *UpToDate*. Walters

Kluwer. <https://www.uptodate.com/contents/clinical-presentation-diagnosis-and-course-of-primary-vesicoureteral-reflux?search> (Accessed 3 March 2022).

Mehta, P. A., & Sharma, G. (2021). Congenital pulmonary airway malformation. In: *StatPearls*. Treasure Island, FL: StatPearls Publishing. <https://www.ncbi.nlm.nih.gov/books/NBK551664/> (Accessed 3 March 2022).

Metry, D. W. (2021). Infantile hemangiomas: management. In: M. L. Levy (Ed.), *UpToDate*. Walters Kluwer. <https://www.uptodate.com/contents/infantile-hemangiomas-management?search> (Accessed 3 March 2022).

Nagy, M. R., & Saleh, A. E. (2021). Hydrocephalus associated with occipital encephalocele: surgical management and clinical outcome. *Egyptian Journal of Neurosurgery, 36*, 6. doi: 10.1186/s41984-021-00101-5.

Nelson, C. P., & Koo, H. P. (2020). Pediatric vesicoureteral reflux workup. In: M. L. Windle & M. D. Bomalaski (Eds.), *Medscape*. <https://emedicine.medscape.com/article/1016439-workup#c4>. (Accessed 3 March 2022).

Nepple, K. G., & Cooper, C. S. (2021). Evaluation and diagnosis of bladder dysfunction in children. In: L. S. Baskin & T. K. Mattoo (Eds.), *UpToDate*. Walters Kluwer. <https://www.uptodate.com/contents/evaluation-and-diagnosis-of-bladder-dysfunction-in-children?search>. (Accessed 3 March 2022).

Netter, F. H. (2019). Abdomen study guide. In: F. H. Netter (Ed.), *Atlas of human anatomy* (7th ed., pp. e62–e81). Philadelphia, PA: Elsevier.

Nguyen, H. T., Herndon, C. D., Cooper, C., Gatti, J., Kirsch, A., Kokorowski, P., et al. (2010). The Society for Fetal Urology consensus statement on the evaluation and management of antenatal hydronephrosis. *Journal of Pediatric Urology, 6*(3), 212–231.

Niaudet, P. (2021). Renal cystic diseases in children. In: T. K. Mattoo (Ed.), *UpToDate*. Walters Kluwer. <https://www.uptodate.com/contents/renal-cystic-diseases-in-children?search>. (Accessed 3 March 2022).

Núñez-Martínez, P. M., García-Delgado, C., Morán-Barroso, V. F., & Jasso-Gutiérrez, L. (2016). Congenital macroglossia: clinical features and therapeutic strategies in pediatric patients. *Boletín Médico Del Hospital Infantil de México (English Edition), 73*(3), 212–216. doi: 10.1016/j.bmhime.2017.08.003.

Okuyama, H. (2016). Intestinal atresia and stenosis. In: T. Taguchi, T. Iwanaks, & T. Okamatsu (Eds.), *Operative general surgery in neonates and infants* (pp. 199–205). Tokyo: Springer Japan.

Ostermaier, K. K. (2020). Down syndrome: management. In: H. V. Firth, & J. E. Drutz (Eds.), *UpToDate*. Walters Kluwer. <https://www.uptodate.com/contents/down-syndrome-management?search=Down%20syndrome:%20management&source=search> (Accessed 3 March 2022).

Parikh, S., & Batra, P. (2022). Achondroplasia. In: F. Talavera, & G. H. Thompson (Eds.), *Medscape*. <https://emedicine.medscape.com/article/1258401-overview#a1> (Accessed 3 March 2022).

Patterson, M. C. (2021). Sturge–Weber syndrome. In: M. L. Levy (Ed.), *UpToDate*. Walters Kluwer. <https://www.uptodate.com/contents/sturge-weber-syndrome?search5Sturge–Weber%20syndrome&source5search> (Accessed 3 March 2022).

Prasad, P., Mori, M., & Toriello, H. V. (2021). Focused revision: policy statement on folic acid and neural tube defects. *Genetics in Medicine, 23*(12), 2464–2466.

Promm, M., & Roesch, W. H. (2019). Recent trends in the management of bladder exstrophy: the Gordian knot has not yet been cut. *Frontiers in Pediatrics, 7*, 110.

Psooy, K., & Collaboration with the Pediatric Urologists of Canada (PUC). (2016). Multicystic dysplastic kidney (MCDK) in the neonate: the role of the urologist. *Canadian Urological Association Journal, 10*(1–2), 18–24. doi: 10.5489/cuaj.3520.

Queremel Milani, D. A., & Chauhan, P. R. (2021). Genetics, mosaicism. In: *StatPearls*. Treasure Island, FL: StatPearls Publishing. <https://www.statpearls.com/ArticleLibrary/viewarticle/22173> (Accessed 3 March 2022).

Ramji, J., & Joshi, R. S. (2021). Laparoscopic pyloromyotomy for congenital hypertrophic pyloric stenosis: our experience with twenty cases. *African Journal of Paediatric Surgery, 18*(1), 14–17. doi: 10.4103/ajps.AJPS_119_20.

Reimer, A., Fliesser, M., & Hoeger, P. H. (2016). Anatomical patterns of infantile hemangioma (IH) of the extremities (IHE). *Journal of the American Academy of Dermatology, 75*(3), 556–563.

Rodgers C.C. (2018). The child with gastrointestinal dysfunction. In: Hockenberry M and Wilson D (eds.) *Wong's Nursing Care of Infants and Children*, 11th ed, pp. 825–882. St Louis: Elsevier Inc.

Rodprasert, W., Virtanen, H. E., Mäkelä, J. A., & Toppari, J. (2020). Hypogonadism and cryptorchidism. *Frontiers in Endocrinology (Lausanne), 15*(10), 906. doi: 10.3389/fendo.2019.00906.

Rosenblum, N. D. (2021). Overview of congenital anomalies of the kidney and urinary tract (CAKUT). In: T. K. Mattoo, & L. S. Baskin (Eds.), *UpToDate*. Walters Kluwer. <https://www.uptodate.com/contents/overview-of-congenital-anomalies-of-the-kidney-and-urinary-tract-cakut?search> (Accessed 3 March 2022).

Sabharwal, S., & Schwarzenberg, S. J. (2021). Cystic fibrosis: overview of gastrointestinal disease. In: G. B. Mallory, & M. B. Heyman (Eds.), *UpToDate*. Walters Kluwer. <https://www.uptodate.com/contents/cystic-fibrosis-overview-of-gastrointestinal-disease?search> (Accessed 3 March 2022).

Sables-Baus S. and Fidanza S. J. (2020) Alterations of digestive function in children. In: Huether S. and McCance K. (eds.) *Understanding Pathophysiology*, 7th ed, pp. 916–932. St Louis: Mosby.

Sawyer C. W. (2020) Hemolytic disorders and congenital anomalies. In: Lowdermilk D., Cashion M. C., Perry S. et al (eds.) *Maternity and Women's Health Care*, 12th ed, pp. 784–804. St Louis: Mosby.

Schendel, S. A. (2019). Beckwith–Wiedemann syndrome. *International Journal of Oral and Maxillofacial Surgery, 48*(12), 1606–1607. doi: 10.1016/j.ijom.2019.05.013.

Shen, S., Xiao, W., Zhang, L., Lu, J., Funk, A., He , J., et al. (2021). Prevalence of congenital microcephaly and its risk factors in an area at risk of Zika outbreaks. *BMC Pregnancy and Childbirth, 21*, 214. doi: 10.1186/s12884-021-03705-9.

Shute, W., Wong, E., Agar, N., & Singh, N. (2021). Unilateral choanal atresia first diagnosed in adulthood and repaired via endoscopic posterior septectomy – a case series and review of the literature. *Australian Journal of Otolaryngology, 4*, 10.21037/ajo-20-63.

Singh, V. (2020). *Textbook of clinical embryology* (2nd ed.). St Louis, MO: Elsevier.

Soliman, N. A., Ali, R. I., Ghobriol, E. E., Habib, E. I., & Ziada, A. M. (2015). Pattern of clinical presentation of congenital anomalies of the kidney and urinary tract among infants and children. *Nephrology, 20*, 413–418.

Stephenson, C. D., Lockwood, C. J., & MacKenzie, A. P. (2021). Gastroschisis. In: L. W. Haug, & D. Levine (Eds.), *UpToDate*. Walters Kluwer. <https://www.uptodate.com/contents/Gastroschisis> (Accessed 3 June 2021).

Sugimoto, K., Enya, T., Joh, K., Miyazaki, K., Miyazawa, T., Ohshima, R., et al. (2021). Pathophysiological clinical features of an infant with hypertension secondary to multicystic dysplastic kidney: a case report. *BMC Nephrology, 22*, 55. doi: 10.1186/s12882-021-02249-6.

Sullivan, M. A., & Adkinson, J. M. (2017). A systematic review and comparison of outcomes following simple syndactyly reconstruction with skin grafts or a dorsal metacarpal advancement flap. *Journal of Hand Surgery – America, 42*(1), 34–40.e6. doi: 10.1016/j.jhsa.2016.11.006.

Sumfest, J. M., Rukstalis, D. B., & Kolon, T. F. (2020). Crypotorchidism. In: E. D. Kim (Ed.), *Medscape*. <https://emedicine.medscape.com/article/438378-overview> (Accessed 3 March 2022).

Tatekawa, Y. (2019). Surgical strategy of urachal remnants in children. *Journal of Surgical Case Reports, 7*, rjz222. doi: 10.1093/jscr/rjz222.

Thompson, A., Thakkar, H., Khan, H., & Yardley, I. E. (2019). Not all neonates with oesophageal atresia and tracheoesophageal fistula are a surgical emergency. *Journal of Pediatric Surgery, 54*(2), 244–246. doi: 10.1016/j.jpedsurg.2018.10.074.

Toi, A., & Levine, D. (2018). The fetal brain. In: C. M. Rumack, & D. Levine (Eds.), *Diagnostic ultrasound* (pp. 1166–1215). Philadelphia, PA: Elsevier.

Tolarova, M. M., Al-Kharafi, L., Tolar, M., & Boyd, C. (2020). Pediatric cleft lip and palate treatment and management. In: R. G. Elluru (Ed.), *Medscape*. <https://emedicine.medscape.com/article/995535-treatment#d11> (Accessed 3 March 2022).

Tomita, T., & Ogiwara, H. (2021). Primary (congenital) encephalocele. In: M. C. Patterson, & L. E. Weisman (Eds.), *UpToDate*. Walters Kluwer. <https://www.uptodate.com/contents/primary-congenital-encephalocele?search> (Accessed 3 March 2022).

van Lennep, M., Singendonk, M. M. J., Dall'Oglio, L., Gottrand, F., Krishnan, U., Terheggen-Lagro, S. W. J., et al. (2019). Oesophageal atresia. *Nature Reviews Disease Primers, 5*, 26. doi: 10.1038/s41572-019-0077-0.

Vic Health. (2022). Gastroschisis in neonates. <https://www.bettersafercare.vic.gov.au/clinical-guidance/neonatal/gastroschisis-in-neonates> (Accessed 3 March 2022).

Wallis, C., Alexopoulou, E., Antón-Pacheco, J. L., Bhatt, J. M., Bush, A., Chang, A. B., et al. (2019). ERS statement on tracheomalacia and bronchomalacia in children. *European Respiratory Journal, 54*(3), 1900382. doi: 10.1183/13993003.00382-2019.

Wesson, D. E. (2021). Intestinal atresia. In: J. A. Garcia-Prats, & M. B. Heyman (Eds.), *UpToDate*. Walters Kluwer. <https://www.uptodate.com/contents/intestinal-atresia?search>. (Accessed 3 March 2022).

Wesson, D. E., & Lopez, M. E. (2021). Congenital aganglionic megacolon (Hirschsprung disease). In: J. I. Singer (Ed.), *UpToDate*. Walters Kluwer. <https://www.uptodate.com/contents/congenital-aganglionic-megacolon-hirschsprung-disease?search> (Accessed 3 March 2022).

Wood, R. J., & Levitt, M. A. (2020). Surgery for pediatric anorectal malformation (imperforate anus). In: E. S. Kim (Ed.), *Medscape*. <https://emedicine.medscape.com/article/933524-overview> (Accessed 3 March 2022).

World Health Organization (WHO). (2016). World Health Organization: congenital anomalies. Geneva: WHO.

Xie, J., Wu, Y., & Wu, C. (2020). Is thoracoscopy superior to thoracotomy in the treatment of congenital lung malformations? An updated meta-analysis. *Therapeutic Advances in Respiratory Disease*. doi: 10.1177/1753466620980267.

Zallmann, M., Leventer, R. J., Mackay, M. T., Ditchfield, M., Bekhor, P. S., & Su, J. C. (2018). Screening for Sturge–Weber syndrome: a state-of-the-art review. *Pediatric Dermatology, 35*(1), 30–42.

Zhang, H., Zhang, L., & Guo, N. (2020). Validation of "urinary tract dilation" classification system: correlation between fetal hydronephrosis and postnatal urological abnormalities. *Medicine (Baltimore), 99*(2), e18707. doi: 10.1097/MD.0000000000018707.

CHAPTER 18

NEONATAL PAIN MANAGEMENT

DENISE HARRISON AND LISA-KIM WRIGHT

Learning objectives

After reading this chapter you will be able to:

- understand sources of pain and the epidemiology of painful procedures and pain management practices
- understand existing evidence for the pathophysiology of pain and short- and long-term adverse effects of pain
- discuss pain assessment using behavioural, physiological and cortical measures and their research application and clinical application
- revise effective strategies to reduce pain and distress
- contribute to improving pain management practices in the clinical setting.

Key words, terms and abbreviations

allodynia
analgesia
analgesics
gestational age (GA)
healthcare provider/professional (HCP)
hyperalgesia
neonatal intensive care unit (NICU)
pain
skin-to-skin care (SSC)

'If a new skin in old people be tender, what is it you think in a newborn Babe? Doth a small thing pain you so much on a finger, how painful is it then to a Child, which is tormented all the body over, which hath but a tender new grown flesh? If such a perfect Child is tormented so soon, what shall we think of a Child, which stayed not in the womb its full time? Surely it is twice worse with him.'

Felix Wurtz (1612). *The children's book*

INTRODUCTION

Neonatal **pain** is increasingly recognised as causing harm in both the short and long term. Short-term effects of pain include behavioural distress and physiological changes, which can lead to physiological compromise. Long-term adverse effects were highlighted in a systematic review of 13 studies, indicating that the number of painful procedures preterm neonates undergo is the strongest predictor of poor outcomes, ranging from structural differences in the brain itself to cognitive, behavioural, emotional and learning disabilities (Valeri et al., 2015). Painful and invasive procedures for monitoring, diagnostic and therapeutic interventions are an inevitable part of care in the neonatal unit; however, the interdisciplinary healthcare team has a responsibility to prevent or minimise pain during these procedures.

Evidence from systematic reviews (Benoit et al., 2017; Harrison et al., 2017; Johnston et al., 2017; Stevens et al., 2016) and clinical practice guidelines (American Academy of Pediatrics (AAP), 2016; Balice-Bourgois et al., 2020) have been distilled into **healthcare provider/professional (HCP)** and parent-targeted knowledge translation tools (Bueno et al., 2020; Gagnon et al., 2020) to inform best newborn pain management practices. Access to effective pain management has been long assumed as a fundamental human right (Brennan et al., 2019). As stated by Brennan and colleagues, 'The ethical responsibility of clinicians to manage pain is well understood and a basic element of ethical codes' (Brennan et al., 2019, p. 62). Our mission as neonatal nurses and midwives is to *use* the knowledge, implement effective evidence-based pain management and support parents to be involved in pain care. Practice changes happen at all levels of an organisation; however, neonatal nurses and midwives are best placed to prioritise pain management and optimise practices. Neonatal clinicians need to partner with each other, interdisciplinary teams, leaders and managers, professional organisations and, most importantly, with parents of the newborns. Facilitating parents' role during painful procedures requires close partnership with neonatal clinicians and organisations, co-development of resources to ensure information is relevant and suitable for parental health literacy, and truly embracing family-centred care. Moving neonatal pain knowledge into action is not only an ethical and professional imperative, but it also has the potential to improve outcomes for the smallest patients. According to the new revised International Association for the Study of Pain definition, pain is defined as 'An unpleasant sensory and emotional experience associated with or resembling that associated with actual or potential tissue damage' (Raja et al., 2020, p. 1977).

Understanding this term and how it applies to all neonates, whether preterm or term, sick or healthy, is important knowledge for this chapter.

HISTORICAL PERSPECTIVE AND SOURCES OF NEONATAL PAIN

Neonatal pain management and research has evolved since the controversial, much cited and what would now be considered unethical, studies by Anand and colleagues (Anand et al., 1987; Anand & Hickey, 1992) in the 1980s and early 1990s. These seminal studies demonstrated that neonates undergoing surgery without anaesthesia or **analgesia** had higher rates of morbidity and mortality compared with infants administered these agents. However, it was the power of a parent's voice that brought unethical treatment of neonatal pain to the world's attention. Jill Lawson (1986), mother of Jeffrey, born at 26 weeks' **gestational age (GA)**, who underwent surgery for ligation of a patent ductus arteriosus without analgesia or anaesthesia, highlighted to the healthcare community and the public, seriously inadequate pain management practices. Following her public lobbying for change, the use of anaesthesia and analgesia became routine for neonatal surgery. However, challenges remain in consistently preventing and treating pain associated with commonly performed procedures, including those considered 'minor'. Such repetitive procedures, including heel lance, venepuncture, airway suctioning, arterial stabs, feeding tube insertion and eye examinations, remain a major source of undertreated pain in this patient population.

CLINICAL PRACTICE 18.1

Pain during repeated painful procedures is under-recognised and under-treated. This burden of under-treated pain places preterm and sick neonates at risk of significant adverse short- and long-term effects.

EPIDEMIOLOGY OF PAINFUL PROCEDURES

A systematic review of 18 epidemiological neonatal pain studies reported that neonates in a **neonatal intensive care unit (NICU)** underwent an average of 7 to 17 painful procedures per day, with minimal or inconsistent use of recommended pain management strategies (Cruz et al., 2016; see Evidence-based Practice Research 18.1). Recommendations for future research included focusing on minimising this burden in partnership with parents and the interdisciplinary healthcare team. For studies reporting more frequent use of pain management strategies, sucrose was the agent used (Courtois et al., 2016; Roofthooft et al., 2014). A study from the Netherlands reported that sucrose is considered a standard of care for all minor procedures (Roofthooft et al., 2014). Minimal to no use of breastfeeding or **skin-to-skin care (SSC)** during painful procedures was reported in all studies. Barriers reported by nurses to performing blood sampling while babies are breastfeeding or being held skin to skin include a lack of knowledge, lack of skill, perception that parents did not want to be there and preferences to complete blood work without having to organise parental participation (Harrison et al., 2015a; Lavin Venegas et al., 2019a).

FAMILY-CENTRED CARE 18.1

Nurses/midwives are in a key position to facilitate and support parents to be present and to participate in comforting their babies during painful procedures.

EVIDENCE-BASED PRACTICE RESEARCH 18.1

A systematic review (Cruz et al., 2016) included 18 studies reporting on the epidemiology of procedural pain in neonates. The studies were published between 1995 and 2014, and were from 13 different countries. The most-performed painful procedure across all studies was heel lances. No treatment for any procedures was reported in these five studies.

Pathophysiology of pain, and short- and long-term adverse effects

Resuscitation of the newborn is now generally considered from 23 weeks' gestation onwards (Mactier et al., 2020). These extremely preterm infants require many weeks to months of neonatal intensive care unit (NICU) and special care baby unit (SCBU) care, including necessary painful procedures for extensive monitoring and care. From these very low gestational ages (GAs) to term (40 weeks) the neonatal brain grows rapidly, undergoing active and complex developmental events. The constant changes during brain maturation render it highly susceptible to injury and effects of pain. In a systematic review including 13 studies, Valeri et al. (2015) reported that the number of painful procedures was the strongest predictor of poor neurological outcomes in the preterm neonate. This highlights that consistent management of pain using effective and recommended interventions is vital for the wellbeing of these extremely preterm neonates. Although less is known about the cumulative effects of painful procedures in the sick term neonate, neonatal clinicians have a responsibility to these more-mature neonates to ensure all pain is minimised using the most effective and evidence-based interventions.

It is over three decades since the seminal paper on nociceptive activity and its resultant physiological stress response was published by Anand and Hickey (1987). Nociception is the anatomical and physiological process of coding noxious stimuli, and involves the peripheral nervous system, spinal cord and brain (Walker, 2019). Nociceptors (pain receptors) are present throughout the body and include A-delta (A-δ) fibres (fast-conducting myelinated fibres) responsible for sharp pain and C fibres (slow-conducting non-myelinated fibres) responsible for transmitting noxious mechanical, thermal and chemical stimuli to the spinal cord. These nociceptive receptors are positioned in the epidermis in preterm neonates, then recede at around term gestation into the dermis. This means that preterm neonates are more sensitive to pain compared with term neonates and with adults, and pain can also be evoked by tactile and non-painful procedures (Fitzgerald, 2015). In addition, the spread of responses is much greater and more disorganised in neonates, especially preterm neonates (Cornelissen et al., 2013). Tissue injury and inflammation caused by repeated stimuli such as heel lance can lead to primary **hyperalgesia** – that is, increased sensitivity of the affected area (Walker, 2014). This may persist for several weeks after the initial injury and can result in **allodynia**, in which a non-noxious stimulus elicits a pain response (Cornelissen et al., 2013). This prolonged response after the initial tissue injury is described by Hatfield et al. (2019) in an overview of the effects of neonatal pain.

CLINICAL PRACTICE 18.2

Nurses' and midwives' competence in neonatal pain treatment in the NICU was studied in connection to knowledge, attitudes, actions and perceptions of competence in a recent systematic review. Nurses and midwives' characteristics, under-utilised pain assessment methods and organisational variables were shown to be barriers to successful neonatal pain management. Clear evidence-based guidelines/protocols, adequate training and the use of appropriate and accurate pain assessment tools were all found to be potential facilitators to effective neonatal pain management. Involvement of parents and a team approach to neonatal pain management were also found to be beneficial.

These findings show that more research is needed to address the barriers to improve newborn pain treatment and increase facilitators (Mala et al., 2021).

Pain inhibition

The neonatal pain experience is intensified by reduced discrimination between noxious and non-noxious stimuli and a lack of pain modulation. Descending inhibitory tracts, which in adults suppress transmission of noxious stimuli, are not fully functional, even at term. This reduced descending inhibition leads to more-widespread responses to pain and may lead to increased sensitivity to acute pain (Fitzgerald, 2015). The most-immature neonates with the least ability to modulate pain are subject to the highest number of painful procedures (Cruz et al., 2016).

When pain is inflicted, there are numerous consequences. These include immediate physiological effects, including sympathetic nervous system stimulation responses. The sympathetic division of the autonomic nervous system is stimulated, which results in increased heart rate, blood pressure, respiration rate and oxygen consumption (Inder et al., 2018). These immediate effects put an increased demand on the cardiorespiratory system in already compromised neonates. Variations in heart rate and blood pressure can lead to an increase in intracranial pressure, predisposing neonates to increased risk of intraventricular haemorrhage. The germinal matrix (most active between 8 and 28 weeks and involuted by 36 weeks) is highly vascular and therefore susceptible to injury (Inder et al., 2018).

CLINICAL PRACTICE 18.3

Be careful of 'clustering procedures' (combining painful procedures and handling) and allow neonates sufficient time to recover between painful stimuli and handling. Stressed neonates may respond to handling the same way they do to painful procedures.

Long-term effects of under-treated pain

It is becoming increasingly evident that there are long-term adverse effects of under-treated pain for infants born preterm. A systematic review examining associations between neonatal pain exposure and developmental outcomes included 13 studies and showed that greater numbers of painful procedures were associated with poor neurodevelopmental outcomes (Valeri et al., 2015). Specifically, results showed that, controlling for confounders such as severity of illness, respiratory support and GA, associations between higher pain exposure and the following were demonstrated (Valeri et al., 2015):

- reduction in grey and white matter
- reduction in postnatal growth
- reduction in cognitive and motor function and reduced visual-perceptual abilities
- persistent alteration to the hypothalamic–pituitary–adrenal axis function, resulting in altered cortisol levels
- hyperalgesia later in childhood.

Five of the included studies measured early developmental outcomes, up to term equivalent, and eight studies measured later developmental outcomes, between 4 months and up to almost 8 years of life. Under-recognised and under-treated pain also has the potential to exacerbate other comorbidities including intracranial haemorrhage. For neonates whose cognition is not compromised, many exhibit detrimental alterations in pain sensitivity in early childhood. Although it is becoming increasingly evident that, for infants born preterm, pain exposure has a negative impact on development throughout infancy and early childhood, less is known about the impact of neonatal pain exposure on sick term infants.

CLINICAL PRACTICE 18.4

The most important 'take-home message' regarding pain exposure in the preterm neonate is that the number of painful procedures is the strongest predictor of poor outcomes (Valeri et al., 2015).

REFLECTION

Consider how you can reduce the burden of pain in neonates for whom you are caring.

Pain assessment

It is incontrovertible that neonates feel pain; however, how to *accurately* assess neonatal pain remains one of the most difficult challenges facing clinicians (Bellieni & Johnston, 2016).

Amid supportive medical equipment and unable to communicate pain verbally, the vulnerable neonate relies on clinicians to identify potentially painful treatments, quantify pain levels and provide and assess the efficacy of pain-relieving strategies. This is a professional and ethical responsibility whereby the proficient nurse 'engages in ethical and lawful practice at all times' (Standard 11, Professional, ethics and legal practice, Council of International Neonatal Nurses (COINN), 2019, p. 262).

REFLECTION

If an adult does not find a procedure painful, does this mean we can assume no pain in a neonate undergoing the same procedure? Consider the presence of pain receptors in the epidermis of preterm neonates and the lack of the pain modulation mechanism.

Routine pain assessment continues to be infrequently performed. A study including 243 NICUs in 18 European countries reported that only 10% of the 6500 included infants had a daily pain assessment (Anand et al., 2017). In a survey of pain assessment and pain management practices conducted in the USA, including 237 nurses, the majority reported that they used pain assessment tools regularly; however, some nurses felt that the assessment tool used in their unit was not an accurate measure of neonatal pain (Cong et al., 2013). This uncertainty and the lack of a 'gold standard' concerning neonatal pain assessment is a key challenge to consistent accurate assessment of neonatal pain. Over 50 measures for neonatal and infant pain have been developed over the past three decades (Giordano et al., 2019), yet there is no consensus on how best to assess neonatal pain. Despite this lack of consensus, the following points, based on current knowledge, are recommended (AAP, 2016):

- Use standardised pain assessment tools to provide a common language and reduce subjectivity.
- Perform pain assessments with vital signs.
- Re-assess pain following treatment – to determine the effectiveness, or otherwise, of the intervention.

A more detailed guide to using a pain assessment tool is included in the Australian-produced evidence-based clinical practice guideline (CPG) for management of newborn pain (Spence et al., 2010). Optimising care includes working together as an interdisciplinary team to consistently assess pain and to use pain assessment scores in order to make decisions regarding pain management. The team needs to include parents, who are a constant at the bedside over weeks of care and can contribute valuable information about the comfort preferences of their infant.

The following sections describe individual and composite indicators of pain used in the clinical and/or research setting.

Behavioural indicators of pain

The most specific, sensitive and commonly used indicators of acute procedural pain in neonates are behavioural responses, facial expressions and crying. The most frequently observed facial expressions in response to pain are brow bulge, eye squeeze, naso-labial furrow and stretched open mouth. These facial expressions of crying were first described by Charles Darwin (1872), and have since been categorised into a subset of the Neonatal Facial Coding System (Grunau et al., 1998). These facial expressions, considered as reflexive reactions to painful stimuli, are the indicators used in nearly all composite pain assessment tools developed for the neonatal population (Harrison et al., 2015b). These facial actions can be expressed by even the most preterm neonates in response to heel lance (Johnston et al., 1995) (Fig. 18.1), although they may occur more subtly in preterm neonates and neonates with neurological impairment than in more-mature healthy neonates (Johnston et al., 1999). Challenges in clearly viewing the neonate's face arise from equipment and tape present on the face as well as eye protection, low lighting or phototherapy lights and methods used to promote a dimly lit environment for the neonate, such as blankets placed over the incubators. All these factors lead to reduced visibility of the neonate's face, with the risk of missing subtle signs of facial expressions of pain.

Crying incidence and duration are relatively objective, and measurable indicators of pain and are included as an indicator in many newborn neonatal pain assessment tools (Table 18.1). Audible crying is, however, altered or non-existent in some sick hospitalised newborns (Harrison et al., 2015a). For this reason, crying characteristics are not included in pain assessment tools developed specifically for measurement of pain in preterm neonates, such as the Premature Infant Pain Profile and its revised versions (Gibbins et al., 2015; Stevens et al., 2014). Some neonates are so clinically compromised they may be unable to mount a behavioural response – for example, neonates with neurological impairment (Stevens et al., 2010).

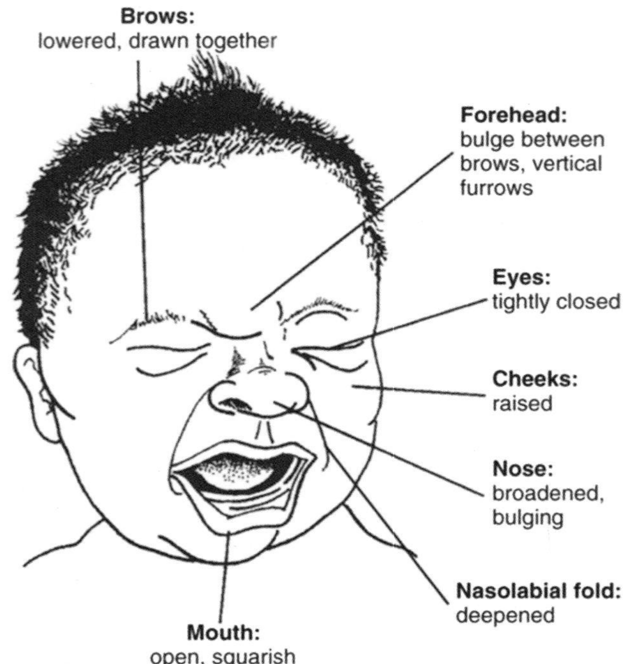

FIGURE 18.1 **Facial expression of physical distress**
Source: Wilson and Hockenberry (2011, Fig. 3-1).

CLINICAL PRACTICE 18.5

Although neonates display other recognisable signals of distress, intubated neonates cannot cry audibly, so it is especially important to recognise their other signals of distress using a validated pain assessment tool.

REFLECTION

Consider whether distress signals may go unheeded if crying is inaudible and/or the neonate's face is not visible. Equipment and tape covering the face, eye protection, low lighting and phototherapy lights lead to reduced visibility of the neonate's face, with the risk of missing subtle signs of facial expressions of pain.

Consider altered crying in sick term neonates following extubation, or with conditions such as subglottic stenosis or tracheomalacia.

Physiological indicators of pain

Physiological indicators of pain are used as proxy markers of pain, and are included in several composite pain assessment tools. The most included indicators are heart rate, respiratory rate and oxygen saturation.

Several physiological indicators are currently used more in research than in clinical care. This list of indicators is currently being explored in the search for more objective,

TABLE 18.1 **Neonatal pain assessment tools**

Tool	Population	Indicators	Type of pain	Scale	Comments
NFCS (Grunau et al., 1998)	Preterm/ full term	Behavioural: facial expressions	Acute procedural Postoperative/ prolonged pain	Full tool: 0–9 Subset: 0–4 or 0–3	Adapted from FACS
PIPP-R (Stevens et al., 2014)	Preterm/ full term	Behavioural: facial expressions Physiological: HR, SpO_2 Contextual: sleep state, gestational age	Acute procedural	0–21	Revised from PIPP, which has had the most psychometric testing
N-PASS (Hummel et al., 2010)	Preterm/ full term	Behavioural: facial expressions, crying, body tone Physiological: HR, RR, BP, SpO_2 Contextual: behavioural state	Acute procedural	−10 to +10	Negative scores associated with high levels of sedation
BIPP (Holsti & Grunau, 2007)	Preterm	Behavioural: 5 facial expressions, 2 hand actions Contextual: sleep/wake state	Acute procedural	0–9	
DAN (Carbajal et al., 1997)	Preterm/ full term	Behavioural: facial expressions, limb movements, vocal expression/crying	Acute procedural	0–10	
PAT pain (Hodgkinson et al., 1994; Spence et al., 2005)	Preterm/ full term	Behavioural: facial expressions, posture/ tone, cry, sleep pattern Physiological: colour Nurse's perception	Postoperative and at rest (no painful procedure)	0–20	Initially developed for postoperative pain Validated in additional NICU populations

BIPP, Behavioral Infant Pain Profile; BP, blood pressure; DAN, Douleur Aigue du Nouveau; FACS, Facial Action Coding System; HR, heart rate; NFCS, Neonatal Facial Coding System; N-PASS, Neonatal Pain Agitation and Sedation Scale; PAT, Pain Assessment Tool; PIPP, Premature Infant Pain Profile; PIPP-R, Premature Infant Pain Profile Revised; RR, respiratory rate; SpO_2, blood oxygen saturation level.

specific sensitive measures of pain, including 'brain-orientated' approaches (Relland et al., 2019):

- skin conductance (Hu et al., 2019)
- near-infrared spectroscopy (NIRS) (Relland et al., 2019)
- electroencephalography (EEG) and amplitude-integrated electroencephalography (a-EEG) (Relland et al., 2019).

Combining assessment of physiological and behavioural indices of pain with measurements such as ECG, NIRS, EEG and electromyograph (EMG) has potential in the future to measure pain objectively (Relland et al., 2019).

Contextual factors, such as sleep or behavioural states at baseline, previous pain exposure, severity of illness and current therapies, and demographic factors, such as GA and postnatal age, may be important considerations in pain assessment (Gibbins et al., 2015; Sellam et al., 2011). As seen in Table 18.1, such contextual-specific indicators are considered in some, but not all, composite pain assessment tools. A systematic review of contextual factors influencing the pain response to heel lance in preterm neonates concluded that inconsistencies were apparent and recommended further research to better understand relationships between pain responses and specific contextual factors (Sellam et al., 2011).

The AAP Committee on Fetus and Newborns, in their updated statement of prevention and management of procedural pain in the neonate (AAP, 2016), stated that five tools have been subject to the most psychometric testing: the Neonatal Facial Coding System (NFCS) (Grunau et al., 1998), the Premature Infant Pain Profile Revised (PIPP-R) (Stevens et al., 2014), the Neonatal Pain and Sedation Tool (N-PASS) (Hummel et al., 2010), the Behavioral Infant Pain Profile (BIPP) (Holsti & Grunau, 2007) and the Douleur Aigue du Nouveau (DAN) (Carbajal et al., 1997). In addition, the Pain Assessment Tool (PAT), developed by a team of Australian NICU nurses for the purpose of measuring neonatal postoperative pain (Hodgkinson et al., 1994), underwent further reliability and validity testing in additional NICU populations (Spence et al., 2005). See Table 18.1 for a summary of these tools, intended population, type of pain, indicators and scoring tools.

Ongoing challenges to consistently and accurately assessing, documenting and using pain scores to make pain treatment decisions in preterm neonates (Gibbins et al., 2015), all newborn neonates (Bellieni et al., 2015) and in paediatric care in general (von Baeyer & Pasero, 2017) include: workload (nurses report if workload is heavy or staffing short, they do not prioritise pain relief strategies), the unpredictable and subtle nature of pain indicators in preterm neonates, obstruction of the face by support devices and medical equipment precluding HCPs accurately assessing neonates' responses, inconsistencies in performing pain assessments owing to lack of agreement on best measures, lack of knowledge and, finally, the fact that nurses and midwives 'work around' the pain scores and simply score 'pain' or 'no pain' requiring treatment based on pain assessment policies. Moving beyond the challenges includes selecting a recommended pain assessment method/tool that is feasible to use, acceptable for nursing/midwifery staff and the interdisciplinary team, suitable for the population of neonates and is documented and consistently used as part of the decision-making process to guide pain management. We have over three decades of neonatal pain assessment research to guide us; our goals are now to use the research in our everyday practices.

CLINICAL PRACTICE 18.6

Pain assessment is integral to pain management. Pain assessments are part of the decision-making process to guide pain treatment.

NON-PHARMACOLOGICAL STRATEGIES TO REDUCE PAIN AND DISTRESS

The most effective method to reduce pain is to *prevent* pain. Neonatal nurses and midwives in partnership with medical staff are key to making decisions about the need for, and coordination of, procedures. When procedures are required, effective pain management is vital to minimise behavioural distress and physiological changes at the time of the procedures, which may also improve long-term outcomes (Walker, 2014). There are evidence-based effective strategies to reduce pain. Table 18.2 summarises systematic reviews of procedural pain management interventions for newborn neonates published since 2012.

EVIDENCE-BASED PRACTICE RESEARCH 18.2

A systematic review of non-pharmacological strategies for reduction of procedural pain in infants and young children (Pillai Riddell et al., 2015) included touch/massage. Findings showed some evidence of benefits of massage in preterm infants in reducing pain reactivity (two studies, low-quality evidence) but no evidence of benefits of massage in reducing immediate pain regulation in preterm infants (three small studies, low-quality evidence) or term neonates (two studies, low-quality evidence).

The following section will describe the evidence for interventions for reduction of acute procedural pain: breastfeeding (Benoit et al., 2017), SSC (Johnston et al., 2017) and sweet solutions (Harrison et al., 2017; Stevens et al., 2016). Following this discussion, pharmacological interventions recommended for procedural pain, postoperative and prolonged pain, including opioid **analgesics**, paracetamol and topical and regional anaesthetics, will be discussed.

Breastfeeding

An update to the Cochrane systematic review of breastfeeding and breast milk for procedural pain reduction (Shah et al., 2012) included an additional 21 trials: 15 of direct breastfeeding and 6 of expressed breast milk (Benoit et al., 2017). Compared with no treatment, oral water, sucrose, holding by the mother or swaddling and positioned in a crib, breastfeeding reduced behavioural indicators (crying time, facial expressions), heart rate and composite pain scores. The mechanisms of effects are considered multifactorial, and encompass SSC, sound, sight, sound and smell of the mother, sucking, slightly sweet taste of the breast milk, movement and, possibly, endogenous opioids present in breast milk (Harrison et al., 2015b). This combination of factors is important, and explains why giving newborns small volumes of breast milk (containing 7% lactose – the least sweet of all sugars) to suck prior to a heel lance procedure is *not* effective (Harrison et al., 2016a).

For the best effects, breastfeeding should commence around 5 minutes prior to the procedure, long enough for the neonate to be well latched and sucking at the time of the intervention. Analgesic effects of breastfeeding also extend beyond the newborn period. Harrison et al. (2016a) included 10 studies evaluating breastfeeding during immunisation in neonates from 1 month to 12 months, and showed that breastfeeding resulted in reduced duration of crying and pain scores.

FAMILY-CENTRED CARE 18.2

A mother asks you if she can breastfeed during her baby's routine blood tests. However, the blood collection is usually completed at 05:00 and the mother cannot be present at this time. How can you facilitate the mother to breastfeed her infant during the procedure as she requests?

Skin-to-skin care (SSC)

A Cochrane systematic review of SSC for pain reduction in newborns (Johnston et al., 2017) included 25 studies and showed that SSC during heel lance and intramuscular injections reduced behavioural indicators and composite pain scores. The mechanisms of effects of SSC are considered multifactorial, and encompass the feel of the mother's heartbeat, warmth, sound, and sight, sound and smell of the mother. In most of the studies, the person providing the SSC was the neonate's mother. As reported in the

TABLE 18.2 **Systematic reviews of neonatal pain reduction strategies published since 2015**

Title (Author)	Year	Review findings	No. of studies (no. of neonates)
A systematic review of behavioural and environmental interventions for procedural pain management in preterm infants (Hatfield et al.)	2019	A combination of behavioural and environmental interventions can be used with preterm infants to reduce pain during painful procedures	14 (888)
Pain-relieving interventions for retinopathy of prematurity: a meta-analysis (Disher et al.)	2018	Combined use of topical anaesthetics, oral sucrose and other interventions (swaddling, etc.) as well as excluding use of a speculum, results in reduction in pain scores	29 (1487)
Sweet solutions to reduce procedural pain in neonates: a meta-analysis (Harrison et al.)	2017	From the first few studies published, evidence of analgesic effects of sweet solutions existed. Studies published since this time have served only to strengthen the evidence	168
Topical anaesthesia for needle-related pain in newborn infants (Foster et al.)	2017	Insufficient evidence to support efficacy and safety	8 (506)
SSC for procedural pain in neonates (Johnston et al.)	2017	SSC reduced behavioural responses to pain in preterm neonates during HL, VP and IM injections	25 (2001)
Breastfeeding analgesia in infants: an update on the current state of evidence (Benoit et al.)	2017	BF reduced pain in term (15 studies) and preterm (6 studies) during HL, VP and IM injections No evidence of analgesic effects of EBM	21 (2336)
Sucrose for analgesia in newborn infants undergoing painful procedures (Stevens et al.)	2016	Sucrose reduced behavioural responses and composite pain scores during HL, VP, gastric tube insertion	74 (7049)
Non-pharmacological management of infant and young child procedural pain (Pillai Riddell et al.)	2015	NNS was the most studied and effective intervention to reduce pain during HL and IM injections. In addition, some evidence for preterm neonates of the efficacy of environmental modification, swaddling/facilitated tucking and for term neonates of swaddling/facilitated tucking	63 (4905)
Paracetamol (acetaminophen) for prevention or treatment of pain in newborns (Ohlsson & Shah)	2020	Paracetamol was ineffective in reducing pain following heel lance, ROP examination and vaginal deliveries Paracetamol may reduce total requirement for morphine following major surgery	9 (728)

Note: Systematic reviews published in this period covered 2015–20.
BF, breastfeeding; EBM, expressed breast milk; HL, heel lance; IM, intramuscular injection; NNS, non-nutritive sucking; ROP, retinopathy of prematurity; SSC, skin-to-skin care; VP, venepuncture.

systematic review, studies of SSC provided by alternative carers, including fathers, non-maternally related women and twins, were also analysed. Although less effective than mothers, SSC provided by fathers and alternative women reduced pain compared with no SSC, whereas co-bedding twins during heel lancing did not result in reduced pain for the twin undergoing the procedure. For the best effects, SSC should be commenced around 15 minutes prior to the painful procedure, long enough for the care giver and neonate to be settled, comfortable and relaxed. See Chapter 21 for further discussion of SSC, and how to facilitate it in diverse neonatal care settings.

CLINICAL PRACTICE 18.7

Parental presence can result in increased use of effective pain management interventions and reduced pain (Courtois et al., 2016). Organise and advocate for non-urgent blood tests to be performed when the parent(s) can be present.

CLINICAL PRACTICE 18.8

Facilitate mothers to breastfeed during procedures if feasible, or facilitate SSC with the mother, father or other family or friend care giver.

Sweet solutions

Three systematic reviews, one of sucrose (Stevens et al., 2016) (74 studies), one of non-sucrose solutions (Bueno et al., 2013) (38 studies) and one which included all sweet solutions (Harrison et al., 2017) (168 studies), showed that sweet solutions consistently reduced behavioural responses and composite pain scores when given in small volumes before painful procedures. In addition, Gao et al. (2016) included eight studies in a systematic review of repeated use of sweet solutions, and reported that sucrose reduced behavioural pain responses and composite pain scores during repeated episodes of procedural pain.

Mechanisms of analgesic effects are primarily due to a sweet-taste-mediated endogenous opioid response – common in all young mammals (Harrison et al., 2017). The solutions must therefore be given orally; installation of sweet solutions via a gastric tube has no analgesic effects. Only small volumes are required, just a drop – or around 0.1 mL (Stevens et al., 2018) – and for best effects, especially for neonates beyond the newborn period and for procedures of prolonged duration, the dose needs to be given in small aliquots over the duration of the procedure (Harrison et al., 2015a). There is no evidence on what is considered a maximum safe daily dose and there is no evidence of harm in the short or long term. However, nurses/midwives need to be cognisant of the risk of inadvertently giving substantial volumes of sweet solutions, if they are used repeatedly for ongoing comforting for irritable/unsettled neonates.

FAMILY-CENTRED CARE 18.3

Consider whether you would encourage a father to hold his baby in SSC during a routine heel lance, or ask him to leave the unit while you do the procedure, and give sucrose for pain management.

PHARMACOLOGICAL STRATEGIES TO REDUCE PAIN AND DISTRESS

Appropriate use of analgesia during painful procedures is important to reduce short-term pain and distress and to reduce risks of long-term adverse outcomes; however, the use of analgesics in this population is challenging. HCPs need to balance the ethical responsibility to provide humane pain management with the gaps in knowledge about risks and benefits of currently available analgesics. Drug elimination in neonates may be delayed owing to the immature renal and hepatic systems; however, there is wide variability in pharmacokinetics and pharmacodynamics amongst this heterogeneous population.

Opioid analgesics

Opioid analgesics work primarily by stimulating mu (μ) receptors in the spinal cord and brain, resulting in a reduction in nociceptive input to the brain (Hathway, 2014). Morphine is the most comprehensively studied opioid analgesic in neonates. It is naturally occurring, isolated from the opium poppy (*Papaver somniferum*) and an agonist (a substance that acts at a receptor site to produce an effect similar to an endogenous messenger) at μ and κ receptors (Yaksh & Wallace, 2018). The onset of action following intravenous administration is approximately 5 minutes (Ainsworth, 2015). The use of opioid analgesics in the care of sick preterm and term newborn neonates is an essential aspect of their care. However, due to uncertainties in short- and longer-term outcomes following its use (Gao et al., 2020), and controversies, its use continues to be questioned.

CLINICAL PRACTICE 18.9

Morphine infusions may not provide sufficient pain relief for acute procedural pain in ventilated infants (Bellù et al., 2020).

Fentanyl is a synthetic selective μ-receptor agonist and is 50–100 times more potent than morphine. It has increased lipid solubility (Yaksh & Wallace, 2018), does not stimulate histamine release and has a rapid onset of action. Fentanyl is associated with greater haemodynamic stability and is less sedating than morphine (Ainsworth, 2015).

Risk of adverse effects of opioids

All neonates receiving opioid analgesics should receive continuous cardiorespiratory monitoring to detect potential side effects. The following are potential adverse effects of opioids:

- respiratory depression – therefore use with caution in spontaneously breathing neonates
- hypotension – morphine may cause histamine release, which induces blood vessel dilation; therefore use with caution in hypovolaemic neonates
- urinary retention – because of effects on smooth muscle
- reduced gastric motility – can delay enteral feeding; observe for ileus
- chest wall rigidity (fentanyl only, especially with rapid administration or large doses) – resulting in inability of the neonate to breathe and difficulties in mechanical ventilation.

Respiratory depression due to opioid effects can be reversed with naloxone. However, this also reverses the analgesic effects and should be used with caution in neonates with opioid infusions as it can trigger withdrawal and possible seizure activity (Ainsworth, 2015).

Opioid tolerance and dependence are a potential risk in the newborn. Tolerance requires dose escalation to sustain sufficient analgesia (Ainsworth, 2015). The Committee on Drug Withdrawal and Committee on Newborn and Fetus notes 'at this time, no optimal pharmacologic regimen for the prevention or treatment of acquired opioid and/or benzodiazepine dependency can be recommended' (Hudak et al., 2012, p. e552). A point to highlight is that neonates who require opioids for more than a few days should be monitored for withdrawal symptoms, and weaned slowly to prevent withdrawal symptoms (Hudak et al., 2012).

CLINICAL PRACTICE 18.10

There are wide variations in the use of analgesics and sedatives in NICUs. In a study covering 243 units in 18 European countries examining the use of these agents in 6680 neonates (mean GA = 35 weeks), the use of sedation and analgesia varied from 0% to 100% between centres (Carbajal et al., 2015).

For details of recommended doses, see the neonatal formulary (Ainsworth, 2015, pp. 344–345).

Sedatives

Sedatives such as midazolam are not analgesic agents and should not be used alone for pain management. They may, however, be associated with improved sedation when used in combination with opioid analgesics. However, a recent Cochrane systematic review including three trials and 148 neonates concluded there were insufficient data to support the use of intravenous midazolam as a sedative for neonates undergoing intensive care (Ng et al., 2017). This evidence from a small number of published trials, which goes against current practices in many NICUs, highlights a problem in providing care that is informed by published evidence. As is the case in many clinical situations in newborn care, evidence-based pain care needs to consider the inclusion of expert opinion and patient (parent) preference, as well as research evidence from high-quality studies.

Mild analgesics

Acetaminophen (paracetamol) is a mild analgesic that is commonly prescribed for the treatment of acute pain in neonates. A Cochrane systematic review determined that paracetamol does not significantly reduce pain associated with acute procedures (e.g. heel lance or ophthalmology examinations) (Ohlsson & Shah, 2020). However, it may reduce morphine requirements postoperatively, although further research is recommended (Ohlsson & Shah, 2020). Paracetamol can be given orally, intravenously or rectally. Absorption by the rectal dose is variable, and the oral route is therefore preferred if possible. The intravenous route is useful for postoperative pain when the oral route cannot be used. There is no evidence that tolerance develops, yet there is an 'analgesic ceiling' where efficacy is not increased by increased dose. In the neonatal population, there is a wide variation in its half-life, from 3.5 hours in term neonates to 5.7 hours in preterm neonates.

For details of recommended doses see the neonatal formulary (Ainsworth, 2015, pp. 391–393).

CASE STUDY 18.1

James is a 27-week gestation neonate with a birthweight of 900 grams. He was delivered by spontaneous vaginal birth. His mother received a partial course of antenatal steroids. He was making some effort to breathe at birth and was electively intubated (not medicated) and given surfactant. During transfer to the neonatal unit, he accidentally extubated and was supported with peak end expiratory pressure (PEEP) via a T-piece circuit. On arrival his oxygen saturations were >92% in 25% FiO_2 so bubble CPAP was commenced at a PEEP of 8.

James now requires insertion of an orogastric tube and umbilical arterial and venous lines.

1. What should nurses/midwives take into consideration so as to optimise comfort and minimise pain and stress?
2. Which strategies/medications would be appropriate in relation to providing analgesia?
3. How can nurses/midwives assess whether James is comfortable?

At 1 week of age and receiving some enteral feeds of expressed breast milk, James becomes unwell; he is pale, and lethargic, with increasing oxygen requirements, apnoeic episodes and desaturations. His abdomen is distended with bile-stained aspirates. An abdominal X-ray is suggestive of necrotising enterocolitis. His condition deteriorates and he requires intubation and ventilation.

4. Which medications should the nurse/midwife anticipate will be required for intubation?
5. If James requires surgery, which interventions (pharmacological and non-pharmacological) should be used to provide adequate pain relief postoperatively?

James is now 8 weeks' postnatal age and doing well. He is receiving some NGT feeds and is increasingly breastfeeding. He is due for his 2-month vaccinations.

6. What pain management strategies may be used for James' vaccinations? What factors will you base your decision on?

Topical and local anaesthetics

While there are several topical anaesthetics available for neonatal use (including lidocaine 2.5%-prilocaine 2.5% (Eutectic Mixture of Local Anaesthetics – EMLA®)), tetracaine 4% gel (Ametop®, Pontocaine®) and liposomal lidocaine 4% cream (LMX4®), most neonatal research has been conducted with EMLA (Carbajal, 2020).

The evidence for anaesthetic creams (liposomal lignocaine 4% (LMX4) and lignocaine (lidocaine) 2.5% and prilocaine 2.5% (EMLA: eutectic mixture of local anaesthetic)) in the management of procedural pain in neonates, in particular preterm neonates, is limited. A Cochrane systematic review of eight randomised controlled trials concluded that there was insufficient information to support clinical recommendations (Foster et al., 2017). The risk of methaemoglobinaemia in neonates associated with the use of EMLA/Numit® (2.5% lidocaine/2.5% prilocaine) has been identified (Woo et al., 2021).

Local infiltration of 1% lignocaine injected subcutaneously at a maximum dose of 0.4 mL/kg (4 mg/kg) has been recommended for lumbar puncture and intrathoracic chest drain insertion, particularly in emergencies when the application of topical anaesthesia is not possible (Lago et al., 2009). Local topical anaesthetics, combined with oral sucrose, are recommended to reduce pain and distress during eye examination (Disher et al., 2018).

Environmental factors can also play a role in the comfort of neonates; therefore, ensuring appropriate noise and light levels, to protect sleep and promote optimal neurodevelopmental outcomes, is important in the care of sick and preterm neonates.

PROMOTING EVIDENCE-BASED PAIN MANAGEMENT PRACTICES

The implementation of pain reduction strategies has been variable across different settings and across the world. An Australian knowledge translation project did result in an increase in use of pain assessment tools and an increase in use of sucrose and breastfeeding for procedural pain; however, breastfeeding during painful procedures remained extremely low, occurring for only 4% of procedures in special care units and 1.5% of procedures in NICUs. The use of SSC for procedural pain management was not even included in the study (Foster et al., 2013). This use of breastfeeding, SSC or sucrose was only slightly higher in studies conducted in Canada (Harrison et al., 2015a; Lavin Venegas et al., 2019b), highlighting that practice globally is slow to change. Although routine use of sucrose for pain management has been reported (Roofthooft et al., 2014), breastfeeding and SSC have not received the same knowledge translation attention. Consequently, recommended pain management practices for newborns have not routinely been adopted into standard practice. Reported barriers to implementing these recommendations include misconceptions, lack of knowledge about pain management strategies and lack of knowledge on how to implement evidence, as well as perceived barriers to workflow, perceived difficulties with accessing the infant for the blood sample while the infant is being held and cultural and organisational barriers (Harrison et al., 2015b; Lavin Venegas et al., 2019a).

Neonatal nurses and midwives are central in partnering with parents and the neonatal unit interdisciplinary team in order to facilitate and support parents to help minimise their baby's pain during procedures. Knowledge translation strategies used to support parents include parent-targeted and -mediated videos and booklets (Fig. 18.2; see also links to these in Online Resources). Whether such patient(parent)-targeted activity can successfully improve the use of recommended pain management interventions is yet to be evaluated (Harrison et al., 2016b). However, what is known is the importance of partnering and supporting parents to be present and to advocate for their babies during painful procedures (Courtois et al., 2016). To optimise a coordinated approach to improving pain management, commitment from individual nurses and midwives at the frontline, in partnership with parents, leaders at all levels of the organisations and professional associations, is warranted (Harrison et al., 2015b).

REFLECTION

Examine your unit's pain management policies. Do they include partnering with parents to facilitate breastfeeding and skin-to-skin contact, where feasible, during non-urgent painful procedures? Consider your unit's practices. Are parents asked to leave the unit when their baby requires blood sampling, *or* are they encouraged to stay, and shown how they can comfort their baby during the procedure?

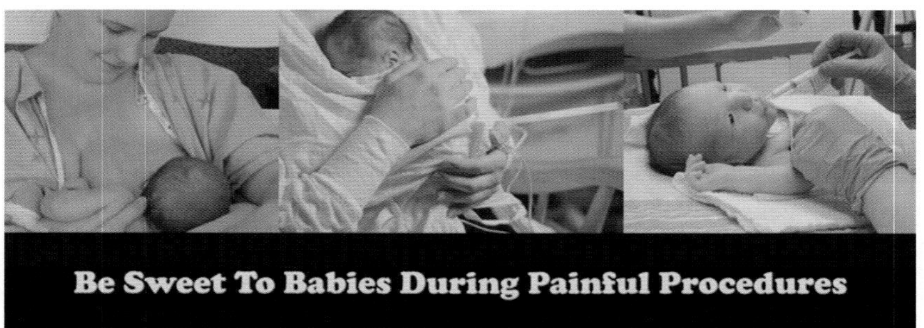

FIGURE 18.2 **Assessing pain in the preterm neonate**

Source: Children's Hospital of Eastern Ontario (CHEO) (n.d.). Courtesy of Denise Harrison.

CONCLUSION

Optimal neonatal pain management is not an isolated practice; it cannot be additional to what neonatal clinicians do, but must be core to their practice. There exists a plethora of evidence highlighting inadequacies (Cruz et al., 2016); however, quintessential to nursing/midwifery care is the relief of suffering and provision of comfort. If neonatal clinicians consider environmental impacts (noise and light) and practices necessary throughout each 24-hour period to monitor and support neonates, they realise how this needs to be integrated into minute-to-minute care, with nurses/

midwives uniquely placed to improve patient outcomes. Nurses/midwives cannot abdicate responsibility, but rather should reflect on practice: how loud their voices are when they converse near the neonate, how much care they take to gently manipulate nasal prongs, how they facilitate parental partnership in all aspects of care, how they reduce the burden of pain, and how they advocate for this defenceless population in the face of challenging medical decisions.

There are significant gaps in knowledge including a lack of a 'gold standard' for pain assessment (Cong et al., 2013; Giordano et al., 2019; Relland et al., 2019), a lack of consensus on the effects of morphine and dosing (Steinhorn et al., 2015) and how to best translate knowledge into action. In a review of 45 clinical trials of analgesic interventions for 'minor' interventions, 64% of neonates in the control group received no treatment or placebo, thus subjecting neonates to unnecessary pain in the face of existing high-quality evidence (Bellieni & Johnston, 2016). There is no justification for this unethical practice and neonatal clinicians need to question such research designs.

There are many strategies that are known to alleviate pain, and vulnerable preterm and sick neonates rely on the bedside nurse/midwife, as the constant carer in partnership with parents and the interdisciplinary team, to do the right thing.

'Now we know better we should do better.'

Jacob Bronowski, 1974

Online Resources

BSweet2Babies video (Dr Denise Harrison, BeSweet2Babies Team, University of Ottawa and Children's Hospital of Eastern Ontario): <https://www.youtube.com/watch?v=L43y0H6XEH4&feature=youtu.be>.

Comforting Your Baby in Intensive Care (Professor Linda S. Franck, University of California, San Francisco): <www.familynursing.ucsf.edu/sites/familynursing.ucsf.edu/files/wysiwyg/Comfy%20PDF%20ENGLISH%20Dec%2017.pdf>

Power of a Parent's Touch video (Dr Marsha Campbell-Yeo, It Doesn't Have to Hurt Team, IWK Health Centre and Dalhousie University): <https://www.youtube.com/watch?v=3nqN9c3FWn8>

Royal Children's Hospital Clinical Practice Guidelines – Pain: <https://www.rch.org.au/clinicalguide/#tab-P>

References/Acknowledgements

Ainsworth, S. B. (Ed.). (2015). *Neonatal formulary: drug use in pregnancy and the first year of life* (7th ed.). Chichester, UK: John Wiley.

American Academy of Pediatrics (AAP). (2016). Prevention and management of procedural pain in the neonate: an update. *Pediatrics, 137*(2), 1–13.

Anand, K. J., & Hickey, P. R. (1987). Pain and its effects in the human neonate and fetus. *New England Journal of Medicine, 317*(21), 1321–1327.

Anand, K. J., & Hickey, P. R. (1992). Halothane-morphine compared with high-dose sufentanil for anaesthesia and postoperative analgesia in neonatal cardiac surgery. *New England Journal of Medicine, 326*(1), 1–9.

Anand, K. J., Sippell, W. G., & Aynsley-Green, A. (1987). Randomised trial of fentanyl anaesthesia in preterm babies undergoing surgery: effects on the stress response. *Lancet, 1*(8524), 62–66.

Anand, K. J. S., Eriksson, M., Boyle, E. M., Avila-Alvarez, A., Andersen, R. D., Sarafidis, K., et al. (2017), Assessment of continuous pain in newborns admitted to NICUs in 18 European countries. *Acta Paediatrica, 106*, 1248–1259. doi: 10.1111/apa.13810.

Balice-Bourgois, C., Jaques, C., Newman, C. J., & Simonetti, G. D. (2020). A systematic review of clinical practice guidelines for acute procedural pain on neonates. *Clinical Journal of Pain, 36*, 390–398. doi: 10.1097/AJP.0000000000000808.

Bellieni, C. V., & Johnston, C. C. (2016). Analgesia, nil or placebo to babies, in trials that test new analgesic treatments for procedural pain. *Acta Paediatrica, 105*(2), 129–136.

Bellieni, C. V., Tei, M., & Buonocore, G. (2015). Should we assess pain in newborn infants using a scoring system or just a detection method? *Acta Paediatrica, 104*(3), 221–224.

Bellù, R., Romantsik, O., Nava, C., Waal, K. A., Zanini, R., & Bruschettini, M. (2020). Opioids for newborn infants receiving mechanical ventilation [protocol]. *Cochrane Database of Systematic Reviews, 9*, CD013732. doi: 10.1002/14651858.CD013732.

Benoit, B., Martin-Misener, R., Latimer, M., & Campbell-Yeo, M. (2017). Breast-feeding analgesia in infants. *Journal of Perinatal and Neonatal Nursing, 31*, 145–159. doi: 10.1097/JPN.0000000000000253.

Brennan, F., Lohman, D., & Gwyther, L. (2019). Access to pain management as a human right. *American Journal of Public Health, 109*, 61–65. doi: 10.2105/AJPH.2018.304743.

Bueno, M., Yamada, J., Harrison, D., Kahn, S., Adams-Webber, T., Beyene, J., et al. (2013). A systematic review and meta-analyses of non-sucrose sweet solutions for pain relief in neonates. *Pain Research and Management, 18*(3), 153–161.

Bueno, M., Stevens, B., Rao, M., Riahi, S., Lanese, A., & Li, S., (2020). Usability, acceptability, and feasibility of the Implementation of Infant Pain Practice Change (ImPaC) resource. *Paediatric Neonatal Pain, 2*, 82–92. doi: 10.1002/pne2.12027.

Carbajal, R. (2020). Neonatal pain. In: E. M. Boyle & J. Cusack (Eds.), *Emerging topics and controversies in neonatology* (pp. 485–501). Cham, Switzerland: Springer Nature.

Carbajal, R., Paupe, A., Hoenn, E., Lenclen, R., & Olivier-Martin, M. (1997). APN: evaluation behavioral scale of acute pain in newborn infants. *Archives de Pédiatrie, 4*(7), 623–628.

Carbajal, R., Eriksson, M., Courtois, E., Boyle, E., Avila-Alvarez, A., Andersen, R., et al. (2015). Sedation and analgesia practices in neonatal intensive care units (EUROPAIN): results from a prospective cohort study. *Lancet Respiratory Medicine, 3*(10), 796–812.

Children's Hospital of Eastern Ontario (CHEO). (n.d.) Reduce your infant's pain during newborn blood tests [video]. Ottawa: CHEO Research Institute, University of Ottawa Be Sweet to Babies team. Courtesy of Denise Harrison.

<https://www.youtube.com/watch?v=L43y0H6XEH4&feature=youtu.be> (Accessed 22 February 2022).

Cong, X., Delaney, C., & Vazquez, V. (2013). Neonatal nurses' perceptions of pain assessment and management in NICUs: a national survey. *Advances in Neonatal Care, 13*(5), 353–360.

Cornelissen, L., Fabrizi, L., Patten, D., Worley, A., Meek, J., Boyd, S., et al. (2013). Postnatal temporal spatial and modality tuning of nociceptive cutaneous flexion reflexes in human infants. *PLoS One, 8*(10), 1–10.

Council of International Neonatal Nurses (COINN). (2019). *Standard 11, Professional ethics and legal practice* (p. 262). Yardley, PA: COINN.

Courtois, E., Droutman, S., Magny, J. F., Merchaoui, Z., Durrmeyer, X., Roussel, C., et al. (2016). Epidemiology and neonatal pain management of heelsticks in intensive care units: EPIPPAIN 2 a prospective observational study. *International Journal of Nursing Studies, 59*, 79–88.

Cruz, M. D., Fernandes, A. M., & Oliveira, C. R. (2016). Epidemiology of painful procedures performed in neonates: a systematic review of observational studies. *European Journal of Pain, 20*(4), 489–498.

Darwin, C. (1872). *The expression of the emotions in man and animals*. Chicago, IL: The University of Chicago Press.

Disher, T., Cameron, C., Mitra, S., Cathcart, K., & Campbell-Yeo, M., 2018. Pain-relieving interventions for retinopathy of prematurity: a meta-analysis. *Pediatrics, 142*, e20180401. doi: 10.1542/peds.2018-0401.

Fitzgerald, M. (2015). What do we really know about newborn infant pain? *Experimental Physiology, 100*(12), 1451–1457.

Foster, J., Spence, K., Henderson-Smart, D., Harrison, D., & Gray, P. (2013). Procedural pain in neonates in Australian hospitals: a survey update of practices. *Journal of Paediatrics and Child Health, 49*(1), E35–E39.

Foster, J., Taylor, C., & Spence, K. (2017). Topical anaesthesia for needle-related pain in newborn infants. *Cochrane Database of Systematic Reviews, 2*, CD010331, doi: 10.1002/14651858.CD010331.pub2.

Gagnon, M. M., Hadjistavropoulos, T., McAleer, L. M., & Stopyn, R. J. N., (2020). Increasing parental access to pediatric pain-related knowledge. *Clinical Journal of Pain, 36*, 47–60. doi: 10.1097/ajp.0000000000000770.

Gao, H., Gao, H., Xu, G., Li, M., Du, S., Li, F., et al. (2016). Efficacy and safety of repeated oral sucrose for repeated procedural pain in neonates: a systematic review. *International Journal of Nursing Studies. 62*, 118–125. doi: 10.1016/j.ijnurstu.2016.07.015.

Gao, H., Gao H., Li, M., Zhang, H., Wang, D., & Wang, B. (2020) Morphine use in the neonatal period and later neuropsychological development: a systematic review. *Developmental Medicine & Child Neurology, 63*(1), 22–28. doi: 10.1111/dmcn.14703.

Gibbins, S., Stevens, B., Dionne, K., Yamada, J., Pillai Riddell, R., McGrath, P., et al. (2015). Perceptions of health professionals on pain in extremely low gestational age infants. *Qualitative Health Research, 25*(6), 763–774.

Giordano, V., Edobor, J., Deindl, P., Wildner, B., Goeral, K., Steinbauer P., et al., (2019). Pain and sedation scales for neonatal and pediatric patients in a preverbal stage of development: a systematic review. *JAMA Pediatrics, 173*, 1186–1197. doi: 10.1001/jamapediatrics.2019.3351.

Grunau, R. E., Oberlander, T., Holsti, L., & Whitfield, M. F. (1998). Bedside application of the Neonatal Facial Coding System in pain assessment of premature neonates. *Pain, 76*(3), 277–286.

Harrison, D., Reszel, J., Wilding, J., Abdulla, K., Bueno, M., Campbell-Yeo, M., et al. (2015a). Neuroprotective core measure 5: neonatal pain management practices during heel lance and venepuncture in Ontario, Canada. *Newborn and Infant Nursing Review, 15*, 116–123.

Harrison, D., Bueno, M., & Reszel, J. (2015b). Prevention and management of pain and stress in the neonate. *Research and Reports in Neonatology, 5*, 9–16.

Harrison, D., Reszel, J., Bueno, M., Sampson, M., Shah, V., Taddio, A., et al. (2016a). Breastfeeding for procedural pain in infants beyond the neonatal period. *Cochrane Database of Systematic Reviews, 10*, CD011248.

Harrison, D., Wilding, J., Bowman, A., Fuller, A., Nicholls, S. G., Pound, C. M., et al. (2016b). Using YouTube to disseminate effective vaccination pain treatment for babies. *PLoS One, 11*(10), e0164123.

Harrison, D., Larocque, C., Bueno, M., Stokes, Y., Turner, L., Hutton, B., et al. (2017). Sweet solutions to reduce procedural pain in neonates: a meta-analysis. *Pediatrics, 139*(1), e20160955. doi: 10.1542/peds.2016-0955.

Hatfield, L. A., Murphy, N., Karp, K., & Polomano, R. C. (2019). A systematic review of behavioral and environmental interventions for procedural pain management in preterm infants. *Journal of Pediatric Nursing, 44*, 22–30. doi: 10.1016/j.pedn.2018.10.004.

Hathway, G. (2014). Developmental pharmacology of opioids. In: P. J. McGrath, B. J. Stevens, S. M. Walker, & W. T. Zempsky (Eds.), *Oxford textbook of paediatric pain* (pp. 449–456). Oxford: Oxford University Press.

Hodgkinson, K., Bear, M., Thorn, J., & van Blaricum, S. (1994). Measuring pain in neonates: evaluating an instrument and developing a common language. *Australian Journal of Advanced Nursing, 12*(1), 17–22.

Holsti, L., & Grunau, R. E. (2007). Initial validation of the Behavioral Indicators of Infant Pain (BIIP). *Pain, 132*(3), 264–272.

Hu, J., Modanloo, S., Squires, J. E., Harrold, J. A., & Harrison, D. (2019). The validity of skin conductance for assessing acute pain in infants: a scoping review. *Clinical Journal of Pain, 35*, 713–724. doi: 10.1097/AJP.0000000000000721.

Hudak, M., Tan, R., & The Committee on Drugs, The Committee on Fetus and Newborn. (2012). Neonatal drug withdrawal. *Pediatrics, 129*(2), e540–e560 (Reaffirmed February 2016).

Hummel, P., Lawlor-Klean, P., & Weiss, M. G. (2010). Validity and reliability of the N-PASS assessment tool with acute pain. *Journal of Perinatology, 30*(7), 474–478.

Inder, T. E., Perlman, J. M., & Volpe, J. J. (2018). Preterm intraventricular hemorrhage/post hemorrhagic hydrocephalus. Unit V. In: J. J. Volpe (Ed. in chief), *Neurology of the newborn* (6th ed., Ch 24, pp. 644–698). Philadelphia, PA: Elsevier.

Johnston, C. C., Stevens, B. J., Yang, F., & Horton, L. (1995). Differential response to pain by very premature neonates. *Pain, 61*(3), 471–479.

Johnston, C. C., Stevens, B. J., Franck, L. S., Jack, A., Stremler, R., & Platt, R. (1999). Factors explaining lack of response to heel stick in preterm newborns. *Journal of Obstetric, Gynecologic, and Neonatal Nursing, 28*(6), 587–594.

Johnston, C. C., Campbell-Yeo, M., Disher, T., Benoit, B., Fernandes, A., Streiner, D., et al. (2017). Skin-to-skin care for procedural pain in neonates. *Cochrane Database of Systematic Reviews, 2*, CD008435.

Lago, P., Garetti, E., Merazzi, D., Pieragostini, L., Ancora, G., Pirelli, A., et al.; Pain Study Group of the Italian Society of Neonatology. (2009). Guidelines for procedural pain in the newborn. *Acta Paediatrica, 98*(6), 932–939.

Lavin Venegas, C., Taljaard, M., Reszel, J., & Harrison, D. (2019a). Barriers and facilitators to using pain treatment during newborn screening blood tests at a mother-baby unit. *Journal of Neonatal Nursing, 25*, 139–144. doi: 10.1016/j.jnn.2018.08.005.

Lavin Venegas, C., Taljaard, M., Reszel, J., Dunn, S., Graham, I. D., Harrold, J., et al. (2019b). A parent-targeted and mediated video intervention to improve uptake of pain treatment for infants during newborn screening: a pilot randomized controlled trial. *Journal of Perinatal and Neonatal Nursing, 33*, 74–81. doi: 10.1097/JPN.0000000000000386.

Lawson, J. (1986). Letter to the Editor. *New England Journal of Medicine, 318*(21), 1398.

Mactier, H., Bates, S. E., Johnston, T., Lee-Davey, C., Marlow, N., Mulley, K., et al.; British Association of Perinatal Medicine (BAPM) Working Group, (2020). Perinatal management of extreme preterm birth before 27 weeks of gestation: a framework for practice. *Archives of Disease in Childhood. Fetal and Neonatal Edition, 105*, 232–239.

Mala, O., Forster, E. M., & Kain, V. J. (2021). Neonatal nurse and midwife competence regarding pain management in neonates: a systematic review. *Advances in Neonatal Care,* doi: 10.1097/ANC.0000000000000911. [Online ahead of print.]

Ng, E., Taddio, A., & Ohlsson, A. (2017). Intravenous midazolam infusion for sedation in the neonatal intensive care unit. *Cochrane Database of Systematic Reviews, 1*, CD002052. doi: 10.1002/14651858.CD002052.pub3.

Ohlsson, A., & Shah, P. S. (2020). Paracetamol (acetaminophen) for prevention or treatment of pain in newborns. *Cochrane Database of Systematic Reviews, 6*, CD011219. doi: 10.1002/14651858.CD011219.pub4.

Pillai Riddell, R., Racine, N., Gennis, H., Turcotte, K., Uman, L., Horton, R., et al. (2015). Non-pharmacological management of infant and young child procedural pain. *Cochrane Database of Systematic Reviews, 12*, CD00627.

Raja, S. N., Carr, D. B., Cohen, M., Finnerup, N. B., Flor, H., Gibson, S., et al. (2020). The revised International Association for the Study of Pain definition of pain. *Pain, 161*, 1976–1982.

Relland, L. M., Gehred, A., & Maitre, N. L. (2019). Behavioral and physiological signs for pain assessment in preterm and term neonates during a nociception-specific response: a systematic review. *Pediatric Neurology, 90*, 13–23. doi: 10.1016/j.pediatrneurol.2018.10.001.

Roofthooft, D. W., Simons, S. H., Anand, K. J., Tibboel, D., & van Dijk, M. (2014). Eight years later are we still hurting newborn infants? *Neonatology, 105*(3), 218–226.

Sellam, G., Cignacco, E. L., Craig, K. D., & Engberg, S. (2011). Contextual factors influencing pain response to heel stick procedures in preterm infants: what do we know? A systematic review. *European Journal of Pain, 15*(7), 661.e1–661.e15.

Shah, P. S., Herbozo, C., Aliwalas, L. I., & Shah, V. S. (2012). Breastfeeding or breast milk for procedural pain in neonates. *Cochrane Database of Systematic Reviews, 12*, CD004950.

Spence, K., Gillies, D., Johnston, L., Harrison, D., & Nagy, S. (2005). A reliable pain assessment tool for clinical assessment in the neonatal intensive care. *Journal of Obstetric, Gynecologic, and Neonatal Nursing, 34*(1), 80–86.

Spence, K., Henderson-Smart, D., New, K., Evans, C., Whitelaw, J., & Woolnough, R. (2010). Evidenced-based clinical practice guideline for management of newborn pain. *Journal of Paediatrics and Child Health, 46*(4), 184–192.

Steinhorn, R., McPherson, C., Anderson, P. J., Neil, J., Doyle, L. W., & Inder, T. (2015). Neonatal morphine exposure in very preterm infants: cerebral development and outcomes. *Journal of Pediatrics, 166*(5), 1200–1207.e4.

Stevens, B., McGrath, P., Ballantyne, M., Yamada, J., Dupuis, A., Gibbins, S., et al. (2010). Influence of risk of neurological impairment and procedure invasiveness on health professionals' management of procedural pain in neonates. *European Journal of Pain, 14*(7), 735–741.

Stevens, B., Gibbins, S.,Yamada, J., Dionne, K., Lee, G., Johnston, C., et al. (2014). The premature infant pain profile-revised (PIPP-R): initial validation and feasibility. *Clinical Journal of Pain, 30*(3), 238–243.

Stevens, B., Yamada, J., Ohlsson, A., Haliburton, S., & Shorkey, A. (2016). Sucrose for analgesia in newborn infants undergoing painful procedures. *Cochrane Database of Systematic Reviews, 7*, CD001069.

Stevens, B., Yamada, J., Campbell-Yeo, M., Gibbins, S., Harrison, D., Dionne, K., et al. (2018). The minimally effective dose of sucrose for procedural pain relief in neonates: a randomized controlled trial. *BMC Pediatrics, 18*, 1–8. doi: 10.1186/s12887-018-1026-x.

Valeri, B. O., Holsti, L., & Linhares, M. B. (2015). Neonatal pain and developmental outcomes in children born preterm: a systematic review. *Clinical Journal of Pain, 31*(4), 355–362.

von Baeyer, C. L., & Pasero, C. (2017). What nurses' workarounds tell us about pain assessment. *International Journal of Nursing Studies, 67*, A1–A2.

Walker, S. M. (2014). Neonatal pain. *Paediatric Anaesthesia, 24*(1), 39–48.

Walker, S. M. (2019) Long-term effects of neonatal pain. *Seminars in Fetal and Neonatal Medicine, 24*(4), 101005. doi: 10.1016/j.siny.2019.04.005.

Wilson, D., & Hockenberry, M. J. (2011). Pain assessment and management. In: D. Wilson & M. J. Hockenberry (Eds.), *Wong's clinical manual of pediatric nursing* (8th ed., pp. 187–206). St Louis, MO: Mosby.

Woo, N.L., Cherian, S., Heaney, M., & Wahl, G. (2021). Methaemoglobinaemia secondary to topical prilocaine toxicity: a cautionary circumcision tale. *Journal of Paediatric Child Health, 57*, 149–150. doi: 10.1111/jpc.14841.

Yaksh, T. L., & Wallace, M. S. (2018). Opioids, analgesia, and pain management. In: L. Brunton, R. Hilal-Dandan, & B. Knollman B. (Eds.), *Goodman and Gilman's the pharmacological basis of therapeutics* (13th ed., pp. 353–386). New York: McGraw Hill Medical.

CHAPTER 19

NEONATAL SKIN AND WOUND CARE

DEANNE AUGUST AND VICTORIA KAIN[a]

Learning objectives

After reading this chapter you will be able to:

- describe the embryological and fetal development of the skin and its implications for neonatal nursing and midwifery practice
- describe factors that affect the skin integrity of the term and preterm neonate
- describe the stages of skin injuries (including the various aetiologies) and wound healing
- discuss preventative strategies to reduce and manage neonatal skin injury
- discuss neonatal skin injury risk and risk assessment scales.

Key words, terms and abbreviations

adhesive
chemical burns
chlorhexidine
collagen
continuous positive airway pressure (CPAP)
dermis
emollients
epidermal stripping
epidermis
epidermolysis bullosa
extravasation
friction
hyaluronidase/hyalase
hydrocolloids
hyperosmolar (extremely concentrated)
hypodermis
incubator humidification
medical adhesive-related skin injury (MARSI)
non-vesicant solutions
pressure
shearing
silicone
stratum corneum
transepidermal water loss (TEWL)
ultraviolet (UV) radiation
vernix caseosa
vesicant solution

[a]The authors would like to acknowledge James Marceau and Judith Benton, co-authors of this chapter in the 1st edition of this book.

INTRODUCTION

Care of neonatal skin is usually the responsibility of the neonatal nurse/midwife, in contrast to the multidisciplinary approach taken to other organ systems. While the skin may seem insignificant compared with the lungs or the brain, neonatal skin is vital to the overall survival and health of the neonate, playing an important role in:

- thermoregulation
- barrier function
- receptor for sensory information (pain, touch, temperature)
- chamber for fat storage
- preventing ultraviolet (UV) absorption
- facilitating vitamin D production (after the neonatal period) (Marieb & Hoehn, 2018).

Neonatal skin was previously believed to be structurally complete at approximately 37 weeks' gestation; however, it is now understood that skin continues to mature for up to 1–2 years of age (Blume-Peytavi et al., 2012).

Neonatal nurses and midwives should protect and assess the neonate's skin throughout their hospitalisation, which for preterm neonates may be months. This chapter will focus on promoting appropriate nursing and midwifery practices and utilising evidence-based skin care. Neonatal skin injuries have immediate effects on morbidity (owing to the risk of infection), as well as a financial health burden and an impact on quality of life and cosmetic implications later in life (Meszes et al., 2016).

CLINICAL PRACTICE 19.1

Skin health is dependent on visual assessment for recognition, diagnosis and treatment.

Photographs of many skin conditions and the assessment of skin can be found at: DermNet New Zealand: DermNet New Zealand Trust (2017), <https://dermnetnz.org/>.

EMBRYOLOGICAL AND FETAL DEVELOPMENT

Mature skin consists of three tissue structures, the **epidermis** being the outer, the **dermis** the middle and the **hypodermis** (containing subcutaneous tissue) the innermost layer (Marieb & Hoehn, 2018). Stratification (building of layers) and desquamation (shedding of layers) is an ongoing process throughout fetal development, and indeed throughout the life span. Ectodermal embryological cells become the fetal epidermis that eventually stratifies to include the lower stratified structures of the epidermis, which include the stratum basale, spinosum, granulosum, lucidum and corneum (the uppermost layer). The dermis arises from mesodermal cells that, when fully developed, are similar to connective tissue, containing a rich supply of nerves, blood vessels and lymphatic structures (Marieb & Hoehn, 2018). These layers form a network of tissues that develop over time during fetal life, into the neonatal period and in early childhood. Table 19.1 describes this development.

TABLE 19.1 **Stages of fetal development of the skin**

Weeks 3–4	Ectoderm, single-cell layer divides into two: basal cell and periderm
Week 8	Capillary network, sensory nerve endings exist within early dermal and epidermal structures
Weeks 8–12	Three layers (periderm, intermediate and basal) Keratinisation and embryonic epidermal stratification has begun
Week 12	Merkel cells present in hand and feet tissues
Weeks 11–13	Epidermal ridges (digits) develop
Weeks 11–17	Langerhans cells develop from precursors in bone marrow and invade embryonic/fetal epidermis
Weeks 22–24	Periderm sloughs away, contributing to vernix caseosa
Weeks 23–28	Lipids released from epidermal cells to form vernix, contributing to water-impermeable barrier Stratification of fetal cells into thin, definitive layers recognisable as postnatal epidermis Lower stratified structures of the epidermis develop
Weeks 28–34	Increase in brown adipose tissues (subcutaneous)
Week 40	Stratum corneum consists of 10–20 layers of dead skin cells

Source: adapted from Carlson (2014); Hoath and Mauro (2014).

PRETERM AND TERM SKIN

Structural differences of the skin are dependent on gestational age; understanding these differences can assist nurses/midwives to care for the skin appropriately. Fig. 19.1 demonstrates the differences between the dermal layers of adult (**a** and **b**), term (**c** and **d**) and 28-week gestation (**e** and **f**) skin. Thickness of the total skin structure is only 0.9 mm at less than 37 weeks' gestation and 1.2 mm in a term neonate, compared with 2.1 mm in an adult (Mathes & Williams, 2014). A useful comparison is to consider that 1 millimetre is equivalent to the thickness of a paperclip or a credit card. Thickening of the **stratum corneum** accelerates when a neonate is born preterm, but the bonds between layers or tissues themselves do not mirror this accelerated growth (Visscher & Narendran, 2014a). Neonatal skin, therefore, is particularly vulnerable to the damage caused by the traction on skin from medical devices, **adhesive** agents, or monitoring equipment, such as those used on monitoring leads.

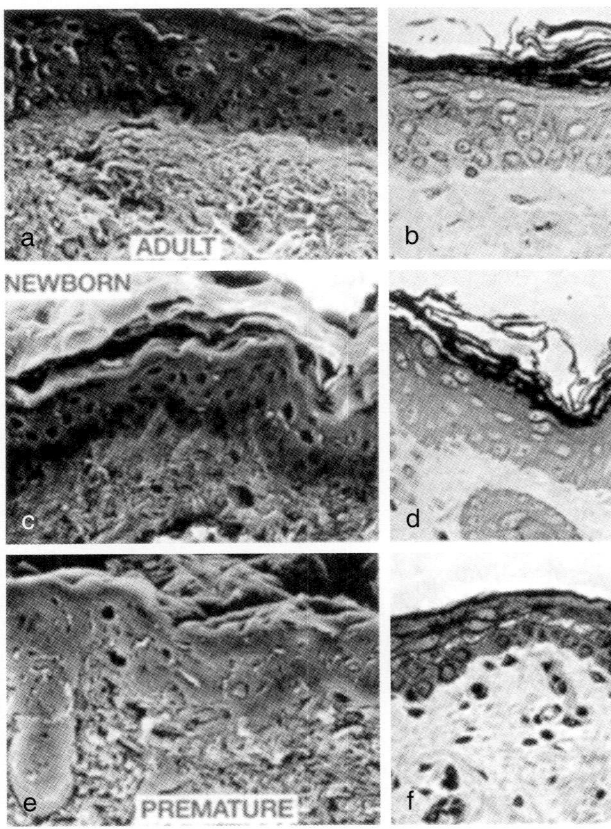

FIGURE 19.1 **Pictograph of human skin**

a, b Adult skin; **c, d** term newborn; **e, f** 28 weeks' gestation.

Source: Holbrook (1982, p. 9), reproduced by permission of Taylor and Francis Group, LLC, a division of Informa plc.

Distinctions between preterm, term and adult skin include the following:

- The term neonatal stratum corneum is 30% thinner than in adults (Almutairi, 2019).
- The neonatal dermis contains fewer **collagen** and elastin fibres and structural proteins, affecting the strength of the skin (Visscher & Narendran, 2014a).
- The junction between the epidermis and dermis is weaker in preterm and term skin, causing layers of skin to separate from each other easily (Lund et al., 2013).

FUNCTIONS OF THE SKIN

Barrier

Although neonatal skin may structurally reflect the mature organ, neonatal skin functions are immature. The skin is more complex than a simple covering; its properties present chemical, physical (mechanical) and biological barriers.

Chemical barrier functions include the following:

- Low pH skin secretions, known as the acid mantle, prevent bacteria on the skin from multiplying.
- Melanin forms a pigment shield to protect against the effects of UV radiation in sunlight.

Physical (mechanical) barrier functions:

- Skin blocks the diffusion of water through **transepidermal water loss (TEWL)** and chemical substances.

Biological barrier properties:

- Dendritic cells (Langerhans cells) ingest foreign substances, activate the immune response and cooperate with T lymphocytes in the skin to initiate cellular responses against foreign antigens.
- Dermal macrophages present a second immunological response (Marieb & Hoehn, 2018).

While the efficacies of these barrier properties are unclear in the neonate, the neonate's susceptibility to infection due to a developing immune system is well documented. Skin integrity impacts on neonatal mortality and morbidity, requiring nurses/midwives to consider skin care a significant part of their role (Visscher & Narendran, 2014a).

Thermoregulation

The skin's role is to assist in maintaining thermal homeostasis, but immaturity and minimal cell layers leave the neonate vulnerable to heat loss (see Chapter 8).

The role of vernix

Vernix caseosa acts as a fetal protective barrier against amniotic fluid. It is a cheese-like substance that consists of 80% water, 10% protein and 10% lipids. Vernix is seen in abundance in the last trimester, where it is thought to facilitate the formation of the stratum corneum (Visscher & Narendran, 2014b). Fig. 19.2 demonstrates the cellular and structural components of vernix.

Vernix is produced from 20 weeks' gestation and is visible from 33–34 weeks (it is not seen on the skin of preterm neonates or post-term neonates beyond 41 weeks owing to desquamation). This substance protects the integrity of the developing skin from exposure in utero to amniotic fluid, and in the perinatal period plays an important role in skin hydration (Visscher & Narendran, 2014b). It contains proteins that are thought to have both immunological and antibacterial properties (Bamalan & Menezes, 2020).

Touch, pain and temperature

Neonatal skin contains receptors that detect pain (nociceptors) (Cornelissen et al., 2013), temperature (thermoreceptors) and touch (mechanoreceptors and Merkel cells) (Ma, 2009). The understanding of the effects of preterm birth on these receptors is uncertain (see chapters on thermoregulation (Chapter 8) and neonatal pain management (Chapter 18) for further information).

Ultraviolet protection

Ultraviolet (UV) radiation is emitted by the sun and has wavelengths of 100–400 nanometres (nm). UV radiation has been shown to damage and age adult skin cells, resulting in a cumulative effect that produces carcinogenic mutations (Suman & Suman, 2019). Avoidance of direct sunlight is advised until a newborn is 6 months of age, and

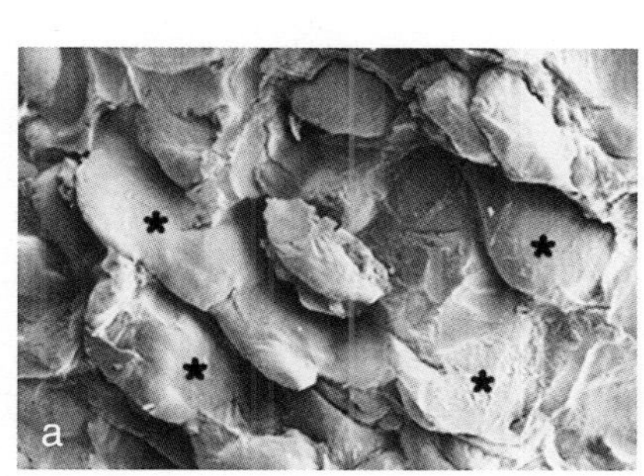

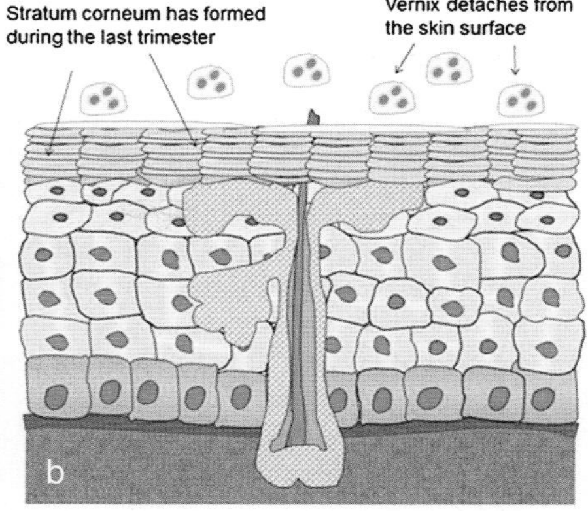

FIGURE 19.2 **Vernix**

a Vernix structure of cells and lipids; **b** process of detachment from skin near term age.

Source: Visscher and Narendran (2014b).

the use of sunscreens should be avoided as clinical trials of sunscreen are limited to infants who are older than 6 months (Li et al., 2019).

EVIDENCE-BASED PRACTICE RESEARCH 19.1

The neonatal microbiome

The neonatal microbiome is the beginning of a symbiotic relationship with a microbiota that has been passed to the neonate before, during and after the birth. These microbiota are estimated to be composed of 1 trillion (10^{12}) microorganisms and constitute the largest living organ in the body (Meropol & Edwards, 2015). A healthy symbiotic interaction between the neonate and the microbiota is paramount for a healthy metabolic and immunological system. The dysbiosis of the neonatal microbiome is associated with neonatal gastrointestinal diseases such as necrotising enterocolitis (NEC) and has been reported to be also involved in inflammatory diseases such as coeliac disease (Giles & Couper, 2020).

PRINCIPLES OF NEONATAL SKIN CARE

Risk of absorption

The immaturity of neonatal skin, coupled with a higher body surface area-to-weight ratio, increases the risks of percutaneous absorption and toxicity from agents applied to the skin (Danby et al., 2014). Absorptive toxicity is a historical finding first recognised as a complication of topical agent application through the reviewing of case studies and data in Rutter's seminal work (Rutter, 2000). Table 19.2 outlines the compounds that have the potential to cause toxicity including neurotoxicity, nephrotoxicity, ototoxicity and skin necrosis. Caution should be taken before any compound is applied to preterm/term skin as both active ingredients and inactive ingredients can result in complications (Danby et al., 2014).

Maintaining moisture

Hydration of neonatal skin is important to the integrity of the stratum corneum (Visscher & Narendran, 2014b). Currently, interventions to promote hydration are limited to **incubator humidification** and the application of oils and **emollients**.

Incubator humidity

Humidification has long been touted to assist in maintaining skin hydration, yet no evidence for this has been established. Incubator humidification, however, remains 'best practice' for improved growth and thermal stability as well as to decrease fluid and electrolyte imbalances (including TEWL) for neonates of less than 34 weeks' gestation. Guidelines for incubator humidification are discussed in more detail in Chapter 8.

TABLE 19.2 **Compounds that may be absorbed via the neonatal skin**

Type of product	Chemical compounds
Clinical/hospital products	• Standard antiseptics (see Table 19.3) • Hexachlorophene (antiseptic) • Adhesive remover solvents • Methylene blue
Infant care products	• Urea containing emollients • Boric acid (baby powders and nappy pastes) • Mercuric chloride (nappy rinses and teething preparations) • Aniline dyes (laundry dye)
Pharmacological products	• Lindane (lice and scabies treatment) • Neomycin • Adrenaline • Corticosteroids • Lignocaine • Oestrogen • Silver sulfadiazine

Source: Danby et al. (2014).

Oils and emollients

The use of emollients (e.g. lotions or ointments) and oils is controversial owing to the lack of studies measuring short-term and long-term outcomes (Pupala et al., 2019). Recently, oils such as sunflower oil have become the preferred choice for practices such as infant massage (Salam et al., 2015). Early research demonstrated that emollient application improved skin condition scores without increasing the risk of infection (Lund et al., 2001). However, a Cochrane review concluded that there is no current evidence that emollient treatment decreases the risk of infection, but it may increase the relative risk of coagulase-negative staphylococcal infection for preterm neonates in high-income countries (Cleminson & McGuire, 2016).

Current evidence comparing moisturising agents for neonatal use is of low quality, and these results cannot be extrapolated for widespread clinical adoption. Furthermore, many neonatal units do not have current guidelines for oil/emollient application, so their use is often at the clinician's or family's discretion. When considering the use of moisturisers, the clinician should consider the product being applied, ingredients, interaction with other treatments and the optimal volume for application. Even the recommended volumes of emollients/oils vary greatly in clinical trials (Pupala et al., 2019).

Review Clinical Practice 19.2 and Family-centred Care 19.1 in this chapter for further information. In summary, there is not enough evidence to suggest that the benefits of emollients or oils outweigh the risks associated with their use, such as toxicity or as a possible vector of infection.

CLINICAL PRACTICE 19.2

Considerations for oils and emollients

- May affect adhesives (e.g. monitoring devices).
- Limited or nil application concurrently with phototherapy or radiant heater use.
- Few published cases of hyperthermic burns but may remain standard practice.
- No increased infection:
  - sunflower seed oil compared with emollient (Salam et al., 2015)
  - coconut oil compared with routine skin care (Nangia et al., 2015; Salam et al., 2015)
  - oils containing high oleic acid content (including apricot seed, olive and sesame oil) are more drying and degrading to the skin (Danby et al., 2014; Visscher & Geiss, 2014).

Adverse outcomes

- Single-use containers prevent product contamination.
- Preservatives: creams manufactured without preservatives can be at risk for contamination, compared with possible risk of preservative absorption (Danby et al., 2014).
- Oils can oxidise when opened or decanted, leading to chemical changes or degradation (i.e. purchasing cooking oils for use as skin care owing to cost-saving and knowledge deficit) (Blume-Peytavi et al., 2016).
- Mustard seed, olive and soya bean oils show detrimental effects to skin cells and would therefore not be recommended for neonates (Danby et al., 2013).
- Mineral oil: little evidence to provide recommendations.
- Oils and emollients containing fragrances remain controversial, yet fragranced nappy wipes are discouraged for infants less than 1 year (Blume-Peytavi et al., 2016).

FAMILY-CENTRED CARE 19.1

There are many reasons why families may wish to apply skin care products, including moisturisers. Culturally, a newborn massage is just as important as the nightly bath for many parents, who believe that these activities are beneficial for their baby and promote attachment (Blume-Peytavi et al., 2016). Additionally, some parents wish to minimise their newborn's exposure to toxins and believe that natural or non-preservative-based products are safer. As in all areas of neonatal nursing/midwifery, provision of known evidence about all options can assist families in maximising their newborn's skin health and making informed decisions.

Natural or non-preservative-based products are not always a harmless alternative to commercially available products (Pupala et al., 2019). Emphasising the lack of evidence comparing commercial products and natural products, as well as cases of infections spreading from contaminated hand lotion, are important teaching points. Certain food oils have been associated with increased water loss and infection, and these points may help families to reconsider their moisturising and bathing practices. Additionally, both food-based skin care products and cooking products/oils being used for skin care are equally controversial. Skin care products with food-based ingredients may increase the risk of sensitisation and possible food allergy in later development. Many healthcare institutions have begun to caution their use, yet high-quality evidence around these recommendations is lacking.

BATHING

Two evidence-based guidelines currently exist to provide information for healthcare professionals regarding a wide range of newborn skin care topics including bathing, nappy care and skin product use for *full-term* newborns.

The first bath should occur only when the newborn's temperature is stable, and should not exceed 10 minutes' duration in a water temperature of around, but not exceeding, 38°C. According to the aforementioned guidelines, important considerations for bathing while in hospital include the following:

- The bath equipment should be disinfected prior to use to prevent the transmission of nosocomial infection (Blume-Peytavi et al., 2016).

- Bathing is a time for the parents to bond with their new baby and for staff to teach and reassure parents, meaning that parents should be present and involved in bath time.
- In terms of frequency, while in hospital the newborn needs to be bathed only every other day; however, some cultures prefer to bathe and massage their baby daily. Education should support that daily bathing is unnecessary for hygiene but is an important bonding activity (Blume-Peytavi et al., 2016). See Family-centred Care 19.1 for further information.
- Immersion bathing (rather than using a damp face washer) is preferred as a bathing practice for preterm neonates as it is less likely to cause physiological stress (Blume-Peytavi et al., 2016) (Fig. 19.3).
- Bathing methods should be dependent on the neonate's age and clinical condition. Refer to Box 19.1 for

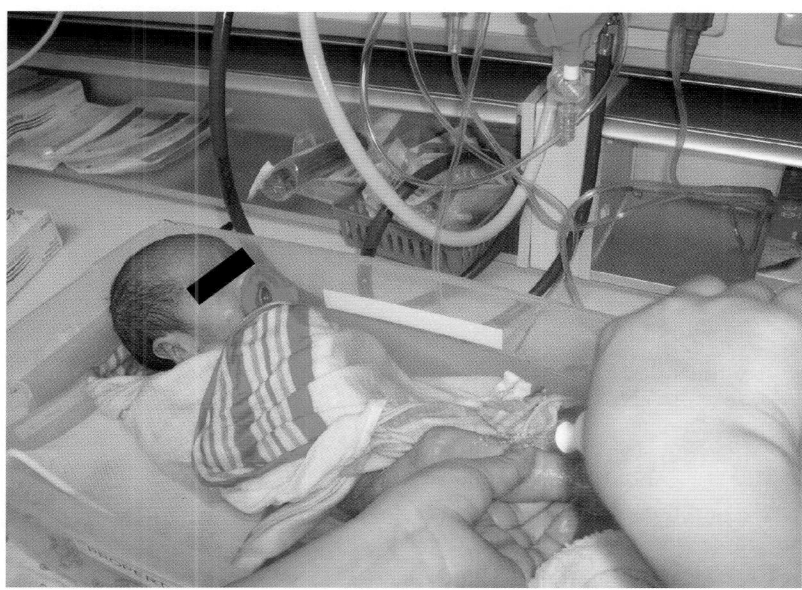

FIGURE 19.3 **Swaddled tub bath technique**
Source: Quraishy et al. (2013).

BOX 19.1 **Bathing considerations**

The first bath

- Where possible *vernix should remain on the skin* as it will benefit development of the neonate's stratum corneum (Visscher et al., 2011).
- Healthcare workers should use standard precautions, including the wearing of disposable gloves.
- The first bath should be postponed after birth for at least 6 hours to enable time for infant bonding and successful breastfeeding (Kuller, 2014).

Preterm (<32 weeks' gestation) bathing considerations

- Avoid bathing during the first week of life, when the preterm neonate of less than 32 weeks' gestation should only be wiped gently with a warm, damp cloth and gently patted dry.

Types of bathing

Sponge/cloth bath

- Use warm water, a face washer and dish/basin.
- Expose one limb or body part at a time: completely exposing the newborn can cause distress and hypothermia.
- Thoroughly and gently pat the neonate dry to prevent heat loss.

Immersion tub bath

- Greater physiological stability is indicated by tub bathing compared with sponge bathing in neonates of greater than 36 weeks' gestation (Loring et al., 2012).
- Hypothermia is limited when the torso and limbs are immersed in water that is between 38°C and 40°C (Kuller, 2014).
- Consider the size of the tub and ensure that term newborns fit in the tub and the upper body is not exposed to the air.
- Due to the risk of hypothermia, the duration of the bath should not exceed 10 minutes.
- Immersion tub bathing without swaddling is not recommended for preterm neonates because it can cause physiological stress.

Swaddled immersion tub bath

- This technique is suited to the neonate in the neonatal intensive care unit (NICU): the limbs are swaddled, as this is less likely to cause physiological stress (see Fig. 19.3).
- The neonate is lowered into the bath; each limb is removed from the swaddled position, washed and re-swaddled (Quraishy et al., 2013).

TABLE 19.3 **Disinfectants used in neonatal care**

Disinfectant	Mechanism of action	Disadvantages and precautions	Available concentrations
Chlorhexidine	Disrupts the cytoplasmic membrane of bacterial cells Denatures proteins	Not effective against *Mycobacterium* Can cause local erythema/skin irritation/chemical burns in preterm neonates	0.25%, 0.5%, 1%, 2%, 4% (aqueous- and alcohol-based)
Alcohols	Damages the cell membrane Denatures proteins	Not active in the presence of organic material Not recommended as less effective and contraindicated in neonates	Ethanol, isopropyl alcohol, methanol
Povidone or iodine	Penetrates bacterial cells causing denaturation of proteins, nucleotides, and fatty acids	Excessive use may cause hypothyroidism If solution is used, the residue should be removed from the skin after the procedure	10% povidone–iodine
Octenidine	Binds to cell membranes and destroys the cell walls of microorganisms	Currently unavailable outside Europe Requires 2 minutes of contact time to achieve antisepsis	Octisept: octenidine dihydrochloride, 2-phenoxy-ethanol

Source: Danby et al. (2014); Ponnusamy et al. (2014).

special considerations for preterm bathing, types of bathing products and recommended frequency.

- Bathing with **chlorhexidine** wipes/chlorhexidine solution to decrease hospital-acquired infection has been investigated in neonates >1000 g and 28 weeks' gestation (Quach et al., 2014). Yet the practice remains controversial owing to concerns of absorption of the active agent (discussed further under 'Procedural skin disinfectants', Table 19.3). While the practice is endemic and well substantiated by evidence in the adult/paediatric intensive care populations, its efficacy in the neonatal setting remains unsubstantiated (Paternoster et al., 2017).

CLINICAL PRACTICE 19.3

Bathing products

A suitable bathing product should have either a neutral or a mildly acidic pH (in the reference range of 6.1–6.5) to avoid irritation of the newborn's skin (Association of Women's Health, Obstetric and Neonatal Nurses (AWHONN), 2018). When parents are shown how to bathe their neonate, they should be advised to avoid purchasing products with fragrance and strong surfactants as they can irritate newborn skin (refer to Evidence-based Practice Research 19.1) (Blume-Peytavi et al., 2016).

How would you discuss bathing product choices with families?

CLINICAL PRACTICE 19.4

Bathing the preterm infant

According to research, frequent daily bathing for preterm newborns can have a number of negative impacts on the infant's physiological responses and comfort/discomfort. Tambunan and Mediani (2019) reported the current evidence for bathing preterm infants in order to improve neurodevelopmental care by utilising an atraumatic strategy. This research found that several of the processes actually lessened the detrimental impacts of bathing on preterm infants' health. Swaddle bathing was shown to be the best and safest technique of bathing for preterm infants during hospitalisation, resulting in fewer changes in physiological and behavioural distress. The use of a swaddling bathing for preterm infants while hospitalised was advised and should be regarded as a standard operating procedure in the perinatology unit and NICU.

REFLECTION

When you next visit your local store or chemist, review the ingredients section for newborn washes and emollients.

1. How many contain irritants, fragrances or one of the following surfactants: lauryl sulfate, dodecyl sulfate, alkyl sulfate, cocoate, tallowate, palmitate, stearate, olefin sulfonate, benzalkonium, bromide, dodecyl trimethyl ammonium, triethanolamine laurate, linear alkyl benzene sulfate?
2. Did any of the ingredients surprise you?

UMBILICAL CORD CARE

Between 5 and 15 days after birth, the cord usually separates. Before the separation, the residual stump might be considered a healed wound and thus a possible path for infection into the neonate's bloodstream via the vessels.

Cord care methods may directly contribute to newborn infections, with neonatal sepsis accounting for more than

15% of the 3.3 million neonatal deaths globally (Basiouny & Lassy, 2019). An estimated one million neonates die each year owing to a bacterial infection in the umbilical cord during the healing process. To reduce morbidity and death, the World Health Organization (WHO) recommends enhancing newborn care procedures at birth. These procedures are known as essential neonatal care (ENC). Clean cord care is one of these key practices, which is critical in reducing early newborn infections. According to social, cultural, economic and geographic variables, methods of caring for the umbilical stump differ widely between countries and healthcare settings (Basiouny & Lassy, 2019).

The underlying principle of umbilical cord care is to keep it clean and dry by allowing the cord to be exposed to the air (AWHONN, 2018). If the remnant stump is thoroughly dried and left uncovered, it will heal within 12–15 days. Care includes cleaning the remnant cord with water if it becomes contaminated with faeces or urine and educating parents that the cord may not detach while the neonate is in hospital owing to current lengths of stay.

PROCEDURAL SKIN DISINFECTANTS

The neonate is extremely vulnerable to nosocomial infections that, if undetected or untreated, can result in sepsis and death (Chan & Smith, 2018). (See Chapter 16 for further information.) To reduce the incidence of central line-associated bloodstream infections (CLABSI), topical antiseptic solutions should be used for all such invasive procedures. However, due to the immature nature of the skin, neonates are highly vulnerable to absorption and irritation (including burns) from disinfectants (Vanzi & Pitaro, 2018). Solutions have been known to cause contact complications (most often in preterm skin), ranging from contact dermatitis to **chemical burns** with catastrophic consequences. Selection of the best disinfectant with the fewest side effects can be challenging.

The choice of a skin disinfectant solution should consider the risks versus the potential benefits of the solution, with side effects and precautions requiring careful consideration (AWHONN, 2018). Recommendations for disinfectants are summarised in Clinical Practice 19.5 and Table 19.3.

Chemical burns in the preterm and term neonate are primarily due to residual cleansing solutions left on the skin following procedures. Errors in solution selection are also possible and can include the use of a 0.5% aqueous chlorhexidine and 70% alcohol solution instead of sterile water or 2% aqueous chlorhexidine (Vanzi & Pitaro, 2018). It is important to verify the identification of the cleansing solution at the start of any procedure, as one would double check the administration of a medication to a neonate. Care should be taken not to pool the solution around the neonate's umbilicus, back or flank, thereby partially immersing the skin, before or during the procedure – see Clinical Practice 19.5.

CLINICAL PRACTICE 19.5

Chemical spillage or contact burns in preterm neonates usually occur as a result of overzealous application of procedural disinfectant solutions. Prolonged exposure of the skin from even the lowest percentage of chlorhexidine can result in skin contact injuries (Vanzi & Pitaro, 2018). Cleansing the skin with sterile water after applying the disinfectant can reduce this risk. Early examination of the neonate's skin, including the back and flanks, is paramount as disinfectant solutions may pool in these areas.

Because the neonatal population lacks the established traits present in older patient cohorts, certain traditional wound care treatments should not be used on neonates just because they are effective in adult patients. Although the use of adhesives, alginates or collagen dressings on neonatal wounds may be necessary in some circumstances, the great majority of neonatal patients would benefit by substituting products with specifically demonstrated efficacies. Hydrocolloids, hydrogels, foams, barrier films and barrier creams are currently recommended as first-line therapies for neonatal wounds based on existing data (Steen et al., 2020).

SKIN INJURY AND WOUNDS

Skin injury is an alteration in the structure and integrity of the skin. Skin injury is a broad term that includes damage from mechanical force (e.g. **pressure** or tearing), chemical/thermal burns or **extravasation** of parenteral fluids into tissues. Skin injuries are often the result of an adverse event combined with preterm physiology, whereas neonatal 'wounds' are more classically associated with surgical sites or extravasations. Both a skin injury and a wound will result in a 'wound bed'. Recognising the cause of the injury may assist in prevention of future incidences and may also direct the treatment that is necessary. There are multiple assessment tools for skin integrity: some for types of skin injury (extravasation stages or pressure injury stages), some for generalised skin conditions (Neonatal Skin Risk Assessment Scale (NSARS)) and others for wound phases. These tools may assist in determining the management and dressing choice for injuries and wounds. Box 19.2 demonstrates the physiological process of uncompromised wound healing, which can be divided into four phases. The differences between uncompromised adult and neonatal wound healing are unknown, and variations between adult and fetal wounds include inflammatory markers, collagens, fibrins and elastin content, as well as the documentation of scar-less healing in fetal models (Karppinen et al., 2019).

Skin injuries from force

Skin injuries from mechanical force are classically referred to as 'pressure injuries' but can be a result of pressure and **shearing** forces and/or pressure and **friction** (Edsberg et al., 2016). Neonatal skin injuries are most often related to medical devices, for example injury to the nose from **continuous positive airway pressure (CPAP)** interfaces

BOX 19.2 **Wound phases, concepts and considerations**

Wound phases

1. *Haemostasis:* vasoconstriction, clot formation and biochemical response
2. *Inflammatory:* increased blood flow, erythema, swelling, heat, probable discomfort
3. *Reconstruction:* granulation (new tissue and blood vessel formation), fibroblasts (produce collagen) contract around wound margin and pull edges together; epithelial cells multiply and migrate, producing a film across the wound bed
4. *Maturation:* fibroblasts remodel collagen, which increases the strength of connective tissues; can occur after the wound appears healed

Wound bed/tissue assessment with corresponding phase

- *Red:* inflammation, tissue is usually still 'healthy'
- *Pink:* healthy granulation, new epithelium
- *Dull pink:* non-healthy epithelisation (granulation or stressed, decreased perfusion)
- *Yellow (grey):* slough with possible infection (slough: mixture of fibrin, exudate, leucocytes and bacteria)
- *Green:* clinical sign of infection, purulence
- *Black/brown:* necrotic or avascular tissue
- *White/pale:* macerated skin, exposed to excessive moisture, possibly avascular

Other considerations

- Wound beds may present as a mixed presentation of phases
- Elements that may prolong healing include:
  - chemicals
  - infection
  - dryness
  - mechanical force (e.g. friction)

Source: adapted from: Carville (2017); Visscher et al. (2011).

(August et al., 2018) or **medical adhesive-related skin injuries (MARSI)** (de Oliveira Marcatto et al., 2021). Staging and prevention of neonatal skin injuries is an evolving field (August et al., 2018). Injuries such as MARSI and pressure injury were previously considered 'unavoidable complications' of preterm birth and referred to as 'scars of prematurity' (Prizant et al., 1996).

Refer to Clinical Practice 19.6 for further information about skin injury forces.

CLINICAL PRACTICE 19.6

Skin injury forces

- **Pressure:** force or compression exerted on/against the skin from another contact source – for example, a neonate lying on an intravenous cannula hub or creased sheet for a prolonged period
- **Friction:** two surfaces moving across/against each other creating resistance between skin and surface – for example, knee rubbing in the prone position
- **Shear:** parallel load, when the outer layers of skin remain still while deeper layers move in a transverse plane, generating distortion of the dermis, fascia, etc. – for example, intrapartum injuries such as forceps or vacuum injury
- **Stripping:** removal of adhesive tape or securement devices, when the adhesive bond to the skin is stronger than the epidermal/dermal bond – for example, red patches after tape removal

Sources: August et al. (2018); de Oliveira Marcatto et al. (2021).

Neonatal skin injuries are dissimilar to adult injuries as they rarely occur over bony prominences, but instead occur over bone or soft tissue such as cartilage. Furthermore, injuries more commonly involve the face, chest, lower and upper extremities (Meszes et al., 2016; Visscher & Taylor, 2014) and are most often related to medical devices rather than bed surfaces or mattress types (August et al., 2014). These devices are necessary components of neonatal survival; therefore diligent implementation and management for the application or removal of devices is required of neonatal teams. Studies continue to investigate the relationship of skin injury types and other risk factors but known associations include (but are not limited to) (August et al., 2018):

- endotracheal tubes, including tapes and fixatives
- CPAP interfaces (masks and prongs), hats or securement devices
- intravenous lines, cannulas and hubs
- leads, probes and monitoring equipment
- identification bands
- plastic and fabric-backed tapes
- gestational age (not limited to birth gestation).

Examples of skin injuries can be seen in Figs 19.4 and 19.5 and the current skin injury classifications applicable to neonates can be found in Table 19.4.

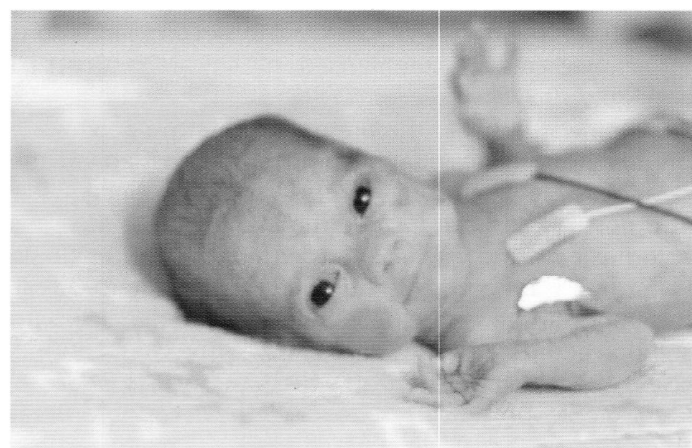

FIGURE 19.4 **Epidermal stripping to cheeks due to medical adhesive-related skin injury**

TABLE 19.4 **Skin injury types and classifications found in neonatal populations**

Type of injury	Characteristics
Suspected deep tissue injury (discoloured; intact)	Darker area of skin, usually intact, may blister (purple or maroon in colour)
Stage 1 (non-blanchable erythema)	Altered skin tone, intact, presents as erythema (redness)
Stage 2 (partial thickness)	Shallow, open wound, pink wound bed without slough (may be intact or open blister)
Stage 3 (full thickness)	Deeper than superficial, depending on injury location subcutaneous fat may be visible (bone/ muscle not exposed)
Stage 4 (full-thickness loss)	Full thickness loss with extensive damage (muscle or bone visible, slough and necrosis/eschar may be present)
Unstageable (unknown depth)	Base of injury is covered by slough and/or eschar, stage undetermined until base is visible
Epidermal stripping (MARSI)	• Tape-related, adhesive-to-skin bond stronger than skin-to-skin layer • Epidermal layers separate from each other or from dermis altogether • Can occur without visual evidence of trauma

Source: adapted from: Lund (2014); Schindler et al. (2013).

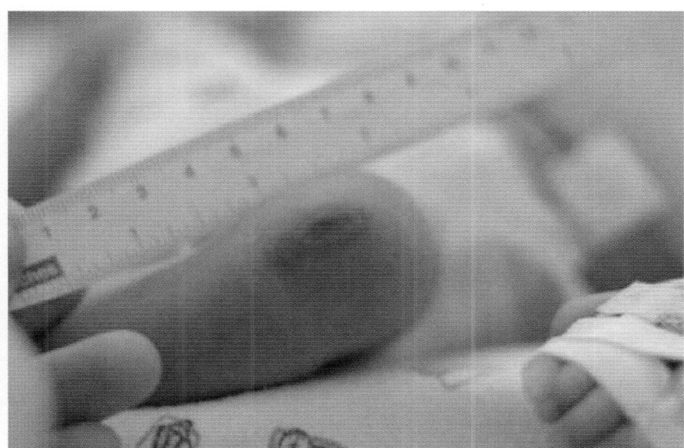

FIGURE 19.5 **Skin injury from pressure, friction and/or shear, stage 1 surrounding suspected deep tissue injury**

Management of skin injury from force

The primary responsibility of the neonatal nurse/midwife is to identify, assess, report and investigate preventative measures for neonatal skin injuries. The uses of risk assessment tools will be discussed at a later stage in this chapter. In general, manufacturers have greater recognition of the fragility of skin and are developing products specific for this population. This includes non-adhesive saturation probes, small electrocardiograph (ECG) leads and non-adhesive straps for cannula stabilisation. Neonatal nurses and midwives should also be diligent in rotation of medical devices and probes (approximately every 4–6 hours). Prolonged periods of supine positioning may increase the risk for heel, ear and occiput injuries (particularly in postoperative or muscle-relaxed neonates). Sheepskin mattresses are associated with reduced risks of pressure injury in healthy adults; however, they have been found to increase risk of SIDS, so are not recommended for neonatal settings (Duncan & Byard, 2018). Gel pads or mattresses may be suggested to prevent pressure-related injuries, while evaluation of their use has yet to be confirmed.

Strategies to minimise MARSIs are equally complicated and the neonatal nurse/midwife should learn about medical adhesive application and removal best practices; the technique described in this chapter is based on the work of Lund (2014) and de Oliveira Marcatto et al. (2021) and is demonstrated in Table 19.5 and Fig. 19.6.

Skin injuries related to respiratory interfaces (CPAP, SIPPV, HHF)

While generalised prevention strategies for skin injury remain complex, skin injury risks related to respiratory support modalities are better understood. Studies have investigated nasal mask and prong interfaces (Imbulana et al., 2018) and identified significant indicators for injury. Strategies shown to reduce nasal injury included:

- nasal barrier dressings
- nasal high-flow therapy as an alternative to binasal prong CPAP
- nasal masks rather than binasal prongs.

Thermal burns

Thermal burns are less common in neonates compared with chemical burns and may occasionally still occur from:

- spillage of hot fluids (Mohamadzadeh et al., 2020)
- therapeutic cooling/heating mats (Strohm et al., 2011)
- transcutaneous oxygen/carbon dioxide monitoring probes (Jensen & Galbraith, 2014)
- gloves filled with hot water (Jensen & Galbraith, 2014).

Historically, events have occurred with ice packs to the facial area during sinus venous tachycardia treatment (Diamantis et al., 2006) and intra- and postoperative heating sources (i.e. Bair Hugger and fan heater).

TABLE 19.5 **Adhesive selection, application and removal**

Product	Action/precaution
Gel and silicone adhesives	Softer than other adhesives but may not be robust enough to adhere to medical devices (especially under heat and humidity)
Pectin/plastic/fabric adhesives	Increased stripping reactions occur compared with gel adhesives
Bonding agents (benzoin tincture)	Solution NOT advised owing to increased stripping result upon adhesive removal
Removal of adhesive	Minimise stripping during removal: • Consult manufacturer guidelines for removal techniques • Remove in parallel/horizontal direction, NOT 90° angle, except for film/occlusive dressing • Slow removal may reduce injury • One hand supports skin while the other pulls away (two-handed technique) • Tabbed edges may assist in lifting the edges of tapes at the start of removal
Adhesive removers (solution or wipe)	• Silicone-based removers • Sterile water • Petrolatum or citrus-based helpful, but can make reapplication difficult and may cause dermal reactions • Alcohol-derived removers • NOT recommended for neonates
Second-skin/hydrocolloid sheets[a]	• Protect skin when tapes need frequent replacement (subnasal oxygen or endotracheal tubes) • Protective layer when harsh adhesive products are used
Adhesive securement devices	• Available for various medical devices (endotracheal tubes, chest tubes and lines) • Ascertain the type of adhesive in individual devices to remove appropriately
Skin barrier wipes	Consider under tapes or areas of fragile skin: • Contain silicone (dimethicone) and may protect from superficial breakdown • One study evaluated efficacy of wipes (found fewer TEWL with wipes compared with standard emollient (Lund et al., 2013))
All adhesives	Increased susceptibility of epidermal stripping for neonates <28 weeks (Boswell & Waker, 2016)

[a] Note: removal can also result in epidermal stripping (equivalent to tape removal).

Source: adapted from de Oliveira Marcatto et al. (2021); Lund (2014).

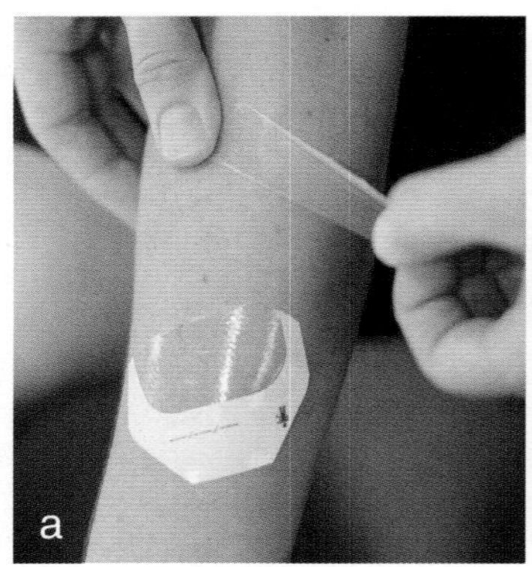

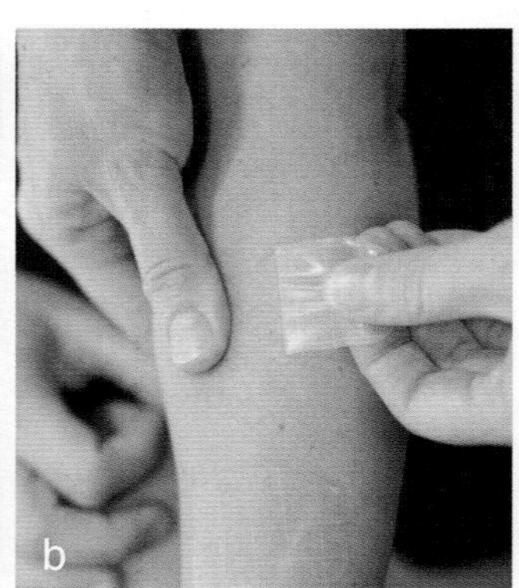

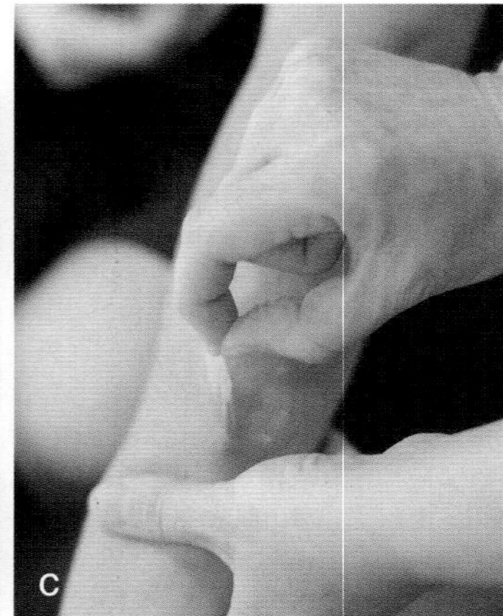

FIGURE 19.6 **Adhesive removal: best practice and poor removal techniques**

Best practice: Removal of polyurethane (**a**) and pectin/hydrocolloid (**b**) demonstrates removal with second hand supplying tension and support. When the skin is unsupported during adhesive removal, such as in **c**, there is a greater chance of causing skin tear/shearing injury.

While thermal injuries are more infrequent, a nurse may be the first to discover the presence of the injury, identify associated factors and communicate and document these complications. The neonatal nurse/midwife must advocate caution in pre/postoperative situations with the surgical team, who may be unfamiliar with the potential risks of thermal injury.

Extravasation injuries

Extravasation injuries (also known as infiltration injuries) occur when an intravenous solution leaks into the extravascular space and can cause debilitating and catastrophic injuries, including skin necrosis and vascular compromised limbs (Cho et al., 2019). Extravasation injuries are more commonly reported in the literature for peripheral cannulas; less common are cases of central extravasation (Ratchagame & Prabakaran, 2021). Injuries can be related to vesicant or **non-vesicant solutions** in the neonatal population. Non-vesicants are IV solutions and medications that do not cause ischaemia or necrosis, whereas vesicants are those that do lead to ischaemia and necrosis. Vesicants are extremely acidic or basic (pH less than 5 or greater than 9), **hyperosmolar (extremely concentrated)** or vasoconstrictive (i.e. cause the blood vessels to constrict). Clinical presentation of an extravasation injury from a **vesicant solution** is more severe and needs immediate attention to prevent further damage. See Box 19.3 for a list of potential solutions.

The veins of a preterm neonate are fragile and sometimes extravasation is unavoidable. Neonates born less than 26 weeks are thought to have increased risk for extravasation. Early identification and intervention at the first sign or symptom of extravasation is crucial, in order to circumvent any adverse outcome. Unassuming reddening and swelling may change within a few hours to a stageable extravasation injury. See Fig. 19.7 for examples of extravasation injuries during recovery. A validated extravasation staging scale should be used to document the extent of the injury at initial assessment (see an example in Table 19.6).

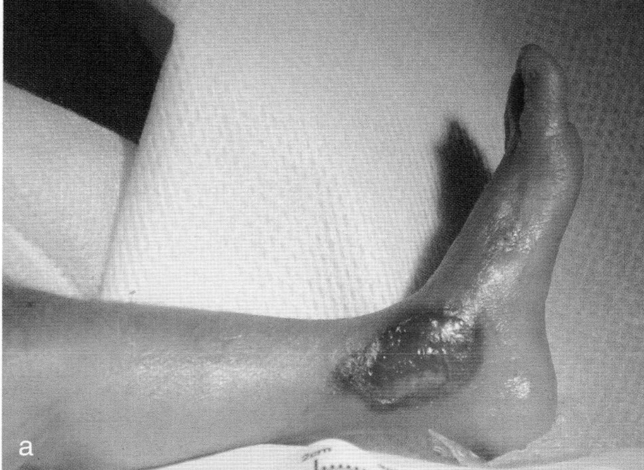

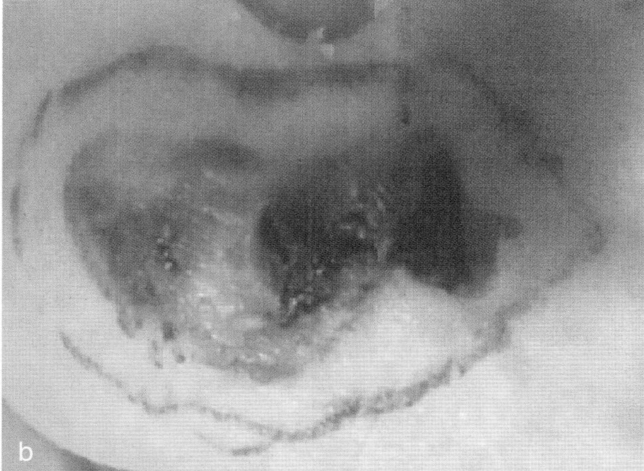

FIGURE 19.7 **Extravasation injuries**
a Extravasation injury to ankle, 24 hours after cannula removal; **b** extravasation injury to forearm, day 10 (with silicone wound gel treatment initiated).

BOX 19.3 **Vesicant and non-vesicant solutions associated with extravasations**

Vesicant:

- Aciclovir
- Dobutaminea
- Dopamine[a]
- Total parenteral infusion (TPN)[a]
- Vancomycin
- Sodium bicarbonate[a]
- Trometamol; tris-hydroxymethyl aminomethane (THAM)[a]
- Dextrose concentrations >12.5%[a]

Non-vesicant:

- Erythromycin
- Gentamicin
- Digoxin
- Calcium-containing solutions[a]

[a] The peripheral administration of these solutions should be avoided.
Sources: Beall et al. (2013); Restieaux et al. (2013).

Peripheral line intravascular extravasations can be minimised by adoption of the following principles:

- The cannula insertion site as it enters the skin should always be visible (e.g. not covered with tapes).
- All intravenous cannula insertion sites should be frequently assessed for potential infiltration (e.g. redness and swelling) (Restieaux et al., 2013).
- Evidence-based unit guidelines on the management of extravasation injuries and a dedicated extravasation kit including dispersal agent and/or antidote treatment should be used (Restieaux et al., 2013).

Extravasation treatment

Treatment of an identified extravasation injury from a vesicant or hyperosmolar solution is a medical emergency and needs urgent intervention. The neonatal nurse/

TABLE 19.6 **Stages of extravasation injury**

Stage	Characteristics
I	The intravenous device flushes with difficulty Discomfort at site, but no indication of injury
II	Minimal inflammation with redness and discomfort at site Pulse and perfusion normal distal to access site
III	Minimal inflammation with redness, blanching and discomfort at site Skin cool to touch Pulse and perfusion normal distal to access site
IV	Severe inflammation on top of and underneath access site Discomfort and blanching at site with cool skin Evidence of skin breakdown and/or necrosis Decreased or absent pulse and perfusion distal to access

Source: adapted from Restieaux et al. (2013).

midwife must act immediately to prevent further injury. They should:

- stop the infusion of the solution
- organise an immediate review by a senior clinician for possible treatment options (for extensive extravasations consultation with plastics/surgical team should be considered)
- leave the cannula in so the senior clinician can aspirate the vesicant fluid if possible
- elevate the affected limb.

Practices that are *discouraged* in the neonatal population include:

- topical application of silver sulfadiazine cream (sulfur-containing medication)
- application of heat or cold (due to risk of thermal injury).

Interventions for extravasation management may include multiple puncture sites for expelling extravasated fluid, subcutaneous irrigation with saline (also known as dispersal or clysis technique), specific dispersal agent and/or antidote treatment. **Hyaluronidase/hyalase** is a mucolytic enzyme that breaks down the vesicant solution, and the timely administration of hyaluronidase is suggested to decrease the severity of tissue damage; hence, it remains the favoured treatment for extravasation (Corbett et al., 2019). However, there is a lack of published evidence to suggest whether saline irrigation ± prior hyaluronidase improves tissue healing in neonates when compared with no intervention or normal wound care (Gopalakrishnan et al., 2017). The evidence basis of some treatment options has not been established, and, as such, an experienced clinician should select from the following options:

- Saline irrigation by a senior clinician who will make puncture holes around the swelling to express the extravasated fluid using aseptic technique (Gopalakrishnan et al., 2017).
- Two percent nitroglycerine ointment (or phentolamine), for the treatment of catecholamine-induced extravasations (dopamine) (Plum & Moukhachen, 2017).
- Hyaluronidase injected into the affected cannula to deliver directly to the site of extravasation. Hyaluronidase (15 units/mL) can be ordered and dispensed into five syringes of 0.2 mL. After cleansing the site, inject these doses at five separate sites around the area of extravasation. The enzyme will assist in dissolving the solution in the localised tissue area and re-dispersing it to a larger surface area (Corbett et al., 2019).
- Medical-grade honey has been recommended for treating extravasation wounds in preterm infants because it possesses antimicrobial, anti-inflammatory and antioxidative activity, enhancing wound healing. Medical-grade honey has been found to be safe and effective for treating extravasation-induced injuries, independent of location and severity (Smaropoulos et al., 2021).

More information about hyaluronidase can be found in Table 19.7, whereas phentolamine (Regitine) is not readily available in Australia but may be ordered through the Therapeutic Goods Administration, via the Special Access Scheme.

EVIDENCE-BASED PRACTICE RESEARCH 19.2

Non-contact vital sign monitoring

Khanam et al. (2021) undertook a single-centre study of non-contact vital sign monitoring on seven neonates in a NICU. An awareness of the fragility of the neonatal skin and potential damage caused by the bond between the dermis and attached monitoring electrodes led them to investigate the possibility of non-contact monitoring using visible light video cameras. A colour-based method was used to detect heart rate (HR), and a motion-based method was used to detect respiratory rate (RR). They found a strong correlation between their measured data and the ECG data for both HR and RR, and concluded that the technique has potential as a non-contact, economical and easily deployable monitoring system in a clinical environment.

TABLE 19.7 **Extravasation guideline: hyaluronidase/hyalase drug profile**

Drug	Mucolytic enzyme
Indications	Used to enhance the diffusion of irritating or vesicant drugs
Presentation	1500 IU dry powder
Reconstitution	Dissolve the powder in 1.5 mL of sterile water for injection Take 0.2 mL (200 IU) and dilute with normal saline to 1 mL
Administration	Inject 0.2 mL aliquots of the reconstituted solution subcutaneously into several (5) sites around the perimeter of the extravasation
Compatibility	5% dextrose, 10% dextrose, normal saline
Adverse effects	Local skin irritation, infection, bleeding and bruising from the injections

Source: Beaulieu (2012).

Birth injuries

Birth injuries have the potential to occur during the antenatal and intrapartum periods. They may present after intrauterine interventions – for example, amniocentesis, intrauterine transfusions and laser ablation for twin-to-twin transfusion, or from assisted deliveries. More specific examples include the following:

- Monitoring:
  - fetal scalp monitor resulting in minor lacerations (Kawakita et al., 2016).
- Instrumental injury:
  - instruments for artificial rupture of membranes (suggested to increase risk of sepsis)
  - misapplication of forceps causing lacerations to the face and scalp (Jensen & Galbraith, 2014)
  - altered skin integrity associated with application of vacuum appliance (or re-positioning of vacuum cup/repeated application), which has potential to cause laceration and abrasion (Jensen & Galbraith, 2014).
- Surgical injury:
  - laceration(s) related to sharp surgical instruments during caesarean section (Jensen & Galbraith, 2014).

There is no current consensus for the management or treatment of birth injuries, so diligent observation, documentation and communication with medical staff is considered best practice.

Heel lancet complications

Heel lancets make a small incision into the heel to access capillary blood and are a necessary component of neonatal care. Although it is an intentional break to the skin, improper application of lancets can cause complications. Lancets are available in multiple sizes and provide various depths of penetration. The correct size needs to be used and it is under the neonatal nurse's/midwife's discretion to consider the following when applying a heel lancet:

- Adult lancets create larger incisions and should not be used.
- Automatic, retractable lancets should be used (the incision is shallow compared with a manual lancet).
- The blade should be applied in one direction for all sampling; avoid overlapping or lancing a previously lanced area.
- The medial and lateral surfaces of the heel are sampled (purple areas); avoid the calcaneus region to prevent nerve damage and osteomyelitis (orange section of V-shape; Fig. 19.8).
- Pain relief including a breastfeed, oral sucrose or non-pharmacological techniques should be implemented prior to and during the procedure (refer to Chapter 18).
- Gentle intermittent pumping should be applied to the incision site to encourage blood flow; pumping rather than squeezing will cause less trauma (Krleza et al., 2015).
- Automatic lancets have been found to be less painful than the needle puncture in neonatal heel-prick blood sampling with no significant difference in blood sampling time (Goto et al., 2020).

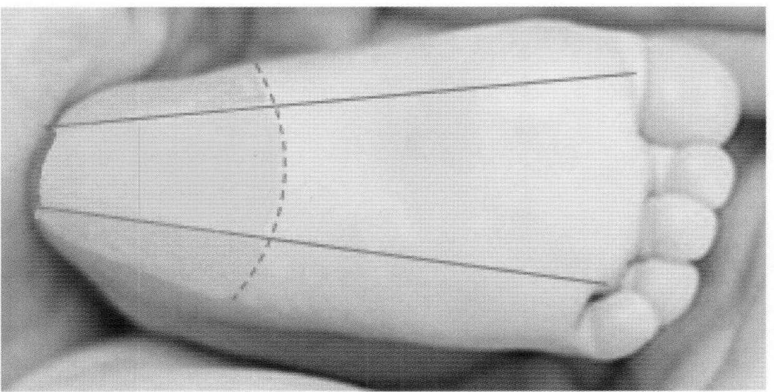

FIGURE 19.8 **Capillary heel sampling locations**
Source: Krleza et al. (2015).

CLINICAL PRACTICE 19.7

Iatrogenic injury reporting

New Zealand

Iatrogenic skin injuries are reportable to the New Zealand Accident Compensation Corporation (ACC), which will deliver injury prevention initiatives and no-fault personal injury cover to the injured party (<https://www.acc.co.nz/>).

Initiatives could include rehabilitation and follow-up treatment including physiotherapy and plastic surgery; all are free of cost. Skin injuries could include burns, extravasations or mechanical force injuries. Check with your healthcare facility for correct reporting procedures.

Australia

Standard 5, *Comprehensive care*, from the National Safety and Quality Health Service (NSQHS), includes the prevention and management of pressure injuries (previously Standard 8; <https://www.safetyandquality.gov.au/>). This standard mandates that facility-acquired injuries are reportable and advanced stages of facility-acquired injury may incur financial penalty. Registered nurses are required to complete compressive skin assessments on admission and each shift thereafter. However, due to the emerging nature of this subspecialty, check with your healthcare facility for correct reporting procedures, which may differ from the adult population.

Dressings

Dressing products have not been thoroughly investigated for neonatal wound healing and hence evidence from adult and paediatric populations currently guides selection. Table 19.8 provides an overview of possible dressing types. Wound beds should be kept 'appropriately moist', which contrasts with the construct of 'healthy skin' assessment being dry and intact (Carville, 2017). Therefore, decision making about dressing selection will centre on factors of the wound bed including presence of exudates, dryness and tissue health. Dressing management will alter at different phases of wound healing (refer to Table 19.8). Occasionally, a dry wound bed may need to be debrided or chemically moistened to promote healing. This is

TABLE 19.8 **Types of dressings**

Wound bed assessment	Covering	Filler	Infection[a]
Dry	• Transparent film dressing • Silicone contact	• Hydrogels[a]	
		• Amorphous sheets • Paraffin gauze	
Moist	• Hydrocolloid (sheets and wafers)	• Hydrocolloid (paste and powder)	
		• Collagen sheets	
		• Alginates • Fibrous absorbent sheets	
Wet	• Silicone foam • Foam • Combination dressings		Silver[a] Honey[a]

[a] Seek advice if an organisational guideline is unavailable.

Source: adapted from: Fox (2011); Kempf et al. (2011).

done in consultation with a wound or surgical team. With an increasing survival of the neonatal population, skin injuries are being more commonly treated with dressings containing active agents and, hopefully, future studies will identify best practice.

Current recommendations for wound care dressings include the following (Steen et al., 2020):

- **Hydrocolloids:** a type of mouldable dressing made from a carbohydrate base that is mildly sticky (commonly gelatine, pectin, or cellulose). This carbohydrate foundation reacts with the fluid in the wound to generate a moisturising gel that absorbs excess moisture and keeps the wound and surrounding skin from drying out. Hydrocolloids hydrate the wound while also acting as a barrier, preventing infection and protecting the skin from other sticky agents. For a variety of reasons, hydrocolloids are a particularly important wound care tool in the neonatal population.
- **Hydrogels:** water, propylene glycol and carboxymethylcellulose are cross-linked to form a three-dimensional hydrophilic polymer. This combination hydrates the wound bed by providing water to the application site while minimising ambient water loss, reducing discomfort and allowing for selective autolytic debridement of nonviable tissue. Because both granulation tissue creation and re-epithelialisation need wound debridement, these phases are especially important during the proliferative stage of wound healing. The most prevalent side effect of using hydrogels is maceration. As a result, neonatal nurses/midwives must check the dressing's placement and integrity, as well as the surrounding skin, on a regular basis. If not adequately protected by an overlying secondary dressing, the dressing can migrate or dry out if left untreated. Although hydrogel-based dressings can typically repair neonatal skin sufficiently while also delivering acceptable aesthetic effects, the aforementioned inefficiencies of hydrogels have the potential to obstruct effective wound healing in some situations.
- **Foams:** natural (cellulose-based) or synthetic (polyurethane blends) materials can be used to make foam dressings, but they all have a spongy architecture that allows them to absorb excess exudate. They can also be cut to shape, making them useful for wounds with uneven shapes. Foam dressings also act as a physical barrier and cushion and can be used as a primary dressing for protection, absorption and pressure injury protection. Foam dressings are frequently used as secondary dressings to protect neonates with **epidermolysis bullosa** from movement injury and to prevent rubbing tissue fusion. Foam dressings must, however, be changed when saturated, just like any other dressing used in exudative wounds, to avoid injuring the healthy skin around the dressing. Another disadvantage of foams is that they are often non-adhesive and may not stay in place without the use of an additional stabilising treatment (and again, adhesives present a clinical challenge when dealing with fragile skin). Foam-based solutions with a **silicone** adhesive are better for preterm neonatal skin because they do not cause harm when applied.
- **Barrier creams and barrier films:** barrier films are a type of semipermeable synthetic bandage that comes in a variety of shapes and sizes. Barrier films provide protection and a measure of soft adhesion. To minimise **epidermal stripping** during dressing removal, some clinicians use liquid barrier films before applying adhesives. Barrier films, though semipermeable, are often non-absorptive, so when treating exudative wounds the neonatal nurse/midwife should investigate alternatives or use them in conjunction with other products.
- **Alginates:** these are very viscous hydrophilic gels or gums made from pure brown algal polysaccharide chain-forming polysaccharides. Alginates, which absorb water from their surroundings, are effective in exudative wounds in older children and adults. Although alginate-derived products are commonly used on neonates, applying them to large mucosal wounds on neonates might dry the wound bed to the point of

electrolyte shortage. Seizures might result from subsequent hyponatraemia and hypocalcaemia. As a result, clinicians should choose these dressings with extreme prudence.

- **Wound therapy with negative pressure:** a foam dressing is applied to the wound site in negative pressure wound therapy (NPWT) to contain the vacuum suction provided by a small electric pump. NPWT eliminates excess wound drainage and oedema from the wound without desiccating the tissue on a macroscopic scale. Unfortunately, because most NPWT research and publications focus on adult patients, there is insufficient evidence to recommend NPWT as a first-line treatment for neonatal wounds. Despite this, due to the high prevalence of severe pressure injuries, abdominal wall abnormalities and necrotising enterocolitis in this population, newborn patients are the most likely paediatric patients to benefit from postoperative wound treatment using NPWT. Further research is required in this area (Steen et al., 2020).

Irritant nappy dermatitis

Irritant nappy dermatitis (also known as diaper dermatitis) is a non-specific acute inflammatory condition in the perianal and groin regions (Hebert, 2021). Dermatitis is caused by excessive hydration that macerates the skin and leads to increased permeability. In combination with alkaline urine, the pH of the skin changes and these effects combine with the action of faecal enzymes that can cause skin breakdown (Hebert, 2021). Cases of dermatitis are believed to be rare in the neonatal period but are believed to occur in 25% of neonates during the first few months of life (Burdell et al., 2019). Presentations may include a combination of erythema (reddening), inflamed skin, blistering, erosive areas, peeling, raw patches and/or small ulcers (see Fig. 19.9 for a photograph of nappy dermatitis).

To prevent nappy dermatitis, the area should be kept cool and dry, with limited faeces and urine contact. Commercial wipes are comparable with water and cotton wool in terms of skin hydration, transepidermal water loss, skin surface pH, erythema and the presence of microbial skin irritants (Burdell et al., 2019). Friction in the nappy area should also be avoided (gentle cleansing), and the absorbent properties of disposable nappies are helpful to keep the area dry and clean (Blume-Peytavi et al., 2014). Frequent nappy changes (every 2 hours) may be required for at-risk neonates or those suffering from ongoing cases of dermatitis. Specifically, short gut or post-stoma patients will be at increased risk because of loose stool consistency. Table 19.9 provides information regarding the characteristics of nappy dermatitis.

Topical ointments continue to be the treatment of choice for the many forms of dermatitis. There are few studies that have reviewed the choice of cream application in comparison with non-intervention (Blume-Peytavi & Kanti, 2018; Sharifi-Heris et al., 2018):

- water-based creams:
  - protectant, apply thinly, easily removed with water and a soft cloth
- non-water-based creams/barrier preparations (zinc creams with petrolatum (white soft paraffin)):
  - protectant against moisture, apply thickly, remove only soiled or top layer
  - petrolatum (occlusive layer) can be applied to the nappy, in addition to a barrier cream on the skin; this can prevent cream adhering to the nappy.
- dimethicone (silicone) products (wipes and creams) have not been studied for neonates and are not currently recommended.

Once the skin is broken, it may take days or weeks to heal completely (Beeckman & Global IAD Expert Panel, 2015). At present, no evidence exists to support the application of heat, oxygen, or antibacterial nappy powder products; therefore, they are not recommended.

Table 19.10 summarises the treatment of nappy dermatitis according to the degree of skin breakdown.

The key to healing nappy dermatitis is consistent treatment, but this may often be challenging, as each nurse/family will have individual impressions regarding treatment

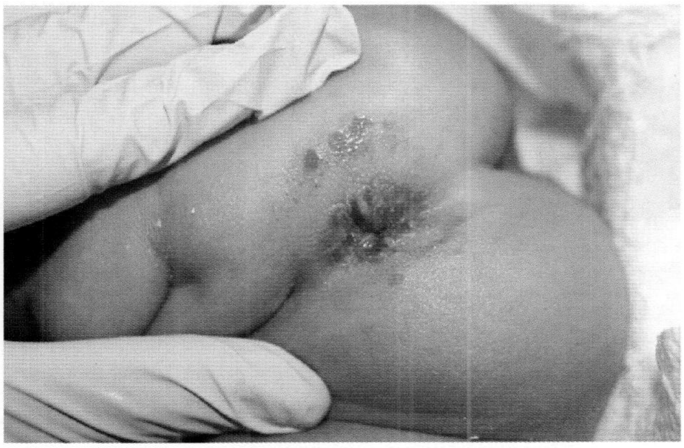

FIGURE 19.9 **Moderate-to-severe nappy dermatitis with erosive areas**

TABLE 19.9 **Dermatitis presentation findings**

Problem	Characteristics
Erythema (skin intact)	Redness forms in skin creases and in the direct perianal area
Erythema (broken areas)	Broken skin areas, ulcers, blistering, peeling
Candida	Red skin with red inflamed papules scattered at edges (± satellite lesions) Develops beyond perianal area (including fissures)
Breakdown and *Candida*	Broken skin areas, ulcers, blistering, peeling with satellite lesions

Source: adapted from Heimall et al. (2012).

TABLE 19.10 **Treatment of nappy dermatitis**

Degree of skin breakdown	Treatment
Erythema (skin intact)	• Frequent nappy changes • Time without nappy and a barrier cream (either water- or non-water-based)
Erythema (broken areas)	As above with: • thickly applied non-water-based barrier cream • only soiled cream removed during nappy change • submersion baths for mildly eroded areas (daily maximum)
Severe breakdown (see Fig. 19.9)	'Crusting': • Pectin powder (stoma adhesive powder) or Orobase • Layer with alcohol-free skin protectant, let dry • Petrolatum or zinc cream on top
Candida	• Antifungal cream/treatment alone • Antifungal cream and then barrier cream
Breakdown and *Candida*	• First two steps of 'crusting' to broken skin • Antifungal treatment (to satellite regions)

Source: adapted from: Blume-Peytavi et al. (2016, 2014); Heimall et al. (2012).

efficiency. Nurses/midwives should check the unit guidelines and care plan, and discuss with senior clinicians before changing treatment plans. Removing creams/compounds and applying another prematurely will increase friction to the area of concern. Partnerships of nurses and parents should maintain consistent therapy for a minimum of 3 days to allow for effective evaluation of one treatment plan (Beeckman & Global IAD Expert Panel, 2015).

Atopic dermatitis

Atopic dermatitis (AD; atopic eczema) is an inflammatory skin condition characterised by dry and scaly skin, redness, blistering and itching (Cooke et al., 2014). Although the initial signs of AD usually develop by 6 or 12 months of age, diagnosing AD in the first year of life can be difficult because of a lack of itch and uncertainty about the severity of eczema (Endre et al., 2022). Additionally, neonates/infants of parents who have a similar allergy or sensitivity may be more prone to the condition; this is called *'parental atopy'* (Kelleher et al., 2015). Early assessment and identification of neonates with the condition can facilitate appropriate dermatological referrals. Evidence suggests emollient use is known to decrease the symptoms of AD with twice-daily application for term newborns (after 3 weeks of life) (Simpson et al., 2014). One study found that infants may be asymptomatic at 2 months but may be later diagnosed with AD at 12 months (Kelleher et al., 2015). Nurses should educate parents that recurrent cases of dry and flaky areas may suggest potential AD diagnosis.

NEONATAL SKIN ASSESSMENT TOOLS

Currently, there is no comprehensive system for reporting skin injuries, wounds and/or complications to neonatal skin. Neonatal risk assessment and pressure injury tools are numerous. Few are evidence based. Risk factors are extrapolated from adult skin injuries and the efficiency of tools is insignificant in many studies without concurrent education and reporting systems (Moore & Cowman, 2014). Current neonatal scoring tools/scales do not change or alter standard neonatal skin care practices, unlike those used for adult populations (Ottinger et al., 2016). Your healthcare facility may elect to enhance skin assessment and prevention skills with a tool that can be found in Tables 19.11 and 19.12.

TABLE 19.11 **Skin injury assessment scales and tools**

Scale	Measurement	Detail
Neonatal Skin Condition Score (NSCS) (Lund et al., 2001)[a,b]	• Dryness • Erythema • Breakdown/ excoriation	Numeric representation of assessment finding
Skin Condition Grading Scale (Lane & Drost, 1993)[a]	• Dryness • Visual assessment • Erythema	Categorical assessment of skin condition
Grading key (erythema) (Visscher, 2014)	• Erythema • Rash • Dryness	Colour and percentage of area notes

[a] Utilised in follow-up studies and guidelines.
[b] Statistically validated and tested for the neonatal population.

TABLE 19.12 **Skin risk assessment scales: pressure injuries (ulcers)**

Scale	Detail
Braden Q (Quigley & Curley, 1996)[a]	Children: 21 days–8 years (used up to 18 years)
Neonatal Skin Risk Assessment Scale (NSARS) (Dolack et al., 2013)[b]	Adapted from paediatric Braden Q
Neonatal/Infant Braden Q (McLane et al., 2004)[a]	Adapted from Braden Q
Glamorgan (Anthony et al., 2010)[a]	Paediatric population (1 day–17 years)
SRAMT (Broom et al., 2017)[b]	Single site validation, neonatal population Assists in awareness of injury risk potential

[a] Utilised in follow-up studies and guidelines.
[b] Statistically validated and tested for the neonatal population.

CLINICAL PRACTICE 19.8

In a 2019 study, August et al. developed a metric graduated colour tool for use in the assessment of neonatal skin injuries. The metric graduated colour tool comprised of 15 colours, measured up to 60 mm, displayed metric dimensions and offered a discernible reference for clinical images and injury/wound bed comparison.

This metric and colour tool can be used in conjunction with digital photographs to enhance objective assessment of neonatal skin injuries/wounds. The metric and colour tool provides the foundation for vital skin injury assessment and documentation essentials including injury bed colour, size and consideration of depth of damage.

CLINICAL PRACTICE 19.9

In addition to the six assessment scales in Tables 19.11 and 19.12, neonatal units have developed individualised skin assessment tools:

- Pressure Ulcer Trigger Tool (Schumacher et al., 2013)
- Tissue Viability Assessment Tool (Ashworth & Briggs, 2011)
- Northampton Skin Assessment Tool (McGurk et al., 2004).

These tools are available in peer-reviewed articles, yet fewer than 30 neonates were assessed in each article and none of the tools was psychometrically evaluated. The tools are applicable in the unit in which they were developed.

- Are the tools appropriate in other neonatal environments?
- What challenges might arise if an unvalidated tool was used for skin injury practice?

STOMA CARE

The reasons for stoma (e.g. ostomies) creation are discussed in Chapter 17. The primary role of stoma care is to protect the skin from effluent output that contains highly acidic pH levels and liquid enzymes that may irritate peristomal skin. Additionally, stoma care will minimise trauma to the stomal mucosa. Peristomal skin trauma is one of many complications that may arise post stoma placement and can be related to adhesives, appliances, improper adhesive removal, inappropriate cleansing and the nature of the effluent output (Tielemans & Voegeli, 2019). Appliances can be two part (bag and base plate/wafer) or single item, but products and techniques for children/adults may be ineffective in the neonatal population. Management of neonatal appliance(s) is often challenging owing to the proximity of stoma to the umbilicus/groin, rounded abdomen and increased complexity of neurodevelopment positioning to maintain containment of stoma losses (Forest-Lalande, 2019). Bowel stomas pose additional challenges related to large gas volumes from swallowing air during sucking.

Collaboration with the surgical team and the local wound care specialist or stoma nurse is essential to achieve consistency for a plan of care. When choosing an appliance for a neonate, considerations include: the size of the abdomen; the diameter, profile and number of stoma(s); the proximity of stomas to each other; the consistency of the output and the enzyme content; the volume of stool/effluent and gas; the presence of scars; and the availability of the appliance/product. Any neonate who has an ileostomy, colostomy or urostomy must have an individualised plan of care, for which considerations are provided in Table 19.13.

FAMILY-CENTRED CARE 19.2

Parents are the primary carers for their neonate, often observing procedures done by a variety of methods. To improve the consistency of stoma care, some neonatal units teach parents how to care for the ostomy before discharge to assist with the transition to home. Two organisations exist to assist parents of neonates with a stoma with supplies and registering families before discharge can be helpful. These websites are also a useful information source for staff and parents:

- Australian Council of Stoma Association Inc.: <https://www.australianstoma.com.au>
- The Federation of New Zealand Ostomy Society Inc.: <https://ostomy.org.nz/>.

CASE STUDY 19.1 SKIN INJURY AND INFECTION

Baby Gerard was the first of twins delivered at 24+[5] weeks at 750 grams, via caesarean section, after a history of ruptured membranes for 2 weeks prior to birth, with minimum antibiotic and antenatal steroid coverage. Apgar scores were assessed as 6 at 1 minute and 7 at 5 minutes. Baby Gerard was ventilated for 3.5 weeks, received 7 weeks of CPAP and was treated for a staphylococcal infection in week 3 of life. On day 33 of age (29+[2]), he was assessed to have a stage 1 skin breakdown on his nose, but no other breaks to the skin were documented.

At day 49 of age (31+[4]) he was receiving caffeine, on full feeds, supported by humidified high flow (HHF) and had stage 2, zone 2 retinopathy of prematurity, with a history of a grade 1 intraventricular haemorrhage. Upon HHF circuit change, removal of the prong attachment pad revealed an obvious break to the skin under the previous adhesive (Fig. 19.10). The team initially assessed it as a skin tear (a form of epidermal stripping) where skin layers peel away from one another. A protective silicone dressing was placed over the lesion and a photograph taken to assist in injury assessment/treatment and document the event. Upon review of the image on a larger scale, the team noticed shallow intact circles

TABLE 19.13 **Stoma care considerations**[a]

Action	Rationale
JELONET (paraffin-soaked gauze) to fistula (stoma head) when unable to fit appliance[a]	Prevent rubbing from nappy and/or sheets
Use adhesive remover (silicone or non-alcohol-based)	Alcohol-containing removers can irritate/dry peristomal skin
During appliance change, clean surrounding skin with warm water and allow area to dry completely	Soap may irritate skin
Follow individualised measure guide and SAVE measuring guide	Limit effluent leaking onto healthy skin from ill-fitting appliance
Use curved scissors to shape appliances	Reduces creation of sharp edges in appliance/flange during trimming
Warming of appliance (base plate) for 1–2 min	Improves adhesive properties and increases ability to mould to abdomen
Minimise touching products that will have direct contact with peristomal skin	Avoids transfer of oils from hands
Ensure 1–2 mm gap between wall of fistula head and appliance	>1–2 mm gap = effluent leaking onto healthy skin from ill-fitting appliance <1–2 mm gap = appliance may rub stoma and protrusion of stoma may be inadequate
Minimise use of emollients and oils between appliance changes	Reduces adhesive properties of appliance
Avoid changing appliance if it is not leaking	Products designed for 2–3-day periods but maximum 1 week
Empty bag or appliance when ⅓–½ full of effluent	Reduce risk of detachment of devices
Empty bag or appliance when full of air	
Record ointments, barriers, products, of skin complications noted from procedure	

[a] Review with surgical team for ur/iliostomy.

Source: adapted from Chandler (2014); Ilhan and Toruner (2015); Lund et al. (2013).

surrounding the broken skin. The injury was swabbed, and the neonate was treated for a possible fungal infection, most likely ringworm (a form of dermatophyte). While the swab returned a negative result, the area healed and baby Gerard was able to progress onto subnasal oxygen and was subsequently discharged into his parent's care.

Skin injuries are often the result of mechanical forces and fragile skin, but it is important to exclude possible bacterial and fungal infections. Ringworm (tinea) is a common dermatophyte and has been described to occur at epidemic levels in some Aboriginal communities (Warren et al., 2017). The infection may have come from the family; however, the mother had no obvious lesions. The fungus is common in non-Aboriginal populations, being identified as the most common cause of tinea capitis in North America (Sproul et al., 2009).

1. Besides familial exposure, what else could have put this infant at risk for entry of this fungus?
2. Consider the anatomical location and the previous respiratory support used. What would have been on this neonate's cheeks for 7 weeks?

DermNet New Zealand Trust (2017) provides examples of common infections from the neonatal period, which can include fungi (*Candida*, ring worm), bacteria (staphylococcal scaled skin syndrome, syphilis or impetigo), viruses (herpes simplex) and infestations (scabies).

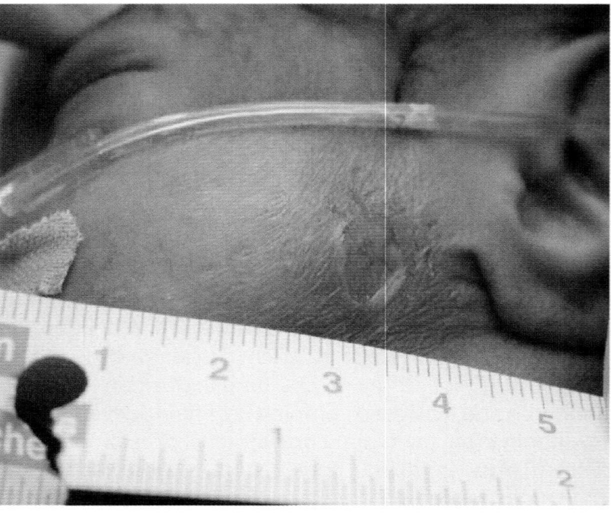

FIGURE 19.10 **Neonatal skin lesion**

CONCLUSION

Care of neonatal skin is frequently the responsibility of the neonatal nurse/midwife caring for the family unit. This chapter has discussed the development of the skin from the ectoderm layer, identifying the structural differences between preterm, neonatal and adult skin, and the functions and roles the skin plays in maintaining homeostasis. We have sought to identify the associated risks for skin injury and implement principles for promoting skin care. Learning points have included environmental considerations, product guides and evaluations, as well as evidence-based guidelines and practices. Neonatal skin health is evaluated by an assessment often initiated by the neonatal nurse/midwife. Additionally, skin integrity assessment in the neonatal period may identify precursors for acute or chronic dermatological conditions in later stages in life.

Neonatal skin care has undergone a revolution in the past 20 years, as previously skin injury or complications were secondary to emergent care. Current tools are non-specific, based on the adult tools, often descriptive in nature rather than predictive and leave room for interpretation. The foundations of neonatal skin injury identification and best-practice wound management are being evaluated through ongoing research, which will hopefully modify future practice. There is an immediate effect on the morbidity, mortality and financial responsibility related to neonatal skin conditions and injury. Evidence-based skin care is one of the areas in which neonatal nurses/midwives have made significant contributions to science, many of which are referenced in this chapter.

References/Acknowledgements

Almutairi, N. (2019). Basic structure and function of the neonatal, infantile, and childhood skin. In: K. Nouri, L. Benjamin, J. Alshaiji, & J. Izakovic (Eds.), *Pediatric Dermatologic Surgery*, pp. 13–21.

Anthony, D., Willock, J., & Baharestani, M. (2010). A comparison of Braden Q, Garvin and Glamorgan risk assessment scales in paediatrics. *Journal of Tissue Viability, 19*(3), 98–105.

Ashworth, C., & Briggs, C. (2011). Design and implementation of a Neonatal Tissue Viability Assessment Tool on the newborn intensive care unit. *Infant, 7*(6), 191–194.

Association of Women's Health, Obstetric and Neonatal Nurses (AWHONN). (2018). *Neonatal skin care: evidence-based clinical practice guideline* (3rd ed.). Washington, DC: Johnson & Johnson.

August, D. L., Edmonds, L., Brown, D. K., Murphy, M., & Kandasamy, Y. (2014). Pressure injuries to the skin in a neonatal unit: fact or fiction. *Journal of Neonatal Nursing, 20*(3), 129–137.

August, D. L., New, K., Ray, R. A., & Kandasamy, Y. (2018). Frequency, location, and risk factors of neonatal skin injuries from mechanical forces of pressure, friction, shear, and stripping: a systematic literature review. *Journal of Neonatal Nursing, 24*(4), 173–180.

August, D., Hitchcock, I., Tangney, J., Ray, R. A., Kandasamy, Y., & New, K. (2019). Graduated colour tape measure: development and demonstration of this tool in a case series of neonatal skin injuries. *Journal of Tissue Viability, 28*(3), 133–138.

Bamalan, O. A., & Menezes, R. G. (2020). Vernix caseosa. *StatPearls*.Treasure Island, FL: StatPearls Publishing. <http://europepmc.org/abstract/MED/32644664> (Accessed 20 February 2022).

Basiouny, N., & Lassy, R. (2019). Effect of three selected antiseptic solutions on umbilical cord infection among neonates. *International Journal of Novel Research in Healthcare and Nursing, 6*(1), 543–552.

Beall, V., Hall, B., Mulholland, J. T., & Gephart, S. M. (2013). Neonatal extravasation: an overview and algorithm for evidence-based treatment. *Newborn and Infant Nursing Reviews, 13*, 189–195.

Beaulieu, M. J. (2012). Hyaluronidase for extravasation management. *Neonatal Network, 31*(6), 413–418.

Beeckman, D., & Global IAD Expert Panel. (2015). Proceedings of the Global IAD expert panel. Incontinence associated dermatitis: moving prevention forward. *Wounds International*, 1–21.

Blume-Peytavi, U., & Kanti, V. (2018). Prevention and treatment of diaper dermatitis. *Pediatric Dermatology, 35*, s19–s23.

Blume-Peytavi, U., Hauser, M., Stamatas, G. N., Pathirana, D., & Garcia Bartels, N. (2012). Skin care practices for newborns and infants: review of the clinical evidence for best practices. *Pediatric Dermatolology, 29*(1), 1–14.

Blume-Peytavi, U., Hauser, M., Lünnemann, L., Stamatas, G. N., Kottner, J., & Garcia Bartels, N. (2014). Prevention of diaper dermatitis in infants – a literature review. *Pediatric Dermatology, 31*(4), 413–429.

Blume-Peytavi, U., Lavender, T., Jenerowicz, D., Ryumina, I., Stalder, J. F., Torrelo, A., et al. (2016). Recommendations from a European roundtable meeting on best practice healthy infant skin care. *Pediatric Dermatology, 33*(3), 311–321.

Boswell, N., & Waker, C. L. (2016). Comparing 2 adhesive methods on skin integrity in the high-risk neonate. *Advances in Neonatal Care, 16*(6), 449–454.

Broom, M., Burton, W., Ehrlich, L., Dunk, A., & Abdel, M. E. (2017). Developing an Australian skin risk assessment and management tool for neonates. *Wounds Practice and Research, 25*(1), 15–22.

Burdall, O., Willgress, L., & Goad, N. (2019). Neonatal skin care: developments in care to maintain neonatal barrier function and prevention of diaper dermatitis. *Pediatric Dermatology, 36*(1), 31–35. doi: 10.1111/pde.13714.

Carlson, B. M. (2014). *Human embryology and developmental biology* (5th ed.). Philadelphia, PA: Saunders.

Carville, K. (2017). *Wound care manual* (7th ed.). Osborne Park, WA: Silver Chain Foundation.

Chan, M. Y., & Smith, M. A. (2018). Infections in pregnancy. *Comprehensive Toxicology, 2018*, 232–249. doi: 10.1016/B978-0-12-801238-3.64293-9.

Chandler, P. (2014). Management of paediatric ileostomies: selecting suitable appliances. *Gastrointestinal Nursing, 12*(8), 34–40.

Cho, K. S., Ahn, H. C., Lee, J. H., Lim, S. Y., Lee, H. J., & Park, H. K. (2019). Extravasation wound care in the neonatal intensive care unit. *Journal of Wound Management and Research, 15*(1), 17–22.

Cleminson, J., & McGuire, W. (2016). Topical emollient for preventing infection in preterm infants. *Cochrane Database of Systematic Reviews, 1*, CD001150. doi: 10.1002/14651858.CD001150.pub3doi: 10.1002/14651858.CD001150.pub3.

Cooke, A., Victor, S., Cork, M., & Lavender, T. (2014). Topical oils for the prevention or treatment of dry skin in term infants. *Cochrane Database of Systematic Reviews, 5*, CD011100.

Corbett, M., Marshall, D., Harden, M., Oddie, S., Phillips, R., & McGuire, W. (2019). Treating extravasation injuries in infants and young children: a scoping review and survey of UK NHS practice. *BMC Pediatrics, 19*(1), 1–7.

Cornelissen, L., Fabrizi, L., Patten, D., Worley, A., Meek, J., Boyd, S., et al. (2013). Postnatal temporal, spatial and modality tuning of nociceptive cutaneous flexion reflexes in human infants. *PLoS One, 8*(10), e76470.

Danby, S. G., AlEnezi, T., Sultan, A., Lavender, T., Chittock, J., Brown, K., et al. (2013). Effect of olive and sunflower seed oil on the adult skin barrier: implications for neonatal skin care. *Pediatric Dermatology, 30*(1), 42–50.

Danby, S. G., Bedwell, C., & Cork, M. (2014). Neonatal skin care and toxicology. In: L. Eichenfield, I. Frieden, E. F. Mathes, & A. L. Zaenglein (Eds.), *Neonatal and infant dermatology* (3rd ed., Ch 5, pp. 46–56). Philadelphia, PA: Saunders Elsevier.

de Oliveira Marcatto, J., Santos, A. S., Oliveira, A. J. F., Costa, A. C. L., Regne, G. R. S., da Trindade, R. E., et al. (2021). Medical adhesive-related skin injuries in the neonatology department of a teaching hospital. *Nursing in Critical Care, Mar 25*. doi: 10.1111/nicc.12621. [Online ahead of print.]

DermNet New Zealand Trust. (2017). All about skin. DermNet New Zealand Trust. <https://dermnetnz.org/> (Accessed 20 February 2022).

Diamantis, S., Bastek, T., Groben, P., & Morrell, D. (2006). Subcutaneous fat necrosis in a newborn following icebag application for treatment of supraventricular tachycardia. *Journal of Perinatology, 26*(8), 518–520.

Dolack, M., Huffines, B., Stikes, R., Hayes, P., & Logsdon, M. C. (2013). Updated neonatal skin risk assessment scale (NSRAS). *Kentucky Nurse, 61*(4), 6.

Duncan, J. R., & Byard, R. W. (Eds.) (2018). *SIDS sudden infant and early childhood death: the past, the present and the future*. Adelaide, SA: University of Adelaide Press.

Edsberg, L. E., Black, J. M., Goldberg, M., McNichol, L., Moore, L., & Sieggreen, M. (2016). Revised National Pressure Ulcer Advisory Panel Pressure Injury Staging System: Revised Pressure Injury Staging System. *Journal of Wound, Ostomy, and Continence Nursing, 43*(6), 585–597.

Endre, K. M. A., Landrø, L., LeBlanc, M., Gjersviki, P., Lødrup Carlsen, K. C., Haugen, G., et al. (2022). Diagnosing atopic dermatitis in infancy using established diagnostic criteria: a cohort study. *British Journal of Dermatology, 186*, 50–58.

Forest-Lalande, L. (2019). Best-practice for stoma care in children and teenagers. *Gastrointestinal Nursing, 17*(suppl5), S12–S13.

Fox, M. D. (2011). Wound care in the neonatal intensive care unit. *Neonatal Network, 30*(5), 291–303.

Giles, E. M., & Couper, J. (2020). Microbiome in health and disease. *Journal of Paediatrics and Child Health, 56*(11), 1735–1738.

Gopalakrishnan, P., Goel, N., & Banerjee, S. (2017). Saline irrigation for the management of skin extravasation injury in neonates. *Cochrane Database of Systematic Reviews, 2*, CD008404, doi: 10.1002/14651858.CD008404.pub2.

Goto, T., Inoue, T., Kamiya, C., Kawabe, H., Higuchi, M., Suyama, M., et al. (2020). Neonatal pain response to automatic lancet versus needle heel-prick blood sampling: a prospective randomized controlled clinical trial. *Pediatrics International, 62*(3), 357–362.

Hebert, A. A. (2021). A new therapeutic horizon in diaper dermatitis: novel agents with novel action. *International Journal of Women's Dermatology, 7*(4):466–470. doi: 10.1016/j.ijwd.2021.02.003.

Heimall, L. M., Storey, B., Stellar, J. J., & Davis, K. F. (2012). Beginning at the bottom: evidence-based care of diaper dermatitis. *America Journal of Maternal Child Nursing, 37*(1), 10–16.

Hoath, S., & Mauro, T. (2014). Fetal skin development. In: L. F. Eichenfield, I. J. Frieden, E. F. Mathes, & A. L. Zaenglein (Eds.), *Neonatal and infant dermatology* (3rd ed., Ch 1, pp. 1–13). Philadelphia, PA: Elsevier Saunders.

Holbrook, K. A. (1982). A histological comparison of infant and adult skin. In: H. Maibach (Ed.), *Neonatal skin: structure and function* (pp. 3–31). New York: Marcel Dekker.

Ilhan, T., & Toruner, E. K. (2015). Assessment of knowledge and skills of neonatal nurses on peristomal skin care. *Journal of Neonatal Nursing, 21*(1), 18–25.

Imbulana, D. I., Manley, B. J., Dawson, J. A., Davis, P. G., & Owen, L. S. (2018). Nasal injury in preterm infants receiving non-invasive respiratory support: a systematic review. *Archives of Disease in Childhood. Fetal and Neonatal Edition, 103*(1), F29–F35.

Jensen, C. B., & Galbraith, S. S. (2014). Iatrogenic and traumatic injuries. In: L. F. Eichenfield, I. J. Frieden, E. F. Mathes, & A. L. Zaenglein (Eds.), *Neonatal and infant dermatology* (3rd ed., Ch 8, pp. 77–93). Philadelphia, PA: Elsevier Saunders.

Karppinen, S. M., Heljasvaara, R., Gullberg, D., Tasanen, K., & Pihlajaniemi, T. (2019). Toward understanding scarless skin wound healing and pathological scarring. *F1000Research*, 8, F1000 Faculty Rev-787. doi: 10.12688/f1000research.18293.1.

Kawakita, T., Reddy, U. M., Landy, H. J., Iqbal, S. N., Huang, C. C., & Grantz, K. L. (2016). Neonatal complications associated with use of fetal scalp electrode: a retrospective study. *British Journal of Obstetrics and Gynaecology, 123*(11), 1793–1803.

Kelleher, M., Dunn-Galvin, A., Hourihane, J. O., Murray, D., Campbell, L., McLean, W. H., et al. (2015). Skin barrier dysfunction measured by transepidermal water loss at 2 days and 2 months predates and predicts atopic dermatitis at 1 year. *Journal of Allergy and Clinical Immunology, 135*(4), 930–935.e1.

Kempf, M., Kimble, R. M., & Cuttle, L. (2011). Cytotoxicity testing of burn wound dressings, ointments, and creams: a method using polycarbonate cell culture inserts on a cell culture system. *Burns, 37*(6), 994–1000.

Khanam, F.-T.-Z., Perera, A. G., Al-Naji, A., Kim Gibson, K., & Chahl, J. (2021). Non-contact automatic vital signs monitoring of infants in a neonatal intensive care unit based on neural networks. *Journal of Imaging, 7*(8), 122. doi: 10.3390/jimaging7080122.

Krleza, J. L., Dorotic, A., Grzunov, A., & Maradin, M. (2015). Capillary blood sampling: national recommendations on behalf of the Croatian Society of Medical Biochemistry and Laboratory Medicine. *Biochemia Medica, 25*(3), 335–358.

Kuller, J. M. (2014). Update on newborn bathing. *Newborn and Infant Nursing Reviews, 14*(4), 166–170.

Lane, A. T., & Drost, S. S. (1993). Effects of repeated application of emollient cream to premature neonates' skin. *Pediatrics, 92*(3), 415–419.

Li, H., Colantonio, S., Dawson, A., Lin, X., & Beecker, J. (2019). Sunscreen application, safety, and sun protection: the evidence. *Journal of Cutaneous Medicine and Surgery, 23*(4), 357–369.

Loring, C., Gregory, K., Gargan, B., LeBlanc, V., Lundgren, D., Reilly, J., et al. (2012). Tub bathing improves thermoregulation of the late preterm infant. *Journal of Obstetric, Gynecologic, and Neonatal Nursing, 41*(2), 171–179.

Lund, C. (2014). Medical adhesives in the NICU. *Newborn and Infant Nursing Reviews, 14*(4), 160–165.

Lund, C. H., Osborne, J. W., Kuller, J., Lane, A. T., Lott, J. W., & Raines, D. A. (2001). Neonatal skin care: clinical outcomes of the AWHONN/NANN evidence-based clinical practice guideline. Association of Women's Health, Obstetric and Neonatal Nurses and the National Association of Neonatal Nurses. *Journal of Obstetric, Gynecologic, and Neonatal Nursing, 30*(1), 41–51.

Lund, C. H., Brandon, D., Holden, A., Kuller, J., & Hill, C. M. (Eds.) (2013). *Neonatal skin care* (3rd ed.) Evidence based clinical practice guideline. Washington, DC: Association of Women's Health, Obstetric and Neonatal Nurses.

Ma, Q. (2009). RETouching upon mechanoreceptors. *Neuron, 64*(6), 773–776.

Marieb, E. N., & Hoehn, K. (2018). *Human anatomy and physiology* (11th ed.) Boston, MA: Pearson.

Mathes, E. F., & Williams, M. L. (2014). Skin of the premature infant. In: L. F. Eichenfield, I. J. Frieden, E. F. Mathes, & A. L. Zaenglein (Eds.), *Neonatal and infant dermatology* (3rd ed., Ch 4, pp. 36–45). Philadelphia, PA: Elsevier Saunders.

McGurk, V., Holloway, B., Crutchley, A., & Izzard, H. (2004). Skin integrity assessment in neonates and children. *Paediatric Nursing, 16*(3), 15–18.

McLane, K. M., Bookout, K., McCord, S., McCain, J., & Jefferson, L. S. (2004). The 2003 national pediatric pressure ulcer and skin breakdown prevalence survey: a multisite study. *Journal of Wound, Ostomy, and Continence Nursing, 31*(4), 168–178.

Meropol, S. B., & Edwards, A. (2015). Development of the infant intestinal microbiome: a bird's eye view of a complex process. *Birth Defects Research. Part C. Embryo Today: Reviews, 105*(4), 228–239.

Meszes, A., Tálosi, G., Máder, K., Orvos, H., Kemény, L., & Csoma, Z. R. (2016). Lesions requiring wound management in a central tertiary neonatal intensive care unit. *World Journal of Pediatrics, 13*(2), 1–8.

Mohamadzadeh, A., Farhat, A., Saeidi, R., & Vaezi, A. (2020). Thermal injury in newborns and infants within the first 6 months of life. *Iranian Journal of Neonatology, 11*(2), 40–42.

Moore, Z. E., & Cowman, S. (2014). Risk assessment tools for the prevention of pressure ulcers. *Cochrane Database of Systematic Reviews, 2*, CD006471.

Nangia, S., Paul, V. K., Deorari, A. K., Sreenivas, V., Agarwal, R., & Chawla, D. (2015). Topical oil application and trans-epidermal water loss in preterm very low birth weight infants: a randomized trial. *Journal of Tropical Pediatrics, 61*(6), 414–420.

Ottinger, D., Hicks, J., Wilson, S., Sperber, S., & Power, K. (2016). The pressure is on: neonatal skin and nasal continuous positive airway pressure. *Advances in Neonatal Care, 16*(6), 420–423.

Paternoster, M., Niola, M., & Graziano, V. (2017). Avoiding chlorhexidine burns in preterm infants. *Journal of Obstetric, Gynecologic and Neonatal Nursing, 46*(2), 267–271.

Plum, M., & Moukhachen, O. (2017). Alternative pharmacological management of vasopressor extravasation in the absence of phentolamine. *Pharmacy and Therapeutics, 42*(9), 581.

Ponnusamy, V., Venkatesh, V., & Clarke, P. (2014). Skin antisepsis in the neonate: what should we use? *Current Opinion on Infectious Diseases, 27*(3), 244–250.

Prizant, T. L., Lucky, A. W., Frieden, I. J., Burton, P. S., & Suarez, S. M. (1996). Spontaneous atrophic patches in extremely premature infants. Anetoderma of prematurity. *Archives of Dermatology, 132*(6), 671–674.

Pupala, S. S., Rao, S., Strunk, T., & Patole, S. (2019). Topical application of coconut oil to the skin of preterm infants: a systematic review. *European Journal of Pediatrics, 178*(9), 1317–1324. doi: 10.1007/s00431-019-03407-7.

Quach, C., Milstone, A. M., Perpete, C., Bonenfant, M., Moore, D. L., & Perreault, T. (2014). Chlorhexidine bathing in a tertiary care neonatal intensive care unit: impact on central line-associated bloodstream infections. *Infection Control and Hospital Epidemiology, 35*(2), 158–163.

Quigley, S. M., & Curley, M. A. (1996). Skin integrity in the pediatric population: preventing and managing pressures. *Journal of the Society of Pediatric Nurses, 1*(1), 7–18.

Quraishy, K., Bowles, S. M., & Moore, J. (2013). A protocol for swaddled bathing in the Neonatal Intensive Care Unit. *Newborn and Infant Reviews, 13*, 48–53.

Ratchagame, V., & Prabakaran, V. (2021). Comparison of risks from central venous catheters and peripheral intravenous lines among term neonates in a tertiary care hospital, India. *Journal of Caring Sciences, 10*(2), 58.

Restieaux, M., Maw, A., Broadbent, R., Jackson, P., Barker, D., & Wheeler, B. (2013). Neonatal extravasation injury: prevention and management in Australia and New Zealand, a survey of current practice. *BMC Pediatrics, 13*, 34.

Rutter, N. (2000). Clinical consequences of an immature barrier. *Seminars in Neonatology, 5*(4), 281–287.

Salam, R. A., Darmstadt, G. L., & Bhutta, Z. A. (2015). Effect of emollient therapy on clinical outcomes in preterm neonates in Pakistan: a randomised controlled trial. *Archives of Disease in Childhood. Fetal and Neonatal Edition, 100*(3), F210–F215.

Schindler, C. A., Mikhailov, T. A., Cashin, S. E., Malin, S., Christensen, M., & Winters, J. (2013). Under pressure: preventing pressure ulcers in critically ill infants. *Journal for Specialists in Pediatric Nursing, 18*(4), 329–341.

Schumacher, B., Askew, M., & Otten, K. (2013). Development of a pressure ulcer trigger tool for the neonatal population. *Journal of Wound, Ostomy, and Continence Nursing, 40*(1), 46–50.

Sharifi-Heris, Z., Farahani, L. A., Haghani, H., Abdoli-Oskouee, S., & Hasanpoor-Azghady, S. B. (2018). Comparison the effects of topical application of olive and calendula ointments on children's diaper dermatitis: a triple-blind randomized clinical trial. *Dermatologic Therapy, 31*(6), e12731.

Simpson, E. L., Chalmers, J. R., Hanifin, J. M., Thomas, K. S., Cork, M. J., McLean, W. H., et al. (2014). Emollient enhancement of the skin barrier from birth offers effective atopic dermatitis prevention. *Journal of Allergy and Clinical Immunology, 134*(4), 818–823.

Smaropoulos, E., Cremers, N. A., & Newberry, D. M. (2021). Medical-grade honey for the treatment of extravasation-induced injuries in preterm neonates: a case series. *Advances in Neonatal Care, 21*(2), 122–132.

Sproul, A. V., Whitehall, J., & Engler, C. (2009). *Trichophyton tonsurans*: ringworm in an NICU. *Neonatal Network, 28*(5), 305–308.

Steen, E. H., Wang, X., Boochoon, K. S., Ewing, D. C., Strang, H. E., Kaul, A., et al. (2020). Wound healing and wound care in neonates: current therapies and novel options. *Advances in Skin and Wound Care, 33*(6), 294–300.

Strohm, B., Hobson, A., Brocklehurst, P., Edwards, A. D., Azzopardi, D., & UK TOBY Cooling Register. (2011). Subcutaneous fat necrosis after moderate therapeutic hypothermia in neonates. *Pediatrics, 128*(2), e450–e452.

Suman, G., & Suman, S. (2019). Ultraviolet radiation-induced immunomodulation: skin ageing and cancer. In: A. Dwivedi, N. Agarwal, L. Ray, & A. Tripathi (Eds.), *Skin aging and cancer* (pp. 47–58). Singapore: Springer. doi: 10.1007/978-981-13-2541-0_5.

Tambunan, D. M., & Mediani, H. S. (2019). Bathing method for preterm infants: a systematic review. *KnE Life Sciences*, 1–11.

Tielemans, C., & Voegeli, D. (2019). Silicone-based adhesive removers for preventing peristomal skin complications caused by mechanical trauma. *Gastrointestinal Nursing, 17*(suppl 9), S22–S28.

Vanzi, V., & Pitaro, R. (2018). Skin injuries and chlorhexidine gluconate-based antisepsis in early premature infants: a case report and review of the literature. *Journal of Perinatal and Neonatal Nursing, 32*(4), 341–350.

Visscher, M. (2014). A practical method for rapid measurement of skin condition. *Newborn and Infant Nursing Reviews, 14*(4), 147–152.

Visscher, M., & Geiss, S. (2014). Emollient therapy for newborn infants: a global perspective. *Newborn and Infant Nursing Reviews, 14*(4), 153–159.

Visscher, M., & Narendran, V. (2014a). The ontogeny of skin. *Advances in Wound Care, 3*(4), 291–303.

Visscher, M., & Narendran, V. (2014b). Vernix caseosa: formation and functions. *Newborn and Infant Nursing Reviews, 14*(4), 142–146.

Visscher, M., & Taylor, T. (2014). Pressure ulcers in the hospitalized neonate: rates and risk factors. *Scientific Reports, 4*, 7429.

Visscher, M. O., Barai, N., LaRuffa, A. A., Pickens, W. L., Narendran, V., & Hoath, S. B. (2011). Epidermal barrier treatments based on vernix caseosa. *Skin Pharmacology and Physiology, 24*(6), 322–329.

Warren, L. J., Tilakaratne, D., & Seth, R. (2017). Neonatal tinea corporis. *Medical Journal of Australia, 207*(8), 324.

CHAPTER 20

NEONATAL ABSTINENCE SYNDROME

ANNDREA FLINT AND JUDITH NEEDHAM

Learning objectives

After reading this chapter you will be able to:

- discuss the aetiological factors related to families and neonates affected by illicit and licit drug use and abuse in Australia, New Zealand and internationally
- describe the epidemiology of drug use/abuse that commonly cause neonatal abstinence syndrome in Australia, New Zealand and internationally
- identify key aspects of antenatal care to maximise perinatal outcomes
- identify the clinical features of neonatal abstinence syndrome, according to maternal drug use/abuse patterns
- understand commonly utilised scoring tools for neonatal drug withdrawal
- develop and implement a plan for the management of neonatal abstinence syndrome, including pharmacological treatment and non-pharmacological management
- utilise a family-centred model of care when supporting and educating families who are affected by substance use disorder.

Key words, terms and abbreviations

neonatal abstinence syndrome (NAS)
neonatal opioid withdrawal syndrome (NOWS)
scoring tools
selective serotonin reuptake inhibitors (SSRIs)
serotonin and noradrenaline (norepinephrine) reuptake inhibitors (SNRIs)
withdrawal

INTRODUCTION

Neonatal abstinence syndrome (NAS) is defined as a condition where neonates have experienced in utero exposure to opioids or other substances used by the mother, causing **withdrawal** symptoms 24–72 hours post birth (Joseph et al., 2020; Lisonkova et al., 2019). More commonly, babies withdrawing from opioids are now described as having **neonatal opioid withdrawal syndrome (NOWS)** (Patrick & Barfield, 2020). This chapter will consider the effects of a wide range of drugs and substances that have been prescribed or abused during pregnancy. Clinical manifestation of NAS will be outlined, including nursing care and management. Key aspects of nursing management and education for mothers will be outlined during antenatal care, to identify and decrease the potential risks of NAS in the neonate. The drugs and substances that are abused or prescribed during pregnancy vary and are dependent on current trends, geographical locations and availability. This chapter will provide an overview of the common **scoring tools** available for assessment of NAS and the use of these tools within the neonatal unit.

EVIDENCE-BASED PRACTICE RESEARCH 20.1

As a neonatal nurse/midwife, you must be familiar with the terminology associated with how medications affect newborns.

Withdrawal versus acute toxicity versus permanent drug effect

- Some drugs neonates are exposed to in utero cause *acute toxicity*. Signs and symptoms lessen with drug elimination (time). Most commonly seen in neonates exposed to SSRIs.
- Some drugs neonates are exposed to in utero cause *withdrawal*. Signs and symptoms of withdrawal worsen with drug elimination (time) – for example, methadone.
- Some drugs neonates are exposed to in utero cause a *permanent effect on the developing fetus*. Signs and symptoms are the result of a permanent drug effect, for example, fetal alcohol syndrome.

Source: Wang & Cosci (2021).

PATHOPHYSIOLOGY OF NAS

Neonatal abstinence syndrome is the result of sudden discontinuation of prolonged fetal exposure to opioids or other drugs of abuse and is associated with withdrawal behaviours including central nervous system hypersensitivity, respiratory distress, gastrointestinal disturbances and autonomic nervous system dysfunction (Lacaze-Masmonteil & O'Flaherty, 2018).

Opioids act by binding to opioid receptors. Opioid receptors are G protein-coupled receptors and there are three types of opioid receptors: μ, κ and δ (Shang & Filizola, 2015). These receptors are distributed across the central nervous system, and within the peripheral nervous system, gastrointestinal system and various other systems (Kocherlakota, 2014), hence the diversity of NAS symptoms. As opiates and CNS drugs can easily cross the placenta owing to their lipophilic nature, the fetus in utero will be stimulated chronically by these drugs and will be influenced by their pharmacological effects. Therefore, following birth, the sudden cessation of receiving these drugs through the placenta and the drop in plasma concentration of opiates in the neonate will increase the activity of opioid receptors, which leads to super-activation of adenyl cyclase enzyme. Activation of this enzyme results in an increased level of cyclic adenosine monophosphate (cAMP) and increased protein kinase activity. Ultimately, this results in the altered (increase or decrease) production of various neurotransmitters (Kocherlakota, 2014) as follows:

- ↑ **corticotrophin**: causes stress and hyperphagia
- ↑ **noradrenaline (norepinephrine)**: causes hyperthermia, hypertension, tremors and tachycardia
- ↑ **acetylcholine**: causes diarrhoea, vomiting, yawning, sneezing and sweating
- ↑ **other receptors**: cause hyperalgesia and allodynia
- ↓ **serotonin**: causes sleep deprivation and sleep fragmentation
- ↓ **dopamine**: causes hyperirritability and anxiety.

EPIDEMIOLOGY

Globally the number of infants born to mothers who use substances that may lead to NAS is increasing every year. Current data from the Australian Institute of Health and Welfare (AIHW) indicates that 2.2% of pregnant women have used an illicit drug such as marijuana, 0.9% misused prescription analgesics, a further 42% used alcohol and 15% smoked tobacco (Australian Institute of Health and Welfare (AIHW), 2020; Department of Health, 2020). More commonly, mothers reported using a combination of licit, illicit drugs and alcohol, and the use of amphetamines has doubled (Department of Health, 2020). Alcohol and tobacco use continued during pregnancy in up to 36% of women. Unfortunately, even though these trends are increasing across both countries, statistical data are sparse. The Australian and New Zealand Neonatal Network report no information about neonatal sequelae as a result of maternal substance use disorder (Chow et al., 2019).

In the United States (US), the current use of illicit and prescribed substances has been reported as a national crisis; Heintzelman et al. (2020, p. 4) identified that in one Colorado community hospital substance use increased from 33.4% to 50.2% between 2013 and 2017 ($p < 0.001$). Another study published in 2018 identified that the cost to the US health system to care for NAS babies was an estimated $1.5 billion in 2012 alone (Lemon et al., 2018). The study by Heintzelman et al. (2020) further highlighted the increased costs of caring for NAS/NOWS babies in comparison with normal newborns, with increased length of stay for NAS babies impacting 'an already overburdened healthcare system' (McQueen et al., 2015, p. 1763). The

Colorado Department of Health developed the 2016–20 Maternal Child Health (MCH) priorities in the state of Colorado to assist with the increased trend of substance use and highlighted the incidence of reported NAS cases in the community (Colorado Department of Public Health and Environment (CDPHE), 2019). The reported cases of NAS in Colorado in 2018 were 5.4 per 1000 hospital births (National Institute on Drug Abuse (NIDA), 2020).

The rising figures of substance abuse in pregnancy have been reflected globally, with 5% of the global population using some sort of illicit drug (Tavella et al., 2020). Further statistics revealed a self-reported rate of illicit drug use during pregnancy of 1.65%, though toxicology reports revealed a much higher rate, at 12.8% (Tavella et al., 2020). This poses major challenges worldwide, both socially and economically, particularly while caring for mothers during their pregnancy and their subsequent babies.

KEY ASPECTS OF ANTENATAL CARE

The management of substance use disorder in pregnancy can be highly complex for nursing, midwifery, allied health and medical staff owing to the environmental, social, financial and psychological needs of the expecting mother and her partner (Joseph et al., 2020; McQueen et al., 2015). Women who use drugs during their pregnancy and prior are less likely to attend antenatal care than are women who do not use drugs (Lisonkova et al., 2019). Given the negative potential effects on the fetus, such as preterm birth and reduced intrauterine growth leading to small for gestational age babies (McQueen et al., 2015), optimal antenatal care provides the ideal opportunity for improved pregnancy outcomes (Chasnoff & Gardner, 2015; Williamson, 2020); therefore, women should be informed about the benefits of antenatal care and encouraged to attend early in the pregnancy.

Comprehensive models of care facilitated by a multidisciplinary team allow the opportunity to thoroughly assess the woman with substance use disorder and her fetus. This multidisciplinary team should include a paediatric consultant or neonatal nurse practitioner, particularly during the antenatal period, to discuss potential risks to the newborn, including treatment of NAS. The model of care should include support for the minimisation or cessation of drug and alcohol use, including enrolment in opioid treatment programs, counselling support and the development of strategies to prevent relapse, and psychosocial and environmental assessments (Department of Health, 2020; Queensland Health, 2021). The woman with substance abuse disorder should not be forced to make a commitment to reducing or abstaining during the pregnancy. Rather, there should be an emphasis on support and engagement for both the woman and her family, as many experience very high levels of psychological distress, including depression and anxiety. This can also be accompanied by homelessness, domestic violence, financial difficulties, relationship breakdown and unemployment. This support provides the opportunity for nursing and midwifery staff to assess the woman and her family to identify risks to both her and her fetus, and the needs required to provide the best possible care. The midwife/nurse also has a responsibility to the unborn child to identify and ensure that they are protected once they are delivered. Notification to the appropriate authority should be made when antenatal documentation is evident in the chart requiring this action. All staff should be aware of their mandatory reporting requirements.

PSYCHOSOCIAL ASPECTS OF POSTNATAL CARE

The types of illicit substances used by women influence the treatment that may be required by the neonate at birth. Care should be developed in negotiation with the woman and, where appropriate, her partner/family, including what treatment is to be provided, by whom and the expected outcomes of care. The nurse/midwife relationship with the mother is crucial; trust needs to be developed as the mother may be suspicious of healthcare workers. Honest, open communication, explaining that all interactions are confidential with safety of the mother and baby paramount, should be implemented. About 10% of these neonates are removed from the mother's care under the child protective services systems (AIHW, 2020). Although there is an initial financial burden on the healthcare system because of the needed neonatal support and possible admission to the neonatal unit if treatment is required, infants with NAS also require additional long-term support including healthcare post discharge and extra education for parents and carers (Maguire et al., 2016). The role of the social worker and, where applicable, the perinatal mental health team is integral to multidisciplinary care of the woman with substance use disorder.

Following birth, the neonate should be transferred with the mother to the postnatal ward (Boucher, 2017; Vogel, 2018). Neonates usually require admission to the neonatal unit only when:

- the neonate requires medical attention
- the mother's drug use is unknown or not controlled; this should be assessed on an individual basis
- the withdrawal score begins to increase, and the neonate can no longer be managed on the postnatal ward.

CLINICAL MANIFESTATIONS OF NAS

Most neonates of substance use disorder women appear stable at birth, but usually manifest signs of drug withdrawal within 24–72 hours of birth depending on the drug amount and pattern of use. At birth, it is recommended that naloxone is not given to neonates with respiratory depression as this may cause an immediate withdrawal (Bailey & Diaz-Barbosa, 2018). Neonates do not withdraw from drugs in the same way as do adults.

The most common signs that the registered nurse/midwife may observe in the neonate with NAS fall within the areas outlined in Table 20.1.

When assessing neonates, nursing and midwifery staff must remember that some of these signs may be seen in neonates with other medical conditions; therefore the neonate may need to undergo tests to exclude other medical conditions. The most common differential diagnoses include infection, hypoglycaemia, hypocalcaemia and metabolic disorders (Lacaze-Masmonteil & O'Flaherty, 2018). Assessments will commence depending on the type of tool used for the assessment of the neonate; most commonly, this occurs 2 hours after birth and continues 3–4 hourly. The assessment is completed 1–1½ hours after a feed and reflects the whole time period from one feed to the next, usually 3–4 hours. Some tools are best used when two staff members assess together, so there is added consistency of scoring (Abbett & Greenwood, 2012). The most common mistake a clinician can make while assessing for withdrawal is to consider only one time point, rather than a whole time period.

MATERNAL DRUGS THAT CONTRIBUTE TO NAS

There are many different types of substances, including alcohol, that can be used and misused that may affect the fetus in utero, and potentially contribute to NAS. Some of these drugs include alcohol, opiates (heroin, oxycodone, codeine), methadone, marijuana, phenobarbitone, **selective serotonin reuptake inhibitors (SSRIs)** and **serotonin and noradrenaline (norepinephrine) reuptake inhibitors (SNRIs)**, although are not limited to these. SSRIs and SNRIs are relatively new drugs to consider in relation to NAS and the risks have been identified in recent years. They can lead to toxicity, withdrawal or permanent neurological disorders. The recommendations on specific substance toxicity change frequently, and new substances are being added, so clinicians are advised to access current guidelines and recommendations related to these.

TABLE 20.1 **Common clinical manifestations and nursing interventions for neonatal abstinence syndrome**

Manifestation	Treatment/support
Central nervous system:	
• Hypertonicity – tense arms, legs and back • Continuous high-pitched cry • Sleeping difficulties • Irritability • Hyperactivity – tremors, jitters, myoclonic activity and potentially seizures	• Wrapping • Wrapping, quiet area, use of volunteer • Wrapping, quiet, darkened area • Wrapping, facilitate midline orientation, use of a sling or swing, deep bath while wrapped with light wrap • Wrapping, quiet area, observation and monitoring
Autonomic:	
• Pyrexia and increased sweating • Skin mottling • Wakefulness, yawning, diaphoresis • Skin care	• Regular temperatures, use of light wraps such as muslin wraps • Regular skin assessment • Daily baths • Regular skin assessment, preventative treatment with zinc-based cream or use of silicone-based covers • For severe excoriation, a 'crusting method' can be used to support healing[a]
Respiratory:	

• Rhinorrhoea, nasal congestion, sneezing
• Respiratory distress:
  • Tachypnoea
  • Nasal flaring
  • Subcostal recession
	• Observation and vital signs
	• Observation and vital signs
	• Observation and vital signs care must be taken to observe for a medical illness; may need to be transferred to a neonatal nursery and be observed in an incubator

Gastrointestinal:	
• Often very hungry babies who want to feed a lot • Excessive and uncoordinated sucking • Vomiting • Diarrhoea • Weight loss or failure to gain weight	• Regular breastfeeds; if artificial feeding – small regular feeds • Use of a dummy/pacifier • Small frequent feeds • Maintenance of skin integrity through observation and prevention • Regular breastfeed, plotting of growth on appropriate growth chart, regular follow-up

[a]Skin specific.

Sources: Association of Women's Health Obstetric and Neonatal Nurses (2018); Cook and Fantasia (2019); Queensland Health (2021).

FETAL ALCOHOL SPECTRUM DISORDER

Fetal alcohol spectrum disorder is a term used to describe a range of effects to the fetus from prenatal alcohol exposure and is often referred to as the 'hidden disability' (Schölin et al., 2021).

The range of diagnoses includes:

- fetal alcohol syndrome (FAS)
- partial FAS
- alcohol-related birth defects (ARBD)
- alcohol-related neurodevelopmental disorder (ARND) (Williams & Smith, 2015).

These babies may present with birth defects or be diagnosed with neurocognitive and behavioural problems later in childhood (Moder et al., 2021). This spectrum of disorders requires further reading and has only been included here to highlight to the nurse/midwife that there may be potential for withdrawal with this group of babies.

The incidence of alcohol consumption in pregnancy worldwide has been documented as 9.8% irrespective of the amount of alcohol consumed (Demiguel, 2021; Moder et al., 2021).

SCORING TOOLS AVAILABLE FOR ASSESSMENT OF NAS

Timing of withdrawal symptoms will occur depending on the type of drug misused and the timing of the last use; the most common are:

- heroin – onset within 24–72 hours
- methadone/buprenorphine – may be delayed until 3–7 days after birth
- SSRI/SNRI – variable in onset and may occur within 2 days of birth, but may not begin until late in the first week of life
- cocaine/methamphetamine – short-acting substances such these may cause withdrawal symptoms closer to birth.

Clinicians should also be aware that withdrawal symptoms may be iatrogenic if a baby has received postoperative pain management and/or sedation (Coyle et al., 2018; Williamson, 2020).

EVIDENCE-BASED PRACTICE 20.2

Read the current evidence-based guidelines on substance abuse for your hospital, state or country. Here are some examples:

Australia

- New South Wales: <https://www.health.nsw.gov.au/aod/Pages/default.aspx>
- Queensland: <www.health.qld.gov.au/qcg/documents/g-psumat.pdf>

New Zealand

- Ministry of Health Manatu Hauora: <https://www.health.govt.nz/your-health/healthy-living/addictions/alcohol-and-drug-abuse>

United Kingdom

- NICE Guidelines: <https://www.evidence.nhs.uk/search?ps=250&q=drug+misuse+in+pregnancy>

United States of America

- CDC: <https://www.cdc.gov/reproductivehealth/maternalinfanthealth/substance-abuse/substance-abuse-during-pregnancy.htm>

World Health Organization

- <https://www.who.int/publications-detail-redirect/9789241548731>

Three of the most frequently used tools in the assessment of NAS include the Finnegan Neonatal Abstinence Scoring Tool (FNAST) (Finnegan et al., 1975) (Box 20.1 and Fig. 20.1), the Lipsitz Neonatal Drug Withdrawal Scoring System (Lipsitz, 1975) (Box 20.2 and Fig. 20.2) and the Neonatal Withdrawal Inventory (Box 20.3 and Fig. 20.3). These tools identify the severity of withdrawal signs and help to guide clinicians when a pharmacological agent may be indicated for use. Most recently, the Eat, Sleep, Console has been utilised to score withdrawal from opioids. This approach focused on

BOX 20.1 Finnegan Neonatal Abstinence Scoring Tool (FNAST)

- The Finnegan system is the most widely used of the NOWS assessment tools (Finnegan et al., 1975).
- This approach, first published by Dr Loretta P. Finnegan, considers various symptoms of NOWS to identify clinical severity and the necessity for pharmaceutical intervention (Finnegan et al., 1975).
- Since the original Finnegan assessment tool was published and implemented, various studies have updated and modified it to make it more accessible. While the original Finnegan scoring instrument had 32 items, recent improvements resulted in creation of a 21-item modified Finnegan assessment.
- Each item in this modified scoring system indicates a symptom that manifests in the central nervous system, the gastrointestinal or respiratory tract, or in conjunction with metabolic or vasomotor processes.
- Each clinical indicator is assessed every 3–4 hours and scored on a scale of 0 to 5, using the same scoring algorithms and cut-off points as the original Finnegan instrument.
- Two consecutive scores of 12 or higher, or three consecutive scores of 8 or higher, suggest that pharmaceutical treatment is required.

Dose modifications and discharge indications are based on how the individual scores evolve over time (Oji-Mmuo, et al. 2021).

System	Sign	Score										
Central nervous system disturbances	High pitch/excessive cry Continuous (high pitched) cry	2 3										
	Sleeps less than 1 hour after feeds Sleeps less than 2 hours after feeds Sleeps less than 3 hours after feeds	3 2 1										
	Hyperactive Moro reflex Markedly hyperactive Moro reflex	2 3										
	Mild tremors disturbed* Mod/severe tremors disturbed* Mild termors undisturbed* Mod/severe tremors undisturbed*	1 2 3 4										
	Increased muscle tone	2										
	Excoriation*	1										
	Myoclonic jerks	3										
	Generalised convulsions	5										
Gastrointestinal disturbances	Excessive sucking	1										
	Poor feeding*	2										
	Regurgitation* Projectile vomiting	2 3										
	Loose stools Watery stools	2 3										
Respiratory/vasomotor disturbances	Sweating	1										
	Fever 37.8° to 38.3°C Fever 38.4°C and above	1 2										
	Frequent yawning (>3–4 in ½ hr)	1										
	Mottling	1										
	Nasal stuffiness	1										
	Sneezing (>3–4 in ½ hr)	2										
	Nasal flaring	1										
	Respiratory rate >60/min Respiratory rate >60/min and retractions	1 2										
	Total score											
	Scorer's initials											

FIGURE 20.1 **Example of the Finnegan Neonatal Abstinence Scoring Tool (FNAST)**
Source: Finnegan et al. (1975).

BOX 20.2 **Lipsitz Neonatal Drug Withdrawal Scoring System**

- The Lipsitz scoring system takes 11 symptoms of newborn withdrawal into account and assesses the severity of the clinical indicators on a scale of 0 to 3 (Lipsitz, 1975).
- Certain symptoms, such as tremor or irritability, are seen to be more crucial in the development of NOWS and are given more weight than less-serious symptoms, such as vomiting.
- While the maximum potential score is 20, a score of 4 or higher indicates that the neonate is experiencing withdrawal symptoms.
- The Lipsitz scoring method is not frequently utilised, and the only known validation was published as part of the initial study 45 years ago.

Source: Oji-Mmuo et al. (2021).

including the family and assessing duration of sleep, eating and difficulty in consoling the infant (Casavant et al., 2021; Miller & Willier, 2021). The challenge when using any scoring tool is to ensure that all midwives and registered nurses are educated in the use of the tool to ensure consistency, and that the scores are not flawed through subjectivity (Casavant et al., 2021). With the increasing prevalence of polydrug use, the FNAST is being used for substance abuse that it was not designed for, and, as such, future research needs to examine the use of these tools and how they can best be utilised in the contemporary clinical setting.

NON-PHARMACOLOGICAL INTERVENTIONS FOR NAS

With the increasing cases of NAS on postnatal wards and possible subsequent admission to neonatal nurseries, nurses and midwives have the responsibility of initiating

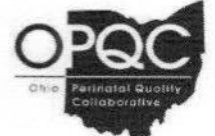

Neonatal Drug Withdrawal: Lipsitz Scoring Tool

Instructions: Score each category with the highest score in that time interval. Score every 3 hours for first 72 hours (if exposed to narcotics or opiates) or for first 96 hours (if exposed to Methadone or Suboxone).

A total score of 4 is recommended for initiation of pharmacologic treatment.

Name:

DOB:

MR#:

Patient Identification Label

Date: Day of Life: (DOB=DOL #1)

	SCORING CATEGORIES				INTERVALS (NOTE TIME in column)								COMMENTS
SIGNS	Score 0	Score 1	Score 2	Score 3									Time and Initial
Tremors (muscle activity of limbs)	Normal	Minimally increased when hungry or disturbed	Moderate/marked increase when undisturbed; stop when fed or cuddled	Marked increase or continuous even when undisturbed, going on to seizure-like movements									
Irritability (excessive crying)	None	Slightly increased	Moderate to severe irritability when disturbed or hungry	Marked irritability even when undisturbed									
Reflexes	Normal	Increased	Markedly increased										
Stools	Normal	Explosive, but frequency ≤8/day	Explosive, > 8 per day										
Muscle tone	Normal	Increased	Rigidity										
Skin abrasions	No	Redness of elbows, heels, pressure points when supine	Breakdown of skin at pressure points										
Respiratory rate (bpm)	<55	55–75	76–95										
Repetitive sneezing	No	Yes											
Repetitive yawning	No	Yes											
Forceful vomiting	No	Yes											
Fever >38°C or >100.4°F	No	Yes											
TOTAL SCORE													
Signatures with initials	Nurse Signatures												

FIGURE 20.2 **Example of Lipsitz Neonatal Drug Withdrawal Scoring System**

Source: Lipsitz (1975).

BOX 20.3 **Neonatal Withdrawal Inventory**

- The NWI is a simplified and rapid-scoring approach developed in the late 1990s to identify neonatal opioid withdrawal.
- On a predetermined weighted scale, the NWI screens for indicators of CNS irritability and autonomic arousal, as well as gastrointestinal and behavioural abnormalities.
- The NWI system has a score range of 0–19, with an intervention threshold of 8 specified.
- While no published educational or training resources are available for nurses and clinicians, the NWI is easy to administer and has been shown to have good sensitivity, specificity and inter-observer reliability.

Source: Oji-Mmuo et al. (2021).

non-pharmacological interventions when caring for these infants (Nelson, 2016). See Box 20.4 and Fig. 20.4 for information about 'Eat, Sleep, Console'. Volunteers have also been utilised to support these babies – they are often called 'cuddle mums' (Shannon et al., 2021) allowing parents self-care time (Hignell et al., 2020).

Routine and comfort cares provided by nurses and midwives include:

- swaddling
- quiet room
- talking gently/singing or playing soft music to the infant
- a darkened room
- dummy/pacifier
- warmed blanket to the infant's abdomen over a thin layer of clothing.

These cares promote sleep and provide comfort for the infant (Nelson, 2016). Other techniques employed to decrease irritability include:

- the infant cared for in a baby sling or swing with gentle rocking
- a stroller for parents/carers to walk the infant.

Decreasing over-stimulation of NAS infants improves their growth and development. The mother and other carers are provided with in-hospital education (as described in Family-centred Care 20.1) during the admission phase of the infant's care and receive ongoing follow-up education and support post discharge (Nelson, 2016). The research by Shannon et al. (2021) promotes continuity of care for NAS infants, identifying that 'best practice is for senior registered nurse/midwife to care for these infants due to specialised knowledge required' (p. 4).

Hypertonicity	Hyperactive Moro reflex	Tremors when disturbed	or	Tremors when undisturbed
2	2	3		4

Sneezing or yawning (>2 per session)	Sweating or mottling	Regurgitation	Loose, watery stools
1	2	2	2

Irritability (restlessness, even after intervention)	or	Crying or frantic fist-sucking	or	Fresh excoriation of limbs (w or w/out crying)	or	Continuous crying
1		2		3		4

Total:

Comments: ____________________

Temperature ____________ Respirations per minute ____________

Withdrawal inventory.

Observation of infant (1 min)
Unswaddling and gentle wakening
Determination of respiratory rate (1 min)
Measurement of axillary temperature
Inspection for signs of excoriation
Assessment of tone and Moro reflex
Nappy change
Reswaddling and positioning
Observation of infant (1 min)

FIGURE 20.3 **Example of Neonatal Withdrawal Inventory**
Source: Zahorodny et al. (1998).

BOX 20.4 **Eat, Sleep, Console**

- Family-centred approach, inclusive of the family unit
- Based on non-instrusive functional assessment
- Observation of the baby's eating, sleeping and consoling patterns

Source: Grossman et al. (2018).

FAMILY-CENTRED CARE 20.1

Parent education – comfort/supportive care

- Midwives and neonatal nurses provide education to mothers/parents/carers in ways to comfort and settle the baby, developing a trusting, respectful relationship between the parents and healthcare providers (Shannon et al., 2021). Explaining to parents what their baby may experience increases their awareness of their baby's symptoms. Teaching parents how and when to use these techniques to settle a baby helps the parent to learn how to confidently care for their baby after discharge at home.
- Parents are shown how to hold the baby close to the body, wrapped in a blanket or sheet (swaddling). Explaining to parents the requirement of reducing loud noises, bright lights and excessive handling will help them decrease the level of stimulus the baby receives when settling for a sleep. This technique will assist parents to decrease prolonged crying in their baby and facilitate growth and development.

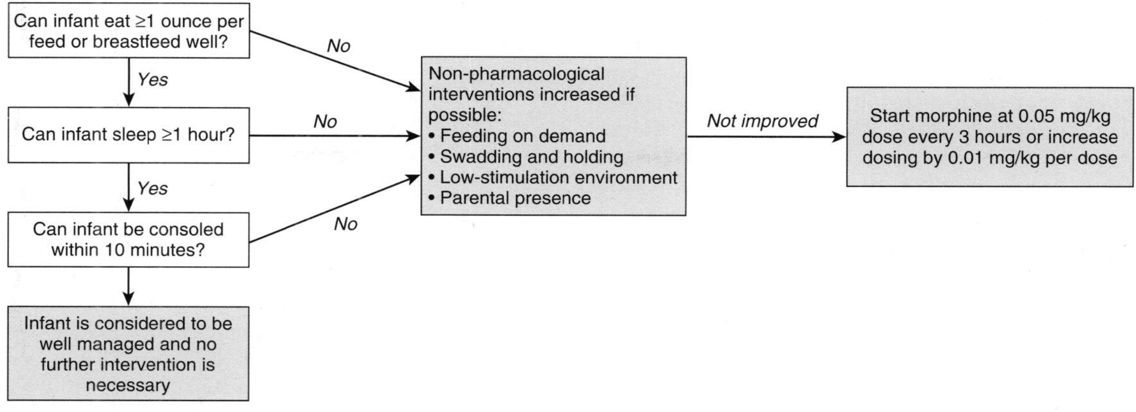

FIGURE 20.4 **Example of Eat, Sleep, Console**
Source: Grossman et al. (2018).

- Teach the parents to use soft flannel blankets around the baby for comfort. Explain that they should speak softly to their baby and play soothing music.
- Complementary therapies and identifying the optimal environment in which to care for newborns with NAS and their families are two areas of emerging interest for supportive care. Aromatherapy, massage therapy, music therapy and skin-to-skin contact have all been shown to be effective in the preterm population (Artigas, 2014).
- Preventative skin care of the perianal region should be commenced immediately post birth with the application of a thick layer of petroleum-based ointment; this may prevent breakdown of the skin of an infant with NAS (Association of Women's Health, Obstetric and Neonatal Nurses, 2018).
- If the skin does break down, a thick layer of zinc oxide should be applied to aid healing through protection. A process called crusting may also be required if there is severe excoriation and first-line measures have been utilised (Association of Women's Health, Obstetric and Neonatal Nurses, 2018).
- Hepatitis B vaccination should be given prior to discharge, and if the mother is hepatitis B positive then immunoglobulin should be given within 12 hours and certainly by 48 (Australian Technical Advisory Group on Immunisation (ATAGI), 2018).

staff. The benefits to both baby and mother include better bonding and attachment.

- If a breastfeeding mother smokes, advise her to smoke straight after a breastfeed as the nicotine levels are halved in about 97 minutes after a cigarette (Australian Breast Feeding Association, 2021). Breastfeeding helps to protect the infant from the harmful effects of cigarette smoke.
- Breastfeeding is not contraindicated for a hepatitis C-positive mother; if the nipples are cracked and bleeding, expressing and discarding of the breast milk should take place until the nipples have healed (Hughes et al., 2017).
- Midwives and nurses should educate mothers and carers about expressing breast milk, providing tips on how to make breastfeeding a little easier – including positioning of baby.
- Educate parents regarding difficult or poor feeding, including feeding in quiet, calm surroundings with minimal noise and disturbance to decrease irritation.
- Provide guidance to parents and carers about bottle feeding, such as use of a slow teat, feeding baby slowly and allowing time for resting between sucking intervals.
- If the baby is bottle fed, giving smaller feeds of a high-caloric formula more often may help.
- Explain to the mother to keep her baby in a semi-sitting position, and well supported, including supporting the chin well to encourage sucking.

FAMILY-CENTRED CARE 20.2

Parent education – feeding

- Breastfeeding is recommended for all babies. It is especially important for babies with NAS as it is thought to help with withdrawal symptoms. Breastfeeding provides mother and baby an opportunity for close contact and skin-to-skin care. Breastfeeding requires commitment from the mother and support from her partner and nursing

BIOMARKERS FOR TESTING SUBSTANCE ABUSE IN NEONATES

Routine testing in neonates is not generally recommended and if required can be collected only with informed maternal consent and in a non-judgemental approach (Grossman & Berkwitt, 2019). Care should be taken with this discussion as it may affect the therapeutic relationship.

Forms of specimen collection utilised are urine, meconium, umbilical cord tissue and hair. Urine and meconium have been most commonly utilised by clinicians, but both can lead to false-positive results (Casavant et al., 2021; Grossman & Berkwitt, 2019; MacMillan, 2019). Clinical presentation is the most important aspect in diagnosing neonatal abstinence syndrome; testing may further complement the clinical presentation and diagnoses.

PHARMACEUTICAL MANAGEMENT OF NAS/NOWS

Refer to Table 20.2 for a summary of the most common pharmacological options for the treatment of neonatal abstinence syndrome.

Morphine

- The most commonly used treatment modality for NAS due to maternal opioid use is morphine hydrochloride; it enables greater stabilisation for improved feeding and less neurological symptoms (Cook & Fantasia, 2019). For specific administration guidelines refer to Evidence-based Practice 20.2.
- Although morphine is most commonly used for the treatment of NOWS worldwide, rigid dosing regimens may actually increase length of stay (Wijekoon et al., 2021). More satisfactory for the care of these neonates may be individualised dosing regimens.
- Frameworks are being developed and tested to stratify risk and predict outcome while providing individualised treatment programs (Patrick et al., 2021; Wijekoon et al., 2021).

EVIDENCE-BASED PRACTICE RESEARCH 20.3

Non-pharmacological therapies (e.g. skin-to-skin contact, holding) can be useful in reducing NAS-related distress. The goal of a study by Williams et al. (2020) was to see whether infant carrying, often known as 'babywearing' (holding a newborn on one's body with fabric), could minimise the distress associated with NAS in infants and care givers.

Heart rates were monitored in newborns and adults (parents versus other adults) in a neonatal intensive care unit (NICU) before (no touching), during and after (5 minutes later) 20 minutes of being worn in a carrier.

Researchers discovered that babywearing reduced infant and care giver heart rates using a 3-level hierarchical linear model at three time points (before, mid and post babywearing). Heart rates of newborns 'worn' by a parent reduced by 15 beats per minute (bpm) over a 30-minute period, compared with 5.5 bpm for infants 'worn' by an unfamiliar adult, and those of adults decreased by 7 bpm (parent) and approximately 3 bpm (unfamiliar adult).

According to the findings of this study, babywearing is a non-invasive and accessible technique that can bring comfort to newborns diagnosed with NAS. Babywearing is a low-cost parenting tool that can be performed by non-parent care givers (e.g. nurses, volunteers).

Close physical contact, such as babywearing, may enhance outcomes in NICU newborns with NAS and potentially lessen the need for pharmaceutical treatment.

Methadone

- In many countries, morphine is the first-line treatment for NOWS.
- This is in contrast to the United States/United Kingdom, where alternatives such as methadone/buprenorphine are accepted options for the treatment of NOWS (Disher et al., 2019; Frazier et al., 2022).
- There have been two randomised controlled trials in recent years comparing morphine with methadone for the treatment of NOWS.
- Brown et al. (2015) compared the use of methadone with morphine in a prospective randomised trial. The study enrolled 78 eligible neonates; of these, 31 were treated: 13 with methadone and 18 with morphine. Although a small study, the results indicated that

TABLE 20.2 **Pharmacological options for the treatment of neonatal abstinence syndrome**

Drug	Clinical application	Currently used	Level of evidence
Morphine	• Currently used for opioid-dependent infants • Used in combination therapy	Yes	I
Methadone	• Currently used for opioid-dependent infants	Yes	II Small study only
Phenobarbitone	• Used in combination therapy • Occasionally used as first-line therapy in cases of polydrug use	Yes	I
Clonidine	• Used in combination therapy	Yes	II Small studies only
Buprenorphine	• Currently used for opioid-dependent infants	Yes	11 Small studies only

Source: National Health & Medical Research Council (1999).

methadone treatment resulted in a shorter length of stay compared with morphine by 7 days.

- Davis et al. (2018) recruited 183 infants; from these 117 required treatment. Primary short-term outcome was length of stay; this was 2.9 days shorter in the methadone group. Unfortunately, long-term outcomes were not included in the study design.
- The lack of rigorous large multicentre studies advocating methadone as first-line treatment for neonatal withdrawal has led to its exclusion in many clinical guidelines.

Phenobarbitone

- Phenobarbitone (phenobarbital) is not advocated as first-line treatment for opioid withdrawal in neonates but can be utilised as a concurrent therapy if the maximum dose of morphine is reached or polydrug use is suspected (Patrick et al., 2020).
- Many studies are conflicting as to whether phenobarbitone is the better adjunct to morphine than clonidine, but a Cochrane review comparing sedatives for opioid withdrawal determined that there was low-certainty evidence of an increase in days' hospitalisation and days' treatment with clonidine and opioid compared with phenobarbital and opioid (Zankl et al., 2021).
- A recent retrospective study reported that, when phenobarbitone is used as a adjunct therapy to morphine, the length of stay in hospital and morphine treatment was shorter but length of treatment on a secondary medication was longer (Merhar et al., 2021).

Clonidine

- Clonidine is regularly used as an adjunct therapy for the management of NOWS in many countries, and the evidence is promising.
- A randomised controlled trial, investigating the efficacy of clonidine versus phenobarbitone, randomised 68 neonates suffering neonatal withdrawal symptoms. The use of either medication was used as an adjunct therapy to morphine to decrease the number of days on treatment (Surran et al., 2013). The use of phenobarbitone decreased the length of treatment, but not significantly, when compared with clonidine (Surran et al., 2013). In the morphine/clonidine arm, 2 out of 32 neonates failed treatment compared with none in the morphine/phenobarbitone arm (Surran et al., 2013). The one notable outcome in the trial was that phenobarbitone treatment often continued post discharge but clonidine did not; some neonates were still receiving phenobarbitone at 8 months of age (Surran et al., 2013).
- Clonidine has been demonstrated to be a far superior supplementary therapy to phenobarbitone in terms of lowering morphine treatment days (Ghazanfarpour et al., 2019).
- In some cases, studies were aimed at using clonidine as primary treatment. A study by Bada et al. published in 2015 investigated clonidine versus morphine for better neurobehavioural performance (Bada et al., 2015). Infants >35 weeks' gestation and suffering from symptoms of neonatal withdrawal were recruited; 14 were randomised to the morphine group and 16 in the clonidine group (Bada et al., 2015). Results indicated that treatment length was of shorter duration, by 11 days, in the clonidine group (Bada et al., 2015). Numbers were small in the trial though results were favourable (Bada et al., 2015).
- A larger multicentre trial is required before advocating the use of clonidine over morphine for first-line treatment for neonatal withdrawal symptoms (Bada et al., 2015).

For specific administration guidelines, refer to Evidence-based Practice 20.2.

Buprenorphine

- A systematic review of pharmacological treatments concluded that sublingual buprenorphine was considered to be the optimal treatment for NOWS, reducing length of treatment days and length of stay, but not the requirement for adjunct therapy (Disher et al., 2019).
- Randomised controlled trials have been undertaken to assess the safety, effectiveness and efficacy for sublingual buprenorphine in neonates suffering neonatal opioid withdrawal (Kraft et al., 2011, 2017).
- In 2011, Kraft conducted a randomised open label, active-control trial which supported earlier findings reconfirming the potential efficacy for the use of sublingual buprenorphine over standard care (Kraft et al., 2011).
- In 2017, Kraft conducted a single-site, double-blind, double-dummy clinical trial, randomly assigning 63 infants displaying signs of NOWS to receive sublingual buprenorphine or oral morphine. Results again concluded that those neonates treated with sublingual buprenorphine underwent a shorter treatment time and had a shorter length of stay (Kraft et al., 2017).

Results must be interpreted as, additionally, a large multicentred trial needs to be undertaken with comparison also with methadone (Wachman & Werler, 2019).

Pharmacology

Morphine

Morphine is an opioid analgesic that induces analgesia, respiratory depression, drowsiness and constipation by activating opioid receptors in the central and peripheral nervous systems. Morphine reduces the pain impulse by modulating the pathways from the brain and spinal cord (Ritter et al., 2019). In neonatal pharmacopeia, oral morphine is used for pain relief, sedation and the minimisation of symptoms in NAS (Cook & Fantasia, 2019; Patrick et al., 2020).

Methadone

Methadone has commonly been used for opioid replacement programs, particularly in pregnant women where the effects of intoxication and withdrawal can adversely affect the fetus (Ritter et al., 2019). It is also being utilised when women are suffering severe pain during pregnancy (Johnson, 2016). Methadone is an opioid analgesic but has a much longer half-life, making dose adjustment difficult (Ritter et al., 2019). Methadone acts directly on the N-methyl-d-aspartate receptor antagonist, inhibiting glutamate, the key excitatory neurotransmitter involved with heroin euphoria (Oji-Mmuo et al., 2021).

Phenobarbitone

Phenobarbitone is a barbiturate '... prolonging the postsynaptic potential by increasing the mean chloride channel opening time hence the duration of gamma-aminobutyric acid (GABA)-induced cell membrane hyperpolarisation' (*Australian medicines handbook*: <https://amhonline.amh.net.au/>). Phenobarbitone has sedative, anticonvulsant and hypnotic properties (Shann, 2014). The medication has a long half-life and takes 2–4 weeks to reach a steady state; therapeutic monitoring must be undertaken while this drug is being administered. Side effects can include respiratory depression and shock (*Australian medicines handbook*, 2021).

Clonidine

Clonidine is predominantly used for the management of hypertension and menopausal flushing, also indicated for use in anaesthetics, pain management and opioid withdrawal in adults (*Australian medicines handbook*: <https://amhonline.amh.net.au/>). It is an alpha$_2$-antagonist, which is helpful in relieving withdrawal symptoms originating from the autonomic nervous system (*Australian medicines handbook*, 2021).

Buprenorphine

Buprenorphine is a partial agonist at μ-opioid receptors and has antagonist effects at opioid receptors (Hakomäki et al., 2020). Due to high affinity and low dissociation rate from the opioid receptors, buprenorphine is classified as a long-acting opioid (Hakomäki et al., 2020).

PREPARATION FOR DISCHARGE

Prior to discharge, parents should be prepared by completing a series of education sessions focusing on normal discharge issues and specific issues related to neonatal withdrawal. The length of stay required in hospital has a significant impact on education provided. Nurses and midwives must also be aware that this education may also involve a foster carer and that individualised discharge planning is necessary. The most commonly addressed topics include:

1. smoking and management in the home
2. sudden unexpected infant death and strategies to minimise the risk
3. immunisation and family pertussis status
4. blood tests if maternal hepatitis C is present, usually at 12–18 months of age; this should be documented in the discharge information for the general practitioner
5. exposing babies to undue risk of infection, such as colds, viruses, etc.
6. if maternal HIV is present, a follow-up plan will be devised involving administration of medications and specific multidisciplinary requirements.

Topics specific to a baby with withdrawal symptoms are:

1. discussion about ongoing symptoms
2. further education about supportive therapies
3. discussion on when to re-present to the hospital
4. the importance of a regular general practitioner
5. expected follow-up.

Parenting programs should be made available to parents who have identified the need to improve their skills around parenting. These support groups or classes should be available in differing formats, including face to face and online. Education is available for first-time parents of all babies, including NAS babies and those who have toddlers and teens who require extra support. The ability to call a parent line which provides counselling and support for parents during stressful times is beneficial and available through government agencies.

HOME WEANING

Outpatient management has been shown to decrease length of stay by 50%, though treatment may continue longer (Cook & Fantasia, 2019). There are only small studies around the effectiveness of home weaning; these have reported that length of treatment is longer, but re-admissions for the exacerbation of symptoms are decreased (Cook & Fantasia, 2019). Further thought must be given to how this can be facilitated more regularly in the current healthcare environment.

FOLLOW-UP

All neonates who are admitted to a neonatal unit for NAS monitoring or treatment are required to be followed up long term. Current evidence suggests that long-term problems may include vision, motor and behavioural/cognitive problems, as well as sleeping disturbances, ear infections, child abuse and neglect (Maguire et al., 2016). Close surveillance, therefore, by a paediatrician is required following discharge. Current models in the US have also advocated that neonatal nurse practitioners may be in the best position to follow up babies who have suffered from NAS in the immediate discharge period (Watson, 2017). Community child health nurses should also be involved in the neonate's ongoing follow-up to assess growth, family interaction, signs of neglect and attainment of milestones. The family should also be encouraged to develop a relationship with a general practitioner who is consulted for ongoing assessment; an example of a follow-up plan is shown in Box 20.5.

BOX 20.5 **Example of a follow-up plan**

1. Neonatal nurse practitioner up to 6 weeks of age
2. Lactation consultant to support breastfeeding for the first 6 weeks of life
3. Paediatrician until at least 2 years of age
4. Community child health from 6 weeks till 4–5 years
5. General practitioner from 6/52 for immunisation, then as per the schedule, and for further blood testing, if required, due to maternal hepatitis C

Sources: Cook and Fantasia (2019); Queensland Health (2021).

CASE STUDY 20.1

Reason for admission

Treatment of neonatal abstinence syndrome.

History of present illness

Spontaneous vaginal delivery at a regional hospital. Significant history with the Department of Child Safety; a care agreement has been negotiated.

Past medical history: maternal

- 30-year-old gravida eight, para seven
- Indigenous
- Normal BMI
- Minimal antenatal care
- Pathology:
  - Blood group-A negative antibodies – negative
  - Hepatitis B – negative
  - Hepatitis C – positive
  - RPR-TPHA – negative
  - HIV – negative
  - Rubella – immune
  - GTT – nil
- Medical issues:
  - Maternal depression and anxiety
- Medications:
  - Buprenorphine
- Recreational drug use:
  - Methamphetamine – last used 6 months ago
  - Cannabis – regular use
- Ultrasound scan:
  - Normal morphology

Social

- Unplanned pregnancy
- Maternal smoker
- Partner not present
- No transport
- Homeless since 2015; no fixed address
- Extensive child protection history: physical harm, emotional harm and neglect in the context of parental substance misuse and previous domestic violence
- All other children in the care of the Department of Child Safety

Neonatal

- Born at 1838 hours
- Apgar:
  - Nine at 1 minute
  - Nine at 5 minutes
- Resuscitation:
  - Nil resuscitation required at birth
  - Birthweight – 3550 grams

Objective information

Baby appears settled; wakes for feeds and settles quite well.

Vital signs	Patient values
Temperature	37.4°C
Heart rate	128 beats per minute
Respiratory rate	66 breaths per minute
Oxygen saturation	97% in air
Finnegan scores	7, 6, 8 last three scores

Plan

Non-pharmacological management

- Care of the family in consultation with social workers and child safety staff
- Organisation of supervised visits
- Discussion with family about course of symptoms and possible interventions
- Discussion with family about supportive therapies:
  - Wrapping/swaddling
  - Quiet environment
  - Early intervention when baby is crying

Pharmacological management

Drugs

- Treatment choice if required is morphine

Other treatments

- Supportive therapies

Patient/family education

- Discussion with mother about change in condition and possible causes of increasing scores
- Explanation of planned interventions, such as medication if required

Follow-up

- Currently in hospital

Referrals

- Social work referral to support the family
- Child safety department/protective services

Investigations

- Finnegan scoring

REFLECTION

Imagine yourself as the neonatal nurse/midwife caring for the family outlined in Case Study 20.1. Are there any other factors you need to consider? For example:

- non-pharmacological management
- pharmacological management
- family support
- feeding
- follow-up.

CONCLUSION

Substance use disorder in pregnancy and NAS in newborns is currently among the fastest growing healthcare challenges in Australia and New Zealand and internationally.

The education of parents/guardians in techniques of feeding and in non-pharmacological interventions for NAS babies provides families with a tool kit to support their baby's ongoing needs. Parents learning how and when to use techniques that best suit their baby will help them feel more comfortable and confident to care for them at discharge. These techniques reflect current safe-sleeping guidelines and will be helpful for settling or comforting the NAS infant. Often the most junior staff care for these babies in a neonatal nursery because they are generally term, yet consideration must be given to the complexity of caring for these babies. Education is imperative for staff and families to achieve the best possible outcome for the baby.

Online Resources

Australian Breastfeeding Association: Is this safe when breastfeeding?: <https://www.breastfeeding.asn.au/bf-info/safe-when-breastfeeding>

Australian Standards for Neonatal Nurses: <https://www.acnn.org.au/resources/australian-standards-for-neonatal-nurses/; https://www.health.qld.gov.au/__data/assets/pdf_file/0018/140814/g-psuneo.pdf>

NIH National Institute on Drug Abuse: Substance use while pregnant and breastfeeding (USA): <https://www.drugabuse.gov/publications/research-reports/substance-use-in-women/substance-use-while-pregnant-breastfeeding>

Queensland Clinical Guidelines. (2021). Supplement: Perinatal substance use: neonatal guideline No. MN21.38-V3-R21. Queensland Health: <https://www.health.qld.gov.au/__data/assets/pdf_file/0018/140814/g-psuneo.pdf>

RANZCOG. Substance use in pregnancy statement: <https://ranzcog.edu.au/RANZCOG_SITE/media/RANZCOG-MEDIA/Women%27s%20Health/Statement%20and%20guidelines/Clinical-Obstetrics/Substance-use-in-pregnancy-(C-Obs-55)-March-2018.pdf?ext=.pdf>

Triple P Positive Parenting Program: <https://www.triplep.net/>

References

Abbett, H., & Greenwood, S. (2012). Nursing infants with neonatal abstinence syndrome: time to change practice? *Journal of Neonatal Nursing, 18*(6), 194–197. doi: http: 10.1016/j.jnn.2012.08.006.

Artigas, V. (2014). Management of neonatal abstinence syndrome in the newborn nursery. *Nursing for Women's Health, 18*(6), 509–514. doi: 10.1111/1751-486X.12163.

Association of Women's Health Obstetric and Neonatal Nurses. (2018). *Neonatal skin care: evidenced based neonatal skin care* (4th ed.). Washington, DC: AWHONN.

Australian Breastfeeding Association. (2021). Is this safe when breastfeeding? <https://www.breastfeeding.asn.au/bf-info/safe-when-breastfeeding> (Accessed 22 February 2022).

Australian Institute of Health and Welfare. (2020). *National Drug Strategy Household Survey detailed report 2020*. Canberra: AIHW. <https://www.aihw.gov.au/about-our-data/our-data-collections/national-drug-strategy-household-survey> (Accessed 22 February 2022).

Australian Medicines Handbook Pty. (2021). *Australian Medicines Handbook 2021 (online)*. Adelaide, SA: Australian Medicines Handbook Pty. <https://amhonline.amh.net.au/> (Accessed 22 February 2022).

Australian Technical Advisory Group on Immunisation (ATAGI). (2018). *Australian immunisation handbook*. Canberra, ACT: Australian Government Department of Health. <https://immunisationhandbook.health.gov.au> (Accessed 22 February 2022).

Bada, H. S., Sithisarn, T., Gibson, J., Garlitz, K., Caldwell, R., Capilouto, G., et al. (2015). Morphine versus clonidine for neonatal abstinence syndrome. *Pediatrics, 135*(2), e383–e391. doi: 10.1542/peds.2014-2377.

Bailey, N. A., & Diaz-Barbosa, M. (2018). Effect of maternal substance abuse on the fetus, neonate and child. *Pediatrics in Review, 39*(11), 550–559. doi: 10.1542/pir,2017-0201.

Boucher, A.-M. (2017). Nonopioid management of neonatal abstinence syndrome. *Advances in Neonatal Care, 17*(2), 84–90. doi: 10.1097/ANC.0000000000000371.

Brown, M. S., Hayes, M. J., & Thornton, L. M. (2015). Methadone versus morphine for treatment of neonatal abstinence syndrome: a prospective randomized clinical trial. *Journal of Perinatology, 35*(4), 278–283. doi: 10.1038/jp.2014.194.

Casavant, S. G., Taylor, M., Fleming, M., Hussain, N., Gork, S. & Cong, X. (2021). Integrated review of the assessment of newborns with neonatal abstinence syndrome. *Journal of Obstetric, Gynecologic and Neonatal Nursing, 50*(5), 539–548.

Chasnoff, I. J., & Gardner, S. (2015). Neonatal abstinence syndrome: a policy perspective. *Journal of Perinatology, 35*(8), 539. doi: 10.1038/jp.2015.53.

Chow, S. S. W., Creighton, P., Chambers, G. M., & Lui, K. (2019). *Report of the Australian and New Zealand Neonatal Network 2017*. Sydney, NSW: ANZNN.

Colorado Department of Public Health and Environment (CDPHE). (2019). FY 16-20 MCH priorities. <https://cdphe.colorado.gov/prevention-and-wellness/maternal-and-child-health/fy-16-20-mch-priorities> (Accessed 22 February 2022).

Cook, C. E., & Fantasia, H. C. (2019). Interventions for the treatment of neonatal abstinence syndrome. *Nursing for Women's Health, 23*(4), 357–365. doi: 10.1016/j.nwh.2019.05.006.

Coyle, M. G., Brogly, S. B., Ahmed, M. S., Patrick, S. W. & Jones, H. E. (2018). Neonatal abstinence syndrome. *Nature Reviews, 4*(47), 1–17. doi: 10.1038/s41572-018-0045-0.

Davis, J. M., Shenberger, J., Terrin, N., Breeze, J. L., Hudak, M., Wachman, E. M., et al. (2018). Comparison of safety and efficacy of methadone vs morphine for treatment of neonatal abstinence syndrome: a randomized clinical trial. *JAMA Pediatrics, 172*(8), 741–748.

Demiguel, V., Laporal, S., Quatremere, G., Barry, Y., Canu, I. G., Goulet, V., et al. (2021). The frequency of severe Fetal Alcohol Spectrum Disorders in the neonatal period using data from the French hospital discharge database between 2006 and 2013. *Drug and Alcohol Dependency,* 225, 108748. doi: 10.1016/j.drugalcdep.2021.108748.

Department of Health. (2020). *Clinical practice guidelines: pregnancy care*. Canberra, ACT: Australian Government; Department of Health. <https://www.health.gov.au/resources/pregnancy-care-guidelines> (Accessed 22 February 2022).

Disher, T., Gullickson, C., Singh, B., Cameron, C., Boulos, L., Beaubien, L., et al. (2019). Pharmacological treatments for neonatal abstinence syndrome: a systematic review and network meta-analysis. *JAMA Pediatrics, 173*(3), 234–243.

Finnegan, L. P., Connaughton, J. F., Kron, R. E., & Emich, J. P. (1975). Neonatal abstinence syndrome: assessment and management. *Addictive Diseases, 2*(1), 141–158.

Frazier, L. M., Bobby, L. E., & Gawronski, K. M. (2022). Emerging therapies for the treatment of neonatal abstinence syndrome. *Journal of Maternal–Fetal and Neonatal Medicine, 35*(5), 987–995.

Ghazanfarpour, M., Najafi, M. N., Roozbeh, N., Mashhadi, M. E., Keramat-Roudi, A., Mégarbane, B., et al. (2019). Therapeutic approaches for neonatal abstinence syndrome: a systematic review of randomized clinical trials. *DARU Journal of Pharmaceutical Sciences, 27*(1), 423–431.

Grossman, M., & Berkwitt, A. (2019). Neonatal abstinence syndrome. *Seminars in Perinatology, 43*(3), 173–186.

Grossman, M. R., Lipshaw, M. J., Osborn, R. R., & Berkwitt, A. K. (2018). A novel approach to assessing infants with neonatal abstinence syndrome. *Hospital Pediatrics, 8*(1), 1–6.

Hakomäki, H., Kokki, H., Lehtonen, M., Ranta, V., Räsänen, J., Voipio, H., et al. (2020). Substance use during pregnancy: impact on Colorado community hospital. *Journal of Cannabis Research, 2*(39), 2–9. doi: 10.1186/s42238-020-00047-9.

Heintzelman, J., Persons, L., & Melnykov, I. (2020). Substance use during pregnancy: impact on Colorado community hospital. *Journal of Cannabis Research, 2*(1), 39. doi: 10.1186/s42238-020-00047-9.

Hignell, A., Carlyle, K., Bishop, C., Murphy, M., Valenzano, T., Turner, S., et al. (2020). The Infant Cuddler Study: evaluating the effectiveness of volunteer cuddling in infants with neonatal abstinence syndrome. *Paediatrics and Child Health, 25*(7), 414–418. doi: 10.1093/pch/pxz127.

Hughes, B. L., Page, C. M., & Kuller, J. A. (2017). Hepatitis C in pregnancy: screening, treatment, and management. *American Journal of Obstetrics and Gynecology, 217*(5), B2–B12. doi: 10.1016/j.ajog.2017.07.039.

Joseph, R., Bradley, E., Hudson, M. E., & Moran, M. M. (2020). Perinatal substance exposure and long-term outcomes in children: a literature review. *Pediatric Nursing, 46*(4), 163–173.

Kocherlakota, P. (2014). Neonatal abstinence syndrome. *Pediatrics, 134*(2), e547–e561. doi: 10.1542/peds.2013-3524.

Kraft, W. K., Dysart, K., Greenspan, J. S., Gibson, E., Kaltenbach, K., & Ehrlich, M. E. (2011). Revised dose schema of sublingual buprenorphine in the treatment of the neonatal opioid abstinence syndrome. *Addiction, 106*(3), 574–580.

Kraft, W. K., Adeniyi-Jones, S. C., Chervoneva, I., Greenspan, J. S., Abatemarco, D., Kaltenbach, K., et al. (2017). Buprenorphine for the treatment of the neonatal abstinence syndrome. *New England Journal of Medicine, 376*(24), 2341–2348.

Lacaze-Masmonteil, T., & O'Flaherty, P. (2018). Managing infants born to mothers who have used opioids during pregnancy. *Paediatrics and Child Health, 23*(3), 220–226 doi: 10.1093/pch/pxx199.

Lemon, L. S., Naimi, A., Caritis, S. N., Platt, R. W., Venkataramanan, R., & Bodnar, L. M. (2018). The role of preterm birth in the association between opioid maintenance therapy and neonatal abstinence syndrome. *Paediatric and Perinatal Epidemiology, 32*(2), 213–222. doi: 10.1111/ppe.12443.

Lipsitz, P. J. (1975). A proposed narcotic withdrawal score for use with newborn infants: a pragmatic evaluation of its efficacy. *Clinical Pediatrics, 14*(6), 592–594. doi: 10.1177/000992287501400613.

Lisonkova, S., Richter, L. L., Ting, J., Muraca, G. M., Wen, Q., Mehrabadi, A., et al. (2019). Neonatal abstinence syndrome and associated neonatal and maternal mortality and morbidity. *Pediatrics, 144*(2), 1–11. doi: 10.1542/peds.2018-3664.

MacMillan, K. D. L. (2019). Neonatal abstinence syndrome: review of epidemiology, care models, and current understanding of outcomes. *Clinics in Perinatology, 46*(4), 817–832.

Maguire, D. J., Taylor, S., Armstrong, K., Shaffer-Hudkins, E., Germain, A. M., Brooks, S. S., et al. (2016). Long-term outcomes of infants with neonatal abstinence syndrome. *Neonatal Network, 35*(5), 277–286. doi: http://dx.doi.org/10.1891/0730-0832.35.5.277.

McQueen, K. A., Murphy-Oikonen, J., & Desaulniers, L. (2015). Maternal substance use and neonatal abstinence syndrome: a descriptive study. *Maternal and Child Health Journal, 19*(8), 1756–1765. doi: 10.1007/s10995-015-1689-y.

Merhar, S. L., Ounpraseuth, S., Devlin, L. A., Poindexter, B. B., Young, L. W., Berkey, S. D., et al. (2021). Phenobarbital and clonidine as secondary medications for neonatal opioid withdrawal syndrome. *Pediatrics, 147*(3), e2020017830.

Miller, P. A., & Willier, T. (2021). Baby STRENGTH: Eat, Sleep, Console for infants with neonatal abstinence syndrome. *Advances in Neonatal Care, 21*(2), 99–106.

Moder, J. E., Ordenewitz, L. K., Schlüter, J. A., Weinmann, T., Altebäumer, P., Jung, J., et al. (2021). [Fetal alcohol spectrum disorders – diagnosis, prognosis, and prevention.] *Bundesgesundheitsblatt, Gesundheitsforschung, Gesundheitsschutz, 64*(6): 747–754.

National Health & Medical Research Council. (1999). A guide to the development, implementation and evaluation of clinical practice guidelines. Canberra, ACT: Australian Government. <https://www.nhmrc.gov.au/sites/default/files/images/a-guide-to-the-development-and-evaluation-of-clinical-practice-guidelines.pdf> (Accessed 22 February 2022).

National Institute on Drug Abuse (NIDA). (2020). Colorado: opioid-involved deaths and related harms. <https://nida.nih.gov/drug-topics/opioids/opioid-summaries-by-state/colorado-opioid-involved-deaths-related-harms> (Accessed 22 February 2022).

Nelson, M. M. (2016). NICU culture of care for infants with neonatal abstinence syndrome: a focused ethnography. *Neonatal Network, 35*(5), 287–295. doi: 10.1891/0730-0832.35.5.287.

Oji-Mmuo, C. N., Jones, A. N., Wu, E. Y., Speer, R. R., & Palmer, T. (2021). Clinical care of neonates undergoing opioid withdrawal in the immediate postpartum period. *Neurotoxicology and Teratology, 86*, 106978.

Patrick, S. W., & Barfield, W. D. (2020). Neonatal opioid withdrawal syndrome. *Pediatrics, 146*(5), e2020029074.

Patrick, S., Slaughter, J., Harrell, F. E., Martin, P. R., Hartmann, K., Dudley, J., et al. (2021). Development and validation of a model to predict neonatal abstinence syndrome. *Journal of Pediatrics, 229*, 154–160.e156.

Queensland Health. (2021). Perinatal substance abuse: neonatal. Queensland Maternity and Neonatal Clinical Guideline. <https://www.health.qld.gov.au/__data/assets/pdf_file/0018/140814/g-psuneo.pdf> (Accessed 22 February 2022).

Ritter, J. M., Flower, R. J., Henderson, G., Loke, Y. K., MacEwan, D. & Rang, H. R. (2019). *Rang & Dale's pharmacology* (9th ed.). London: Elsevier.

Schölin, L., Mukherjee, R. A. S., Aiton, N., Blackburn, C., Brown, S., Flemming, K. M., et al. (2021). Fetal alcohol spectrum disorders: an overview of current evidence and activities in the UK. *Archives of Disease in Childhood, 106*(7), 636–640. doi: 10.1136/archdischild-2020-320435.

Shang, Y., & Filizola, M. (2015) Opioid receptors: structural and mechanistic insights into pharmacology and signalling. *European Journal of Pharmacology, 763*, 206–213. doi: 10.1016/j.ejphar.2015.05.012.

Shann, F. (2014). *Drug doses* (16th ed.). Melbourne, Vic: The Royal Children's Hospital.

Shannon, J., Blythe, S., & Peters, K. (2021). The complexities associated with caring for hospitalised infants with neonatal abstinence syndrome: the perspectives of nurses and midwives. *Children, 8*, 152. doi: 10.3390/children8020152.

Surran, B., Visintainer, P., Chamberlain, S., Kopcza, K., Shah, B., & Singh, R. (2013). Efficacy of clonidine versus phenobarbital in reducing neonatal morphine sulfate therapy days for neonatal abstinence syndrome. A prospective randomized clinical trial. *Journal of Perinatology, 33*(12), 954. doi: 10.1038/jp.2013.95.

Tavella, R. A., De Abreu, V. O. M., Muccillo-Baisch, A. L., Flavio M. R., & Da Silva, F. (2020). Prevalence of illicit drug use during pregnancy: a global perspective. *Anais da Academia Brasileira de Ciências, 92*(4), e20200302. doi: 10.1590/0001-3765202020200302.

Vogel, L. (2018). Newborns exposed to opioids need mothers more than NICU, say pediatricians. *Canadian Medical Association Journal, 190*, E123. doi: 10.1503/cmaj.109-5550.

Wachman, E. M., & Werler, M. M. (2019). Pharmacologic treatment for neonatal abstinence syndrome: which medication is best? [Comment] *American Medical Association Pediatrics, 173*(3), 221–223. doi: 10.1001/jamapediatrics.2018.5029.

Wang, J., & Cosci, F. (2021). Neonatal withdrawal syndrome following late in utero exposure to selective serotonin reuptake inhibitors: a systematic review and meta-analysis of observational studies. *Psychotherapy and Psychosomatics,* 90(5), 299–307. doi: 10.1159/000516031.

Watson, L. R. (2017). Neonatal abstinence syndrome: inpatient and outpatient diagnosis. *Journal for Nurse Practitioners, 13*(7), e355–e356.

Wijekoon, N., Wijekoon, N., Aduroja, O., Biggs, J. M., El-Metwally, D., & Gopalakrishnan, M. (2021). Model-based approach to improve clinical outcomes in neonates with opioid withdrawal syndrome using real-world data. *Clinical Pharmacology and Therapeutics, 109*(1), 243–252.

Williams, J. F., & Smith, V. C. (2015). Fetal alcohol spectrum disorders. *Pediatrics, 136*(5), 1395–1406.

Williams, L. R., Gebler-Wolfe, M., Grisham, L. M., Bader, M. Y., & Cleveland, L. M. (2020). "Babywearing" in the NICU: an intervention for infants with neonatal abstinence syndrome. *Advances in Neonatal Care, 20*(6), 440–449.

Williamson, L. (2020). Neonatal abstinence syndrome: a literature review. Saskatoon, Canada: Saskatchewan Prevention Institute.

Zahorodny, W., Rom, C., Whitney, W., Giddens, S., Samuel, M., Maichuk, G., et al. (1998). The Neonatal Withdrawal Inventory: a simplified score of newborn withdrawal. *Journal of Developmental and Behavioural Pediatrics, 19*(2), 89–93. doi: 10.1097/00004703-199804000-00005.

Zankl, A., Martin, J., Davey, J. G., & Osborn, D. A. (2021). Sedatives for opioid withdrawal in newborn infants. *Cochrane Database of Systematic Reviews, 5*(5), CD002053. doi: 10.1002/14651858.CD002053.pub4.

CHAPTER 21

FAMILY-CENTRED CARE IN THE NEONATAL CARE UNIT

SUZA TRAJKOVSKI AND TRUDI MANNIX

Learning objectives

After reading this chapter you will be able to:

- understand the concepts of family-centred care and family-integrated care, strategies for their implementation, barriers and enablers
- understand normal attachment and bonding between the family and the neonate, and short- and long-term adverse effects of their separation
- discuss the effect that admission of a newborn to a neonatal unit has on the family, health professionals and healthcare delivery
- understand the impact of preterm birth on Indigenous families, fathers, adolescent parents and other vulnerable groups, and consider ways to reduce this impact.

Key words, terms and abbreviations

attachment
bonding
developmental care (DC)
family-integrated care (FIC)
family-centred care (FCC)
kangaroo care (KC)
skin-to-skin care

INTRODUCTION

The birth of an infant is usually a joyful time for parents but, for the parents of a preterm or sick infant, emotions are mixed. Hospitalisation of the neonate can be a highly traumatic experience for both infants and their families. Parental processes through pregnancy and preparation for parenthood are disrupted and parents are often not prepared physically or psychologically for these unexpected events.

Family-centred care (FCC) is an approach to care that has been developed to support and meet the needs of neonates and their families while in the neonatal unit, and empower families to care for their infant during their stay in the neonatal unit as an integral part of the care-giving team. This chapter will discuss parents' experiences in the neonatal unit, the philosophy of FCC, the importance of, and strategies for, supporting and developing partnerships with families, and facilitators and barriers to FCC. Certain vulnerable groups, such as fathers and adolescent parents, require extra support to make the transition into the parenting role, and a therapeutic approach to these issues is described here. Neonatal nurses/midwives are at the core of a system that coaches and encourages parents to feel confident and skilled in caring for their fragile newborn during admission and after discharge.

During pregnancy, women develop **attachment** to their baby that continues and develops further after the baby is born. Expected development of interactive skills for parents and the infant are disrupted when the infant is admitted to the neonatal unit, and there is less time to plan for parenthood. Preterm infants often spend weeks, even months, in hospital, which makes them particularly vulnerable to the effects of separation from their parents. Research suggests families with infants in the neonatal unit are at greater risk for disturbances in the development of maternal and paternal newborn attachment (Bonacquisti et al., 2020).

EVIDENCE-BASED PRACTICE RESEARCH 21.1

Recent work in the area of epigenetics suggests that the impact of prenatal maternal stress can be transferred to the next generation. Chronic stress in utero affects the fetus's developing neural system, and neonates born to mothers who experience high levels of anxiety while pregnant are more reactive to stress. This can have a detrimental effect on the temperament of the child and school performance at age 6, and lead to poorer health outcomes in later life. However, there is good news. Although genes cannot be changed, epigenetic markers can be. Exposure to positive environments, optimal nutrition and stress management can ameliorate the effects of chronic stress in utero.

Source: based on Moore, T. G., Arefadib, N., Deery, A., & West, S. (2017). The first thousand days: an evidence paper. Parkville, Vic; Centre for Community Child Health, Murdoch Children's Research Institute.

NORMAL ATTACHMENT AND BONDING AND THE EFFECTS OF SEPARATION

The survival and development of newborn infants are dependent on the presence of an affectionate bond between them and their parents. **Bonding** and attachment theories suggest that forming a strong bond or physical or emotional attachment between a parent and their infant is critical to personal development, positive parenting behaviours and improved cognitive and neurobehavioural development of a child (Ainsworth et al., 1978; Klaus & Kennell, 1976). Failure to establish a bond or connection with the infant soon after birth may have serious long-term effects on the mother–child relationship and can affect the child's social, emotional, intellectual and physical development (Klaus & Kennell, 1976). Poor bonding may result in a lack of maternal feelings, hostility, avoidance, neglect, rejection and infant abuse (Kinsey & Hupcey, 2013). These seminal works highlight family as an essential part of the infant's life and, therefore, their need to have close contact with, and be included in, their infant's care in the neonatal unit.

PARENTS' EXPERIENCES IN THE NEONATAL UNIT

Infant admission to a neonatal unit can be a traumatic experience for many parents, resulting in psychological distress and altered parenting roles (Bonacquisti et al., 2020). Mothers describe feelings of relief and happiness along with shock, fear, grief, sadness and guilt when first seeing their infant (Loewenstein, 2018). The mother may grieve not having a term baby and feel fearful of the fragile preterm infant. Parents often struggle with the highly technical, busy, overcrowded and noisy environment in the neonatal unit (Dicky et al., 2020). Witnessing painful procedures being performed on their baby causes further distress, and they fear for their baby's survival.

Mothers report feeling distressed at the inability to care for and protect their infant and struggle in making the transition to the parenting role while in the neonatal unit (Govindaswamy et al., 2019). Stress, depression, helplessness, powerlessness and alienation have been reported by the parents of hospitalised neonates. Some parents expressed feeling a loss of control that shifted between feeling included and then excluded in their infant's care (Loewenstein, 2018), while others reported feeling like a spectator to their infant's care, experiencing 'uselessness and clumsiness' (Dicky et al., 2020, p. 230). Mäkelä et al. (2018) reported that parents were thrown onto a 'rollercoaster' of closeness and separation with little time to prepare for the ride. Sleep disturbances, anxiety, high levels of fatigue and reduced feelings of wellbeing have also been reported in parents with infants in a neonatal unit (Nieves et al., 2021).

Research suggests these experiences may have long-term health impacts on parents and overall family functioning (Schecter et al., 2020). Studies report that families in the neonatal unit experience emotional stress, depressive symptoms, feeling like an intruder in their baby's life and having added financial burden following their baby's discharge (Grunberg et al., 2019).

Factors such as stress caused by the infant's hospitalisation has led to symptoms of acute stress disorder (ASD), which may lead to post-traumatic stress disorder (PTSD) (Bonacquisti et al., 2020). Research indicates mothers in the neonatal unit experience a 40% rate of postpartum depression, compared with 11.5% in the general population, and fathers in the neonatal unit are also at risk of depression (Loewenstein et al., 2019; Schecter et al., 2020). The altered parental role was most strongly associated with the symptoms of ASD. Reported outcomes of disrupted parenting included increased risk of child abuse, financial difficulties and family breakdown (Govindaswamy et al., 2019). Parents require education to recognise their infant's behavioural cues that indicate whether the infant is ready for, or not ready for, coping with, or not coping with, their interaction, and how to support their infant when the neonate is overwhelmed.

Parents have reported the need to receive accurate, timely information, be involved in decision-making processes and have individualised care and unlimited contact with their infant, with opportunities to practise hands-on care (Lakshmanan et al., 2019). Additionally, parents want to be positively perceived by neonatal nurses and midwives, develop a therapeutic relationship with staff and feel included and empowered in their infant's care (He et al., 2021).

PRINCIPLES OF FAMILY-CENTRED CARE

Family-centred care was originally developed for children in paediatric settings and was later introduced into neonatal units. FCC is now considered a central standard for practice when providing care for neonates and their families (Australian College of Neonatal Nurses (ACNN), 2019; Jones, 2019; New Zealand Nurses Organisation, 2015). FCC focuses on the health and wellbeing of the newborn and their family through the development of respectful partnerships between healthcare professionals and parents. This model of care aims to improve the health and wellbeing of the neonate while also recognising the significant role that family members play in the care of their hospitalised infant. FCC puts the infant at the centre of care and promotes individualised, flexible care underpinned by information sharing, effective communication and support with the infants' parents. The term is frequently accompanied by terms such as 'partnership', 'collaboration', 'negotiation' and families as 'experts' to describe the process of care delivery. The Institute for Patient and Family Centred Care (IPFCC) was formed in 1992 to develop strategies and resources to facilitate an FCC approach. They define FCC as '... an approach to the planning, delivery and evaluation of healthcare that is grounded in mutually beneficial partnerships among healthcare providers, patients and families' (IPFCC, 2021). FCC acknowledges the emotional, social and developmental needs of infants and the family and promotes health and wellbeing by restoring dignity and control (IPFCC, 2021).

EVIDENCE-BASED PRACTICE RESEARCH 21.2

Family-centred care has been recognised as a central tenet in providing care for infants and their families in the neonatal unit; however, despite widespread endorsement, FCC continues to be insufficiently implemented into clinical practice (Mendizabal-Espinosa & Warren, 2020).

The nine elements for FCC according to the IPFCC are listed in Box 21.1.

The core concepts of FCC are demonstrating *respect and dignity* by listening to and honouring family perspectives, knowledge, choices, values, beliefs and cultural needs; *sharing information* with families that is unbiased, timely, accurate and complete through effective communication to ensure effective participation in care and informed decision making; encouraging *participation* of families in care delivery and decision-making processes at the level they feel comfortable with; and *collaboration* by working with families on policy and program development/implementation/evaluation, healthcare facility design, education and delivery of healthcare (IPFCC, 2021).

BOX 21.1 **Elements of family-centred care**

- Recognising the family as a constant in the child's life
- Facilitating parent–professional collaboration at all levels of healthcare
- Honouring the racial, ethnic, cultural and socioeconomic diversity of families
- Recognising family strengths and individuality and respecting different methods of coping
- Sharing complete and unbiased information with families on a continuous basis
- Encouraging and facilitating family to develop family support and networking
- Responding to child and family developmental needs as part of healthcare practices
- Adopting policies and practices that provide families with emotional and financial support
- Designing healthcare that is flexible, culturally competent and responsive to family needs

Source: Shields et al. (2006, p. 1318).

EVIDENCE-BASED PRACTICE RESEARCH 21.3

While it seems intuitive that addressing family needs improves neonatal healthcare and outcomes, the evidence regarding the effectiveness of FCC remains limited. A lack of clarity exists on how FCC is defined or operationalised, and there is an absence of studies that include all principles of FCC, making it difficult to determine the impact (Vetcho et al., 2020).

FAMILY-INTEGRATED CARE

Family-integrated care (FIC) is an *extension* of the principles of FCC and integrates families as partners in the neonatal unit care team. FIC is an actionable model by which parents are considered true partners in their infant's care when in the neonatal unit. FIC considers families as an integral part of the neonatal unit team, and not as passive onlookers to their infant's care (Soni & Tscherning, 2021). In this program, parents provide all care except that associated with technical procedures such as nasogastric tube insertion, intravenous fluids and medication administration and continuous positive airway pressure (CPAP)/ventilation. Neonatal nurses/midwives educate and coach parents while parents provide the care their infant needs. The primary carer commits to providing 7–8 hours of care per day between 7 am and 8 pm, attends medical rounds and daily educational sessions, administers feeds, performs basic charting, dresses and bathes their baby and provides skin-to-skin care.

FIC has been shown to increase breastfeeding rates and infants' weight gain, and reduce not only the number of adverse incidents that occur in the neonatal unit, but also length of stay, infections and the incidence of retinopathy of prematurity (Banerjee et al., 2020). Parents engaged in FIC report greater involvement in the medical care of their infant, increased confidence and reduced stress levels (Franck & O'Brien, 2019).

EVIDENCE-BASED PRACTICE RESEARCH 21.4

Despite a lack of rigorous research to assess the effectiveness of FCC, no direct harm of implementing FCC principles have been reported. However, high-quality evidence is needed to support healthcare system changes and policies that facilitate FCC practices (Benzies et al., 2019; Vetcho et al., 2020).

DEVELOPMENTAL CARE, KANGAROO CARE AND SKIN-TO-SKIN CARE

Developmental care (DC), **kangaroo care (KC)** and **skin-to-skin care** were introduced to reduce the potential negative impacts of the environment on the infant and to support infant neuro-maturation (Als, 1986; see also Chapter 22). DC initially focused on the infant's physical needs and later acknowledged parents' contribution to the development of their infant. DC includes interventions such as skin-to-skin contact, breastfeeding and support for mothers and infants. The reported benefits of KC and skin-to-skin care include improved infant vital signs, digestion and weight gain along with increased maternal milk supply, bonding and interaction (Cunningham et al., 2021).

Despite the reported benefits, neonatal nurses/midwives tend to focus on meeting the medical and technological needs of the infant rather than encouraging positive interactions between infants and their parents. Barriers such as lack of privacy, opportunity, access, space, support and time have been identified (Coutts et al., 2021). Other reported factors that discourage neonatal nurses/midwives from implementing KC and skin-to-skin practices are a lack of policies and guidelines, a lack of staff, education and training, insufficient knowledge about the importance of KC, parental anxiety, difficulty in defining sociocultural constructs of gender and parent roles, and a lack of clear practice guidelines (Coutts et al., 2021).

EVIDENCE-BASED PRACTICE RESEARCH 21.5

Kenaley et al. (2020) initiated a bundle approach to care in order to reduce the time to the parents' first hold of their infant who required respiratory support in the neonatal unit. Among strategies, they developed educational pamphlets for parents and staff, a checklist for nurses, a unit policy that defined medical 'stability for holding' and a visual display board with an appointment time for holding. They reduced the time to the first hold of the infant from 6.4 days to 1.2 days ($p < 0.01$), and percentage of infants held in the first 24 hours after birth from 6% to 35%.

In recent years, there has been a greater focus on the design of a neonatal unit trending from traditional, multi-patient, open-plan 'baby barn' style neonatal units to single-room/pod and double-room/pod designs so as to accommodate infant and family needs. Reported benefits of the single/double-room pods are less parental stress, more parental engagement and empowerment, less over-stimulation of the infant, quieter more spacious rooms and a private environment for the neonate and the family to implement practices such as DC, KC and FCC (van Veenendaal et al., 2020). Although having a newly designed and built neonatal care unit is ideal, it is unlikely that all neonatal units will be redesigned in the near future. Therefore, neonatal unit staff experience obstacles on a daily basis pertaining to poor neonatal unit design, limited resources and a lack of space. Despite this, however, there are strategies that neonatal nurses/midwives can implement to assist in the layout and flow of work in their neonatal unit, such as controlling lighting, limiting noise levels, supporting families and removing clutter (Box 21.2). Additionally, staff can advocate for changes in neonatal unit design, be active on advisory boards and meet with architectural firms should a renovation or new design be proposed.

BOX 21.2 **Strategies to enhance family-centred care (FCC)**

The neonatal unit

- Develop a vision/mission statement for the neonatal unit that has a strong focus on FCC
- Establish clearly defined roles for neonatal nurses/midwives and parents (considering parents' level of ability to be involved)
- Provide photo boards in the neonatal unit with before and after baby pictures, with a story line attached written by parents
- Limit visitor numbers and display signs that visitors are not to walk around and look at other babies
- Remind parents to also look after themselves (i.e. advice on diet, exercise, sleep and general wellbeing)
- Provide a neonatal nurse/midwife to advocate for infants and families in difficult situations
- Provide well-qualified staff 24 hours a day, including neonatologists after hours and support for medical fellows/ neonatal nurse practitioners
- Establish consistency in neonatal nursing/midwifery practices
- Provide consistency in neonatal nurses/midwives looking after the same baby (dedicated team for consistency in care) and ensure that the parents/family know the name of the neonatal nurse/midwife caring for their baby

The environment

- Create a welcoming environment (visitor-friendly reception area, greeting on arrival, directions to the neonatal unit, welcoming décor, wall colouring and furnishings)
- Provide a single room, pods or cubicles that can be opened or closed (allowing privacy yet not being completely separated and isolated)
- Provide more space in between cots (for skin-to-skin care, visitors, etc.)
- Keep infants in the same bed location throughout hospitalisation
- Never place a newborn infant in the same bed space as the one where the family had previously lost an infant
- Remove excessive signs/posters displayed on walls as they look unattractive, and parents report they do not read them
- Provide a designated room for privacy during times such as baptism or for parents and infants receiving palliative care
- Provide facilities for siblings (e.g. crèche within close proximity to the neonatal unit) to allow parents to spend one-on-one time with their newborn
- Provide a cafeteria (decent meal options for parents after hours)
- Provide parking that is free or affordable (or breast milk drop-off area to avoid parking fees)

Equipment

- Provide equipment that is current and working
- Provide a hand wash basin installed at the entrance of the neonatal unit (for everyone entering/exiting the neonatal unit to wash hands regardless of whether they are/are not handling an infant)
- Provide shelving for parents to store belongings, and provide a small display area to personalise infant bed area
- Provide individual lighting for babies and families with dimming features
- Provide music therapy for babies (or parents' recorded reading placed in the isolette/cot for baby to hear)
- Provide comfortable seating arrangements for families when in the neonatal unit (lightweight chairs that are easy to move)
- Provide sufficient privacy screens for mothers who are breastfeeding or for families who want privacy with their baby

The family

- Provide parent information during the antenatal period (e.g. neonatal nursing/midwifery and medical staff visiting the high-risk mother in the antenatal ward, offering parents a tour of the unit)
- Encourage families to be involved in the infant's care (including fathers)
- Educate and share information with parents (e.g. development of pamphlets, LCD slide shows (on continuous rotation) displaying relevant information throughout the neonatal unit and developing educational videos for parents in the antenatal period and throughout the different stages of the neonatal journey)
- Refer parents to appropriate support services (e.g. social workers, counsellors or psychologists)
- Encourage parents to collect mementos and keepsakes (e.g. hand and feet moulds, photos, the cord clamp, to keep a journal and record milestones)
- Facilitate parents being able to phone the neonatal unit 24/7
- Provide access for parents to a live cot-side camera
- As parents are not allowed to eat by their baby's cot, provide meals in a dining room that all parents share so they eat together and therefore socialise
- Provide easy access to lactation consultants
- Provide access to parent support groups (linking parents with similar situations)
- Allow parents to sleep next to their babies
- Provide separate toilet and shower facilities for families
- Allow parents to be involved in ward rounds
- Provide parents with swipe cards to enter, rather than having to seek permission to enter, their baby's room

Source: adapted from Trajkovski et al. (2015).

Neonatal nurses/midwives are in a unique position to assist parents and infants throughout the neonatal unit experience. Their roles include delivering individualised care to neonates and their families that is specific to family needs, preferences, situation and individual ability. Strategies such as education of staff and parents, building a trusting relationship between neonatal nurses/midwives and parents, and developing systematic, consistent and standardised care practices are required. Neonatal nurses/midwives have a responsibility to adapt and implement practices designed to deliver high-quality therapeutic and supportive care for infants and their families (Reid et al., 2021).

REFLECTION

Despite the advantages of skin-to-skin care, neonatal nurses/midwives cite a variety of barriers to its implementation, such as lack of time, space and the acuity of the patient. Most of the obstacles can be overcome. Think about the barriers that exist in your workplace, and how you can increase the opportunities for parents to practise skin-to-skin care.

MEETING THE CULTURAL, RELIGIOUS AND SPIRITUAL NEEDS OF FAMILIES

Recognising the newborn's place within the family emphasises the cultural, religious and spiritual dimensions of families' lives, which may highlight significant diversity within these areas. In a multicultural society, parents and clinicians are unlikely to have the same beliefs, value contexts, family experiences and perspectives, and these differences may offer substantial challenges to healthcare professionals during times of stress.

It is critical to acknowledge, comprehend and respect parents' and families' cultural, religious and spiritual views and values. Suboptimal patient outcomes can result from misperceptions caused by a lack of sensitivity. Cultural competence involves more than simply acknowledging cultural norms that differ from one's own. Cultural competence is the ability to interact effectively with people from diverse cultures (Laventhal & Fanaroff, 2020). Cultural diversity may also result in communication challenges. When parents do not have a sound enough grasp of English to communicate with healthcare professionals, interpreters need to be utilised to facilitate a two-way understanding between clinicians and the family. Ideally, interpreters should be booked in advance and the parents given time to formulate their questions prior to the meeting. It is important that the clinician focus on the parents when they are talking, rather than the interpreter, and that the interpreter repeats the information to be shared with the parents prior to translation to ensure the content is accurate. Communicating empathically with parents of any culture when they are feeling stressed and anxious is important, and neonatal nurses/midwives may benefit from formal communication training to better respond to parents' feelings and facilitate FCC (Kasat et al., 2020).

The FCC approach seeks to respect ethnic, cultural, religious and social diversity in families. A systematic review published in 2019 highlighted some of the issues associated with access to health services for women in vulnerable populations (Jesuthasan et al., 2019). They found that language barriers, a lack of respect for cultural differences and family separation lead to a deterioration in women's health status. Knowledge of different cultural rites and ceremonies and accommodation of specific cultural requests is one example of how a neonatal nurse/midwife can demonstrate respect for diverse beliefs, values and ways of living.

CARING FOR VULNERABLE FAMILIES

Global trends in the movement of vulnerable populations show that 82.4 million people were forcibly displaced at the end of 2020 due to 'persecution, conflict, violence, human rights violations or events seriously disrupting public order' (UNHCR, 2021). Childbearing women in this cohort have poor access to antenatal care, malnutrition, higher rates of diarrhoea, malaria, hepatitis B and anaemia, and their rate of obstetric complications is higher (Rawal et al., 2021). Vulnerable families from these countries need interpreters and translated resources when their baby is admitted to the neonatal unit. While each family must be assessed individually, the neonatal nurse/midwife caring for their infant should be alert to the potential need for a range of support services coordinated by a social worker.

The inequalities in health status and outcomes and barriers to access to healthcare faced by the Indigenous populations of the world are comparable (Sarfati et al., 2018). While Indigenous peoples represent less than 5% of the world's population, they account for 15% of the poorest (D'Angelo et al., 2020). Using the example of Australia and New Zealand's Indigenous populations, the prevalence of low birthweight in New Zealand is slightly higher for Māori than for non-Māori (New Zealand Ministry of Health, 2018). In New Zealand in 2010–14, the mortality rate for Māori infants was 6.9% and that for babies of Pacific ethnic groups was 7.0%, while the rate for Europeans was 5.3% (Edmonds et al., 2021). Preterm birth rates are significantly higher for Māori babies than for non-Māori non-Pacific babies (Edmonds et al., 2021). Australian Aboriginal women are also at increased risk of adverse pregnancy outcomes, especially for preterm birth (14% versus non-Indigenous 8%) (AIHW, 2021) and low birthweight. Indigenous mothers are more likely to be teenagers, to be obese, to have pre-existing diabetes or hypertension, to live in remote or disadvantaged areas, to undertake risk behaviours including smoking and drug-taking, and to receive less antenatal care (AIHW, 2021) in the first 20 weeks of their pregnancy, compared with non-Indigenous mothers.

There is a tendency to assume that all Aboriginal women are alike, but they often have different origins, languages, traditional beliefs and lifestyles. In seminal research, Hancock and the Ngaanyatjarra Health Service (2006) reported that Aboriginal women perceived a lack of sensitivity to their needs, values and customs, and a lack of respect for, and trust in, their abilities compared with mothers in many mainstream healthcare settings. Culturally competent neonatal nurses/midwives recognise that it is the inadequacy of the healthcare system that impacts on the compliance of Aboriginal women with hospital protocols and procedures, and not their negligence (Kildea et al., 2021).

If Māori and Aboriginal women feel safe and respected in the neonatal unit environment, they are more likely to be receptive to advice and education about how best to care for their infants using a positive parenting approach. Staff who have undergone cultural sensitivity training are more aware of the increased need for respect, confidentiality, negotiation and feedback for these mothers. As with any new family in the neonatal unit, staff members need to be welcoming and friendly, involve the parents in care, be non-judgemental and supportive, and focus on building relationships and trust. Open visiting, the provision of timely and de-jargonised information and involving these parents in decision making all work to empower these families to take their preterm babies home with more confidence and skills. Continuity of carer is helpful in the neonatal unit to focus on communication, respectful relationship building and the development of trust (Gallagher et al., 2018).

While the concept of 'family' is significant in all cultures, it is especially so in the Māori society, where family (*whanau*) is the most fundamental unit of Māori society and may include several generations. Whanau is not restricted to parents but rather includes whoever is identified by the parents in this role. This often sees family representatives as key spokespersons or carers, and it is important for neonatal nurses/midwives to include these spokespersons in multidisciplinary meetings. In the Māori culture, the family is responsible for supporting the new mother, to teach her how to look after her baby, be responsive to the baby's needs and bond with her baby. The Treaty of Waitangi principles of partnership, protection and participation are synonymous with FCC (Richardson et al., 2017).

Within the philosophy of FCC is the need to honour the cultural, ethnic and socioeconomic diversity of families and to ensure that culturally competent care is delivered. The diverse population in Australia and New Zealand and rising numbers of new immigrant and refugee families in the neonatal unit require care that is delivered in a culturally sensitive and respectful manner. Culturally sensitive FCC provides a setting in which the family is encouraged to support the care their baby requires, as the constant caretakers from admission onwards until discharge. This also prepares them for better handling and care of the baby at home after discharge (Toivonen et al., 2020).

REFLECTION

In Australia, Indigenous childbearing women are a widely dispersed population, and only 38% live in major cities compared with 71% of non-Indigenous women (Australian Bureau of Statistics (ABS), 2020). As a result, Aboriginal babies are often transferred out of their local hospital when their healthcare needs escalate. Mothers cannot always be transferred with their babies, although this is obviously ideal.

Consider the impact this separation has on the mother, and extended family, specifically due to their Aboriginality.

CASE STUDY 21.1

A 29-week gestation female infant was born via caesarean section for breech presentation and preterm labour and subsequently admitted to the neonatal unit because of prematurity and respiratory distress. The infant weighed 1250 g, and she commenced ventilatory support with nasal continuous positive airway pressure (CPAP) in 25% oxygen. Her vital signs were temperature of 37.2°C under radiant heat, blood pressure 58/44 mmHg, heart rate 119 bpm, oxygen saturation 97% and blood glucose level 3.7 mmol/L. She was non-dysmorphic, centrally pink and well perfused. An intravenous (IV) cannula was inserted and IV fluids commenced. At 4 hours of age, the midwife brought the mother into the unit in a wheelchair with her husband to see their infant. The parents were of Asian appearance with limited English, but managed to ask in their broken English how their baby was, what was happening with their baby and whether they could touch their baby. You are the neonatal nurse/midwife looking after their infant, and note that the parents appear scared and anxious.

1. How will you reassure them? What information do they need at this stage, and how will you provide it?

ADOLESCENT PARENTS IN THE NEONATAL UNIT

Adolescent parents are a vulnerable group, transitioning to parenthood at a time of their own physical, emotional and cognitive development. While rates of adolescent pregnancy have declined since the mid 1970s globally, rates remain high in developed countries such as Canada, the United States, New Zealand and Western European countries (Wong et al., 2020). Risks of teenage birth to the neonate include low Apgar score at 5 minutes, prematurity, small for gestational age and low birthweight (Rexhepi et al., 2019). While smoking is related to poorer perinatal outcomes such as low birthweight, being small for gestational age, preterm birth and perinatal death, teenage mothers were the most likely to smoke in Australia in 2019 (33%) (AIHW, 2021).

The National Health and Medical Research Council (NHMRC) infant-feeding guidelines recommend exclusive breastfeeding to around 6 months of age (McGuire et al., 2018). However, in 2017–18 in Australia, only 29% of Australian infants were exclusively breastfed at 6 months of age (ABS, 2018). The breastfeeding rate among adolescent mothers is even lower, with a study in a large regional Australian sample showing that the rate of initiation of breastfeeding in mothers aged 19 or less was 4.2%, compared with 76.8% of mothers aged 20–34 (Bish et al., 2021).

Adolescent mothers experience higher levels of psychological distress and are at risk of 'double jeopardy,' in which the mother suffers long-term repercussions such as depression and rapid repeat pregnancies (Wong et al., 2020). Neonatal nurses/midwives must be prepared to assess for trauma and be open to listening to their experiences. Principles of strengths-based and trauma-informed care can support these young mothers. Adolescent parents might be at increased risk of intimate partner violence, inadequate partner support, perceived parenting criticism and financial difficulties (Thomas et al., 2019). Improving the outcomes for babies of adolescent mothers can be achieved by implementing the strategies associated with FCC (see Box 21.2), treating these young parents with respect and facilitating bonding with their newborn. Encouraging young mothers to breastfeed, teaching them to express their breast milk and enlisting their parents as support persons also improve neonatal outcomes. They can benefit from pre- and postnatal education programs aimed specifically at their age group, and from peer counselling, peer support and telephone support to motivate them to breastfeed and encourage their engagement with their baby (Buckland et al., 2020). Adolescent mothers typically acknowledge their own mother as their principal source of support (Lee et al., 2020), but when the infant's father is a significant support person then neonatal nurses/midwives must ensure his involvement is fully facilitated.

REFLECTION

Young parents need extra support to cope with having a preterm infant. What support could you offer to them, and how can you act as a role model to other neonatal nurses/midwives, showing respect and a non-judgemental approach to these young parents as they learn to care for their baby?

FATHERS IN THE NEONATAL UNIT

Although fathers are usually the first parent to meet the preterm newborn, they are considered the 'forgotten parent' in the neonatal unit, and neonatal nurses/midwives need to work harder to involve fathers more fully in the care of their baby (Baldoni et al., 2021). Gender role stereotyping leaves fathers feeling excluded from the care of their infant, when most are ready to be involved and look forward to the new relationship with their babies (Mäkelä et al., 2018). If the mother is also unwell and hospitalised, the father is anxious about her wellbeing while juggling multiple responsibilities, such as caring for their other children and serving as the household provider. The father may face, or fear, job loss because of shifting responsibilities and duties and, once the mother does come home, marital discord may result from the change in family routines as parents maintain visits to the hospitalised infant (Baldoni et al., 2021). New fathers may be required to make decisions about the hospitalised infant, and to update concerned family and friends. Involving fathers in the care of their babies, and offering skin-to-skin care with their babies, reduces fathers' stress and anxiety, facilitates bonding with their baby and improves the relationship with their spouse (Lian et al., 2021). Fathers also benefit from contact with a psychologist, peer-to-peer communication such as men-only support groups, and being provided with comprehensive written and verbal information about their baby's problems and behaviour directly (not via the mother) (Fisher et al., 2018).

FAMILY-CENTRED CARE 21.1

Some fathers may be *more* involved with their preterm infants than fathers of full-term infants, as they have a unique responsibility and need to embrace a supporting role, especially when their partner is still recovering from the pregnancy and delivery, and their baby is admitted to the neonatal unit.

SOCIAL AND PSYCHOSOCIAL CHALLENGES IN THE NEONATAL UNIT

When a medically fragile infant is born into a family with significant social challenges, such as domestic violence, mental illness or substance abuse, the infant is at risk of both poor developmental outcomes and neglect. Tenets of FCC hold the family as the central player in the care of their infant during hospitalisation and beyond, in order to promote the best long-term outcomes. Families with these difficulties already face significant stress, and it is vital that contact is established and maintained with them, in order to support them throughout this vulnerable period. Sensitive, respectful conversations can determine the extent of issues facing the family that are resulting in stress, anxiety and depression. Referrals to agencies and relevant support staff to meet the parents' emotional, psychological, social and financial needs can be made by the neonatal nurses/midwives who best know them.

Intimate partner violence (IPV) is an international public health issue, affecting one-quarter of mothers globally (Román-Gálvez et al., 2021). IPV has been found to increase the rate of preterm birth, uterine rupture, low birthweight, stillbirth, perinatal depression, haemorrhage and reduced rates of breastfeeding (Román-Gálvez et al., 2021). Nurses/midwives in all Australian states and territories are mandated to report suspected cases of child abuse and neglect to government authorities. Neonatal nurses/midwives working in neonatal units are ideally placed to observe the parents' and siblings' demeanour and physical appearance while visiting the unit. Rogers and Nurse (2019) say that preterm infants are more than twice as likely to be placed on an at-risk register, and that neonatal nurses/midwives can increase their knowledge on potential indicators for infant abuse and prevention. Once the infant goes home, staff providing follow-up services need to be aware of, and manage, stressors in the family to prevent harm.

EVIDENCE-BASED PRACTICE RESEARCH 21.6

Increased parental visitation, interactions and holding/cuddling infants have been associated with more-mature and fluid infant motor skills and a calmer, more predictable affect. The more parents visit and hold their baby, the better are the neurobehavioural outcomes (Pineda et al., 2018).

REFLECTION

What are the core concepts of family-centred care? How may these be implemented in the clinical environment in which you work?

CONCLUSION

Various programs around the world have been devised to facilitate FCC in the neonatal unit, with many common features including peer support from other parents, the provision of educational material about small babies, their capacities and their care; the positive impact parents can have by being actively engaged with the care of their baby; and specific information about how they can provide that care. Neonatal nurses/midwives are core in the promotion of these facets of FCC, and helping parents build their confidence and skills to take their small baby home. There are extra costs associated with the provision of programs that support FCC, but the long-term benefits outweigh those costs. Parents are the architects of their baby's brain, and neonatal nurses/midwives are available around the clock to support and coach them.

Recommended Reading

Cunningham, C., Patton, D., Moore, Z., O'Connor, T., Dhani Bux, D., & Nugent, L. (2021). Neonatal kangaroo care – what we know and how we can improve its practice: an evidence review. *Journal of Neonatal Nursing*. doi: 10.1016/j.jnn.2021.10.004.

Loewenstein, K., Barroso, J., & Phillips, S. (2019). The experiences of parents in the neonatal intensive care unit: an integrative review of qualitative studies within the transactional model of stress and coping. *Journal of Perinatal and Neonatal Nursing, 33*(4), 340–349. doi: 10.1097/JPN.0000000000000436.

Nieves, H., Clements-Hickman, A., & Davies C. C. (2021). Effect of a parent empowerment program on parental stress, satisfaction, and length of stay in the neonatal intensive care unit. *Journal of Perinatal and Neonatal Nursing, 35*(1), 92–99.

Online Resources

Family-centred care in the NICU. This resource for parents describes FCC, and what they can do to facilitate FCC with their baby: <https://raisingchildren.net.au/newborns/premature-babies/neonatal-intensive-care/nicu-family-centred-care>

World Prematurity Day (WPD) – the global theme for WPD in 2021 was 'zero separation'. You can read about it here: <https://www.efcni.org/activities/campaigns/wpd/>

References/Acknowledgements

Ainsworth, M. D. S., Blehar, M. C., Waters, E., & Wall, S. (1978). *Patterns of attachment: a psychological study of the strange situation*. Hillsdale, NJ: Lawrence Erlbaum Associates.

Als, H. (1986). A synactive model of neonatal behavioural organization. Part 1: Framework for the assessment and support of the neurobehavioral development of the premature infant and his parents in the environment of the neonatal intensive care unit. *Physical and Occupational Therapy in Pediatrics, 6*(3–4), 3–53. doi: 10.1080/J006v06n03_02. [Online.]

Australian Bureau of Statistics. (2018). Breastfeeding. <https://www.abs.gov.au/statistics/health/health-conditions-and-risks/breastfeeding/latest-release#endnotes> (Accessed 3 March 2022).

Australian Bureau of Statistics. (2020). Births, Australia. <https://www.abs.gov.au/statistics/people/population/births-australia/2020> (Accessed 12 March 2022).

Australian College of Neonatal Nurses (ACNN). (2019). *Australian standards for practice* (4th ed.). <https://www.acnn.org.au/resources/resources/ACNN-Standards-for-Practice-4th-Ed.pdf> (Accessed 3 March 2022).

Australian Institute of Health and Welfare. (2021). *Australia's mothers and babies*. Perinatal statistics series no. 33. Cat no. PER 101. Canberra, ACT: AIHW. <https://www.aihw.gov.au/getmedia/bba093ef-a623-4cfd-818b-1bb5af9f0d20/Australia-s-mothers-and-babies.pdf.aspx?inline=true> (Accessed 12 March 2022).

Baldoni, F., Ancora, G., & Latour, J. M. (2021). Being the father of a preterm-born child: contemporary research and recommendations for NICU staff. *Frontiers in Pediatrics, 9*, 947. doi: 10.3389/fped.2021.724992.

Banerjee, J., Aloysius, A., Mitchell, K., Silva, I., Rallis, D., Godambe, S. V., et al. (2020). Improving infant outcomes through implementation of a family integrated care bundle including a parent supporting mobile application. *Archives of Disease in Childhood. Fetal and Neonatal Edition, 105*(2), 172–177.

Benzies, K. M., Shah, V., Aziz, K., Lodha, A., & Misfeldt, R. (2019). The system is making 'too much noise' to provide family-centred care in neonatal intensive care units: perspectives of health care providers and hospital administrators. *Intensive and Critical Care Nursing, 50*, 44–53. doi: 10.1016/j.iccn.2018.05.001.

Bish, M. R., Faulks, F., Amir, L. H., Huxley, R. R., McIntyre, H. D., James, R., et al. (2021). Relationship between obesity and lower rates of breast feeding initiation in regional Victoria, Australia: an 8-year retrospective panel study. *BMJ Open, 11*, e044884. doi: 10.1136/ bmjopen-2020-044884.

Bonacquisti, A., Geller, P. A., & Patterson, C. A. (2020). Maternal depression, anxiety, stress, and maternal–infant attachment in the neonatal intensive care unit. *Journal of Reproductive and Infant Psychology, 38*(3), 297–310. doi: 10.1080/02646838.2019.1695041.

Buckland, C., Hector, D., Kolt, G. S., Fahey, P., & Arora, A. (2020). Interventions to promote exclusive breastfeeding among young mothers: a systematic review and meta-analysis. *International Breastfeeding Journal, 15*, 102. doi: 10.1186/ s13006-020-00340-6.

Coutts, S., Woldring, A., Pederson, A., de Salaberry, J., Osiovich, H., & Brotte, L. A. (2021). What is stopping us? An implementation science study of kangaroo care in British Columbia's neonatal intensive care units. *BMC Pregnancy Childbirth, 21*, 52. doi: 10.1186/s12884-020-03488-5.

Cunningham, C., Patton, D., Moore, Z., O'Connor, T., Dhani Bux, D., & Nugent, L. (2021). Neonatal kangaroo care – what we know and how we can improve its practice: an evidence review. *Journal of Neonatal Nursing*. doi: 10.1016/j.jnn.2021.10.004. [Online.]

D'Angelo C. S., Hermes A., McMaster C. R., Prichep, E., Richer, É., van der Westhuizen, F. H., et al. (2020). Barriers and considerations for diagnosing rare diseases in Indigenous populations. *Frontiers in Pediatrics, 8*, 797. <https://www.frontiersin.org/article/10.3389/fped.2020.579924> (Accessed 3 March 2022).

Dicky, O., Kuhn, P., Akrich, M., Reynaud, A., Caeymaex, L., Tscherning, C.; the GREEN Committee (Groupe de Réflexion et d'Evaluation de l'Environnement du Nouveau-né de la Société Française de Néonatologie). (2020). Emotional responses of parents participating for the first time in caregiving for their baby in a neonatal unit. *Paediatric Perinatal Epidemiology, 35*, 227–235. doi: 10.1111/ppe.12718.

Edmonds, K. L., Sibanda, N., Geller, S., Cram, F., Robson, B., Filoche, S., et al. (2021). He Tamariki Kokoti Tau: tackling preterm incidence and outcomes of preterm births by ethnicity in Aotearoa New Zealand 2010–2014. *International Journal of Gynecology and Obstetrics, 155*(2), 239–246. doi: 10.1002/ijgo.13855.

Fisher, D., Khashu, M., Adama, E. A., Feeley, N., Garffield, C. F., Ireland, J., et al. (2018). Fathers in neonatal units: improving infant health by supporting the baby–father bond and mother-father coparenting. *Journal of Neonatal Nursing, 24*(6), 306–312. doi: 10.1016/j.jnn.2018.08.007.

Franck, L. S., & O'Brien, K. (2019). The evolution of family-centred care: from supporting parent-delivered interventions to a model of family integrated care. *Birth Defects Research, 111*(15), 1044–1059.

Gallagher, K., Shaw, C., Aladangady, N., & Marlow, N. (2018). Parental experience of interaction with healthcare professionals during their infant's stay in the neonatal intensive care unit. *Archives of Disease in Childhood-Fetal and Neonatal Edition, 103*(4), F343–F348.

Govindaswamy, P., Laing, S., Waters, D., Walker, K., Spence, K., & Badawi, N. (2019). Needs and stressors of parents of term and near-term infants in the NICU: a systematic review with best practice guidelines. *Early Human Development, 139*, 104839. doi: 10.1016/j.earlhumdev.2019.104839.

Grunberg, V. A., Geller, P. A., Bonacquisti, A., & Patterson, C. A. (2019). NICU infant health severity and family outcomes: a systematic review of assessments and findings in psychosocial research. *Journal of Perinatology, 39*, 156–172.

Hancock, H., & Ngaanyatjarra Health Service. (2006). *Aboriginal women's perinatal needs, experiences and maternity services: a literature review to enable considerations to be made about quality indicators.* Alice Springs, NT: Ngaanyatjarra Health Service.

He, F. B., Axelin, A., Ahlqvist-Björkroth, S., Raiskila, S., Löyttyniemi, E., & Lehtonen, L. (2021). Effectiveness of the Close Collaboration with Parents intervention on parent–infant closeness in NICU. *BMC Pediatrics, 2*(1), 28. doi: 10.1186/s12887-020-02474-2.

Institute for Patient- and Family-Centred Care (IPFCC). (2021). Patient- and family-centred care. <https://ipfcc.org/about/index.html> (Accessed 3 March 2022).

Jesuthasan, J., Witte, Z., & Oertelt-Prigione, S. (2019). Health-related needs and barriers for forcibly displaced women: a systematic review. *Gender and the Genome, 3*, 247028971989528.

Jones, T., on behalf of the Council of International Neonatal Nurses, Inc. (COINN) Working Group. (2019). International neonatal nursing competency framework. *Journal of Neonatal Nursing, 25*, 258–264.

Kasat, K., Stoffels, G., & Ellington, M. (2020). Improving communication with parents: the Neonatal Intensive Care Unit Empathy Workshop. *Journal of Perinatology, 40*, 1423–1432. doi: 10.1038/s41372-020-0742-x.

Kenaley, K. M., Rickolt, A. L., Vandersteur, D. A., Ryan, J. D., & Stefano, J. L. (2020). An intervention to decrease time to parents' first hold of infants in the Neonatal Intensive Care Unit requiring respiratory support. *Journal of Perinatology, 40*, 812–819. doi: 10.1038/s41372-019-0569-5.

Kildea, S., Gao, Y., Hickey, S., Nelson, C., Kruske, S., Carson, A., et al. (2021). Effect of a Birthing on Country service redesign on maternal and neonatal health outcomes for First Nations Australians: a prospective, non-randomised, interventional trial. *The Lancet, 9*(5), E651–659. doi: 10.1016/S2214-109X(21)00061-9.

Kinsey, C. B., & Hupcey, J. E. (2013). State of the science of maternal–infant bonding: a principle-based concept analysis. *Midwifery, 29*, 1214–1320. doi: 10.1016/j.midw.2012.12.019.

Klaus, M. H., & Kennell, J. H. (1976). *Maternal–infant bonding.* Saint Louis, MO: CV Mosby.

Lakshmanan, A., Kubicek, K., Williams, R., Robles, M., Vanderbilt, D. L., Mirzaian, C. B., et al. (2019). Viewpoints from families for improving transition from NICU-to-home for infants with medical complexity at a safety net hospital: a qualitative study. *BMC Pediatrics, 19*(1), 223. doi: 10.1186/s12887-019-1604-6.

Laventhal, N. T., & Fanaroff, J. M. (2020). Medical ethics in neonatal care. In: R. J. Martin, A. A. Fanaroff, & M. C. Walsh (Eds.), *Fanaroff and Martin's neonatal–perinatal medicine* (pp. 25–46). Elsevier Health Sciences. <https://www.elsevier-elibrary.com/product/fanaroff-martins-neonatalperinatal-medicine> (Accessed 3 March 2022) [e-book].

Lee, H. Y., Edwards, R. C., & Hans, S. L. (2020). Young first-time mothers' parenting of infants: the role of depression and social support. *Maternal and Child Health Journal, 24*, 575–586. doi: 10.1007/s10995-019-02849-7.

Lian, B. X., Amin, Z., Sensaki, S., & Aishworiya, R. (2021). An active pursuit of reassurance – coping strategies of fathers with infants in the Neonatal Intensive Care Unit. *Journal of Perinatology, 41*(8), 2019–2027. doi: 10.1038/s41372-020-00853-2.

Loewenstein, K. (2018). Parent psychological distress in the neonatal intensive care unit within the context of the social ecological model: a scoping review. *Journal of the American Psychiatric Nurses Association, 24*(6), 495–509. doi: 10.1177/1078390318765205.

Loewenstein, K., Barroso, J., & Phillips, S. (2019). The experiences of parents in the neonatal intensive care unit. *Journal of Perinatal and Neonatal Nursing, 33*(4) 340–349. doi: 10.1097/JPN.0000000000000436.

Mäkelä, H., Axelin, A., Feeley, N., & Niela-Vilén, H. (2018). Clinging to closeness: the parental view on developing a close bond with their infants in a NICU. *Midwifery, 62*, 183–188. doi: 10.1016/j.midw.2018.04.003.

McGuire, J., Gallegos, D., & Irvine, S. (2018). Infant feeding nutrition policies in Australian early childhood education and care services: a content and qualitative analysis. *International Journal of Child Care and Education Policy, 12*, 14. doi: 10.1186/s40723-018-0053-2.

Mendizabal-Espinosa, R. M., & Warren, I. (2020). Non-evidence-based beliefs increase inequalities in the provision of infant and family centred neonatal care. *Acta Paediatrica, 109*(2), 314–320. doi: 10.1111/apa.14972.

Moore, T. G., Arefadib, N., Deery, A., & West, S. (2017). The first thousand days: an evidence paper. Parkville, Vic: Centre for Community Child Health, Murdoch Children's Research Institute.

New Zealand Ministry of Health. (2018). Infant health. Wellington, NZ: Ministry of Health. <https://www.health.govt.nz/our-work/populations/maori-health/tatau-kahukura-maori-health-statistics/nga-mana-hauora-tutohu-health-status-indicators/infant-health> (Accessed 3 March 2022).

New Zealand Nurses Organisation. (2015). *NNCA standards for neonatal nursing practice*. Wellington: New Zealand Nurses Organisation. <https://www.nzno.org.nz/Portals/0/Files/Documents/Groups/Neonatal%20Nurses/2016-05-11%20Final%20draft%20Neonatal%20Nursing%20Standards%202015.pdf> (Accessed 3 March 2022).

Nieves, H., Clements-Hickman, A., & Davies C. C. (2021). Effect of a parent empowerment program on parental stress, satisfaction, and length of stay in the neonatal intensive care unit. *Journal of Perinatal and Neonatal Nursing, 35*(1), 92–99.

Pineda, R., Bender, J., Hall, B., Shabosky, L., Annecca, A., & Smith, J. (2018). Parent participation in the neonatal intensive care unit: predictors and relationships to neurobehavior and developmental outcomes. *Early Human Development, 117*, 32–38. doi: 10.1016/j.earlhumdev.2017.12.008.

Rawal, L. B., Kanda, K., Biswas, T., Tanim, M. I., Dahal, P. K., Islam, M. R., et al. (2021). Health problems and utilization of health services among forcibly displaced Myanmar nationals in Bangladesh. *Global Health Research Policy. 6*, 39. doi: 10.1186/s41256-021-00223-1.

Reid, S., Bredemeyer, S., & Chiarella, M. (2021). The evolution of neonatal family centred care. *Journal of Neonatal Nursing, 27*(5), 327–333. doi: 10.1016/j.jnn.2021.03.002.

Rexhepi, M., Besimi, F., Rufati, N., Alili, A., Bajrami, S., & Ismaili, H. (2019). Hospital-based study of maternal, perinatal and neonatal outcomes in adolescent pregnancy compared to adult women pregnancy. *Open Access Macedonia Journal of Medical Science, 7*(5), 760–766. doi: 10.3889/oamjms.2019.210.

Richardson, A., Yarwood, J., & Richardson, S. (2017). Expressions of cultural safety in public health nursing practice. *Nursing Inquiry, 24*(1), e12171. doi: 10.1111/nin.12171.

Rogers, A., & Nurse, S. (2019). Child protection in the neonatal unit. *Journal of Neonatal Nursing, 25*(2), 99–101. ISSN 1355–1841. doi: 10.1016/j.jnn.2018.09.007.

Román-Gálvez, R. M., Martín-Peláez, S., Fernández-Félix, B. M., Zamora, J., Khan, K. S., & Bueno-Cavanillas, A. (2021). Worldwide prevalence of intimate partner violence in pregnancy. A systematic review and meta-analysis. *Frontiers in Public Health, 9*, 1278.

Sarfati, D., Robson, B., Garvey, G., Goza, T., Foliaki, S., Millar, E., et al. (2018). Improving the health of Indigenous people globally. *Lancet Oncology, 19*, e276. doi: 10.1016/S1470-2045(18)30336-X.

Schecter, R., Pham, T., Hua, A., Spinazzola, R., Sonnenklar, J., Li, D., et al. (2020). Prevalence and longevity of PTSD symptoms among parents of NICU infants analysed across gestational age categories. *Clinical Pediatrics (Philadelphia), 59*(2), 163–169. doi: 10.1177/0009922819892046.

Shields, L., Pratt, J., & Hunter, J. (2006). Family centred care: a review of qualitative studies. *Journal of Clinical Nursing, 15*(10), 1317–1323. doi: 10.1111/j.1365-2702.2006.01433.x.

Soni, R., & Tscherning, C. (2021). Family-centred and developmental care on the neonatal unit. *Paediatrics and Child Health, 31*(1), 18–23. doi: 10.1016/j.paed.2020.10.003.

Thomas, J. L., Lewis, J. B., Martinez, I., Cunningham, S. D., Siddique, M., Tobin, J. N., et al. (2019). Associations between intimate partner violence profiles and mental health among low-income, urban pregnant adolescents. *BMC Pregnancy Childbirth, 19*, 120. doi: 10.1186/s12884-019-2256-0.

Toivonen, M., Lehtonen, L., Löyttyniemi, E., Ahlqvist-Björkroth, S., & Axelin, A. (2020). Close collaboration with parents intervention improves family-centred care in different neonatal unit contexts: a pre–post study. *Pediatric Research, 88*, 421–428. doi: 10.1038/s41390-020-0934-2.

Trajkovski, S., Schmied, V., Vickers, M., & Jackson, D. (2015). Using appreciative inquiry to bring neonatal nurses and parents together to enhance family-centred care: a collaborative workshop. *Journal of Child Health Care, 19*(2), 239–263. doi: 10.1177/1367493513508059.

UNHCR. (2021). Figures at a glance. <https://www.unhcr.org/en-au/figures-at-a-glance.html> (Accessed 3 March 2022).

van Veenendaal, N. R., van Kempen, A., Franck, L. S., O'Brien, K., Limpens, J., van der Lee, J. H., et al. (2020). Hospitalising preterm infants in single family rooms versus open bay units: a systematic review and meta-analysis of impact on parents. *EClinicalMedicine, 23*, 100388. doi: 10.1016/j.eclinm.2020.100388.

Vetcho, S., Cooke, M., & Ullman, A. J. (2020). Family-centred care in dedicated neonatal units: an integrative review of international perspectives. *Journal of Neonatal Nursing, 26*(2), 73–92. doi: 10.1016/j.jnn.2019.09.004.

Wong, S. P. W., Twynstra, J., Gilliland, J. A., Cook, J. L., & Seabrook, J. A. (2020). Risk factors and birth outcomes associated with teenage pregnancy: a Canadian sample. *Journal of Pediatric and Adolescent Gynecology, 33*(2) 153–159. doi: 10.1016/j.jpag.2019.10.006.

CHAPTER 22

DEVELOPMENTALLY FOCUSED NEONATAL CARE

NADINE GRIFFITHS AND KIM PSAILA

Learning objectives

After reading this chapter you will be able to:

- identify the overall goals of family-centred, developmentally supportive care
- describe neonatal neurodevelopment and outline neuroprotective strategies in the neonatal setting
- identify the key components of individualised, developmentally supportive care
- examine techniques for building collaborative care relationships with parents of sick neonates
- discuss the relationship between developmental care and improving quality and outcomes
- explore evidence-based guidelines for the provision of developmental support to high-risk neonates and their families.

Key words, terms and abbreviations

Assessment of Preterm Infants' Behaviour (APIB)
developmental care
early developmental care (EDC)
Family and Infant Neurodevelopmental Education (FINE)
family-centred care
Family Integrated Care program (FICare)
individualised care
Neonatal Integrative Developmental Care Model (NIDCM)
Newborn Individualized Developmental Care and Assessment Program (NIDCAP)

INTRODUCTION

Developmental care refers to a range of strategies designed to modify the neonatal care-giving environment and care giving to reduce the stressors on the developing brain. Approaches include minimising noise and light, cue-based cares and promotion of sleep and rest (Soleimani et al., 2020). Developmental care is also a philosophy of care requiring a rethinking of the relationships that exist in the neonatal setting among neonates, families and healthcare professionals and extends further than modifying the environment to **individualised care** giving based upon the neonate's unique needs (Bruton et al., 2018). Early researchers such as Brazelton (1973) recognised the capacity of neonates for social relationships, and developed an observational scale, the Neonatal Behavioural Assessment Scale (NBAS), to score the abilities of a neonate and then utilise the score to support care (Gardner & Niermeyer, 2021). The NBAS identified the neonate as a highly developed individual, acknowledging their strengths, adaptive responses and potential vulnerabilities, and aimed to teach parents about their individual infant's cues for interaction and distance to help them better relate to their infant (Gardner & Niermeyer, 2021).

The concept of developmental care evolved from Heidelise Als' work based on the synactive theory of infant development (Fig. 22.1). The synactive model proposes that 'development proceeds through the continuous balancing of approach and avoidance behaviours, yielding a spiral potentiation of continuous intraorganism subsystems interaction' (Als, 1982, p. 234). This model represents the way in which the infant's subsystems (autonomic, motor, state and attention/interaction) interact with one another to achieve homeostatic balance. Infants actively respond to the inputs they receive from the environment to support their own balance. If infants experience environmental inputs as overwhelming, they will use avoidance behaviours to minimise their exposure to the stimulus. However, if the stimulus is appropriate and tolerable, neonates will utilise a range of approach behaviours to elicit information from the environment to support them to move on to the next developmental step (Als, 1982). Hence, opportunities exist for care givers to manipulate environmental inputs to support the neonate's ongoing development.

Lammertink et al. (2021) believe that the exposure of the preterm infant's immature neurobiological system to stress in the NICU exceeds their capacity to cope, and so, although survival rates of preterm infants have increased in the last few decades, deficits in attention, executive functioning and emotional symptoms have worsened.

Als also developed the **Assessment of Preterm Infants' Behaviour (APIB)** based on Brazelton's Neonatal Behavioural Assessment Scale (Brazelton, 1973). APIB is a newborn neurobehavioural assessment tool that identifies the infant's self-regulatory efforts and thresholds for disorganisation as viewed through aspects of the neonate's behaviours referred to as 'subsystem interactions'. APIB findings are used clinically for behavioural intervention and to direct individually appropriate developmentally supportive care. The synactive theory of development provides a framework to understand the behaviour of preterm and sick neonates (Spruill, 2021).

A range of supportive strategies designed to modify the neonatal care-giving environment to reduce the stressors on the developing brain are included in a developmentally supportive care plan.

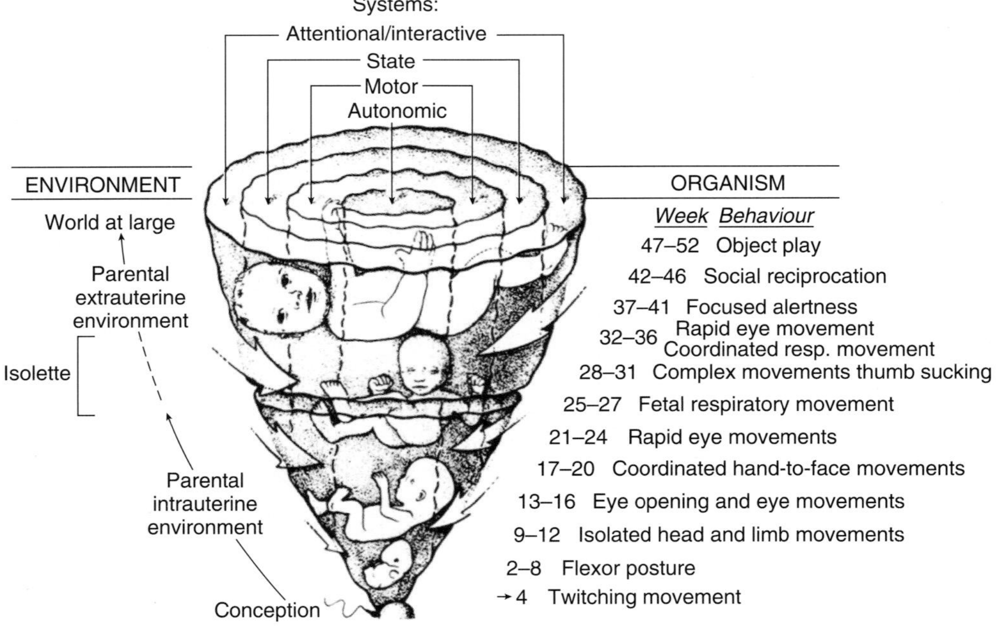

FIGURE 22.1 **Synactive theory of behavioural development**
Source: Als (1982).

EVIDENCE-BASED PRACTICE RESEARCH 22.1

Benefits of developmental care (systematic reviews)

- Reduced heart rate, cortisol levels, improved sleep states, reduced stress-related behaviours and reduced respiratory rate (Silva et al., 2018)
- Improved mental developmental index and improved psychomotor index (Soleimani et al., 2020)
- Positive effects on language, IQ, motor and cognitive development (Burke, 2018)

Developmental outcomes in high-risk neonates

Advancements in technology and care provided in neonatal units over the past three decades include surfactant use, aggressive resuscitation, mechanical ventilation, antenatal corticosteroids and parenteral nutritional support. This has resulted in the survival of extremely preterm neonates and sick neonates who previously may have died. Despite improved survival, improvements in developmental outcomes have not been reported (Korska et al., 2020).

Studies of children exposed to high stress levels in the early stages of development have demonstrated an association between the experience of adversity with disrupted maternal–infant attachment and negative neurodevelopmental trajectories, particularly those associated with emotion and cognition (Manzari et al., 2019). In addition, neonates born preterm or unwell face many potential risk factors that may contribute to abnormal brain development. For example, neonates admitted to a neonatal unit are more likely to have been resuscitated at birth and have a higher prevalence of respiratory distress, retinopathy of prematurity, patent ductus arteriosus, chronic lung disease, late-onset sepsis, necrotising enterocolitis, intraventricular haemorrhage and periventricular leucomalacia (Mandy et al., 2019). More recently, focus has been directed towards the cognitive, behavioural and psychological problems that arise for preterm survivors – for example, cognitive delay, cerebral palsy, hearing deficits, visual impairment, attention-deficit disorder, depression, obsessive–compulsive disorder and anxiety (Wilson-Costello & Payne, 2021). However, unhealthy stress responses may be mitigated through positive maternal–infant interactions. Changes in neonatal neurobiological processes and brain structure and function can be shaped to trigger adaptive healthy stress responses (Lavallee et al., 2019).

Neurosensory development of the sick or preterm neonate

Three interrelated elements affect neonatal development: genetics, relationships and the environment. Genes are responsible for physical characteristics through brain structure, initial connections and brain framework, growth and development sequences, composition of muscle fibres and sensory organisation. The developing maternal–infant relationship plays a critical role in development beginning in the prenatal period. During social interaction, the brain circuitry is stimulated. Stimulation of adequate intensity, time and regularity creates and maintains neuronal connections. This relationship between neonate and primary care giver has been referred to as the active ingredient for brain development (Knight & Smith, 2016).

Environmental (intra- and extrauterine) factors support the normal developmental trajectory of gene expression. A nurturing environment provides stimulation required for normal healthy brain development. During this period, which extends from the antenatal period through to the late childhood stage of development (Fitzgerald et al., 2020), differentiation of major brain structures is occurring, resulting in a high sensitivity to negative environmental factors. Exposure to environmental stressors in utero or during early postnatal development may trigger reprogramming of tissue structure and function.

Normal development is therefore an interactive process between the individual and the environment, beginning within the uterine environment. The increased health and disease risk that results from the short- and long-term effects of the environment on the developing fetus and neonate forms the foundation of the Developmental Origins of Health and Disease (DOHaD) research hypothesis, which asserts that stress in the antenatal period can have long-term effects on the health trajectory of the offspring (Fitzgerald et al., 2020). Just as the rapid development of the fetal brain provides the foundation for further development, the vulnerability of the developing brain to long-term neurodevelopmental and neuropsychiatric disorders is also increased.

While acute activation of the body's stress response systems is thought to be an adaptive process that mobilises resources to boost chances of survival, persistent or high levels of stress can disrupt brain development and damage mental health (Pechtel & Pizzagali, 2011). The adverse impact on fetal and neonatal brain architecture from exposure to toxic stress shapes how circuits are activated and managed. The result may be poorly controlled stress response systems, which are either overly reactive or alternatively slow to shut down. In the extreme, especially during early, sensitive periods of brain development, the regions of the brain involved in fear, anxiety and impulsive responses may over-produce neural connections, while those regions dedicated to reasoning, planning and behavioural control may produce fewer neural connections (National Scientific Council on the Developing Child, 2020).

The role of prenatal stress in creating a negative uterine environment has been identified. Animal and human research evidence demonstrating the adverse effects of maternal psychosocial stress during pregnancy on fetal development, resulting in poorer long-term developmental outcomes, is accumulating (Lautarescu et al., 2020). Outcomes such as delayed neurodevelopment and infant cognitive, motor and emotional development (Schechter et al., 2017) have been described. An increased risk for disrupted neurodevelopment has been linked to maternal pathogenesis and, more recently, to maternal stressors (death of a loved one, unwanted pregnancy, natural disaster, depression and/or anxiety).

Pregnancy-specific stress refers to the woman's concerns about the health of the unborn child and fears regarding the birth. An association between pregnancy-specific stress and shorter gestation has been established. Pregnancy-specific stress is also a predictor of longer-term age-related diseases such as hypertension and type 2 diabetes (Van den Bergh et al., 2020). The belief that pregnancy-specific stress may be a more sensitive predictor of adverse fetal and neonatal outcomes than maternal general stress is gaining momentum (Levine et al., 2017); however, many of the biological mechanisms underlying these outcomes remain unclear. Pregnancy-specific stress and its outcomes are particularly relevant to families whose neonates are admitted to the neonatal unit. Neurosensory development and its trajectory within fetal development are outlined in Fig. 22.2.

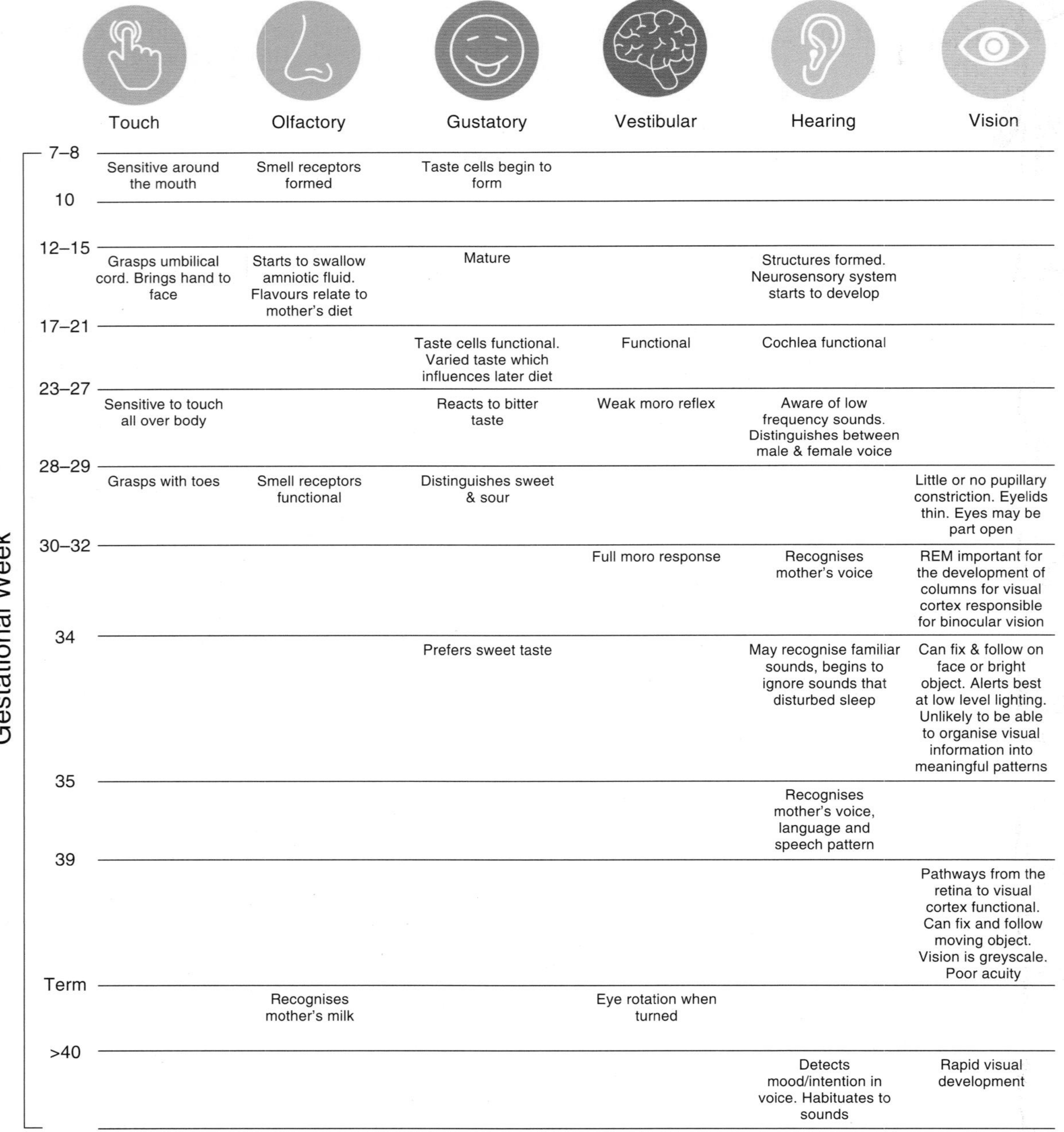

FIGURE 22.2 **Neurosensory development**

Source: developed by Nadine Griffiths and Bonnie Dorise; images from Piktochart.

Risk of admission to the neonatal unit

Recent research has highlighted that it is not only premature infants who require care in a neonatal unit, with more than 80% of admissions to the NICU of infants born at 34 or more weeks' gestation (Braun et al., 2021). Unwell neonates irrespective of gestational age confront numerous physiological and environmental stressors in the neonatal unit that may potentially lead to altered neurodevelopment (pain, thermal changes and olfactory, auditory, vestibular and visual stimuli) (Nist et al., 2019). Alterations in the developing brains of neonates admitted to the neonatal unit and SCBU may result from repeated exposure and their own physiological response to these stressors (D'Agata et al., 2018). In order to successfully manage their adaptation to the stressors of the neonatal unit or SCBU environment, the neonate works towards the maintenance of physiological and motor homeostasis (stability) (Schechter et al., 2017). These allostatic processes are necessary for adequate short-term adaptation; however, when these processes are repeatedly induced or prolonged, the allostatic load for the neonate becomes overwhelming (Casavant et al., 2019).

The recent marked improvement in technology, and neonatal surgical and medical treatment, has increased neonatal survival rates with a subsequent increase in the number of vulnerable neonates who survive to be admitted for neonatal care (Mandy, 2021). These advances have inadvertently led to increased patient acuity levels within neonatal units. Very little has been written regarding the overall burden of morbidity related to admission to the NICU (D'Ágata et al., 2018). However, Inder et al. (2019) have made some inroads into measuring the related stress imposed on vulnerable neonates resulting from admission to the neonatal unit and SCBU and its effect on brain development.

Along with technological and clinical management advances, a change in clinical practice moving away from task-orientated care to the provision of developmentally sensitive family-focused care has occurred throughout the world. The philosophy underlying this change is the provision of an environment that supports the psychological and developmental needs of families and their neonates (Bruton et al., 2018). One of the most important objectives of this change in clinical practice is to support care givers in becoming more responsive to the neonate's stress cues, enhancing interactions between the care giver and the neonate. This will result in care givers being more attuned to the neonate's needs, enabling them to provide appropriate levels of stimulation. Positive interaction between parent and neonate is expected to continue after discharge, enhancing the parent–infant relationship. It is this evolution of change in clinical practice that focuses on the interaction between the newborn and parent that has provided the impetus for the development of several models of practice that advocate developmental care practices (Table 22.1). These programs are based on a philosophy built on the recognition of the family as key to the neonate's ongoing development, and are further described in the next section.

Neurodevelopmental care models

Newborn Individualized Developmental Care and Assessment Program

The best known of these models is the **Newborn Individualized Developmental Care and Assessment Program (NIDCAP)**, developed by Aita et al. (2021a). NIDCAP provides a comprehensive approach to care that

TABLE 22.1 **Attributes of neonatal unit models of care**

Attribute	NIDCAP	FINE	UDC	Wee Care	FiCare
Recognised philosophy of care	✓	✓	✓	✓	✓
Staff education sessions	✓	✓	×	✓	✓
Formalised training curriculum for health professionals	✓	✓	×	✓	×
Accreditation process	✓	✓	×	×	×
Early developmental care (EDC) intervention component	✓	✓	✓	✓	×
Family-centred care philosophy	✓	✓	✓	✓	✓
Parent sensitivity component	✓	✓	✓	✓	✓
Parent educational sessions	✓	✓	×	✓	✓
Newborn neurodevelopmental assessment	✓	✓	×	×	×
Program outcomes reported	✓	✓	×	✓	✓
Program to implement nursery-wide change	✓	✓	×	✓	✓
Training currently available in Australia	✓	✓	×	✓	✓

FiCare, Family Integrated Care; FINE, Family and Infant Neurodevelopmental Education; NIDCAP, Newborn Individualized Developmental Care Assessment Program; UDC, Universe of Developmental Care Model; Wee Care, neuroprotective NICU program based on the Neonatal Integrative Developmental Care Model. Developed by K. Psaila.

is developmentally supportive and individualised to the neonate's goals and level of stability, which includes the provision of support for family and professionals caring for sick and preterm neonates. Currently NIDCAP is the only program based on individual neonatal observations. Care and therapeutic interventions are organised according to the neonate's individual tolerance, as opposed to being planned according to staff preference. Specific recommendations regarding support strategies are planned according to the neonate's needs: non-nutritive sucking, grasping, facilitated tucking and appropriate positioning or skin-to-skin care. Professionals collaborate with parents to support them in their role as primary care givers (Aita et al., 2021a).

The scientific evidence on the positive effects of NIDCAP on cognitive and motor development in preterm neonates is limited. Currently, there is no evidence on the effects of NIDCAP in other populations of sick neonates. Each of the studies appraised was rated as having medium quality and internal validity. In outcome variables where significant difference was found between the intervention and control groups, all of the studies showed better cognitive and psychomotor development results for the NIDCAP group. Notably, the longest follow-up period reported in the studies was just over 5 years. A major criticism of this model is the ongoing costs related to the specialised training of clinicians and continuous behavioural observations undertaken on neonates. Research recommendations include the need for well-designed studies with extended follow-up of standardised outcome variables (Lien, 2020).

The Family and Infant Neurodevelopmental Education program

The framework for **Family and Infant Neurodevelopmental Education (FINE)** comes from the synactive theory of newborn behavioural organisation and development and draws on the NIDCAP program. The FINE program involves the training of the entire neonatal care team in **family-centred care** and promotes learning through experience, hence bridging the gap between theory and practice. The curriculum focuses on topics such as fetal and preterm brain development, the family's journey, observing neonates, stress, pain, sleep, sensory development, comfort and early intervention strategies. Neonatal units in countries across Europe, such as the Netherlands, UK and Germany, have successfully adopted the FINE framework. Developed and delivered by a team of experienced UK NIDCAP professionals, FINE has been endorsed by the NIDCAP Federation International, and is supported by Bliss, a UK charity, and the European Foundation for the Care of Newborn Infants (EFCNI). A mixed-method evaluation of FINE has been undertaken with results indicating improved confidence in participant professional ability or role, and positive staff perceptions across a range of impact factors related to the program themes (Warren et al., 2019). The results indicate confidence in the FINE program as a means to achieve common goals across neonatal services, namely enhancement of the wellbeing and safety of infants, as well as parent engagement in their care (Warren et al., 2019).

The Universe of Developmental Care model

The Universe of Developmental Care model (UDC) is a reformulation of the neonatal developmental care theory introduced in 2008, which expands on the work of Als with the concept of a shared surface interface. This model assumes that the 'skin' is a representation of the surface of the brain conceived to incorporate all sensory systems, recognising the integration of the neonate's senses (visual, auditory, vestibular and so forth) with the care giver and the environment (Spruill, 2021). This approach thus provided a basis for formulating individualised neonatal care plans, and at the same time took into account the crucial role of family in the neonate's hospital experience (Spruill, 2021).

The Neonatal Integrative Developmental Care Model (NIDCM)

The **Neonatal Integrative Developmental Care Model (NIDCM)** was developed to simplify aspects of the UDC and incorporates the core measures of neonatal developmental care to guide clinical practice. They include partnering with families, positioning and handling, safeguarding sleep, minimising pain and stress, protecting skin and optimising nutrition (Bruton et al., 2018).

The Wee Care Neuroprotective NICU program

Phillips Healthcare and Altimier et al. (2015) developed the Wee Care Neuroprotective NICU program for neonates (Wee Care), an 18-month developmental care training program based on the NIDCM. The training program aims to provide comprehensive, neuroprotective, family-centred developmental care education and training for any healthcare professionals who care for high-risk neonates and their families on a daily basis. The program is delivered via online eLearning, didactic education and hands-on interactive workshops.

EVIDENCE-BASED PRACTICE RESEARCH 22.2

Altimier et al. (2015) reported findings from a pre–post implementation quality improvement project of the Wee Care Neuroprotective NICU training program in 81 NICUs in the US, Belgium and the Netherlands. Findings demonstrated a statistically significant improvement ($p < 0.001$) in the composite scores of the core measures of neonatal developmental care of partnering with families, minimising stress and pain, the healing environment, safeguarding sleep, optimising nutrition and positioning and handling (Altimier et al., 2015). Although the authors recommended further research in the area, no further studies evaluating the Wee Care program have since been published.

The Family Integrated Care program (FICare)

The **Family Integrated Care program (FICare)** is based on the Humane Neonatal Care model and includes (1) education of nurses and midwives on how to teach parents to provide safe care in a NICU, so that parents become the main care givers, and not the nurse/midwife, (2) parents spending at least 6 hours a day in the NICU and attending group classes on how to care for their infant in NICU, (3) parents being explicitly incorporated into the medical rounds, reporting on their infant and sharing in clinical decisions and (4) trained 'alumni' parents of former NICU infants who support the current NICU parents (Franck et al., 2019). A prospective cohort study of 123 FICare infants compared with standard care controls demonstrated better self-regulation skills at 18–21 months corrected age ($p < 0.01$), with the researchers also concluding that FICare parents were less stressed than controls because they spent more time with their babies, facilitating the development of organised attachment (Church et al., 2020).

EVIDENCE-BASED PRACTICE RESEARCH 22.3

The results of the first randomised controlled trial on the effectiveness of the FICare program undertaken by the Alberta group between December 2015 and July 2018 have recently been reported. This trial reported on the effectiveness of FICare with regard to length of stay (Benzies et al., 2020). Ten level II NICUs were randomised to provide Alberta FICare™ ($n = 5$) or standard care ($n = 5$). Intention-to-treat analysis included 353 infants/308 mothers in the Alberta FICare™ group and 365 infants/306 mothers in the standard care group. Infants were born at gestational ages between 32 weeks and 34 weeks 6 days. The unadjusted difference between groups in infant hospital late-onset sepsis (LOS) (1.96 days) was not statistically significant. Accounting for site geographic area and infant risk factors, infant hospital LOS was 2.55 days shorter (95% CI, −4.44 to −0.66) in the Alberta FICare™ group than in the standard care group ($p < 0.02$). Secondary outcomes were not significantly different between groups.

RELATIONSHIP-BASED CARE AND CO-REGULATION

Physical closeness and emotional closeness are considered crucial to the physical, emotional and social wellbeing of both the parent and infant (Thomson et al., 2020). The ability to form bonds through cues (infant to mother, mother to infant) is controlled by a complex physiological mechanism, developed during evolution, in order to maximise the species' chances of survival (Widström et al., 2019). Preterm birth alters these cues, and therefore bonding, in many ways. Preterm neonates' cues are often unrecognisable as, due to their physical immaturity, they are not capable of expressing their internal states in the way that term neonates can (Feldman et al., 2014). The physical fragility of the infant, combined with medical complications that may lead to physical separation from one or both parents, interrupts the normal process of parent–infant connection, and disrupts the start of co-regulation and the reciprocal emotional relationship between parent and infant (Erdei et al., 2019).

Recent findings suggest that early life conditions evolve to be either harmful or protective, dependent on the context of the infant's later life environment (Kommers et al., 2016). This implies that early life conditions might prepare the infant for their future life through glucocorticoid programming and phenotypic plasticity that matches future environmental demands (Kommers et al., 2016). Optimised parent–infant bonding is reported to overcome the negative impacts of preterm birth, which supports any efforts to strengthen bonding in neonatal settings (Welch, 2016). Co-regulation between mothers and neonates occurs during close physical contact such as holding and breastfeeding, with benefits of homeostasis observed in both (Welch, 2016). A recent pan-European study highlighted that the global aspirations of neonatal care should embrace a more humanising agenda, with specific emphasis on closeness between parents and neonates, and with skin-to-skin contact considered central in keeping the family together (Dykes et al., 2016). The absence of maternal buffering and co-regulation has been described as acutely distressing for the infant (Bergman et al., 2019). Frequent or continuous skin-to-skin contact is viewed as an intervention that directly supports neural connections for emotion development, creating both a physical and a social environment that connects infant and parent (Bergman et al., 2019). Given that the impact of adverse early life experiences can be reversed by improving the care-giving context and by optimising parent–infant bonding, attention on adequate bonding in neonatal units should be increased. Recognition that the place or environment in which development occurs is fundamentally more important than was previously appreciated (Bergman et al., 2019), highlighting the importance of neonatal unit design.

THE CHANGING NEONATAL UNIT ENVIRONMENT

The layout of the neonatal unit has evolved over the past two decades, moving away from open-bay design, with current global trends suggesting single family room (SFR) design as the gold standard in design. SFR design provides a private space for parents and neonates to have their first interactions, with the rooms designed to facilitate parent presence through the provision of sleeping facilities (EFCNI et al., 2018). The importance of maternal input in infant physiological, nutritional and emotional regulation or stability is presented as a case to care for the infant and mother simultaneously in the neonatal setting (Browne et al., 2020). Physical proximity between parents and infants through frequent feeding, holding and other interactions reinforces parental roles and increases parental perceptions of closeness. SFR unit layout is a means by which closeness and minimising parental separation may be achieved. The interest in SFRs has progressed in response to an increasing awareness of the importance of the sensory environment during a period of critical brain growth and development (Pineda et al., 2016). In the third trimester of pregnancy, the infant's brain increases in mass by 400%, comparable to the 400% growth seen in the entire period from term birth to adulthood (White, 2010). Shielding the neonate from some of the activity, noise and light experienced in an open-bay neonatal unit design is viewed positively from a developmental perspective and has been shown to improve neurobehavioural organisation and growth in preterm neonates (Lester et al., 2016). The European Standards of Care for Newborn Health project includes a specific NICU design standard. Based on a review of current evidence and consensus among content experts the recommendations advocate for unit designs that promote family-centred care, and facilitate skin-to-skin and parental involvement through the physical environment (European Foundation for the Care of Newborn Infants (EFCNI) et al., 2018). A number of components are recommended for European neonatal units moving forward; they are outlined in Table 22.2.

Family perspectives

International studies concluded that, when the space constructs of a neonatal unit create separation between a mother and an infant, it can make the mother feel unimportant by reducing her to the status of visitor (Flacking & Dykes, 2013). These findings highlight the impact of the spatial configuration of neonatal units on parental experiences, parent–infant attunement, neonatal feeding practices and ways and degrees of socialising with other parents (Dykes et al., 2016). In the context of SFR designs, research exploring parents' perspectives identified (Broom & Kecskes, 2020; Stichler, 2012):

- an ability to spend more time with their infants
- increased privacy and space for personal items
- facilitated parental involvement in skin to skin and breastfeeding
- enabled parents to attend to their infant's care with minimal interruptions and privacy
- a perception of less over-stimulation for their infants from noise and light
- increased access to nursing, midwifery and medical staff
- feeling more informed by the team than in previous room designs.

Staff perspectives

Calls to support the creation of a nurturing environment for both families and staff reflect evolving global shifts in the focus of infant- and family-centred care within SFR design (Broom et al., 2017). Yet, transitioning to an SFR environment has been reported to impact on midwifery staff more than other healthcare professionals (Swanson et al., 2018). Nurses' and midwives' perceptions of SFR design are that it puts the neonate at risk as they cannot be directly observed, that there is an increased walking distance and workload due to unit layout and more staff are required to provide care (Broom et al., 2017; Stichler, 2012). Neonatal nurses and midwives have reported a sense of isolation and perception of an increased workload in SFR unit designs (Hogan et al., 2016). Yet, there was no evidence of an effect on burnout, turnover intentions or

TABLE 22.2 **EFCNI unit design recommendations**

Component	Recommendations
Core principles of NICU design to promote family-centred care	• Incorporate SFR concept in national guidelines • Facilitate parental presence in SFRs • Provide SFR adequately sized to care for multiple births
Facilitation of skin-to-skin care and parental involvement through the physical environment	• Provide facilities to commence skin to skin in the delivery unit and during transfer for stable NICU infants • Provide SFR or adequately protected patient treatment areas to promote undisturbed skin to skin • Optimise the use of wireless monitoring • Provide adequately sized beds for parents with high-quality electrically adjustable mattresses • Provide separate bathrooms for parents • Provide flexible mounting of equipment to prevent disconnection during transfer • Provide a suitable area for visiting siblings and promote sibling access to the neonatal unit • Ensure space for both parents
General layout	• Facilitate the provision of couplet care • Incorporate space for infant, family and staff • Incorporate evidence-based lighting and acoustic recommendations • Provide access to protected gardens, balconies or atriums

Source: developed by N. Griffiths from EFCNI document EFCNI (2018).

job satisfaction and, overall, nurses/midwives supported the move to the SFR design owing to the perceived benefits for parents and infants (Hogan et al., 2016).

Research has found a nurse's/midwife's level of experience and length of employment influences their perception of overall infant safety and work level (Brand et al., 2021); after moving to a new SFR, increased stress occurs for between 9 months and 1 year, with perceptions shifting to a more-favourable view the longer they worked in the SFR design and being mostly resolved at 2 years (Brand et al., 2021). Adequate communication and staffing are recommended to assist staff during the transition (Brand et al., 2021). From a hospital administrator perspective, SFR designs are favoured as patients are admitted to one room for the duration of their admission, which is associated with fewer clinical incidents and a reduced potential for drug errors.

Environmental perspectives

A transition to SFR design unit layout has been shown to decrease noise, yet increase light owing to the number and configuration of windows in the newer units allowing for more daylight entry (Aita et al., 2021b). This suggests that, even in SFR designs, modifications are required to meet individual infant needs.

Neurodevelopmental outcome concerns

Several studies have identified concerns that preterm neonates cared for in SFRs may have less-favourable developmental language trajectories than those cared for in open-bay units (Chow & Shellhaas, 2016). However, other research comparing preterm infants cared for in an SFR with an open bay found those cared for in an SFR NICU had higher Bayley language and cognitive scores and received more human milk (Vohr et al., 2017). Exposure to language and parental presence may account for the differences in the studies. Research comparing exposure to meaningful adult words and mechanical noise in an SFR with open ward areas found there was more silence in the SFR than in the open ward, with an average of 1.9 hours more silence in a 16-hour period (Pineda et al., 2016). Medical interventions were related to more noise in the environment, particularly in the early weeks of hospitalisation associated with life-saving treatments (Pineda et al., 2016). Experts in neonatal unit redesign have suggested that the overall context of these studies requires review, with settings required to facilitate neonates and their parents being together frequently and for extended periods of time. In the absence of their family, a combination of unit design that includes open settings should be available for infants who do not receive adequate stimuli (Barton & White, 2016). Recent research identified that NICU noise levels are not driven by conversations among care givers, and interventions should continue to focus on reducing ambient noise of equipment and general NICU activity (Chow & Shellhaas, 2016). Unsurprisingly, neonates are exposed to more adult spoken words when parents are present (Chow & Shellhaas, 2016). Further studies are needed evaluating the effects of language exposure on short-term clinical and physiological parameters and on longer-term neurodevelopmental outcomes including language and cognition (Best et al., 2018). The ideal neonatal unit environment consists of positive language and protection from environmental sound (Pineda et al., 2016). Recommendations to enrich exposure to spoken language include reading of books and encouraging staff to role model speaking to infants during interactions, and to continue this practice when parents are not present (Newnam & Muñoz, 2021).

Unit design: European standards of care for newborn health recommendations

Following a review of international guidelines and policies, EFCNI has determined a consensus opinion regarding the size of bed spaces in the neonatal setting (EFCNI et al., 2018). Recommendations include the following:

- Multiple-bed rooms have a minimal space of 18 m^2 per patient.
- Single-family rooms have a minimal space of 24 m^2, taking into account family integrity and privacy and providing enough room for:
  - at least one comfortable and reclining chair
  - hospital bed
  - lockable wardrobe
  - easy access to restrooms and bathroom
  - technical equipment
  - ability for multiple care staff staying in the room at the same time.
- A barrier-free room with a window is available within the NICU, providing:
  - sinks with equipment (soap, towel and disinfectant dispenser)
  - comfortable chairs
  - tables.
- Bereavement space with window and space to stay with the infant after death, including a cooling facility, is provided in a culturally and spiritually appropriate design.
- The organisation of the NICU is decentralised, with distributed support spaces, medication, disinfection and storage, etc.
- Acoustically separate rooms for professional, administrative and personal needs provide privacy and reduce noise in the NICU.
- Wall colours radiating comfort and homeliness are used, adapted to cultural values.

Room size recommendations vary between global regions, with bedspaces in neonatal units in Australia differing significantly from the EFCNI recommendation. Rooms in Australia are noted to vary based on acuity, with 12.5m^2 allocated in a special care nursery to 16.5m^2 for NICU/high-dependency beds (Australasian Health Infrastructure Alliance, 2019).

An example of an infant- and family-centred NICU room design is shown in Fig. 22.3.

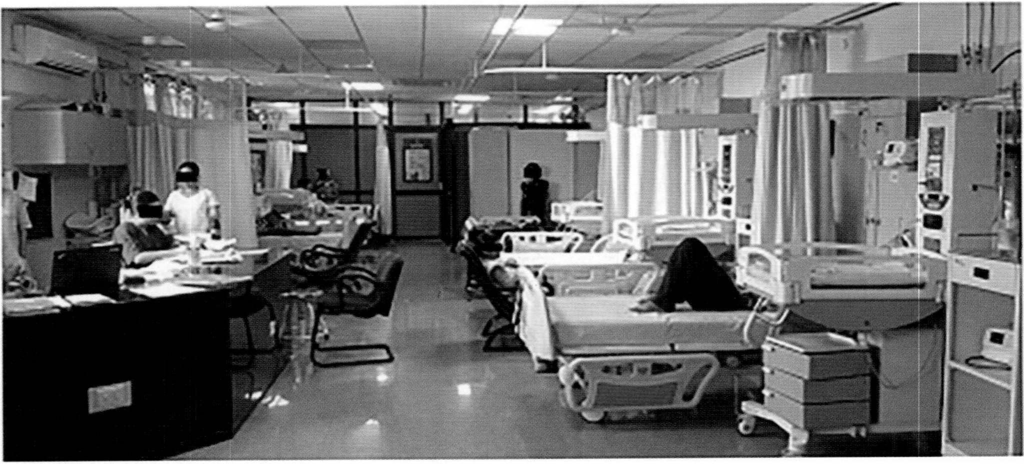

FIGURE 22.3 **An example of an infant- and family-centred NICU room design**

Source: Reproduced with permission from Chellani H., Arya S., Mittal P., Bahl R. (2022). Mother-Newborn Care Unit (MNCU) Experience in India: A Paradigm Shift in Care of Small and Sick Newborns. Indian Journal of Pediatrics, 89(5), 484–489. doi.org/10.1007/s12098-022-04145-9.

CARE-GIVING STRATEGIES TO ENHANCE BEHAVIOURAL DEVELOPMENT

One of the challenges for healthcare professionals is modifying care-giving interactions and the environment to provide individualised developmentally supportive care that promotes neurodevelopmental outcomes (see Table 22.3 for examples of best-practice, developmentally supportive strategies). Research has identified that extremely preterm infants (<29 weeks' gestation) spend a considerable amount of time alone during hospitalisation, with nursing care comprising the majority of human interaction (Gonya et al., 2018). Human interaction and isolation in the NICU were associated with social competence and dysregulation outcomes in extremely preterm infants, with infants who experienced greater human interaction demonstrating better outcome scores (Gonya et al., 2018). Consistency in the application of nurse/midwife-delivered care giving in the NICU remains a challenge (Gonya et al., 2019). Care giving is not innocuous, with immediate effects of altered infant physiological and behavioural responses and non-optimal infant developmental outcomes identified (Griffiths et al., 2021). Care-giving strategies to enhance infant behavioural development that provide an evidence-based framework in which to apply care are necessary when delivering care to neonates, irrespective of the clinical setting.

Skin-to-skin care

Skin-to-skin care, also known as kangaroo mother care, was initiated as an alternative method to care for low birthweight

TABLE 22.3 **Summary of best-practice infant- and family-centred developmental care recommendations**

Recommendations	Supporting evidence
Parent/infant separation recommendations	

• Facilitate 24 h/day parent/carer access to their infant(s)
• Sensitive care practices, procedures and the physical environment need to be organised to support:
  • parent–infant closeness
  • early and prolonged skin-to-skin contact
  • family-centred care
  • family rooms
  • optimisation of space during unit redesign
• Support parents in their skills to observe and interpret their infant's behaviour has been associated with improved cognition in later life and should be incorporated in clinical practice
• Provide families with education and support to improve parent/care giver–child interactions through play, reading and positive interactions, supporting bonding and attachment
• Provide parents with education to assist in the recognition of infant behavioural cues
	Dykes et al., 2016; Roué et al., 2017; Sutton & Darmstadt, 2013

TABLE 22.3 **Summary of best-practice infant- and family-centred developmental care recommendations—cont'd**

Recommendations	Supporting evidence
Sensory environment recommendations	

• Implement early positive sensory exposures such as tactile, auditory, visual, kinaesthetic, gustatory and olfactory, which have been identified as being safe and potentially important for optimising infant and parent outcomes in the NICU
• Interventions should continue to focus on reducing ambient noise of equipment and general NICU activity
• SFRs are recommended as they can improve outcomes for preterm neonates, with increasing parental involvement and better control of the environment, resulting in fewer inappropriate stimulations such as high levels of noise and illumination
• SFRs may be considered for vulnerable infants as they help parents and staff focus on the importance of the sensory environment during a period of critical brain growth and development
• In the absence of their family, a combination of unit design that includes open settings should be available for infants who do not receive adequate stimuli
• Appropriately timed sensory interventions that place the parents at the centre of the infant's care should be provided within the context of developmental care
• Sound-activated noise meters should be considered in NICUs as part of the effort to provide an appropriate sound environment for fragile infants
• Adjusted to the sensitivity of the infant and their developmental and medical stages, human voice can assist in reducing infant stress, promoting attachment with parents, and/or facilitating neurological, communication and social development
• It is recommended the background sound level is 45 dBA; the hourly equivalent sound level does not exceed 50 dBA more than 10% of the time, with transient maximum sounds to 65 dBA
• Cycled lighting over 24 h appears preferable to continuous bright lights and should be individually implemented based on an infant's state and time of day:
  • Ambient lighting in infant care area: 10–600 lux with adjustable/manual controls to limit direct sunlight; access to daylight is incorporated in unit design
  • Procedure lighting in infant care area: 2000 lux for critical areas shielding the infant's eyes when this level of lighting is used
  • Illumination of support areas: 300 lux
• Reading to infants in the NICU should be encouraged as it can have a positive impact on parenting behaviours and attitudes and the infant's cognitive development
	Braid & Bernstein, 2015; Filippa et al., 2017; Morag & Ohlsson, 2016; Pineda et al., 2017; Rea & Figueiro, 2016; Rodríguez & Pattini, 2016; Servel & Rideau Batista Novais, 2016; Wang et al., 2014; White et al., 2013

Sleep recommendations	
• Promotion and protection of sleep should be taught as a cornerstone of neonatal care for the treatment of patients in the NICU via integrated teaching programs targeted to nurses, medical staff, parents and other care givers • Sleep measurements should be incorporated into daily ward rounds to increase awareness of sleep as a key factor in neonatal health and to improve sleep outcomes • Elective care procedures should be postponed during sleep • Cyclical lighting should be used to assist in the establishment of a daily melatonin rhythm • Completing care giving as a neonate transitions to sleep is not recommended as preterm infants are unable to display the various overt behaviours associated with differing sleep–wake states, and responses may consequently be misinterpreted • Avoid sleep interruption as a relationship has been established between quantity and quality of sleep in preterm infants and neurocognitive and socio-emotional outcomes. The interruption of normal sleep can lead to the modification of the expression of several genes that can reduce the brain plasticity	Allen, 2012; Roué et al., 2017; van den Hoogen et al., 2017; Vásquez-Ruiz et al., 2014; White, 2015
Pain and stress recommendations	
• Minimise exposure to painful, stressful stimuli related to care • Minimise invasive procedures in very preterm infants as those who have a greater number of invasive procedures during their hospital stay have been shown to have an altered brain microstructure and poorer cognitive outcome at 18 months' corrected age • Minimise neonatal procedural pain/stress exposure as it has been identified as being significantly associated with specific changes in brain development in the premature infant • Adverse sensory experiences such as noise, light and repeated activities are known to influence brain development, potentially resulting in abnormal neurodevelopment and need to be kept to a minimum	Harrison et al., 2015; Roué et al., 2017; Shah et al., 2012; Smith et al., 2011; Stevens et al., 2016

Continued

TABLE 22.3 **Summary of best-practice infant- and family-centred developmental care recommendations—cont'd**	
Recommendations	Supporting evidence
• Regular pain assessment using an appropriate assessment tool should be used as standard practice in the NICU • Non-pharmacological pain interventions such as breastfeeding, breast milk, sucrose or glucose, as well as positioning, swaddling, non-nutritive sucking and odour should be used for potentially painful interventions such as heel lance and venepuncture in both term and preterm infants, depending on the infant's medical condition • Pharmacological interventions such as morphine or fentanyl should be titrated according to the infant's pain scores following developmental care interventions and a risk–benefit assessment • Parents should be given information and education about their baby's pain so they can be better prepared to take an active role in their infant's pain care	
Feeding recommendations	
• Nutrition is closely linked to neurodevelopmental outcomes, with breastfeeding identified as the optimal method of infant feeding to reduce risks of infant morbidity and mortality and improve long-term cognitive functioning • Promote safe and efficient feeding by considering the infant's arousal, physiological regulation, posture, oropharyngeal structure and function, in addition to suck–swallow–breathe patterns • A focus on cue-based individualised feeding experiences should be implemented as it has been demonstrated to lead to earlier achievement of full-suck feeds • Responsive sensitive feeding is associated with the parent or care giver's capacity to respond to the infant's physiological and behavioural communication. The transition from tube to suck feeds should be undertaken according to the infant's behavioural cues for readiness • Advice and support for mothers initiating breastfeeds in premature infants needs to be consistent	Belfort et al., 2016; Brown & White, 2011; Hallowell et al., 2016; Roué et al., 2017
Skin-to-skin recommendations	
• SSC increases breast milk supply and breastfeeding. Facilitating SSC for at least 1 h a day increases the length of breastfeeding after discharge and should be offered to mothers where the infant's medical condition allows • SSC can support physiological regulation of temperature and heart rate and is used to promote physiological stability in infants • SSC should be offered during painful procedures where practical to help minimise stress and behavioural responses • Ensuring staff are competent and confident in supporting infants and parents during transfers can assist to facilitate skin-to-skin episodes • SSC has been shown to be feasible and safe in the NICU in stable infants as young as 26 weeks' gestation, with benefits for both parents and infants; healthcare professionals are encouraged to offer SSC frequently as a part of routine care	Bailey, 2015; Boundy et al., 2016; Roué et al., 2017
Care-giving recommendations	
• Healthcare professionals require extensive education and support to implement developmentally supportive care giving • Age-appropriate individualised care giving should be implemented as it enhances the developing competencies of the infant • Timing of care giving should be optimised to support sleep and paced to minimise stress and promote stability	Griffiths et al., 2021; Lizarondo, 2016
Positioning recommendations	
• There is insufficient evidence to determine effects of body positioning on apnoea, bradycardia and oxygen saturation in preterm infants; however, positioning should be considered when trying to optimise an infant's condition • Prone positioning slightly improves oxygenation in neonates undergoing mechanical ventilation and can be considered as an alternate position to supine • Swaddling preterm infants should be promoted as it can decrease physiological distress and improve self-regulation attempts • Support infants with motoric containment in a side-lying position after a painful procedure as it reduces crying and sleep disruption	Ballout et al., 2017: Long Khanh Dao Le, 2017; Rivas-Fernandez et al., 2016; Roué et al., 2017

TABLE 22.3 **Summary of best-practice infant- and family-centred developmental care recommendations—cont'd**

Recommendations	Supporting evidence
• Physiological stability can be promoted by moving the preterm infant slowly and maintaining alignment and flexion • The use of postural supports can aid in ensuring functional support. Extra consideration should be taken when altering body position from horizontal to head-tilt so as to decrease the impact on cerebral perfusion • Preventive positioning (i.e. alternating positions) should be implemented to avoid the likelihood of preterm infants acquiring postural deformations which can decrease body movement and limit exploration of the infant's environment	
Continuity in care-giving recommendations	
• Involving parents in their baby's care in the neonatal unit empowers and enables their competence and confidence as care givers in the NICU and beyond • In collaboration with parents, a case management plan should be made in order to efficiently plan and coordinate required investigations and procedures and follow-up planning, as well as to ensure the acquisition of needed parental competences • Parenting education is considered a key intervention component to decrease maternal anxiety • Parents of preterm and vulnerable infants should be trained and provided with sufficient instructions to perform tasks associated with developmental care • Staff who are trained and experienced in mental healthcare and psychological screening for stress, depression and other forms of emotional distress, should be utilised to support the delivery of family-centred care in the neonatal unit • Supportive interventions that include psychosocial support should be provided as they result in better outcomes for mothers of preterm infants	Ingram et al., 2017; Lizarondo, 2016; Roué et al., 2017
Education and training recommendations	
• Developmental care education should be included in the orientation of all new staff to the neonatal setting • In order to effectively support parents, staff require extensive and ongoing training to understand infant behavioural responses and role model supportive care • Information regarding expected infant development and the influence of the neonatal setting should be provided to all staff • Developmental care training should be offered in postgraduate and advanced practice courses in neonatal care	D'Agata et al., 2017; Dykes et al., 2016; Griffiths et al., 2021; Lizarondo 2016; Milette et al., 2017

NICU, neonatal intensive care unit; SFR, single family room; SSC, skin to skin.

Source: adapted from Griffiths et al. (2019), compiled by N. Griffiths.

infants in resource-limited countries, where neonatal mortality and infection rates are high owing to overcrowding, inadequate staffing and lack of equipment (Bailey, 2015). It is recognised as one of the most well-researched and frequently applied components of neurosupportive developmental care, with benefits for neurosensory development, bonding and attachment, thermoregulation, weight gain and improved breastfeeding outcomes (Roué et al., 2017).

INTERPRETATION OF NEONATAL BEHAVIOUR

Crucial to supporting parents is having staff who can understand neonatal cues and teach parents the same (Dykes et al., 2016). Each neonate has their own unique patterns of behaviour that will vary and change over time depending on their gestational age, underlying clinical condition and other clinical or environmental variables (Als, 1982). Tables 22.4–22.6 highlight behaviour that indicates defence/avoidance (red) or approach/coping (green) behaviours, concepts first explained here:

- Defence behaviours include signs of stress, fending off or withdrawing actions. They indicate that the neonate requires support, time-out or a change in approach (Bond, 2002).
- Avoidance behaviours usually appear in clusters or may be a repetition of a single behaviour (i.e. three yawns in a row (Bond, 2002)). If the stimulation is reduced when the first avoidance behaviours are observed, the neonate is helped to maintain a balance that avoids overstimulation or tipping into stronger avoidance behaviour (i.e. loss of tone, apnoea).
- Approach or coping behaviours indicate the neonate's ability to settle themselves, calm their movements or seek to interact and look for contact. When neonates demonstrate these behaviours, they can either maintain balance or require little help to do so.

TABLE 22.4 **Autonomic system behaviours**

	Respiratory	Colour	Visceral
Approach/coping	• Respiratory rate within normal range • No signs of respiratory distress	• Normal colour	• Reduced tremors or twitches
Defence/avoidance	• Irregular • Respiratory pauses • Tachypnoea • Gasping	• Pale • Mottled • Dusky • Cyanotic • Marked colour changes	• Gagging • Grunting • Spitting up • Hiccups • Straining • Tremors • Startles • Twitches • Coughing • Sneezing • Sighing • Yawning

Source: adapted from Als and Lawhon (2010).

TABLE 22.5 **Motor system behaviours**

	Tone	Posture	Activity
Approach/coping	• Ability to maintain tone • Ability to reduce flaccidity, hypertonicity or hyperflexion	• Maintenance of flexed posture • Ability to clasp hands • Attempts to tuck trunk	• Smooth movements • Attempts to brace leg or foot • Ability to control when hands are brought together
Defence/avoidance	• Flaccidity of trunk extremities or face • Hypertonicity	• Hypertonicity • Hyperextension of legs, arms, fingers and trunk • Splaying of fingers • Hyperflexion of trunk and extremities	• Frantic diffuse activity

Source: adapted from Als and Lawhon (2010).

TABLE 22.6 **State system regulation**

	Sleep	Drowsy	Quiet alert	Active	Crying
Approach/coping	• Movement between light and deep sleep	• Minimal activity • Awake and quiet	• Alert and bright • Focuses on stimuli • Minimal activity	• Considerable activity • Well-defined fussing • Cooing • Smiles with interactions • Animated face	• Lusty cry • Rhythmic • Vigorous
Defence/avoidance	• Diffuse sleep states • Grimacing • Twitching • Whimpering • Irregular breathing • Jerky movements	• Eyes half open • Eyes open; glazed/dull look	• Hyper-alert • Eyes wide open • Fixate intensely • Staring • Panicked, worried look	• Mildly distressed face • Grimacing • Diffused fussing • Gaze aversion	• Intense grimace • Very strained weak cry or sounds

Source: adapted from Als and Lawhon (2010).

State system regulation

States are clusters of behaviours that tend to occur together and represent the neonate's level of arousal, their response to external stimulation and the underlying activation of the central nervous system (Als & Lawhon, 2010). Refer to Table 22.6 for more information about state system regulation.

Self-regulation

Self-regulatory behaviours are attempts to deal with stress and regain control within the environment. These behaviours are seen more often as the neonate matures, closer to 40 weeks' gestation (Als & Lawhon, 2010). The earlier the gestation, the fewer self-regulatory behaviours the neonate has available and the more the neonate relies on external support to help regulate themselves (Als et al., 2003). Parents and healthcare providers are therefore required to recognise and support self-regulation attempts.

IMPLEMENTING DEVELOPMENTAL CARE IN THE CLINICAL SETTING

When implementing practice changes, a systematic approach is considered the most effective strategy for identifying potential problems and translating policy meaningfully to front-line clinicians and patient care (Altimier et al., 2015). The development and implementation of a local evidence-based guideline is recommended to assist clinicians in the standardised application of developmentally supportive interventions (Griffiths et al., 2019). A position statement from the Canadian Association of Neonatal Nurses, Canadian Association of Perinatal and Women's Health Nurses, National Association of Neonatal Nurses and Council of International Nurses formed the basis of the *Guidelines for the institutional implementation of developmental neuroprotective care in the NICU* document, which may assist clinicians to determine local developmental care implementation needs (Milette et al., 2017). The document provides guidance in the areas of clinical care, education, management and research; steps in the guideline are recommended to be operationalised over different, sometimes parallel, time points, with a focus on outcomes measurable for quality improvement and research purposes (Milette et al., 2017). Five phases are suggested:

1. planning
2. education
3. prioritisation
4. evaluation
5. ensuring stability.

The individual steps within each phase are outlined in Fig. 22.4.

CASE STUDY 22.1

Sofia is a 28-week gestation neonate admitted to the neonatal unit for respiratory, nutrition and thermoregulation management.

1. Given Sofia's gestational age, what developmentally supportive care-giving strategies could you implement?
2. How would you orientate and incorporate Sofia's family into the care-giving practices in the neonatal unit?
3. What types of behaviour would you expect Sofia to demonstrate?
4. How would you explain her behaviour to her family?
5. What strategies would you recommend to her family to help support Sofia during behaviour demonstrating avoidance or not coping?

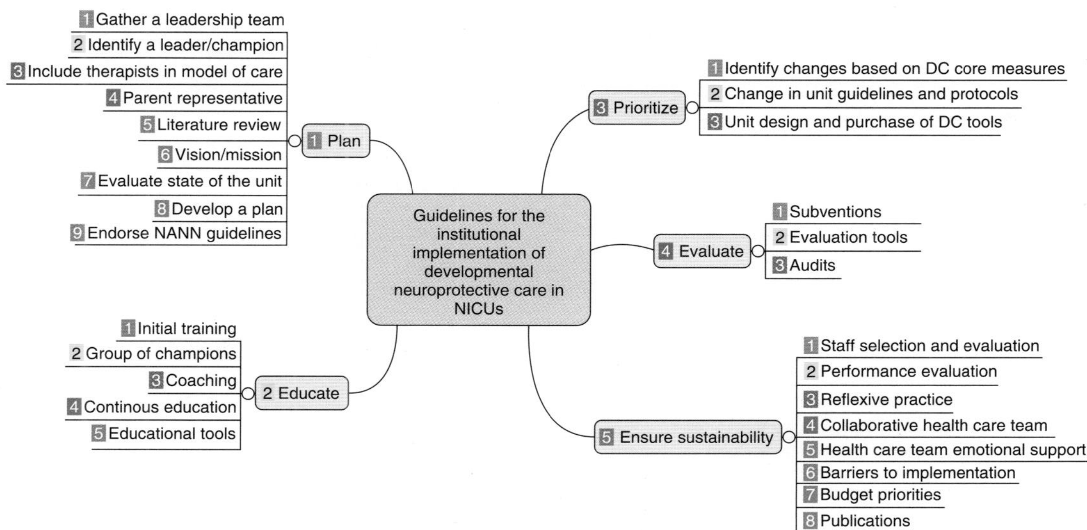

FIGURE 22.4 **Algorithm version of the guidelines for the institutional implementation of developmental neuroprotective care in the NICU**

Source: Milette et al. (2017).

CONCLUSION

Over the past 20 years, developmentally supportive care has become the guiding philosophy of clinical practice in the neonatal setting. Challenges remain for healthcare professionals, with the concept of developmental care represented by a range of interchangeable terms and differing levels of understanding. The fundamental objective of developmental care giving is to support brain development of the neonate. It consists of various activities designed to manage the stress of the environment and promote healthy growth and development of the infant and family, based on a shared understanding of neurosensory development and neuroprotective and neuropromotive strategies (Knudsen et al., 2021). The future of developmental care and its link to neurodevelopmental outcomes are dependent upon promoting consistency in the application of developmental care, staff trained in the application of developmental care in the clinical setting and clinical environments that promote parent–infant interactions. Neonatal nurses/midwives have a major role and responsibility to understand and meet the developmental needs of the neonates in their care, and to teach parents to do the same. For infants and families, life beyond the neonatal unit can be complex and overwhelming. The area of infant mental health is an area of increasing focus, with neonatal units required to consider how we can extend the provision of supportive care beyond the intensive care setting.

Online resources

Bliss: <https://www.bliss.org.uk>
European Foundation for the Care of Newborn Infants: European Standards of Care for Newborn Health: <https://newborn-health-standards.org/>
Family and Infant Neurodevelopmental Care Education Program UK: <https://finetraininguk.com/>
NIDCAP Federation International: <https://nidcap.org>
The European Foundation for the Care of Newborn Infants (EFCNI): <https://www.efcni.org/>

References

Aita, M., De Clifford Faugère, G., Lavallée, A., Feeley, N., Stremler, R., Rioux, É., et al. (2021a). Effectiveness of interventions on early neurodevelopment of preterm infants: a systematic review and meta-analysis. *BMC Pediatrics, 21*, 210. doi: 10.1186/s12887-021-02559-6.

Aita, M., Robins, S., Charbonneau, L., Doray-Demers, P., & Feely, N. (2021b). Comparing light and noise levels before and after a NICU change of design. *Journal of Perinatology, 41*(9), 2235–2243. doi: 10.1038/s41372-021-01007-8.

Allen, K. (2012). Promoting and protecting infant sleep. *Advances in Neonatal Care, 5*, 288–291.

Als, H. (1982). Toward a syntactive theory of development: promise for the assessment and support of infant individuality. *Infant Mental Health Journal, 3*, 229–243.

Als, H., & Lawhon, G. (2010). Theoretic perspective for developmentally supportive care. In: C. Kenner, & J. M. McGrath (Eds.), *Developmental care of newborns and infants: a guide for health professionals* (2nd ed.). St Louis, MO: Mosby.

Als, H., Gilkerson, L., Duffy, F. H., McAnulty, J. B., Buehler, D. H., Vandenberg, K., et al. (2003). A three-center, randomized, controlled trial of individualized developmental care for very low birth weight preterm infants: medical, neurodevelopmental, parenting, and caregiving effects developmental and behavioural. *Pediatrics, 24*, 399–408.

Altimier, L., Kenner, C., & Damus, K. (2015). The Wee Care Neuroprotective NICU Program (Wee Care): the effect of a comprehensive developmental care training program on seven neuroprotective core measures for family-centered developmental care of premature neonates. *Newborn and Infant Nursing Reviews, 15*(1), 6–16.

Australasian Health Infrastructure Alliance. (2019). *Australasian health facility design: part B health facility briefing and planning*. <https://aushfg-prod-com-au.s3.amazonaws.com/HPU_B.0390_7.pdf> (Accessed 2 March 2022).

Bailey, J. (2015). Skin-to-skin care for term and preterm infants in the neonatal ICU. *Pediatrics, 136*, 593–596.

Ballout, R. A., Foster, J. P., Kahale, L. A., & Badr, L. (2017). Body positioning for spontaneously breathing preterm infants with apnoea. *Cochrane Database of Systematic Reviews, 1*, CD004951. doi: 10.1002/14651858.CD004951.pub3.

Barton, S. A., & White, R. D. (2016). Advancing NICU care with a new multi-purpose room concept. *Newborn and Infant Nursing Reviews, 16*, 222–224.

Belfort, M. B., Anderson, P. J., Nowak, V. A., Lee, K. J., Molesworth, C., Thompson, D. K., et al. (2016). Breast milk feeding, brain development, and neurocognitive outcomes: a 7-year longitudinal study in infants born <30 weeks' gestation. *Journal of Pediatrics, 177*, 133–139. doi: 10.1016/j.jpeds.2016.06.045.

Benzies, K. M., Shah, V., Faris, P., Isaranuwatchai, W., Scotland, J., Larocque, J., et al. (2020). Effectiveness of Alberta Family Integrated Care on infant length of stay in level II neonatal intensive care units: a cluster randomized controlled trial. *BMC Paediatrics, 20*, 535.

Bergman, N. J., Ludwig, R. J., Westrup, B., & Welch, M. G. (2019). Nurture science versus neuroscience: a case for rethinking perinatal mother–infant behaviours and relationship. *Birth Defects Research, 111*, 1110–1127. doi: 10.1002/bdr2.1529.

Best, K., Bogossian, F., & New, K. (2018). Language exposure of preterm infants in the neonatal unit: a systematic review. *Neonatology, 114*(3), 261–276. doi: 10.1159/000489600.

Bond, C. (2002). Positive touch and massage in the neonatal unit: a British approach. *Seminars in Neonatology, 7*(7), 477–486.

Boundy, E. O., Dastjerdi, R., Spiegelman, D., Fawzi, W. W., Missmer, S. A., Lieberman, E., et al. (2016). Kangaroo mother care and neonatal outcomes: a meta-analysis. *Pediatrics, 137*, 26702029. doi: 10.1542/peds.2015-2238.

Braid, S., & Bernstein, J. (2015). Improved cognitive development in preterm infants with shared book reading. *Neonatal Network, 34*, 10–17. doi: 10.1891/0730-0832.34.1.10.

Brand, M. C., Shippey, H., Hagan, J., Hanneman, S. K., Levy, B., Range, S., et al. (2021). Comparison of psychological and physiological stress in NICU nurses: effects of unit design and shift. *Advances in Neonatal Care, 21*(4), E93–E100. doi: 10.1097/ANC.0000000000000837.

Braun, D., Edwards, M. E., Schulman, J., Profit, J., Pursley, D. M., & Goodman, D. C. (2021). Choosing wisely for the other 80%: what we need to know about the more mature newborn and NICU care. *Seminars in Perinatology, 45*(3), 151395. doi: 10.1016/j.semperi.2021.151395.

Brazelton, T. B. (1973). *Neonatal Behavioural Assessment Scale*. Clinics in Developmental Medicine. London: William Heinemann Medical.

Broom, M., & Kecskes, K. (2020). Exploring the impact of a dual-occupancy NICU design on parental experience. *Journal of Neonatal Nursing, 26*(4), 217–221. doi: 10.1016/j.jnn.2020.01.007.

Broom, M., Gardner, A., Keceskes, Z., & Kildea, S. (2017). Transition from an open plan to a two-cot neonatal intensive care unit: a participatory action research approach. *Journal of Clinical Nursing, 26*(13–14), 1939–1948. doi: 10.1111/jocn.13509.

Browne, J. V., & White, R. D. (2011). Clinics in perinatology: foundations in developmental care. *Clinical Perinatology, 38*, 591–758.

Browne, J. V., Jaeger, C. B., Kenner, C.; Gravens Consensus Committee on Infant and Family Centered Developmental Care. (2020). Executive summary: standards, competencies, and recommended best practices for infant- and family-centered developmental care in the intensive care unit. *Journal of Perinatology, 40*(suppl 1), 5–10. doi: 10.1038/s41372-020-0767-1.

Bruton, C., Meckley, J., & Nelson, L. (2018). NICU nurses and families partnering to provide neuroprotective, family-centered, developmental care. *Neonatal Network, 37*(6), 351–357.

Burke, S. (2018). Systematic review of developmental care interventions in the neonatal intensive care unit since 2006. *Journal of Child Health Care, 22*(2), 269–286. doi: 10.1177/1367493517753085.

Casavant, S. G., Cong, X., Fitch, R. H., Moore, J., Rosenkrantz, T., & Starkweather, A. (2019). Allostatic load and biomarkers of stress in the preterm infant: an integrative review. *Biological Research for Nursing, 21*(2), 210–223.

Chow, V. Y., & Shellhaas, R. A. (2016). Acoustic environment profile of the neonatal intensive care unit: high ambient noise and limited language exposure. *Journal of Neonatal Nursing, 22*(4), 159–162. doi: 10.1016/j.jnn.2016.03.003.

Church, P. T., Grunau, R. E., Mirea, L., Petrie, J., Soraisham, A. S., Synnes, A., et al. (2020). Family Integrated Care (FICare): positive impact on behavioural outcomes at 18 months. *Early Human Development, 151*, 105196–105202.

D'Agata, A. L., Sanders, M. R., Grasso, D. J., Young, E. E., Cong, X., & McGrath, J. M. (2017). Unpacking the burden of care for infants in the NICU. *Infant Mental Health Journal, 38*(2), 306–317.

D'Ágata, A. L., Coughline, M., & Sanders, M. R. (2018). Clinician perceptions of the NICU infant experience: is the NICU hospitalization traumatic? *American Journal of Perinatology, 35*, 1159–1167. doi: 10.1055/s-0038-1641747.

Dykes, F., Thomson, G., Gardner, C., Moran, V. H., & Flacking, R. (2016). Perceptions of European medical staff on the facilitators and barriers to physical closeness between parents and infant in neonatal units. *Acta Paediatrica, 105*, 1039–1046.

Erdei, C., Inder, T. E., Dodrill, P., & Woodward, L. J. (2019). The Growth and Development Unit. A proposed approach for enhancing infant neurodevelopment and family-centered care in the Neonatal Intensive Care Unit. *Journal of Perinatology, 39*, 1684–1687. doi: 10.1038/s41372-019-0514-7.

European Foundation for the Care of Newborn Infants (EFCNI), & Kuhn, P., Westrup, B., Bertoncelli, N., Filippa, M., Huppi, P., & Warren, I. (2018). *European standards of care for newborn health: supportive sensory environment*. <https://www.efcni.org/wp-content/uploads/2018/11/2018_11_16_ESCNH_Report_final.pdf> (Accessed 4 March 2022).

Feldman, R., Rosenthal, Z., & Eidelman, A. I. (2014). Maternal–preterm skin-to-skin contact enhances child physiologic organization and cognitive control across the first 10 years of life. *Biology of Psychiatry, 75*(1), 56–64.

Filippa, M., Panza, C., Ferrari, F., Frassoldati, R., Kuhn, P., Balduzzi, S., et al. (2017). Systematic review of maternal voice interventions demonstrates increased stability in preterm infants. *Acta Paediatrica, 106*, 1220–1229. doi: 10.1111/apa.13832.

Fitzgerald, E., Hor, K., & Drake, A. J. (2020). Maternal influences on fetal brain development: the role of nutrition, infection and stress, and the potential for intergenerational consequences. *Early Human Development, 150*, 105190. doi: 10.1016/j.earlhumdev.2020.105190.

Flacking, R., & Dykes, F. (2013). 'Being in a womb' or 'playing musical chairs': the impact of place and space on infant feeding in NUs. *BMC Pregnancy and Childbirth, 13*, 179.

Gardner, S. L., & Niermeyer, S. (2021). Immediate newborn care after birth. In: S. L. Gardner, B. S. Carter, M. I. Enzman-Hines, & S. Niemeyer (Eds.), *Merenstein & Gardner's handbook of neonatal intensive care: an interprofessional approach* (9th ed., pp. 93–136). St Louis, MO: Elsevier.

Gonya, J., Feldman, K., Brown, K., Stein, M., Keim, S., Boone, K., et al. (2018). Human interaction in the NICU and its association with outcomes on the Brief Infant-Toddler Social and Emotional Assessment (BITSEA). *Early Human Development, 27*, 6–14. doi: 10.1016/j.earlhumdev.2018.08.010.

Gonya, J., Harrison, T., Feldman, K., Stein, M., & Chawla, N. (2019). Nursing networks in the NICU and their association with maternal stress: a pilot study. *Journal of Nursing Management, 27*, 442–449. doi: 10.1111/jonm.12679.

Griffiths, N., Spence, K., Loughran-Fowlds, A., & Westrup, B. (2019). Individualised developmental care for babies and parents in the NICU: evidence-based best practice guideline recommendations. *Early Human Development, 139*, 104840.

Griffiths, N., Laing, S., Spence, K., Foureur, M., & Sinclair, L. (2021). The effects of nurse-delivered caregiving in the neonatal setting: an integrative review. *Journal of Neonatal Nursing, 27*(5), 317–326. doi: 10.1016/j.jnn.2021.03.005.

Hallowell, S. G., Rogowski, J. A., Spatz, D. L., Hanlon, A. L., Kenny, M., & Lake, E. T. (2016). Factors associated with infant feeding of human milk at discharge from neonatal intensive care: cross-sectional analysis of nurse survey and infant outcomes data. *International Journal of Nursing Studies, 53*, 190–203. doi: 10.1016/j.ijnurstu.2015.09.016.

Harrison, D., Bueno, M., & Reszel, J. (2015). Prevention and management of pain and stress in the neonate. *Research and Reports in Neonatology, 5*, 9–16, doi: 10.2147/RRN.S52378.

Hogan, C., Jones, L., & Saul, J. (2016). The impact of special care nursery design on neonatal nurses. *Journal of Neonatal Nursing, 22*, 74–80.

Ingram, J., Redshaw, M., Manns, S., Beasant, L., Johnson, D., Fleming, P., et al. (2017). Giving us hope: parent and neonatal staff views and expectations of a planned family-centered discharge process (train-to-home). *Health Expectations, 20*, 751–759. doi: 10.1111/hex.12514.

Knight, A. K., & Smith, A. K. (2016). Epigenetic biomarkers of preterm birth and its risk factors. *Genes, 7*(4), 15.

Knudsen, K., McGill, G., Waitzman, K., Powell, J., Carlson, M., Shaffer, G., et al. (2021). Collaboration to improve neuroprotection and neuropromotion in the NICU: team education and family engagement. *Neonatal Network, 40*(4), 212–223.

Kommers, D., Oei, G., Chen, W., Feijs, L., & Bambang Oetomo, S. (2016). Suboptimal bonding impairs hormonal, epigenetic and neuronal development in preterm infants, but these impairments can be reversed. *Acta Paediatrica, 105*, 738–751.

Korska, M., Petersen, M., Lund Andersen, B., & Brodsgaard, A. (2020). Supporting families on their journey towards a normal everyday life – facilitating partnership in an early discharge program for families with premature infants. *Journal for Specialists in Pediatric Nursing, 25*(1), e12274. doi: 10.1111/jspn.12274.

Lammertink, F., Vinkers, C. H., Tataranno, M. L., & Benders M. J. N. L. (2021). Premature birth and developmental programming: mechanisms of resilience and vulnerability. *Frontiers in Psychiatry, 11*, 1515–1539. doi: 10.3389/fpsyt.2020.531571.

Lautarescu, A., Craig, M. C., & Glover, V. (2020). Prenatal stress: effects on fetal and child brain development. *International Review of Neurobiology, 150*, 17–40. doi: 10.1016/bs.irn.2019.11.002.

Lautarescu, A., Hadaya, L., Craig, M. C., Makropoulos, A., Batalle, D., Nosarti, C., et al. (2021). Exploring the relationship between maternal prenatal stress and brain structure in premature neonates. *PLoS One, 16*(4), e0250413. doi: 10.1371/journal.pone.0250413.

Lavallee, A., De Clifford-Faugere, G., Garcia, C., Fernanadez Oviedo, A. F., Heon, M., & Aita, M. (2019). Part 1: Narrative overview of developmental care interventions for the preterm newborn. *Journal of Neonatal Nursing, 25*, 3–8.

Lester, B. M., Salisbury, A. L., Hawes, K., Dansereau, L. M., Bigsby, R., Laptook, A., et al. (2016). 18-Month follow-up of infants cared for in a single-family room neonatal intensive care unit. *Journal of Pediatrics, 134*, 754–760.

Levine, T. A., Grunau, R. E., Segurado, R., Daly, S., Geary, M. P., Kennelly, M. M., et al. (2017). Pregnancy-specific stress, fetoplacental haemodynamics, and neonatal outcomes in women with small for gestational age pregnancies: a secondary analysis of the multicentre Prospective Observational Trial to Optimise Paediatric Health in Intrauterine Growth Restriction. *BMJ Open, 7*(6), e015326. doi: 10.1136/bmjopen-2016-015326.

Lien, R. (2020). Neurocritical care of premature infants. *Biomedical Journal, 43*(3), 259–267. doi: 10.1016/j.bj.2020.03.007.

Lizarondo, L. (2016). Evidence summary. Developmental care: preterm or ill neonates. The Joanna Briggs Institute EBP Database; JBI@Ovid: JBI16368.

Long Khanh Dao Le, B. (2017). Evidence summary. Positioning of preterm infants. The Joanna Briggs Institute EBP Database. JBI3701.

Mandy, G. T. (2021). Incidence and mortality of the preterm infant. In: L. Weisman (Ed.), Preterm birth: definitions of prematurity, epidemiology, and risk factors for infant mortality. *UpToDate*. Walters Kluwer. <https://www.uptodate.com/contents/preterm-birth-definitions-of-prematurity-epidemiology-and-risk-factors-for-infant-mortality> (Accessed 2 March 2022).

Mandy, G. T., Martin, R. & Kim, M. S. (2019). Short-term complications of the preterm infant. In: R. Martin (Ed.), *UpToDate*. Walters Kluwer. <https://www.uptodate.com/contents/short-term-complications-of-the-preterm-infant?search> (Accessed 2 March 2022).

Manzari, N., Matvlenko-Sikar, K., Baldoni, F., O'Keefe, G. W., & Khashan, A. S. (2019). Prenatal maternal stress and risk of neurodevelopmental disorders in the offspring: a systematic review and meta-analysis. *Social Psychiatry and Psychiatric Epidemiology, 54*, 1299–1309. doi: 10.1007/s00127-019-01745-3.

Milette, I., Martel, M. J., da Silva, M. R., & Coughlin McNeil, M. (2017). Guidelines for the institutional implementation of developmental neuroprotective care in the NICU. Part B: recommendations and justification. A joint position statement from the CANN, CAPWHN, NANN, and COINN. *Canadian Journal of Nursing Research, 49*(2), 63–74.

Morag, I., & Ohlsson, A. (2016). Cycled light in the intensive care unit for preterm and low birth weight infants. *Cochrane Database of Systematic Reviews, 8*, CD006982.pub4. doi: 10.1002/14651858.CD006982.pub4.

National Scientific Council on the Developing Child. (2020). Connecting the brain to the rest of the body: early childhood development and lifelong health are deeply intertwined. Working paper no. 15. <https://developingchild.harvard.edu/resources/connecting-the-brain-to-the-rest-of-the-body-early-childhood-development-and-lifelong-health-are-deeply-intertwined/> (Accessed 2 March 2022).

Newnam, K. M., & Muñoz, L. R. (2021). Purposeful language exposure by neonatal nurses and caregivers in the NICU. *Advances in Neonatal Care, 21*(5), 407–417. doi: 10.1097/ANC.0000000000000833.

Nist, M. D., Pickler, R. H., Steward, D. K., Harrison, T. M., & Shoben, A. B. (2019). Inflammatory mediators of stress exposure and neurodevelopment in very preterm infants: protocol for the stress neuro-immune study. *Journal of Advanced Nursing, 75*, 10, 2236–2245.

Pechtel, P., & Pizzagali, D. A. (2011). Effects of early life stress on cognitive and affective function: an integrated review of human literature. *Psychopharmacology Bulletin, 214*(1), 55–70. doi: 10.1007/s00213-010-2009-2.

Pineda, R., Durant, P., Mathur, A., Inder, T., Wallendorf, M., & Schlaggar, B. L. (2016). Auditory exposure in the neonatal intensive care unit: room type and other predictors. *Journal of Pediatrics, 183*, 56–63.

Pineda, R., Guth, R., Herring, A., Reynolds, L., Oberle, S., & Smith, J. (2017). Enhancing sensory experiences for very preterm infants in the NICU: an integrative review. *Journal of Perinatology, 37*, 323–332. doi: 10.1038/jp.2016.179.

Rea, M. S., & Figueiro, M. G. (2016). The NICU lighted environment. *Newborn Infant Nursing Reviews, 16*(4), 195–202. doi: 10.1053/j.nainr.2016.09.009.

Rivas-Fernandez, M., Roqué i Figuls, M., Diez-Izquierdo, A., Escribano, J., & Balaguer, A. (2016). Infant position in neonates receiving mechanical ventilation. *Cochrane Database of Systematic Reviews, 11*, CD003668. doi: 10.1002/14651858.CD003668.pub4.

Rodríguez, R. G., & Pattini, A. E. (2016). Neonatal intensive care unit lighting: update and recommendations. *Archivos Argentinos de Pediatría, 114*(4), 361–367.

Roué, J. M., Kuhn, P., Maestro, M. L., Maastrup, R. A., Mitanchez, D., Westrup, B., et al. (2017). Eight principles for patient-centered and family-centered care for newborns in the neonatal intensive care unit. *Archives of Disease in Childhood. Fetal and Neonatal Edition, 102*(4), F364–F368.

Schechter, J. C., Brennan, P. A., Smith, A. K., Stowe, Z. N., Newport, D. J., & Johnson, K. C. (2017). Maternal prenatal psychological distress and preschool cognitive functioning: the protective role of positive parental engagement. *Journal of Abnormal Child Psychology, 45*(2), 249–260.

Servel, A. C., & Rideau Batista Novais, A. (2016). Single-family rooms for neonatal intensive care units impacts on preterm newborns, families, and health-care staff. A systematic literature review. *Archives de Pédiatrie, 23*, 921–926. doi: 10.1016/j.arcped.2016.04.022.

Shah, P. S., Herbozo, C., Aliwalas, L. I., & Shah, V. S. (2012). Breastfeeding or breast milk for procedural pain in neonates. *Cochrane Database of Systematic Reviews, 12*, CD004950. doi: 10.1002/14651858.CD004950.pub3.

Silva, N. d. F., Linhares, M. B. M., & Gaspardo, C. M. (2018). Developmental care approaches for mitigating stress in preterm neonates in the neonatal intensive care unit: a systematic review. *Psychology and Neuroscience, 11*(2), 117–131. doi: 10.1037/pne0000119.

Smith, G. C., Gutovich, B. A., Smyser, C., Pineda, R., Newnham, C., Tjoeng, T. H., et al. (2011). Neonatal intensive care unit stress is associated with brain development in preterm infants. *Annals of Neurology, 70*, 541–549.

Soleimani, F., Azari, N., Ghiasvand, H., Shahrokhi, A., Rahmani, N., & Fatollahierad, S. (2020). Do NICU developmental care improve cognitive and motor outcomes for preterm infants? A systematic review and meta-analysis. *BMC Pediatrics, 20*, 67. doi: 10.1186/s12887-020-1953-1.

Spruill, C. T. (2021). Developmental support. In: M. T. Verklan, M. Walden, & S. Forest (Eds.), *Core curriculum for neonatal intensive care nursing* (6th ed.). St Louis, MO: Elsevier.

Stevens, B., Yamada. J., Ohlsson, A., Haliburton, S., & Shorkey, A. (2016). Sucrose for analgesia in newborn infants undergoing painful procedures. *Cochrane Database of Systematic Reviews, 7*, CD001069. doi: 10.1002/14651858.CD001069.pub5.

Stichler, J. F. (2012). The new standard: single family room design. *Journal of Nursing Administration*, 42(10), 447–450.

Sutton, P. S., & Darmstadt, G. L. (2013). Preterm birth and neurodevelopment: a review of outcomes and recommendations for early identification and cost-effective interventions. *Journal of Tropical Pediatrics, 59*, 258–265. doi: 10.1093/tropej/ fmt012.

Swanson, J. R., Peters, C., & Lee, B. H. (2018). NICU redesign from open ward to private room: a longitudinal study of parent and staff perceptions. *Journal of Perinatology, 33*(6), 466–469.

Thomson, G., Flacking, R., George, K., Feeley, N., Haslund-Thomsen, H., De Coen, K., et al. (2020). Parents' experiences of emotional closeness to their infants in the neonatal unit: a meta-ethnography. *Early Human Development, 149*, 105155. doi: 10.1016/j.earlhumdev.2020.105155.

Van den Bergh, B. R. H., van den Heuvel, M. I., Lahti, M., Braeken, M., de Rooij, S. R., Hoyer, D., et al. (2020). Prenatal developmental origins of behaviour and mental health: the influence of maternal stress in pregnancy. *Neuroscience and Biobehavioral Reviews, 117*, 26–64.

van den Hoogen, A., Teunis, C. J., Shellhaas, R. A., Pillen, S., Benders, M., & Dudink, J. (2017). How to improve sleep in a neonatal intensive care unit: a systematic review. *Early Human Development, 113*, 78–86.

Vásquez-Ruiz, S., Maya-Barrios, J. A., Torres-Narváez, P., Vega-Martínez, B. R., Rojas-Granados, A., Escobar, C., et al. (2014). Light/dark cycle in the NICU accelerates body weight gain and shortens time to discharge in preterm infants. *Early Human Development, 90*, 535–540. doi: 10.1016/j.earlhumdev.2014.04.015.

Vohr, B., McGowan, E., McKinley, L., Tucker, R., Keszler, L., & Alksninis, B. (2017). Differential effects of the single-family room neonatal intensive care unit on 18-to-24 month Bayley scores of preterm infants. *Journal of Pediatrics, 185*, 42–48.e1. doi: 10.1016/j.jpeds.2017.01.056.

Wang, D., Aubertin, C., Barrowman, N., Moreau, K., Dunn, S., & Harrold, J. (2014). Reduction of noise in the neonatal intensive care unit using sound-activated noise meters. *Archives of Disease in Childhood. Fetal and Neonatal Edition, 99*, F515–F516. doi: 10.1136/archdischild-2014-306490.

Warren, I., Mat-Ali, E., Green, M., & Nyathi, D. (2019). Evaluation of the Family and Infant Neurodevelopmental Education (FINE) programme in the UK. *Journal of Neonatal Nursing, 25*(2), 93–98. doi: 10.1016/j.jnn.2018.11.004.

Welch, M. (2016). Nurture in the neonatal intensive care unit. *Acta Paediatrica, 105*, 730–737.

White, R. (2010). Single-family room design in the neonatal intensive care unit: challenges and opportunities. *Newborn and Infant Nursing Reviews, 10*(2), 84–86.

White, R. D. (2015). Core measure 4: safeguarding sleep – its value in neuroprotection of the newborn. *Newborn and Infant Nursing Reviews, 15*(3), 114–115.

White, R. D., Smith, J. A., & Shepley M. (2013). *Recommended standards for newborn ICU design* (8th ed.). Committee to establish recommended standards for newborn ICU design. *Journal of Perinatology, 33*, S2–S16. doi: 10.1038/jp.2013.10.

Widström, A-M., Brimdyr, K., Svensson, K., Cadwell, K., & Nissen, E. (2019). Skin-to-skin contact the first hour after birth, underlying implications and clinical practice. *Acta Paediatrica, 108*(7), 1192–1204.

Wilson-Costello, D., & Payne, A. (2021). Long-term neurodevelopmental outcome of preterm infants: epidemiology and risk factors. In: R. Martin, & M. Augustyn (Eds.), *UpToDate*. Walters Kluwer. <https://www.uptodate.com/contents/long-term-neurodevelopmental-impairment-in-infants-born-preterm-epidemiology-and-risk-factors?search> (Accessed 2 March 2022).

CHAPTER 23

LEGAL AND ETHICAL ISSUES IN THE NEONATAL UNIT

LYN FRANCIS AND JANET GREEN

Learning objectives

After reading this chapter you will be able to:

- identify the main legal issues that may arise in neonatal units
- recognise professional accountability issues for health professionals working in neonatal units
- understand ethical principles as they apply to neonatal care
- identify ethical issues related to providing nursing and midwifery care in neonatal units
- discuss the necessity for ethical decision making in neonatal units
- examine the role of the neonatal nurse/midwife in ethical decision making and outline a framework for ethical decision making in neonatal units that can be used by neonatal nurses/midwives.

Key words, terms and abbreviations

assault
battery
civil law
consent
criminal law
ethical decision making
ethical principles
law
legal
negligence
neonatal intensive care unit (NICU)
quality of life (QOL)
trespass
vicarious liability

INTRODUCTION

This chapter will provide an overview of **legal** and **ethical principles** and some common issues that may confront a neonatal nurse or midwife working in a neonatal unit. Although the focus on this chapter is based on law in Australia, the concepts raised are similar to other countries. As discussed by Jones on behalf of the Council of International Neonatal Nurses (COINN, 2019), the role and scope of practice of nurses and midwives who work in neonatal units is complex and varies across the globe, as do the law and ethical standards. As outlined by COINN (2019), guiding framework principles for nurses and midwives working in neonatal units internationally include the inherent requirement to engage continuously in ethical and legal practice.

Neonatal nurses/midwives work in an increasingly complex and litigious work environment and must comply with constantly changing and evolving evidence-based practices. Health professionals in the neonatal unit often make complex decisions that include choices that the neonatal nurse/midwife may morally and ethically disagree with, such as withdrawal of active treatment. Neonatal nurses/midwives need to be aware of possible legal and ethical challenges that may arise in the neonatal setting, and this chapter will provide information and frameworks to assist in this decision making. It is important to understand and reflect upon the impact that ethical dilemmas can have on the ability of the neonatal nurse/midwife to continue working in the neonatal area (Green et al., 2018).

The main legal issues that can occur in the neonatal care unit include:

- a knowledge deficit of law, as applicable to nurses/midwives in the neonatal unit
- medication errors
- privacy and confidentiality
- documentation in healthcare records
- professional accountability issues
- child protection laws and obligations
- viability
- knowledge deficit of criminal law issues and the role and function of the coroner.

COMMON LAW AND CIVIL LAW TORTS APPLICABLE TO NEONATAL NURSES/MIDWIVES

There are two types of **law** in Australia: **criminal law** and **civil law**. Criminal law involves punishing conduct when the rules of behaviour as determined by legislation are breached. Criminal law may apply in the healthcare setting where behaviour is clearly unacceptable and warrants punishment – for example, murder or theft (Forrester & Griffiths, 2015). Civil law involves resolving disputes regarding payment of damages (compensation, usually in the form of money) sought by a person who is claiming personal or property loss or damage (Staunton & Chiarella, 2020).

Sources of law derive from laws made and passed by elected governments (referred to as *legislation* or *statutes*) and judgements handed down from the courts (referred to as *common law*) (Staunton & Chiarella, 2020). In Australia, common law, also referred to as *'judge made law'*, includes civil wrongs to people and property (referred to as *torts*) that include negligence and trespass to the person, such as civil assault (Allan, 2019). In Australia, each state has created legislation (e.g. the *Civil Liability Act* 2002 (NSW)) that has modified common law.

Although health professionals including neonatal nurses and midwives aim to provide the best healthcare available, errors occur that can result in civil action, action by regulatory authorities, coronial inquiries and, occasionally, criminal prosecution. In addition, action may be taken by the professional's employer and professional bodies including the Nursing and Midwifery Board of Australia (NMBA), the Nursing and Midwifery Councils (NMC) in Australia, the Nursing or Midwifery Councils of New Zealand (NCNZ, MCNZ) or similar international councils and boards. Australian civil law evolved from English common law. Civil matters relevant to neonatal nurses/midwives may include professional negligence, lack of consent resulting in **trespass** to a person comprising civil assault, battery or false imprisonment (also referred to as *wrongful imprisonment*).

Consent and trespass to person

In neonatal units, the people from whom **consent** is sought to deliver care to the neonate are usually the parents. Competent adults (those who have the capacity to make their own decisions, which generally does not include minors aged less than 18 years) have the right to make their own autonomous decisions regarding whether they consent, or refuse to consent, to healthcare (Kerridge et al., 2013). The word 'consent' comes from the Latin word *consensure* meaning 'to agree'. The term 'consent', rather than 'informed consent', is more consistent with terminology used in Australian law (Kerridge et al., 2013), although neither term fully describes the complexity inherent in decision making between healthcare professionals and patients (Kerridge et al., 2013). In situations when parents are emotional and/or under considerable stress, providing written information, or recording conversations, is useful so they can digest complex information and make considered decisions. Swaney et al. (2021, p. 1172) believe that if parents are at risk of not understanding the information they need in order to make a difficult decision about their baby, due to such stressors, then 'uncontested paternalism' may result, and informed consent may just be a token. If no consent is obtained (whether verbal, oral or implied) prior to a procedure, action may be taken for civil assault or battery.

Assault is the deliberate and unlawful touching of another person. This may be even the slightest touch, and it does not have to be hostile in intent. **Battery** is when the person is touched without their consent. This would include touch to the neonate when consent is not obtained from the parent or guardian. There does not need to be actual harm caused to the patient for legal action to be taken for torts alleging 'trespass to the person' (Allan, 2019).

Consent is a legal defence to allegations regarding assault, battery or false imprisonment (Staunton & Chiarella, 2020). Consent is not generally required in an emergency or urgent situation if the treatment provided is needed to save that person's life or prevent severe and long-lasting damage (Allan, 2019). For consent to be considered valid, it must be given by the parent(s) or guardian without coercion, fraud or pressure applied by the members of the healthcare team. In addition, adequate information about the risks associated with the proposed procedure must be provided to a parent or legal guardian so that an informed decision may be made (Staunton & Chiarella, 2021). Parental decision making in relation to the neonate must be in the infant's best interests and, if there is disagreement between parents and health practitioners treating the neonate, the issue may be taken to court (Forrester & Griffiths, 2015).

CASE STUDY

23.1

Olivia is a neonatal nurse with 5 years' experience practising in the neonatal unit. Liam was born preterm at 23 weeks' gestation and has been progressing reasonably well. Olivia has been caring for Liam for the fortnight since he was born. Liam's mother, Katrina, has no current partner. Liam develops necrotising enterocolitis (NEC), and his entire large bowel is affected. Liam requires urgent surgery for a perforated bowel.

Katrina does not agree with the decision for surgical intervention, and is fearful Liam may require a blood transfusion, which she is opposed to as she is a Jehovah's Witness.

Consider the following:

1. What are the legal and ethical issues regarding Liam?
2. In Olivia's professional capacity as Liam's neonatal nurse/midwife, how might she approach this issue in order to provide support to Liam and his mother?

In Case Study 23.1 Liam, as a neonate, lacks the capacity to understand the nature and consequences of any decisions regarding his healthcare, so his mother, Katrina, as his legal guardian (we can assume Katrina has been identified as the decision maker) (Forrester & Griffiths, 2015), needs to be provided with adequate information to make an *informed decision* about whether to consent to Liam's surgery and the need for a blood transfusion. Katrina has the right to withhold consent to treatment. However, if Liam's condition is rapidly deteriorating and he urgently requires surgery and a blood transfusion to save his life or prevent further deterioration, *consent may not be required*. The 'doctrine of emergency' essentially provides the health professional with a justification *against* assault and battery for the treatment given at the time of the emergency (Allan, 2019; Staunton & Chiarella, 2020).

Negligence

Nurses/midwives are increasingly held accountable for their practice and must justify and accept accountability for their actions. **Negligence** may be intentional or unintentional and can be described as an absence of due care that was a departure from the standards of accepted practice at the time the incident occurred (Foley & Christensen, 2016). For example, a nurse or midwife in the neonatal unit could be accused of being negligent when they fail to identify that an intravenous cannula has dislodged, resulting in infiltration of medication into the surrounding tissues causing a third-degree burn to a neonate in their care. The neonatal nurse, or midwife, is unlikely to be negligent if found to be practising at a level that was widely accepted, by a significant group of other respected nurses or midwives, as competent professional practice under the circumstances (Langslow, 2014).

Negligence is a distinctly different civil tort than the torts of trespass to a person previously discussed. When a neonate suffers damage following a medical procedure, then the parents may seek legal advice regarding a potential negligence claim. In civil cases, including negligence, the person *seeking a claim* for damages is referred to as the 'plaintiff' and the person alleged to have *caused* the harm is referred to as the 'defendant' (Staunton & Chiarella, 2020).

Four basic elements need to be established before negligence can be proven. Firstly, it needs to be established by the plaintiff (e.g. the neonate's parent or guardian on behalf of the neonate who would usually seek a lawyer to represent them) that there was a duty of care owed. Secondly, that the appropriate standard of care was breached. Thirdly, that the breach caused harm or damage to the neonate. Lastly, that the damage resulting was reasonably foreseeable with no defences that may excuse the negligent behaviour of the defendant (Allan, 2019).

Regarding Case Study 23.1, Olivia has a duty of care to Liam, Katrina and to others who may be impacted by any of her actions, or inactions. In Australia the common-law position regarding duty of care is cited in the *Rogers versus Whitaker* case (1992) 175 CLR 479, where it was stated: 'The law imposes ... a duty to exercise reasonable care and skill in the provision of professional advice and treatment'. The context of the standard of care will vary according to whether the situation relates to treatment or providing information.

In most cases it is accepted by the court that all health professionals owe a duty of care to their patient. In a hypothetical situation as in Case Study 23.1 where negligence may be alleged against Olivia, the court would determine whether the standard of care by Olivia was below the standard expected of a registered nurse who has been practising in a neonatal unit for 5 years. To determine the standard of care, expert witnesses (who would include other respected neonatal nurses or midwives) may be called to provide evidence in court. The court will determine whether it was reasonable for Olivia to have acted as she did at that point in time, or whether the care provided was below the standard that would be expected of a neonatal nurse/midwife practising in a neonatal unit (Miller, 2016).

If a health practitioner, including a nurse such as Olivia outlined in Case Study 23.1, was found to be negligent, the hospital, being her employer, will usually be held *vicariously* liable for any harm caused.

The doctrine of '**vicarious liability**' is a common-law doctrine that imposes legal liability on a person or organisation for the wrongdoing of another, although how this is applied varies across jurisdictions. If vicarious liability does apply, the liability and financial consequences may be transferred to the hospital, resulting in the hospital's insurance company paying out any successful damage claims to the plaintiff (i.e. Katrina, the mother, in the hypothetical case study). However, this does not mean that the health practitioner will not still be held *personally* liable for any wrongdoing (Staunton & Chiarella, 2020). The hospital would most probably act to discipline and possibly terminate the health practitioner's employment and make a report to professional bodies including the NMBA or NMC (see professional issues below).

MEDICATION ERRORS

Medication errors occur more commonly in neonatal units than in adult wards, with the neonate particularly vulnerable to further risk of harm following such errors (Antonucci & Porcella, 2014). As suggested by Antonucci and Porcella (2014), the increased risk of medication errors is due to the neonatal environment itself, with current prevention strategies based on those used in adult wards rather than being tailored to the neonatal care environment. Smaller medication doses, unfamiliar equipment and distractions have been reported to increase medication errors (Hewitt et al., 2015) relevant to the busy and noisy neonatal unit.

Hospitalised neonates are at greater risk of harm caused by medication errors owing to their small size, physiological immaturity and poor medication metabolism and excretion by the immature liver and kidneys (Antonucci & Porcella, 2014). Failure to follow protocols resulting in incorrect or missed doses of medications and errors in documentation, often due to factors in the working environment, have also been linked to incidents involving neonatal units (Alghamdi et al., 2021). For example, protocols for administration of medications via peripheral intravenous catheters (PIVCs) are inconsistent, which increases the risks of infection and skin complications in neonates (August et al., 2019).

EVIDENCE-BASED PRACTICE RESEARCH 23.1

A literature review reported that the most common medication errors in neonatal units were incorrect doses (over-dosing or under-dosing), followed by medications given to the incorrect patient (Krzyaniak & Barjorek, 2016). As Currie (cited by Langslow, 2014, p. 199) stated, 'Drug errors are usually caused by failure to monitor a highly routine action'.

Medication errors are one of the most reported health events in Australia and internationally (Isaacs et al., 2020). While nurses/midwives have a duty to update and maintain their medication knowledge (Langslow, 2014), nurse/patient ratios and high workloads have been associated with medication errors in recent research (Isaacs et al., 2020). There are various legislative and policy requirements that must be followed by nurses/midwives regarding safe management and administration of medications. Nurses/midwives must have a thorough understanding of potential problems and how to minimise the risk of errors and the resulting damage caused by potential medication issues (Staunton & Chiarella, 2020). The Australian Commission on Safety and Quality in Health Care develops standards and guidelines regarding healthcare provided to the Australian public, with action plans that include protecting the public from medication errors. Protection of the public includes maintaining the privacy and confidentiality of the neonates and their families cared for in neonatal units.

PRIVACY AND CONFIDENTIALITY

It is a professional requirement and common-law duty that neonatal nurses/midwives respect confidential information disclosed to them by parents in the neonatal unit, and indeed in all areas of nursing and midwifery practice. There are also legislative provisions in place that provide for the protection of confidential healthcare records. There are exceptions to the rule where confidential information may be lawfully disclosed, including situations requiring mandatory reporting of notifiable diseases, child protection or where the disclosure may be held by the court to be in the public interest (Forrester & Griffiths, 2015). There may be a request by third parties for access to healthcare records – for example, a request for a healthcare report on a neonate you are caring for by a court or relatives. In all cases the patient or, in the context of the neonate, the parent or guardian needs to consent to providing this information (Staunton & Chiarella, 2020).

The NMBA (2018) provides clear guidelines regarding the requirement to uphold the duty of confidentiality, which is included in the code of conduct for nurses (2018) principle 3.5 'The requirement for nurses to have ethical and legal obligations to protect the privacy of people', similarly the code of conduct for midwives (2018) principle 3.5, which includes ethical and legal obligations to protect the confidentiality and privacy of women in their care. The domain for nurses and midwives under the applicable codes of conduct to abide with principle 3 regarding cultural practice and respectful practice for nurses and midwives also includes the legal obligation to abide by social media policies and standards for practice regarding use of social media (NMBA, 2016, 2018).

Green (2017) discussed the critical issues surrounding nurses' online behaviour. Being conscientious of the information we document and the manner in which we record it about the neonates for whom we provide care is a critical component of neonatal nursing and midwifery care.

Nurses and midwives have a professional obligation to promote health and prevent disease, and therefore have an essential role to play in vaccination promotion. However, some nurses and midwives have adopted an anti-vaccination stance and promulgate misinformation about vaccines. Facebook is now considered to be the main vehicle by which these 'anti-vax' groups spread mistruths and misinformation (Smith & Graham, 2019). Some nurses and midwives have also joined these anti-vaccine groups on Facebook, offering advice and discouraging vaccination. Nurses and midwives are not qualified to offer a medical opinion, and they have a clear role in health promotion and education. A recent publication by Green et al. (2022) outlined examples of medical advice given by nurses and midwives on Facebook and included a nurse who stated, 'she identified herself as a midwife and told mothers in a premature baby group that vaccinating prem [premature] babies could ruin their immune system'. In another example, 'she urged mothers of prem [premature] babies to avoid all vaccines'. In another Facebook post, a midwife stated that a fellow midwife in a group for pregnant women 'spoke of avoiding the influenza vaccine during pregnancy, as well as declining vitamin K and the hepatitis B vaccine consent for the baby. I'll be honest, I considered reporting her.' (S431). Regulatory authorities such as the NMBA have taken disciplinary action against nurses and midwives who have promoted anti-vaccination via social media, considering it a breach of their professional obligations.

BOX 23.1 **Guidelines for writing progress reports in case notes**

- Always write your own reports and *never* write on behalf of another health practitioner.
- Reports should always be accurate, concise and brief.
- Only write what you personally observed – write what you saw, not what you *think* you saw.
- Record whether a parent or guardian refuses treatment.
- Write legibly, and always check if you do not understand what someone else has written – also check with computerised programs as typographical errors can still occur and auto spell checks may create problems.
- Record the actual time an incident occurs, or a treatment is given – it is not acceptable to make the time up later.
- Be careful of using acronyms, medical jargon and abbreviations.
- Ensure you write in the correct neonate's record.
- Do not use liquid correcting fluid for errors but put a line through the incorrect entry and then initial it before continuing (e.g. 'sleeping[LF] not sleeping at 22:00 when oxygen saturations recorded').
- It is important to remember when using electronic health documents that, if you change any notes written by you or someone else, it will be recorded with your name. Electronic systems can be taken back to the original notes and a comparison can be made between the original notes and the changed notes.

Sources: Forrester (2011); Langslow (2014); Staunton and Chiarella (2020).

CASE STUDY

23.1 (...CONTINUED...)

Olivia posts a photo of Liam on Facebook and Instagram and says 'Liam's a fighter. I love looking after this little cutie'.

A few days later a man arrives at the hospital demanding to see his son, Liam, who he had not seen since birth. Katrina (Liam's mother) is furious with Olivia for posting the photo of Liam on the internet. Apparently, Liam's father saw the photo through a friend's Facebook account.

Olivia did not obtain consent from Katrina to post the photo.

3. Consider some of the professional issues regarding this situation. The publication by Green (2017) will be helpful as the issues have been explored in that paper.

DOCUMENTATION IN HEALTHCARE RECORDS

The critical nature of communication, including written documentation, cannot be overstated, with research indicating that inadequate documentation contributes to medication errors (Hewitt et al., 2015). Effective documentation of patient records is also critical for providing an account of neonatal care and treatment and may be used as evidence in pending or future legal action or in complaints to regulatory bodies (Forrester, 2011).

Box 23.1 contains a summary of tips that may be useful in guiding documentation practice.

PROFESSIONAL ACCOUNTABILITY ISSUES IN THE NEONATAL UNIT

In Australia the *Health Practitioner Regulation National Law Act* 2009 (Qld) (the 'National Law Act') is the law governing the regulation of health professionals and has been enacted in each participating jurisdiction in Australia. The Australian Health Practitioner Regulation Authority (AHPRA) (2020a) under the National Law Act has responsibilities that include supporting the operation of the NMBA (Forrester & Griffith, 2015). Other countries have similar laws in place governing the regulation of health practitioners.

Professional regulation of nurses/midwives in Australia is administered by the NMBA. The primary role of regulatory bodies in Australia is keeping the public safe, a role that includes the regulation of nursing and midwifery education and requirements for registration.

If a nurse or midwife does not adhere to the procedures, actions and processes within their own scope of practice, action may be taken by their employer and the regulating authority. The Australian College of Neonatal Nurses (ACNN) (2019) also provides competency standards and ethical guidelines expected of nurses/midwives working in neonatal units.

Unsatisfactory professional conduct and professional misconduct

The role of regulatory bodies in Australia and other countries includes registration standards, ongoing development of codes and guidelines, accreditation of training providers and handling complaints and notifications about nurses and midwives. Complaints and notifications may include concerns about the conduct of a nurse or midwife if there is a risk to public safety, health issues that may impair the ability of a nurse or midwife to practise safely or where there are concerns about clinical practice or competence (Staunton & Chiarella, 2020).

In Australia, complaints may be reported by anyone including the general public, or other health workers, to the AHPRA (2020b) directly or to local co-regulatory bodies such as the Health Care Complaints Commission in NSW or the Health Ombudsman in Queensland (Forrester & Griffiths, 2015). Under the National Law Act (section 140), health practitioners are mandated to report certain notifiable events including unsafe practice such as intoxication while on duty, placing the public at risk of substantial harm due to impairment, practising below accepted professional standards (Staunton & Chiarella, 2020) and sexual misconduct (AHPRA, 2020b). When a registered health practitioner practises below the standard acceptable to the profession, disciplinary action may be commenced (Forrester & Griffiths, 2015). The disciplinary process may include further investigation, no further action, immediate action to protect public safety or referral to applicable bodies such as tribunals or health panels (Forrester & Griffiths, 2015). If nurses/midwives are accused of serious professional misconduct, this may result in the loss of their professional registration. In 2019–20 the most common complaints regarding nurses were in relation to inadequate clinical care, health impairment and other issues including medications (AHPRA, 2020b). Another mandatory reporting role required of nurses/midwives working with neonates includes reporting infants who are at risk of significant harm from their parents or guardians.

CASE STUDY

23.1 (...CONTINUED)

Olivia, a registered nurse, has been late for work and was observed by her RN colleague Susan, to be somewhat vague and forgetful on some of her shifts in the neonatal unit.

Susan witnesses Olivia taking medications surreptitiously out of her locker during lunch break. Olivia later makes an incorrect medication calculation for a routine medication – fortunately, Susan was checking the dose with Olivia and promptly corrected the error.

4. Does Susan have an obligation to report Olivia's behaviour?
5. Consider who might be at risk, as well as the mandatory reporting obligations.

CHILD PROTECTION

There are various statutes in Australia – for example, the *Children and Young Persons (Care and Protection) Act* 1998 in NSW) – regarding protection of the child including the neonate. There are situations when children need to be removed from their parents without consent. Consent for children who are subject to care and protection orders is made by the relevant government minister or delegated person and is usually managed by Family and Community Services in Australia. If a neonatal nurse holds a reasonable suspicion that a neonate is at risk of significant harm, including neglect or abuse, there is a requirement to notify the relevant government department (Staunton & Chiarella, 2020). There is limited research regarding neonatal units and their role in child protection; however, Saltmarsh and Wilson (2017) reported that nurses working in neonatal units have a significant role in identifying and referring neonates at risk of harm, particularly preterm and sick neonates, who spend a considerable period of time in the neonatal unit. Research has identified that removal of infants from their mothers following a report to child protection agencies may be traumatic for the mother and family, as well as the nurse or midwife involved (Marsh et al., 2019).

Viability

When a neonate is born between the ages of 23 weeks and 0 days and 24 weeks and 6 days, it is generally accepted that the decision whether or not to resuscitate the neonate should be made in consultation with parents and consultant specialists; however, this issue is complex particularly if there is no consensus between parents and health professionals (Gillam et al., 2017). It is beyond the scope of this chapter to fully debate the issues; however, there are cases when it is determined that treatment should not be started (be withheld), such as neonates at the borderline of viability deemed too young, too immature or too unwell to survive. Alternatively, it has been suggested that a decision to withhold treatment may be postponed until a collaborative decision is made to either provide active treatment or withdraw life support, once it has been determined that the neonate will or will not survive, or will be damaged from treatment (Syltern et al., 2021). This issue is relevant to neonatal nursing and midwifery staff, who may be involved in discussions with neonatal specialists and the parents regarding the assessment of gestational age and decision making regarding resuscitation (Wilkinson et al., 2009). Options for neonates born in the 'grey zone' include providing comfort only (for infants at 22 weeks' gestation), providing full **neonatal intensive care unit (NICU)** support (from 24 weeks), or a trial of management adjusted to the response to resuscitation and intensive care (at 23 weeks' gestation), depending on the parents' wishes (Department of Health, 2019). Providing meaningful outcome data to parents is a challenge, and ethical issues associated with beneficence and non-maleficence come into play. In addition, there may be a requirement for a neonatal nurse/midwife to provide evidence to a coronial investigation following the death of a neonate in the neonatal unit. For example, there has been a coronial investigation of a neonate born alive after a termination of pregnancy at 21–22 weeks' gestation where a midwife was called to give evidence following the death of the infant after 80 minutes of life (Langslow, 2014; Office of the State Coroner, 2000). Although this matter involved a midwife in a labour ward, it may be relevant to future care in neonatal units.

CRIMINAL LAW ISSUES

Civil law as discussed in relation to torts (*civil wrongs*) is about personal or property issues between citizens. The standard of proof is the balance of probability and, if successful, the plaintiff may be awarded damages, usually financially. On the other hand, criminal law is a legal action between the state (represented by the 'prosecution') and a citizen, with punishment including a fine or possible jail term if the accused is found to be guilty beyond reasonable doubt. In criminal actions the police or prosecution needs to prove that the neonatal nurse/midwife not only committed the criminal act but also *intended* to do that act. In most cases where nursing actions result in harm to a patient, this is done negligently with no intention to do so and is dealt with under civil law (Staunton & Chiarella, 2020).

THE ROLE OF THE CORONER

The Coroner's Court investigates reportable deaths, which include those where the identity of the deceased is unknown, the death happened in suspicious, violent or unnatural circumstances, the death occurred in care (including police custody or during police operations) and/or the death was related to healthcare (Staunton & Chiarella, 2020). This would include 'reportable' deaths that occur in the neonatal unit. Once a death is reported, the coroner must investigate the circumstances of the death to establish the identity of the deceased, details of when, where and how they died and the medical cause of death (Staunton & Chiarella, 2020). The legislation varies in each state and territory of Australia (Staunton & Chiarella, 2020) but, where a neonate in the neonatal unit dies unexpectedly, and/or the cause was unknown, this would be a 'reportable death', and the coroner would be notified. The coroner may investigate the death depending on the circumstances and then may hold a 'coronial inquest'. A coronial inquest will attempt to find out what happened and will make recommendations based on findings following this investigation to avoid similar issues recurring. The coroner will also consider whether there is any public interest to be served in holding an inquest and provide recommendations to improve patient care and to help prevent future accidents – for example, revised guidelines for use and correct positioning of umbilical venous catheters following the death of a premature infant in a neonatal unit in the United Kingdom (Dyer, 2021).

The role of the coroner is not to apportion blame or guilt (Langslow, 2014). If a nurse or midwife is called to be a witness for a coronial inquest, the healthcare record will also be used to substantiate what is said by the witness. It is essential that documentation include a clear description of clinical problems as they arise, in addition to actions taken or not taken and the reasons why. It is also suggested that the most pertinent points of discussions with the parents be recorded (Langslow, 2014). If a neonatal nurse/midwife is called to be a witness or requested to provide a statement regarding their role in circumstances regarding a death, it is suggested that legal advice be sought (Forrester & Griffiths, 2015).

Ethical principles

To practise neonatal nursing and midwifery in an ethically sound professional manner, it is necessary to balance ethical considerations with professional values, common law and relevant legislation. Ethical principles provide a generalised framework within which particular ethical dilemmas may be analysed; therefore, these principles can provide guidance in resolving ethical issues.

Autonomy

The ethical principle of *autonomy* refers to self-determination. Neonates in the neonatal unit do not have the ability to make choices; therefore, they require a surrogate, usually their parents. In order for parents to take their legitimate place in the decision-making framework, they require the provision of the best-available evidence-based information in a format and language they can understand. The disclosure of objective and truthful information is important for valid consent. The law gives parents much scope in decision making for their infants; however, parental autonomy is not absolute. Parents are expected to make decisions based on the best interests of their infant; however, at times conflicts arise between parents and clinicians about what constitutes the infant's best interest. Parents and clinicians have complex value systems, which may clash, with all parties believing that their alternative is the most compelling. Clinicians need to consider the cultural and religious values of the families in their care, and work with families to help them determine the best care for the neonate and family (Hendson et al., 2015).

Beneficence

Beneficence is action that is performed for the benefit of others, or acts guided by compassion (Stanak, 2019). In relation to neonatal care, beneficence involves balancing the benefits of treatment against the risks of harm. Clinicians need to consider beneficence from the perspective of the family and their cultural and religious beliefs. An example would be the case of the extremely preterm neonate who has suffered a grade IV intraventricular haemorrhage (IVH). The evidence (Hinojosa-Rodríguez et al., 2017) suggests that ultrasound and functional MRI (fMRI) technology used by expert clinicians can predict the outcome for neonates; therefore, this grade of haemorrhage is significant and would be grounds to consider withdrawal of curative treatment (Sheehan et al., 2017). Giving parents the best-available information on the long-term consequences of a grade IV IVH demonstrates beneficence towards the family and its situation. A confounder of beneficence is the unpredictability and uncertainty associated with the outcomes of extreme prematurity (Green et al., 2015a). Outcome data provide an understanding of outcomes for cohort groups, but not individual neonates; therefore, determining the outcome for an individual neonate is difficult (Green et al., 2018). Neonatal clinicians need to support and respect parents' decisions even when disagreements occur. Healthcare workers must be skilled and work within their scope of practice in order to deliver high-quality, safe care befitting their qualifications and experience.

Non-maleficence

Non-maleficence means non-harming or inflicting the least harm possible to reach a beneficial outcome for the neonate in the neonatal unit. The problematic part of non-maleficence is that harm, though unintentional, often accompanies life-saving treatment in the neonatal unit. Consider again the extremely preterm neonate of 23 weeks' gestation who will undergo multiple painful procedures in the course of their treatment. The long-term effects of unrelieved pain have been well documented (Riddell et al., 2015), and the effects of inflicting pain on these neonates have also been documented by Green et al. (2016) as being a source of distress for neonatal nurses and midwives. It is important to balance the principles of beneficence and non-maleficence by determining the best interest of the neonate considering the iatrogenic effects of the treatment provided in the neonatal unit. Working within scopes of practice, reporting the negligent care performed by others and not coming to work when excessively tired, or sick, also protects the vulnerable neonate from harm.

Futile care in the neonatal unit refers to care that either prolongs suffering of the neonate, does not improve his or her quality of life or fails to achieve a good outcome (Borhani et al., 2015). Schneiderman (2011) defines 'futility' as the unacceptable likelihood of achieving an effect that the patient has the capacity to appreciate. Consider the case of the extremely preterm neonate with a grade IV IVH who is unresponsive but on full life support. In this case, where the prognosis is poor, prolonging treatment is a violation of the principle of non-maleficence, while the withdrawal of treatment and the institution of palliative care and allowing a peaceful death would be in keeping with the principle of non-maleficence. Withdrawing curative treatment minimises harm to the infant and prevents prolongation of treatment that could burden the neonate.

Justice

Justice refers to fairness, entitlement and equality. Clinicians in the neonatal unit may question the principle of justice when confronted with neonates of parents whose values and lifestyles bring them into conflict with those of the treating team. Consider the desperate parents of an extremely preterm neonate who have had 9 years of infertility and multiple in-vitro fertilisation (IVF) cycles (Green et al., 2015b). Their infant might not survive and is nursed in an isolette next to a robust neonate whose mother is addicted to cocaine. This neonate is suffering severe withdrawal and is under a care and protection order from community services. In this situation, clinicians experience conflict and question the ethical principle of justice. It needs to be emphasised that the treating team, regardless of the circumstances, must provide quality, compassion and humane care to both neonates and treat both families with dignity and respect. Neonatal care is expensive, and the principle of justice is supported by impartial decision making when it comes to a fair distribution of resources.

Ethical issues arising in neonatal care

Parents and neonatal staff as individuals are made up of complex value systems, and this individual approach to how they live their lives and make decisions can make conflict inevitable. It also means that parents and clinicians may differ in how they approach and respond to ethical dilemmas, interpret medical data and statistics and what they consider to be in the best interests of the neonates in the neonatal unit. Clinicians should reflect on their own moral and ethical beliefs to help them discover the potential issues of conflict, while remembering that their own moral beliefs are not necessarily important when trying to determine the best interests of others. It is important that clinicians avoid bringing their value systems to discussions about the best interests of others (Green et al., 2018).

Withholding versus withdrawing treatment

Making decisions regarding neonatal survival requires a consistent and coordinated approach to individual cases by obstetric and neonatal teams and parents. Despite some confusion, ethically, the withholding and the withdrawal of life-sustaining treatment are equivalent (Ursin, 2019), inasmuch as a determination has been made that survival is not in the neonate's best interest, and the neonate will die. However, there is a difference *medically* between withholding and withdrawing treatment. It is common practice to resuscitate a neonate at birth and then make decisions after the neonate's response to treatment is determined. There might also be situations when decisions are made by the healthcare team not to resuscitate the neonate; therefore, treatment is withheld. However, if the neonate is resuscitated, following resuscitation, diagnostics and investigations, the clinical picture evolves so more information is available to make decisions. A decision might be made to then withdraw treatment.

There is a lack of consistent clinical guidelines available in Australia to guide parents or health professionals in end-of-life decision making regarding severely disabled or critically ill neonates (Bhatia, 2015a; Bhatia & Tibballs, 2015). Each jurisdiction has different legal requirements and there is not a national or international approach to this issue. If parents and the healthcare team, which may include the hospital ethics committee, do not agree on the best treatment options for a neonate, the intervention of the court may be sought (Bhatia & Tibballs, 2015). Generally, when parents and medical practitioners agree regarding withdrawal or withholding of life-sustaining treatment, the courts are reluctant to intervene (Bhatia & Tibballs, 2015). In 2011 a set of twins were born with one neonate (given the pseudonym of 'Baby D' by the court) having severe irreversible brain damage (Family Court of Australia, 2011). A decision was made by the court to support withdrawal/withholding treatment as being in the 'best interests' of Baby D (Family Court of Australia, 2011).

Although there are general entitlements under the *Family Law Act* 1975 (Cth) (cited by Skene, 2008), there are limits on parental decisions that are not legally sanctioned, including withdrawal or withholding treatment and euthanasia. Parents cannot demand their infant be given particular medical treatments. Parental decisions regarding refusal of consent for treatments that are held to be in the infant's best interests are usually overruled by the courts. While problematic, the courts will determine the best interests of the neonate, and this does not always require that a neonate will undergo treatment even when that may prolong their life (Skene, 2008).

REFLECTION

Charlie Gard was born in 2016 in the United Kingdom and was diagnosed with a rare genetic condition called mitochondrial depletion syndrome, resulting in brain damage and the need for mechanical ventilation to breathe. Charlie's situation became public all over the world as his parents sought funding in January 2017 via the crowdfunding website, GoFundMe, to take their critically ill son to the USA for an experimental treatment that some medical experts suggested might improve his quality of life. Charlie's parents raised over 1.3 million pounds. Charlie's parents challenged the decision by medical experts not to allow Charlie to go to the USA for this untested yet arguably innovative treatment (Wilkinson & Savulescu, 2017). Several court cases followed, with the High Court of Justice (Family Division) finally affirming the decision that it was *not* in Charlie's best interests to undergo the experimental nucleoside therapy, nor for artificial ventilation to be continued (*Great Ormond Street Hospital v Yates & Gard*, 2017). The court held it *was* in Charlie's best interests for artificial ventilation to be withdrawn, allowing Charlie to be given palliative care only. Charlie died 4 days after the lawful withdrawal of treatment just before his first birthday. Charlie's parents were quoted in the media as saying, 'Mummy and Daddy love you so much, Charlie, we always have and we always will and we are so sorry that we couldn't save you' (Australian Broadcasting Corporation (ABC), 2017).

If you were the neonatal nurse or midwife caring for Charlie, would you have supported Charlie's parents in seeking a treatment that may (or may not) have enhanced his quality of life? On reflection, think about how you may have dealt with this situation and some of the challenges here.

PROVIDING DETAILED INFORMATION AND OPTIONS

The provision of detailed information and options is important when having conversations with prospective parents, before the birth of neonates with potentially poor or unknown outcomes (Stanak, 2019). Janvier et al. (2014, p. 38) suggested that the mnemonic SOBPIE might be useful to guide these difficult discussions with families:

S – What is the **S**ituation? Is the infant's death imminent? Should withholding or withdrawing life-sustaining interventions be considered?

O – **O**pinions and options: what are the personal biases of healthcare professionals, and how can their impact be minimised? What are the alternative options for the infant's care?

B – **B**asic human interactions (such as level of parental support).

P – **P**arents – what are their story, their concerns, their needs and their goals?

I – **I**nformation – meeting parental informational needs and providing balanced information.

E – **E**motions – relational aspects of decision making, which include the following: emotions, social supports, coping with uncertainty, adaptation and resilience.

Emotionally, the decision to withhold treatment rather than withdraw it may be harder for parents to accept. When treatment is withdrawn, parents may believe that everything possible has been done to save their infant's life. There is evidence that neonatologists, neonatal nurses, midwives and parents can work together to make compassionate decisions to withhold or withdraw treatment when the burdens of treatment and existence will outweigh the benefits. Examples of when treatment might not be started, discontinued or withdrawn include:

- non-resuscitation of a neonate at birth with a congenital abnormality that is incompatible with survival (e.g. anencephaly)
- non-resuscitation of a neonate born with a confirmed gestational age of 22 weeks or less, where the neonatologist is of the opinion that survival would be associated with severe neurological impairment
- withdrawal of artificial ventilation from a neonate who has suffered birth asphyxia and in whom investigation has revealed profound brain damage (Brecht & Wilkinson, 2015).

It is important for the family to understand that withholding or withdrawing life support does not imply that their infant will not receive comfort and care. The decision should signal a change in focus from active treatment to palliative care, ensuring the neonate is comfortable and pain free. See Chapter 24 for further discussion. The role of nurses and midwives in these circumstances is to provide comfort for the neonate, relieve suffering and help the grieving family (Swaney et al., 2021, p. 1180).

Uncertainty

Major improvements in neonatal care mean that extremely preterm and critically ill neonates have better chances of survival and making a good recovery. However, it can be difficult to predict which neonates will live or die, develop minor or major disabilities or suffer ongoing health problems. The risks of immediate treatment need to be balanced against the uncertainty of the future. As Paris (2005, p. 1415) stated: 'the best one can do ... is to make a human judgement based on probabilities'. The difficulty of uncertainty is that, for many neonates nursed in the neonatal unit, it is not known at the time of resuscitation and commencement of aggressive treatment whether the neonate will benefit by intensive care or be harmed by it (Lantos, 2018). One can only look back retrospectively.

Discussions with families and guiding them to make decisions about whether or not to initiate or continue their infant's treatment are mostly based on predictions of estimated prognosis for mortality and long-term physical and neurodevelopmental outcomes using population-based studies. Recent evidence suggests that predicting a single infant's future based on population statistics is fraught with difficulties (Shinwell, 2015). Parents struggle with uncertainty (Krick et al., 2020), and dealing with the uncertainty of a neonate's prognosis and outcome has been shown to be difficult for neonatal nurses (Green et al., 2015a).

Quality of life

The ability to save the lives of critically ill neonates has increased substantially over the past three decades. This survival, however, can be associated with unfavourable outcomes for both neonate and family (Green et al., 2017). Questions are now being asked about **quality of life (QOL)** for survivors of neonatal intensive care and their families. Use of the term 'quality of life' is almost always controversial (Green et al., 2017). Diminished QOL is a frequent consideration in shaping the boundaries of medical intervention. Quality of life is rightly deemed to be an important consideration in high-technology neonatal care, yet it is notoriously difficult to determine or predict. QOL is a broad multidimensional concept that usually includes subjective evaluations of both positive and negative aspects of life (Green et al., 2017). The purpose of QOL determinations is to decide when a life lacks sufficient quality that it ought not to be lived. QOL is both objective and subjective, and one of the major problems with considering QOL is the question of how this is defined and by whom (Green et al., 2017). It should be remembered that QOL should not be about making judgements regarding the value or worth of a particular life (Green et al., 2017).

When considering the outcomes of neonates in the neonatal unit, it is important that the families are provided with truthful and balanced information. Message framing has been discussed by Marmion (2018), who showed that neonatologists may impart information to parents that frames the message of potential survival in positive terms so that parents will be guided to choose resuscitation or continued treatment as being in their infant's best interest. The author used a vignette of an extremely immature neonate (Marmion, 2018). Alternatively, they may be given a message from the neonatologist that potential survival of their infant will have negative outcomes (Marmion, 2018). Families should receive balanced information about their infant's survival and long-term outcome. Parents should be given an opportunity to ponder what a diagnosis means for them, their family and their future and the integration of their infant and child into society (Janvier et al., 2016). Families should be told about the positives as well as the negatives. Midwives and neonatal nurses have a key role in helping families during these difficult times. One of the best ways that they can provide help is to ensure the family has access to the most up-to-date information that is currently available and that involves directing parents to reputable internet sites.

Best interests

At its most basic, the 'best-interests' standard has an ethical and legal basis for decision making involving neonates, infants, children and other 'incompetent' persons (persons who lack capacity, e.g. minors) who cannot make their own decisions. Despite the best-available treatment, some neonates will survive neonatal intensive care with multiple and severe disabilities. When considering the withdrawal of treatment, decisions need to be made to determine the benefits and burdens for the infant. Decisions will impact on the family so a contemporary definition of best interests must include the family, as they have the most to gain and the most to lose from the impact of these decisions (Collura & Wolfe, 2015).

Our current society is pluralistic, and it is inevitable that health professionals will encounter families whose views about childbearing and rearing differ widely; however, this does not necessarily make them wrong. When considering best interests, medical professionals have been given the legitimate position of arbiters of what is best for a neonate; however, the family may see the situation differently. A commitment to the best interests of the neonate without considering the needs, values and perspectives of the family, may put medical professionals into conflict with the neonate's family (Raho, 2016). A non-judgemental approach and understanding of how the parents' values shape their decisions will be helpful for neonatal nurses and midwives.

Treatment versus experimentation

Research has allowed neonatology to push forwards successfully during the past 20 years. Research outcomes have enabled many extremely preterm neonates and other sick neonates to live; however, questions need to be asked about where the line between research and experimentation begins and ends (Green, 2007). There has been a historical reluctance on the part of neonatologists to insist that every new treatment be subjected to rigorous clinical trials before adopting it (Silverman, 1987). The use of a promising treatment spreads rapidly and widely, but the formal testing follows far behind, by which time the damage has been done (Silverman, 1987). There is no doubt that research and experimentation are essential because contemporary neonates nursed in the neonatal unit have reaped the benefits of research on previous generations of sick neonates. Candee et al., as early as 1982, found that neonatologists' attitudes towards unsalvageable cases in the neonatal unit were influenced by the possibility of potential research. Green (2007) found that research that was likely to benefit a particular infant, as opposed to future infants, was acceptable to the neonatal nurses in her study. Herein lies the difference between therapeutic research and non-therapeutic research. Therapeutic research is designed to benefit the subjects under investigation, while non-therapeutic research might benefit similar patients in the future (Kaye, 2019).

Parents of neonates diagnosed with a complex congenital heart anomaly, such as hypoplastic left heart syndrome (HLHS), are faced with the challenge of choosing the best treatment option for their infants. Parents must decide among options of compassionate care, palliative reconstructive surgery or neonatal cardiac transplantation and, additionally, after an antenatal diagnosis, must decide whether to continue the pregnancy (Sullivan et al., 2015; Wei et al., 2015).

With experimentation and ongoing research, a treatment regimen can become accepted practice, and HLHS is a case in point. HLHS is a complex and rare congenital heart defect present at birth where the left side of the heart is critically underdeveloped. Fifteen years ago, parents were advised to either terminate the pregnancy or be provided with compassionate palliative care. A three-stage repair (Norwood, Glenn and Fontan procedures) is now offered (Kane, 2015).

Although this three-stage procedure is now fairly standard, ethical concerns continue to be raised about the short- and long-term outcomes. Mortality associated with the Norwood procedure remains the highest among common congenital heart procedures, ranging from 5% to 20% (Kaplinski et al., 2020), and resource utilisation for HLHS is associated with the highest cost and the third longest length of stay. Between discharge after hospitalisation for the Norwood procedure and re-admission for the stage II procedure, the interstage mortality was 10.8% (Kaplinski et al., 2020). The outcomes for neonates are concerning, with infants at 1 year of age having a significant incidence of neurodevelopmental and motor functioning disabilities (Davidson et al., 2015).

Parents of children with HLHS reported more-negative impacts of the child's illness on the family and more parenting stress. These children and their families experience the stress of multiple surgical procedures spaced over 2–4 years. These children are at higher risk of behavioural problems, which may make them more challenging to parents (Davidson et al., 2015).

CASE STUDY 23.2

Emily, a term infant born with HLHS, has had a Norwood procedure and is being cared for in the special care neonatal unit, with an aim to send her home with her parents. Emily's parents have relocated from the country to the city, which has taken them away from their support network. They are now living in a unit near the children's hospital. The cardiac surgical team want the family to be close to the hospital because, after the Norwood procedure, infants still have an inefficient parallel circulation and risk sudden death due to inadequate cardiac output, particularly in the early postoperative period (Alghamdi et al., 2011). The staff members are teaching Emily's parents about the unique needs of the infant with HLHS in relation to minimising energy expenditure and providing the appropriate nutrition to meet Emily's needs for energy and growth. They are also helping Emily's parents to recognise the signs and symptoms that would require her re-hospitalisation.

1. Olivia, the RN from the first case study, wonders whether Emily's parents were aware of the treatment for HLHS and what it entails – extensive hospitalisation after the Norwood procedure, a high mortality rate within the first year of life and a high risk of poor neurodevelopmental outcome – and thus whether they really gave informed consent to surgery. What are your thoughts?
2. Olivia also thinks that it would be a good idea for Emily's parents to talk to other parents to appreciate what they will be facing, and what their baby will be going through, before choosing the staged surgical interventions for HLHS. Despite improvements, the surgery is still referred to as palliative and not curative.

Do the outcomes justify the means?

Allocation of scarce resources provokes much discussion, mostly because all countries have finite resources for their health budget, making it inevitable that increasing demands for high-technology care are not able to be met. In countries like Australia and New Zealand, taxation contributes to a basic level of healthcare. However, an ageing population contributes to decreasing levels of available taxation (Bhatia, 2015b).

The neonatal unit costs are relatively small in the big picture of Australia's and New Zealand's healthcare costs. Research has focused nearly exclusively on the costs of the initial hospitalisation of the neonate, with less research conducted on the financial outlay to support ongoing care beyond hospitalisation (Cheah, 2019). These added costs associated with providing the medical, educational and social needs of extremely preterm neonates and term newborns with ongoing needs are often not discussed with parents early in the infant's care (Muraskas & Parsi, 2008). This cost does not consider the possible lifetime care required by some of these children, or the economic cost to the family and on society (Cheah, 2019). Extant research has shown that families of a severely disabled infant are less likely to have other children (Reichman et al., 2008). The burden incurred by these families can be substantial (Shahat & Greco, 2021) and the ongoing overall costs to the household can be ten times higher compared with those for a normal term neonate (Gibson & Harrison, 2010).

Hope for a good outcome means that families may be drawn to the 'feel good' miracle infant stories in the popular press (Green et al., 2015c). 'Miracle baby' stories in the popular press are a regular occurrence and these reports are often the first source from which the general public learns about advances in medicine (Green et al., 2015c) and the outcomes of extremely preterm neonates and other neonates cared for in the neonatal unit. Green et al. (2015c) outlined that, unless the journalist has a science or medical background, the reports might encourage false hope and unfounded optimism for the survival and outcome. The use of sensationalist language implying breakthroughs and cures has the potential to influence the behaviour, beliefs and expectations of the public, without providing a full understanding of the implications of the extremely preterm infant's survival on the family and society (Green et al., 2015c). The article by Green et al. (2015c) provides an understanding of these implications for neonatal nurses and midwives and how they should approach 'miracle baby' stories.

ROLE OF THE NEONATAL NURSE/MIDWIFE IN ETHICAL DECISION MAKING

Ethical issues in the neonatal unit can be complex and challenging for clinicians. Clinicians can help families with **ethical decision making** by being familiar with the current best evidence for treatment and outcomes and the legal guidelines. Being up to date with treatment options and outcomes data helps to provide families with the best information available so they take part in the discussions. Høye and Severinsson (2010) explored intensive care nurses' experiences of conflicts related to situations when they encountered culturally diverse families of critically ill patients. Extrapolation of this research shows that consideration and respect of the cultural and religious beliefs of families is important, as is staff members recognising their own inherent beliefs and biases and ensuring that such beliefs and biases do not cloud their judgement. This type of objectivity could help to reduce ethical conflicts in the neonatal unit. Nurses and midwives are advocates for the neonate, providing care that minimises suffering and avoids unnecessary pain. They are a voice for parents, and must respect parents' decisions as long as they are rational and defensible.

Moral distress as a consequence of ethical decision making

Many neonatal nurses and midwives have at times felt that they were caring for a sick neonate in the neonatal unit when it may not have been in the neonate's best interests to continue aggressive therapy, and that life support should be withdrawn. At these times, neonatal nurses and midwives have felt that their ethical and moral principles were confronted (Janvier et al., 2007). The professions of nursing and midwifery were both founded on the moral obligation to care for others, and nurses and midwives are guided by moral decision making in their daily practice (Haddad & Geiger, 2021). Their failure to live up to their moral obligations results in moral distress, and every episode of moral distress is assumed to leave 'moral residue' (Hardingham, 2004), which is the emotional and physical response that remains with nurses and midwives after dealing with a moral dilemma. The concept of moral distress was originally defined by Jameton (1984, p. 6) as 'painful feelings and/or psychological disequilibrium that occurs when nurses are conscious of the morally appropriate action a situation requires but cannot carry out that action because of institutionalized obstacles'. Moral distress 'occurs when nurses are unable to translate their moral choices into moral action' (Hylton Rushton, 2006, p. 161). Accumulated moral distress can have a profound effect on nurses and can be responsible for their seeking alternative employment (Hylton Rushton, 2006). Hylton Rushton (2016) has proposed that moral resiliency is essential when nurses are managing moral distress.

A FRAMEWORK FOR ETHICAL DECISION MAKING

One approach to consider in ethical decision making has been provided by Kerridge et al. (2013), and this could be used by the neonatal nurse/midwife faced with an ethical dilemma.

1. Clearly state the problem – recognise the ethical issue and differentiate it from medical, social, cultural and legal issues.
2. Get the facts – what are the relevant facts of the case? What are the results of investigations? What facts are not known? What is important for the neonate/family?
3. Consider the fundamental ethical principles – autonomy, beneficence, non-maleficence, justice.
4. Identify ethical conflicts.
5. Evaluate alternative options – how would the problem look from another perspective? (Which option will yield the 'most good' and do the 'least harm', respects the rights of those involved, treats people equally or is proportionate to their needs? Which options serve the community rather than an individual?)
6. What does the law say?
7. Make the ethical decision – justify how you came to your decision, document your decision.
8. Reflect on and evaluate the decision and the outcome – what have I learned from this situation?

Another useful model called the 'Zone of Parental Discretion (ZPD)' (McDougall et al., 2016) might also be considered, particularly when parents and health professionals disagree about medical treatment options for a sick neonate. This ethical tool focuses on decision making and subsequent potential harms to the infant (McDougall et al., 2016). The ZPD is a welcome alternative model of decision making that also incorporates a range of factors including long-term prognosis rather than focusing on the gestational age (McDougall et al., 2016).

Caring for the care givers

It is inevitable that neonatal nurses and midwives will experience ethical dilemmas when caring for neonates in the neonatal unit. Decreased viability and burgeoning technology have contributed to these dilemmas (Green, 2007). Neonatal nurses/midwives could benefit from the opportunity to explore their experience of ethical dilemmas through the provision of clinical supervision. Clinical supervision is the process of two or more professionals meeting formally with the aim of supporting clinicians and helping them learn from their experience. Through a process of reflection and education, the neonatal nurse/midwife can also discuss difficult situations and ethical dilemmas. The benefits of clinical supervision have been documented as improved clinical competence and increased job satisfaction and confidence (Cruz et al., 2015).

Resilience is also needed to help care-giving staff to recover from setbacks and distressing situations such as ethical and moral dilemmas. Hart et al. (2014) outline strategies used by nurses to build resilience, which include cognitive reframing, toughening up, emotional toughness and emotional detachment, grounding connections and work–life balance, critical reflection and reconciliation. A focus on the positive rather than the negative aspects helped the nurses stay focused on the bigger picture in relation to patient care, and what constituted a good outcome.

CONCLUSION

This chapter has provided an overview of some of the legal and ethical issues that may be experienced by a neonatal nurse or midwife in a neonatal unit in Australia or other common-law countries. An understanding of the legal and ethical issues associated with neonatal care is essential for neonatal nurses and midwives. The complexity of the legal and ethical issues in neonatal medicine means that neonatal nurses/midwives who care for sick neonates and their families will be confronted with, and experience, ethical and legal dilemmas as their own values are challenged. Consequently, they need a working knowledge of the relevant law and ethics as they contribute to, and implement, decisions about initiation, withdrawing and withholding of treatment, and support the family in the process.

Recommended Reading

Australian Commission on Safety and Quality in Health Care. Medication safety: <http://www.safetyandquality.gov.au/our-work/medication-safety>

Australian Health Practitioner Regulation Agency (AHPRA) and related guidelines: <https://www.ahpra.gov.au/Search.aspx?q=Guidelines>

Australian Health Practitioner Regulation Agency (AHPRA) (2020). Guidelines: Mandatory notifications about registered health practitioners: <https://www.ahpra.gov.au/Search.aspx?q=Mandatory+notifications+about+registered+health+practitioners>

Australian Institute of Family Studies, Legislation in Australia and children at risk (2021). <https://aifs.gov.au/cfca/publications/australian-legal-definitions-when-child-need-protection>.

Negligence and nursing case study (based on Australian law): Foley, M., & Christensen, M. (2016). Negligence and the duty of care: a case study discussion. *Singapore Nursing Journal, 43*(1), 7–11.

Patient documentation: Forrester, K. (2011). A nuts and bolts' guide to effective patient documentation. *The Queensland Nurse, 30*(2), 26–27.

Perils and pitfalls of social media for nurses: Green, J. (2017). Nurses' online behaviour: lessons for the nursing profession. *Contemporary Nurse, 53*(3), 355–367. doi: 10.1080/10376178.2017.1281749.

Online Resources

Legal advice for nurses and midwives

See, for example, the Nurses Association of NSW, <https://www.nswnma.asn.au/> (or your local or international association or union.

References/Acknowledgements

Alghamdi, A. A., Baliulis, G., & Van Arsdell, G. S. (2011). Contemporary management of pulmonary and systemic circulations after the Norwood procedure. *Expert Review of Cardiovascular Therapy, 9*(12), 1539–1546.

Alghamdi, A. A., Keers, R. N., Sutherland, A., Carson-Stevens, A., & Ashcroft, D. M. (2021). A mixed-methods analysis of medication safety incidents reported in neonatal and children's intensive care. *Pediatric Drugs, 23*(3), 287–297.

Allan, S. (2019). *Law and ethics for practitioners*. Sydney, NSW: Elsevier.

Antonucci, R., & Porcella, A. (2014). Preventing medication errors in neonatology: is it a dream? *World Journal of Clinical Pediatrics, 3*(3), 37–44.

August, D., Ullman, A. J., Rickards, C. M., & News, K. (2019). Peripheral intravenous catheter practices in Australian and New Zealand neonatal units: a cross-sectional survey. *Journal of Neonatal Nursing, 25*, 240–244.

Australian Broadcasting Corporation (ABC). (2017). Charlie Gard: 'Beautiful little boy' at heart of UK legal dispute dies, 29th July. <www.abc.net.au/news/2017-07-29/charlie-gard-beautiful-little-boy-at-heart-of-dispute-dies/8755714> (Accessed 22 February 2022).

Australian College of Neonatal Nurses (ACNN). (2019). *Australian standards for neonatal nurses* (4th ed.). Camperdown, NSW: Australian College of Neonatal Nurses.

Australian Health Practitioner Regulation Agency. (2020a). *Annual report 2019/2020*. <https://www.ahpra.gov.au/Publications/Annual-reports/Annual-Report-2020.aspx> (Accessed 22 February 2022).

Australian Health Practitioner Regulation Agency (AHPRA). (2020b). Guidelines: Mandatory notifications about registered health practitioners. <https://www.ahpra.gov.au/Search.aspx?q=Mandatory+notifications+about+registered+health+practitioners> (Accessed 22 February 2022).

Bhatia, N. (2015a). *Critically impaired infants and end of life decision making: resource allocation and difficult decisions*. Abingdon, Oxon: Routledge.

Bhatia, N. (2015b). Cutting the cord: can society over-invest in extremely premature and critically impaired neonates? *Journal of Law and Medicine, 23*(2), 443–456.

Bhatia, N., & Tibballs, J. (2015). Deficiencies and missed opportunities to formulate clinical guidelines in Australia for withholding or withdrawing life-sustaining treatment in severely disabled and impaired infants. *Bioethical Inquiry, 12*, 449–459. doi: 10.1007/s11673-014-9572.

Borhani, F., Mohammadi, S., & Roshanzadeh, M. (2015). Moral distress and perception of futile care in intensive care nurses. *Journal of Medical Ethics and History of Medicine, 8*, 2.

Brecht, M., & Wilkinson, D. J. (2015). The outcome of treatment limitation discussions in newborns with brain injury. *Archives of Disease in Childhood. Fetal and Neonatal Edition, 100*(2), F155–F160.

Candee, D., Sheehan, T. J., Cook, C. D., Husted, S. D. R., & Bargen, M. (1982). Moral reasoning and decisions and dilemmas of neonatal care. *Pediatric Research, 16*, 846–850.

Cheah, I. G. S. (2019). Economic assessment of neonatal intensive care. *Translational Pediatrics, 8*(3), 246.

Collura, C., & Wolfe, J. (2015). From goals of care to improved family outcomes in the neonatal intensive care unit: determining the intervention. *Journal of Palliative Medicine, 18*(2), 94–95.

Council of International Neonatal Nurses (COINN). (2019). News page. *Journal of Neonatal Nursing, 25*(5), 258–264.

Cruz, S., Carvalho, A. L., & Sousa, P. (2015). Clinical supervision and emotional intelligence capabilities: e excellence in clinical practice. *Procedia-Social and Behavioural Sciences, 171*, 153–157.

Davidson, J., Gringras, P., Fairhurst, C., & Simpson, J. (2015). Physical and neurodevelopmental outcomes in children with single-ventricle circulation. *Archives of Disease in Childhood, 100*(5), 449–453.

Department for Health and Wellbeing, Government of South Australia. (2019). South Australian perinatal practice guideline. Perinatal care at the threshold of viability. <https://www.sahealth.sa.gov.au/wps/wcm/connect/8ddf798042ac004d9f11bfad100c470d/Perinatal+Care+at-+the+Threshold+of+Viability_PPG_v2_0.pdf?MOD=AJPERES&CACHEID=ROOTWORKSPACE-8dd-f798042ac004d9f11bfad100c470d-nGEP68S> (Accessed 28 February 2022).

Dyer, C. (2021). Coroner calls for new guidance on umbilical venous catheters after baby's death. *British Medical Journal, 372*, n290. doi: 10.1136/bmj.n290.

Family Court of Australia. (2011). *Re: Baby D (No. 2)* [2011] FamCA 176. <http://www.austlii.edu.au/au/cases/cth/FamCA/2011/176.html> (Accessed 28 February 2022).

Foley, M., & Christensen, M. (2016). Negligence and the duty of care: a case study discussion. *Singapore Nursing Journal, 43*(1), 7–11.

Forrester, K. (2011). A nuts and bolts' guide to effective patient documentation. *Queensland Nurse, 30*(2), 26–27.

Forrester, K., & Griffiths, D. (2015). *Essentials of law for health professionals* (4th ed.). Sydney, NSW: Elsevier.

Gibson, A. T., & Harrison, C. M. (2010). The consequences for society of intensive care for babies born at less than 30 weeks' gestation. *Paediatrics and Child Health, 20*(4), 167–170.

Gillam, L., Wilkinson, D., Xafis, V., & Isaacs, D. (2017). Decision-making at the borderline of viability: who should decide and on what basis? *Journal of Paediatrics and Child Health, 53*, 105–111.

Great Ormond Street Hospital v Yates and Gard [2017] EWHC 1909 (Fam). <www.judiciary.gov.uk/judgments/great-ormond-street-hospital-v-yates-and-gard-24-july-2017/> (Accessed 28 February 2022).

Green, J. (2017). Nurses' online behaviour: lessons for the nursing profession. *Contemporary Nurse, 53*(3), 355–367. doi: 10.1080/10376178.2017.1281749.

Green, J., Darbyshire, P., Adams, A., & Jackson, D. (2015a). Balancing hope with reality: how neonatal nurses manage the uncertainty of caring for extremely premature babies. *Journal of Clinical Nursing, 24*(17–18), 2410–2418. doi: 10.1111/jocn.12800.

Green, J., Darbyshire, P., Adams, A., & Jackson, D. (2015b). Desperately seeking parenthood: neonatal nurses reflect on parental anguish. *Journal of Clinical Nursing, 24*(13–14), 1885–1894. doi: 10.1111/jocn.12811.

Green, J., Darbyshire, P., Adams, A., & Jackson, D. (2015c). The myth of the miracle baby: how neonatal nurses interpret media accounts of babies of extreme prematurity. *Nursing Inquiry, 22*(3), 273–281. doi: 10.1111/nin.12095.

Green, J., Darbyshire, P., Adams, A., & Jackson, D. (2016). It's agony for us as well: neonatal nurses reflect on iatrogenic pain. *Nursing Ethics, 23*(2), 176–190. doi: 10.1177/0969733014558968.

Green, J., Darbyshire, P., Adams, A., & Jackson, D. (2017). Quality versus quantity: the complexities of quality-of-life determinations for neonatal nurses. *Nursing Ethics, 24*(7), 802–820. doi: 10.1177/0969733015625367.

Green, J., Darbyshire, P., Adams, A., & Jackson, D. (2018). Neonatal nurses' response to a hypothetical premature birth situation: what if it was my baby? *Nursing Ethics, 25*(7), 880–896. doi: 10.1177/0969733016677871.

Green, J., Petty, W., Whiting, L., Orr, F., Smart, L., Brown, A.-M., et al. (2022). 'Blurred boundaries': when nurses and midwives give anti-vaccination advice on Facebook. *Nursing Ethics, Feb 10*, 9697330211041749. doi: 10.1177/09697330211041749. [Online ahead of print.]

Green, J. A. (2007). Balancing hope with reality: caregiving dilemmas for neonatal nurses in caring for extremely premature babies. (PhD thesis.) Adelaide, SA: Flinders University.

Haddad, L. M., & Geiger, R. A. (2021). Nursing ethical considerations. *StatPearls*. Treasure Island, FL: StatPearls Publishing. <https://www.statpearls.com/articlelibrary/viewarticle/92/>. (Accessed 28 February 2022).

Hardingham, L. (2004). Integrity and moral residue: nurses as participants in a moral community. *Nursing Philosophy, 5*, 127–134.

Hart, P. L., Brannan, J. D., & De Chesnay, M. (2014). Resilience in nurses: an integrative review. *Journal of Nursing Management, 22*(6), 720–734.

Hendson, L., Reis, M. D., & Nicholas, D. B. (2015). Health care providers' perspectives of providing culturally competent care in the NICU. *Journal of Obstetric, Gynecologic and Neonatal Nursing, 44*(1), 17–27. doi: 10.1111/1552-6909.12524.

Hewitt, J., Tower, M., & Latimer, S. (2015). An education intervention to improve nursing students' understanding of medication safety. *Nurse Education in Practice, 15*, 17–21.

Hinojosa-Rodríguez, M., Harmony, T., Carrillo-Prado, C., Van Horn, J. D., Irimia, A., Torgerson, C., et al. (2017). Clinical neuroimaging in the preterm infant: diagnosis and prognosis. *NeuroImage: Clinical, 16*, 355–368. doi: 10.1016/j.nicl.2017.08.015.

Høye, S., & Severinsson, E. (2010). Professional and cultural conflicts for intensive care nurses. *Journal of Advanced Nursing, 66*(4), 858–867.

Hylton Rushton, C. (2006). Defining and addressing moral distress: tools for critical care nursing leaders. *AACN Advanced Critical Care, 17*, 161–168.

Hylton Rushton, C. (2016). Moral resilience: a capacity for navigating moral distress in critical care. *AACN Advanced Critical Care, 27*(1), 111–119.

Isaacs, A., Ch'ng, K., Delhiwale, N., Taylor, K., Kent, B., & Raymond, A. (2020). Hospital medication errors: a cross-sectional study. *International Journal for Quality in Health Care, 33*(1), mzaa136. doi: 10.1093/intqhc/mzaa136.

Jameton, A. (1984). *Nursing practice: the ethical issues* (p. 8). Englewood Cliffs, NJ: Prentice Hall.

Janvier, A., Nadeau, S., Deschenes, M., Couture, E., & Barrington, K. J. (2007). Moral distress in the neonatal intensive care unit: caregiver's experience. *Journal of Perinatology, 27*(4), 203–208.

Janvier, A., Barrington, K., & Farlow, B. (2014). Communication with parents concerning withholding or withdrawing of life-sustaining interventions in neonatology. *Seminars in Perinatology, 38*(1), 38–46.

Janvier, A., Farlow, B., Baardsnes, J., Pearce, R., & Barrington, K. J. (2016). Measuring and communicating meaningful outcomes in neonatology: a family perspective. *Seminars in Perinatology, 40*(8), 571–577.

Kane, J. M. (2015). Surgical and non-surgical management trends for neonates with hypoplastic left heart syndrome. In: 2015 American Academy of Pediatrics National Conference and Exhibition. <https://aap.confex.com/aap/2015/webprogrampress/Paper30259.html> (Accessed 28 February 2022).

Kaplinski, M., Ittenbach, R. F., Hunt, M. L., Stephan, D., Natarajan, S. S., Ravishankar, C., et al. (2020). Decreasing interstage mortality after the Norwood procedure: a 30-year experience. *Journal of the American Heart Association, 9*(19), e016889. doi: 10.1161/JAHA.120.016889.

Kaye, D. K. (2019). The ethical justification for inclusion of neonates in pragmatic randomized clinical trials for emergency newborn care. *BMC Pediatrics, 19*(1), 1–8. doi: 10.1186/s12887-019-1600-x.

Kerridge, I., Lowe, M., & Stewart, C. (2013). *Ethics and law for the health professions* (4th ed.). Leichhardt, NSW: Federation Press.

Krick, J. A., Weiss, E. M., Snyder, A., Haldar, S., Campelia, G. D., & Opel, D. J. (2020). Living with the unknown: a qualitative study of parental experience of prognostic uncertainty in the neonatal intensive care unit. *American Journal of Perinatology, 38*(8), 821–827. doi: 10.1055/s-0039-3402722.

Krzyaniak, N., & Barjorek, B. (2016). Medication safety in neonatal care: a review of medication errors among neonates. *Therapeutic Advances in Drug Safety, 7*(3), 102–119.

Langslow, A. (2014). *Keep out of court: a medico-legal casebook for midwifery and neonatal nursing*. Malmsbury, Vic: Health Law Education.

Lantos, J. D. (2018). Ethical problems in decision making in the neonatal ICU. *New England Journal of Medicine, 379*(19), 1851–1860.

Marmion, P. (2018). Refusing to examine extremely premature newborns. *Linacre Quarterly, 85*, 9–10. doi: 10.1177/0024363918756390.

Marsh, C. A., Browne, J., Taylor, J., & Davis, D. (2019). Making the hidden seen: a narrative analysis of the experiences of assumption of care at birth. *Women and Birth, 32*(1), e1–e11. doi: 10.1016/j.wombi.2018.04.009.

McDougall, R., Delaney, C., & Gillam, L. (Eds.). (2016). *When doctors and parents disagree: ethics, paediatrics and the zone of parental discretion*. Annandale, NSW: Federation Press.

Miller, L. A. (2016). Offering expert testimony: tips for success. *Journal of Perinatal and Neonatal Nursing, 30*(2), 93–94.

Muraskas, J., & Parsi, K. (2008). The cost of saving the tiniest lives: NICUs versus prevention. *Virtual Mentor, 10*(10), 655.

Nursing and Midwifery Board of Australia (NMBA). (2016). *Registered nurse standards for practice*. <https://www.nursingmidwiferyboard.gov.au/codes-guidelines-statements/professional-standards.aspx> (Accessed 28 February 2022).

Nursing and Midwifery Board of Australia (NMBA). (2018). *Code of conduct for midwives and Code of conduct for nurses*. <https://www.nursingmidwiferyboard.gov.au/codes-guidelines-statements/professional-standards.aspx> (Accessed 28 February 2022).

Office of the State Coroner. (2000). Inquest into the death of Jessica Jane. NTMC 37. <https://justice.nt.gov.au/__data/assets/pdf_file/0017/206702/baby-j.pdf> (Accessed 28 February 2022).

Paris, J. J. (2005). Resuscitation decisions for 'fetal infants'. *Pediatrics, 115*, 1415.

Raho, J. A. (2016). In whose best interests? Critiquing the "family-as-unit" myth in pediatric ethics. In: P. A. Clark (Ed.), *Bioethics: medical, ethical and legal perspectives* (pp. 145–160). Rijeka, Croatia: InTech. doi: 10.5772/66715.

Reichman, N. E., Corman, H., & Noonan, K. (2008). Impact of child disability on the family. *Maternal and Child Health Journal, 12*(6), 679–683.

Riddell, R. R. P., Racine, N. M., Gennis, H. G., Turcotte, K., Uman, L. S., Horton, R. E., et al. (2015). Non-pharmacological management of infant and young child procedural pain. *Cochrane Database of Systematic Reviews, 2015*(12), CD006275. doi: 10.1002/14651858.CD006275.pub3.

Rogers versus Whitaker (1992) 175 CLR 47. <https://staging.hcourt.gov.au/assets/publications/judgments/1992/051—ROGERS_v._WHITAKER—(1992)_175_CLR_479.html> (Accessed 28 February 2022).

Saltmarsh, T., & Wilson, D. (2017). Dancing around families: neonatal nurses and their role in child protection. *Journal of Clinical Nursing, 26*(15–16), 2244–2255.

Schneiderman, L. J. (2011). Defining medical futility and improving medical care. *Journal of Bioethical Inquiry, 8*(2), 123–131.

Shahat, A. R. S., & Greco, G. (2021). The economic costs of childhood disability: a literature review. *International Journal of Environmental Research and Public Health, 18*(7), 3531.

Sheehan, J. W., Pritchard, M., Heyne, R. J., Brown, L. S., Jaleel, M. A., Engle, W. D., et al. (2017). Severe intraventricular haemorrhage and withdrawal of support in preterm infants. *Journal of Perinatology, 37*(4), 441–447. doi: 10.1038/jp.2016.233.

Shinwell, E. S. (2015). Ethics of birth at the limits of viability: the risky business of prediction. *Neonatology, 107*(4), 317–320.

Silverman, W. A. (1987). Human experimentation in perinatology. *Clinics in Perinatology, 14*, 403.

Skene, L. (2008). *Law and medical practice: rights, duties, claims and defences* (3rd ed.). Chatswood, NSW: LexisNexis Butterworths.

Smith, N., & Graham, T. (2019). Mapping the anti-vaccination movement on Facebook. *Information Communication and Society, 22*, 1310–1327.

Staunton, P., & Chiarella, M. (2020). *Law for nurses and midwives* (9th ed.). Sydney, NSW: Elsevier.

Stanak, M. (2019). Professional ethics: the case of neonatology. *Medicine, Health Care, and Philosophy, 22*(2), 231–238.

Sullivan, J., Gillam, L., & Monagle, P. (2015). Parents and end-of-life decision-making for their child: roles and responsibilities. *BMJ Supportive and Palliative Care, 5*(3), 240–248.

Swaney, J. R., English, N. K., & Carter, B. S. (2021). Ethics, values and palliative care in neonatal intensive care. In: S. L. Gardner, B. S. Carter, M. Enzman-Hines, & S. Niermeyer (Eds.), *Merenstein & Gardner's handbook of neonatal intensive care* (pp. 1167–1190). Philadelphia, PA: Elsevier.

Syltern, J., Ursin, L., Solberg, B., & Støen, R. (2021). Postponed withholding: balanced decision-making at the margins of viability. *American Journal of Bioethics, May 17*, 1–12. doi: 10.1080/15265161.2021.1925777. [Online ahead of print.]

Ursin, L. Ø. (2019). Withholding and withdrawing life-sustaining treatment: ethically equivalent? *American Journal of Bioethics, 19*(3), 10–20. doi: 10.1080/15265161.2018.1561961.

Wei, H., Roscigno, C. I., Hanson, C. C., & Swanson, K. M. (2015). Families of children with congenital heart disease: a literature review. *Heart & Lung, 44*(6), 494–511.

Wilkinson, A. R., Ahluwalia, J., Cole, A., Crawford, D., Fyle, J., Gordon, A., et al. (2009). Management of babies born extremely preterm at less than 26 weeks of gestation: a framework for clinical practice at the time of birth. *Archives of Disease in Childhood. Fetal and Neonatal Edition, 94*(1), 2–5.

Wilkinson, D., & Savulescu, J. (2017). After Charlie Gard: ethically ensuring access to innovative treatment. *Lancet, 390*(10094), 540–542.

CHAPTER 24

END-OF-LIFE CARE IN THE NEONATAL UNIT

VICTORIA KAIN AND REBECCA MAY

Learning objectives

After reading this chapter you will be able to:

- discuss the status of neonatal end-of-life care within Australia, New Zealand and globally
- identify the leading causes of neonatal death
- define neonatal 'palliative care', 'end-of-life care' and 'hospice care'
- discuss the comfort needs of the neonate who is dying, including assessing and managing pain, care options and considerations, including environmental, cultural and religious factors
- discuss the support needs of the dying neonate's family, including the facilitation of end-of-life care discussions and preparing families when death is imminent
- describe the support needs of neonatal nurses/midwives and other care givers
- identify the long-term care considerations for families, including bereavement care.

Key words, terms and abbreviations

end-of-life care (EoLC)
life-limiting condition (LLC)
life-threatening condition (LTC)
neonatal palliative care (NPC)
perinatal palliative care (PPC)
quality of life (QoL)

INTRODUCTION

Despite breakthroughs in newborn care that have resulted in a marked reduction in infant mortality, a significant number of babies born with a **life-limiting condition (LLC)** will not survive (Chin et al., 2021). The highly technological environment of the modern neonatal unit with its abundance of life-sustaining medical equipment has allowed the boundaries of viability to increase, and even blur. Despite these technological advances, the increase in margins of viability and care provided by highly skilled health professionals, some neonates will die in the neonatal unit (Kain & Chin, 2020). The care of dying neonates presents health professionals with many practical and ethical challenges. However, withdrawal or withholding of life-sustaining curative treatment should be considered when there is little hope of survival, or when **quality of life (QoL)** is deemed to be unacceptably poor (Soltani Gerdfaramarzi & Bazmi, 2020).

In the latest Australian and New Zealand Neonatal Network report (ANZNN) (Chow et al., 2021) 96.3% of ANZNN registrants survived to be discharged home. These data include babies who were transferred to level II or level I units, as well as those who were transferred to another level III unit and to a children's hospital.

There were 416 newborn deaths in 2019, with 192 occurring in the early neonatal period (within 7 days of delivery). The mortality rate was highest for babies born before 30 weeks' gestation, with the discharge rate increasing week by week from 62.5% for babies born before 24 weeks to 95.2% for babies born at 27 weeks. A lethal congenital abnormality resulted in the death of 0.9% of registrants, with the majority of deaths occurring in babies delivered between 35 and 39 weeks' gestation (Chow et al., 2019). This suggests that there are a number of neonates who are born with LLCs, or at the lowest margins of viability, who would benefit from early intervention neonatal palliative care (NPC).

Definitions

To explore palliative care, it is first necessary to examine the operational definitions and commonly used terminology in this field.

Neonatal palliative care

The neonatal period is defined from birth to 28 days; however, many neonates requiring palliative care exceed this age period. **Neonatal palliative care (NPC)** should be considered in cases where an LLC or **life-threatening condition (LTC)** (see Clinical Practice 24.1) is suspected or diagnosed at birth, because of birth trauma or after failed efforts to sustain life in the neonatal unit. Palliative care may be considered when a neonate is deteriorating despite intensive resuscitation efforts or when ongoing treatment is considered to be burdensome and prolonging suffering.

NPC is an active and comprehensive approach that is an essential component of the neonatal care delivery model. Once a life-limiting, terminal or uncertain condition is identified, this active form of care begins before, during or after birth. It includes a well-planned treatment approach with a multidisciplinary team and collaborative decision making with the family. As the infant's health deteriorates, the benefits of curative therapy are carefully reviewed and weighed against the benefits of transitioning to palliative care. The preferences of the parents are crucial in the decision-making process and are the deciding factor in determining the appropriateness of treatments, whether curative or palliative in nature.

The importance of sustaining QoL while providing ethical and humane treatment that enables a 'good death' is at the heart of NPC. Support for the family, which addresses their spiritual, cultural and emotional needs, is a key component of a palliative care paradigm. The infant's care comprises the relief of suffering through appropriate pain assessment and medication-managed treatment, as well as the management of distressing symptoms during the dying process (Kain & Chin, 2020).

Palliative care includes support for the family both during and after their infant's death. NPC includes memory-making exercises that will aid in the grief process later on. Follow-up care, such as referrals to support groups and bereavement groups, is critical to the grieving process and the family's long-term mental and physical health.

CLINICAL PRACTICE 24.1

When referring to conditions from which a neonate is unlikely to survive, terms such as 'lethal' or 'incompatible with life' for which treatment is 'futile' are often used. It is, however, recommended that clinicians avoid using such terms and suggested that counselling should focus on salient prognostic features instead (Wilkinson et al., 2014).

The following terminology is recommended:

Life-limiting condition (LLC): a condition with no reasonable hope of cure and from which the neonate will be likely to die prematurely (Larcher et al., 2015).

Life-threatening condition (LTC): a condition with a high probability of death due to severe illness, but a chance of long-term survival exists (Larcher et al., 2015). Curative treatment may be considered feasible with the recognition it may fail. LTCs can be further divided into four groups:

- Group 1: conditions in which curative treatment may be feasible but can fail. Palliative care should be offered alongside cure-focused treatment. Such conditions may include neonatal cancers.
- Group 2: conditions in which premature death is inevitable, such as a diagnosis of hypoplastic left heart.
- Group 3: a progressive condition without curative treatment options; treatment should be exclusively palliative care.
- Group 4: irreversible, but non-progressive conditions with complex healthcare needs leading to complications and likely preterm death. Includes conditions such as cerebral palsy and hypoxic ischaemic encephalopathy (HIE) (Larcher et al., 2015).

Dying: the terminal phase of life where death is imminent and likely to occur in hours, days or weeks (Alsuhail et al., 2020).

Quality of life: QoL is critical in any palliative care strategy across the life cycle continuum. The neonatal palliative care literature is replete with the notion that sustaining QoL is the essence of good NPC. QoL encompasses the entire family and must include emotional, spiritual, social and physical aspects of care. It is concerned with alleviating suffering, and hence is a significant component when examining the conceptual definition of NPC and improving the life and dying conditions of the newborn (Kain & Chin, 2020).

Life-sustaining treatment/intervention: treatment or intervention that has the potential to prolong life.

Perinatal palliative care

Perinatal palliative care (PPC) encompasses the care of the fetus/neonate diagnosed with an LLC or LTC during pregnancy. It is a coordinated care plan that includes choices for obstetric and newborn care, with a focus on optimising quality of life and comfort for newborns with a variety of diseases that are considered life limiting in early infancy.

PPC is one of several alternatives along a continuum of care that should be provided to pregnant women with pregnancies complicated by an LLC or LTC, including pregnancy termination and comprehensive newborn resuscitation and treatment. Perinatal palliative care programs are encouraged to be developed by healthcare providers and institutions and may include the following: a formal prenatal consultation, the development of a birth plan, access to other neonatal and paediatric specialties as needed, and support and care during the prenatal, birth and postnatal periods, including bereavement counselling. Once an LTC is suspected antenatally, the principles of informed consent require that pregnant women and their partners/families be provided with information that is comprehensive enough to allow them to make an informed decision about their care (American College of Obstetricians and Gynaecologists (ACOG), 2021).

End-of-life care

End-of-life care (EoLC) is a term generally used for the final stages of palliative care when the illness is prolonged (Kain, 2021). EoLC focuses on preparing for the anticipated death and managing the end stage of a terminal illness, including care during and around the time of death and immediately after the death, and continues into bereavement. EoLC should be instituted when the goals of treatment change and the neonate is recognised as dying (Together for Short Lives, 2017).

Hospice care

Hospice care is the care of the family and the neonate who is no longer receiving life-prolonging curative treatment (Lefkowits & Solomon, 2016). Hospice care can be provided in any place, including the home, assisted living facility or inpatient hospital, and begins after disease treatment has been discontinued and the person is not expected to survive the illness. Hospice care is often provided only when a person's life expectancy is 6 months or less (Kain & Chin, 2020).

THE GOALS OF END-OF-LIFE CARE

The goals of EoLC are to achieve a so-called 'good death' by minimising suffering and optimising QoL for the neonate and the family, regardless of the stage of illness or length of life (Stokowski, 2014). A more comprehensive definition of a good death includes the following: the person receives holistic EoLC; the dying person is treated with dignity and respect; the death is not sudden and unexpected; people are prepared and, ideally, have done some advance care planning; people are aware that someone is dying and openly discuss this; all involved are to work towards achieving the dying person's preferences; the place of death is important; and the person's family are involved (Borgstrom, 2020). These goals can be achieved through open and honest communication; collaboration among the healthcare team and family; access to a qualified interdisciplinary team trained in providing palliative care; effective management of pain and discomfort; environmental changes to facilitate dying with dignity; participation in rituals to meet the spiritual, cultural and religious preferences of the family; and facilitation of memory making and psychosocial support for the parents, siblings and family (Falck et al., 2016; Together for Short Lives, 2017).

Consultation with a dedicated palliative care team can support the neonatal team in providing optimal care for the neonate and ongoing guidance to the family. Discussions with the family should be clearly documented, outlining the goals of care, wishes of the family and any limitations of treatment to alleviate staff anxiety and ensure a good death is achieved in line with the family's wishes and beliefs (Larcher et al., 2015). When death is imminent, treatment goals should be revised to focus on comfort care. The neonate's family requires information, choices, guidance and the reassurance that they will not be abandoned and that the decisions they make will be supported by the healthcare team (Cortezzo & Meyer, 2020).

The family should be educated about what to expect, their role and involvement, with the focus on 'doing' rather than 'stopping' or 'not doing'. Using the words 'death' and 'dying' and avoiding misleading and confusing euphemisms assists the family in coming to terms with the reality of the situation (Rawlings et al., 2017).

Hope is a powerful and important element of palliative care for families; however, hope needs to be balanced and realistic, without giving false hope (Kishimoto et al., 2021). It should be considered appropriate to hope for the best, while planning for the worst.

END-OF-LIFE CARE MANAGEMENT

Palliative care protocols

Evidence-based protocols are available to inform a high standard of palliative care for neonates who are not expected to survive yet, in reality, provision of palliative care to neonates using an evidence-based protocol is ad hoc (Kain, 2016). Although neonatal units may have guidelines in place to manage newborns at the EOL, it is important that these guidelines are based on evidence, and that nurses and midwives have opportunities to access palliative care education (Chin et al., 2021).

EVIDENCE-BASED PRACTICE RESEARCH 24.1

Kyc et al. (2020) investigated institutional and individual barriers to and facilitators of infant palliative care from both a medical and nursing standpoint.

Six facilitators of neonatal palliative care were identified: (1) healthcare team support for palliative care, (2) medical and nursing discipline support for palliative care, (3) agreement that palliative care is as important as curative care, (4) parental involvement in decision making, (5) recognition of the importance of palliative care education and (6) prioritisation of pain relief. Three hurdles to neonatal palliative care were identified: (1) an unsuitable physical setting for delivering palliative care, (2) technical demands and parental demands and (3) the societal notion that babies should not die.

Furthermore, there were disparities in opinions between medical and nursing staff on a number of themes.

PALLIATIVE CARE IN PRACTICE

Palliative care should always be a treatment consideration when it is recognised that aggressive and invasive therapy may not be in the neonate's best interest (Larcher et al., 2015). The individual context for applying palliative care requires that each case for each family in each healthcare setting be explored individually (Embleton & Stephenson, 2020). The way in which health professionals introduce palliative care has a major impact on the way it is perceived by the family. It is often offered as a final option or an alternative to treatment, rather than a specialised field available *alongside* treatment-focused care. Stigma exists within society and healthcare about palliative care, as it is often associated with the end-of-life and terminal phase (Shen & Wellman, 2019). This stigma and confusion makes the idea of palliative care difficult for the family to accept and prevents them from gaining access to therapies and support designed to alleviate symptoms and improve QoL. The term *withdrawal* or *cessation of care* should *never* be used as this can be misinterpreted by parents as giving up or not caring at all (Kain & Chin, 2020). The focus of palliative care is on providing comfort care measures to manage symptoms, minimise suffering and optimise QoL (Kenner et al., 2015).

Palliative care may be considered when the neonate is not responding to intensive therapy and is deteriorating despite all appropriate efforts or in combination with a life-threatening acute event, including non-responsiveness to aggressive resuscitation, repeated resuscitation, severe perinatal brain injury, severe asphyxia, hypoxic ischaemic encephalopathy (HIE), multi-organ failure, overwhelming sepsis, necrotising enterocolitis with subsequent short gut syndrome or inability to wean from extracorporeal membranous oxygenation (ECMO).

Neonates with LLCs should have palliative care measures introduced early *alongside* treatment-focused care. LLCs include:

- chromosomal aneuploidies with complex and life-threatening prognoses:
  - severe metabolic, storage or mitochondrial abnormalities
  - severe types of skeletal dysplasia
- organ system issues:
  - severe CNS malformations (neural tube defects, migrational disorders)
  - hypoxic–ischaemic encephalopathy
  - spinal muscular atrophy type 1 and myotonic dystrophies
  - epidermolysis bullosa
  - Potter's syndrome, fetal oligohydramnios sequence, fetal–neonatal chronic renal failure
  - short-gut syndrome with parenteral nutrition dependence
  - multivisceral organ transplant under consideration (e.g. liver)
- infections and immunological problems:
  - perinatal HIV infection and acquired immune deficiency syndrome (HIV/AIDS)
  - severe combined immune deficiency (SCID)
  - severe perinatal herpes simplex virus (HSV), cytomegalovirus (CMV), toxoplasmosis, or Zika virus with meningoencephalitis or severe encephalopathy
- periviable pregnancy
- severe intraventricular haemorrhage (IVH, grade IV) or periventricular leucomalacia (PVL)
- refractory respiratory failure
- ventilator-dependent BPD
- severe necrotising enterocolitis (NEC) with short gut
- liver failure (Carter, 2018).

Decision making and conflict resolution

There is much debate about the extent and/or appropriateness of parents' involvement in decision making about their baby. Evidence suggests that parents wish to be involved in decision making as they are historically considered the natural surrogate decision makers for the care of their children (Kain & Chin, 2020). It is essential that prospective parents of extremely preterm newborns are informed of the expectations for neonatal survival and outcome, and the risks and benefits of the various approaches to care, as they are responsible for the emotional and financial consequences of the birth (Kain & Chin, 2020). However, Lantos (2018, p. 1852) wrote about the complexity of decision making, and suggested that presenting parents with a standard set of facts does not consider that 'understanding risk information is dependent on relationships, trust, balances between cognitive and affective elements, life experiences, subjective interpretations of decisional outcomes, tolerance of risk/uncertainty and other personal factors'.

Neonatal nurses/midwives play a key role in facilitating decision making, and should be involved in conversations between parents and doctors (Kain & Chin, 2020).

Conflict may arise when there are differing opinions between the staff and parents about decisions being made on behalf of the marginally viable and critically ill newborn (Kain & Chin, 2020).

Empowering parents as the key decision makers on behalf of their infant and ensuring that they are kept up to date on their infant's condition at all times may assist in assuaging conflict between parents and the healthcare team.

Tension may be inevitable when decisions are being made about whether or not treatment is in the neonate's best interests (Kain & Chin, 2020). However, it is imperative for health professionals caring for the neonate and family to utilise best-interest principles as a standard for decision making. Decision making has evolved in ways that have made treatment decisions more, rather than less, difficult. The legal system, health system and technological factors all form this social context for resolving decisions about withholding or withdrawing curative treatment for fragile newborns (Kain & Chin, 2020).

Managing symptoms

Symptom management is the cornerstone of practice in palliative care. The assessment, early recognition and management of symptoms are paramount in improving QoL and achieving a 'good death' for the neonate and family. Symptom assessment and management can be challenging in the neonatal period as the neonate is not able to describe the experience of the symptoms, and the signs of distress and suffering are often subtle (Marc-Aurele & English, 2017). The neonate should be continuously assessed for signs and symptoms of distress and discomfort, and the appropriate management/treatment initiated to provide an optimal level of comfort. Symptom management involves non-pharmacological and pharmacological interventions while providing support to the family.

Pain

Pain is common at the end of life. The neonate should be assessed regularly using a validated pain assessment tool and the appropriate management initiated (Marc-Aurele & English, 2017) (see Chapter 18 for more information).

Non-pharmacological pain control strategies are safe and essential therapies in the NICU for mild to moderate pain. Swaddling, kangaroo (skin-to-skin) care, non-nutritive sucking and massage are among non-pharmacological choices. Following acute episodes of moderate discomfort, such as heel sticks, or oral gastric tube insertion, non-nutritive sucking, with or without the addition of sucrose, can improve pain scores and decrease distress. This effect is produced by boosting endogenous endorphin release. Additionally, a reduction in noxious stimuli – irritant touch, bright lights and noise – should be pursued to alleviate pain and agitation in dying babies. Non-pharmacological pain treatment in the NICU should consider how procedures are performed, when they are performed and whether they are necessary. Following a shift in treatment priorities towards palliation, interventions should be reduced or avoided unless they actually provide comfort or symptom relief for dying neonates. At the EOL, parents should be permitted to hold their newborn as they like (swaddled or skin-to-skin) and should be assisted in providing calming touch, sounds and suckling if deemed beneficial (Carter & Brunkhorst, 2017).

Informed clinicians who have been trained in pain evaluation and management as well as palliative care principles can more confidently support and reassure parents that their loved one is not being abandoned. When treatment aims shift from life sustaining to palliative, professionals should assist parents in understanding and anticipating changes in the baby's tone, colour, perfusion, temperature and attentiveness. It is crucial to explain anticipated changes in the baby's breathing rhythm, and promoting parental use of oral or pharyngeal suction is generally valued. Parents who are followed through this time by staff who can support them in delivering EOL care frequently express gratitude and exhibit less-complicated grieving.

Care givers may express anxiety or feel anxious about delivering various analgesics to a dying infant, especially if palliative care is not 'routine'. There may be an underlying fear that the care giver is contributing to or facilitating the infant's death. In this context, the rule of double effect applies – as long as the aim is to do good, foreseen but unfavourable effects are permissible. If the purpose is to alleviate the dying neonate's pain and suffering, subsequent and inadvertent respiratory depression is ethically permissible. The rule (or doctrine) of double effect derives from the Catholic moral philosophy and theology tradition. Its usefulness in specific palliative care circumstances is not universally agreed upon by doctors and ethicists. While some clinicians remain concerned about pharmaceutical dosing that risks respiratory depression – even at the end of life – it is critical for parents that their dying baby or young infant not experience discomfort (Carter & Brunkhorst, 2017).

REFLECTION

Consider the doctrine of 'double effect': have you been in the situation of administering morphine to a neonate with intractable pain who is not expected to live? You know that by administering the morphine you will alleviate suffering, but you are also concerned that it may hasten the neonate's death.

The doctrine of double effect means that, if doing something morally beneficial for the neonate (alleviating pain) has a morally 'undesirable' side effect (it may hasten death), it would be considered ethically sound to do this, provided that the 'undesirable' side effect was not intended. This is considered true even if you foresee that the 'undesirable' effect will probably ensue (Wholihan & Olson, 2017).

The doctrine of double effect is often used to justify the use of high doses of drugs such as morphine for the purpose of relieving suffering in terminally ill patients, even though it is known that the drugs are likely to cause the patient to die sooner.

Fluids and hydration

Feeding neonates who are dying is emotive and presents challenges in neonatal EoLC. The goal of feeding is to reduce distress from hunger and provide comfort. The benefits versus risks of feeding should be weighed when considering initiating or withholding feeds. Oral feeds should be withheld only if it is believed that the feeds are causing pain or discomfort, or the neonate is at risk of aspiration (Larcher et al., 2015).

If the neonate is demanding feeds, breastfeeding, bottle or small volumes of nasogastric feeds should be offered for comfort. If vomiting is an issue, the feed volume should be reduced.

The administration of parenteral/enteral nutrition/ hydration is rarely indicated as it is considered a medical form of life support (Willems et al., 2014). If the duration between the transition to a palliative approach to care and death is expected to be short, it is reasonable to cease feeds and stop intravenous hydration if it is felt that feeding could cause distress. When withholding of feeds is indicated, the family needs to be reassured that this is done in the best interest of the neonate (Larcher et al., 2015).

Respiratory symptoms

Respiratory distress, irregular breathing and gasping are common in neonates at the end of life. Morphine can be administered to prevent signs and symptoms of air hunger, provide comfort to the neonate and reduce the distress experienced by the family (Foster & Monterosso, 2012). Supplemental oxygen may be considered for comfort. Respiratory secretions are common at the end of life and should be treated only if they are causing distress to the neonate and/or family. Gentle suction should be initiated only if required, and not as routine care. It may be appropriate to consider reducing or stopping feeds to reduce respiratory secretions if the neonate is not demanding feeds. Medications such as hyoscine or glycopyrrolate bromide may be used to manage excessive secretions if other management techniques fail (Mancini et al., 2014).

Other end-of-life symptoms

Medication to control seizures should be continued. The oral or intranasal route is preferred. Constipation commonly occurs as a result of the administration of opioid analgesia. The neonate should be ordered regular aperients such as lactulose or glycerine suppositories (Friedrichsdorf et al., 2022). Gentle passive movements of the lower limbs or abdominal massage can be effective in treating constipation. Urinary retention occurs as a result of opioids administered. Catheters are rarely required. The neonate's bladder should be gently expressed regularly to avoid urinary retention.

Refer to Table 24.1 for suggested medications and dosages that are commonly used for NPC.

Invasive cardiorespiratory monitoring and investigations should be ceased unless the monitoring leads to treatment that improves QoL or assists with diagnosis and symptom management (Foster & Monterosso, 2012). Heart rate can be assessed regularly by auscultating the chest, temperature can be monitored through touch, and the neonate should be observed for changes in condition and signs of distress. Only reversible symptoms should be treated in order to reduce discomfort. All other symptoms should be managed with appropriate assessment and non-pharmacological and pharmacological interventions (Willems et al., 2014).

Supportive care is extremely important in palliative care. All measures should be taken to maintain the comfort of the neonate and reduce distress of the neonate and family. Positioning, pressure area care with the use of an air mattress, gel pillows, skin care, mouth care, basic hygiene, warm wraps, neurodevelopmental care, human contact and skin-to-skin contact should continue.

Symptoms at the end of life are distressing not only for the neonate but also for the family and the staff caring for the neonate. The staff caring for the neonate should understand the signs and symptoms of discomfort and distress. Non-pharmacological and supportive care should be initiated to manage symptoms and make pharmacological management readily available as required. The family should be actively involved in symptom management, and management should be done in accordance with their wishes, goals of care and ethical values (Kenner & Loser, 2016).

Care options, cultural and environmental considerations

Neonatal nurses/midwives have a unique role in integrating the family in care.

Seminal research found that the location of care is equally as important as the *mindset* of the staff caring for the neonate and family (Catlin & Carter, 2002). The attitude of the staff, desire to care for the neonate and family, training, support from management and knowledge of bereavement have a significant impact on the experience of the family (Larcher et al., 2015). It is vital for the healthcare setting to have institutional policies in place that allow staff the flexibility to respond to the parents' wishes. Families should be enabled to have the opportunity to spend time with their infant in the environment that best suits their needs, including staying overnight. The location of care may include remaining within the neonatal unit, relocating to a purpose-built EoLC space, relocating to maternal or paediatric inpatient wards, relocating to a hospice facility

TABLE 24.1 **Suggested medications and dosages commonly used for NPC**			
Medication	Uses	Dosage	Suggested route
Chloral hydrate	Long-term sedation	20–30 mg/kg up to 50 mg/kg 4 times daily	Oral/rectal
Clonazepam	Seizures Status epilepticus	100 μg/kg over 2 min, repeated after 24 h if required	Intravenous injection
Diazepam	Seizures	0.5–1.0 mg/kg repeated after 5 min if necessary	Rectal
Domperidone	Gastro-oesophageal reflux and stasis	100–300 μg/kg 4–6 times daily before feeds	Oral
Glycopyrronium bromide	Control of airway secretions and hypersalivation	40–100 μg/kg 3–4 times daily	Oral
Hyoscine hydrobromide	Control of airway secretions and hypersalivation	250 μg (quarter of a patch to skin) every 72 h	Transdermal patch applied to hairless area of skin behind ear
Loperamide	Diarrhoea	100–200 μg/kg twice daily 30 min before feed. Increase as necessary up to 2 mg/kg in divided doses	Oral
Midazolam	Status epilepticus	300 μg/kg single dose	Buccal
		150–200 μg/kg	Intravenous injection
		1 μg/kg/min, increasing by 1 μg/kg/min every 15 min until seizure is controlled (max dose 5 μg/kg/min)	Continuous intravenous infusion
Morphine	Acute pain/ postoperative	Preterm infant: initially by intravenous injection over at least 5 min, 25–50 μg/kg, then by continuous infusion 5 μg/kg/h adjusted according to response	Intravenous injection and infusion
		Term neonate: initially by intravenous injection over at least 5 min, 50–100 μg/kg, then by continuous intravenous injection 10–20 μg/kg/h adjusted according to response up to 40 μcg/ kg/h	Intravenous injection and infusion
		10 μcg/kg/h	Subcutaneous infusion
	Chronic pain	80 μcg/kg every 4 h adjusted according to response	Oral/rectal
		150–200 μcg/kg every 4 h adjusted according to response	Subcutaneous injection
Omeprazole	Gastro-oesophageal reflux	700 μg/kg once daily orally, increased if necessary, after 7–14 days to 1.4 mg/kg Some neonates may require up to 2.8 mg/kg once a day	Oral
Paracetamol	Pain Pyrexia	Neonate 28–32 weeks' postmenstrual age: 20 mg/kg single dose, then 10–15 mg/kg every 8–12 h as necessary (max dose 30 mg/kg in divided doses)	Oral
		Neonate >32 weeks' postmenstrual age: 20 mg/kg single dose, then 10–15 mg/kg every 6–8 h as necessary (max dose 60 mg/kg daily in divided doses	Oral
		Neonate 28–32 weeks' postmenstrual age: 20 mg/kg single dose, then 15 mg/kg every 12 h as necessary (max dose 30 mg/kg in divided doses)	Rectal
Paraldehyde	Seizures Status epilepticus	0.2–0.3 mL (of pure paraldehyde)/kg (this volume of paraldehyde must be diluted before administration) as single dose, maximum 0.5 mL	Rectal
Phenobarbitone	Seizures Status epilepticus	20 mg/kg	Slow intravenous injection
		Then: 2.5–5 mg/kg once daily Dose and frequency adjusted according to response	Oral/slow intravenous injection
Phenytoin	Seizures Status epilepticus	Initially 20 mg/kg as loading dose, then 2.5–5 mg/kg twice daily, adjusted according to response	Slow injection or infusion
Ranitidine	Gastro-oesophageal reflux	2 mg/kg 3 times daily (max 3 mg/kg 3 times daily)	Oral
		0.5–1 mg/kg every 6–8 h	Slow intravenous injection

Source: data From British National Formulary for Children (BNFc). 2016–2017.

or transferring home. For families who do not want to leave the hospital, relocating to a private, home-like environment within close proximity of the neonatal unit is preferred.

See Box 24.1 for suggestions for this environment; Fig. 24.1 shows examples of a dedicated room for palliative care purposes.

However, some families may not want to leave the neonatal unit and may feel isolated in a private space. If the family wishes to remain in the neonatal unit, measures can be taken to improve privacy including closing curtains, moving to a quieter area or making attempts to reduce the noise level (Zadeh et al., 2018). If transitioning out of the neonatal unit, staff members need to handle this gently and compassionately and demonstrate that care and support in the new environment will continue. For some families, discharge home may be the goal. This can be facilitated with the support of a specialised palliative care team who can put ongoing community supports in place.

Continuity of care is important at the end of life: all efforts should be made to ensure that the neonate and family are cared for by staff with whom they are familiar, and with whom a therapeutic relationship has been built (Falck et al., 2016). Regardless of the location of care, health professionals should foster a positive environment for care in order to reduce the stress level of the family. The surroundings at time of death create powerful memories and can have a lasting impact on the family (Chambers, 2019). Individual institutions need to put standards, policies and guidelines in place to support the provision of family-centred palliative care (Chambers, 2019).

Cultural and religious differences affect communication styles, beliefs, roles, views on death and illness and

BOX 24.1 **Custom built end-of-life care space requirements**

- Home-like environment (warm, welcoming)
- Adjustable lighting
- Adjustable temperature control
- Access to natural light
- View outside
- Items to assist with memory making (music, aromatherapy oils, fragrant room spray)
- Written resources for parents, siblings, extended family
- Play/activity area for siblings
- Bassinette/cot/Moses basket
- Suction/oxygen/air outlets (fixed or portable)
- Large enough to accommodate extended family
- Double bed
- Kitchenette with basic facilities (food, drinks, storage of breast milk)
- Camera with printer
- Library with books about grief and bereavement
- Bath and bath/body products
- Cushions and blankets for family to keep as mementos
- Access to 24/7 staff support

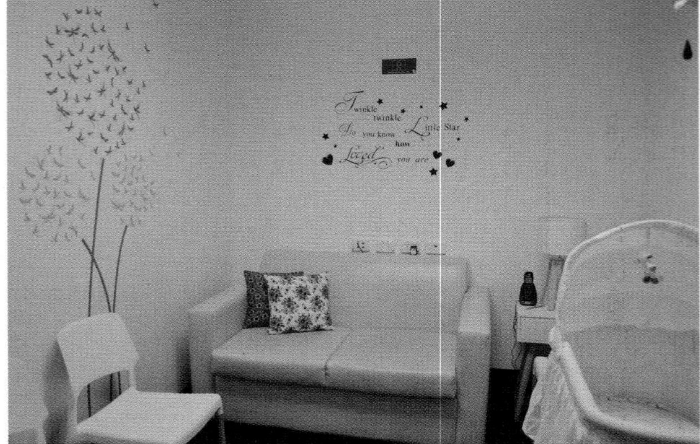
Twinkle
twinkle
Little Star
Do you know
how
Loved
you are
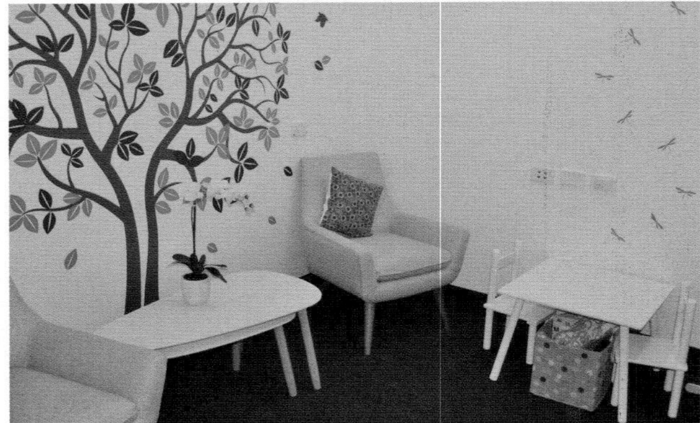
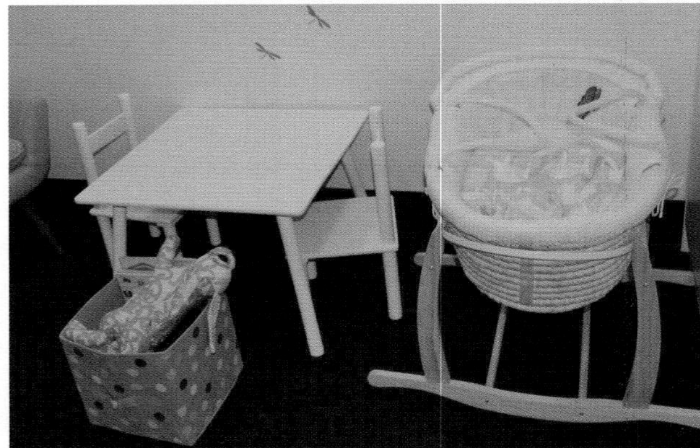

FIGURE 24.1 **Features of a palliative care room**

decision-making approaches (Kain, 2021). Staff caring for the neonate and family need to be mindful of cultural and religious differences and provide culturally sensitive care in order to respect the spiritual needs of the family. Asking open-ended questions can assist nurses/midwives in exploring the specific cultural and religious beliefs and practices important to the individual family (Furtado-Eraso et al., 2021). All families should have access to cultural and spiritual support and the opportunity to practise rituals and ceremonies in line with their beliefs including baptisms and blessings (Carter, 2016).

Historically, some social and ethnic groups view palliative care as a denial of care, and withholding or withdrawing technical support may be considered unacceptable (Catlin & Carter, 2002). Health professionals should handle this compassionately, sensitively and be respectful of the family's beliefs and wishes for their infant. It may be beneficial to offer the family the opportunity to call upon spiritual and cultural leaders to assist with decision making. Health professionals should never make assumptions based on ethnicity or previous experiences with other families (Ryan et al., 2015). Each individual family has very unique cultural and spiritual beliefs and values and these should be explored on an individual basis, free from judgement (Ryan et al., 2015).

Health professionals working in NICU are used to providing sophisticated care using high levels of technology and skill. They may feel challenged when asked to provide palliative care and support the family of the dying neonate (Cortezzo & Meyer, 2020). The culture of intensive care is focused on treatment with the goal of cure, whereas the goal of palliative care is to provide comfort and optimise QoL (Kain & Chin, 2020). However, the neonate receiving palliative care requires highly intensive care focused on comfort and enabling the family to spend time together and build memories in an environment free from the technological demands of the neonatal unit.

IMMEDIATE POST-DEATH CARE OF THE NEONATE

Memory making

Memory making is an important element of EoLC. Seeing, holding and creating memories are important for the family, as mementos are valuable in assisting the family in validating the neonate's life and coping with their grief (Furtado-Eraso et al., 2021; Marchuk, 2016). See Fig. 24.2

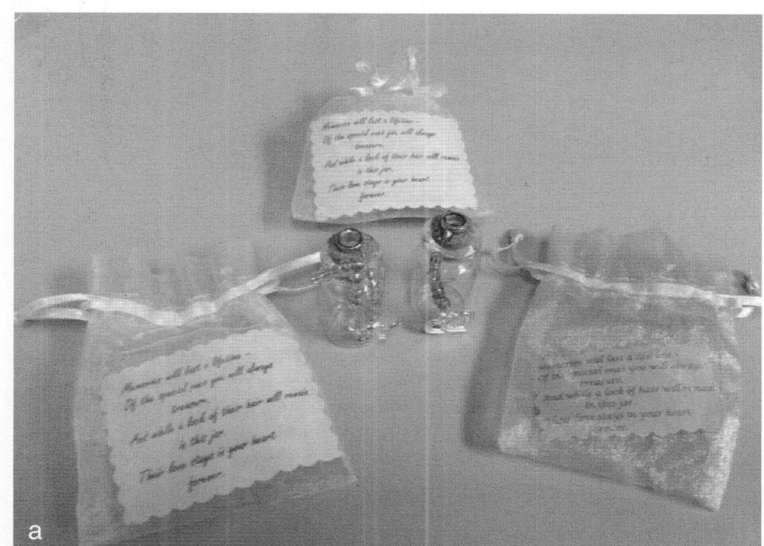

a

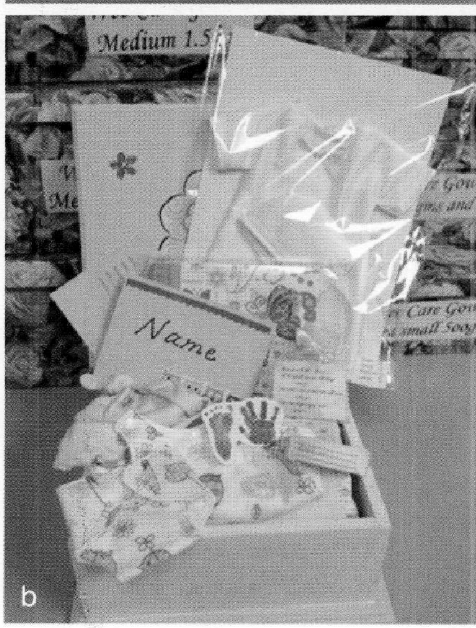

b

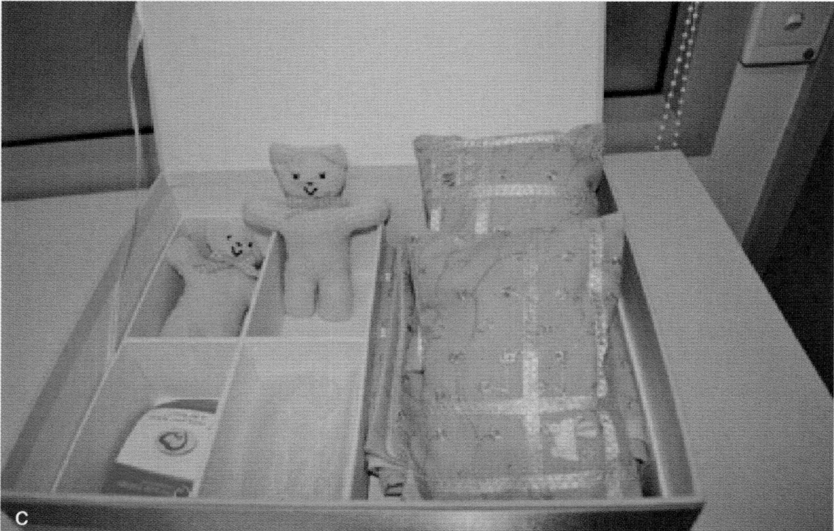

c

FIGURE 24.2 **Examples of memory-making mementos**

for examples of memory-making mementos. The goal of memory making is to focus on the neonate's life, rather than on the death. Memory making should be a positive experience for the family and staff involved and should be integrated throughout the palliative care process, not just at the end of life when death becomes imminent. Healthcare professionals need to facilitate memory making by explaining options available and providing the family with the opportunity to create memories (Chambers, 2019; Marchuk, 2016). With the guidance of the health professionals, families can determine what is valuable and meaningful to them. Memory making is not just about the final product or items, but it is about the process and bond between the neonate and family. Health professionals need to be respectful of this time and enable the family the privacy and space to value this time as a family (Together for Short Lives, 2017). All opportunities should be embraced to create a space for memory making, not only in the physical form but also in the visual form and experiences.

FAMILY-CENTRED CARE 24.1

Memory making includes:

- allowing the family to parent their infant (e.g. nappy changing, bathing, dressing, breastfeeding, massage)
- professional photography
- photographs of the family, experiences, features on the neonate (ears, feet), items in the environment (e.g. cot card, blanket)
- hand and footprints (coloured ink is preferred to black and white)
- hand and footprints on canvas with family members
- hand and foot casts
- hand casts integrating the family – joined hands with neonate and parents
- lock of hair (consider cultural implications)
- neonatal unit memorabilia (e.g. cot card, name tags, clothing worn)
- memory box to store items
- essential oils (aromatherapy)
- music
- experiences (e.g. going outside, zoo, beach)
- cultural and spiritual wishes (e.g. baptism, christening)
- naming ceremony
- photos and experiences with siblings and extended family
- if a multiple birth, time spent with sibling(s)
- diaries and scrapbooking
- special clothing worn (e.g. angel gowns)
- items in the room (e.g. flowers, pictures, scent)
- music and art therapy.

Parental permission is required for memory making. If parents decline, it is recommended that photos be taken and stored in the case notes in the event the family would like them in the future (Furtado-Eraso et al., 2021). In some cultures, memory making is not acceptable; if the family decline for this reason, their beliefs and wishes should be respected at all times (Kenner et al., 2015).

CASE STUDY 24.1

Baby Alex has been in your neonatal unit for several weeks.

He was born at 28 weeks and had an antenatal diagnosis of severe hydronephrosis, an enlarged bladder, polyhydramnios and requiring insertion of a vesico-amniotic shunt. Since birth, he has suffered an intestinal perforation, a recurrent bowel obstruction, numerous suprapubic bladder catheterisations and has had a jejunostomy. He has also been diagnosed with periventricular leucomalacia, bilateral sensorineural hearing loss and chronic lung disease.

After weeks of feed intolerance, he had biopsies that revealed a diagnosis of congenital bladder and bowel myopathy. Other than 0.25 litres of oxygen via a nasal cannula, he no longer requires any other respiratory support, but he is dependent on parenteral nutrition administered through a central line.

After consultation with the team, the decision is made to cease further invasive tests and to cease monitoring as it becomes clear that Alex is dying.

Alex's parents' wish is to spend time with their infant away from the neonatal unit. Discussions between the parents and the medical staff resulted in a decision to continue with parenteral nutrition although it was acknowledged that this could prolong life and delay death.

After 5 and a half months in a neonatal intensive care unit, and following discussion with his parents, he is transferred, still receiving parenteral nutrition, to a children's hospice. This approach allows the parents time with him, with the focus of care on his comfort and QoL.

Alex dies 2 weeks after transfer to the hospice.

1 Explain the philosophy of the hospice model of care

Supporting parents and families

Throughout the palliative and EoLC process, the family should be acknowledged as a crucial part of the interdisciplinary team (Falck et al., 2016). The family should continue to maintain control and be offered choices following their infant's death (Chambers, 2019; Larcher et al., 2015). They may wish to spend time with their infant in the hours following the death, and this should be accommodated and supported by the staff. They should be reassured that almost anything realistic that they wish to do is possible, and that their infant will continue to be cared for with dignity and respect (Chambers, 2019). Conversations and information about preparing for the neonate's death and the time following the death should be initiated early and decisions made documented on an EoLC plan (Together for Short Lives, 2017). A needs assessment can assist in determining the level of support required by the family including the psychosocial, physical, practical and financial needs.

The family should be reassured that they will not be abandoned after the death and that ongoing support for families is available and will be provided for the duration they require (Catlin & Carter, 2002). Parents benefit from discussing the grief process, the way in which it may be expressed and the bereavement process. A spiritual assessment can assist in identifying what gives the family strength at difficult times, and staff should validate the deep feeling of loss experienced by the family.

Verbal and written resources should be provided to parents including for parents, siblings, grandparents and family and friends. Parents could be provided with a teddy bear when departing the neonatal unit as a symbol of not leaving with empty arms. Families may be referred to government and not-for-profit support services and agencies for ongoing bereavement support and follow-up. The type and level of support should be tailored to the needs of the family (Stokowski, 2014). Mothers who have been breastfeeding and/or expressing milk require written and verbal information about lactation suppression and the support of a lactation consultant.

In the months following the death, the family should be provided with the opportunity to meet with the neonatal consultant and a nursing/midwifery staff member who cared for the neonate. This provides the family with the opportunity to ask questions and seek comfort and support from the healthcare staff who cared for their infant. A bereavement card sent from staff in the neonatal unit, a follow-up phone call and health professionals' attendance at funeral services are important ways of validating the neonate's life to the family (Cortezzo et al., 2015).

The social worker is a key member of the multidisciplinary team, and can assist families with financial and emotional support, funeral planning and access to government benefits. The family doctor should be notified of the death by the healthcare team. The interdisciplinary team offers support to the family following the neonate's death, including chaplain and spiritual support, grief and loss counsellor, infant mental health services and specialised palliative care teams.

A mother who remains an inpatient following her infant's death may have a blue butterfly or similar placed on the door to her room and medical charts as a sensitive way to notify staff of the neonatal death (Furtado-Eraso et al., 2021). The surviving sibling(s) of a multiple birth could have a symbol placed on the cot as a sensitive way of identifying a multiple loss. Siblings require ongoing support tailored to their age and developmental stage (Embleton & Stephenson, 2020). Books about death and dying are a helpful way of assisting parents to talk to their children. Referral to art or music therapy and siblings' support groups could be considered.

Support for the healthcare team

Healthcare professionals also require support following the death of the neonate. Neonatal nurses/midwives have reported variable experiences when providing EoLC to neonates and their families. Although all healthcare professionals in the neonatal team will gain confidence with experience, ongoing support is also necessary. Working alongside experienced staff has been demonstrated as highly effective, as have regular debrief sessions (Banaka et al., 2016).

Providing EoLC to neonates and their families can be very intense. It is therefore essential that the healthcare team participating in this form of care have both ongoing support and debriefing after difficult cases from outside experts. Given the stress and potential for grief associated with caring for these neonates, seminal research suggests that care assignments should be voluntary (Catlin & Carter, 2002). Furthermore, research has found that neonatal nurses/midwives deal with grief and feelings of loss routinely, and that senior staff within organisations need to be equipped to assist the healthcare team in understanding the grief process, and to guide appropriate interventions for ongoing staff support (Kain, 2013).

BEREAVEMENT CARE

Long-term considerations

The grief and bereavement journey is unique for each individual. It is an ever-changing phenomenon, experienced and expressed differently by each individual, and can vary in intensity over time (Chambers, 2019). The death of a neonate has a significant impact not only on the parents but also on the entire family, the wider community and the staff providing care to the neonate. Parents grieve for many months and years following the death.

Bereavement following a neonatal death can vary in comparison with the death of a child or adult, in that there is usually less time for anticipatory grief owing to the often-rapid onset and nature of the death (Boyle et al., 2020). This can predispose parents to be at increased risk of developing complicated grief, a type of grief that leads to a chronic, heightened state of mourning (Ravaldi et al., 2018). Everyone views death differently; some families will continue the relationship with the infant after death, while others view death with finality (Ravaldi et al., 2018). Offering the family choices about the type of bereavement support available is vital. The supports offered should be tailored to the individual needs of the family and be flexible to change over time as the needs of the family change. A key worker allocated to support the family in bereavement is essential for assessing and planning bereavement support and connecting the family with appropriate support services. This should continue for as long as the support is required.

Conceiving and child rearing is a central role of human existence and the bond between the neonate and parents is formed well before the birth, with hopes, dreams and goals for the future developed (Kishimoto et al., 2021). The death of a neonate not only has a physical and emotional impact but also impacts on relationships and finances. For some families it can strengthen their relationships and they can find meaning in supporting each other and helping others through fundraising and support groups. Other families can experience a negative response to bereavement if there is conflict, anger or blame, communication breakdowns, discordant coping and a change in intimacy (Boyle et al., 2020).

Furthermore, lack of bereavement support increases the risk of complicated grief and adverse health outcomes for the family. Siblings require unique support and inclusion in the grief experience of the family because strong emotions, including sadness, anger, fear guilt and confusion, can be difficult for children to manage on their own (Nguyen, 2019).

The family should be provided with access to support from a range of interdisciplinary services including social work, chaplain/spiritual care, grief and loss counsellor, not-for-profit organisations, qualified counsellors and psychologists, art and music therapists, a multiple birth coordinator and specialised paediatric palliative care services (Furtado-Eraso et al., 2021). The family should be empowered through awareness of supports available and guided by their key worker throughout their bereavement journey.

FAMILY-CENTRED CARE 24.2

Not-for-profit organisations providing bereavement support include:

- SIDS and Kids, <https://rednosegriefandloss.com.au>:
  - assistance for those who experienced a sudden and unexpected death of a neonate or child during birth, pregnancy or infancy regardless of the cause
  - counselling, parent and family support, peer support, siblings' support, grandparents' support groups, group activities, annual memorial service, telephone counselling and national 24-hour free call bereavement support line.
- SANDS, <https://www.sands.org.au> or <www.sands.org.nz>:
  - miscarriage, stillbirth and neonatal death charity
  - volunteers of bereaved parents supporting bereaved parents. Supports include national phone support line, men's support line, online support (chat service), local group support, email support, quarterly newsletter and annual memorial service.
- Pillars of strength, <https://pillarsofstrength.com.au>:
  - respite and support for fathers
  - support includes access to events for time out, practical and peer support rather than counselling.
- Bears of Hope, <https://www.bearsofhope.org.au>:
  - pregnancy and infant loss
  - parents receive a Bear of Hope prior to discharge donated by another bereaved family to ensure they do not leave the hospital with empty arms; this allows a family to give their infant a lasting legacy while filling the arms of another family as they leave the hospital without their infant
  - support includes written information, parent-led support groups, psychologist-facilitated support groups, private online groups, phone and email counselling, annual community events, access to hope and healing resource library.
- March of Dimes, <https://www.marchofdimes.org>:
  - educate healthcare professionals and the public about best practices
  - support lifesaving research and provide comfort and support to families in NICUs, and advocate mothers and babies.

CONCLUSION

Neonatal nurses/midwives need to continue to strive to improve care for neonates who are not expected to survive, and their families. The healthcare professionals in the neonatal unit need to work together to make a difference in the lives of the neonates they care for who are approaching the end of life. Having a protocol to support evidence-based NPC is imperative in the neonatal unit, and the information in this chapter can assist in the development of such a protocol.

Online Resources

The Butterfly Project: <https://www.neonatalbutterflyproject.org/>:

The butterfly project grew out of a number of research investigations, other projects and clinical experience, including honest feedback from parents. This research investigates the experiences of parents whose infant died, and the health professionals who cared for them, as well as their experiences when one or more babies from a multiple pregnancy died but there was still at least one surviving baby.

Together for Short Lives: <https://www.togetherforshortlives.org.uk/>:

Support healthcare professionals who care for babies, children and young people with life-limiting conditions, and their families. They bring professionals together, share practice and offer resources and tools to support the work with children and families.

The Neonatal Comfort Care Program <http://www.neonatalcomfortcare.com/education>:

The Neonatal Comfort Care Program conducts annual workshops, teaching theory and methods related to the management of newborns diagnosed with life-limiting conditions. It is geared primarily toward nurses.

References/Acknowledgements

Alsuhail, A. I., Duraisamy, B. P., Alkhudhair, A., Alshammary, S. A., & Al Rehaili, A. (2020). The accuracy of imminent death diagnosis in a palliative care setting. *Cureus, 12*(8), e9503. doi: 10.7759/cureus.9503.

American College of Obstetricians and Gynaecologists (ACOG). (2021). Perinatal palliative care. ACOG Committee Opinion (786). <https://www.acog.org/clinical/clinical-guidance/committee-opinion/articles/2019/09/perinatal-palliative-care> (Accessed 27 February 2022).

Banaka, M., Barrington, H., & Holland, N. (2016). Are we looking after our neonatal nursing colleagues? Experiences from an end-of-life care support study. *Archives of Disease in Childhood. Fetal and Neonatal Edition, 101*, A243–A244.

Borgstrom, E. (2020). What is a good death? A critical discourse policy analysis. *British Medical Journal Support Palliative Care, 2020 Jul 6*, bmjspcare-2019-002173. doi: 10.1136/bmjspcare-2019-002173. [Online ahead of print.]

Boyle, F. M., Horey, D., Middleton, P. F., & Flenady, V. (2020). Clinical practice guidelines for perinatal bereavement care – an overview. *Women and Birth, 33*(2), 107–110.

British National Formulary for Children (BNFc). 2016–2017. (2018). London: British Medical Journal, RCPCH Publications /Royal Pharmaceutical Society of Great Britain. © BMJ Group.

Carter, B. S. (2016). More than medication: perinatal palliative care. *Acta Paediatrica, 105*(11), 1255–1256.

Carter, B. S. (2018). Pediatric palliative care in infants and neonates. *Children, 5*(2), 21.

Carter, B. S., & Brunkhorst, J. (2017). Neonatal pain management. *Seminars in Perinatology, 41*(2), 111–116. doi: 10.1053/j.semperi.2016.11.001.

Catlin, A., & Carter, B. S. (2002). Creation of a neonatal end-of-life palliative care protocol. *Journal of Perinatology, 22*(3), 184–195.

Chambers, L. (2019). *Caring for a child at end of life – a guide for professionals on the care of children and young people.* Together for Short Lives. <https://www.togetherforshortlives.org.uk/resource/guide-end-life-care/> (Accessed 22 February 2022).

Chin, S. D. N., Paraszczuk, A. M., Eckardt, P., & Bressler, T. (2021). Neonatal nurses' perceptions of palliative care in the neonatal intensive care unit. *American Journal of Maternal/Child Nursing, 46*(5), 250–257. doi: 10.1097/nmc.0000000000000738.

Chow, S. S. W., Creighton, P., Chambers, G. M., & Lui, K. (2019). *Report of the Australian and New Zealand Neonatal Network 2017*. Sydney, NSW: ANZNN.

Chow, S. S. W., Le Marsney, R., Hossain, S., Haslam, R., & Lui, K. (2021). *Report of the Australian and New Zealand Neonatal Network 2019*. Sydney, NSW: ANZNN.

Cortezzo, D. E., & Meyer, M. (2020). Neonatal end-of-life symptom management [review]. *Frontiers in Pediatrics, 8*, 574121. doi: 10.3389/fped.2020.574121.

Cortezzo, D. E., Sanders, M. R., Brownell, E. A., & Moss, K. (2015). End-of-life care in the neonatal intensive care unit: experiences of staff and parents. *American Journal of Perinatology, 32*(8), 713–724. doi: 10.1055/s-0034-1395475.

Embleton, N. D., & Stephenson, S. (2020). Care of twins, multiple births and support for the family: The Butterfly Project. In: A. Mancini, J. Price, & T. Kerr-Elliott (Eds.), *Neonatal palliative care for nurses* (pp. 171–175). Champaign, IL: Springer.

Falck, A. J., Moorthy, S., & Hussey-Gardner, B. (2016). Perception of palliative care in the NICU. *Advances in Neonatal Care, 16*(3), 191–200.

Foster, C., & Monterosso, L. (2012). The ventilator-dependent infant requiring palliative care in the neonatal intensive care unit: a literature review. *Neonatal, Paediatric, and Child Health Nursing*, 15(1), 8–19.

Friedrichsdorf, S. J., Khalid, F., & Noah, N. (2022). Pediatric population. In: N. Dimitrov & K. Kemle (Eds.), *Palliative care medicine for physician assistants: fostering resilience and managing seriously ill patients* (p. 285). New York: Oxford University Press.

Furtado-Eraso, S., Escalada-Hernández, P., & Marín-Fernández, B. (2021). Integrative review of emotional care following perinatal loss. *Western Journal of Nursing Research, 43*(5), 489–504. doi: 10.1177/0193945920954448.

Kain, V. J. (2013). An exploration of the grief experiences of neonatal nurses: a focus group study. *Journal of Newborn Nursing, 19*(2), 80–88. doi: 10.1016/j.jnn.2012.04.001.

Kain, V. J. (2016). The Praecox Program: pilot testing of an online educational program to improve neonatal palliative care practice. *Journal of Newborn Nursing, 23*(4). doi: 10.1016/j.jnn.2016.11.003.

Kain, V. J. (2021). Perinatal palliative care: cultural, spiritual and religious considerations for parents – what clinicians need to know. *Frontiers in Pediatrics, 9*, 597519. doi: 10.3389/fped.2021.597519.

Kain, V. J., & Chin, S. D. (2020). Conceptually redefining neonatal palliative care. *Advances in Neonatal Care, 20*(3), 187–195. doi: 10.1097/ANC.0000000000000731.

Kenner, C., & Loser, C. K. (2016). The role of neonatal nurses in palliative care. *Newborn and Infant Nursing Reviews, 16*(2), 74–77. doi: 10.1053/j.nainr.2016.03.009.

Kenner, C., Press, J., & Ryan, D. (2015). Recommendations for palliative and bereavement care in the NICU: a family-centred integrative approach. *Journal of Perinatology, 35*, s19–s23. doi: 10.1038/jp.2015.145.

Kishimoto, M., Yamaguchi, A., Niimura, M., Mizumoto, M., Hikitsuchi, T., Ogawa, K., et al. (2021). Factors affecting the grieving process after perinatal loss. *BMC Women's Health, 21*(1), 1–6.

Kyc, S. J., Bruno, C. J., Shabanova, V., & Montgomery, A. M. (2020). Perceptions of neonatal palliative care: similarities and differences between medical and nursing staff in a level IV Neonatal Intensive Care Unit. *Journal of Palliative Medicine, 23*(5), 662–669. doi: 10.1089/jpm.2019.0523.

Lantos, J. (2018). Ethical problems in decision making in the neonatal ICU. *New England Journal of Medicine, 379*(19), 1851–1860.

Larcher, V., Craig, F., Bhogal, K., Wilkinson, D., & Brierley, J. (2015). Making decisions to limit treatment in life-limiting and life-threatening conditions in children: a framework for practice. *Archives of Disease in Childhood, 100*(2), s1–s23. doi: 10.1136/archdischild-2014-306666.

Lefkowits, C., & Solomon, C. (2016). Palliative care in obstetrics and gynecology. *Obstetrics and Gynecology, 128*(6), 1403–1420. doi: 10.1097/AOG.0000000000001739.

Mancini, A., Uthaya, S., Beardsley, C., Wood, D., & Modi, N. (2014). Practical guidance for the management of palliative care on neonatal units. London: Royal College of Paediatrics and Child Health. <https://www.sands.org.uk/sites/default/files/NICU-Palliative-Care-Feb-2014.pdf> (Accessed 27 February 2022).

Marc-Aurele, K. L., & English, N. K. (2017). Primary palliative care in neonatal intensive care. *Seminars in Perinatology, 41*(2), 133–139.

Marchuk, A. (2016). End-of-life care in the neonatal intensive care unit: applying comfort theory. *International Journal of Palliative Nursing, 22*(7), 317–323.

Nguyen, M. R. (2019). Helping siblings connect, relate, and say goodbye. In: R. Limbo, C. Wool, & B. S. Carter (Eds.), *Handbook of perinatal and neonatal palliative care: a guide for nurses, physicians, and other health professionals* (pp. 81–102). New York: Springer.

Ravaldi, C., Levi, M., Angeli, E., Romeo, G., Biffino, M., Bonaiuti, R., et al. (2018). Stillbirth and perinatal care: are professionals trained to address parents' needs? *Midwifery, 64*, 53–59.

Rawlings, D., Tieman, J. J., Sanderson, C., Parker, D., & Miller-Lewis, L. (2017). Never say die: death euphemisms, misunderstandings and their implications for practice. *International Journal of Palliative Nursing, 23*(7), 324–330.

Ryan, A., Bernhard, B. S., & Fahlberg, B. (2015). Best practices for perinatal palliative care. *Nursing, 45*(10), 14–16.

Shen, M. J., & Wellman, J. D. (2019). Evidence of palliative care stigma: the role of negative stereotypes in preventing willingness to use palliative care. *Palliative and Supportive Care, 17*(4), 374–380. doi: 10.1017/S1478951518000834.

Soltani Gerdfaramarzi, M., & Bazmi, S. (2020). Neonatal end-of-life decisions and ethical perspectives. *Journal of Medical Ethics and History of Medicine, 13*, 19. doi: 10.18502/jmehm.v13i19.4827.

Stokowski, L. (2014). Palliative care and neonatal loss. *Medscape*. <www.medscape.org/viewarticle/494959> (Accessed 27 February 2022).

Together for Short Lives. (2017). Care pathways. Bristol, UK: Together for Short Lives. <http://www.togetherforshort-lives.org.uk/professionals/care_provision/care_pathways> (Accessed 27 February 2022).

Wholihan, D., & Olson, E. (2017). The doctrine of double effect: a review for the bedside nurse providing end-of-life care. *Journal of Hospice and Palliative Nursing, 19*(3), 205–211. doi: 10.1097/njh.0000000000000348.

Wilkinson, D., Xafis, V., & De Crespigny, L. (2014). Ethical language and decision-making for prenatally diagnosed lethal malformations. *Seminars in Fetal and Neonatal Medicine, 19*(5), 306–311.

Willems, D. L., Verhagen, E., & van Wijlick, E. (2014). Infants' best interests in end-of-life care for newborns. *Pediatrics, 134*(4), e1163–e1168.

Zadeh, R. S., Eshelman, P., Setla, J., Kennedy, L., Hon, E., & Basara, A. (2018). Environmental design for end-of-life care: an integrative review on improving the quality of life and managing symptoms for patients in institutional settings. *Journal of Pain and Symptom Management, 55*(3), 1018–1034.

CHAPTER 25

DISCHARGE PLANNING AND FOLLOW-UP CARE

TRUDI MANNIX AND VICTORIA KAIN[a]

Learning objectives

At the completion of this chapter, you will be able to:

- plan a tailored approach to the discharge of a neonate from a neonatal unit, including the coordination of ongoing follow-up care
- assess parents' readiness for the discharge of their infant and communicate with, educate and support them towards a seamless transition to discharge
- discuss the components of effective partnerships and professional relationships across all discharge and follow-up services
- discuss the inclusion criteria for neonatal long-term follow-up programs
- describe the timing and format of assessments and outcome measures needed in quality longitudinal follow-up programs
- explain the results of aggregated data of health and developmental outcomes that have arisen from neonatal long-term follow-up studies in Australia and New Zealand and link these data with the specialist care neonates require in follow-up programs after discharge.

Key words, terms and abbreviations

cerebral palsy (CP)
chronic lung disease (CLD)
congenital heart disease (CHD)
discharge coordinator
discharge planning
early discharge
long-term follow-up
neonatal early discharge (NED) teams
neonatal outreach team
oral aversion
retinopathy of prematurity (ROP)
return transfer

[a]The authors would like to acknowledge Robyn Richards, co-author of this chapter in the 1st edition of this book.

INTRODUCTION

Preparation for discharge from the neonatal unit begins at admission to allow parents to gradually assimilate the information required to meet their infant's needs and to develop parenting skills while the infant is still in the unit. Adequately prepared, confident parents, who have gained skills throughout their infant's stay in the neonatal unit, can enable a smooth transition from hospital to home. Appropriate preparation for discharge and well-organised follow-up care reduces neonatal morbidity and mortality and re-admission rates (Walter & Robb, 2019). The risk of re-admission to the neonatal unit is reduced because parents feel more skilled and confident in the care of their baby, knowing when to seek timely support and/or medical intervention.

EVIDENCE-BASED PRACTICE RESEARCH 25.1

In a concept analysis of the transition from neonatal unit care to home, Shillington and McNeil (2021) found that the defining characteristics for parents were 'a mix of emotions', 'uncertainty' and 'coming into parenthood'. Working with parents in partnership to gradually increase their involvement in their baby's care and plan their discharge reduced their uncertainty. The researchers developed a visual tool for parents with images that represented each step towards discharge and encouraged them to journal their thoughts, feelings and questions along the way.

Every year, over 10,000 newborns in Australia and New Zealand are admitted to a neonatal intensive care or special care unit and meet the Australian and New Zealand Neonatal Network (ANZNN) registration criteria (Chow et al., 2021). The ANZNN criteria for inclusion of neonates in the register are a gestational age <32 weeks, or a birthweight <1500 g, or assisted ventilation (intermittent positive pressure ventilation (IPPV)) or continuous positive airway pressure (CPAP) for 4 hours or more, or major surgery or therapeutic hypothermia (Chow et al., 2021). Much of the information in this chapter is based around the process of discharge and follow-up of neonates represented in the most recently published ANZNN data. While neonates included in this data set are obviously in a high-risk category, it should be noted that late preterm neonates (those born between 34 and 37 weeks' gestation) also demonstrate considerably higher rates of medical complications and prolonged hospital stays than full-term neonates (Karnati et al., 2020), and their **discharge planning** and follow-up care are equally important.

DISCHARGE PLANNING

Discharge home with a new infant should be a joyful experience, but it is often extremely stressful for parents of a preterm or previously sick infant being discharged from a neonatal unit. Relationships with their baby should be strengthened and supported from the start, and parents' confidence must be gradually increased so that they feel self-sufficient and ready to take their baby home (Aloysius et al., 2018). Parents must be able to care for their infant without the support and advice of a plethora of health professionals on whom they have previously relied heavily. Therefore, the process needs to be as streamlined as possible, with expert coordination and integration strategies to make the move to community paediatric services as stress free for the parents as possible. As a general rule, most neonates should go home by their due date or earlier, mostly depending on their sucking maturity. As the neonate progresses from intensive to special care, supportive technology and interventions should be gradually decreased to reduce parental anxiety (e.g. reduced levels of monitoring and increased time between feeds). The neonates most at risk of taking longer to achieve readiness for discharge are those of extreme prematurity, with a surgical, genetic or cardiac condition or who contract a nosocomial infection during their stay.

Discharge readiness is usually determined by the neonate demonstrating functional maturation rather than weight or postmenstrual age criteria. In the extremely preterm neonate, there is individual variability with length of stay, depending on illness severity. Once physiological maturity is attained, and when the parents are more confident, rooming in can occur to provide focused education to build parents' skills and knowledge prior to discharge. In the uncomplicated neonate the period of rooming in required should be assessed on an individual basis, to ensure the parents are confident with their skills prior to discharge. In most cases, one to two nights is an adequate amount of time for rooming-in, although this may increase for the technology-dependent neonate or for the family who needs additional emotional and educational support.

The most important skills the mother/parents need to master during this period are breastfeeding, settling the neonate and general care routines. Parents also need education to recognise their infant's behavioural cues, which indicate whether the infant is ready for, or not ready for, coping with, or not coping with, their interaction and how to support their infant when he/she is overwhelmed.

Preparation for discharge should include pulse oximetry screening. Approximately half of all newborns with **congenital heart disease (CHD)** are asymptomatic in the first few days of life. There is now a significant body of evidence to support pulse oximetry screening in apparently healthy neonates when used as an adjunct to physical examination, because it can improve detection of medical problems including critical CHD and other respiratory or sepsis-related pathology requiring medical intervention, with the potential for improved outcomes for the affected neonate (Lemyre et al., 2018). Timely identification of this small percentage of neonates can prompt early intervention and improve outcomes by reducing the risk of cardiovascular compromise in the postnatal ward or at home. To this end, in some states of Australia and in some district health boards in New

Zealand, pre-discharge evaluation of oxygen saturation to detect CHD occurs routinely, either in the postnatal ward in the case of the well term infant, or in the neonatal unit for a preterm neonate or sick neonate prior to discharge.

In addition to pulse oximetry screening, all neonates in the neonatal unit should have audiology screening prior to discharge. Hearing screening is undertaken by a trained technician in the hospital setting for neonates of >34 weeks' gestation, when the neonate is quiet or asleep. The screening tools used are currently the transient evoked otoacoustic emissions (TEOAE) test and the automated auditory brainstem response (AABR). The AABR detects impairment at the level of the cochlea, auditory nerve and auditory pathways in the brainstem (Wroblewska-Seniuk et al., 2017). The screening takes approximately 20 minutes and is usually completed just prior to discharge, ensuring screening is completed by no later than 4 weeks of age. The technician attaches the electrodes to the neonate's head and the back of their neck with sticky pads. Small earphone cups are then placed over the ears. Clicking sounds are generated and the responses from the ears are measured in terms of brain wave activity. If a strong response is received from the ears, this indicates that it is unlikely the neonate has any hearing loss. Once the hearing screening is completed, the technician will discuss the findings with the relevant clinicians and document them in the neonate's personal health record (Wroblewska-Seniuk et al., 2017).

CLINICAL PRACTICE 25.1

Parents of infants with complex needs, especially those who have been born extremely preterm and have developed chronic lung disease, will need to develop skills to manage feeding a fussy baby, giving oral medications, using oxygen, managing all aspects of home monitoring and what to do in an emergency before taking their baby home.

FAMILY-CENTRED CARE 25.1

The rates of early breast expression, first attempt at a breastfeed and exclusive breastfeeding were found to be higher in Norwegian mothers whose babies were cared for in single family rooms (SFRs) in the neonatal unit (Grundt et al., 2021). Similarly, in an observational cohort study in Canada, researchers found that parents spent significantly more time in the neonatal unit when their babies were in SFRs although increased time spent in the neonatal unit did not translate to more involvement in care activities (Campbell-Yeo et al., 2021). In literature reviewed by Campbell-Yeo et al. (2021), it was found that greater parental presence and involvement in the neonatal unit was associated with increased parental confidence and self-efficacy on discharge.

Prior to discharge, the baby may be transferred to a neonatal unit closer to home for continued care. The four most important 'physiological competencies' the neonate needs to be able to achieve prior to discharge include:

1. the ability to maintain thermoregulation while fully clothed in a normal, open cot
2. respiratory stability
3. feeding
4. appropriate weight gain.

Table 25.1 lists additional neonatal milestones indicating preparedness for discharge.

The discharge process for all neonates is heavily task and skills oriented, with parents often overwhelmed by the knowledge and information they need to acquire before taking their infant home. The prerequisites for the standard discharge from a neonatal unit include the following:

- The family has appropriate transport (e.g. a pram, a correct fitted car seat/capsule, etc.).
- All ongoing appointments have been made.
- The neonate's newborn assessment has been completed and documented.
- Feeding is well established.
- Parenting skills have been established.
- Any questions from the family regarding discharge and ongoing management have been answered.
- Parent and general practitioner contact details are correct on all documentation.

Boykova (2016) identified a number of characteristics that influence parental role development and parenting style in preterm newborn parents, as well as their preparedness to take their infant home. The issue of the mother being discharged without her infant created a feeling of 'not being a parent' (Boykova, 2016, p. 329). Many other factors identified in the literature that hamper parenting include anxiety and depression, grief and guilt, the development of post-traumatic stress disorder and the complex task of having to learn how to be a parent. Mothers also identified that they felt unprepared and wanted more hands-on experience before discharge. Parents must be present in the neonatal unit and actively participate in care as early as possible for a strong emotional bond to develop between the parent and the infant. This can be improved by encouraging parents to spend more time gradually participating in all parts of newborn care, with assistance and encouragement from the neonatal unit nursing/midwifery team. Many parents report that the transition from the organised routine of the neonatal unit to home is chaotic as they adjust to their infant's needs, and they should be advised that the transfer may not be seamless (Fig. 25.1).

Table 25.2 outlines the goals that should be met by the family and healthcare providers prior to discharge.

Discharge of the high-risk neonate

Discharge of the high-risk neonate who may be technology dependent at discharge is more complicated and should be anticipated and planned. In addition to meeting standard prerequisites for discharge as previously described, parents of these infants are provided with a checklist of the specific educational support they have received prior to discharge to ensure that they have learnt

TABLE 25.1 **Readiness for hospital discharge – infant goals**

Infant goal	Strategies for achievement
Appropriate immunisations have been administered	All members of the family, including grandparents, should be fully immunised. This is of particular importance in the neonate with chronic lung disease who is discharged in the months when respiratory syncytial virus (RSV) is prevalent. Some centres supply RSV immunisations to these high-risk infants The 2-month vaccinations should generally be given at 6–8 weeks chronological age If the 2-month vaccination has been delayed because the neonate was deemed medically unstable or is <32 weeks and/or <2 kg, the subsequent vaccination can be given 1 month later. For example, if the neonate receives the 2-month vaccines at 3 months, then the 4-month vaccines should still be given at 4 months of age
Universal newborn hearing screening is performed on all infants prior to discharge, and referrals made as necessary	Infants who fail their hearing screening test in hospital will be referred to follow-up audiology services
Retinopathy of prematurity examination has been completed and therapies instituted as indicated (Doyle et al., 2014)	Post discharge, some neonates will require ongoing treatment
Some centres will offer a safety car seat challenge test before discharge. This is a period of oxygen saturation/heart rate monitoring for 1–2 hours (about the duration of the car ride home) to ensure the neonate's wellbeing while positioned in the car seat	This is especially beneficial in the extremely low birthweight neonate who may be difficult to position safely in the car seat due to low discharge weight and poor head control

Source: adapted from Verklan and Walden (2021).

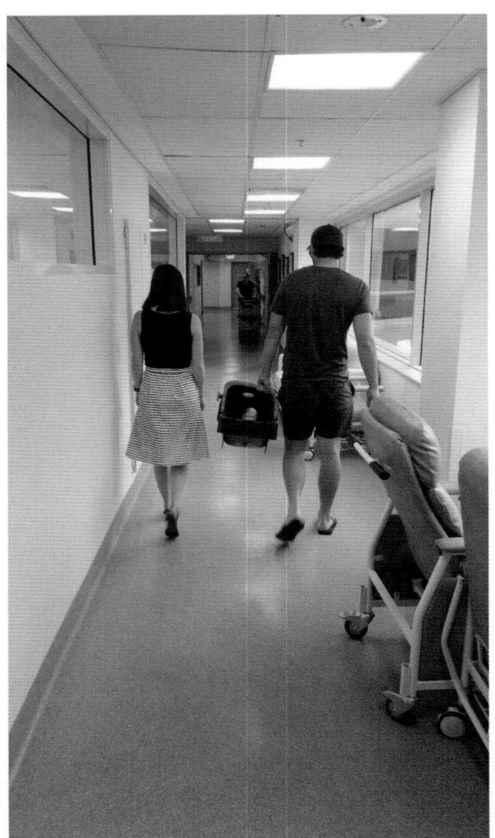

FIGURE 25.1 **Taking the preterm baby home**
© Miracle Mumma (2016).

the skills to care for their infant at home with confidence. An interdisciplinary discharge-planning meeting should occur with the family at least 1 week prior to discharge to ensure they are well prepared. Additional discharge prerequisites for these families may include the ordering and installation of home technology prior to discharge (e.g. home oxygen or apnoea-monitoring devices). In addition to the discharge requirements stated in Fig. 25.2, parents who take home a newborn who still requires oxygen need additional education, supplies, community resources and referrals as outlined in Box 25.1.

The family will need to go through basic resuscitation training and may require ongoing social work support after they are discharged. Prior to the infant's discharge, every parent–infant relationship should be evaluated in order to understand the challenges that parents face and to reinforce the protective aspects in the home environment (South Australia (SA) Health, 2018). Parents of high-risk infants experience more stress, which increases the risk of child abuse, financial difficulties and family breakdowns (Chamberlain et al., 2019). Before discharge, a multi-agency discharge-planning team should discuss safety plans established in the home for families in these high-risk situations, and there should be planned ongoing surveillance for these high-risk infants.

Safe-sleeping guidelines such as placing the infant flat on their back to sleep, with the face clear of bedding, without pillows, toys or extra bedding, should be role modelled in the neonatal unit during the neonate's hospitalisation, and reinforced upon discharge (see Chapter 2). It is also important to avoid deformational

TABLE 25.2 **Readiness for hospital discharge – family goals**

Family/provider goal	Strategies for achievement
Parents as partners in care	Parents are equal members of their infant's care team. Two-way communications between the interdisciplinary team and the family are pivotal for easing anxiety and frustration
A family that is confident and competent in providing the necessary care to their infant at home with appropriate support services in the community	Start the discharge process on admission, giving an estimated date of discharge to work towards Promote gradual skills development in the parents/family, supplying parents with appropriate information at regular intervals and maintaining open communication with all members of the interdisciplinary team Parent education sessions should be parent/carer appropriate, varied, coordinated and factual and be reviewed regularly to assess whether they meet parents' needs. These should include the importance of touch, stress cues with over-stimulation, positioning and exercise, understanding growth charts, corrected vs chronological age, infant developmental milestones, settling techniques, early childhood centre/community or other resources
Any unresolved medical problems have been identified, plans for follow-up monitoring and treatment have been instituted or organised for post-discharge completion	Arrange planned, timely, appropriate interventions, seeking early consultation with nursing, medical and allied health as necessary
A primary care provider (paediatrician, general practitioner) who is nominated and prepared to assume responsibility for ongoing care with the appropriate backup is engaged with the family unit prior to discharge	The primary care provider should be conveniently located to the family's home, and contacts may have been previously established with the care of an older sibling
If there are any issues with language as a barrier, they are addressed early and appropriately with interpreter services and at every critical point prior to discharge	Every non-English-speaking family unit needs to be offered early, regular interpreter services. No hospital should use family members, nursing or medical staff as interpreters
An individualised home care plan has been developed with input from the family and the appropriate interdisciplinary team and this has been forwarded to the selected primary care provider	This will reduce anxiety and allow for a smoother transition to home. Good communication networks between healthcare providers will ensure a smoother transition for parents
If there is ongoing need for technology in the home (e.g. home oxygen or monitoring, etc.) this is installed and the family adequately educated in its use prior to the day of discharge. This will include education regarding oxygen use safety and instruction in basic resuscitation skills for parents	This will be managed by the nurse/midwife organising the discharge process
If there are child and wellbeing protection issues, alternative care arrangements may need to be organised prior to discharge	This needs to be managed by the interdisciplinary team sensitively, in a private area away from the neonatal unit. Security services may be required if there are safety issues for staff and neonate

Source: adapted from Verklan and Walden (2021).

plagiocephaly by alternating the position of the neonate's head between the left and right side each time they sleep, both in the neonatal unit and after discharge (American Academy of Pediatrics (AAP), 2021).

Fig. 25.2 provides an exemplar checklist of criteria to be met prior to discharge of the high-risk neonate. This checklist should ideally be completed in stages and in a timely manner so that parents are not overwhelmed. Every neonatal nurse/midwife in the neonatal unit should assume responsibility for the newborn and family for whom they are caring from the day of admission, by actively completing tasks on the checklist rather than delaying this process until the final days before discharge. It is critical to mark off the checklist and document the completion of discharge activities in the neonate's progress notes as well as in the infant's health records that parents take home to ensure that the discharge procedure is communicated to the team.

Neonatal early discharge, outreach and ongoing programs

As part of a structured '**early discharge**' program, some newborns can be discharged home from a neonatal unit early, while still receiving the support of the neonatal healthcare team. Eligibility criteria vary from unit to unit in Australia and New Zealand, but usually include neonates who are stable, around 2 kg in weight, but who

Expected discharge date____________________	**Date checked**	**Initial**

Parent meeting
Discuss upcoming discharge date and preparation for discharge
Review medical criteria for discharge
Review sleep study
Review growth chart and discuss expected growth
Review parent education requirements
 	
Nutrition
Establish and document discharge feeding plan whether by breast or bottle
Discuss feeding amounts, frequency and duration
Review breastfeeding or bottle feeding techniques
Organise breastfeeding review by lactation specialist
Supply information on breast pump hire/rental
Discuss and organise medications for mothers with low breast milk supply
Review recipe for higher kilojoules formula preparation if needed
 	
Oxygen saturation screening
Check before discharge to identify congenital heart disease and to allow early intervention and treatment
 	
Hearing
Organise screening and review results
Discuss the possibility of rescreening with parents if required
Make a referral for hearing screen failure if appropriate
 	
Immunisations
Administer initial dose of vaccine at 6–8 weeks. This is a combined primary immunisation against diphtheria, tetanus, pertussis, hepatitis B, poliomyelitis and *Haemophilus influenzae* B
Rotavirus vaccine between 8 and 14 weeks PMA
Pneumococcal vaccine for at-risk infants:
  Indigenous infants
  Infants with a medical condition associated with an increased risk of invasive pneumococcal disease
  Preterm infants of <28 weeks' gestation with severe chronic lung disease (CLD)
Provide a record of upcoming schedule to parents
Discuss the need for parents to have influenza injections
Organise protection against respiratory syncytial virus (RSV) with monthly injections of synthetic antibodies for infants with CLD when there are other siblings
Discuss the need for **blood pressure** assessment
 	
Eye examination
Organise a follow-up eye examination if required for retinopathy of prematurity
 	
Medications
Ensure parents can perform administration of ongoing oral medications to infant
Discuss potential side effects of medications
Provide parents with oral syringes appropriate for home use
Adjust timing of medication doses for home use; avoid the middle of the night
Discuss how to obtain medications and refills
Discuss the importance of using a consistent pharmacy		

FIGURE 25.2 **Discharge checklist for the high-risk infant**

Source: Richards (2017a).

Home monitoring Review the need for an apnoea monitor, and when to use the monitor Discuss safe sleep/back to sleep procedures Assist parents to organise home monitoring rental 1 week prior to discharge Ensure parents and support caregivers attend CPR workshop Ensure parents attend home safety class and learn about alarm limits, settings, application of leads, false alarms, responding to alarms, keeping a record of alarms, response for apnoea		
Home oxygen use Discuss home oxygen prescription Review reasons for home oxygen Review normal breathing patterns (rate, effort, colour), signs of distress Review when to call the GP Discuss current laboratory test findings and the implications for their infant (e.g. haematocrit) Discuss RSV and illness prevention Discuss expected developmental milestones Review correct age calculations Discuss the transition from hospital to home and parents' expectations Discuss the possibility of hospital readmissions Discuss the signs and symptoms of illness Safe sleeping guidelines		
Review oxygen equipment Provide parents with the manufacturing company name and phone number Discuss home safety issues Ensure parents contact their home insurance company Organise portable oxygen tanks Discuss the use of stationary oxygen tanks at home Discuss setting up oxygen gauges/regulator and adjusting oxygen flows Review the need for extra supplies – adaptors/tubing		
Oxygen cannula use Discuss the positioning of a cannula Discuss the frequency and technique for changing the cannula Ensure parents know how to obtain additional supplies		
Travelling with oxygen Discuss methods of securing oxygen tanks to a vehicle Describe methods of securing oxygen tanks to a stroller or car seat Discuss the importance of having extra supplies available		
Documentation All treatments should be recorded in the 'Blue book' and in the discharge summary to enable appropriate continuity of care with the attending paediatrician or general practitioner		
Resources Identify community resources: • Early childhood centres • Centres that cater for babies and mothers with settling and feeding issues • Breastfeeding clinics Provide advice regarding credible internet resources		
Follow-up appointments Schedule appointments prior to discharge and review with parents **Discuss what to expect**		

FIGURE 25.2, cont'd

BOX 25.1 **Preparation for parents to take home a neonate on oxygen**

Education

- Parents should understand why their baby requires home oxygen and they also need to be given the opportunity to discuss their baby's general health and respiratory status.
- Parents should be familiar with the equipment being delivered to their home including nasal prongs and tubing, know how to check that prongs are patent and in the correct position, be confident in changing nasal prongs and know the cleaning procedures. Prongs should be changed weekly or if blocked.
- Parents should be shown how to check and adjust oxygen flow rates and increase oxygen requirements as needed, according to saturation monitoring or neonatal condition prior to seeking medical advice.
- Parents should be instructed on safe usage of oxygen, including fire safety issues.
- Parents should be taught to assess their baby for signs of cyanosis or respiratory distress (e.g. colour changes, increased respiratory effort, poor feeding, lethargy, etc.).
- Parents should attend a paediatric airway management demonstration provided by the discharge coordinators. Parents are also taught how to use the apnoea monitor if supplied.

Equipment

- Parents will be provided with a sufficient supply of adhesive tape for nasal prong changes at home.
- Parents need to be able to assess when an oxygen cylinder requires changing and know how and when to order additional oxygen supplies.
- The oxygen supplier company will provide parents with the safety guidelines for the use of oxygen therapy at home.
- Parents must notify the relevant local fire brigades about their 'use of medical oxygen in domestic premises' and can request a home visit by the Fire Prevention Officer, if required.

Referrals and community resources

- The family GP, paediatrician, early childhood centre or any other community support services should be notified of discharge plans, and appointments made prior to discharge.

Source: Richards (2017b).

may still be tube fed, are oxygen dependent, require apnoea monitoring, have major congenital abnormalities and require end-of-life care, or late preterm infants who need support to fully establish feeds. Neonatal nurses and midwives in these **neonatal early discharge (NED) teams** support parents as they care for their infant at home, weaning them from oxygen or transitioning their infant from tube feeds to full sucking feeds, sometimes over a period of weeks. Alternatively, parents can return to the hospital or attend clinics several times a week with their infant until their needs are met – this is sometimes referred to as 'reverse NED'. Larger neonatal units may also offer the services of a '**neonatal outreach team**' where parents receive frequent and regular visits from neonatal nurses/midwives after their infant is discharged, until parents are confident they can manage without this level of support. During home visits, neonatal nurses/midwives in these outreach teams may teach parenting techniques, design and revise feeding regimens, weigh and physically assess the newborn, refer the infant to other health experts as needed and provide emotional support to parents.

Mannix et al. (2019) conducted a case-controlled study and found that neonates in such programs had a shorter length of stay by approximately 11 days, reflecting a cost saving for the health service. These neonates are also at less risk of nosocomial infection although further research is required to test other assertions regarding breastfeeding outcomes and weight gain.

Once the neonatal outreach team members have concluded their support of the family, they hand over to other government services, such as child and family health nurses in Australia and the Well Child/Tamariki Ora program in New Zealand (Australian Government Department of Health, 2013; New Zealand Ministry of Health, 2021). Both services offer free and universal healthcare based on the principles of primary healthcare and aim to meet the needs of families and children until the child is 5 years of age.

EVIDENCE-BASED PRACTICE RESEARCH 25.2

In an ethnographic study of parents' perspective on the neonatal unit discharge process, Berman et al. (2019) found that the system could have better prepared them and connected them with essential services. Parents would have preferred continuity of care from both medical and nursing/midwifery staff during the admission in order to provide consistent information, as well as more information on how to balance the needs of the baby with self-care once discharged, particularly managing sleep deprivation and fatigue. The sudden removal of monitoring made parents anxious, as did the idea of managing breathing problems on their own at home. Several parents wished they had the option to take their babies home early, and said '"Here's another option, would you be comfortable taking this and getting out of here and going home [early]?" We could have gone home sooner, had I known … .' (Berman et al., 2019, p. 102).

TRANSFER OF THE NEONATE BETWEEN NEONATAL UNITS

Neonates are often transferred from a tertiary referral centre to a neonatal unit closer to the parents' home address; this is referred to as a 'back' or 'return' transfer. This has a number of benefits:

- proximity of the neonate to home, enabling more frequent visiting
- a reduction in the intensity of care to reduce the stress levels for parents
- linkage with local services for ongoing care after discharge
- improved utilisation of neonatal unit beds at the tertiary centre.

In New Zealand, a **return transfer** takes place from a tertiary unit to a level 2 unit when an infant is more than 32 weeks' gestation. A return transfer to a level 1 unit takes place when the infant is capable of almost all sucking feeds. See Chapter 1 for a description of the levels of care.

Specialised discharge and follow-up care

Some neonates admitted to a neonatal unit require increased intervention and support prior to discharge, and specialised follow-up care after discharge. They include neonates with:

- cardiac disorders
- genetic disorders
- some surgical conditions, including orofacial clefts
- long-term morbidities associated with prematurity, such as **chronic lung disease (CLD)**, feeding and growth difficulties and sensory losses (hearing and vision).

While the pathophysiology of these conditions is discussed in other chapters, discussion will now concentrate on the increased intervention required to prepare infants with these problems and their families for discharge, and the follow-up required after discharge.

Cardiac disorders

Approximately half of all infants diagnosed with CHD will require surgery. Some infants will be transported to a specialist cardiac centre for surgery shortly after birth, while others may be allowed home to gain weight until surgery can be scheduled. Each tertiary cardiac centre offers a follow-up clinic for continued monitoring of the newborn and family, including coordination of care for neonates with non-surgical cardiac issues such as congestive cardiac failure or arrhythmias. Referral pathways to ongoing cardiac specialists would be considered as part of discharge planning from the cardiac tertiary centre.

These neonates may also require ongoing support from occupational therapists, physiotherapists and speech therapists. Discharge-planning priorities of surgical patients include ensuring the provision of adequate nutrition for growth, development and wound healing. Infants going home prior to surgery have high caloric needs due to low energy and feeding reserves, and they are often described as poor feeders. They may give fewer feeding cues, and are at risk of growth failure due to the following:

- congestive heart failure
- dyspnoea
- hypermetabolism
- delayed gastric emptying
- poor oral intake
- increased protein and energy requirements
- cyanosis
- complicated recovery of surgical wounds.

Prior to discharge, parents of these vulnerable neonates need to be made aware of the signs and symptoms of cardiorespiratory compromise, the interventions required and where to seek help if they are concerned about their infant. Cheung et al. (2021) reinforced the need for high-quality **long-term follow-up** of critically ill preterm neonates who have undergone cardiac surgery to detect neurodevelopmental concerns in a timely fashion, so that early intervention programs can help them reach their full potential.

EVIDENCE-BASED PRACTICE RESEARCH 25.3

Setiawan et al. (2019) conducted a literature search on the effects of a neonatal early discharge program and found that, while such a program enhanced bonding between parents and their preterm babies, they also found the burden of responsibility of taking their preterm infant home early very stressful.

The around-the-clock care required for their infant, sleep deprivation and balancing work and family commitments affected both parents. Parents wanted more practical and emotional support prior to and after taking their baby home, to help ease the stress of the transition to early discharge.

FAMILY-CENTRED CARE 25.2

Pineda et al. (2020) developed the 'Baby Bridge' program to support high-risk infants and their parents after discharge from the neonatal unit. A specialised licensed therapist saw the neonate and family in the neonatal unit prior to discharge to complete a neurodevelopmental assessment in collaboration with the multidisciplinary neonatal team, and followed up with visits in the home within a week of discharge, and weekly thereafter. They provided targeted education to parents about strategies to support their infant's neurodevelopment. They found that infants ≤30 weeks' gestation received early therapy services an average of 85 days earlier than historical controls.

Surgical conditions

Due to improvements in antenatal diagnosis, the majority of infants with a major surgical condition will be birthed in a perinatal centre attached to a surgical centre. There will be some infants with minor conditions (e.g. cleft lip and palate, hydrocele, limb deformities, congenital hip dysplasia or simple congenital heart defects not requiring urgent treatment) who will be managed at the perinatal centre while awaiting ongoing diagnosis and bed availability at the surgical centre. If the neonate presents with an undiagnosed severe congenital defect, they will be transferred to a surgical centre at the earliest convenience once stabilised by the neonatal team. Following recovery from surgery in a tertiary surgical centre, neonates will be returned to their referring neonatal unit or to a neonatal unit offering a lower level of care closer to home. Discharge planning will depend on the specific condition, the need for prosthesis, splints, special feeding aids or modifications to diet and physical activity.

Appropriate education of the parents/carers will be required to ensure they are confident in the care of their neonate and any equipment that may be utilised in their care. There may also be the need to prepare parents for the demands of caring for a special-needs or chronically ill infant who may require palliative care options, including the viable options for respite care.

Extremely preterm neonates

Many prematurity-related problems often continue throughout the neonate's hospitalisation and after discharge from the neonatal unit. CLD, feeding and development challenges and sensory (vision and hearing) losses are the most prevalent issues faced by the extremely preterm infant and must be considered when preparing the parents and infant for discharge.

CHRONIC LUNG DISEASE

Extremely preterm neonates may acquire CLD (also known as bronchopulmonary dysplasia (BPD)) after birth as a result of the side effects of supplemental oxygen and/or assisted ventilation after birth. As a consequence, they may have an ongoing oxygen dependency and may be discharged home on oxygen, which may continue for up to 12 months. Prior to discharge at-risk neonates should have an overnight oxygen saturation (SpO_2) test to ascertain oxygen requirements, and after discharge this is repeated every 2–3 months to allow weaning of oxygen. Best-practice guidelines recommend at least 6 hours of evaluation of the infant using overnight oximetry, incorporating sleeping and eating – the two most vulnerable daily activities (Wong et al., 2020). Infants who cannot meet the $\geq$93% mean SpO_2 target, or who spend $>$10% of the study time with SpO_2 $<$90% but are otherwise ready for discharge, are considered candidates for home oxygen (Starship, 2020). Regular reviews after discharge will be necessary to ensure correct maintenance of oxygen saturations, feed tolerance and growth parameters, and the neonate will also need to have an apnoea monitor. Oxygen therapy will need to continue until the neonate consistently demonstrates normal oxygen saturations, positive growth velocity and sufficient stamina during feeding and activity without tachypnoea, retractions or other evidence of ongoing respiratory distress. Oxygen will then be gradually weaned as dictated by appropriate oxygen saturations.

Wong et al. (2021) found that neonates with a $PCO_2 \leq 55$ mmHg at discharge had a median time to oxygen weaning of 6.3 months (95% CI, 5.7–7.0), whereas patients with $PCO_2 > 55$ mmHg had a median time of 8.4 months (95% CI, 7.7–9.1). Despite the stresses of taking their infant home on oxygen, most parents choose home oxygen to a prolonged stay in the neonatal unit because of the comfort of home, the reduced expenditures and inconvenience of travel and the enhanced bonding (Lau et al., 2019).

In some centres, parents are supplied with a home oxygen monitor with functionality to download data to the neonatal unit. The monitor is then returned to the discharge coordinators where a computer download is performed. The results are discussed with the medical officer, who will then inform the parents of the neonate's ongoing oxygen requirements. For more detail about CLD, see Chapter 9. A recent position statement from the Thoracic Society of Australia and New Zealand was not in favour of routine monitoring with an oximeter at home (Kapur et al., 2020, p. 883).

CLINICAL PRACTICE 25.2

Some neonatal units advocate the use of the 'air test' prior to discharge to establish the risk that might occur if the oxygen is accidentally switched off at home. Neonates are assessed to determine if they can maintain an SpO_2 $>$80% during an episode of inadvertent disconnection from supplemental oxygen over 4 hours (Kapur et al., 2020, p. 883).

FEEDING AND GROWTH ISSUES

The extremely preterm neonate experiences relatively slow growth compared with the term neonate. These neonates lose more weight initially and take longer to regain their birthweight; consequently, their weight is mostly less than the 10th percentile on the growth chart. Nutritional complications are also more severe in neonates with CLD as they have increased work of breathing and often require 150–200 kcal/kg/day for satisfactory weight gain. They often require increased feed volumes or supplemental calories in order to maintain satisfactory weight gain. A dietitian should be consulted to provide advice on the nutritional needs of all oxygen-dependent neonates.

A number of these neonates will develop **oral aversion** (the reluctance, avoidance or fear of eating, drinking or accepting sensation in or around the mouth) and will push or turn away from anything that comes near their face, even a dummy, bottle or their mother's breast (Jones et al., 2021). This will require patience and a concentrated effort on the part of the neonatal nursing/midwifery and lactation staff, the speech pathologist and occupational therapist, to develop strategies to work with the family in assisting gradual positive experiences with breast or bottle feeding. Neonatal nurses/midwives must be aware that a number of issues cause oral aversion. These include ignoring the infant's behavioural and physiological cues which signal stress during suck feeding (Morag et al., 2019), as well as the noxious stimuli that occurred regularly for this neonate during the early period of his/her admission to the neonatal unit, such as placement of either nasal or oral endotracheal tubes, insertion of nasal cannulae such as CPAP prongs or mask, placement of oral or nasal feeding tubes and oral or nasal suctioning. It is therefore imperative that measures to reduce these noxious experiences are part of everyday care, including cue-based feeding rather than volume-driven feeding (Morag et al., 2019), pain management with sucrose or sedation, the use of a pain score, minimal handling strategies and teaching neonatal nurses/midwives and parents to recognise cues for engagement. Morag et al. (2019) showed that avoiding intrusiveness, initiating suck feeding when signs of hunger appear, terminating feeding with signs of satiety and then supplementing the feed with 65–75% of the maximum via a feeding tube was safe, and infants were discharged sooner. Oral aversion may also be reduced using oropharyngeal therapy, where 0.2 mL of colostrum/expressed breast milk is applied to the oral buccal mucosa with an oral syringe as soon as colostrum is available (Wetzel et al., 2020). In the few cases of severe oral aversion, infants may be discharged with long-term feeding tubes such as a transpyloric or gastrostomy tube, and these infants are often managed in a feeding clinic attached to a hospital. In any case, after discharge, the neonatal outreach team must focus their attention on supporting the mother in her continued efforts to breastfeed and may need to involve the continued help of the interdisciplinary team.

Early breastfeeding establishment, support and education are vital in developing a confident, exclusively breastfeeding mother–baby dyad. Neonatal nurses/midwives provide early education and support regarding breastfeeding and breast expression to mothers wishing to breastfeed. If there are issues with supply of breast milk, early support from a lactation specialist is imperative, and medication may be required. Information on the safe storage of expressed breast milk is vital for mothers who have preterm or sick neonates in the neonatal unit. There is further information on breastfeeding the normal newborn in Chapter 2 and the preterm infant in Chapter 5.

SENSORY LOSSES (HEARING AND VISION)

Congenital hearing deficits occur in approximately 350 babies in Australia (Sung & Carew, 2019) and up to 170 newborns in New Zealand (Health Navigator New Zealand, 2021) each year. Neonatal illness and younger maternal age at birth, but not shorter gestational age, have been found to be risk factors for hearing impairment in children (Butcher et al., 2020). Neonatal risk factors include prematurity, birthweight <1250 g, hypoxia, jaundice, seizures, ventilation, hypoglycaemia, meningitis, asphyxia and treatment with aminoglycosides and frusemide (Hardani et al., 2020). Universal audiology screening is now also implemented in 40 European countries, as well as Russia, Malawi, Rwanda, India and China, but because programs are diverse, research comparisons between them are difficult (Bussé et al., 2021). It is important that parents of infants with a hearing impairment receive early support to understand their baby's socio-emotional development, as language deprivation has been shown to lead to delays in empathy-related skills (Wright et al., 2021). Parents also need information regarding the need for speech and language therapy, hearing amplification to ameliorate hearing loss, an evaluation by an otorhinolaryngologist and early-intervention services. In infants less than 12 months old, cochlear implantation provides an opportunity for children to develop more positive expressive and receptive language outcomes, with some children achieving normal language skills by the time they start school (Purcell et al., 2021).

Evaluation of vision impairment in neonates at risk takes place prior to discharge from the neonatal unit. The eye starts to develop at about 16 weeks of gestation, and the blood vessels of the retina begin to form at the optic nerve on the back of the eye, and branch outward towards the edges of the developing retina. **Retinopathy of prematurity (ROP)** is a leading cause of visual impairment in preterm neonates that occurs when the normal process of vascularisation of the retina is interrupted, around 31–32 weeks of gestation (Fraser & Diehl-Jones, 2021). Being gestation dependent, 80% of neonates born under 26 weeks' gestation develop some form of ROP, whereas only 50% have the same outcomes at 29 weeks (Fraser & Diehl-Jones, 2021). ROP develops in five stages, and is also classified in zones and further using indicators of activity called 'pre-plus' and 'plus' (Fraser & Dielh-Jones, 2021, p. 698). Hyperoxia and fluctuating hypo/hyperoxia from the period immediately after birth is the most significant risk factor for ROP, as hyperoxygenation interrupts normal vascularisation of the retina (Azad et al., 2020). A period of rapid vasoproliferation then occurs which forms an abrupt ridge between the vascular retina and the avascular retina (stage 1 ROP). These new vessels are weak, and leak blood and fluid into the eye which can cause scarring, and can pull on the retina and lead to detachment (stage V ROP). Most infants with stage I and II will improve with no treatment and eventually go on to have normal vision, but infants with stage III with 'plus' disease, and stage IV and V need treatment to avoid visual impairment and permanent blindness (National Eye Institute, 2019).

Screening for ROP occurs in all neonates born at less than 31 weeks' gestation, or less than 1250 g, or those born to mothers with suspected intrauterine infections. The first screening should occur at 32 weeks' gestation and the ongoing further assessments will be dictated by the treating ophthalmologist. Prevention of ROP includes attention to neonatal nutrition and infection control, while the greatest potential to reduce the risk occurs when oxygen saturation levels are targeted (Darlow & Husain, 2019). In high-income settings with established programs to screen for and treat ROP, a SpO_2 target of 90–94% is recommended, and in low-income settings the WHO recommends settings of 88–94% (Darlow & Husain, 2019). Treatment with laser therapy to ablate the avascular retina has largely replaced cryotherapy to treat ROP, but still results in permanent loss to the peripheral visual field.

EVIDENCE-BASED PRACTICE RESEARCH 25.4

Recent trials comparing laser/cryotherapy with intravitreal injections of antivascular endothelial growth factor (VEGF) antibodies have found that, while the risk of refractive errors (high myopia) in childhood was reduced, there was no effect on the risk of retinal detachment or the recurrence of ROP (Sankar et al., 2018). Further studies are needed in this area.

EVIDENCE-BASED PRACTICE RESEARCH 25.5

Numerous trials to target optimal SpO_2 targets have been conducted over the years, including SUPPORT, COT, BOOST-NZ, BOOST II UK and BOOST II Aus. The outcome of the trials confirms that too little oxygen increases the risk of mortality in very preterm infants, while too much oxygen increases the risk of ROP. Studies recommend an oxygen saturation target of 90–94% in this cohort, with the upper alarm limit set at 95% (Darlow & Husain, 2019).

FAMILY-CENTRED CARE 25.3

The neonate with extreme prematurity and chronic lung disease will be in the neonatal unit for an extended period of time. Neonatal nurses/midwives need confidence in caring for these infants' physiological needs, while supporting the families during a protracted and difficult stay. Establishing a trusting relationship with these parents as they prepare to take their at-risk infant home involves coming to know their strengths, limitations, fears and anxieties.

Emotional, cognitive and neurobehavioural issues

Increasing rates of neurodevelopmental disability in preterm infants lead to increased use of special need education, with learning difficulties in reading and mathematics in particular. Children and adolescents born preterm have been found to be two to four times more at risk of psychopathology compared with those born at term, and the risk of a diagnosis of psychopathology increases with every weekly decrease in gestational age at birth (Fitzallen et al., 2020). Extremely preterm infants have higher rates of autism spectrum disorder, hyperactivity, poor peer interaction, anxiety and depression, being withdrawn, and difficulties in attention as children. Subtle deficits with motor coordination, social interactive skills, working memory, problem solving and planning have been found to impact on the completion of daily activities and quality of life in school age children who were born extremely or very preterm. In one systematic review, adults born preterm were less likely to experience romantic and sexual partnerships and parenting (Wilson-Costello & Payne, 2021).

THE ROLE OF THE DISCHARGE COORDINATOR

The role of the **discharge coordinator** is to collaborate with the interdisciplinary team and families of neonates to provide a coordinated, seamless transition from the neonatal unit to home or to accepting hospitals for ongoing care. The neonatal nurse/midwife in this role needs the ability to liaise with a wide range of interdisciplinary team members as well as deal with parents who have been in crisis for an extended period of time. Other roles include education of the family and nominated support persons, and support and education of the neonatal nursing/midwifery staff in the neonatal unit regarding the preparation for discharge and information required by parents. Discharge coordinators also liaise with external supply companies for equipment parents may need, such as oxygen if it is required in the home, including ensuring the home environment is safe. They may perform oxygen saturation downloads and teach neonatal resuscitation skills to parents. Referrals to early childhood services should also be managed, and in some centres the discharge coordinator will also undertake transfers of infants to other neonatal units closer to the family home. The incumbent should be a highly skilled neonatal nurse, preferably with midwifery and lactation qualifications. By the time the parents leave the neonatal unit to take their infant home (Fig. 25.3), they should be feeling confident to care for their infant with resources in place to support them in the transition to parenthood at home.

EVIDENCE-BASED PRACTICE RESEARCH 25.6

Discharge criteria from neonatal units vary. Preterm infants can be discharged safely while weighing less than 2 kg, in a car seat that can safely accommodate their size. To be discharged, neonates must be physiologically stable, with resolution of the problems that required hospitalisation. They should be gaining weight on enteral feeds, able to control their temperature within the normal range and have mature respiratory control. Parents should be trained and ready psychologically to take their baby home, and follow-up services planned. Neonates should be immunised, have had their hearing tested and oximetry performed (Lauriello & Aylward, 2021).

LONG-TERM FOLLOW-UP

Inclusion criteria for neonatal long-term follow-up programs

In the United Kingdom, of those neonates who are alive at birth and receiving care, 35% born at 22 weeks survive, 38% at 23 weeks and 60% at 24 weeks (Mactier et al., 2020), while the ANZNN data of infants born between 2013 and 2016 shows that 51.3% of neonates born <24

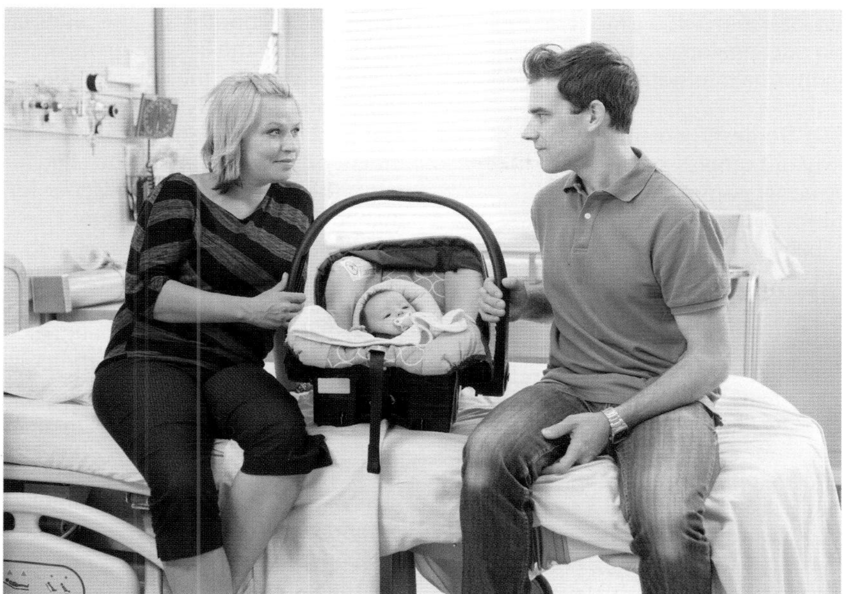

FIGURE 25.3 **Parents taking their infant home from the neonatal unit**
Source: Shutterstock/Tyler Olson.

weeks survive to discharge, 69.8% at 24 weeks and 83.4% at 25 weeks (Chow et al., 2021). These infants would qualify for enrolment in formal follow-up programs to monitor their growth and development, either in a designated clinic or by their local primary healthcare provider. Most developed countries have national networks that collect and then pool data from neonatal units, and analyse it to benchmark, monitor and improve outcomes. For example, there is the ANZNN, the Canadian Neonatal Network and similar neonatal networks in the UK, Europe and the USA.

REFLECTION

Neonatal nurses/midwives caring for neonates in a neonatal unit continuously record any interventions and the neonate's responses, test results and complete other significant documentation on progress sheets or in the neonate's case notes. Remember that the data may be collected in the future for follow-up purposes and, for documentation to have integrity, it needs to be complete and accurate.

Despite the need for a consistent approach to neonatal follow-up programs in order to be able to compare and contrast outcomes, or even to aggregate the data, programs vary widely across the world. There are differences in inclusion criteria, the timing of assessments, the outcome measures and the use of appropriate control groups. Without consistency, it is difficult to be able to provide parents with reliable information about the probable outcomes for their neonate, and what to look for in terms of milestones at certain ages.

FAMILY-CENTRED CARE 25.4

Outcome statistics are needed to counsel families about their infant's likely course, and so that parents know at what ages specific problems may emerge.

Doyle et al. (2014) developed a framework to follow neonates at higher risk for long-term health problems, particularly neurosensory impairments, and included neonates from the following categories:

- preterm (PT; gestational age <37 weeks); higher risk – very preterm (VPT; <32 weeks); highest risk – extremely preterm (EPT; <28 weeks)
- low birthweight (LBW; birthweight <2500 g); higher risk – very low birthweight (VLBW; <1500 g); highest risk – extremely low birthweight (ELBW; <1000 g)
- small for gestational age (SGA – <3rd percentile or <−2 SD weight for gestational age and sex): infants who are also at higher risk, but would also usually fall into one of the LBW categories
- neonatal encephalopathy (including seizures), regardless of cause
- term neonates who have received positive pressure ventilation for >24 hours
- congenital brain or heart malformations, genetic syndromes or inborn errors of metabolism that affect neurodevelopmental outcomes
- failed newborn hearing screening
- neonatal central nervous system infections – meningitis/encephalitis
- requiring major surgery (e.g. brain, cardiac, other thoracic or abdominal)

- hyperbilirubinaemia (bilirubin >400 μmol/L or clinical evidence of bilirubin encephalopathy)
- neurobehavioural abnormalities noted in the newborn period
- at high social risk (e.g. domestic violence, previous child abuse, severe poverty or homelessness)
- substance abuse by either parent
- major psychiatric history in either parent
- developmental disability in either parent.

Timing and format of follow-up programs

High-risk neonates need follow-up appointments at regular intervals. These are generally held soon after discharge, at 4 months, 8 months, 12 and 24 months of age. Some infants may be recommended for longer-term follow-up, up to 8 years of age, if developmental difficulties arise and the infant needs additional support to strive to meet their milestones (Lauriello & Aylward, 2021). Appointment dates are adjusted for prematurity – for example, a neonate born 3 months early will have the 12-month developmental check at 15 months of age, although this correction is made for only the first few years of the infant's life.

In many cases, the needs of the neonate will determine the personnel involved. Infants with few concerns can be assessed by their primary care provider, such as a general practitioner or a maternal and child health nurse, who then refers the neonate to specialists for further assessment and management when necessary. The assessments may be much more detailed if data are being collected for research, or if infants have multiple areas of concern, and involve many other health professionals, such as the '... physician, nurse practitioner, occupational therapist, physical therapist, audiologist, psychologist, ophthalmologist, speech and language specialist, respiratory therapist, nutritionist, neurologist, and subspecialists' (Hummel & Naber, 2021, p. 342). Late preterm infants also require specific follow-up services as they have been shown to have higher rates of developmental delay, behavioural and emotional disorders, as well as **cerebral palsy (CP)** than term infants (Reymundo et al., 2019).

The parameters set out in Table 25.3 will be assessed.

TABLE 25.3 **Parameters assessed in a long-term follow-up program**

Parameter	Measurement
Physical health	Physical examination and standard history taking with parents about any health issues
Growth	Height, weight and head circumference compared with WHO standards
Feeding	Discussion with parents or questionnaire about any feeding issues
Special senses	Eye examination; universal hearing screening
Neurological	Motor function, tone and tendon reflexes (checking for evidence of cerebral palsy)
Motor skills	Fine and gross motor skill development and coordination (e.g. Bayley Scales (see Fig. 25.4), Prechtl's General Movement Assessment)
Cardiovascular health	Vital signs including blood pressure
Respiratory health	Auscultation and vital signs, 6-minute walk test, lung volumes
Learning and cognition	Examples include the Bayley Scales of Infant and Toddler Development, Griffiths Mental Development Scales, Wechsler scales, IQ tests
Language	Speaking and understanding (e.g. the Rosetti Infant Toddler Language Scale, Pre-School Language Scale)
Pre-academic skills	As school age approaches, assessment of school readiness such as cognitive ability, communication and emotional wellbeing (e.g. Pre-School Screening Test)
Academic progress	At school age, numeracy and literacy (e.g. Wechsler Individual Achievement Test)
Behaviour	Neurobehavioural evaluation, crying, settling, sleeping, interaction with family members, social withdrawal, anxiety
Social skills	Smiling, eye contact, vocalisation – interaction with the environment
Daily functioning	1–2 years of age – taking more responsibility in their own care (e.g. feeding, dressing and toileting themselves)
Self-esteem and wellbeing	Ability to form and maintain relationships (e.g. Preschool Age Psychiatric Assessment, the Modified Checklist for Autism in Toddlers)
Parents' mental health	Parents' mental wellbeing is needed to allow them to nurture their infant
Carer–child interaction	Understanding their infant's needs, cues and behaviours, scaffolding the child's learning, fostering successful social behaviour
Social support	Ensuring parents are not isolated (e.g. interview questions, Parenting Stress Index)
Siblings	Ensuring siblings are not adversely affected (e.g. Depression Anxiety Stress Scales)

Source: adapted from Doyle et al. (2014).

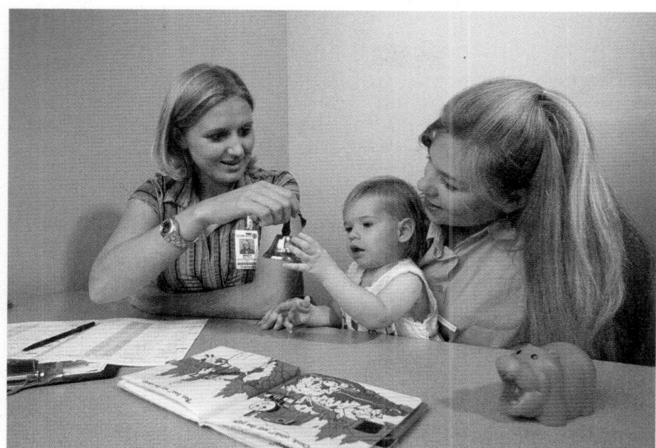

FIGURE 25.4 **Infant undergoing the Bayley Scales assessment**

Source: USDA/Stephen Ausmus.

FAMILY-CENTRED CARE 25.5

Families of high-risk neonates need the support of high-quality follow-up programs after discharge so they can be reassured that their child is healthy and growing and developing normally. They also need to know whether any health problems are likely to be encountered in the future. Ideally, this follow-up care should be coordinated by a case worker who is responsible for coordination of care, at least until school entry.

Problems after discharge requiring follow-up

High-risk neonates discharged from neonatal units may suffer from a range of difficulties and/or disabilities owing to their gestational age and illness. As a result, their ongoing care is an interdisciplinary effort that may include medical evaluation, physiotherapy, occupational therapy, developmental psychology, audiology, ophthalmology, speech pathology, neurology, nutritionists/dietitians and social workers, with the support of specialists from the areas of cardiology, ophthalmology, neurology and otorhinolaryngology (Hummel & Naber, 2021). A neonatal nurse has the appropriate background and skills to coordinate these services for the family and is recognised as the facilitator of the process of constructing the family's autonomy in taking care of the preterm neonate after discharge from hospital. The most frequently encountered disorders and the relevant follow-up considerations are explained below.

Cerebral palsy

Cerebral palsy (CP) is characterised by abnormal muscle tone and impaired motor function and control, and is not an uncommon neurological outcome among extremely preterm and/or extremely low birthweight infants. The prevalence of CP varies from country to country, and in high-income countries it occurs in approximately 2/1000 live births. Interestingly, while CP rates increase as gestational age falls, the prevalence of CP in preterm infants is actually declining (Haataja, 2020). The cause of CP is still unknown, but it is associated with comorbidities, and various underlying genetic variants. Risk factors include prematurity (in these neonates CP is related to periventricular leucomalacia, intraventricular haemorrhage and bronchopulmonary dysplasia), IUGR, intrauterine infection, antepartum haemorrhage, severe placental pathology and multiple pregnancy. Only a few cases of CP are attributed to perinatal hypoxia and/or ischaemia (Barkoudah & Glader, 2021). The ANZNN collects data on CP in infants assessed at 18 months' corrected age or older, as mild CP may be difficult to diagnose prior to this age (Chow et al., 2021). Of the 3611 infants with a follow-up assessment at 18–42 months of corrected age in the ANZNN report published in 2019, 200 (5.7%) had a diagnosis of CP (Chow et al., 2021, p. 43). Accompanying the motor impairments associated with CP are spastic diplegia and intellectual disability. Due to the complex needs of infants with CP, follow-up and coordination of their ongoing care is critical to their long-term outcomes. Some children's motor milestones will catch up to their peers, while others will need ongoing care from a physiotherapist or occupational therapist. A paediatric rehabilitation specialist may be needed on the interdisciplinary team for the care of these children.

Early diagnosis of CP is paramount for commencing early intervention. There is now compelling evidence that assessing infants' general movements (GMs) by video can be a very predictive indicator of CP. In the period from 3 to 5 months after term, so-called 'fidgety movements' are tiny movements of the neck, trunk and limbs in all directions and of variable acceleration. If fidgety movements are present and normal, the motor outcome will be normal, whereas absent or abnormal fidgety movements are predictive of CP with 95–98% accuracy, and when these findings are combined with brain MRI the sensitivity and specificity can be as high as 100% in extremely preterm infants (Haataja, 2020). The best age to take the video is 12–14 weeks after the neonate's due date. General movements are assessed with an awake, alert and calm neonate lying on their back. The neonate is then videoed for 3–5 minutes and the assessment is then scored. These assessments are now being undertaken routinely in many neonatal units, and there is a push to train neonatal nurses/midwives in GM assessment.

EVIDENCE-BASED PRACTICE RESEARCH 25.7

Family-centred discharge preparation and planning is important to facilitate parental confidence and competence. Walter and Robb (2019) addressed a problem of inadequate family discharge readiness in a neonatal unit with implementation of a quality improvement project where neonatal nurses undertook a 30-minute educational session focused on family-centred care followed by 4 weeks of mentoring. They concluded that 'family-centred discharge preparation improves parental confidence through bonding and hands-on skills acquisition which empowers parents to transition to home successfully' (Walter & Robb, 2019, p. 136).

The late preterm neonate

The late preterm neonate being discharged from a neonatal unit may not be included in a formal follow-up program but should be monitored by a community-based healthcare provider, who should see the neonate within 48 hours of discharge (Currie et al., 2018). These neonates are particularly at risk of re-admission with hyperbilirubinaemia, feeding difficulties, weight loss, apnoea or acute life-threatening events, suspected sepsis, respiratory problems and hypothermia (Currie et al., 2018). Until weight gain without jaundice is assured, these neonates should be monitored for the first 10 days of life, particularly with first-time mothers. Guidelines to prevent sudden infant death should be communicated to the parents taking home a late preterm neonate. To minimise the stress in parents taking home later preterm neonates, and in fact any neonate from a neonatal unit, neonatal discharge needs to be flexible and reversible.

FAMILY-CENTRED CARE 25.6

With the recent introduction of the National Disability Insurance Scheme in Australia (based on the model in New Zealand), decisions regarding the funding or resources and programs to manage the needs of high-risk neonates are now in the hands of parents and care givers. This means that it is even more imperative that parents understand the need for follow-up care and make informed decisions about the care their neonate needs now and in the long term, and that the care provided is evidence based.

CONCLUSION

A relatively trouble-free course in the neonatal unit usually results in a preterm neonate being discharged to home close to their due date. The stress associated with taking home a preterm neonate, even without the added complications of the neonate needing home oxygen or feeding through nasogastric or gastrostomy tubes, cannot be underestimated. Neonatal nurses/midwives understand this journey and are well placed to plan a smooth transition leading up to discharge and to coordinate the services required in the community to support these families. While the introduction of exogenous surfactant, less barotraumatic ventilation strategies and improved targeting of oxygen saturations has improved the outcomes of preterm neonates, they remain at high risk of neurodevelopmental impairment and need follow-up programs into early childhood to monitor and meet their developmental, learning, behavioural and social needs. Follow-up programs need to be well funded to enable them to track high-risk infants at least until school age. This process of evaluation after discharge must be organised, systematic, well documented, continuous, flexible and dialogic. Parents' opinions of their infant's progress must be included in the evaluation. Various tests measuring the infant's development, growth and general health should be evidence based, and the results should contribute to a shared database for use in audit and benchmarking.

Online Resources

Cerebral Palsy Society (Australia): <http://www.cpaustralia.com.au>

Cerebral Palsy Society (New Zealand): <https://cerebral-palsy.org.nz>

Down Syndrome Australia: <https://heartkids.org.nz>

New Zealand Down Syndrome Association: <https://nzdsa.org.nz>

The Neonatal Trust (New Zealand): <https://www.neonataltrust.org.nz>

References/Acknowledgements

Aloysius, A., Kharusi, M., Winter, R., Platonos, K., Banerjee, J., & Deierl, A. (2018). Support for families beyond discharge from the NICU. *Journal of Neonatal Nursing, 24*(1), 55–60.

American Academy of Pediatrics (AAP). (2021). When a baby's head is misshapen: positional skull deformities. <https://tinyurl.com/52v2ae3z> (Accessed 28 February 2022).

Australian Government Department of Health. (2013). *Australia's child and family health service system*. <https://www1.health.gov.au/internet/publications/publishing.nsf/Content/nat-fram-ucfhs-html,background,australia-child> (Accessed 28 February 2022).

Azad, R., Gilbert, C., Gangwe, A. B., Zhao, P., Wu, W-C., Sarbajna, P., et al. (2020). Retinopathy of prematurity: how to prevent the third epidemics in developing countries. *Asia-Pacific Journal of Ophthalmology. 9*(5), 440–448. doi: 10.1097/APO.0000000000000313.

Barkoudah, E., & Glader, L. (2021). Cerebral palsy: epidemiology, aetiology and prevention. In: M. Patterson (Ed.), *UpToDate*. Walters Kluwer. <https://www.uptodate.com/contents/cerebral-palsy-epidemiology-etiology-and-prevention#!> (Accessed 28 February 2022).

Berman, L., Raval, M. V., Ottosen, M., Mackow, A. K., Cho, M., & Goldin, A. B. (2019). Parent perspectives on readiness for discharge home after neonatal intensive care unit admission. *Journal of Pediatrics, 205*, 98–104. doi: 10.1016/j.jpeds.2018.08.086.

Boykova, M. (2016). Transition from hospital to home in parents of preterm infants. *Perinatal Neonatal Nursing, 30*(4), 327–348. doi: 10.1097/JPN.0000000000000211.

Bussé, M. L., Mackey, A. R., Carr, G., Hoeve, H. L. J., Uhlén, I. M., Goedegebure, A., et al. for the EUS€REEN Foundation.

(2021). Assessment of hearing screening programmes across 47 countries or regions III: provision of childhood hearing screening after the newborn period. *International Journal of Audiology, 60*(11), 841–848. doi: 10.1080/14992027.2021.1897170.

Butcher, E., Dezateux, C., & Knowles, R. L. (2020). Risk factors for permanent childhood hearing impairment. *Archives of Disease in Childhood, 105*(2), 187.

Campbell-Yeo, M., Kim, T., Disher, T., Richardson, B., Dol, J., Bishop, T., et al. (2021). Do single-family rooms increase parental presence, involvement, and maternal well-being in neonatal intensive care? *Journal of Perinatal Neonatal Nursing, 35*(4), 350–361. doi: 10.1097/JPN.0000000000000600. PMID: 34726653.

Chamberlain, C., Gee, G., Harfield, S., Campbell, S., Brennan, S., Clark, Y., et al. (2019). Parenting after a history of childhood maltreatment: a scoping review and map of evidence in the perinatal period. *PLoS One*. doi: 10.1371/journal.pone.0213460.

Cheung, P-Y., Hajihosseini, M., Dinu, I. A., Switzer, H., Joffe, A. R., Bond, G. Y., et al. (2021). Outcomes of preterm infants with congenital heart defects after early surgery: defining risk factors at different time points during hospitalization. *Frontiers in Pediatrics, 8*, 925. doi: 10.3389/fped.2020.616659.

Chow, S. S. W., Le Marsney, R., Haslam, R., & Lui, K. (2021). *Report of the Australian and New Zealand Neonatal Network 2014*. Sydney, NSW: ANZNN. <https://anznn.net/Portals/0/AnnualReports/Report%20of%20the%20Australian%20and%20New%20Zealand%20Neonatal%20Network%202019.pdf> (Accessed 28 February 2022).

Currie, G., Dosani, A., Premji, S. S., Reilly, S. M., Lodha, K. L., & Young, M. (2018). Caring for late preterm infants: public health nurses' experiences. *BMC Nursing, 17*, 16. doi: 10.1186/s12912-018-0286-y.

Darlow, B. A., & Husain, S. (2019). Primary prevention of ROP and the oxygen saturation targeting trials. *Seminars in Perinatology, 43*(6), 333–340. doi: 10.1053/j.semperi.2019.05.004.

Doyle, L. W., Anderson, P. J., Battin, M., Bowen, J. R., Brown, N., Callanan, C., et al. (2014). Long term follow up of high-risk children: who, why and how? *BMC Pediatrics, 14*(279), 1–15. doi: 10.1186/1471-2431-14-279.

Fitzallen, G. C., Taylor, H. G., & Bora, S. (2020). What do we know about the preterm behavioural phenotype? A narrative review. *Frontiers in Psychiatry, 11*, 154. doi: 10.3389/fpsyt.2020.00154.

Fraser, D., & Diehl-Jones, W. (2021). Ophthalmologic and auditory disorders. In: M. T. Verklan, M. Walden, & S. Forest (Eds.), *Core curriculum for neonatal intensive care nursing* (6th ed., pp. 691–780). St Louis, MO: Elsevier.

Grundt, H., Tandberg, B. S., Flacking, R., Drageset, J., & Moen, A. (2021). Associations between single-family room care and breastfeeding rates in preterm infants. *Journal of Human Lactation, 37*(3), 593–602. doi: 10.1177/0890334420962709.

Haataja, L. (2020). Early diagnosis of cerebral palsy. *Pediatric Medicine, 1*. doi: 10.21037/pm-20–53. doi: 10.21037/pm-20-53.

Hardani, A. K., Goodarzi, E., Delphi, M., & Badfar, G. (2020). Prevalence and risk factors for hearing loss in neonates admitted to the neonatal intensive care unit: a hospital study. *Cureus, 12*(10), e11207. doi: 10.7759/cureus.112.

Health Navigator New Zealand (2021). Hearing loss in babies and children. <https://www.healthnavigator.org.nz/health-a-z/h/hearing-loss-in-babies-and-children/> (Accessed 28 February 2022).

Hummel, P., & Naber, M. M. (2021). Discharge planning and transition to home. In: M. T. Verklan, M. Walden, & S. Forest (Eds.), *Core curriculum for neonatal intensive care nursing* (6th ed., pp. 329–345). St Louis, MO: Elsevier.

Jones, C., Desai, H., Fogel, J., Negrin, K., Torzone, A., Willette, S., et al. (2021). Disruptions in the development of feeding for infants with congenital heart disease. *Cardiology in the Young, 31*(4), 589–596. doi: 10.1017/S1047951120004382.

Kapur, N., Nixon, G., Robinson, P., Massie, J., Prentice, B., Wilson, A., et al. (2020). Respiratory management of infants with chronic neonatal lung disease beyond the NICU: a position statement from the Thoracic Society of Australia and New Zealand. *Respirology, 25*(8), 880–888.

Karnati, S., Kollikonda, S., & Abu-Shaweesh, J. (2020). Late preterm infants – changing trends and continuing challenges. *International Journal of Pediatrics and Adolescent Medicine, 7*(1), 36–44. doi: 10.1016/j.ijpam.2020.02.006.

Lau, R., Crump, R. T., Brousseau, D. C., Panepinto, J. A., Nicholson, M., Engel, J., et al. (2019). Parent preferences regarding home oxygen use for infants with bronchopulmonary dysplasia. *Journal of Pediatrics, 213*, 30–37. doi: 10.1016/j.jpeds.2019.05.069.

Lauriello, N. F., & Aylward, G. P. (2021). Follow-up of the NICU patient. In: T. Rosenkrantz (Ed.), *Medscape*. <https://emedicine.medscape.com/article/1833812-overview#a1> (Accessed 28 February 2022).

Lemyre, B., Jefferies, A. L., & O'Flaherty, P. (2018). Facilitating discharge from hospital of the healthy term infant. *Paediatrics and Child Health, 23*(8), 515–522. doi: 10.1093/pch/pxy127.

Mactier, H., Bates, S. E., Johnston, T., Lee-Davey, C., Marlow, N., Mulley, K., et al.; BAPM Working Group. (2020). Perinatal management of extreme preterm birth before 27 weeks of gestation: a framework for practice. *Archives of Disease in Childhood. Fetal and Neonatal Edition, 105*, 232–239.

Mannix, T., Tan, A., Morris, S., & Marshall, P. (2019). Cost effectiveness of a neonatal early discharge programme. *Journal of Paediatrics and Child Health, 55*(S.1), 56–115.

Morag, I., Hendel, Y., Karol, D., Geva, R., & Tzipi, S. (2019). Transition from nasogastric tube to oral feeding: the role of parental guided responsive feeding. *Frontiers in Pediatrics, 7*, 190. doi: 10.3389/fped.2019.00190.

National Eye Institute. (2019). Retinopathy of prematurity. <https://www.nei.nih.gov/learn-about-eye-health/eye-conditions-and-diseases/retinopathy-prematurity> (Accessed 28 February 2022).

New Zealand Ministry of Health. (2021). The Well Child/Tamariki Ora Program. <https://www.health.govt.nz/publication/well-child-tamariki-ora-review-report> (Accessed 28 February 2022).

Pineda, R., Heiny, E., Roussin, J., Nellis, P., Bogan, K., & Smith, J. (2020). Implementation of the baby bridge program reduces timing between NICU discharge and therapy activc. *Journal of Early Intervention, 42*(3), 275–296. doi: 10.1177/1053815119900241.

Purcell, P. L., Deep, N. L., Waltzman, S. B., Roland, J. T. Jr, Cushing, S. L., Papsin, B. C., et al. (2021). Cochlear implantation in infants: why and how. *Trends in Hearing, 25*, 23312165211031751. doi: 10.1177/23312165211031751.

Reymundo, M. C., Suazo, J. A. H., Aguilar, M. J. C., Faura, F. J. S., Galiana, G. G., Peinador, Y. M., et al. (2019). Follow-up recommendations for the late preterm infant. *Annals of Pediatrics, 90*(5), 318.e1–318.e8. doi: 10.1016/j.anpedi.2019.01.008.

Richards, R. (2017a). Discharge checklist for the high-risk infant. Sydney, NSW [Unpublished].

Richards, R. (2017b). Preparation for parents to take a neonate home on oxygen. Sydney, NSW [Unpublished].

Sankar, M. J., Sankar, J., & Chandra, P. (2018). Anti-vascular endothelial growth factor (VEGF) drugs for treatment of retinopathy of prematurity. *Cochrane Database of Systematic Reviews, 1*, CD009734. doi: 10.1002/14651858.CD009734.pub3.

Setiawan, J., Mannix, T., & Sweet, L. (2019). Understanding the effects of neonatal early discharge on parents: a literature review. *Journal of Perinatal and Neonatal Nursing, 33*, 170–188. doi: 10.1097/JPN.0000000000000395.

Shillington, J., & Deborah McNeil, D. (2021). Transition from the neonatal intensive care unit to home: a concept analysis. *Advanced Neonatal Care, 21*(5), 399–406. doi: 10.1097/ANC.0000000000000835.

South Australia (SA) Health. (2018). Assessing parent infant relationship. SA Maternal and Clinical Network. <https://www.sahealth.sa.gov.au/wps/wcm/connect/1d2582004ee1d8d1ac7badd150ce4f37/Assessing+parent+infant+relationship_PPG_v2_0.pdf?MOD=AJPERES&CACHEID=ROOTWORKSPACE-1d2582004ee1d8d1ac7badd-150ce4f37-nKKxb7Z> (Accessed 28 February 2022).

Starship. (2020). Home oxygen – care of babies following discharge from NICU. <https://starship.org.nz/guidelines/home-oxygen-care-of-babies-following-discharge-from-nicu/> (Accessed 28 February 2022).

Sung, V., & Carew, P. (2019). Hearing loss still a challenge for kids. Melbourne, Vic: University of Melbourne. <https://pursuit.unimelb.edu.au/articles/hearing-loss-still-a-challenge-for-kids> (Accessed 28 February 2022).

Verklan, M. T., & Walden, M. (Eds.). (2021). *Core curriculum for neonatal intensive care nursing* (6th ed.). St Louis, MO: Elsevier.

Walter, L., & Robb, M. (2019). Promoting croach. *Journal for Nurses in Professional Development, 35*, 132–136. doi: 10.1097/NND.0000000000000519.

Wetzel, C., Davis, L., Grohler, N., Oprondek, D., Ruff, D., Lowery, K., et al. (2020). A quality improvement project to improve the use of mother's own milk (MOM) with precision oropharyngeal therapy. *Advances in Neonatal Care, 20*, E19–E30. doi: 10.1097/ANC.0000000000000691.

Wilson-Costello, D., & Payne, A. (2021). Long-term neurodevelopmental outcome of preterm infants: epidemiology and risk factors. In: R. Martin & M. Augustyn (Eds.), *UpToDate*. Walters Kluwer. <https://www.uptodate.com/contents/103308#!> (Accessed 28 February 2022).

Wong, M. D., Chung, H., & Chawla, J. (2020). Using continuous overnight pulse oximetry to guide home oxygen therapy in chronic neonatal lung disease. *Journal of Paediatric Child Health, 56*, 309–316. doi: 10.1111/jpc.14606.

Wong, M. D., Neylan, M., Williams, G., Zahir, S. F., & Chawla, J. (2021). Predictors of home oxygen duration in chronic neonatal lung disease. *Pediatric Pulmonology, 56*, 992–999. doi: 10.1002/ppul.25257.

Wright, B., Hargate, R., Garside, M., Carr, G., Wakefield, T., Swanwick, R., et al. (2021). A systematic scoping review of early interventions for parents of deaf infants. *BMC Pediatrics, 21*, 467. doi: 10.1186/s12887-021-02893-9.

Wroblewska-Seniuk, K., Dabrowski, P., Szyfter, W., & Mazela, J. (2017). Universal newborn hearing screening: methods and results, obstacles, and benefits. *Pediatric Research, 81*, 415–422. doi: 10.1038/pr.2016.250.

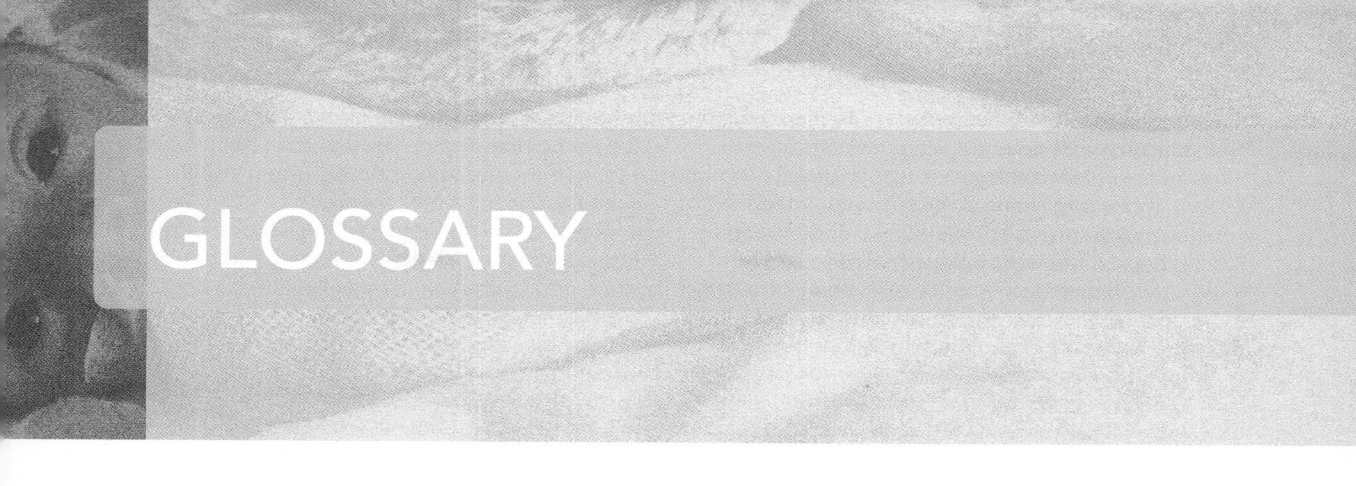

GLOSSARY

Aboriginal Community Controlled Health Service (ACCHS) An incorporated Aboriginal organisation initiated by and based in a local Aboriginal community. Delivers a holistic and culturally appropriate health service to the community.

activated partial thromboplastin time (APTT) An assay used as a screening test to evaluate the overall integrity of the intrinsic/common coagulation pathway.

acute renal failure (ARF) Also known as acute kidney injury (AKI), ARF is defined as an abrupt or rapid decline in renal filtration function.

acyanotic Characterised as the absence of cyanosis. Acyanotic heart defects, also known as non-cyanotic heart defects, are a class of congenital heart defects whereby blood is shunted from the left side of the heart to the right side of the heart owing to a structural defect in the interventricular septum.

adenosine triphosphate (ATP) An energy-carrying molecule found in all living organisms' cells. ATP extracts chemical energy from the breakdown of food molecules and uses it to generate other cellular processes.

adipose tissue An anatomical term for loose connective tissue composed of adipocytes. Its main role is to store energy in the form of fat.

analgesia A class of drugs that relieve pain without causing loss of consciousness.

antenatal hydronephrosis (ANH) The most common urological abnormality detected in pregnancy. ANH includes various urological conditions from transient dilatation of the renal collecting system to severe obstructive uropathy requiring surgical intervention.

arrhythmia Any change from the normal sequence of electrical impulses, such as atrial fibrillation, bradycardia, tachycardia, conduction disorders, rhythm disorders, ventricular fibrillation, premature contractions, etc.

assessment of preterm infant's behaviour (APIB) A newborn neurobehavioural assessment appropriate for preterm, at-risk and full-term newborns, from birth to 1 month after the expected due date.

atrial septal defect (ASD) A hole in the wall between the atria. The condition is congenital. Small defects may never cause a problem and may be found incidentally.

atrioventricular septal defect (AVSD) A heart defect in which there are holes between the chambers of the right and left sides of the heart, and the valves that control the flow of blood between these chambers may not be formed correctly.

Australian and New Zealand Neonatal Network (ANZNN) A collaborative network established in 1994 that monitors the care of high-risk newborn infants by pooling data to provide quality assurance for this resource-consuming care.

Australian Bureau of Statistics (ABS) Australia's official statistical organisation; it assists and encourages informed decision making, research and discussion within governments and the community, by providing high-quality, objective and responsive national data.

Australian College of Neonatal Nurses (ACNN) A national, not-for-profit organisation that serves as the peak professional body for neonatal nurses in all states of Australia.

Australian Health Practitioner Regulation Agency (AHPRA) The organisation responsible for the registration and accreditation of health professions across Australia, including nursing and midwifery.

back transfer A back transfer occurs when babies have graduated from intensive care to special care, whereby they are returned to their local base hospital's special care unit via a back-transfer team. Also known as 'return transfer' or 'step down'.

birth suite A birthing area designed to keep the baby and mother together. Emergency equipment should be available, but the design should be more 'homely' than 'medical'.

blood culture (BC) A culture performed to test the blood for bacteria, fungi and other microorganisms. A positive BC means a pathogen has been detected in the blood.

blood pressure (BP) The pressure of circulating blood on the walls of blood vessels.

bowel obstruction Bowel obstruction, also referred to as intestinal obstruction, is a mechanical or functional obstruction of the intestines that prevents the normal movement of the products of digestion. Either the small intestine or the large intestine may be affected.

brown adipose tissue (BAT) A uniquely mammalian tissue that protects neonatal body temperature around the time of birth by combusting triglycerides in the numerous mitochondria to emit heat.

bundle approach A set of evidence-based practices that, when performed collectively and reliably, improve patient outcomes. Many bundle elements are well-established practices, combined in a structured protocol that is agreed upon and is the responsibility of the whole clinical team.

carbon dioxide (CO_2) A gas produced by all aerobic organisms when they metabolise carbohydrates and lipids to produce energy by respiration.

cardiac output (CO) CO is the product of the heart rate (HR), or the number of heart beats per minute (bpm), and the stroke volume (SV), which is the volume of blood pumped from the ventricle per beat; hence, $CO = HR \times SV$.

cardiopulmonary bypass (CPB) CPB replaces the function of the heart and lungs while the heart is arrested to provide a bloodless, stable surgical field.

central line-associated bloodstream infection (CLABSI) Central line-associated bloodstream infections are defined as a laboratory-confirmed bloodstream infection (not related to an infection at another site) where a central line was in place within a 48-hour period before the development of a bloodstream infection.

cerebral blood flow (CBF) CBF is defined as the volume of blood passing through a given amount of brain tissue per unit of time, most commonly millilitres of blood per minute per 100 g of brain tissue.

cerebral palsy (CP) An umbrella term that refers to a group of disorders affecting an individual's ability to move. It is due to damage to the developing brain either during pregnancy or shortly after birth.

cerebrospinal fluid (CSF) A clear, colourless body fluid found in the brain and spinal cord. It is produced by the specialised ependymal cells in the choroid plexuses of the ventricles of the brain, and absorbed in the arachnoid granulations.

chemical burn An extravasation chemical burn is the process by which any liquid (fluid or drug) accidentally leaks into the surrounding subcutaneous or subdermal tissues surrounding the intravenous or intra-arterial administration site.

chlorhexidine A disinfectant and antiseptic that is used for skin disinfection. It is active against gram-positive and gram-negative organisms, facultative anaerobes, aerobes and yeasts.

chronic lung disease (CLD) CLD results from the effects of positive pressure ventilation on a structurally and functionally immature lung. Chorioamnionitis and an inflammatory cascade have also been implicated in the pathogenesis of CLD, but their precise role is uncertain. It is characterised primarily by prolonged need for ventilatory support, O_2 requirements, need for home oxygen and re-admission with respiratory illness in the first year of life. Also referred to as bronchopulmonary dysplasia (BPD).

clinical governance A system by which managing bodies, managers, clinicians and staff share responsibility and accountability for the quality of care, continuously improving and minimising risks and fostering an environment of excellence in patient care.

coarctation of the aorta (COA) A congenital condition whereby the aorta is narrow, usually in the area where the ductus arteriosus (ligamentum arteriosum after regression) inserts. Also known as aortic narrowing.

cold stress Cold stress is the result of prolonged hypothermia. Prolonged, unrecognised cold stress may divert calories to produce heat, impairing growth. Neonates have a metabolic response to cooling that involves chemical (non-shivering) thermogenesis by sympathetic nerve discharge of noradrenaline (norepinephrine) in the brown fat.

collagen The main structural protein in the extracellular space in the various connective tissues. As the main component of connective tissue, it is the most abundant protein in mammals. It consists of amino acids wound together to form triple helices that form elongated fibrils. It is mostly found in fibrous tissues such as tendons, ligaments and skin.

complete heart block (CHB) Third-degree atrioventricular block (AV block), also known as complete heart block, is a condition in which the nerve impulses generated in the sinoatrial (SA) node in the atrium do not propagate to the ventricles.

computed tomography (CT) A CT scan uses a computer-processed combination of many X-ray measurements taken from different angles to produce cross-sectional (tomographic) images (virtual 'slices') of specific areas of a scanned object, allowing the user to see inside the object. Other terms include computed axial tomography (CAT scan) and computer-aided tomography.

congenital diaphragmatic hernia (CDH) CDH is a birth defect of the diaphragm. The most common type is a Bochdalek hernia; other types include Morgagni hernia, diaphragm eventration and central tendon defects of the diaphragm. It is a serious congenital abnormality associated with pulmonary hypoplasia (generally worse on the ipsilateral side); structural and functional lung immaturity; a reduction in pulmonary arteriolar cross-sectional area; muscular hyperplasia of the remaining pulmonary arterioles; and an association with other major anomalies, chromosomal and non-chromosomal, in up to 20% of cases.

congenital heart disease (CHD) A congenital heart defect, also known as a congenital heart anomaly or congenital heart disease, is a problem in the structure of the heart that is present at birth.

congestive heart failure (CHF) CHF refers to a clinical state of systemic and pulmonary congestion resulting from the inability of the heart to pump as much blood as is required for the adequate metabolism of the body. Signs and symptoms of CHF in a newborn include tachycardia, respiratory distress, feeding intolerance, irritability and a weak cry. The neonate with CHF will usually have hepatosplenomegaly.

Congress of Aboriginal and Torres Strait Islander Nurses and Midwives (CATSINaM) The sole representative body for Aboriginal and Torres Strait Islander nurses and midwives in Australia.

continuous positive airway pressure (CPAP) A type of positive airway pressure ventilator which applies mild air pressure on a continuous basis to keep the airways continuously patent. It is an alternative to positive end expiratory pressure (PEEP). Both modalities stent the lungs' alveoli open and thus recruit more of the lungs' surface area for ventilation.

convection Heat is transferred by convection when air currents carry heat away from the body surface. If the infant's body surface is warmer than the surrounding air, heat is first conducted into the air and then carried away by the convective air currents.

core temperature The core temperature is the physical state at which the internal organs and bodily systems function at an optimal level. Core body temperature is an aspect of thermoregulation, the body's ability to control its operating temperature within a constant range.

Council of International Neonatal Nurses (COINN) An organisation which represents nurses who specialise in the care of newborn infants and their families or have a special interest in this area of nursing. COINN is part of the growing international community of nurses that represents a resource for nurses who want to form a national or local organisation, create guidelines for care or professional standards or want advice on neonatal nursing issues.

culture Culture is the sum of attitudes, customs and beliefs that distinguishes one group of people from another. Culture is transmitted through language, material objects, ritual, institutions and art, from one generation to the next.

cyanosis Cyanosis is defined as the bluish or purplish discoloration of the skin or mucous membranes due to the tissues near the skin surface having low oxygen saturation.

dermis The thick layer of living tissue below the epidermis which forms the true skin, containing blood capillaries, nerve endings, sweat glands, hair follicles and other structures.

developmental care (DC) An approach to care that individualises care of infants to maximise neurological development and reduce long-term cognitive and behavioural problems.

dextrose gel Oral dextrose (glucose) gel is a popular therapy for neonatal hypoglycaemia. Dextrose gel (administered buccally) is non-invasive, inexpensive and effective for treatment of neonatal hypoglycaemia in neonates who meet eligibility criteria.

dimercaptosuccinic acid (DMSA) scan The DMSA renal scan is a method for assessing kidney function.

direct antiglobulin test (DAT) The DAT, also known as the direct Coombs test, is used primarily to help determine whether the cause of haemolytic anaemia, a condition in which red blood cells (RBCs) are destroyed more quickly than they can be replaced, is due to antibodies attached to RBCs.

discharge planning A process that involves the family and any staff involved in the neonate's care. The aim of discharge planning is to ensure a safe and smooth discharge from hospital – whether to home, another nursery setting closer to home or another location.

disseminated intravascular coagulation (DIC) DIC is characterised by systemic activation of blood coagulation, which results in generation and deposition of fibrin, leading to microvascular thrombi in various organs and contributing to multiple organ dysfunction.

donor breast milk Excess human milk provided by a mother for use by a recipient who is not the mother's own baby, i.e. a hospitalised preterm or ill infant. The human milk is donated on a voluntary basis. Donor human milk is an alternative to infant formula for special needs infants, not a substitute for the mother's own milk.

ductus arteriosus (DA) In the developing fetus, the ductus arteriosus is a blood vessel connecting the main pulmonary artery to the proximal descending aorta. It allows most of the blood from the right ventricle to bypass the fetus's fluid-filled non-functioning lungs. Upon closure at birth, it becomes the ligamentum arteriosum.

dysrhythmia Dysrhythmias (arrhythmias) are disorders of the electrical properties of the heart. Two major types of disorders can occur: an abnormality in the generation of an electrical impulse (abnormality in automaticity) or an abnormality in impulse conduction after generation of the impulse (abnormality in propagation).

early discharge Early discharge from hospital is generally defined as 6–12 hours following a normal delivery.

early-onset sepsis (EOS) EOS refers to sepsis presenting in the first 7 days of life with some sources referring to EOS as developing within the first 72 hours of life. Group B streptococcus (GBS) is the most common aetiological agent, while *Escherichia coli* is the most common cause of mortality.

electrocardiography (ECG) An ECG records the electrical activity generated by heart muscle depolarisations, which propagate in pulsating electrical waves towards the skin.

electroencephalography/ electroencephalogram (EEG) EEG is an electrophysiological monitoring method to record electrical activity of the brain. It is typically non-invasive, with the electrodes placed along the scalp, although invasive electrodes are sometimes used such as in electrocorticography.

emollients Emollient ointments are commonly used to treat dry skin in all populations as they help the body retain moisture. Emollients have been used to improve the condition of neonatal skin.

end-of-life care (EOLC) EOLC is often referred to as palliative care. EOLC, however, refers to the final days and/or hours of a baby's life for babies with life-limiting conditions. The aim of EOLC is to keep the baby comfortable and to support the parents in caring for their baby according to their wishes and beliefs.

endotracheal tube (ETT) An ETT is a catheter that is inserted into the trachea for the primary purpose of establishing and maintaining a patent airway and to ensure the adequate exchange of oxygen and carbon dioxide.

enteral nutrition Enteral nutrition refers to any method of feeding the neonate that uses the gastrointestinal (GI) tract to deliver part or all of the neonate's caloric requirements.

epidermal stripping Epidermal (skin) stripping is the accidental removal of one or more layers of the stratum corneum following removal of adhesive tape or dressings.

epidermis The epidermis is the outer layer of the three layers of the skin, the inner layers being the dermis and the hypodermis. The epidermal layer provides a barrier to infection from environmental pathogens and regulates the amount of water released from the body through transepidermal water loss.

epidermolysis bullosa (EB) A group of mainly inherited connective tissue diseases that cause blisters in the skin and mucous membranes.

erythropoiesis The process by which red blood cells (erythrocytes) are produced. During human fetal development, erythropoiesis first occurs in the yolk sac, then in the fetal liver and then, in the third trimester and after birth, in the bone marrow.

erythropoietin (EPO) A hormone produced by the kidney that promotes the formation of red blood cells by the bone marrow.

ethical decision making Ethical decision making refers to the process of evaluating and choosing among alternatives in a manner consistent with ethical principles.

ethical principles The two major classifications of ethical principles and ethical thought are utilitarianism and deontology. Deontology requires that both the means and the end goal must be moral and ethical; and the utilitarian school of ethical thought states that the end goal justifies the means even when the means are not moral. The ethical principles that nurses and midwives must adhere to are the principles of justice, beneficence, nonmaleficence, accountability, fidelity, autonomy and veracity.

ethics Ethics, simply defined, is a principle that describes what is expected in terms of 'right' and 'correct' and 'wrong' or 'incorrect' in terms of behaviour. Ethics and ethical practice are integrated into all aspects of nursing and midwifery care.

evaporation The process of losing heat through the conversion of water to gas.

extracellular fluid (ECF) ECF refers to all body fluid outside the cells. The main component of extracellular fluid is the interstitial fluid that bathes cells.

extracorporeal membrane oxygenation (ECMO) ECMO involves the use of an artificial lung (membrane) located outside the body (extracorporeal) that oxygenates the blood. ECMO is an important treatment for infants and children with cardiorespiratory failure. There are several forms of ECMO; the two most common are veno-arterial (VA) ECMO and veno-venous (VV) ECMO.

extremely low birthweight (ELBW) An ELBW infant is defined as one with a birthweight of less than 1000 g. Most ELBW infants are usually born at 27 weeks' gestational age or younger.

family and infant neurodevelopmental education (FINE) An educational pathway in family-centred developmental care for all healthcare professionals working in neonatal care. It has two established courses: a foundation course and a more advanced course for practical skills. A third level is in the planning stages.

family-centred care (FCC) FCC assures the health and wellbeing of newborns and their families through a respectful family–professional partnership. It honours the strengths, cultures, traditions and expertise that everyone brings to this relationship. FCC is the standard of practice that results in high-quality services.

family-integrated care (FIC) A model of neonatal care that supports parents to be primary care givers, as partners with the clinical team.

Family Integrated Care program (FICare) The goal of the FICare program is to support parents in becoming engaged as part of their infant's care team, becoming empowered, comfortable and confident in caring for their baby in the neonatal unit. The components of the program include staff education and support, parent education, NICU environment and psychosocial support.

feeding tolerance Feeding tolerance is demonstrated when the preterm infant is capable of safely ingesting and digesting a prescribed enteral feed without complications associated with aspiration, infection and gastrointestinal dysfunction.

free fatty acids (FFA) The by-products of the metabolism of fat in adipose tissues, FFA can be used as an immediate source of energy by many organs and can be converted by the liver into ketone bodies.

fresh frozen plasma (FFP) FFP, also known as plasma, is the blood component that remains once all the blood cells are removed from whole blood. FFP is indicated in infants with a coagulopathy who are bleeding or at risk of bleeding where a specific therapy such as vitamin K or factor concentrate is not appropriate or available. FFP contains all coagulation factors including factors VIII and V.

full blood count (FBC) An FBC, also known as a complete blood count (CBC), or full blood exam (FBE), is a blood test that measures a broad range of indices, including white cells, red cells, haemoglobin, haematocrit, mean corpuscular volume (MCV), mean corpuscular haemoglobin (MCH), mean corpuscular haemoglobin concentration (MCHC), red cell distribution width (RDW) and platelets.

functional residual capacity (FRC) The resting volume at which the elastic recoil pressure of the lung inwards equals the elastic recoil pressure of the chest wall outwards, alveolar and mouth pressure are both zero and there is no air flow.

gastrointestinal (GI) tract The GI tract includes the oesophagus, stomach, small intestine, large intestine and rectum, and the accessory organs of digestion: the liver, gallbladder and pancreas.

gastro-oesophageal reflux (GOR) The passage of gastric contents into the oesophagus. Its clinical presentation of vomiting or regurgitation is very common in infants and, in the majority of cases, is self-resolving and does not need treatment. It may be associated with irritability but only very few 'crying babies' will have significant GOR as the cause of their irritability. Gastro-oesophageal reflux disease (GORD) is GOR leading to complications.

gastroschisis Gastroschisis is characterised by the herniation of bowel and other abdominal contents through an abdominal wall defect usually located just to the right of the umbilicus. The normal insertion of the umbilical cord into the abdominal wall and the absence of a sac covering the herniated abdominal contents distinguish gastroschisis from exomphalos, the other common abdominal wall defect.

gestational age (GA) The common term used during pregnancy to describe how advanced the pregnancy is. It is measured in weeks, from the first day of the woman's last menstrual cycle to the current date.

gestational diabetes mellitus (GDM) A specific type of diabetes that only occurs during pregnancy. It is defined as any degree of glucose intolerance with onset or first recognition during pregnancy. The definition applies whether insulin or only diet modification is used for treatment and whether or not the condition persists after pregnancy.

glomerular filtration rate (GFR) The GFR describes the flow rate of filtered fluid through the kidney. Specifically, it estimates how much blood passes through the glomeruli each minute.

gluconeogenesis A metabolic pathway that results in the generation of glucose from non-carbohydrate carbon substrates such as lactate, glycerol and glucogenic amino acids.

glycogen A readily mobilised storage form of glucose. It is a very large, branched polymer of glucose residues that can be broken down to yield glucose molecules when energy is needed.

glycogenolysis A process by which glycogen, the primary carbohydrate stored in the liver and muscle cells of animals, is broken down into glucose to provide immediate energy and to maintain blood glucose levels during fasting.

golden hour protocol (GHP) A GHP includes practising evidence-based interventions for term and preterm neonates in the initial 60 minutes of postnatal life (referred to as the golden hour) for better long-term outcomes.

haemangioma A benign tumour of vascular origin usually seen in early childhood; divided into infantile haemangiomas and congenital haemangiomas.

haematocrit (Hct) The haematocrit (Hct or packed cell volume (PCV)) is a measurement of the proportion of blood that is made up of cells. The value is expressed as a fraction of cells in blood.

haematological disorders This group of disorders includes, but is not limited to, various types of anaemia, blood cancers and haemorrhagic conditions. Haematological disorders can affect the central and peripheral nervous systems, producing a wide range of neurological disturbances.

haematopoiesis Haematopoiesis refers to the commitment and differentiation processes that lead to the formation of all blood cells from haematopoietic stem cells. The early stages of mammalian haematopoiesis begin in the blood islands of the yolk sac.

haemoglobin (Hb) The protein molecule in red blood cells that carries oxygen from the lungs to the body's tissues and returns carbon dioxide from the tissues back to the lungs. It is made up of four protein molecules (globulin chains) that are connected together.

hand hygiene Hand hygiene is defined as any method that removes or destroys microorganisms on hands. It is well documented that the most important measure for preventing the spread of pathogens is effective handwashing.

healthcare provider/professional (HCP) A health professional, health practitioner or healthcare provider (sometimes simply 'provider') is an individual who provides preventive, curative, promotional or rehabilitative healthcare services in a systematic way to people, families or communities.

heart rate (HR) The speed of the heartbeat measured by the number of contractions of the heart per minute (bpm).

high-flow nasal cannula (HFNC) (Humidified) HFNC (or prong) therapy is a method of providing continuous positive airway pressure (CPAP) to neonates requiring respiratory support or in respiratory distress. HFNC may act as a bridge between low-flow oxygen therapies (O_2) and nasal continuous positive airway pressure (NCPAP), reducing the need for NCPAP/intubation. At high flows of 2 litres per kilogram per minute, using appropriate nasal prongs, a positive distending pressure of 4–8 cmH_2O may be achieved. This improves functional residual capacity (FRC), thereby reducing the work of breathing. Because flows used are high, heated water humidification is necessary to avoid drying of respiratory secretions. Also referred to as HH (heated humidified) HFNC.

high-frequency oscillatory ventilation (HFOV) A type of mechanical ventilation that uses a constant distending pressure (mean airway pressure (MAP)) with pressure variations oscillating around the MAP at very high rates (up to 900 cycles per minute). This creates small tidal volumes, often less than the dead space. In conventional ventilation, large pressure changes (the difference between PEEP and PIP) create physiological tidal volumes, and gas exchange is dependent on bulk convection (expired gas exchanged for inspired gas). HFOV relies on alternative mechanisms of gas exchange.

hospital-acquired infection (HAI) An HAI, also known as a nosocomial infection, is an infection that is acquired in a hospital or other healthcare facility. To emphasise both hospital and non-hospital settings, it is sometimes called a healthcare-associated infection (HAI or HCAI).

hyaluronidase An enzyme that breaks down hyaluronic acid, a compound best described as the 'glue' that holds cells together. When this extracellular glue is dissolved, cells are separated. The overall effect is to minimise the local damage caused by extravasation. This is helpful in extravasations as it allows for the medication to distribute through a larger area by breaking down the walls that keep it localised.

hydrocolloid A wafer type of dressing that contains gel-forming agents in an adhesive compound laminated onto a flexible, water-resistant outer layer. Some formulations contain an alginate to increase absorption capabilities.

hydronephrosis A condition that typically occurs when a kidney swells owing to urine failing to properly drain from the kidney to the bladder. This swelling most commonly affects only one kidney, but it can involve both.

hyperglycaemia Hyperglycaemia or high blood sugar is an abnormally high blood glucose (blood sugar) level in the blood.

hyperinsulinism Neonatal hyperinsulinism is a clinical syndrome of pancreatic beta-cell dysfunction characterised by failure to suppress insulin secretion in the presence of hypoglycaemia. Although rare, it is the most common cause for persistent hypoglycaemia in the newborn period.

hyperosmolar A hyperosmolar (extremely concentrated) solution is a solution with an abnormally increased concentration of solute (e.g. salt water as opposed to fresh water).

hyperthermia An elevated body temperature due to failed thermoregulation that occurs when the body produces or absorbs more heat than it dissipates.

hypoglycaemia A transient or temporary condition of decreased blood sugar or hypoglycaemia in a neonate. Hypoglycaemia is the most common metabolic problem in neonates. Within the neonatal period, hypoglycaemia is (generally) defined as a blood glucose level less than 2.6 mmol/L.

hypothermia A per axilla temperature less than 36.5°C. Mild hypothermia is defined as a temperature between 36.0°C and 36.4°C, moderate hypothermia as 32.0°C to 35.9°C, and severe hypothermia as less than 32°C.

hypoxic ischaemic encephalopathy (HIE) An acute or subacute brain injury that occurs as a result of perinatal asphyxia, caused by systemic hypoxaemia and/or reduced cerebral blood flow.

immunity The ability of an organism to resist a particular infection or toxin by the action of specific antibodies or sensitised white blood cells.

inborn errors of metabolism (IEM) A large group of rare genetic diseases that generally result from a defect in an enzyme or transport protein which results in a block in a metabolic pathway.

incubator humidification The provision of humidification of the air inside incubators, which helps reduce epidermal water loss and improves the maintenance of body temperature.

infection control The discipline concerned with preventing nosocomial or healthcare-associated infection, a practical (rather than academic) sub-discipline of epidemiology.

inhaled nitric oxide (iNO) An endogenous free radical, synthesised in endothelial cells, that causes vascular smooth muscle relaxation and, hence, vasodilation. Inhaled nitric oxide selectively targets pulmonary vessels, causing a potent and sustained vasodilatation and, therefore, increased pulmonary blood flow.

insulin A hormone produced in the pancreas by the islets of Langerhans, which regulates the amount of glucose in the blood.

intermittent positive pressure ventilation (IPPV) A form of assisted or controlled respiration produced by a ventilatory apparatus in which compressed gas is delivered under positive pressure into the airways until a preset pressure is reached.

interrupted aortic arch (IAA) A rare cardiac anomaly in which the aortic arch is incomplete or interrupted.

intracellular fluid (ICF) The fluid found inside living cells, and is also known as cytosol. It consists of water and anything soluble that is dissolved in it, such as soluble proteins and ions.

intrauterine growth restriction (IUGR) IUGR occurs when a fetus has an estimated weight below the 10th percentile for its gestational age.

intravenous immunoglobulin (IVIG) A sterile solution of concentrated antibodies extracted from healthy people that is administered intravenously to treat disorders of the immune system or to boost the immune response to serious illness.

intraventricular haemorrhage (IVH) Bleeding inside or around the ventricles, the spaces in the brain containing the cerebral spinal fluid.

kangaroo care (KC) Kangaroo care (also known as skin-to-skin care) refers to the method of holding an infant in an upright and prone position, skin to skin, on the parent's chest for a period of time. Also referred to as kangaroo mother care (KMC).

ketogenesis The biochemical process by which organisms produce a group of substances collectively known as ketone bodies through the breakdown of fatty acids and ketogenic amino acids.

large for gestational age (LGA) LGA newborns are those who are larger in size than normal for their gestational age, most commonly defined as a weight above the 90th percentile for their gestational age.

late-onset sepsis (LOS) The presence of at least one episode of systemic sepsis with the initial symptoms occurring among babies aged 48 hours or more.

life-limiting condition (LLC) A condition with no reasonable hope of cure and from which the neonate is likely to die prematurely.

life-threatening condition (LTC) A condition with a high probability of death due to severe illness, but where a chance of long-term survival exists.

lipolysis The breakdown of fats and other lipids by hydrolysis to release fatty acids and produce energy.

low birthweight (LBW) A term used to describe babies who are born weighing less than 2500 grams.

magnetic resonance imaging (MRI) A non-invasive form of imaging that utilises a magnetic field, radio-frequency pulses and a computer to produce detailed pictures of organs, soft tissues, bone and virtually all other internal body structures.

mean cell volume (MCV) A measure of the average volume of a red blood cell. The MCV is attained by multiplying a volume of blood by the proportion of blood that is cellular (the haematocrit), and dividing that product by the number of red cells in that volume.

meconium-stained amniotic fluid (MSAF) MSAF occurs when the fetus passes meconium in utero and the amniotic fluid is stained with it, usually as a result of fetal distress.

medical adhesive-related skin injury (MARSI) An occurrence in which erythema and/or other manifestation of cutaneous abnormality (including, but not limited to, a vesicle, bulla, erosion or tear) persists 30 minutes or more after removal of the adhesive.

metabolic rate (MR) The amount of energy expended by an organism in a given period.

microculture and sensitivity (MCS) A laboratory test whereby a specimen (blood, urine, CSF, etc.) is examined under microscopy to identify organisms (e.g. gram-positive) which are then grown under culture to enable more specific identification (e.g. group B streptococci), and then seeded onto an agar plate containing discs saturated with various antibiotics to identify resistance to antibiotics.

micturating cystourethrogram (MCUG) An MCUG or voiding cystourethrography (VCUG) is a fluoroscopic study of the lower urinary tract in which contrast is introduced into the bladder via a urethral catheter in order to assess the bladder, urethra, postoperative anatomy and micturition to determine the presence or absence of bladder and urethral abnormalities, including vesicoureteral reflux.

minimal enteral feeds (MEF) 'Trophic' feeds, or feeds given at small volumes to stimulate development of the immature gastrointestinal tract. These feeds are not meant to be nutritive, but rather they are meant to prepare the GI tract for later nutritional feedings.

minimally invasive surfactant therapy (MIST) The administration of exogenous surfactant with non-invasive respiratory support, such as intrapharyngeal instillation, nebulisation, a laryngeal mask or a thin catheter.

multicystic dysplastic kidney disease (MCDKD) A congenital maldevelopment in which the renal cortex is replaced by numerous cysts of multiple sizes.

National Aboriginal and Torres Strait Islander Health Plan (NATSIHP) An evidence-based policy framework designed to guide policies and programs to improve Australian Aboriginal and Torres Strait Islander health until 2023.

necrotising enterocolitis (NEC) Damage to the intestinal tract ranging from mucosal injury to full-thickness necrosis and perforation, which typically occurs in the second to third week of life in preterm, formula-fed infants.

negligence A legal term that is described as an absence of due care departing from the standards of accepted practice at the time that the incident occurred.

neonatal abstinence syndrome (NAS) NAS comprises a range of clinical symptoms observed in newborns as a result of withdrawal from intrauterine drug exposure. It is more frequently linked to maternal opioid usage. The prevalence of NAS has increased fivefold in the last decade, driving up healthcare costs. Long-term neurodevelopmental morbidity and mortality are common in NAS newborns.

Neonatal Integrative Developmental Care Model (NIDCM) A specific model of care for neonates that encompasses neuroprotective developmental care utilising a family-centred approach.

neonatal intensive care unit (NICU) An environment built to provide specialised care for critically ill and/or preterm newborn infants, combining advanced technology and trained healthcare professionals.

Neonatal Nurses College of Aotearoa (NNCA) The peak professional body for neonatal nurses in New Zealand, it is a college of the New Zealand Nurses Organisation (NZNO).

neonatal retrieval Neonatal retrieval systems are designed to transport preterm or critically ill neonates from a referral centre to a major hospital using road or air transport.

neural tube defect (NTD) NTDs are a group of birth defects in which there is an opening in the spinal cord or brain because of a defect in the neurulation process.

neurodevelopment Neurodevelopment encompasses the structural and functional development of the brain, which is shaped by genetics, internal, endogenous or hormonal stimulation and external experiences from the environment that stimulate the sensory organs.

neutral thermal environment (NTE) The environmental air temperature at which a neonate can maintain their normal body temperature with a minimal metabolic rate and therefore minimal oxygen consumption.

Newborn Screening Card Originally known as the Guthrie test, the Newborn Screening Card involves the collection of blood, usually around 48 hours of age, via a heel prick. The blood is soaked into four small spots on special filter paper to enable the early diagnosis of certain metabolic disorders.

non-shivering thermogenesis (NST) The production of heat in the newborn by metabolism in brown fat, when the oxidation of fatty acids in the mitochondria produces heat that is then circulated around the body.

non-vesicant solutions Non-vesicant solutions and medications are those that do not cause ischaemia or necrosis when they escape from a vein.

nosocomial infection An infection that is acquired in a hospital or other healthcare facility.

nurse practitioner (NP) A registered nurse (RN) experienced in their clinical specialty, educated at Masters level, and who is endorsed by the Nursing and Midwifery Board of Australia (NMBA) to provide patient care in an advanced and extended clinical role.

oesophageal atresia (OA) A group of congenital anomalies where there is an interruption of the continuity of the oesophagus with or without a persistent communication with the trachea.

oliguria Oliguria in neonates is defined as a urine output less than 1 mL/kg/h.

omphalocele A birth defect in which part of the intestine, covered only by a thin transparent membrane, protrudes outside the abdomen at the umbilicus. It occurs owing to a failure during embryonic development of a section of the midgut to return from outside the abdomen and re-enter the abdomen, as it should around the 9th week of gestation.

oxygenation Oxygenation means to treat, combine or enrich with oxygen.

palliative care The comprehensive, holistic, family-centred care of neonates diagnosed with life-threatening or life-limiting conditions, which involves the prevention and relief of suffering.

parenteral nutrition-associated liver disease (PNALD) Injury to the liver caused by the long-term use of parenteral nutrition.

partial arterial carbon dioxide pressure ($PaCO_2$) Since partial pressure refers to the pressure exerted on the container walls by a specific gas in a mixture of other gases, $PaCO_2$ is the measurement of the carbon dioxide content in arterial blood.

partial arterial oxygen pressure (PaO_2) Partial pressure refers to the pressure exerted on the container walls by a specific gas in a mixture of other gases. PaO_2 is the measurement of the oxygen content in arterial blood.

partial exchange transfusion (PET) A PET involves slowly removing some of the blood volume and replacing the withdrawn blood with fluids to help dilute the red blood cell concentration, usually to treat polycythaemia.

partial oxygen pressure (PO_2) The PO_2 reflects the amount of oxygen gas dissolved in the blood.

patent ductus arteriosus (PDA) A PDA occurs when the ductus arteriosus, a fetal artery, fails to close after birth and there is persisting blood flow between the descending thoracic aorta and the pulmonary artery.

peak inspiratory pressure (PIP) The uppermost level of pressure (in cmH_2O) applied to the lungs in an inspiratory breath during mechanical ventilation.

pelviureteric junction (PUJ) obstruction PUJ obstruction/stenosis, also known as ureteropelvic junction (UPJ) obstruction/stenosis, is one of the causes of obstructive uropathy. It can be congenital or acquired, with a congenital pelviureteric junction obstruction being one of the commonest causes of antenatal hydronephrosis.

perinatal palliative care A model of support for parents who choose to continue their pregnancies following a prenatal diagnosis indicating that their baby has a life-limiting condition and might die before or shortly after birth.

peripheral oxygen saturation (SpO_2) SpO_2, also known as oxygen saturation, is an estimation expressed as a percentage of the overall percentage of binding sites on haemoglobin that are occupied by oxygen in arterial blood, usually measured with a pulse oximeter device.

periventricular leucomalacia (PVL) A form of ischaemic periventricular white matter brain injury that results in the death and decay of injured cells, leaving the brain with cystic changes. Also referred to as leukomalacia.

point-of-care testing (POCT) POCT is defined as medical diagnostic testing performed outside the clinical laboratory in close proximity to where the patient is receiving care, and is usually performed by non-laboratory personnel.

positive end expiratory pressure (PEEP) The pressure in the lungs above atmospheric pressure that exists at the end of expiration. PEEP can also be delivered as a method of ventilation in which airway pressure is maintained above atmospheric pressure at the end of exhalation by means of mechanical impedance, to prevent alveolar collapse between breaths.

positive pressure ventilation (PPV) The delivery of a controlled pressure of a gas by a mechanical respirator to the lungs to assist in ventilation or expansion of the lungs.

posterior urethral valve (PUV) An abnormality of the urethra that occurs when the urethral valves, which are small leaflets of tissue, have a narrow, slit-like opening that partially impedes urine outflow.

post-haemorrhagic hydrocephalus (PHH) PHH occurs after an intraventricular haemorrhage when disturbances in cerebrospinal fluid flow or absorption lead to progressive ventriculomegaly.

pulmonary interstitial emphysema (PIE) PIE occurs when air accumulates outside the normal air space of the pulmonary alveoli, in the connective tissue of the pulmonary interstitium.

pulse oximeter (PO) A sensor usually attached to the foot of a neonate that measures the oxygen saturation of arterial blood, by determining the percentage of oxyhaemoglobin in blood pulsating through a network of capillaries.

quality of life (QoL) A standard described to encompass the general wellbeing of individuals and societies that involves all aspects of the emotional, social, physical wellbeing, intellectual capability and ability of the person to independently perform ordinary tasks of living.

red blood cells (RBC) RBC (or erythrocytes) are red cells that contain haemoglobin, a transport molecule with a red pigment that carries oxygen and carbon dioxide.

respiratory distress syndrome (RDS) Respiratory distress in the preterm newborn (previously referred to as hyaline membrane disease) caused by developmental insufficiency of pulmonary surfactant and structural immaturity in the lungs.

rhesus (Rh) factor An inherited protein (an antigen) found on the surface of red blood cells. Red blood cells with the antigen are said to be Rh positive (Rh+). Those without the surface antigen are said to be Rh negative (Rh−).

rupture of membranes (ROM)/premature rupture of membranes (PROM) A term used during pregnancy to describe a rupture of the amniotic sac. Normally, it occurs spontaneously at full term either during or at the beginning of labour. PROM is a rupture of the amnion that occurs prior to the onset of labour.

sea level (also known as ground level) An average level of the surface of one or more of Earth's oceans from which heights such as elevations may be measured.

selective serotonin reuptake inhibitor (SSRI) A class of commonly prescribed drugs for treating depression. SSRIs affect the chemicals that nerves in the brain use to send messages to one another.

sepsis Life-threatening organ dysfunction caused by a dysregulated host response to infection.

serotonin and noradrenaline reuptake inhibitor (SNRI) A class of medications that are effective in treating depression. They are also sometimes used to treat other conditions, such as anxiety disorders and long-term (chronic) pain, especially nerve pain.

serum bilirubin reading (SBR) An orange–yellow substance made during the normal breakdown of red blood cells. The SBR level reflects the amount of bilirubin in the blood.

servo-control An electronic feedback system which functions as a thermostat to maintain a constant temperature at the site of a thermistor probe attached to the neonate by regulating the heat output of an incubator or radiant warmer.

shear A mechanical force created from parallel loads that causes the body to slide against resistance between the skin and a contact surface. The outer layers of the skin (the epidermis and dermis) remain stationary while deep fascia moves with the skeleton leading to blood-flow disruption, and eventually leading to breakdown. Shear forces are a significant risk for pressure injury formation.

silicone A synthetic material used to protect the neonatal skin, either as a protective film or as a component of an adhesive remover.

skin-to-skin care (SSC) SSC (also referred to as kangaroo care or kangaroo mother care) refers to the method of holding an infant in an upright and prone position, skin to skin, on the parent's chest for a period of time.

small for gestational age (SGA) Small for gestational age newborns are those who are smaller in size than normal for their gestational age, most commonly defined as a weight below the 10th percentile for the gestational age.

special care nursery (SCN)/special care baby unit (SCBU) A nursery or baby unit that provides care for well babies who are catching up on growth and development after a preterm birth, or those who are getting better after more complex treatment.

standard precautions A set of infection control practices that can prevent disease being transmitted by contact with blood, body fluids, non-intact skin and mucous membranes.

stratum corneum The outermost layer of skin, a mechanical barrier to the environment made up of keratins, proteins and a lipid matrix. It protects against toxins, irritants, allergens and pathogens, retains heat and water as well as maintains a normal microbiome.

sudden infant death syndrome (SIDS) SIDS is defined as the sudden and unexpected death of a newborn under 1 year of age with an onset of a fatal episode occurring during sleep, which remains unexplained after a full investigation, including a complete autopsy and assessment of the circumstances of death and the clinical history.

sudden unexpected death in infancy (SUDI) When a newborn dies suddenly and unexpectedly with no apparent cause, this is referred to as sudden unexpected death in infancy (SUDI). Sudden infant death syndrome (SIDS) and fatal sleep accidents are examples of this. A newborn can die of SUDI at any time of day or night, although most die while sleeping.

tandem mass spectrometry (TMS) Mass spectrometers are used to identify metabolic disorders in neonates by electronically weighing molecules in a blood sample. In tandem mass spectrometry, two spectrometers in a series connected by a chamber break a molecule into pieces to sort and weigh the molecules.

teratogen A drug or other substance capable of interfering with the development of a fetus, causing birth defects.

thermogenesis The process of heat production in organisms. Adults shiver when cold, which increases muscle activity, and thus produces heat. Newborns cannot shiver, so they produce heat by 'non-shivering thermogenesis'.

thermoregulation The ability to balance heat production and heat loss in order to maintain body temperature within a certain normal range.

thyroid-stimulating hormone (TSH) A hormone produced by the pituitary gland in response to signals from the hypothalamus gland to promote the growth of the thyroid gland in the neck and stimulate it to produce more thyroid hormones.

tidal volume (TV) Tidal volume (symbol TV or VT) is the volume of air inhaled or exhaled with every respiratory movement. In the term neonate it is normally approximately 6–10 mL/kg and in the preterm infant it is 4–6 mL/kg.

total parenteral (intravenous) nutrition (TPN) A method of supplying nutrients to the body by an intravenous route, it is indicated in neonates with an impaired or non-functioning gastrointestinal tract.

transcutaneous bilirubinometry (TcB) A non-invasive method for measuring serum bilirubin levels by directing light into the skin and measuring the intensity of the wavelength of light that is returned.

transcutaneous monitoring (TCM) TCM devices induce hyperperfusion by local heating of the skin to provide estimates of the partial pressure of oxygen and carbon dioxide electrochemically.

transepidermal water loss (TEWL) The loss of water that passes from inside the body through the epidermal layer of the skin to the surrounding atmosphere by diffusion and/or evaporation processes. It is also known as insensible water loss (IWL).

transfusion-related acute gastrointestinal injury (TRAGI)/transfusion-associated necrotising enterocolitis (TANEC) The occurrence of necrotising enterocolitis within 48 hours of red cell transfusion.

transient tachypnoea of the newborn (TTNB) A common cause of respiratory distress in the immediate newborn period characterised by pulmonary oedema resulting from delayed resorption and clearance of fetal alveolar fluid.

trespass Trespass to a person caused by direct or intentional interference with their body or liberty, in the form of assault, battery or false imprisonment.

undescended testes (UDT) Also known as cryptorchidism, the testicles develop in the abdomen (near the kidneys) and usually descend via the inguinal canal into the scrotum by the time of birth. UDT remain in the inguinal canal.

urinary tract infection (UTI) Any infection of the kidney, ureter, bladder or urethra.

ventilation Assisting or stimulating of pulmonary respiration by any means.

ventilator-associated pneumonia (VAP) Pneumonia that develops 48 hours or longer after mechanical ventilation is given by means of an endotracheal tube or tracheostomy and results from the invasion of the lower respiratory tract and lung parenchyma by microorganisms.

vernix caseosa A white cheesy substance composed of sebum (the oil of the skin) and cells that have sloughed off the fetus's skin that covers and protects the skin of the fetus and may still be present in varying amounts at birth.

very low birthweight (VLBW) Infants born with a birthweight of less than 1500 grams are defined as very low birthweight infants.

vesicant solutions Any medication or fluid capable of causing necrosis or tissue injury when it escapes from the vein.

vesico-ureteric junction (VUJ) The area located where the ureter drains into the bladder.

vesico-ureteric reflux (VUR) VUR occurs when urine flows backwards from the bladder upwards towards the ureter, sometimes extending into the renal pelvis, calyces and collecting ducts.

vitamin K deficiency bleeding (VKDB) A bleeding problem caused by a deficiency of vitamin K that occurs in some newborns during the first few days of life.

white blood cells (WBC) Cells of the immune system that protect the body against infections and foreign matter. They are also called leucocytes.

withdrawal Symptoms of substance withdrawal in infants after birth are caused by in utero exposure to drugs of dependence. Infants may develop the condition called 'neonatal abstinence syndrome'.

APPENDICES

APPENDIX 1 NORMAL NEONATAL VITAL SIGNS

Temperature	36.4–37.4°C per axilla	
Heart rate	120–160 beats per minute	
Respiratory rate	40–60 breaths per minute	
Blood pressure	Preterm: Systolic range: 48–63 mmHg Diastolic range: 24–39 mmHg	Term: Systolic range: 60–80 mmHg Diastolic range: 40–50 mmHg Source: <https://www.safercare.vic.gov.au/clinical-guidance/neonatal/blood-pressure-disorders#goto-normal-neonatal-blood-pressure-values>
Oxygen saturation	91–95%	

Source: The Royal Children's Hospital Melbourne. Oxygen saturation SpO_2 level targeting in neonates. Online. <https://www.rch.org.au/rchcpg/hospital_clinical_guideline_index/Oxygen_Saturation_SpO2_Level_Targeting_Premature_Neonates/>.

APPENDIX 2 NORMAL LABORATORY VALUES REFERENCE RANGES (TERM NEONATES)

Value	Cord	1–24 hours	24–48 hours	48 hours–10 days
Prothrombin time (PT) (seconds)		11–14		
Activated partial thromboplastin time (APTT) (seconds)		23–35		
Capillary refill		<3 seconds		
Platelets ($10^3/mm^3$)	150–350			
Sodium (Na) (mEq/L)	147 (126–166)	143 then 145 (124–159)	148 (134–160)	149 (139–162)
Potassium (K) (mEq/L)	7.8 (5.6–12)	6.4 then 6.3 (5.3–8.9)	6.0 (5.2–7.3)	5.9 (5.0–7.7)
Chloride (Cl) (mEq/L)	103 (98–110)	101 then 103 (80–114)	102 (92–114)	103 (93–112)
Calcium (Ca) (mmol/L)	2.33 (2.1–2.8)	2.1 then 1.95 (1.7–2.4)	2.0 (1.5–2.5)	1.98 (1.5–2.4)
Calcium ionised (Ca I) (mmol/L)		1.05–1.37		1.10–1.44 (48–72 hours) 1.20–1.48 (3–10 days)
C-reactive protein (CRP) (mg/L)	<7			

Continued

APPENDIX 2 NORMAL LABORATORY VALUES REFERENCE RANGES (TERM NEONATES)—cont'd

Value	Cord	1–24 hours	24–48 hours	48 hours–10 days
Phosphate (PO_4) (mmol/L)	1.8 (1.2–2.6)	1.97 then 1.84 (0.9–2.8)	1.91 (1.0–2.8)	1.87 (0.9–2.5)
Magnesium (Mg) (mmol/L)		0.72–1.00 (12–24 hours)		0.81–1.05 (48–72 hours) 0.78–1.02 (3–10 days)
Urea (mmol/L)	10.4 (7.5–14.3)	9.6–11.8 (2.9–22.5)	11.4 (4.6–27.5)	11.1 (5.4–24.3)
Alkaline phosphatase test (ALP) (IU/L)	28–300			
Creatinine (mmol/L)			0.04–0.11	0.01–0.09
Lactate (mmol/L)	1.5–4.5	0.9–2.7 (1–12 hours) 0.8–1.2 (12–24 hours)		0.5–1.4 (3–10 days)
Albumin (g/L)	28–43			30–43 (3–10 days)
Thyroxine (T4)	8.2 (± 1.8)	19.0 (12–24 hours) (± 2.1)	19.0 (± 2.1)	19.0 then 15.9 (± 2.1 – ± 3.0)
Thyroid-stimulating hormone (TSH)		3.0–120 (12–24 hours)	3.0–30	0.3–10 (3–10 days)
Cortisol (nanomol/L)	200–700			
17-Hydroxyprogesterone (17-OHP) (nanomol/L)				0.7–12.4
Neutrophils × 10^9/L	11.1 (6–26)	15.5 then 11.5 (5–28)		5.5 (1.5–10)
Lymphocytes × 10^9/L	5.5 (2–11)	5.5 then 5.8 (2–11.5)		5.0 (2–17)
Monocytes × 10^9/L	1.1	1.2 then 1.1		1.1
Haemoglobin (Hb) (g/L)	168	184 (12–24 hours)		178 then 170
Haematocrit (Hct) (%)	53	58 (12–24 hours)		55 then 54
Mean corpuscular volume (MCV)	107	108 (12–24 hours)		99 then 98
Reticulocytes (%)	3–7	3–7 (12–24 hours)		1–3 then 0–1
White cell count (WCC) × 10^9/L	18.1 (9–30)	22.8 then 18.9 (9.4–38)		12.2 (5–21) (3–10 days)
Eosinophils × 10^9/L	0.4	0.5		0.5

Source: data from Department of Health and Human Services (2017) Consultative Council on Obstetric and Paediatric Mortality and Morbidity. Normal laboratory values for neonates. Neonatal ehandbook: Pathology. *© State of Victoria 2021. Online. <https://www2.health.vic.gov.au/hospitals-and-health-services/patient-care/perinatal-reproductive/neonatal-ehandbook/pathology/normal-laboratory-values>.*

APPENDIX 3 ELECTROLYTES – PRETERM NEONATES (<37 WEEKS) (BY DAY OF LIFE)

Value	Days 1–7			Days 21–49
Calcium ionised (Ca I) (mmol/L)	0.81–1.41 (day 1)	0.72–1.44 (day 3)	1.04–1.52 (day 5)	1.04–1.52
Potassium (K) (mEq/L)	5.6 (4.6–6.7)			5.8 (4.5–7.1) (day 21) 5.5 (4.5–6.6) (day 35) 5.7 (4.6–7.1) (day 49)
Sodium (Na) (mEq/L)	140 (133–146)			136–137 (129–142) then (133–148)
Chloride (Cl) (mEq/L)	108 (100–117)			108–117 (102–116) then (100–115)
Calcium (Ca) (mmol/L)	2.3 (1.5–2.9)			2.4 (2.0–2.8) (day 21) 2.4 (2.2–2.7) (days 35–49)
Phosphate (PO_4) (mmol/L)	2.5 (1.7–3.5)			2.4 (2.0–2.8) (day 21) 2.3 (1.8–2.6) (day 35) 2.2 (1.4–2.7) (day 49)
Magnesium (Mg) (mmol/L)	0.62–1.02 (day 1)	0.66–1.10 (day 3)	0.75–1.00	
Urea (mmol/L)	3.3 (1.1–9.1)			4.8 (0.8–11.2) (day 21) 4.8 (0.7–9.5) (day 35) 4.8 (0.9–10.9) (day 49)

Source: data from Department of Health and Human Services (2017) Consultative Council on Obstetric and Paediatric Mortality and Morbidity. Normal laboratory values for neonates. Neonatal ehandbook: Pathology. *© State of Victoria 2021. Online. <https://www2.health.vic.gov.au/hospitals-and-health-services/patient-care/perinatal-reproductive/neonatal-ehandbook/pathology/normal-laboratory-values>.*

APPENDIX 4 OTHER BIOCHEMISTRY – PRETERM NEONATES (BY GESTATION)

Value	27–29 weeks	31–35 weeks
Creatinine (μmol/L) – day 2	0.08–0.16 then 0.07–0.14	0.07–0.14 (31 weeks) 0.05–0.13 (33–35 weeks)
Creatinine (μmol/L) – day 7	0.05–0.11 then 0.04–0.12	0.04–0.12 (31 weeks) 0.02–0.11 (33–35 weeks)
Creatinine (μmol/L) – day 14	0.04–0.10	0.04–0.10 (31 weeks) 0.02–0.09 (33–35 weeks)
Creatinine (μmol/L) – day 21	0.03–0.09	0.03–0.09 (31 weeks) 0.02–0.09 (33–35 weeks)
Creatinine (μmol/L) – day 28	0.03–0.08 (27 weeks) 0.02–0.09 (29 weeks)	0.02–0.09 (31 weeks) 0.01–0.06 (33–35 weeks)
Albumin (Alb) (g/L)	21–33 (27 weeks) 23–34 (29 weeks)	22–36
Alkaline phosphatase (ALP) (IU/L)	35–604 (27 weeks) 119–465 (29 weeks)	112–450 (31 weeks) 110–398 (33 weeks) 113–360 (35 weeks)

Source: data from Department of Health and Human Services (2017) Consultative Council on Obstetric and Paediatric Mortality and Morbidity. Normal laboratory values for neonates. Neonatal ehandbook: Pathology. *© State of Victoria 2021. Online. <https://www2.health.vic.gov.au/hospitals-and-health-services/patient-care/perinatal-reproductive/neonatal-ehandbook/pathology/normal-laboratory-values>.*

APPENDIX 5 HAEMATOLOGY – PRETERM NEONATES (BY AGE)

Value	Birth	12 hours	24 hours	1 week	2 weeks	1 month
Haemoglobin (Hb) (g/L)	140 (24 weeks)					
	145 (28 weeks)					
	150 (34 weeks)					
White cell count (WCC) × 10^9/L	18.1 (9–30)	22.8 (13–38)	18.9 (9.4–34)	12.2 (5–21)	11.4 (5–20)	10.8 (5–19.5)
Neutrophils × 10^9/L	11.1 (6–26)	15.5 (6–28)	11.5 (5–21)	5.5 (1.5–10)	4.5 (1–9.5)	3.8 (1–9)
Bands (10^3/mm^3)	0.2–2.4		0.2–0.6 (72 hours)			
Lymphocytes × 10^9/L	5.5 (2–11)		5.8 (2–11.5)	5 (2–17)	5.5 (2–17)	6.0 (2.5–16.5)
Monocytes × 10^9/L	1.1	1.2	1.1		1.0	0.7
Eosinophils × 10^9/L	0.4	0.5			0.4	0.3
Basophils (10^3/mm^3)	0–1 (up to 72 hours)					
Platelets (10^3/mm^3)	150–350					

Sources: data from Department of Health and Human Services (2017) Consultative Council on Obstetric and Paediatric Mortality and Morbidity. Normal laboratory values for neonates. Neonatal ehandbook: Pathology. *© State of Victoria 2021. Online. <https://www2.health.vic.gov.au/hospitals-and-health-services/patient-care/perinatal-reproductive/neonatal-ehandbook/pathology/normal-laboratory-values>; Milcic, T. L. (2009). The complete blood count.* Neonatal Network, *28(2), 109–115. <http://www.academyofneonatalnursing.org/NNT/Hematology_CBC.pdf>.*

APPENDIX 6 COAGULATION PROFILE – PRETERM NEONATES (BY AGE)

Value	Days 1–5	Day 30
Prothrombin time (PT) (s)	13–12.5 (10.6–15.3)	11.8 (10–13.6)
Activated partial thromboplastin time (APTT) (s)	53.6–50.5 (27–74)	44.7 (27–62)
Fasting blood glucose (g/L)	2.43 (1.5–3.7) (day 1) 2.8 (1.6–4.2) (day 5)	2.54 (1.5–4.14)

Source: data from Department of Health and Human Services (2017) Consultative Council on Obstetric and Paediatric Mortality and Morbidity. Normal laboratory values for neonates. Neonatal ehandbook: Pathology. *© State of Victoria 2021. Online. <https://www2.health.vic.gov.au/hospitals-and-health-services/patient-care/perinatal-reproductive/neonatal-ehandbook/pathology/normal-laboratory-values>.*

APPENDIX 7 CEREBROSPINAL FLUID (CSF) – TERM AND PRETERM NEONATES (BY AGE OF LIFE)

Value	Term <7 days – >7 days	Preterm <7 days – >7 days
White cell count (WCC) (/mm^3)	5 (0–30) – 3 (0–10)	9 (0–30) – 12 (2–70)
Red cell count (RCC) (/mm^3)	9 (0–50) – <10	30 (0–333)
Protein (g/L)	0.6 (0.3–2.5) – 0.5 (0.2–0.8)	1 (0.5–2.9) – 0.9 (0.5–2.6)
Glucose (mmol/L)	3 (1.5–5.5)	

Source: data from Department of Health and Human Services (2017) Consultative Council on Obstetric and Paediatric Mortality and Morbidity. Normal laboratory values for neonates. Neonatal ehandbook: Pathology. *© State of Victoria 2021. Online. <https://www2.health.vic.gov.au/hospitals-and-health-services/patient-care/perinatal-reproductive/neonatal-ehandbook/pathology/normal-laboratory-values>.*

APPENDIX 8 URINE – TERM AND PRETERM NEONATES

Value	Term <7 days – preterm >7 days
White cell count (WCC) (per HPF[a])	<5
Red cell count (RCC) (per HPF[a])	0–2
Squames (per HPF[a])	<5
Organisms	Nil

[a]Per high power field (HPF) on microscopic urine examination.

Source: data from Department of Health and Human Services (2017) Consultative Council on Obstetric and Paediatric Mortality and Morbidity. Normal laboratory values for neonates. Neonatal ehandbook: Pathology. *© State of Victoria 2021. Online. <https://www2.health.vic.gov.au/hospitals-and-health-services/patient-care/perinatal-reproductive/neonatal-ehandbook/pathology/normal-laboratory-values>.*

APPENDIX 9 ACID–BASE VALUES[a] – TERM AND PRETERM NEONATES (BY AGE OF LIFE)

Value	Cord	1–48 hours
pH	7.33 (UV)	7.30–7.39 (art)
PCO_2 (mmHg)	43 (UV)	39–34
HCO_3 (mEq/L)	21.6 (UV)	18.8–20
PO_2 (mmHg)	28 (± 8) (UV)	62 (± 13.8)–87
Anion gap	<20	

[a]Capillary ranges similar, except PO_2.

Art, arterial specimen; UV, umbilical vein.

Source: data from Department of Health and Human Services (2017) Consultative Council on Obstetric and Paediatric Mortality and Morbidity. Normal laboratory values for neonates. Neonatal ehandbook: Pathology. *© State of Victoria 2021. Online. <https://www2.health.vic.gov.au/hospitals-and-health-services/patient-care/perinatal-reproductive/neonatal-ehandbook/pathology/normal-laboratory-values>.*

INDEX

Page numbers followed by "*f*" indicate figures, "*t*" indicate tables and "*b*" indicate boxes.

B

E

G

H

N

O

Q

T

U